◆ DSM-IV Diagnosis Boxes

Psychiatric-Mental Health Nursing

Adaptation and Growth

FOURTH EDITION

Psychiatric-Mental Health Nursing

Adaptation and Growth

Barbara Schoen Johnson,
PhD, RN, CS
Psychiatric Mental Health Nurse Practitioner and Specialist
The University of Texas at Arlington
School of Nursing
Arlington, Texas

FOURTH EDITION

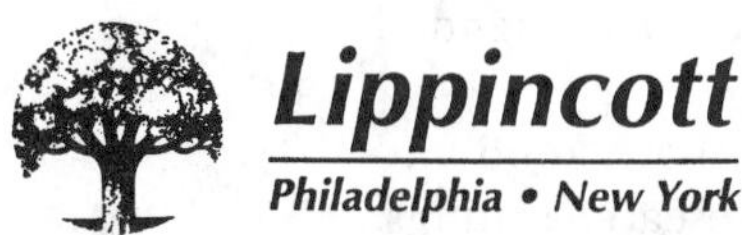

Acquisitions Editor: Margaret B. Zuccarini
Assistant Editor: Emily Cotlier
Project Editor: Erika Kors
Production Manager: Helen Ewan
Production Coordinator: Patricia McCloskey
Design Coordinator: Kathy Kelley-Luedtke
Indexer: Ellen Murray

Edition 4

9 8 7 6 5 4 3 2 1

Library of Congress Cataloging-in-Publications Data

Psychiatric-mental health nursing: adaptation and growth / [edited by] Barbara Schoen Johnson.—4th ed.
p. cm.
Includes bibliographical references and index.
ISBN 0-397-55243-2
1. Psychiatric nursing. I. Johnson, Barbara Schoen.
[DNLM: 1. Mental Disorders—nursing. 2. Psychiatric Nursing. WY 160 P97204 1997]
RC440.P737 1997
610.73'68—dc20
DNLM/DLC
for Library of Congress 96-32247
CIP

To Barry

Did you ever know that you're my hero?

Contributors

Cheryl Ann Lindamood Anderson, MSN, PhD, RN
Adjunct Assistant Professor
University of Texas at Arlington
Arlington, Texas
and
President/Owner
Educational Resources and Services, Inc.
Euless, Texas

Marjorie F. Bendik, DNSc, RN
Associate Professor and Coordinator/San Diego Area
California State University
Carson, California

Virginia Trotter Betts, MSN, JD, RN
President and CEO
HealthFutures, Inc.
Nashville, Tennessee
and
Immediate Past President
American Nurses Association
Washington, DC

Patriciann Furnari Brady, EdD, RN
Assistant Professor
Coordinator of Mental Health Nursing
South Dakota State University
Brookings, South Dakota

Sharon E. Byers, MSN, RN, CS
Clinical Nurse Specialist
Crisis Outreach Team
Hennepin County Family and Children's Mental Health Services
Minneapolis, Minnesota

Sandra Carter Chandler, MS, RN
Coordinator/Instructor, Nursing
El Centro College
Brookhaven College Satellite,
Dallas, Texas

Jeanneane Lewis Cline, MS, RN, CS, LMFT, LCDC
Specialist
School of Nursing
University of Texas at Arlington
Arlington, Texas
and
Psychotherapist, Private Practice
Fort Worth, Texas

Phyllis M. Connolly, PhD, RN, CS
San Jose State University
School of Nursing
San Jose, California

Barbara G. Tunley Crenshaw, MS, RN, CNS
Professor Emeritus
Front Range Community College
Denver, Colorado

Sherill Nones Cronin, PhD, RN.C
Associate Professor of Nursing
Bellarmine College
Louisville, Kentucky
and
Nurse Researcher
at The Jewish Hospital
Louisville, Kentucky

Jan Dalsheimer, MS, RN
Doctoral Candidate
School of Nursing
Texas Woman's University
Denton, Texas

Joy Randolph Davidson, MSN, RN
Instructor, Nursing
El Centro College
Dallas, Texas

Susan D. Decker, PhD, RN
Associate Professor
School of Nursing
University of Portland
Portland, Oregon

Kathleen R. Delaney, DNSc., RN
Practitioner-Teacher and Associate Professor
Rush University
College of Nursing
Chicago, Illinois

Cheryl Detwiler, MSN, RN
Associate Professor
Nursing Department
Jackson State Community College
Jackson, Tennessee

Robin S. Diamond, MSN, JD, RN
Director, Patient Care Services
Huntsville Hospital System
Huntsville, Alabama

Suzanne Doscher, MSN, RN
Associate Professor
Medical University of South Carolina
College of Nursing
Charleston, South Carolina

Peggy J. Drapo, PhD, RN (Retired)
Professor Emerita
College of Nursing
Texas Women's University
Denton, Texas

Delia Esparza, PhD, RN, LMFP
Sexual Trauma Therapist
Department of Veteran Affairs Veteran Center
Austin, Texas

Linda Fischer, MS, RN, FNP
Director of Nursing
Denton State School
Denton, Texas

Sally Francis, MS, MA
Missoula, Montana
Formerly
Assistant Professor
Department of Pediatrics
Children's Medical Center of Dallas
University of Texas Southwestern Medical Center
Dallas, Texas

Judith A. Greene, PhD, RN, CS
Owner-Private Practice
Individual Marital and Family Systems Therapy
Cleveland, Tennessee

Christina R. Hogarth, MS, RN, CS
Consultant
St. Simon's Island, Georgia

Celeste M. Johnson, MSN, RN
Director of Nursing/Psychiatry and Neurology
Children's Medical Center of Dallas
Dallas, Texas

Mary Huggins, MA, RN
Program Specialist, Division of Mental Health
Hennepin County
Minneapolis, Minnesota

Anita G. Hufft, PhD, RN
Campus Dean
School of Nursing
Indiana University Southeast
New Albany, Indiana

Marilyn Jaffe-Ruiz, EdD, RN, CS
Dean and Professor, Lienhard School of Nursing
Pace University
New York, New York

Kathryn Kavanaugh, PhD, RN
Associate Professor
School of Nursing
University of Maryland
Baltimore, Maryland

Nina A. Klebanoff, PhD, RN, CS, LPCC
Independent Practice-Behavioral Health
Carson, New Mexico

Nancy Kupper, MSN, RN
Associate Professor
Tarrant County Junior College District
Fort Worth, Texas

Evelyn Labun, BN, MScN, DNSc(Candidate), RN
Program Coordinator-Nursing
Red River Community College
Winnipeg, Manitoba, CANADA

Donna Lettieri-Marks, PSY.D, RN
Practitioner-Teacher and Instructor
Rush University
College of Nursing
Chicago, Illinois

Patricia Murphey Lucas, MS, RN
School Nurse
Cypress Fairbanks I.S.D.
Houston, Texas

Beverly L. Malone, PhD, RN, FAAN
Dean and Professor
School of Nursing
North Carolina A&T State University
Greensboro, North Carolina

James J. McColgan, Jr, MS, CAES, RN
Lieutenant Colonel, US Army Nurse Corps
Assistant Chief Nurse
405th Combat Support Hospital
West Hartford, Connecticut

Bruce Payne Mericle, MS, RN
Assistant Professor of Nursing
Trenton State College
Trenton, New Jersey

Cynthia Ann Pastorino, MSN, RNC, ONC
Clinical Nurse Specialist
Alliant Health System
Louisville, Kentucky

Geraldine S. Pearson, MSN, RN, CS
Clinical Nurse Specialist
Riverview Hospital for Children and Youth
Middletown, Connecticut
and
Ph.D Student
School of Nursing
University of Connecticut
Storrs, Connecticut

Cindy Ann Peternelj-Taylor, BScN, MSc, RN
Associate Professor
College of Nursing
University of Saskatchewan
Saskatoon, Saskatchewan, CANADA

Kay Peterson, MS, RN, CS
Psychiatric-Mental Health Practitioner
Project Respond
Mental Health Services West
Portland, Oregon

Katherine Pritchett, MS, RN
Curriculum Coordinator and Instructor, Nursing
El Centro College
Dallas, Texas

Juliann Casey Reakes, EdD, RN, CS, LPC, LMFT, LCDC
Director, Baccalaureate Nursing Program
Abilene Intercollegate School of Nursing
Abilene, Texas

Bonnie Louise Rickelman, EdD, RN, CS, LMFT, CGP
Associate Professor
School of Nursing
The University of Texas at Austin
Austin, Texas

Stefan Ripich, MSN, RN, CS
Assistant Chief of Nursing
Palo Alto Veterans Health Care System
Palo Alto, California

Diane M. Snow, PhD, RN, CARN, PMHNP
Faculty and Acting Director
Psychiatric-Mental Health Practitioner Program
University of Texas at Arlington
School of Nursing
Arlington, Texas

Mary Anne Sweeney, PhD, RN
Professor and Project Director, School of Nursing
The University of Texas Medical Branch at Galveston
Galveston, Texas

Cheryl Taylor, PhD, RN
Assistant Professor
School of Nursing
North Carolina A&T State University
Greensboro, North Carolina

Barbara A. Thurston, MS, RN
Professor of Nursing
New Hampshire Technical Institute
Concord, New Hampshire

Susan Mace Weeks, MS, RN
Instructor
Texas Christian University-Harris College of Nursing
Fort Worth, TX

Sylvia Anderson Whiting, PhD, RN, CS
Associate Professor
South Carolina State University
Orangeburg, South Carolina
and
Private Practice
Summerville, South Carolina

Foreword

This fourth edition of *Psychiatric-Mental Health Nursing: Adaptation and Growth* will be published shortly before the beginning of the 21st century. It must serve students of both the old and the new millennia.

Compared with what is known today, 60 years ago psychiatric nursing knowledge was almost nonexistent. Then most psychiatric nursing texts were written by psychiatrists, sometimes with nurse coauthors. More often than not, they were less than two hundred pages long. What they conveyed was mostly a watered-down psychiatry and neurology consisting of piecemeal descriptions of the major psychopathologies, discussions of treatment, and surprisingly sparse commentaries on nursing comportment and procedures.

Today's psychiatric-mental health nursing texts are tightly compressed double-column compendiums of near one thousand, and sometimes more, pages. They are edited and written by a large number of nurse scholar-clinicians who specialize in the wide variety of topics that now epitomize the end-of-century text.

The earlier texts were first used by psychiatric nurses employed in state mental hospitals. Later, nursing students were sent to such hospitals for a three-month period of psychiatric nursing study which, during the middle of the century, was a required element of basic nursing education. They became the primary consumers and the stimulus for the rapid development of these texts. The three months previously devoted to exclusively psychiatric nursing studies has yielded to integrated approaches to nursing studies. Psychiatric-mental health courses are now ordinarily offered along with other courses and, in some schools, with other clinical experiences.

Today, most mental patients, even those with severe disturbances, spend most of their time in the community. At the same time, the range of problems addressed by psychiatric-mental health nursing has expanded. Students must learn not only about severe and chronic mental illness, as in the past, but also about the mental health needs of families, small groups, and communities; about people at risk for violence, suicide, homelessness, and substance abuse; and about the psychosocial aspects of physiological disease and disability, social and economic disadvantage, racial discrimination, cultural differences, sexual and gender issues, age-related problems, and lifestyles such as single parenthood. Thus, clinical experiences in psychiatric-mental health nursing are now offered in general hospitals and community health and social service centers, as well as in psychiatric hospitals.

These changes in the kinds of people served, their needs, and the settings where care is provided reflect profound changes in the culture and structure of our society. No longer do we believe that all mentally ill are so different from other troubled people that they must be confined to mental hospitals for long periods of time. No longer do we ignore psychosocial troubles that do not arise from mental illness. No longer do we confine our assessment and treatment to the individual; rather, we consider family, community, and the broader society as part of our concern. A wide variety of pharmacological, psychological, and sociological treatment strategies are thought to be beneficial, both to the mildly distressed and the severely disturbed.

What changes can we foresee at the end of this century and into the next millennium? The 101st Congress designated the 1990s as the "decade of the brain." This act has focused nursing's attention on the importance of neurobiological research and treatment approaches. Yet, as the decade progresses, increasing attention is being given to violence, already considered a public health problem. Substance abuse, suicide, stress, aging and a host of other social problems are increasingly seen as issues of concern to mental health workers. We can suppose that by the year 2000, the brain will be replaced by some other biological or social priority as the official focus of attention. Yet I am confident that, within the 51 chapters of this text, the student will find more than enough knowledge to prepare for many future developments.

The particular challenge to authors of contemporary psychiatric-mental health nursing texts is that their work reflect the discipline as holistic, comprehensive, and synthesizing. As *holistic,* it must include not only the beliefs and knowledge peculiar to psychiatric-mental health nursing, but also applicable knowledge from other nursing specialties and from associated disciplines, such as social work, psychiatry, pharmacy, neurology, sociology, anthropology, and psychology. As *comprehensive,* it must present information that is complete, accurate, and up to date. As *synthesizing,* it must ensure that this knowledge, brought together from a vast array of different intellectual traditions, makes sense. To meet such extraordinary challenges, this text contains a gold mine of information on a vast array of topics. Of particular note is the editor's and contributors' imaginative use of adaptation and growth as the organizing conceptual framework for the vast amount of information they convey.

Their successful effort presents the student with an equally demanding task: how can you best use this book to your own advantage and that of your patients? I recommend that you think of it as more than a textbook. You cannot hope to absorb and retain all of its information in the short period devoted to a psychiatric-mental health nursing course. In addition to those portions of it which will be used for class assignments, I urge you to browse it to be aware of all it contains, and to keep it at hand as you continue your studies and begin your career. Thus it will become a valued reference work, its knowledge and perspectives informing you as you confront the wide assortment of human problems and possibilities.

Oliver H. Osborne, RN, PhD
Professor Emeritus, Nursing
Adjunct Professor Emeritus, Anthropology and Ethnic Studies
University of Washington
Seattle, Washington

Preface

Preparing this preface to the fourth edition of *Psychiatric Mental Health Nursing: Adaptation and Growth* marks the ten-year anniversary of its publication. And, like any good anniversary celebration, it is a time to reflect on the past and look forward to the future.

Guiding the Text

The first edition was built on a foundation of three goals:

- To compile a book with accurate, comprehensive, and up-to-date material that would stimulate the reader to seek out additional information and experience
- To produce a work of high-quality writing that would communicate clearly, concisely, and in an interesting and understandable manner
- To expose the reader to exciting applications of psychiatric-mental health nursing concepts not ordinarily found within a traditional text

Some things endure; I am proud that these goals still direct each edition and figure prominently in its acceptance and success.

The authors and I wanted readers to enjoy reading this book, to read "for the fun of it," and even to offer it to family and friends who might also enjoy reading it. This is a lofty aim for a college textbook but one which, students tell us, we are achieving and towards which we will continue to strive.

This is more than a textbook about people's mental and emotional problems. It is a book about adaptation, recovery, and growth achieved by working through these problems. It guides nurses to help individuals, families, and communities become stronger through application of effective assessment, planning and outcome identification, and intervention. It encompasses psychiatric and mental health nursing care in many contexts:

- For people with physical or mental disorders
- For children, adolescents, young adults, midlife men and women, or the aged
- In a multiplicity of settings throughout the health care delivery continuum

EXAMINING THE CONTENTS

The textbook is organized into twelve units:

Unit I contains material foundational to the study of psychiatric and mental health nursing—introduction to the field, mental health promotion, conceptual frameworks, nursing theory, therapeutic relationships and communication, and biological bases for care.

Unit II discusses the application of the nursing process—assessment, diagnosis, planning, intervention, and evaluation—to psychiatric-mental health nursing.

Unit III demonstrates the importance of holistic care through consideration of the sociocultural and spiritual aspects of care, sexuality and sexual concerns, and grief and loss issues.

Unit IV describes the interventions of milieu, individual, group, family, behavior, and alternative therapies, and psychopharmacology.

Unit V introduces the developmental issues that affect mental health and includes the mental health concerns of children, adolescents, and the aging.

Unit VI discusses the many mental disorders and illnesses, including anxiety, somatoform and personality disorders, depressive, bipolar, schizophrenic, and dissociative disorders, and aggressive and violent behavior.

Unit VII addresses the issues of addiction—substance abuse, eating disorders, and codependency.

Unit VIII covers the special topics of mental illness in

the homeless population, mental retardation, and forensic psychiatric nursing.

Unit IX discusses crisis theory and intervention, as well as the crises of rape and sexual assault, family violence, and suicide.

Unit X features community-based care, including community mental health, psychosocial home care, and the community support and rehabilitation of those persons with persistent and severe mental illness.

Unit XI focuses on mental health interventions with medical patients, including the psychosocial impact of acute illness, children with physical illness and disability, and clients on the HIV spectrum.

Unit XII approaches the professional issues of the legal implications of, and research in, psychiatric nursing, and features profiles of the careers of nurses from around North America.

NEW TO THIS EDITION

New content assures that the textbook keeps pace with scientific research, the changing health care environment, a complex web of care-delivery sites and the resulting evolving discipline of psychiatric nursing. All chapters have been thoroughly reviewed and revised to reflect current research, DSM-IV classification, treatment and psychiatric nursing practice. In addition, the following chapters are new to the fourth edition:

Chapter 2, Mental Health Promotion—This new chapter presents the important nursing responsibility of health promotion and illness prevention, specifically the role that psychiatric-mental health nurses play in strengthening personal resources to enhance mental health and in diminishing risk factors to prevent mental illness.

Chapter 19, Alternative Therapies—This new chapter presents a selected history and overview of alternative therapies as they pertain to psychiatric disorders and mental health problems. It provides the reader with information about the wide range of alternative therapies available today.

Chapter 32, Dissociative Disorders—This new chapter addresses dissociative disorders. The four types of currently recognized dissociative disorders are explored, as well as nursing process, with a focus on interventions and milieu management.

Chapter 38, Forensic Psychiatric Nursing—This new chapter outlines the tremendous opportunities that exist for nurses to demonstrate leadership in providing mental health care to the varied and complex needs of the forensic client.

Several other chapters have new authors and contain totally new content in the fourth edition:

Chapter 10, Sociocultural Aspects of Care—This chapter addresses the critical need for nurses to be aware of both their own and their client's cultural background and experiences, to know that each person is unique and to plan and implement culturally sensitive care that is shaped by the mental, emotional, and cultural needs and care expectations of each person.

Chapter 20, Psychopharmacology—This chapter describes the principles of medication management with psychiatric clients and presents psychotropic medications according to major classifications, target symptoms, side effects, dosages, and specific nursing interventions.

Chapter 23, Adolescents—This chapter identifies the dynamics of adolescent disorders and applies the nursing process to adolescents with mental and emotional disturbance in adolescents.

Chapter 31, Aggressive and Violent Behavior—This chapter discusses aggressive and violent behavior in persons who have been diagnosed with mental illness and means to intervene in the behaviors.

KEY FEATURES

The text includes key features from previous editions and incorporates new features to highlight, support, and clarify important content:

**Integrated nursing process* helps students focus on the nurse's vital role in the psychiatric care of clients, in the application of a variety of therapies, and in all care delivery settings.

**Current issues and topics,* including biological bases of care, alternative therapies, forensic nursing, continuum of care settings, and psychopharmacology, reflect the rapidly changing scope of psychiatric-mental health nursing.

**Focus on psychopharmacology* throughout the text emphasizes nursing intervention, including teaching, in this biological treatment.

**Entire unit on community-based care* underscores the importance of understanding the role of the psychiatric-mental health nurse in the care of clients in many community-based settings.

SPECIAL FEATURES

***Therapeutic Dialogues** help students integrate therapeutic communication into nurse-client interactions.

***Nursing Care Plans** illustrate concepts and provide realistic clinical examples of *outcome-based application* of the nursing process.

***Case Studies** with questions for discussion provide students with vivid examples of client presentation in a variety of settings, demonstrate nurse-client interaction, and present opportunities for personal reflection and group discussion.

NEW FEATURES

***DSM-IV Diagnostic Criteria Boxes** reflect the need for nurses to understand medical diagnoses and the collaborative nature of psychiatric nursing.

***Clinical Pathways** provide many examples of managed care parameters.

***Review Questions** at the end of each chapter help students focus on learning and reviewing important concepts.

***Critical Thinking Questions** promote reflection, integration, and analysis of content, thereby reinforcing learning.

***Special Boxes** on client and family education about illness and medications demonstrate the scope of client and family information needs.

*FREE COMPUTER DISK presents more than 75 psychopharmacologic agents in a complete software package. The disk enables access to drug information using either a generic or trade drug name. Once selected, a drug can be viewed on screen, a monograph can be printed, or an ASCII file can be created so that drug cards or custom-designed patient teaching printouts can be made.

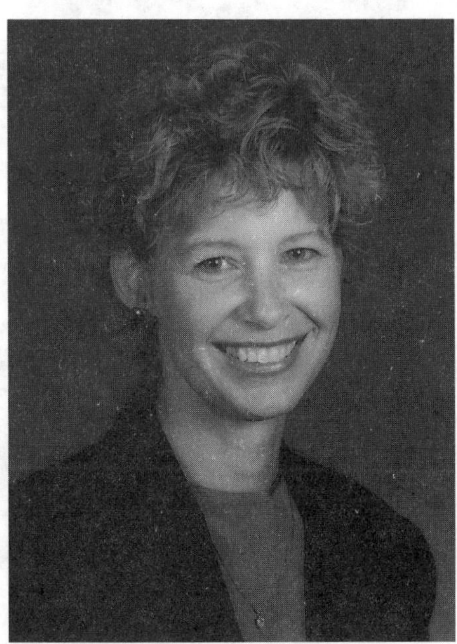

TEACHING-LEARNING PACKAGE

The teaching/learning package that accompanies this edition contains a computerized testbank, a printed testbank, an instructor's manual and overhead transparency masters.

*A Computerized Testbank, based on the ParTEST program, consists of 1000 new questions for this edition and is available free to instructors upon adoption of the text. ParTEST is a sophisticated program that allows instructors to edit the questions in the testbank or add new questions.

*A Printed Testbank, consisting of the questions in the computerized testbank, is available to enable instructors to see the questions for a particular chapter or unit at a glance.

*An Instructor's Manual, completely new, includes a chapter overview, key terms, teaching strategies, additional teaching support materials including electronic product, and overhead transparency masters.

• Videos are available that have been designed for in-classroom use to assist students with the transition to clinical practice. There are four videos in the Basic Mental Status Examination Series, as follows:

Video I: Conducting the Patient Interview

Video II: Evaluating Aspects of Appearance and Mood

Video III: Evaluating Language and Thought Patterns

Video IV: Evaluating Intellectual and Cognitive Function

Together, the contributing authors and I have worked to create an outstanding edition of *Psychiatric-Mental Health Nursing: Adaptation and Growth.* We are proud of the results and believe you will find the text and its accompaniments current, informative, useful, innovative, and inspiring. This is our overriding goal—to inspire psychiatric nurses and *all* nurse-colleagues to find new and more effective ways to help the people entrusted to our care.

Barbara Schoen Johnson
Southlake, Texas

Acknowledgments

Each edition teaches me something new. The first edition (1986) taught me about dedication and sacrifice. The second (1989) about discipline. The third (1993) about cooperation. This, the fourth edition (1997) has taught me about people and what they're made of. It has reminded me to appreciate the goodness in those close to me.

Each edition teaches me, again, something I already know. That the support of my family and friends is limitless. That nothing is more important than treating all people with respect and kindness. That during times of stress, the essence of a person comes shining through (or rushing out). That work, even meaningful work, is never as important as the people we care about and the people who care about us.

These are valuable lessons.

I am surrounded by the caring and laughter of friends. Some I talk with or email every day (JZF), but most others less often. They know, however, that they are in my thoughts daily. I thank these shining, smiling friends—Juanita Zapata Flint, Barbara Burke, Sondra Flemming, Fela Alfaro, Dana Stahl, Margaret Brunett, Wissa Winslow, Marjorie Westberry, Sandy Chandler, Sue McLelland, Linda Camin, Celeste Johnson, Kathy Pritchett, Pattie Lucas, Betty Nelson, Diana Reding, Cheryl Detwiler, Kathy Lee Hakala, and the many others who enrich my life.

A close friend and role model, Margie Slaughter, died since work on the last edition. The original author of the chapter on Sociocultural Aspects of Care and a fellow teacher, Margie taught me to put on a show to grab and hold students' attention. Every time I dress up and perform in class, Margie, I think of you. May you rest in peace.

My family and I live in a town that was once small but is now growing. However, we have maintained friendships with our neighbors and friends, Susan and Charlie Wegman, Bethann and Darwin Scratchard, Barbara and Foster Vernon, Emily and Charlie Williams, and the many others we greet regularly at high school events.

The faculty and staff of The University of Texas at Arlington have become my colleagues and friends. The psychiatric nursing team is loaded with talent—Diane Snow, Jeanneane Cline, and until recently, Rosalyn Tolbert and Pat Gordon—I thank them for their tremendous help and kindness and for stimulating me to think in new, broader ways about our field. I have found the faculty to be a supportive bunch and thank Andi Smith, Karen Heusinkveld, Susan Chappell, Regina Johnson, and the others who smile at me in the halls. Our new dean, Liz Poster, and assistant deans, Mary Lou Bond and Susan Grove, have encouraged me throughout this endeavor.

To the students who have challenged me to look at this material through new eyes, who have asked me questions I could not answer, and who have inspired me to always improve my teaching, I say thank you.

The children, adolescents, adults, and families who battle against mental illness and addictions exemplify courage every day of their lives. I admire the ferocity of your struggle and pray for effective treatments and care. It is for you that this book was and is written.

Good writing springs from good thinking. The authors of this fourth edition are good thinkers. They have drawn on their massive experience and knowledge to put together chapters that reflect up-to-the-minute thinking on their topics. They have gone beyond what is expected of writers to contribute to this edition. At one point Evelyn Labun, the author of the chapter on Spiritual Aspects of Care, said to me, "Barbara, I am not just a person who writes about spirituality; I am a person of prayer. And I pray for you during this difficult work." It brought tears to my eyes. I thank all of the authors for similar words and acts of kindness to me, and for their patience with and dedication to this work. Most of the authors and I have been through life changes together, through degrees and positions, through marriage and children. I feel honored to have shared their lives and work.

This edition marks my 16th year of working with Lippincott. I have learned that editors come and go but the influence of a few remains. Bill initiated me to the rigors of writing. Dave taught me to be forgiving of myself. But, oh, Ellen, how I've missed *you* most of all . . .

Thank you to Erika Kors, the height of tact, graciousness, and professionalism, for managing the thousands of details involved in coordinating the entire production of this book and for listening to my worries and my dreams for it.

My parents, Roy and Marie Schoen, always communicated to me that I was capable of whatever I chose to undertake. And so I thank them for that inestimable gift, belief in oneself, and for their willing ears during times of struggle.

I thank my sisters, brother, sisters- and brothers-in-law, Bobi and Fred Ravagnani (thanks for that unending stream of obnoxious mementos of my fiftieth), Mary Ellen and Don Makkos, Jeff and Angela Schoen, Bonnie and John Weseloh, Bryan and Dee Johnson for their encouragement.

Eric was almost 3 years old and Jessica a newborn when I started to create the ideas that developed into this text. Jessica is now 15 years and Eric, at age 18, will graduate from high school in a few days. They are both stars in our universe. Jessica has shown the same drive for excellence in her studies that motivates her in sports and has taken her to the position of state high jump champion. Eric has persevered in his academics and in tennis and has overcome challenges to succeed in whatever he tries. He is admired by teachers and coaches, and by his family. As he heads to college, we are struck by the honesty and goodness of our son. I am struck by how much he reminds me of his father. The sun (that great Texas sun) rises and sets on these two children-almost-young-adults of ours. They are everything to their father and me.

My life-hero and constant during 28 years of wedded bliss has been Barry. He is truly my hero—I wish I had his patience, his charitable view of the world, his goodness. Even when we were newlyweds and I a mere 22 years old, Barry let me know that his opinion of my ability was higher than my own. He has encouraged, supported, teased, and cared for me, during good times and troubles.

I owe you, Barry, for everything. I thank you for doing the weekly grocery shopping and bringing home much better stuff than I would have, for the romantic late night drives to the post office and FedEx (particularly the party-like excitement of the airport FedEx at 10:30 PM to the sounds of plane engines revving in the night air), for sometimes being both Mom and Dad to our two teens, for tutoring them in chemistry and algebra and history and basketball, for listening to my troubles, my fears, and my hopes with equanimity, for loving me when I'm unlovable and making me laugh when I desperately need to laugh. You *are* the wind beneath my wings. I love you, Barry.

Contents in Brief

VIII

Special Topics in Psychiatric-Mental Health Nursing 725

IX

Crisis 787

X

Community-Based Care 877

XI

Mental Health Intervention With the Medical Client 923

XII

Professional Issues in Psychiatric-Mental Health Nursing 969

Contents

Foundations of Psychiatric-Mental Health Nursing

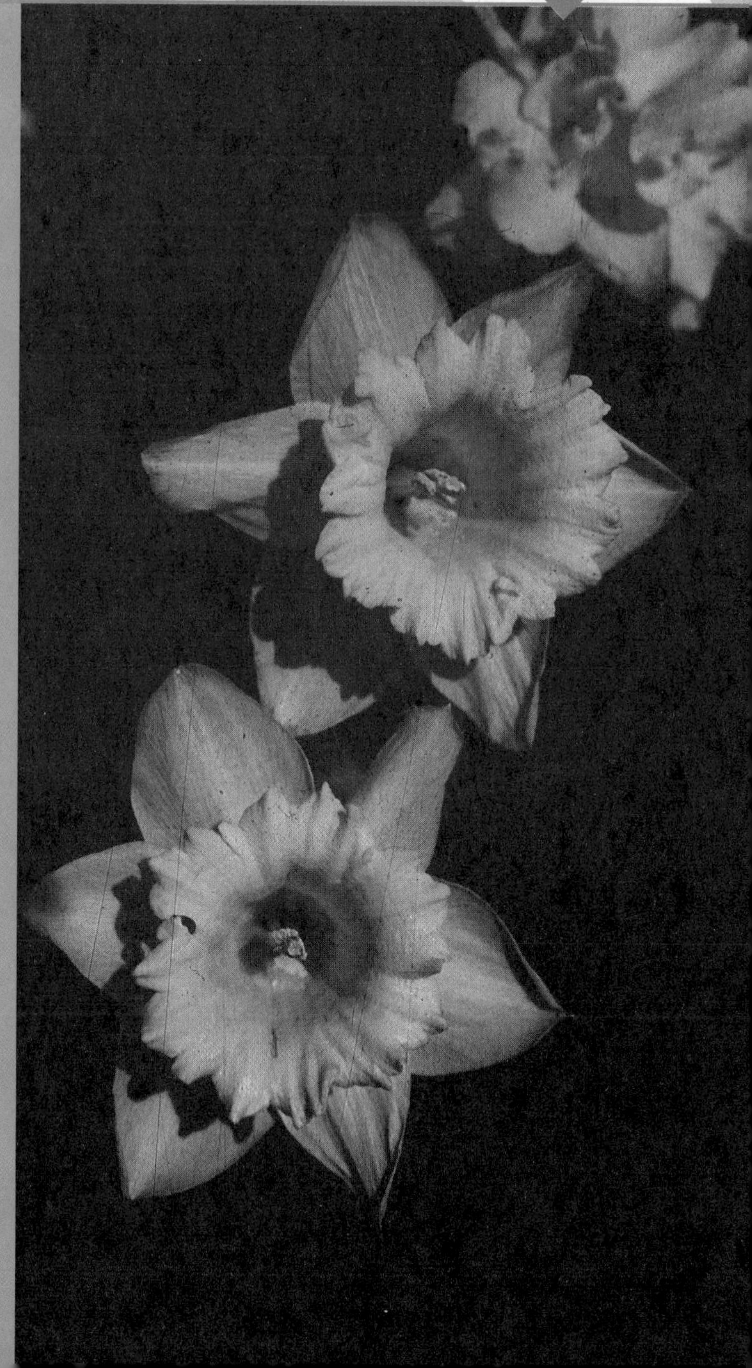

Introduction to Psychiatric-Mental Health Nursing

Barbara Schoen Johnson

1

I do not know what causes insanity or what can cure it, and I don't really believe that anyone else knows either. I do not even think that it is a constant condition, much less an "illness," or that the crazy people live over there on that side of the line, and the rest of us over here. I think that madness is part of all of us, all the time, that it comes and goes, waxes and wanes. . . . I myself don't think that madness can be fully understood, only experienced—in oneself or in one's friends or in the people one sees crumbling at the office or on the streets.

Otto Friedrich,
Going Crazy: An Inquiry into Madness in Our Time, *1976*

This chapter invites the reader to explore the field of psychiatric-mental health nursing. Initially, psychiatric-mental health nursing may seem mystifying or even frightening to the novice, but its foundation is the same nursing process as other areas of nursing. Based in biological, social, and nursing sciences, psychiatric-mental health nursing emerges as a mental health field that provides comprehensive care to clients.

The principles of psychiatric-mental health nursing permeate all areas of nursing practice. Nurses use these principles when they comfort the dying and their family, teach assertiveness skills to adolescents, calm the fears of ill or abused children, coach adults in relaxation techniques, encourage bonding in new parents, and in countless other nursing skills.

This chapter examines mental health and mental illness, functions and roles of psychiatric-mental health nurses, and application of the nursing process to maximize clients' progress toward resolution of their problems. It explores the stress response, adaptation, and use of coping mechanisms. The need for nurses to attend to their own needs is discussed throughout the chapter; the reader is also directed to Chapter 2, Mental Health Promotion

Learning Objectives

On completion of this chapter, you should be able to accomplish the following:

1. *Define the terms mental health and mental illness.*
2. *Identify the issues and challenges facing mental health care and psychiatric-mental health nursing.*
3. *Differentiate between stress and distress.*
4. *Explain the stages of the general adaptation syndrome.*
5. *Give examples of the following coping mechanisms: denial, regression, displacement, projection, reaction formation, repression, suppression, identification, rationalization, fantasy, and intellectualization.*
6. *Describe the steps of the nursing process.*
7. *Describe basic and advanced level roles and functions of psychiatric-mental health nurses.*
8. *Identify measures to prevent or alleviate stress and burnout in psychiatric-mental health nursing.*

◆ Mental Health and Mental Illness

Society defines health and illness according to its beliefs and values. When a person is able to carry out his or her role in society and his or her behavior is adaptive to the environment, we say that person is healthy; when role responsibilities are not met and behavior is maladaptive, we say the person is ill. Culture greatly influences these determinations about health and illness. Behavior that is acceptable in one cultural group may or may not be tolerated in another group. (For more information about cultural variations of behavior, see Chapter 10, Sociocultural Aspects of Care.)

MENTAL HEALTH

The World Health Organization defines *health* as "a state of complete physical, mental, and social well-being, not merely the absence of disease or infirmity." This definition emphasizes the positive, a state of well-being, rather than focusing on the lack of disease or disorder. People in a state of emotional well-being, or *mental health,* function comfortably within society and are satisfied with their achievements.

Menninger defined mental health as "the adjustment of human beings to each other and to the world around them with a maximum of effectiveness and happiness" (p 1).[20] Although no generally accepted definition of mental health exists, we infer the presence or absence of mental health from an individual's behavior.

Components of Mental Health

Mental health implies mastery in the areas of life involving love, work, play, and even happiness. Components of mental health include the following:

1. Self-governance: The person demonstrates autonomy, a sense of detachment, independence, and a tendency to look within for guiding values and rules by which to live. The person acts independently, dependently, or interdependently as the need arises, without permanently losing independence.
2. Growth orientation: The person is willing to depart from the status quo to progress toward self-realization and maximization of capacities.
3. Tolerance of uncertainty: The person faces the uncertainty of living and the certainty of death with faith and hope.
4. Self-esteem: The person's self-esteem is built on self-knowledge and awareness of talents, abilities, and limitations.
5. Mastery of the environment: The person is effective, capable, competent, and creative in dealing with and influencing the environment.
6. Reality orientation: The person distinguishes fact from fantasy, the real world from a dream world, and acts accordingly.
7. Stress management: The person experiences appropriate depression, anxiety, and so forth in daily life and can tolerate high levels of stress, knowing that the feeling is not going to last forever. The person is flexible and can experience failure without self-castigation. Usually the person copes with crises without needing help beyond the support of family and friends.

Many aspects of a person's life indicate signs of mental health. These include meaningful work, enjoyment of life, humor, ability to benefit from rest and sleep, optimism, spontaneity, satisfaction in relationships with others, ability to work well alone and with others, ability to make sound judgments and decisions, acceptance of responsibility for actions, ability to give and receive, demonstration of behavior that is generally accepted by the group, and ability to express emotions, including strong feelings. Humor may be a coping mechanism and an indicator of mental health because it suggests an ability to laugh at one's own troubles and mistakes.[23] (Chapter 2, Mental Health Promotion, provides a more in-depth view of mental health.)

Influences on Mental Health

Biological, psychological, and sociocultural variables influence mental health. *Biological factors* include prenatal and perinatal influences, physical health, neuroanatomy, and physiology. *Psychological factors* include parent, sibling, and infant or child interactions; intelligence quotient; self-concept; skills; talents; creativity; and emotional developmental level. *Sociocultural factors* include family stability, child-rearing patterns, economic level, housing, membership in a minority that may experience the effects of prejudice or inadequate health resources, religious influences, and values.[13,17,28]

MENTAL ILLNESS OR DISORDER

Views of Mental Illness: History and Stigma

In years past, mental illness has been viewed as demonic possession, the influence of ancestral spirits, the result of violating a taboo or neglecting a cultural ritual, and spiritual condemnation. The mentally ill have been ridiculed, neglected, banned, persecuted, and deprived of their freedoms.

The common belief that mental disturbance was related to supernatural phenomena meant that healing, if it took place at all, had to involve supernatural intercession. Other beliefs have held that the passions that interfered with proper reasoning were responsible for mental illness. *Melancholia,* now called depression, at one time was thought to result from an imbalance of body systems causing an excess of bile in the body.

In the 19th century, mental illness was viewed as incurable, and little humane treatment existed. Until 1820, the mentally ill were exhibited as diversion and entertainment for the public. Until 1886, they typically were restrained in iron manacles.[7]

Beginning in the 1950s, pharmacotherapy dramatically changed mental health care. The discovery of neuroleptic and later antidepressant drugs brought new hope to treating mental illness, particularly psychotic disorders. Psychoactive drugs relieve many symptoms of mental illnesses and allow psychotic clients to gain greater benefit from other therapies.

Despite great advances, treatment of mental illness still has far to go. Lewis Judd, past Director of the National Institutes of Mental Health (NIMH), addressing the low priority given to treating mental disorders in the United States, said that in the Middle Ages, the mentally ill were burned at the stake, during the age of enlightenment, they were kept in prisons and chains, and today they are treated with inattention and neglect.[15]

Stigma is experienced by individuals who need or use psychiatric-mental health services. Public education directed at modifying or altering misconceptions about mental illness and people with mental disorders will help to reduce stigma. Toward this end, in 1990, the NIMH set forth a National Mental Health Agenda to focus attention on mental disorders proportional to the level of suffering and disability these disorders cause.[15]

Defining Mental Disorder

Following is the American Psychiatric Association's definition of *mental disorder*:

> A clinically significant behavioral or psychological syndrome or pattern that occurs in an individual and that is associated with present distress (e.g., a painful symptom) or disability (i.e., impairment in one or more important areas of functioning) or with a significantly increased risk of suffering death, pain, disability, or an important loss of freedom.[2]

In addition, the person's behavior must not be an expected and culturally sanctioned response to a life event, such as a loss of a loved one, for it to be classified as a disorder. Deviant behavior is not necessarily a sign of a mental disorder.[2]

General criteria for *mental disorders* include the following:

1. Dissatisfaction with one's characteristics, abilities, and accomplishments
2. Ineffective or unsatisfying interpersonal relationships
3. Dissatisfaction with one's place in the world
4. Ineffective coping or adaptation to the events in one's life and a lack of personal growth

Nevertheless, precise definitions of mental illness or disorder are elusive and impractical. The Diagnostic and Statistical Manual of Mental Disorders, 4th edition (DSM-IV) provides the diagnostic criteria for mental disorders or illnesses. The DSM-IV categorizes disorders, however, not *people.* Nurses are reminded that a person *has* the disorder of schizophrenia or depression or alcoholism; the person *is not* a schizophrenic or depressive or alcoholic.[2]

Incidence of Mental Illness

According to the National Institute of Mental Health, more than 12% of adults in the United States have a diagnosable mental illness at any time, and 22% of adults will experience a mental disorder needing treatment at some point in life.[15] Between 12% and 20% of children younger than 18 years in the United States are believed to have a diagnosable mental disorder. Many of these individuals receive inappropriate, fragmented, or inadequate care or no care at all.

The number of adults with mental illness includes about 10 million people with depressive disorders (80%–85% of whom can be successfully treated) and 1.5 to 2 million people with panic disorders. Between 33,000 and 34,000 people commit suicide each year. The incidence of suicide is escalating, especially in people 14 to 24 years old, in whom the rate has tripled during the last 30 years. Suicide remains the leading cause of death in adolescents.[15]

Attitudes and Myths

Society's attitudes toward mental illness have not progressed dramatically over the centuries.[8] Our approaches to the mentally ill are determined not only by medical and psychiatric theory, but also by the political and social climates of the time. In the mid-1800s, for example, a schoolteacher from New England, Dorothea Lynde Dix, investigated the deplorable conditions in mental institutions in the United States and appealed to state legislatures for better treatment of the mentally ill. Almost single-handedly, she began a revolution in mental health care.[16]

On February 5, 1963, President John F. Kennedy delivered his well-known "bold new approach" address to the United States Congress. The result of this address and subsequent legislation was the creation and growth of the community mental health movement. Unfortunately, after the 1970s, interest in community mental health waned, and currently there are vast unserved and underserved populations in the United States.

The U.S. judicial system has influenced psychiatric-mental health treatment issues. In recent years, court decisions have affirmed individuals' right to treatment, right to refuse treatment, and right to treatment in the least restrictive setting.[8] These rulings influence our attitudes about mentally disturbed people and their rights and responsibilities (see Chapter 49, Legal Implications of Psychiatric-Mental Health Nursing).

Individuals' values and personal beliefs affect attitudes toward mental illness, people with mental disorders, and treatment of mental illness. For example, people who strongly value independence may disdain the apparent dependence or weakness of depressed individuals. People who highly value liberty and personal free dom may fail to appreciate the need for physical or chemical restraint of aggressive clients. Those who value stoicism may find it difficult to understand the usefulness of expressing feelings in restoring or maintaining mental health.

Myths about mental illness are harmful to clients, their families, and their future. Nurses and other mental health care providers are also influenced by these myths, for example, predicting a person's prognosis by diagnosis or symptoms. Rather, sound psychiatric principles encourage caregivers to promote a full life with optimal opportunities for all clients.[22]

PSYCHIATRIC-MENTAL HEALTH CARE

Psychiatric-mental health care involves the interdisciplinary collaboration of psychiatric nurses, psychiatrists, psychiatric social workers, psychologists, activities therapists, chaplains, and other mental health team members with the client and family.

Current Trends in Care

Consumer-focused care in a seamless continuum of therapeutic possibilities is the goal of today's psychiatric-mental health treatment. Community-based care, that is, treatment of the client in his or her community, is emphasized for reasons of quality outcomes and cost. New neurobiological theories and discoveries bring about new treatments for mental illness, including new psychopharmacological agents. Clients receive shorter lengths of stay and are treated with brief therapy and crisis stabilization. Client and family education and health teaching to at-risk populations reflect the philosophy of mental health promotion and illness or symptom prevention.

Unfortunately, many problems face the mental health care system. Psychiatric-mental health treatment is costly, and many medical insurance plans do not cover or inadequately cover treatment of mental disorders. Managed care may dictate treatment decisions. Clients hospitalized in a state institution for the mentally ill are removed from their support systems and often receive little more than custodial care. The lack of governmental support for community mental health centers has hastened the centers' narrowing of services and populations served.

The Decade of the Brain

In the 1990s, the "decade of the brain," mental health professionals are focusing on the connection between mental illness and biological malfunctions in the brain and the neuroendocrine-immune system. This represents a shift away from the traditional psychodynamic view of mental disorder as solely a disturbance of the mind.[2,13]

The biological view holds that biological defects are

responsible for certain serious mental illnesses. In contrast, the psychodynamic view holds that intrapersonal, social, cultural, and environmental factors are instrumental in determining the etiology of mental illness. The optimal approach to psychiatric diagnosis and care considers both viewpoints to provide nurses with the broadest understanding of mental illness and the widest range of therapeutic possibilities.[25]

Primary Mental Health Care

Primary mental health care is the "continuous and comprehensive services necessary for the promotion of optimal mental health, prevention of mental illness, and health maintenance, and includes the management (treatment) of and/or referral for mental and general health problems" (p 155).[12] This model proposes nursing's professional role responsibilities—advocacy, shaping public policy, involvement in professional oragnaizations, and community action—and intervention activities at basic and advanced level functioning. These nursing activities are built around the concept of mental health promotion and preventive intervention programs.[12]

Consumer Advocacy

The United States still has unequal access to health care. Consumer advocate groups, such as the National Alliance for the Mentally Ill (NAMI), have demanded improved mental health care; their voices are strong and are becoming stronger.

All mental health self-help groups have an advocacy base and a dissatisfaction with the present mental health care system. To achieve their aims, the self-help groups have created alternative programs of mutual support.

Care of the Aged

The 1971 White House Conference on Aging acknowledged the need for comprehensive health care (including mental health care) for the elderly.[31] It called for the diagnosis of disorders, treatment or safe transfer to a more adequate site for care, rehabilitation of elderly people with emotional disorders, and their return home to family and community. The conference also recommended alternatives to institutional care: training of mental health care providers to work with the elderly, increased funding of research on treating the elderly, and the development of innovative therapeutic services for institutionalized older people.[31]

Persistent Mental Illness

Deinstitutionalization of state mental hospitals during the 1970s unwittingly created many problems in the delivery of services to those with long-term mental illness. Clients with serious and persistent mental illness typically encounter many barriers that limit their access to services and prevent continuity of care. The development of a mental illness, for example, is a risk factor for becoming homeless (see Chapter 36, The Homeless Mentally Ill).[15]

Challenges

In the 1990s, psychiatric-mental health nursing is facing challenges from the following:

1. The growth in scientific knowledge, which is providing new insights into the biological roots and treatment of mental illness
2. Technological advances allowing more precise examination of the structure and function of the brain than has been possible in the past
3. Changes in the mental health care delivery system, such as deinstitutionalization and the rise in outpatient treatment
4. The increased and increasing numbers of poor, elderly, ethnic people of color, and chronically mentally ill who are uninsured or underinsured
5. The continuing stigmatization of mentally ill people
6. A changing definition of nursing's role in the evolving specialty[18]

Holistic Mental Health Care

Holistic care involves the whole person in the total environment. Holistic mental health care encompasses these concepts:

1. The uniqueness of the client, including the unique life history and personal style of expression and fulfillment
2. The healing partnership between caregiver and client, which alters the traditional authoritarian relationship and empowers the client
3. The healing ability of the caregiver, that is, the use of interpersonal skills and instillation of hope in the client
4. The view that a disorder is an opportunity to grow, not just to recover, and that it is a challenge to understand and overcome, and as a result learn, new, healthier ways of functioning[10]

Nursing and other mental health fields are turning to older and less westernized cultures for a range of therapeutic techniques. For example, very fast deep nasal breathing, an ancient technique from Tibet, can energize depressed individuals. Mantra meditation, a Hindu technique in which a certain sound is silently repeated, can lower anxiety. Healing measures not usually used in traditional psychiatric treatment, such as acupuncture, transcendental meditation, homeopathy, and laying on of hands (therapeutic touch), are powerful concomitant therapies. Increasingly, clients are taught ways to participate in their return to health through diet and exercise.[10]

◆ Stress: Mechanisms and Responses

Hans Selye, a renowned biological scientist, defined *stress* as the "nonspecific response of the body to any demand made upon it."[29] Although *stressors,* or stress-producing factors, vary—such as physical stressors of heat and cold and psychological stressors of failure, success, and a new challenge—they elicit essentially the same biological stress response. Stress is neither a synonym for distress, anxiety, and tension, nor something to be avoided at all costs. The absence of all stress is, according to Selye, death.

Richard Lazarus' definition of stress focuses on the relationship between the person and the environment and the person's appraisal that the environment is taxing or beyond his or her resources and harmful to his or her well-being. Therefore, how the person appraises the situation determines whether it is perceived as stressful.[19]

GENERAL ADAPTATION SYNDROME

To cope with any type of increased demand made on it, according to Selye, the body responds in a stereotyped manner, with identical biochemical changes.[29] These responses, termed the *general adaptation syndrome* (GAS) and commonly called the "fight or flight" response, demonstrates the body's manifestations of stress. The GAS evolves in three stages:

1. *Alarm reaction*: The body begins to respond and adjust to the stressor. The body's resistance is being diminished, and death may occur if the stressor is sufficiently strong.
2. *Stage of resistance*: The body continues to resist the stressor and no longer evidences signs of the initial reaction. The person's level of resistance is greater than usual.
3. *Stage of exhaustion*: The body's ability to resist the stressor, or adaptation energy, becomes exhausted following lengthy exposure to the same stressor. The signs of the initial reaction return but are irreversible, and the person dies.[29]

DISTRESS

According to Selye, damaging stressors (eg, anxiety, frustration, insecurity, aimlessness) may result in various physical and emotional disorders, such as migraine headache, peptic ulcer, myocardial infarction (heart attack), hypertension, suicide, mental illness, and hopeless unhappiness.[29]

What is the ultimate aim of people? Is it, as Selye suggests, to express ourselves as fully as possible, according to our own talents and desires, and to achieve a sense of security? If so, then we must learn how to accomplish this. Selye's solution is to discover our own optimal stress level and then use this adaptive energy at a rate and in a direction adjusted to our own qualifications and preferences. The words of Selye's own philosophy provide a guideline for using adaptive energy:

> Fight for your highest attainable aim
> But never put up resistance in vain.[29]

COPING MECHANISMS

Also called ego-defense mechanisms, mental mechanisms, and defense mechanisms, *coping mechanisms* protect the ego from overwhelming anxiety. For the most part, they operate on an unconscious level and occur in everyday life. The usefulness of these various coping mechanisms lies in their protection of the person from intolerable anxiety. We all use these mechanisms at one time or another, particularly in situations that elicit threatening or painful feelings; however, their value depends on their judicious use. The continuous, exclusive use of these mechanisms inhibits or prevents the learning of more effective ways to cope with, adapt to, and grow in relation to the environment and the challenges of our life.

Denial

In this common coping mechanism, a person denies the existence of some external reality. The person using *denial* is unaware of doing so. For example, someone informed of a medical diagnosis may deny its existence for some time. Denial generally operates as a healthy mechanism, protecting the individual from the immediate shock of reality. In time, denial usually diminishes, and the person gradually begins to face, accept, and deal with the harsh reality of the truth.

There are varying degrees of denial. For example, a man who has been told that he has had a heart attack that caused a great deal of damage to the heart muscle may deny that he has had a heart attack at all. Another man facing the same diagnosis may acknowledge that he has suffered a heart attack and recognize the need for treatment and for modification of his lifestyle but may not believe that the extent of heart damage is as serious as his doctors have described.

Denial also may have treatment implications. For example, a child exhibits overtly disturbed behavior, but the parents deny that a problem exists, will not seek treatment for their child, and may become indignant when a teacher or school nurse recommends psychological assessment of the child.

A person may deny selectively, that is, deny certain facts but accept or seem to accept others. Consider, for example, the following scenario:

> A husband and wife in their early 30s were told by the pediatric neurologist that their son, 10 months old, had static congenital encephalopathy (cerebral palsy) as evidenced by right-sided hemiparesis. While dealing with their shock, anger, and other facets of grief, they began to plan and implement various therapies needed by their son, for example, passive exercising of his right arm and leg and an active swimming program. Eight months after the diagnosis of the child's condition, the couple sat in their living room watching the summer Olympic Games on television. The woman turned to her husband and asked, "Do you think someday our son will be an Olympic athlete?" "What?!" replied the man, looking at his wife in disbelief.

Denial takes many forms and serves many functions. In this situation, it protected the mother from the full force of her grief over the loss of the "ideal child."

Regression

Through *regression,* a person avoids anxiety by returning to an earlier, more comfortable time in life when needs were met more readily. For instance, a 3-year-old child might regress in response to the birth of a sibling and begin again to soil her pants, suck her thumb, engage in baby talk, and ask for a bottle. An adult undergoing physical or emotional stress may regress by becoming irritable, demanding, and whining or may take to the bed for a sick day, thereby giving up responsibilities for the day and allowing others to meet his or her needs.

Play is an important form of regression, a way of voluntarily relinquishing adult concerns and duties and engaging in a childlike state of spontaneity and enjoyment. For children, play serves many functions, including fantasy, learning, and opportunity for mastery of physical and emotional challenges. Like the other coping mechanisms, regression may be a useful and healthy response to stressors, but it may become maladaptive if used excessively or exclusively.

Displacement

Displacement is the transfer of an emotion from its original object to a substitute object. For example, a person angry with a superior at work or school may feel too threatened to confront that individual with the anger; instead, he or she may go home and vent the anger on a family member. The person has displaced the feeling (anger) from its original object (his or her superior) to a substitute object (a family member).

Individuals who displace feelings usually have no awareness of doing so. Later, however, they may look back on the events and realize that, because they were angry with someone to whom they could not comfortably express the feelings, they took it out on a family member.

Projection

Projection involves displacing feelings, usually feelings perceived as negative, onto another individual. If, for example, a person feels guilty (or angry, dependent, aggressive, or hostile) and this feeling is unacceptable, he or she may project it onto another rather than owning up to it. The following statements could indicate projection:

- "I'm not angry, but she's mad at me."
- "I don't have any bad feelings toward him, but he sure hates me."

Individuals with paranoid behavior frequently overuse projection. A person who is fearful of the environment may project those feelings onto the external world and develop the delusion that outside forces, such as the FBI, CIA, or spies, are out to get him or her. This person may believe that others are constantly watching and plotting his or her demise.

Sometimes projection functions as an adaptive mechanism, protecting us from feelings that we find unacceptable in ourselves until we can learn to own them and acknowledge that having positive and negative feelings is part of our humanity.

Reaction Formation

Using *reaction formation,* a person acts in a way opposite to how he or she feels, because the feelings are unacceptable. For example, a person who feels aggressive or hostile toward another might behave very kindly and politely toward the object of those feelings. The person who uses reaction formation is not aware of the great disparity between feelings and actions. Consider this scenario:

> A student seemed to be angry at one particular instructor. She was displeased with her grades on the instructor's examinations and with the criticisms and corrections she received from him. When she interacted with the instructor, however, she wore a frozen, continuous smile on her face, was excessively polite, and talked in a high-pitched, "little girl" tone of voice. She often gave the instructor gifts.

People who cannot acknowledge feelings of dependency may behave in ways that emphasize independence. They may assert that they need no one and verbally and nonverbally drive others away.

Repression

Through *repression,* certain feelings or thoughts are forced into the unconscious. The repressed material, such as painful memories or feelings, remains in the unconscious, although it may surface from time to time in dreams or slips of the tongue. Repression acts as a protective mechanism against overwhelming anxiety. The person involuntarily forgets certain events or feelings that evoke a great deal of anxiety. People who suffered abuse as children, for example, may have little or no recollection of it. Repression helps protect those people from the emotional trauma associated with their abuse.

Suppression

Suppression occurs when certain anxiety-producing thoughts or feelings are consciously excluded from consideration. This coping mechanism operates at the conscious level. A person deciding to "put something out of mind" or "not worry about it until tomorrow" is using suppression. The classic example of suppression is found in *Gone with the Wind* when Scarlett O'Hara faces insurmountable odds with the words, "I won't think about that today. I'll think of it tomorrow."

Identification

Identification involves the unconscious adoption of personality characteristics, attitudes, values, and behaviors of another. Children frequently identify with their parents, aunts, uncles, teachers, and even well-known public figures in sports or entertainment. Adults also use identification as a means of continued growth by adopting attributes of their role models. When this process becomes conscious, it is called *imitation.*

The person using identification is unaware of doing so, although others may recognize it. Overuse of identification may result in low self-esteem and little sense of individuality due to over-reliance on others' advice and support. However, identification with positive role models generally leads to the incorporation of positive traits.

Rationalization

Rationalization refers to the substitution of acceptable reasons for the actual reasons that motivate behavior. Through rationalization, a person justifies behavior or conceals disappointments. For example, a man who interviews for a job but is not hired may rationalize that the interviewer did not spend enough time to get a fair impression of his strengths, that he did not really want the job, or that the job would have required more time than he was willing to devote to it. In each of these rationalizations, real feelings of failure and disappointment are covered to protect the person from the anxiety associated with these feelings.

Fantasy

Fantasy is nonrational mental activity that allows escape from daily pressures and responsibilities. Fantasy temporarily breaks through the boundaries of reality and allows people to daydream about whatever is most pleasurable to them. For example, a person overwhelmed by the pressures of a task he or she has undertaken may imagine completing the task and the feelings of satisfaction and pride this will engender. These feelings may spur him or her to work harder toward a goal.

Children's thinking, especially that of young children, is characterized by fantasy. Often, adults become stifled by the realities of the world and abandon their use of fantasy. The ability to fantasize, however, provides an effective escape valve for people of all ages and promotes childlike creativity. Excessive use of fantasy, on the other hand, reduces contact with reality and may render a person incapable of dealing with the demands of life.

Intellectualization

Through *intellectualization,* a person uses the intellectual powers of thinking, reasoning, and analyzing to blunt or avoid emotional issues that are too threatening or painful. Sometimes a person with significant emotional problems (eg, a severe lack of interpersonal skills) intellectualizes those problems. The person may discuss Sullivan's interpersonal theory and the effect of childhood interpersonal experiences on adult functioning and may weigh the value of one therapeutic intervention over another but will avoid the more difficult discussion of personal feelings. Feelings are often the heart of the issue in psychiatric-mental health nursing, but facing them requires a degree of courage and confidence.

◆ Psychiatric-Mental Health Nursing

Psychiatric-mental health nursing is the diagnosis and treatment of human responses to actual or potential mental health problems.[1] It views people holistically, considering strengths, talents, needs, and problems.

Psychiatric nursing is built on several principles or beliefs about people and the care they deserve:

1. Every person is worthy of dignity and respect.
2. Every person has the potential to change and grow.
3. All people have basic human needs in common with others.
4. All behavior is meaningful and can be understood from the person's perspective.
5. People have the right to participate in decisions about their health and their care.

Psychiatric-mental health nursing has evolved into a unique discipline combining the knowledge, experience, and skills of nursing and biological and social sciences and the art of therapeutic use of self. The term psychiatric-mental health nursing implies two areas of nursing that interact and overlap. *Psychiatric nursing* focuses on the care and rehabilitation of those with identifiable emotional disorders. *Mental health nursing* focuses on well and at-risk populations and intervenes in crisis situations to prevent the development of mental illness or disorder. Together, psychiatric-mental health nursing offers a wide range of preventive and interventive strategies to promote optimal functioning and health.

Through the nursing process, psychiatric-mental health nursing provides comprehensive care to individuals, families, groups, and communities.

NURSING PROCESS

The *nursing process* is a systematic problem-solving approach to client problems. The five steps of the nursing process—assessment, nursing diagnosis, planning, intervention, and evaluation—provide a systematic method for delivering care (Box 1-1). Chapters 8 (Assessment and Nursing Diagnosis) and 9 (Planning, Intervention, and Evaluation) demonstrate the application of the nursing process to client problems.

Assessment

Assessment, the first step of the nursing process, involves systematic collection of comprehensive data about clients and their problems and needs. The nurse explores psychological, social, and cultural influences on the client's functioning.

Nursing Diagnosis

In the second step of the nursing process, *nursing diagnosis,* data are organized into categories. Actual and potential client problems are determined. The causes of problems are explored, if possible, and conclusions are formulated.

Planning

The third step, *planning,* involves determining goals and client outcomes and designing interventions to achieve these goals. Planning is a collaborative process involving the client, family, and other members of the psychiatric treatment team.

Intervention

Intervention, the fourth step of the nursing process, occurs when nursing activities aimed at achieving client goals are implemented.

Evaluation

In *evaluation,* the fifth and final step of the nursing process, the nurse determines the outcomes and effectiveness of nursing interventions and identifies the need for further intervention.

HISTORY OF PSYCHIATRIC-MENTAL HEALTH NURSING

One of the most significant figures in the history of psychiatric care in the United States was Dorothea Lynde Dix (1802–1887). During her lifetime, the standard treatment of the mentally ill ranged from negligence to brutality, with clients sometimes confined in cages and cellars, chained, and beaten.[12] She pioneered the crusade for reforms in the treatment of the mentally ill and gained the support of influential citizens by publicizing the abhorrent conditions in which mental health clients lived.

By 1940, there were only about 4,000 graduate nurses working in state mental hospitals. In some states, psychiatric nursing was not even taught, although those states operated psychiatric hospitals. Nurses may have learned how to care for the mentally ill in a general hospital school of nursing, a psychiatric hospital school of nursing, or through their experience in a psychiatric institution. At this time, some nursing leaders were beginning to recognize that the responsibilities and role of the psychiatric nurse differ from those of a nurse caring for the physically ill. Some nurses began to see the importance of interaction, acceptance, respect for other human beings, and what today would be called the therapeutic use of self.[16]

In July 1946, the U.S. Congress passed the National Mental Health Act, administered by NIMH, to finance mental health research, training programs, and community mental health services. The NIMH traineeship program, begun in 1948, became a significant support for graduate-level education of psychiatric nurses.[16] Unfortunately, as this money disappeared, recruitment into the specialty decreased. Now, however, the growing need for psychiatric nurses in a variety of service settings and roles has focused more attention on the field.

FUNCTIONS AND ROLES OF PSYCHIATRIC-MENTAL HEALTH NURSES

The Statement on Psychiatric-Mental Health Clinical Nursing Practice categorizes nursing functions into basic level and advanced level functions.

Basic Level Functions

Basic level functions include the following:

1. Health promotion and health maintenance, including health assessments, health teaching, pre-

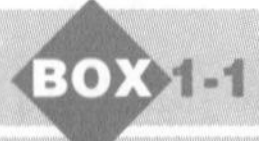
BOX 1-1

Statement on Psychiatric-Mental Health Clinical Nursing Practice and Standards of Psychiatric-Mental Health Clinical Nursing Practice

STANDARDS OF CARE

Standard I. Assessment: The psychiatric-mental health nurse collects client health data.

Standard II Diagnosis: The psychiatric-mental health nurse analyzes the assessment data to determine diagnoses.

Standard III. Outcome Identification: The psychiatric-mental health nurse identifies expected outcomes individualized to the client.

Standard IV. Planning: The psychiatric-mental health nurse develops a plan of care that prescribes interventions to attain expected outcomes.

Standard V. Implementation: The psychiatric-mental health nurse implements the interventions identified in the plan of care.

Standard V-a. Counseling: The psychiatric-mental health nurse uses counseling interventions to assist clients in improving or regaining their previous coping abilities, to foster mental health, and to prevent mental illness and disability.

Standard V-b. Milieu Therapy: The psychiatric-mental health nurse provides, structures, and maintains a therapeutic environment in collaboration with the client and other health care providers.

Standard V-c. Self-Care Activities: The psychiatric-mental health nurse structures interventions around the client's activities of daily living in a goal-directed way to foster self-care and physical and mental well-being.

Standard V-d. Psychobiological Interventions: The psychiatric-mental health nurse uses knowledge of psychobiological interventions and applies clinical skills to restore the client's health and prevent further disability.

Standard V-e. Health Teaching: The psychiatric-mental health nurse, through health teaching, assists clients to achieve satisfying, productive, and healthy patterns of living.

Standard V-f. Case management: The psychiatric-mental health nurse provides case management to coordinate comprehensive health services and ensure continuity of care.

Standard V-g. Health Promotion and Health Maintenance: The psychiatric-mental health nurse uses strategies and interventions to promote and maintain mental health and prevent mental illness.

Advanced Practice Interventions (V-h–V-j)

Standard V-h. Psychotherapy: The certified specialist in psychiatric-mental health nursing uses individual, group, and family psychotherapy; child psychotherapy; and other therapeutic treatments to assist clients in fostering mental health, preventing mental illness and disability, and improving or regaining previous health status and functional abilities.

Standard V-i. Prescription of Pharmacological Agents: The certified specialist uses prescription of pharmacological agents in accordance with the state Nurse Practice Act to treat symptoms of psychiatric illness and improve functional health status.

Standard V-j. Consultation: The certified specialist provides consultation to health care providers and others to influence the plans of care for clients and to enhance the abilities of others to provide psychiatric and mental health care and effect change in systems.

Standard VI. Evaluation: The psychiatric-mental health nurse evaluates the client's progress in attaining expected outcomes.

STANDARDS OF PROFESSIONAL PERFORMANCE

Standard I. Quality of Care: The psychiatric-mental health nurse systematically evaluates the quality of care and effectiveness of psychiatric-mental health nursing practice.

Standard II. Performance appraisal: The psychiatric-mental health nurse evaluates own psychiatric-mental health nursing practice in relation to professional practice standards and relevant statutes and regulations.

continued

venting potential complications, and intervening with at-risk populations. The nurse educates clients through programs, such as parenting classes, stress management techniques, and assertiveness training.

2. Intake screening and evaluation to intervene at the client's point of entry into the mental health care system. The nurse conducts physical and psychosocial assessments, makes nursing diagnoses, and refers the clients for specialized testing if needed.

BOX 1-1 (Continued)

Standard III. Education: The psychiatric-mental health nurse acquires and maintains current knowledge in nursing practice.
Standard IV. Collegiality: The psychiatric-mental health nurse contributes to the professional development of peers, colleagues, and others.
Standard V. Ethics: The psychiatric-mental health nurse's decisions and actions on behalf of clients are determined in an ethical manner.
Standard VI. Collaboration: The psychiatric-mental health nurse collaborates with the client, significant others, and health care providers in providing care.
Standard VII. Research: The psychiatric-mental health nurse contributes to nursing and mental health through the use of research.
Standard VIII. Resource Utilization: The psychiatric-mental health nurse considers factors related to safety, effectiveness, and cost in planning and delivering client care.

(This material has been published by the American Nurses Association and is reprinted with permission.)

(American Nurses Association; American Psychiatric Nurses Association; Association of Child and Adolescent Psychiatric Nurses; Society for Education and Research in Psychiatric-Mental Health Nursing, Washington DC, American Nurses Publishing, 1994. Reprinted with permission.)

3. Case management in inpatient and outpatient settings. The nurse supports the client's highest level of functioning to promote self-sufficiency. Case management activities may include monitoring of the client's functional level and medication efficacy, problem solving and supportive counseling, care planning, and referral to community resources.
4. Milieu therapy, using the resources of mental health care providers, other clients, and supervised therapeutic environments to restore, maintain, or build the client's functional abilities. On behalf of the client's individual needs, the nurse attends to the physical environment, programming, social structure, and interactions.
5. Self-care activities of daily living, such as personal hygiene, eating, leisure activities, and the practical skills needed in life (shopping, using public transportation). The nurse guides, directs, and reinforces the client's progress toward independent functioning.
6. Psychobiological interventions, such as teaching and implementing nutrition, rest, and activity programs; explaining, administering, and evaluating medication effectiveness and side effects; and assisting with electroconvulsive and other somatic therapies. The nurse teaches about and evaluates the client's response to psychobiological interventions.
7. Health teaching of the client and family in relation to promoting mental health or treating mental illness. This teaching is based on sound teaching-learning principles and maximizes the use of experiential learning (that is, learning that is derived from experience). The nurse teaches a psychiatric client and family about, for example, the client's mental illness, its etiology and manifestations, symptom management, information about medications and managing side effects, coping skills, supportive interventions for significant others.
8. Crisis intervention, that is, short-term therapeutic intervention to resolve an immediate crisis or emergency using all available resources
9. Counseling that is directed toward resolution of a health-related problem
10. Home visit or client residence, which may mean a nursing home, prison, halfway house, or homeless shelter. The nurse gathers data from the home setting and encourages the supportive involvement of the client's family members and significant others.
11. Community action or concern for sociocultural factors that adversely affect populations and interventions to reduce those problems. The nurse serves on or interacts with advisory and planning boards and other community-oriented people to address the populations' mental health needs.
12. Advocacy through political processes, consumer and professional groups, and protection of client rights[1]

Advanced Level Functions

Psychiatric-mental health nurses who have achieved additional preparation by means of education and practice also perform the following advanced level nursing functions:

1. Psychotherapy by means of individual, group, family, and couple or marital therapies. The nurse acquires certification credentials and functions autonomously as a primary therapist.

2. Psychobiological interventions that range from relaxation techniques and nutrition counseling to prescription of pharmacological agents. The advanced practice nurse with prescriptive authority functions in accordance with the state practice act and state and federal laws.
3. Clinical supervision of and clinical consultation with other psychiatric-mental health care providers
4. Consultation-liaison activities in which the nurse intervenes directly to promote optimal mental functioning in physically ill or disabled clients and indirectly as consultant and educator with other nurses and health caregivers[1]

Psychiatric-mental health nurses are skilled communicators, role models of adaptive behavior, directors of the therapeutic milieu, advocates for the client and family, members of the mental health care team, primary nurses for specific clients, and therapists with individuals, groups, and families. These roles are explored throughout the chapters of this book.

NURSES' REACTIONS

Like everyone else, nurses are affected by the behavior of the people around them. A nurse working with clients with psychiatric problems may encounter various forms of disturbed behavior—bizarre, aggressive, hostile, suspicious, dependent, and violent. Reaction to these behaviors is likely to reflect the range of the nurses' personal experiences and values.

The nurse reacting to disturbed behavior may be offended, repulsed, threatened, annoyed, angered, surprised, or shocked. These feelings may confuse and frighten the nurse, who may view the feelings as unprofessional and be ashamed of them. If the goal of nursing is to provide the highest quality care for clients, then nurses must first examine their own values, feelings, and reactions. Self-exploration and working through difficult issues, such as how to interpret and deal with manipulation or hostility, are crucial developments in the nurse's professional growth.

There is no one right way to intervene therapeutically in disturbed behavior. Mental health care providers explore their thoughts and feelings, follow guidelines or standards of care, search for more effective interventions, and measure the outcomes of interventions.

NOVICE NURSES

Nurses who are new to psychiatric-mental health nursing face certain impressions, perceptions, and fears that, if unexamined, may hamper the nurse's effectiveness in intervention. Commonly, nursing students facing their first psychiatric nursing experiences feel anxious, fearful of the client's actions and possible rejection, possibly fearful of damaging the client through nontherapeutic communication, or concern for their own mental health or mental symptoms (Box 1-2).

CLIENTS' VIEWS OF MENTAL HEALTH CARE

The client's views and feelings are important to consider. Often clients are frightened or relieved by hospitalization in a psychiatric unit. They may fear that treatment will dehumanize them or that care providers will overmedicate, discount, or neglect them. Clients may be suspicious of the new environment and unfamiliar with mental health professionals.

Clients seeking psychiatric treatment often expect that the care providers will be able to solve their problems for them. They may expect to play a passive role while the psychiatrist, nurse, psychologist, or social worker actively cures them. Mental health care professionals must rectify such misperceptions and provide clients with straightforward information about mental health care and the expected participation of the client as a member of the health care team.

STRESS AND BURNOUT AMONG PSYCHIATRIC-MENTAL HEALTH NURSES

The stressors experienced by psychiatric-mental health nurses are considerable. Intervening daily with individuals whose behavior is disordered or maladaptive requires a great deal of personal and professional resources and exacts a heavy toll.

Nurses should be alert to certain warning signs of increasing job stress. These may take the form of *horizontal violence*—anger, negativity, and sarcasm a nurse directs to peers—or *passive-aggressive* behavior, which undermines other nurses.[5] Nurses may notice that they have lost energy and enthusiasm for their job, feel fatigued, have trouble sleeping, and look for escape through alcohol and drug use. As burnout becomes more severe, nurses may become exhausted, physically ill, moody, withdrawn, obsesssed with their own problems, and increasing their use of drugs and alcohol.

One study found that older, more experienced therapists perceived the work-related issues of maintaining the therapeutic relationship, scheduling, professional doubt, work overinvolvement, and personal depletion less stressful than inexperienced therapists. Regardless of level of experience, however, all therapists experienced stress from working with particularly difficult client behaviors, such as negative affect,

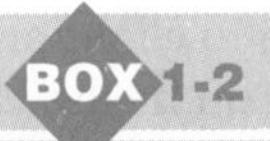

Preparing for Psychiatric-Mental Health Nursing Experiences

Johnnie Bonner, MS, RN, Staff Development Specialist Dallas Veterans Administration Medical Center, Dallas, Texas

During your psychiatric nursing experience, you will discover varying philosophies and theories about the nature of human behavior and what constitutes competent, ethical treatment of individuals with emotional disorders. You may also be exposed to a variety of settings or may realize that your textbook or instructor describes different kinds of treatment from what you observe. If you think of the inconsistencies as differences and refrain from making judgments about "right or wrong," you may be more open to learning.

Sometimes, the structure of daily tasks is not as easy to identify on a psychiatric unit as in other services. This apparent lack of specific tasks may leave you wondering whether you can make any meaningful contribution to clients. Most psychiatric-mental health professionals and agencies believe that contributing to your learning experience is an investment that will pay off directly by adding you to the ranks of clinicians or indirectly by providing you with an awareness of psychiatric nursing. Psychiatric-mental health staff do not expect you to do anything but learn; however, they also know from experience that you will make significant contributions. Your energy and enthusiasm are refreshing. Your relatively unbiased exploration of what staff are doing and why will raise important questions and issues that need to be reviewed in the ongoing process of evaluating care.

You may wonder, particularly during your initial psychiatric nursing experience, "What will I discuss with the client?" The client may choose to keep the process of your interactions superficial, partially due to the dynamics of his or her problems and partially due to the reality of your limited time. Focus initial questions or interview openings on what led to the client's or others' decision to seek treatment. This will help you become acquainted with the client and give him or her an opportunity to reflect on the nature of his or her difficulties or treatment issues. Discussing the decision to seek treatment can be genuinely helpful, even when it is repeated many times, because it is an opportunity to examine the same set of circumstances from different perspectives.

Other areas to explore with clients include their expectations of the treatment facility and services and their responses to them. Thoughtful reflection on progress in the course of treatment can help build the client's self-esteem and hope for change.

The issue of confidentiality assumes an important and perhaps somewhat different perspective within the psychiatric-mental health team. You may be asked by the client not to share some information that he or she has revealed. I can think of *no* situation in which agreeing to this kind of request would be therapeutic. The client will need to be reminded, kindly but firmly, that it is important for all members of the treatment team to share any information that might contribute to treatment. In addition, you might ask the client to explore why he or she is unable to trust the other members of the treatment team.

Another crucial issue in psychiatric-mental health nursing is that of maintaining "separateness" or detachment in the therapeutic role. You may bristle and think that others are suggesting that you develop an attitude of coldness. On the contrary, your values of compassion and empathy are not being challenged; it is impossible to be therapeutic without those qualities. To use your knowledge and skills therapeutically, your compassion and empathy must be expressed in a manner that leaves your personal life separate from the client's. Clients do not need us as friends or companions as much as they need us to teach them how to have friendship and companionship outside of treatment. Identifying your own feelings and attitudes and discussing them with an experienced clinician may help you develop as a professional who is caring and effective in relationships with clients.

As you work with clients, keep in mind that although you may provide an opportunity and an environment in which change may occur, you cannot make a client change. Try to imagine what it would cost the client to make the changes you feel would benefit him. Change is the client's choice. He or she may need our skills, knowledge, and a safe place to work, and although he or she may sometimes borrow our hope, the client makes the choices, does the internal work, and needs to feel the pride and take the credit. The client lives with the choices.

resistance, suicidal threats, psychopathological symptoms, and passive-aggressive behaviors.[14] Whether nurses work as therapists or in other kinds of therapeutic positions with psychiatric clients, they suffer the effects of personal depletion, the stress of maintaining the therapeutic relationship, work overinvolvement, and frustration related to difficult client behaviors.

Factors contributing to professional burnout are not the sole result of internal forces. External forces, such as multiple regulations of the health care system and understaffing of the institution, create a psychologically toxic work environment. Working in such a toxic environment leads nurses to feel devalued, unable to provide quality care without lowering their standards, and dissatisfied with their job.[5]

Positive coping with job stress and burnout requires a concerted effort. Support systems at work and away from work allow the nurse to ventilate feelings and help keep events in perspective. A realistic outlook and expectations regarding the job also are essential. Taking frequent, brief vacations has been found to be more refreshing and relaxing than infrequent, longer vacations. Paying attention to physical health needs, particularly nutrition and exercise, brings great returns in terms of stress management and satisfaction with life (Box 1-3).

In addition, nurses need to evaluate their workplace honestly to determine whether they are blocked from providing excellence in care or forced to lower their standards, situations that are likely to result in burnout. The nurse should avoid assuming responsibility for others' problems; align client care according to priorities; keep own priorities of family, friends, personal goals in order; and search for creative ways to express excellence at work.[5]

NURSING MODELS

All nursing models have some truth or usefulness, given the diverse problems and needs of diverse clients in diverse settings.[4] In every model, nurses explore these issues:

1. Who defines the client problems?
2. Is the client blamed for those problems?
3. Is the client expected to take responsibility for arriving at solutions to problems?
4. Who evaluates the success or failure of the solutions?

Nursing models provide frameworks in which clients assume increased responsibility for solving their own problems, thus developing competence and independence. In contrast, the medical model of helping, wherein the helpers decide the solutions to client problems, promotes the client's dependence on health care providers.

Roy's model of nursing promotes the client's adaptation to a changing environment. The nurse assesses the adaptiveness or maladaptiveness of client behaviors and plans interventions to modify maladaptive behaviors.[4] The goal of nursing intervention may be regained stability for the client, that is, adaptation of the client to the environment. Instead, it may be more dynamic and change oriented, related to an improved level of wellness or mental health.

Traditionally, psychiatric nursing was provided by means of a long-term nurse–client relationship rooted in psychoanalytic and interpersonal theories. Most of today's treatment settings and situations, however, are built on the models of crisis intervention and brief psychotherapy. Within these time-limited and here-and-now frameworks for treatment, the nurse learns to make rapid assessments, formulate realistic plans, and intervene swiftly and appropriately. Eliminating unrealistic goals and plans may also help reduce job frustration and burnout among psychiatric-mental health nurses.

◆ Chapter Summary

This chapter introduced the basic principles of psychiatric-mental health nursing, including the following:

1. Mental health and mental illness are imprecisely defined states.
2. Mental health is characterized by satisfaction with one's characteristics, abilities, and accomplishments; effective and satisfying interpersonal relationships; effective coping or adaptation to life events; and personal growth.
3. Mental health care today is consumer-focused and community-based and incorporates briefer therapies, biological treatments, health teaching, and mental health promotion.
4. Challenges facing psychiatric-mental health nursing include implementing interventions derived from recent biological discoveries and technological advances; changes in the health care delivery system; increased numbers of poor, elderly, and chronically mentally ill in need of services; and stigmatization.
5. Stress is the nonspecific response of the body to any demand made on it; stressors, or stress-producing factors, whether physical or psychological, pleasant or unpleasant, elicit the same biological stress response.
6. The GAS evolves in three stages—alarm reaction, stage of resistance, and stage of exhaustion.

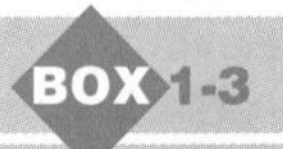

BOX 1-3

Energizing Yourself for Work and Play

Any area of nursing is stimulating and draining. Psychiatric-mental health nurses face the opportunity to make a significant difference in people's lives but also recognize that progress comes neither easily nor readily. They often admit that positive changes in their clients' lives do not occur as frequently and quickly as they would like.

Maintaining hopefulness for their clients, acknowledging the importance of therapeutic skills, and "hanging in there for the long haul" are essential capacities of psychiatric-mental health nurses. Often, psychiatric nursing reminds us of the words of Edmund Burke, "Nobody made a greater mistake than he who did nothing because he could only do a little."

Staying energized in the face of multiple demands and stressors at work and home requires that psychiatric-mental health nurses attend to self-care needs and activities. The attainment and maintenance of physical and mental health should be in the forefront of nurses' career goals. To accomplish this goal, nurses must draw on strategies that promote coping with and managing stress optimally. Some of these strategies follow:

- Do physical activity.
  You don't have to run a marathon to benefit from exercise. Engaging in a physical activity, such as walking, that raises your heart rate for 30 minutes three times per week contributes to cardiorespiratory fitness; builds strength, endurance, and flexibility; aids in weight control; improves mood; and fosters a feeling of well-being.
- Eat right.
  Excess and imbalanced diets are damaging to health. Americans consume too much sugar and fat in their diets. Eat a variety of foods low in fat, saturated fat, and cholesterol and plenty of vegetables, fruits, and grains. Reduce your use of caffeine. Nutrition may be one of the most important determinants of physical and mental health.
- Stay away from tobacco, alcohol, and other drugs.
  Cigarettes are the gateway drug opening the door to the use of many other substances. Find ways to relax that do not require substances—meditation, relaxation techniques, and physical activity balanced with rest.
- Remember to play.
  Play is not just something we do as children. Play refreshes and restores us; it absorbs and relaxes us. It even prepares us to return to our day-to-day responsibilities and pressures. Choose any activity that is enjoyable to you.
- Break from the routine.
  If you find yourself tense and aching, change your posture and concentrate on relaxing those tight muscles. If you find yourself becoming bored, learn a new skill or make a new friend. If you find yourself muttering angry words, hum a favorite tune, and give yourself time to reconstruct a verbal response.
- Learn to plan.
  Anxiety and poor coping can result from feelings of being overwhelmed. Plan your tasks and remember to schedule in personal time for fun and relaxation.
- Keep your priorities straight.
  Although your work may be interesting and satisfying, remember the importance of being connected and loved by family and friends. These are the people who will support you, nourish you, and help you maintain a sense of direction and perspective in your life.
- Don't forget help for yourself.
  When you need help, seek it out. Never believe that because you're a nurse, you don't need others' help. Communicate your needs to your family and friends, and if needed, obtain professional help.

7. Coping mechanisms, such as denial, rationalization, regression, and fantasy, protect the individual from anxiety.
8. The nursing process—assessment, nursing diagnosis, planning, intervention, and evaluation—is a problem-solving approach through which psychiatric-mental health nurses deliver care to clients.
9. Basic and advanced level functions and roles of psychiatric-mental health nurses include advocacy, health promotion and maintenance, case management, screening and evaluation, milieu therapy, health teaching, psychobiological interventions, and membership in the interdisciplinary health team.
10. Stress and burnout in the workplace can be minimized through early detection of stress symptoms; self-care measures, such as nutrition and exercise; involvement in non-nursing activities; and honesty about what can and cannot be changed on the job.

Critical Thinking Questions

1. *What are your views of mental illness?*
2. *Who or what do you think is responsible for a person becoming mentally ill? What did you learn from your family and teachers about mental illness and people who were mentally ill when you were a child growing up?*
3. *How are societal forces affecting the care of people with mental illness today?*
4. *Do you believe that people with mental illness are being treated as they should be in today's mental health care market?*

Review Questions

1. Identify four components of mental health.
2. Discuss current trends in psychiatric-mental health care.
3. Mental illness
   - **A.** is characterized by effective interpersonal relationships.
   - **B.** is present in 5% to 7% of adults and children in the United States.
   - **C.** is perceived by the public through stigma and misconceptions.
   - **D.** is precisely defined.
4. Selye's GAS includes
   - **A.** "fight or flight" mechanism in response to a stressor.
   - **B.** alarm reaction, in which the body adjusts to a stressor.
   - **C.** stage of irrevocable depletion, in which the body resists the stressor.
   - **D.** stage of distress, in which damaging stressors overwhelm the body's resistance.
5. A person who received a "below standards" evaluation rating for job performance tells a coworker that the supervisor doesn't like and "has it in" for him. This behavior is an example of
   - **A.** fantasy.
   - **B.** rationalization.
   - **C.** denial.
   - **D.** displacement.
6. Basic level functions of psychiatric mental health nurses include all of the following except
   - **A.** health promotion and health maintenance.
   - **B.** case management.
   - **C.** psychotherapy.
   - **D.** teaching self-care activities.
7. Nurses can cope positively with job stress and burnout by
   - **A.** taking care of physical health needs.
   - **B.** keeping stress and problems to oneself.
   - **C.** taking infrequent, long vacations.
   - **D.** maintaining the highest possible standards for one's work performance.

◆ References

1. American Nurses Association; American Psychiatric Nurses Association; Association of Child and Adolescent Psychiatric Nurses; Society for Education and Research in Psychiatric-Mental Health Nursing: Statement on Psychiatric-Mental Health Clinical Nursing Practice and Standards of Psychiatric-Mental Health Clinical Nursing Practice. Washington, DC, American Nurses Publishing, 1994
2. American Psychiatric Association: Diagnostic and Statistical Manual of Mental Disorders, 4th ed. Washington, DC, American Psychiatric Association, 1994
3. Babich K: Answers: Professionally Speaking. J Psychosoc Nurs Ment Health Serv 30 (1): 33–35, 1992
4. Cronenwett LR: Helping and Nursing Models. Nurs Res 32 (November/December): 342–346, 1983
5. Cullen A: Burnout: Why Do We Blame the Nurse? Am J Nurs 95 (11): 22–27, 1995
6. Dalsheimer JW: The Mental Health Nurse as Person. In Johnson BS (ed): Psychiatric-Mental Health Nursing: Adaptation and Growth, 3rd ed, pp 17–18. Philadelphia, JB Lippincott, 1993
7. Dolan JA, Fitzpatrick ML, Hermann EK: Nursing in Society: A Historical Perspective, 15th ed. Philadelphia, WB Saunders, 1983
8. Flagg JM: Public Policy and Mental Health: Past, Present, and Future. Nurs Health Care 4 (May): 246–251, 1983
9. Friedrich O: Going Crazy: An Inquiry into Madness in Our Time. New York, Simon and Schuster, 1976
10. Gordon JS: Holistic Medicine and Mental Health Practice: Toward a New Synthesis. Am J Orthopsychiatry 60 (3): 357–370, 1990
11. Gottschalk LA: The Psychotherapies in the Context of New Developments in the Neurosciences and Biological Psychiatry. Am J Psychotherapy 44 (3): 321–339, 1990
12. Haber J, Billings CV: Primary Mental Health Care: A Model for Psychiatric-Mental Health Nursing. Journal of the American Psychiatric Nurses Association 1 (5): 154–163, 1995
13. Hays A: Psychiatric Nursing: What Does Biology Have to Do With It? Archives of Psychiatric Nursing IX (4): 216–224, 1995
14. Hellman ID, Morrison TL, Abramowitz SI: Therapist Experience and the Stresses of Psychotherapeutic Work. Psychotherapy 24 (Summer): 171–176, 1987
15. Judd L: National Mental Health Agenda: The Next Decade. Plenary Session presented to the Fourth Annual Convention of the American Psychiatric Nurses' Association. Washington, DC, October 12, 1990
16. Kalisch PA, Kalisch BJ: The Advance of American Nursing, 2d ed. Boston, Little, Brown & Co, 1986
17. Keefe RSE: The Contribution of Neuropsychology to Psychiatry. Am J Psychiatry 152 (1): 6–15, 1995

18. Lowery BJ: Psychiatric Nursing in the 1990s and Beyond. J Psychosoc Nurs Ment Health Serv 30 (1): 7–13, 1992
19. McCain NL, Smith JC: Stress and Coping in the Context of Psychoneuroimmunology: A Holistic Framework for Nursing Practice and Research. Archives of Psychiatric Nursing VIII (4): 221–227, 1994
20. Menninger KA: The Human Mind, 3rd ed. New York: Alfred A. Knopf, 1945
21. Pardes H, Kaufmann CA, Pincu HA, et al: Genetics and Psychiatry: Past Discoveries, Current Dilemmas, and Future Directions. Am J Psychiatry 146 (4): 435–443, 1989
22. Palmer-Erbs VK, Anthony WA: Incorporating Psychiatric Rehabilitation Principles into Mental Health Nursing: An Opportunity to Develop a Full Partnership Among Nurses, Consumers, and Families. J Psychosoc Nurs 33 (3): 36–44, 1995
23. Pasquali EA: Learning to Laugh: Humor as Therapy. J Psychosoc Nurs Ment Health Serv 28 (3): 31–35, 1990
24. Peplau HE: Interpersonal Relations in Nursing. New York, GP Putnam's & Sons, 1952
25. Peplau HE: Some Unresolved Issues in the Era of Biopsychosocial Nursing. Journal of the American Psychiatric Nurses Association 1 (3): 92–96, 1995
26. Pothier PC, Stuart GW, Puskar K, Babich K: Dilemmas and Directions for Psychiatric Nursing in the 1990's. Archives of Psychiatric Nursing IV (5), 284–291, 1990
27. Rosenhan DL: On Being Sane in Insane Places. In Brink PJ (ed): Transcultural Nursing: A Book of Readings, pp 175–197. Englewood Cliffs, NJ, Prentice-Hall, 1976
28. Ruesch J: Therapeutic Communication. New York, WW Norton, 1973
29. Selye H: Stress Without Distress. New York: New American Library, 1974
30. Tolbert RB: Answers: Professionally Speaking. J Psychosoc Nurs Ment Health Serv 30 (1): 35–38, 1992
31. Toward a National Policy on Aging. Proceedings of the 1971 White House Conference on Aging, vol II. Washington, DC, 1971

Mental Health Promotion

Barbara Schoen Johnson

2

Health is an ability to love, to think critically, and to work and play at our best.

Ashley Montagu, foreword to **Pathways to Peace,** *1996*

Health promotion and illness prevention are critical nursing functions. All nurses, in fact, contribute to mental health promotion and illness prevention in the course of their work with clients, families, and communities. Pediatric nurses who counsel families about ways to deal with a 2-year-old's tantrums are promoting mental health. Obstetrical nurses who foster parental attachment to their newborn are promoting mental health. Medical-surgical nurses who encourage clients to learn to live optimally with a chronic illness or condition are promoting mental health. Hospice nurses who comfort the dying and their loved ones are promoting mental health. Community health nurses who fight against discriminatory practices in their communities are promoting mental health.

Psychiatric-mental health nurses are particularly well prepared for mental health promotion, *that is, intervening with individuals, families, groups, and communities in ways that strengthen personal resources to enhance mental health and diminish risk factors to prevent mental illness.*

Learning Objectives

On completion of this chapter, you should be able to accomplish the following:

1. *Define mental health promotion.*
2. *Differentiate among the three categories of health objectives in Healthy People 2000—health promotion, health protection, and preventive services.*
3. *Discuss characteristics of mentally healthy people.*
4. *Identify the level of prevention, and give examples of each level.*
5. *Explain the concept of primary mental health care.*
6. *Give examples of universal, selective, and indicated preventive interventions.*
7. *Describe self-care measures for nurses to promote their own mental health.*

◆ A Nation's Agenda: Healthy People 2000

The report *Healthy People 2000* offers a new vision of health for the next century by outlining a national agenda to prevent unnecessary disease and disability and achieve a better quality of life. Its broad goals are to increase the span of healthy life for all Americans, reduce health disparities among Americans, and achieve access to preventive services for all Americans.[13]

In Healthy People 2000, health objectives are grouped into three categories: health promotion, health protection, and preventive services.

HEALTH PROMOTION

Health promotion strategies are tied to lifestyle choices that can have a powerful impact on the person's present and future health status. These strategies, which are largely the result of an individual's behavior, include physical activity and fitness, nutrition, tobacco, alcohol and other drugs, mental health and disorders, and violent and abusive behavior. Making an impact in the adoption of health-promoting behaviors requires education of populations at all age levels and across all socioeconomic strata.[13]

Healthy People 2000 has proposed that reductions must take place in the number of suicides and suicide attempts, homicides, and weapon-related violent deaths; the incidence of rape and attempted rape; the abuse of children and women; the prevalence of child, adolescent, and adult mental disorders; and the number of people who suffer adverse health effects from stress.[13]

HEALTH PROTECTION

Health protection strategies are related to environmental or regulatory measures that protect large population groups. Prevention of injuries, occupational safety and health, and reporting of suspected child or elder abuse occur largely through community-wide initiatives.[13]

Risk reduction objectives for the nation, according to Healthy People 2000, are to increase the use of community support programs by people with severe and persistent mental disorders, help people with major depression obtain treatment, and help people seek help to cope with personal and emotional problems. In addition, reducing the incidence of violent behavior among adolescents and adults contributes to health protection.[13]

In 1986, the National Institute of Mental Health began its first major educational campaign, Depression/Awareness, Recognition, Treatment (D/ART), aimed at public and professional groups (Box 2-1).

PREVENTIVE SERVICES

Preventive services include counseling, screening, and prophylactic interventions within clinical settings. Interventions to prevent chronic disabling conditions, human immunodeficiency virus, and sexually transmitted diseases are examples of preventive services.

According to Healthy People 2000, these services could be met by creating worksite programs to teach stress management to employees; primary care providers including emotional and behavioral functioning in health assessments; properly treating and referring victims of suicide attempts, sexual assault, and abuse;

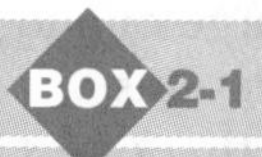

The D/ART Program

Nancy Kupper MSN, RN, Associate Professor of Nursing, Tarrant County Junior College, Fort Worth, Texas

The National Institute of Mental Health (NIMH) launched the first major national educational campaign in its 40-year history late in 1986.

Known as Depression/Awareness, Recognition, Treatment (D/ART), the campaign is intended to be a systematic application of the knowledge gained from years of research. The NIMH views D/ART as a return on the public's investment in mental health research, which in the last 20 years has included research on psychobiology, natural history, epidemiology, and the treatment of affective disorders.

Although NIMH initiated and organized D/ART, its purpose is to create national and local partnerships linking professional and lay mental health agencies and groups, business, government, professional organizations, and service providers to educate the public about the symptoms and treatment of depressive disorders. Local D/ART community partnerships are being organized to parallel the national D/ART group in an education campaign that combines media and community activities.

Project D/ART was developed to disseminate a consistent message.

1. Depression is a disorder that when recognized, can be treated.
2. Effective medications and psychological treatments exist and may be used in combination.
3. Even the most serious forms of depressive disorders respond rapidly to treatment.

Education and training programs encompass the professional and public sectors. The professional education program aims to provide health care providers with the most up-to-date information on the diagnosis and treatment of depressive disorders. Short-term clinical training grants are awarded to medical schools, university psychiatry departments, and nursing, social work, and psychology graduate schools. Brief education courses are also offered at professional meetings and at sites around the nation.

The public education program aims to create changes in the attitudes and behaviors of the general public. This is expected to help people recognize depression in themselves or their friends and families, to understand that it is treatable, and to learn how to seek treatment.

D/ART's Community Partnership program has been established to help implement the education campaign. Lead organizations, chosen by the D/ART Program (typically mental health association state and local affiliates), disseminate electronic and print materials and products developed by D/ART. Media kits with electronic and print materials, including bilingual materials, are being distributed nationally and to participating community partnership programs. By coordinating national and local efforts, using multiple channels for communication, and coordinating community programs with media efforts, NIMH hopes to maximize D/ART's effectiveness. The project's name describes its goals of enhancing public awareness and encouraging help-seeking behavior. Public and professional participation and involvement will help meet these goals by educating individuals, families, employers, school counselors and teachers, the media, and the public.

teaching nonviolent conflict resolution; and offering other nonviolence prevention programs in schools.[13]

◆ Mentally Healthy People

CHARACTERISTICS

Chapter 1, Introduction to Psychiatric-Mental Health Nursing, discusses mental health as a positive concept, that is, more than the absence of illness or disorder. Research continues in the search for characteristics found in mentally healthy individuals.

Psychosocial Resilience

Resilience is the ability of the personality to readily recover from or adjust to difficult, painful situations and events and to mobilize coping resources and strength. Often children are described as resilient because of their ability to "bounce back" quickly from a significant loss or misfortune.

Studies of psychosocial resilience have examined why some people succumb to stress and adversity, whereas others escape its damage. Researchers propose that *protective processes* reduce the impact of risk situations (such as a threatening event), reduce the negative chain reactions stemming from the encounter with the risk situation, promote self-esteem and self-efficacy through secure and supportive relationships and successful task accomplishment, and created opportunities for the individual. Protection resides in the ways in which individuals perceive and deal with life changes and cope with stressful life circumstances.[11]

Freedoms

According to Satir and others, mentally healthy people demonstrate certain "freedoms" in their behavior:

1. The freedom to see and hear what is occurring instead of what was, will be, or should be
2. The freedom to think, feel, and express what one actually thinks and feels rather than what one should think or feel
3. The freedom to ask for what one wants rather than waiting for permission
4. The freedom to take risks rather than choosing to be safe and not "rock the boat"[12]

Hardiness

Hardiness is a personality characteristic that has been identified in healthy individuals. It has been proposed that hardiness allows people under high levels of stress to remain healthy and resist illness. The three components of hardiness follow:

1. Control: feeling in charge of and able to influence one's own life and life events
2. Commitment: feeling that one's life and work are of importance and feeling deeply involved in life activities
3. Challenge: viewing change as normal and obstacles in life as challenges and opportunities[5,6,14]

Androgyny

Androgyny is the interaction and balance of feminine and masculine characteristics in an individual. Sex-role stereotypes, such as, "Men should be strong and not express their feelings" or "It is OK for women to cry and ask for help," are often inflexible and limit a person's adaptive and interpersonal effectiveness. Androgyny, on the other hand, allows a person to adapt behavior according to various situations and needs, rather than gender.

Roles assigned on the basis of gender alone are restricting; new roles based on individual inherent abilities and traits promote actualization of one's potential. The androgynous person integrates so-called masculine and feminine characteristics in an adaptive manner. The person is likely to develop a wider behavioral repertoire, but he or she also risks suffering role strain due to conflicting internal and societal expectations. A person who takes on new roles without resolving the conflict between personal and societal demands and tries to meet all the demands of multiple roles eventually experiences increased stress, role strain, and risk of illness. Instead of adding new behaviors to old ones, the person must relinquish or renegotiate roles that are not personally satisfying.

The result of androgyny may be a greater degree of mental health and personal fulfillment. One study, however, suggests a double standard of mental health for men and women among mental health professionals. In this study, androgynous behavior was seen by professionals as more acceptable in female clients than in male clients.[7]

Balance in Life

Mentally healthy people strive for balance in their lives. Balancing the physical, spiritual, emotional, and social aspects of life requires attention to needs and goals and determination to carry it through.[3] Often, one aspect of a person's life dominates the others to the detriment of one's health. For example, busy adults are often so caught up in the day-to-day struggle of work and care of their children and home that they forget to attend to their own needs for exercise, recreation, or spiritual refreshment.

Without attention to one's physical health needs, however, the other aspects of life and living suffer. Maslow illustrated this idea through his hierarchy of needs, in which one's physiological needs must be met before meeting safety and security needs. Physiological needs and safety and security needs must be met before love and belonging needs can be met; this occurs through esteem and self-actualization needs[8] (Fig. 2-1).

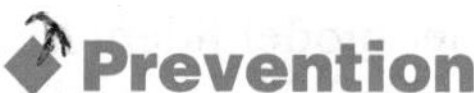

Prevention

Prevention of mental or emotional disorders is a vital topic in mental health care. A decade ago, psychiatric care providers called for action, not additional rhetoric, in the prevention of mental illnesses.[2] Today's neurobiological research is striving to make an impact in the drive to prevent mental illness in the future. Illness or disease prevention is commonly described in terms of three levels—primary, secondary, and tertiary prevention (Table 2-1).

PRIMARY PREVENTION

Primary prevention refers to reducing the incidence of disorder, that is, preventing disorders from occurring in the first place. Primary preventive efforts in mental health include reducing risk factors associated with certain disorders. For example, post-traumatic stress disorder (PTSD) is associated with experiences of being traumatized, such as being abused, raped, or victimized in a violent crime. Reducing the incidence of these traumatic experiences through family abuse and crime prevention programs will lead to a reduction in the incidence of PTSD.

In a variety of community- and hospital-based settings, nurses engage in primary preventive interventions. Whether teaching people stress management and relaxation techniques, instructing parents in effective behavior modification measures to change their child's troublesome behavior, practicing assertiveness or conflict resolution skills with a group of adolescents, or using a number of other strategies, nurses intervene to prevent mental disorder from developing.

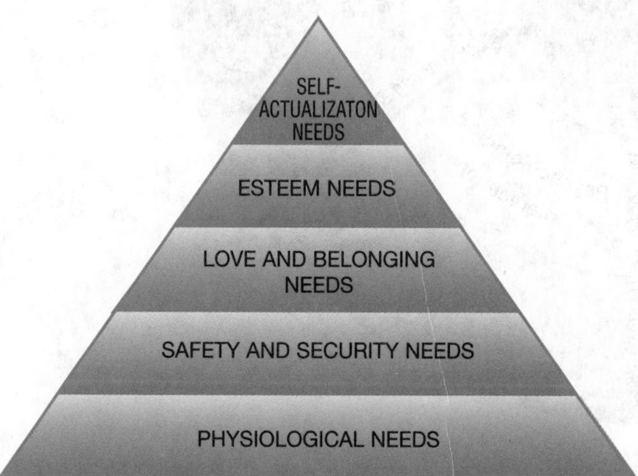

Figure 2-1. Maslow's Hierarchy of Needs (From Maslow AH: Toward a Psychology of Being, 2d ed. New York, Van Nostrand Reinhold, 1968)

Table 2-1

Levels of Prevention

Level of Prevention	Purpose	Example
Primary	Reduce the incidence of mental disorder	Parenting classes for new parents
Secondary	Reduce the prevalence of mental disorder	Early diagnosis and prompt treatment of depression
Tertiary	Reduce the severity of mental disorder	Symptom management education for clients with schizophrenia or bipolar disorder

SECONDARY PREVENTION

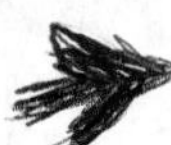

Secondary prevention refers to reducing the prevalence or severity of disorder. Secondary preventive interventions in mental health include screening, early detection or diagnosis, and prompt treatment of mental disorders. Early detection and prompt effective treatment of depression, for example, alleviate depressive symptoms, reduce suicide attempts, and restore productive living. The National Institute of Mental Health's public education campaign is designed to spread the message, "Depression is treatable" (see Box 2-1).

Nurses participate in secondary preventive interventions when they screen for signs and symptoms of disorder, participate in case management activities, and promote crisis stabilization and the development of optimal functioning following crises.

TERTIARY PREVENTION

Tertiary prevention refers to reducing the severity of disorder and associated disability by means of rehabilitative intervention. When mental illness already exists, tertiary preventive efforts are aimed at minimizing or managing symptoms, diminishing the disabling complications of the illness, and providing "wraparound services" to assist in all areas of life, such as housing, employment, and socialization. A person with schizophrenia, for example, would benefit from the tertiary preventive interventions of client and family education to learn about medication, methods of symptom management, social skill development, and job training.

Nurses participate in tertiary preventive interventions by administering medication, teaching self-advocacy skills, assisting with self-care activities, and promoting relapse prevention.

◆ Primary Mental Health Care

Primary mental health care is the "continuous and comprehensive services necessary for the promotion of optimal mental health, prevention of mental illness, and health maintenance, and includes the management (treatment) of and/or referral for mental and general health problems"[4] (p 155). This comprehensive model of care views the person holistically, considering strengths and goals. It is designed to provide seamless, integrated services to individuals who need them.[4]

The primary mental health care model (Fig. 2-2) demonstrates the relationship between psychiatric-mental health nursing practice and mental health care delivery. The outer circle of the model identifies nursing's professional role responsibilities, which include advocacy, involvement in professional organizations, shaping public policy, and community action. The next circle identifies basic and advanced psychiatric nursing interventions, including milieu therapy; self-care activities; psychobiological interventions; consultation-liaison services; counseling and crisis intervention; individual, family, and group psychotherapy; and case management.

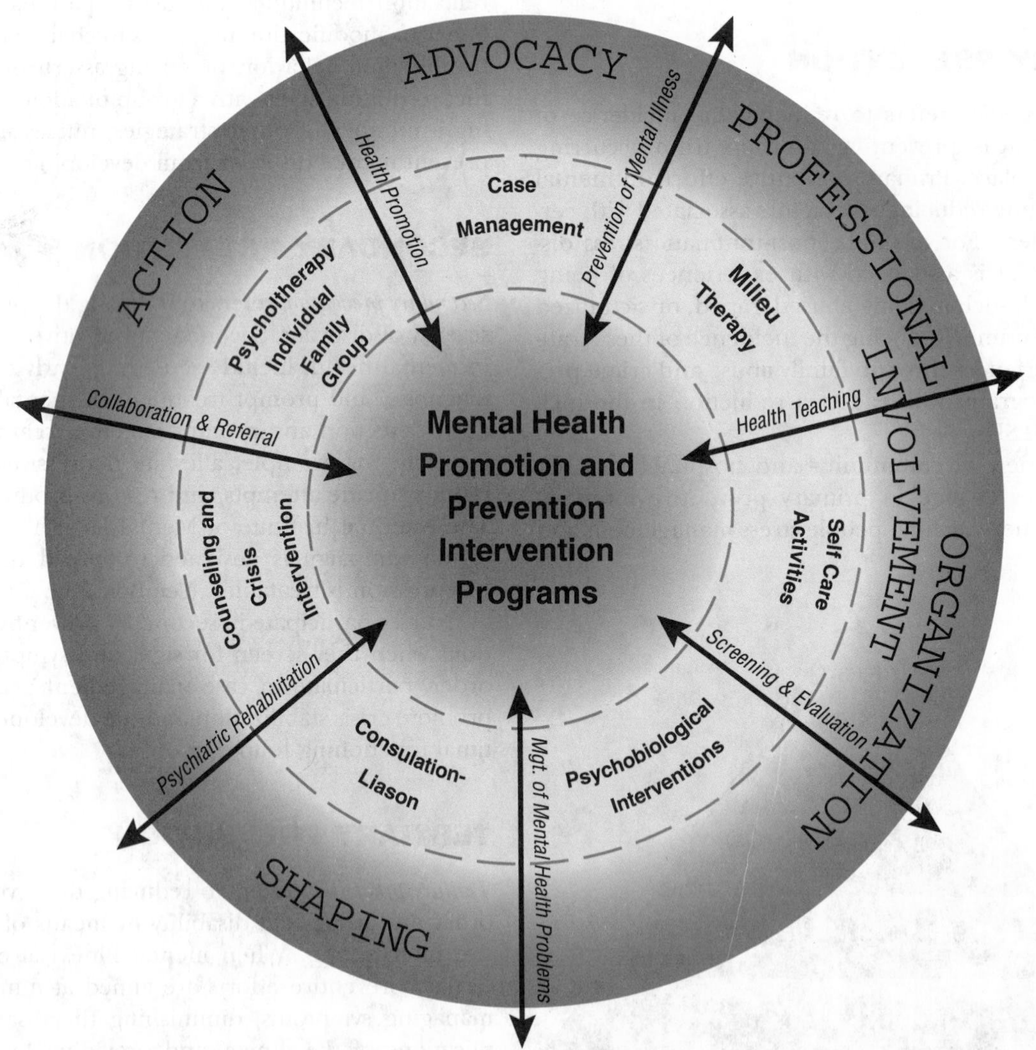

Figure 2-2. Primary Mental Health Care Model (From Haber, J, Billings, CV: Primary Mental Health Care: A Model for Psychiatric-Mental Health Nursing. Journal of the American Psychiatric Nurses Association, *1* (5), 154–163, 1995)

The inner circle places mental health promotion and preventive intervention as the central focus of mental health care. The arrows that intersect the circles represent professional role functions that are needed in the delivery of care, such as health promotion, mental illness prevention, screening and evaluation, health teaching, management of mental health problems, psychiatric rehabilitation, and collaboration and referral.[4]

MENTAL HEALTH PROMOTION

Health is promoted and protected when individuals, families, communities, and larger societal groups participate in activities that foster resilience and well-being and avoid circumstances that increase the likelihood of illness.[10] Box 2-2 identifies some of the possible mental health promotion activities of nurses.

Strategies to promote mental health and prevent mental disorder may be categorized as universal, selective, and indicated preventive interventions.[9] *Universal preventive interventions* are directed to targeted population groups not necessarily at risk for mental health problems. These interventions, such as parenting education for all new parents, enhance the mental health functioning of the individuals.

Selective preventive interventions target individuals or groups at risk for mental health problems. Individuals who are mourning the loss of a loved one, for example, are at risk for depression; selective preventive interventions target healthy grieving and effective coping to deal with the loss. Another example of selective preventive intervention is a community-based program to support high-risk adolescent parents during the early postpartum period.[14]

Indicated preventive interventions target individuals at high risk for disorder who presently show minimal, but detectable, signs that the disorder is developing or who have a biological marker for a disorder. However, these individuals do not meet the Diagnostic and Statistical Manual for Mental Disorders, fourth edition, criteria for disorder.[9] Examples of these interventions are parenting classes and groups for parents of children exhibiting behavior problems and education classes and groups for children with a parent who has schizophrenia.

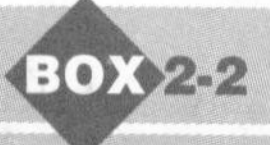

2-2

Nurses Promoting Mental Health

Nurses promote mental health through many preventive interventions. The following is a partial list of these interventions:

- Teaching normal growth and development to parents and teachers
- Fostering bonding behaviors
- Consulting with parents about appropriate disciplinary measures
- Promoting open, healthy communication in families
- Helping parents learn to strengthen their child's self-esteem
- Teaching adolescents peer pressure refusal skills
- Coaching in assertiveness techniques
- Teaching relaxation, imagery, and other stress management techniques
- Helping individuals use cognitive techniques to reframe events and interpretations
- Practicing self-affirmations with depressed individuals
- Supporting caregivers of the elderly
- Working with bereaved individuals to foster grief resolution
- Encouraging the adoption of physical health-promoting behaviors
- Working through political processes to enact mental health legislation

SELF-CARE

Nurses are affected by their stressful work environments in addition to demands of their personal lives. The self-care measures they teach clients provide nurses with significant benefit themselves. Self-care measures, such as peer support, nutrition and exercise, hobbies, and enriching personal relationships, reduce stress and promote optimal effectiveness in psychiatric-mental health nursing.

◆ Chapter Summary

This chapter has discussed the concepts of mental health promotion and illness prevention, which are essential aspects of nursing in every specialty area. The main points of this chapter include the following:

1. The government document, Healthy People 2000, outlines goals for promoting health for the country's citizens and preventing disease and disability.
2. Mental health objectives may be attained through health promotion measures, health protection activities, and preventive services.
3. Mentally healthy people demonstrate resilience, hardiness, androgyny, freedom, and balance.
4. Prevention activities are categorized as primary (ie, reducing the prevalence or severity of the disorder

through early detection and treatment) or tertiary (ie, reducing the severity of the disorder and associated disability through rehabilitation).

5. Primary mental health care offers a comprehensive model of continuous services that promote mental health, prevent mental illness, and treat disorders promptly and effectively.

Review Questions

1. People's health promotion activities are linked with their
   - **A.** genetic predisposition.
   - **B.** family's health.
   - **C.** lifestyle choices.
   - **D.** behavioral experiences.
2. According to Healthy People 2000, environmental and regulatory measures that protect the health of large environmental groups are strategies that are best termed
   - **A.** health promotion.
   - **B.** health protection.
   - **C.** preventive services.
   - **D.** risk reduction.
3. People who recover readily from loss and mobilize their coping resources are described as
   - **A.** resilient.
   - **B.** androgynous.
   - **C.** hardy.
   - **D.** balanced.
4. Secondary preventive interventions are designed to reduce what of a disorder?
   - **A.** Incidence
   - **B.** Length
   - **C.** Type
   - **D.** Prevalence
5. Education of a client with schizophrenia and his or her family about the disorder, symptoms, management, and medication is an example of
   - **A.** primary prevention.
   - **B.** secondary prevention.
   - **C.** tertiary prevention.
6. Which of the following is an example of universal preventive interventions?
   - **A.** A support group for children of parents with schizophrenia
   - **B.** A stress management class for adults at the worksite
   - **C.** A bereavement group for recently widowed individuals
   - **D.** A coping skills class for clients with depression
7. Primary health care is
   - **A.** comprehensive.
   - **B.** crisis oriented.
   - **C.** intermittent.
   - **D.** consultative.

◆ References

1. Knollmueller RM (ed): American Nurses Association, Council of Community Health Nursing. Prevention Across the Life Span: Healthy People for the 21st Century. Washington, DC, American Nurses Publishing, 1993
2. Bower EM: Prevention: A Word Whose Time Has Come. Am J Orthopsychiatry 57 (January): 4–5, 1987
3. Bruenjes SJ: Orchestrating Health: Middle-Aged Women's Process of Living Health. Holistic Nursing Practice 8 (4): 22–32, 1994
4. Haber J, Billings CV: Primary Mental Health Care: A Model for Psychiatric-Mental Health Nursing. Journal of the American Psychiatric Nurses Association 1 (5): 154–163, 1995
5. Jennings BM, Staggers N: A Critical Analysis of Hardiness. Nurs Res 43 (5): 274–281, 1994
6. Kobasa SC: Stressful Life Events, Personality, and Health: An Inquiry into Hardiness. Journal of Personality and Social Psychology 37: 1–11, 1979
7. Kravetz D, Jones LE: Androgyny as a Standard of Mental Health. Am J Orthopsychiatry 51 (July): 502–509, 1981
8. Maslow AH: Toward a Psychology of Being, 2d ed. New York, Van Nostrand Reinhold, 1968
9. Mrazek PJ, Haggerty RJ: Reducing Risks for Mental Disorders. Washington, DC, National Academy Press, 1994
10. O'Connor FW: Health Promotion and Disease Prevention in Psychiatric Mental Health Nursing. In McFarland GK, Thomas MD (eds): Psychiatric Mental Health Nursing: Application of the Nursing Process, pp 97–102. Philadelphia, JB Lippincott, 1991
11. Rutter M: Psychosocial Resilience and Protective Mechanisms. Am J Orthopsychiatry 57 (July): 316–331, 1987
12. Satir V, Bernard YM, Macdonald N: Using the Family Unit for Change. In Beiser M, Krell R, Lin T, Miller M (eds): Today's Priorities in Mental Health: Knowing and Doing, pp 35–39. Miami, Symposia Specialists, 1978
13. U.S. Department of Health and Human Services: Healthy People 2000: National Health Promotion and Disease Prevention Objectives. Boston, Jones and Bartlett Publishers, 1992
14. Wagnild G, Young HM: Another Look at Hardiness. Image 23 (4): 257–259, 1991
15. Williams-Burgess C, Vines SW, Ditulio MB: The Parent-Baby Venture Program: Prevention of Child Abuse. Journal of Child and Adolescent Psychiatric Nursing 8 (3, July-September): 15–23, 1995

Conceptual Frameworks for Care

Judith A. Greene

3

The intimate union of theory and practice aids both.

Alfred North Whitehead

A theory *is a conceptual system that describes and explains selected phenomena. In this way, a theory is a tool to guide and shape human understanding and behavior. To the extent that theories apply to real events, they are considered useful. When theories apply to real nursing events, they guide the understanding and behavior of nurses.*

Nurses use theories of human behavior to understand clients and to intervene therapeutically. Theories commonly used by psychiatric-mental health nurses fall into these five categories:

1. *Psychoanalytic theory*
2. *Interpersonal theory*
3. *Behavioristic theory*
4. *General systems theory*
5. *Natural systems theory*

Each of these theoretical categories views humankind from a different perspective and thus emphasizes or accentuates one aspect of human existence over others. Nevertheless, all of these theoretical perspectives are useful to nurses.

Learning Objectives

On completion of this chapter, you should be able to accomplish the following:

1. *Explain the purpose of theoretical perspectives or frameworks.*
2. *Discuss the basic assumptions underlying the psychoanalytic, interpersonal, behavioristic, and systems theories.*
3. *Apply selected theoretical perspectives to the nursing care of clients.*
4. *Compare selected theoretical perspectives and their applications to nursing.*

◆ Psychoanalytic Theoretical Perspective

Derived from the work of Sigmund Freud and his followers, psychoanalytic theory is deterministic and reflects a pessimistic attitude toward society's and humankind's potential for constructive change.[1,5] The basic assumptions underlying this theoretical perspective include the following:

1. All human behavior is caused and thus is capable of explanation. Slips of the tongue, accidents, dreams, artistic creations, and all other forms of human behavior have meaning and therefore can be explained.[11] In other words, human behavior, however insignificant or obscure, does not occur randomly or by chance; rather, all human behavior is determined by prior life events.
2. All human behavior from birth to old age is driven by an energy called the *libido*. The goal of the libido is the reduction of tension through the attainment of pleasure. The libido is closely associated with physiological or instinctual drives (eg, hunger, thirst, elimination, sex). Release of these drives results in the reduction of tension, resulting in the experience of pleasure. Hence, the *pleasure principle* becomes operative when pleasure-seeking behaviors are used.[16]
3. Human behavior that channels impulsive pleasure-seeking behaviors into creative pursuits (sublimation) is considered the highest form of human expression. Maturity is thus associated with the ability to invent and use substitutive or disguised forms of gratification.[16] This ability to delay pleasure in favor of more acceptable behavior is called the *reality principle.*
4. The personality of the human being can be understood by way of three major hypothetical structures: id, ego, and superego. The *id* represents the most primitive structure of the human personality; it houses the physiological drives or instincts and cannot delay the attainment of pleasure. Human behavior originating from the id is impulsive, pleasure-oriented, disconnected from reality, and consequently often inappropriate. Thought processes deriving from the id are characterized by their illogic, confused form, and preverbal content.[16] Such thought patterns, called *primary process thinking,* are often reflected in verbalizations of psychotic individuals with schizophrenia (see Chap. 30, Schizophrenic Disorders).

   The *superego* is the personality structure containing the values, legal and moral regulations, and social expectations that thwart free expression of pleasure-seeking behaviors. The superego thus functions to oppose the id. Society and the family determine the content of the superego and the kinds of limitations it places on the individual.[11]

   The *ego* represents the part of the human personality in closest contact with reality. Unlike the id, the ego is capable of postponing pleasure until an appropriate time, place, or object is available. Unlike the superego, the ego is not driven to blind conformity with rules and regulations. Rather, the ego, acting as mediator between the id and superego, gives rise to more mature and adaptive behavior.[16]

   With the id and superego constantly at odds with one another, the ego faces the task of maintaining control over instinctual impulses while taking into consideration moral values and injunctions. Understandably, humans occasionally experience anxiety when confronted with situations that challenge the tenuous balance between the id and the superego. At these times, the ego uses defense mechanisms to ward off anxiety.[14] Commonly used defense mechanisms include repression, denial, regression, rationalization, reaction formation, undoing, projection, displacement, sublimation, isolation, and fixation.

5. The human personality functions on three levels of awareness: conscious, preconscious, and unconscious. *Consciousness* refers to the perceptions, thoughts, and feelings existing in a person's immediate awareness. *Preconscious* content, on the other hand, is not immediately accessible to awareness. The person must make an effort to retrieve this content before it reaches awareness. Unlike conscious and preconscious content, *unconscious* material remains inaccessible for the most part.[16]
6. The unconscious affects all three personality structures—id, superego, and ego. Although the id's content resides totally in the unconscious, the superego and the ego have aspects in all three levels of consciousness.[16] Through these three levels of consciousness, the ego maintains contact with reality and with the id and the superego.
7. Human personality development unfolds through five innate psychosexual stages—oral, anal, phallic, latent, and genital—so named because psychoanalytical theory assumes that all pleasure is essentially sexual in nature. Although these stages extend throughout the life span, the theory also holds that the first 6 years of life determine the individual's long-term personality characteristics; that is, early life events, especially with regard to parent–child experiences, determine the individual's behavior throughout life.[16]
8. Despite this theory's deterministic and pessimistic view of human behavior, it assumes that human personality and behavior possess enough flexibility to progress toward change.[12]

THERAPEUTIC APPROACHES

In keeping with these basic assumptions, the psychoanalytic view of human behavior relies on the therapeutic approach of *psychoanalysis,* practiced by psychiatrists, psychologists, and advanced practice psychiatric-mental health nurses formally trained in its use. Psychoanalysis uses strategies such as hypnosis, dream interpretation, and free association. The psychoanalyst attempts to maintain a relatively passive demeanor to create a neutral environment devoid of approval or disapproval and to encourage the client to be natural. When the psychoanalyst interacts with the client, it is usually to make an interpretation of the client's verbal or nonverbal behavior. No touching occurs between the client and psychoanalyst. Usually, the psychoanalyst remains largely out of the client's sight.[12]

The primary goal of psychoanalysis is to create a permissive yet safe situation in which clients can recall past traumas and work through residual conflicts and emotions that have thwarted or fixated their growth and integration as a person. In short, the goal of psychoanalysis is to help clients release their full potential as healthy, well-integrated human beings.

APPLICATION TO NURSING

Psychoanalytic theory has influenced psychiatric-mental health nursing in many ways. This theoretical perspective, perhaps more than any other, has helped mental health professionals understand psychopathology and stress-related behaviors. More importantly, this theory illustrates the importance of not taking human behavior at face value. That is, it helps the psychiatric-mental health nurse to discern and explore the meaning behind human behavior.

◆ Interpersonal Theoretical Perspective

As a derivative of psychoanalytic theory, interpersonal theory has similar basic assumptions. Nevertheless, there are important differences between interpersonal theory and the psychoanalytic perspective.

Unlike Freud and his followers, Harry S. Sullivan, the originator of interpersonal relations theory, viewed humans as essentially social beings. In keeping with this basic premise, Sullivan set forth these assumptions about the interpersonal nature of human life:

1. Human personality is determined in the context of social interactions with other human beings. While biological factors influence personality development, social factors presumably exert a greater influence.
2. Anxiety plays a central role in the formation of human personality by serving as a primary motivator of human behavior. Specifically, anxiety is important in building self-esteem and enabling a person to learn from their life experiences.
3. Unlike psychoanalytic theory, this theoretical orientation asserts that interpersonal experiences, rather than intrapsychic ones, determine the personality organization achieved by human beings.
4. The *self-system* is an important facet of human personality that forms in reaction to the experience of anxiety. Interactions with significant others conveying disapproval or other such negative meanings contribute to self-system formation. In reaction to such interactions, *security mechanisms* are used to reduce or avoid the experience of anxiety. These security mechanisms include sublimation, selective inattention, and dissociation.

In interpersonal theory, *sublimation* refers to an unconscious process whereby socially acceptable behavioral patterns are substituted to satisfy partially the need for a behavioral pattern that would result in increased anxiety. *Selective inattention,* also an unconscious substitutive process, occurs when many important details causing increased anxiety go unnoticed by the individual. *Dissociation,* commonly called the *not me,* is used unconsciously to minimize parts of the individual's experiences to avoid anxiety. Using these security mechanisms can result in a loss of objectivity when evaluating the person's own behavior. Consequently, the self-system can function as a barrier to positive personality change.

5. Early life experiences with parents, especially the mother, influence an individual's development throughout life. This lasting effect is produced by *personifications,* consisting of images that the individual has of the self and other people. These images, composed of feelings, attitudes, and ideas, form as the result of experiences with anxiety and need satisfaction with "the mothering one." For example, a calm, tolerant mother is personified as a good mother, while an anxious, intolerant mother is personified as a bad mother. As a child's development unfolds, these dichotomous personifications become fused. If fusion of these "either-or" personifications does not occur, the individual may go through life with extreme, polarized views of self, others, and situations.

   Three personifications of the self arise from infancy as the result of care given by parents: "good me," "bad me," and "not me." The good me results from experiences of approval and tenderness and is associated with good feelings about the self. Experiences associated with high anxiety situations result in the bad me and are associated with feelings of shame, guilt, and low self-esteem. The not me develops in reaction to overwhelming anxiety arising from situations that provoke feelings of horror or dread. These three personifications also form part of the self-system.

6. Interpersonal theory describes cognitive processes in terms of three experience modes: prototaxic, parataxic, and syntaxic. The *prototaxic* mode is characterized by sensations, feelings, and fleeting images occurring during infancy that are primitive and illogical. They also provide a backdrop for the next level of experience, the parataxic mode. Prototaxic experiences, while considered normal in infancy, are associated with floridly psychotic states when present in other age groups.

   The *parataxic* mode of experience is also illogical in nature. To illustrate, events occurring simultaneously or in close approximation to each other are considered causally related. For example, a child who has experienced losses of several significant others through death could erroneously conclude that all people entering a hospital die. While the parataxic mode of experience may be normal in childhood, it may continue into adulthood. Common parataxic distortions occurring in adult years include racial, sexual, and ethnic stereotypes and prejudices.

   The most developed level of experience, the *syntaxic* mode, is characterized by logical thinking and emerges in the juvenile stage. This mode of experience develops as the young person engages in the process of consensual validation. *Consensual validation* is the process by which people come to agreement about the meaning and significance of specific symbols. Through the syntaxic mode of experience, individuals develop the ability to relate effectively.

7. Human development proceeds through six stages of development: infancy, childhood, juvenility, preadolescence, early adolescence, and late adolescence. According to interpersonal theory, juvenile and preadolescent stages hold the greatest potential for correction of previous behavior and personality difficulties.[17]

THERAPEUTIC APPROACHES

The overall goal of interpersonal theory is to assist the individual toward increased maturity. More specific goals include the following:

- Freeing the individual from previously ineffective interpersonal patterns acquired earlier in life
- Assisting the individual to manage personal anxieties and to be concerned for the welfare of significant others

To meet these goals, the therapist remains active during interpersonal interactions and points out the client's problem areas as they are displayed during the interaction. The client's problem areas and defenses are usually outside the client's awareness at the outset of interpersonal interactions. With time, recognition and integration of problem areas and traumas occur during the therapeutic process. The therapeutic process provides for immediate feedback to the client without increasing anxiety.[17]

APPLICATION TO NURSING

Sullivan's interpersonal theory has been the cornerstone of psychiatric-mental health nursing curricula on the undergraduate and graduate levels. As a result, concepts addressed in such curricula (eg, anxiety, self-esteem, trust, security) derive in large part from Sullivan's work. Additionally, nurse–client, one-to-one interaction, or interpersonal process, is based on Sullivan's interpersonal theory. The use of interpersonal process recordings in the clinical aspect of psychiatric-mental health nursing courses also derives from Sullivan's interpersonal theory.[16] Like psychoanalytic theory, this theoretical perspective is deterministic in nature. Unlike psychoanalytic theory, it is less pessimistic and presents a more hopeful outlook for clients and practitioners using the theory.

◆ Behavioristic Theoretical Perspective

Based on the works of Ivan Pavlov, John Watson, and B. F. Skinner, the behavioristic theoretical perspective is deterministic in nature, like the psychoanalytic and interpersonal theories. Unlike those theories, the behavioristic theoretical perspective is concerned only with observable behavior rather than with intrapsychic or interpersonal processes or the personality itself.[1] Several basic assumptions underlie the behavioristic theoretical perspective:

1. All behavior is a response to a stimulus or to stimuli from the environment.
2. Human beings are passive organisms that can be conditioned or shaped to do anything if correct responses to specific stimuli are rewarded or reinforced.
3. Human beings can control or determine the behavior of others, whether or not they wish to be controlled.
4. The human personality is a pattern of stimulus-response chains or habits.
5. Adaptive and maladaptive behaviors are learned and perpetuated through reinforcements.
6. Maladaptive behaviors can be unlearned and replaced by adaptive behavior if the person receives exposure to specific stimuli and reinforcements for the desired adaptive behavior.[7,15]

THERAPEUTIC APPROACHES

Several therapeutic approaches stem from the behavioristic theoretical perspective:

1. With *token reinforcement,* direct use of reinforcers is delayed through the administration of tokens. When desired adaptive behavioral responses are emitted, tokens are awarded. After a specific number of adaptive behavioral responses occur, the tokens can be redeemed for actual reinforcers, such as an extra cup of coffee or a higher level of privileges.[16]
2. *Shaping* is another behavioral reinforcement technique used to condition close approximations of some desired adaptive behavior. In applying this technique, reinforcement of successively closer approximations occurs until the final adaptive behavioral outcome is reached.[16] Shaping requires careful observation and a great deal of patience to identify and reinforce desired behavior approximations.
3. *Systematic desensitization,* described by Wolfe, is a counter-conditioning technique used to extinguish maladaptive responses. This technique involves helping the client overcome the anxiety aroused by a specific stimulus by evoking a simultaneous response incompatible with anxiety. This is a step-by-step process. Systematic desensitization rests on the premise that a person cannot be frightened and relaxed simultaneously. Hence, increasing the strength of the relaxation response gradually weakens and eventually extinguishes anxiety evoked by the stimulus.[21]

   The step-by-step process by which desensitization is administered occurs in a structured setting. The therapist and client initially construct an anxiety or fear stimulus hierarchy. This hierarchy is an ordered list of situations that cause anxiety to the client, starting from the least and extending to the most frightening situation.

   Deep muscle relaxation is usually used as a response incompatible with anxiety. When the client has been trained to relax, he or she is then asked to imagine the first (least frightening) situation in the hierarchy. If the client can do that without discomfort, the therapist then proceeds to the next situation on the list. If during this process, the client reports even slight anxiety, he or she is asked to relax again. These procedures are repeated until the client is able to imagine all the situations without experiencing even minimal anxiety. In some cases, the therapy includes introduction of the actual situation while practicing relaxation. When the client no longer experiences anxiety in the presence of the anxiety-provoking situation, the therapy is considered complete.[21]

   This technique is highly effective in reducing phobic reactions related to specific situations or objects. Systematic desensitization is much less effective when the client displays generalized anxiety to a number of ill-defined situations.[21]
4. *Rational-emotive therapy,* developed by Albert Ellis, is one type of cognitive behavioral technique. There are four basic assumptions underlying rational-emotive therapy.

   People acquire a basic set of values and beliefs

early in life and are governed by these. Rational and irrational thoughts and behaviors can be identified, understood, and changed once these values and beliefs are specified.

People want to survive and experience happiness, which is defined as need satisfaction and freedom from pain.

People usually strive to belong to and harmonize with a social group or community.

People desire to form more intimate relationships with a few members of this group.[4]

Ellis asserts that behaviors that support these four basic assumptions are rational and those that do not are irrational. Combined with rational-emotive techniques, Ellis uses the ABC theory of personality to assist in eliciting behavior change. In this theory, A is the activating event, B is the person's belief system about A, and C is the emotional consequence. According to Ellis, the person's appropriate or inappropriate emotional response to an event is determined by the person's belief system about the event and not by the event itself.[4] To illustrate, if a student feels depressed (point C) after receiving a failing score on a test (point A), the test failure does not cause the student's depression. Rather, it is the student's beliefs (point B) about the test failure. Rational beliefs, such as, "failing scores can be improved through improving study habits" and "grades are no reflection on a person's worth as a human being," can lead to feelings of acceptance of the score and a commitment to improve study plans and test performance. Thus, rational beliefs and appropriate feelings related to an event can motivate a person to work harder toward achieving goals. Irrational beliefs and inappropriate feelings (eg, believing that someone else was responsible for the poor test performance or blaming and being angry with another) tend to reinforce self-defeating behaviors.

5. Other cognitive therapy techniques include identifying automatic dysfunctional cognitive patterns, using thought stoppage to break the habit of dysfunctional thinking, and replacing dysfunctional thinking with functional cognitive patterns. To implement these techniques, the cognitive therapist actively manipulates the session by using the Socratic method to examine logically the client's thought processes. The therapy is time limited and specifically related to problem areas identified by the client. The overall goal of cognitive therapy is to restructure the client's thought processes. This goal is achieved by discovering the client's basic beliefs and values about people, relationships, and the world so that they may be tested against a more rational set of beliefs and values.[4]
6. Other behavior-change techniques derived from the behavioristic approach include aversion conditioning, implosion, flooding, and assertiveness training. When using these techniques, the therapist usually determines what behavior should be changed and what behavioral approach to use.

APPLICATION TO NURSING

Advanced practice psychiatric-mental health nurses commonly use behavioral techniques in a wide variety of mental health settings. Additionally, nurses who work with clients with physical disability, chronic pain, or chemical dependency in a rehabilitation setting will find behavioristic strategies useful (see Chap. 18, Behavioral Approaches).

◆ General System Theoretical Perspective

This theoretical perspective derives chiefly from the works of Ludwig von Bertalanffy.[19,20] It has influenced the ways in which dyadic, group, family, and organizational behaviors have been analyzed and explained by other theorists of human behavior.[2,18] Some basic assumptions of this theory and others derived from it include the following:

1. The human being is a living, open system consisting of interrelated subsystems.[10,20]
2. These interrelated subsystems are components or parts of the total human organism.[10,20]
3. These subsystems in relation to each other tie the human system together, forming a whole.[10,20]
4. Individual subsystems or subwholes possess attributes in common with each other and with the human system as a whole. Consequently, every part of the human system is related to its fellow parts, and a change in one part or subsystem will cause a change in the remaining parts or subsystems.[20]
5. The human system behaves not as a composite of independent elements, but rather, coherently and as an inseparable whole.[10,20]
6. The human system is surrounded by a boundary that separates it from the surrounding environment. Information may cross this boundary to enter or leave the human system.[20]
7. The five sensory channels plus the verbal and nonverbal behavioral modes of the human system form the boundary separating the human system from the surrounding environment. Information that crosses this boundary provides sensory *input* to the human system. The human system then transforms this sensory input into useful, meaningful forms. This transformation process, called *thruput,* involves feeding the sensory input through thoughts, feelings, mem-

ories, values, attitudes, intelligence, physiological structures, and so forth. In turn, the human system produces information, or *output,* that can be fed back to the human organism or to the environment and other human beings through verbal and nonverbal behaviors. Also called *feedback,* output is not always equivalent or similar to input; consequently, output is not always predictable on the basis of input. The reason for this lack of predictability is that the transformation of input (the thruput process) is unique for each human system.

8. The human system favors a steady state, in which there is an orderly exchange of information within the human system and between the human system and the environment.[10]
9. Disruption of stability results in stress on the total human organism; this stress affects the amount of energy available to activate or maintain the human organism. The amount of available energy in turn affects the quality and quantity of information processing. Finally, the effects of stress and the accompanying change in energy level affect not only informational output and thruput processes, but also the quality and quantity of the human organism's output, that is, its verbal and nonverbal behavior.

APPLICATION TO NURSING

According to general systems theory, the goal of nursing care is to help clients maintain or regain a steady state. This theory also provides the nurse with a holistic theoretical perspective from which to understand the human being. In other words, general systems theory resolves the mind-body dispute by viewing the human organism from a matter-energy-information perspective.

Recognizing that human beings are not simple, passive organisms, this theory can help the nurse observe and understand how clients affect and are affected by the environment, other people, and themselves. In providing such a holistic viewpoint, general systems theory allows the nurse to identify client strengths that can be used to overcome or compensate for weaknesses and limitations. Moreover, this theory views the human being as complex; it acknowledges that human behavior has multiple causes and meanings. Thus, general system theory sheds light on the uniqueness and complexity of human life.

◆ Natural Systems Theoretical Perspective

Family systems theory and therapy, developed by Murray Bowen in the mid-1950s, rests on the assumption that human beings and the human family are more like than unlike other natural biological systems. Another major assumption underlying this theory is that all human behavior is linked to biological functioning. Hence, the human being's emotional functioning is linked in as yet unspecified ways to biological functioning.[8]

According to natural systems theory, two major interacting variables influence human behavior in the relationship system: anxiety and level of differentiation. In this theoretical framework, *anxiety* is the human reaction to stress, not the stress itself. The theory further asserts that the anxiety reaction to stress, not the stressors, give humans problems and symptoms. This assertion is in sharp contrast to Selye's stress theory. These assertions are based on facts and observations revealing that people can be extremely stressed and still not be overly anxious; conversely, people can be mildly stressed and be severely anxious. The theory asserts that this difference can be explained on the basis of the human being's *level of differentiation.*

The level of differentiation describes varying levels of human adaptability. Basically, level of differentiation refers to the degree to which a person defines self in terms of self-chosen beliefs, principles, and convictions versus defining the self by external factors and emotional forces. Level of differentiation also can be viewed as the degree to which a person is defined by extreme anxiety imposed by the surrounding emotional field versus the degree to which the person defines the self in a calm and thoughtful way in the face of such anxiety.[3]

THEORETICAL CONCEPTS

Eight concepts comprise natural systems theory. Three of these concepts apply to overall characteristics of family, and the other five focus on the details of individual and family functioning.

1. The concept of *differentiation of self* stands as the cornerstone of natural systems theory. Differentiation is described in terms of a scale ranging from 1 to 100. People at the lower end of the scale are described as less adaptable, less flexible, and more emotionally dependent on those around them. As a result, these individuals seek togetherness with others to function and tend to fuse their intellectual and emotional functioning. Consequently, their lives are dominated and controlled by the automatic, instinct-oriented emotional system. People at the low end of the scale also tend to become dysfunctional with minor stress and have prolonged recoveries. They seem to have more of life's problems.[3]

   In contrast, people at the higher end of the continuum are clearer on what is intellectual and emotional functioning. As a result, they are more flexible, more adaptable, and more emotionally independent of others. Those at higher levels of differentiation cope more effectively with life's stressors and consequently lead more orderly, successful, and problem-free lives.[3]

Another important aspect of differentiation of self involves levels of solid self and pseudo self. The *solid self* is based on clearly defined, self-chosen beliefs, opinions, convictions, and principles derived through intellectual reasoning. When making decisions, the solid self accepts responsibility for decisions and their consequences.[3] On the other hand, the *pseudo self* is composed of principles, beliefs, philosophies, and knowledge acquired through group pressure and often inconsistent with one another. The individual, however, is unaware of these inconsistencies as he or she strives to relate harmoniously with family members and others.[6]

2. The *triangle* is the basic building block of an emotional system. According to Bowen's theory, a two-person relationship is calm and stable only when anxiety is low. When anxiety increases between the two people, one of the pair automatically will involve a third person, forming a triangle. If anxiety continues to mount, the triangle will involve others. This progressive involvement of others leads to development of a series of interlocking triangles that can transmit anxiety or calmness throughout the family system.[3,13]
3. The concept of the *nuclear family system* describes and explains a family's emotional functioning within a single generation. Patterns of emotional functioning between and among the father, mother, and children are reproduced from past generations. By studying past generations and observing the current generation, predictions about the family's future emotional functioning can be made. According to this concept, people tend to choose spouses whose differentiation levels match their own. During courtship, people are usually more themselves and more open than at any other time in their relationship. Once a firm commitment is made, however, the process of fusion between the partners begins. The lower the differentiation of self, the more intense the emotional fusion between the pair. As a result of the fusion process, one partner becomes the dominant decision maker while the other becomes adaptive or passive. If the two people compete for dominance, marital conflict ensues. On the other hand, if both spouses strive to become adaptive or passive, the couple cannot make decisions. Fusion creates anxiety for both spouses, and the greater the fusion, the greater the anxiety within the spouses.[3]

There are at least four ways of managing anxiety within the nuclear family:

Emotional distancing is the most common way to reduce anxiety in the family. It is present in varying degrees in all marriages and families.

Dysfunction in one spouse results when the undifferentiation within the marital pair is manifested by the passive or adaptive spouse. In such marriages, one spouse overfunctions and dominates the marriage. The other spouse underfunctions and is dependent on the overfunctioning spouse. The spousal dysfunction may be in the form of physical or emotional illnesses. The overfunctioning spouse is usually uncomplaining but may eventually succumb to the burdens of overfunctioning. The fusion in such marriages is usually intense and anxiety ridden, and dysfunction can occur with even mild stress.

Marital conflict is a relationship pattern characterized by spouses who cannot defer or give in to each other. Both strive to become dominant. Conflictual marriages are intense, and both spouses invest a great deal of energy in each other. The relationship goes through periods of intense closeness, conflict, and distance. Such marriages are not harmful to children, as their spousal undifferentiation is bound in the marital relationship. When the projective process is also present, children are adversely affected.[3]

Family projection process is addressed as a separate concept because of its importance in this theory.

4. The *family projection process* occurs when the parents project their own differentiation on to one or more of their children. This projective process operates within the triangle—father, mother, and child. The parent who is the primary caretaker of the child plays a central part in this process. The result of this process is dysfunction in the child. The family projection process exists to some degree (mild to severe) in all father-mother-child triangles. The degree to which the child is impaired depends on the intensity of this projective process.[3]

According to natural systems theory, a certain amount of undifferentiation seems to be bound in marital conflict, spousal dysfunction, and projection of symptoms to the child. Usually, families use all these mechanisms to control anxiety and bind undifferentiation. The more the family varies its use of these methods, the less impairment or dysfunction will occur within the child.[3]

5. *Emotional cutoff* is the concept describing how people cope with their unresolved emotional attachments

to their parents. While all people have some degree of unresolved attachment to their parents, the intensity depends on the level of differentiation of the people involved. For example, people with low levels of differentiation have more intense unresolved attachments, while those with higher differentiation levels have much less intense unresolved attachments to their parents. Methods used to achieve emotional cutoff include geographically relocating to allow for only brief "duty" visits, remaining uninvolved with parents while residing in the same geographical area as the parents, and remaining in the parent's home while psychologically withdrawing from the situation.

Usually, individuals who are distant or uninvolved with their parents describe themselves as independent. These individuals, however, are as driven by togetherness forces with their parents as are individuals who cannot leave their parents. The more intense the cutoff, the more likely these people are to duplicate the relationship pattern they have with their parents in new relationships.[3,9]

6. The concept of *multigenerational transmission process* describes the trajectory of the family projective process. In the nuclear family, one child invariably becomes more involved in the projective process than the other children. As a consequence, this child has a lower level of differentiation than his or her siblings. Because the siblings were less involved in the parents' emotional process, they emerge from the family with a higher level of differentiation. In the multigenerational transmission process, people emerge from their families with differentiation levels higher, lower, or the same as their parents. With all families, there are those with lower differentiation levels who produce descendants with even lower differentiation levels, until dysfunction occurs in one or more people. In the same manner, all families produce individuals with higher differentiation levels who produce descendants with even higher differentiation levels. Through this process, families are able to maintain balance as a system.[3]
7. The concept of *sibling position* provides a way of describing how a specific child is selected to become involved in the family projection process. The extent to which functioning fits a person's sibling position in the family of origin reveals how the level of differentiation and family projective process have operated across generations.[3] For example, the oldest and youngest child tend to be the offspring most often in triangles with the parents.
8. The concept of *societal regression* describes how society is a macrocosm of the emotional problems found in families. Like the human family, society loses contact with intellectually determined principles and resorts increasingly to emotionally determined decisions to decrease anxiety when subjected to chronic, unremitting anxiety. The outcome of this process is the development of symptoms and eventually regression to lower levels of functioning. Societal attempts to alleviate problems through emotionally based legislation tend to increase the problems.[3] Hence, society goes through cycles similar to those of families, which lead to dysfunction.

THERAPEUTIC APPROACHES

Natural systems theory provides a way of understanding behavior of an individual in a family and the family itself. Based on this understanding, the therapist can intervene with the individual in the context of the family, with the marital pair in the context of the marital family, and with the respective families of origin. Since minor children do not hold positions of authority and power in terms of decision-making, they are usually not included in therapy sessions. The therapist does not attempt to enter into the family system but remains outside the family's emotional field and functions similarly to the way a coach relates to players in a ball game.[3] The coach never becomes a player but relates to individual players from a neutral position on the sidelines. Thus, the therapist's ability to remain a differentiated self during therapy is of paramount importance to prevent his or her triangulation into the family system.

From a position of neutrality, the therapist attempts to gain a clear picture of how the client functions as an individual in the family and how the family itself functions. To do so, the therapist uses open questions and refrains from making interpretive statements. Additionally, the therapist provides information about how families function, the nuclear family process, and how individuals are affected by the family projective process and the multigenerational transmission process. The therapist also attempts to coach the individual's efforts to define the self in the face of anxiety aroused by contact with the family.

Efforts to define the self in the presence of anxiety aroused by emotional contact with the family usually take the form of encouraging the individual to identify personal goals that he or she can meet without the cooperation of other family members. The therapist may act as a coach to help the client learn and implement ways of remaining calm when confronted with family opposition to such independent efforts. Acting as a coach, the therapist relies minimally on specific techniques but focuses instead on understanding the client in the context of his or her family and helping the client to do the same. Through this understanding, the client may achieve increased separation of the emotional and intellectual systems and become less emotionally reactive. Being less driven by emotions and more directed by reason increases the client's ability to adapt more effectively to life's demands and stress.[3,13]

APPLICATION TO NURSING

Natural systems theory provides psychiatric-mental health nurses with a means of understanding individual and family behaviors and how they are connected to each other; it is also a tool for assessment, nursing diagnosis, planning, intervention, and evaluation. Unlike other theoretical perspectives, natural systems theory is probabilistic rather than deterministic and provides a basis for providing care to individuals, families, and groups.

◆ Chapter Summary

This chapter has examined various theoretical bases for understanding human behavior and intervening in maladaptive behavior. Some of the major points of the chapter are as follows:

1. Psychoanalytic, interpersonal, and behavioristic theoretical perspectives emphasize that human behavior is largely determined by external forces outside the individual's control.
2. General systems theory acknowledges the effect of external forces on human behavior but maintains that the individual can either influence these outside forces or compensate for them.
3. Natural systems theory also acknowledges the effect of external and internal forces on human development and behavior, while asserting that the individual has the capacity to choose between reacting emotionally to stress or responding reasonably on the basis of self-chosen principles, values, and beliefs. While the theory concedes that the human organism is emotionally governed, it asserts that the intellectual system can be used to reduce the degree of emotional reactivity.
4. Psychoanalytic, interpersonal, and behavioristic theoretical perspectives hold that human behavior has a singular cause.
5. Psychoanalytic and interpersonal theories hold that behavior is determined by early life events with parental figures.
6. Behavioristic theory holds that exposure to given stimuli and reinforcements determines how a person learns to behave.
7. General systems theory holds that human behavior has multiple causes.
8. Natural systems theory holds that the human being and the human family are more like than unlike other natural biological systems.
9. All five theoretical perspectives are useful to nurses in assessing, diagnosing, planning, implementing, and evaluating nursing care.

Review Questions

1. Which of the following statements is a major premise underlying psychoanalytic theory?
   - A. The human personality functions on three levels of awareness.
   - B. Interpersonal not intrapsychic experiences form personality.
   - C. Human personality is acquired through reinforcing experiences.
   - D. Human personality and behavior are complex with multiple causes.
   - E. Human behavior is linked to biological functioning in unspecified ways.
2. Which of the following treatment modalities is derived from behavioristic theory?
   - A. Psychoanalytic therapy
   - B. Psychoanalysis
   - C. Family psychotherapy
   - D. Assertiveness training
3. An adolescent boy rebels against his parents and teachers, gets in fights with his classmates, and threatens to run away from home. His parents have not been successful in persuading him to change. From a family systems perspective, which approach would be indicated to assist this boy and his parents?
   - A. The parents should be referred to marital therapy.
   - B. Token reinforcements should be used to shape the son's behavior.
   - C. The parents should send the son to a psychoanalyst.
   - D. The son needs to engage in consensual validation with his peers.

◆ References

1. Bart PB: Ideologies and Utopias of Psychotherapy. In Roman PM, Trice HM (eds): The Sociology of Psychotherapy, pp 9–55. New York, Aronson, 1974
2. Boulding KE: General Systems Theory: The Skeleton of Science. In Walter B (ed): Modern Systems Research for the Behavioral Scientist, pp 3–10. Chicago, Aldine Publishing, 1968
3. Bowen M: Family Therapy in Clinical Practice. New York, Aronson, 1978
4. Ellis A, Grieger R: Handbook of Rational-Emotive Therapy. New York, Springer Publishing, 1978

5. Freud S: Civilization and Its Discontents. New York, WW Norton, 1961
6. Gilbert R: Extraordinary Relationships: A New Way of Thinking about Human Interactions. Minneapolis: Chronimed Publishing, 1992
7. Hilgard ER, Bower GH: Theories of Learning, 4th ed. Englewood Cliffs, NJ, Prentice-Hall, 1975
8. Kerr ME: Theoretical Base for Differentiation of Self in One's Family of Origin. Washington, DC, Haworth Press, 1984
9. Kerr ME, Bowen M: Family Evaluation. New York, WW Norton, 1988
10. Miller JG: General Living Systems Theory. In Kaplan HI, Freeman AM, Saddock BJ (eds): Comprehensive Textbook of Psychiatry III, vol 1, 3d ed, pp 98–114. Baltimore, Williams & Wilkins, 1980
11. Nye RD: Three Views of Man. Monterey, Brooks-Cole, 1975
12. Offenkrantz W, Tabin A: Psychoanalytic Psychotherapy. In Arieti S (ed): American Handbook of Psychiatry, vol 5, 2d ed, pp 183–205. New York, Basic Books, 1975
13. Papero D: Bowen Family Systems Theory. Boston, Allyn & Bacon, 1990
14. Roberts SL: Behavioral Concepts and Nursing Throughout the Life Span. Englewood Cliffs, NJ, Prentice-Hall, 1978
15. Snelbecker GE: Learning Theory, Instructional Theory, and Psychoeducational Design. New York, McGraw-Hill, 1974
16. Starr BD, Goldstein HS: Human Development and Behavior. New York, Springer, 1975
17. Sullivan HS: Interpersonal Theory of Psychiatry. New York, WW Norton, 1953
18. Sutherland JW: A General Systems Philosophy for the Social and Behavioral Sciences. New York, George Braziller, 1973
19. Von Bertalanffy L: General System Theory. New York, George Braziller, 1968
20. Von Bertalanffy L: General System Theory and Psychiatry. In Arieti S: American Handbook of Psychiatry, vol 1, 2d ed, pp 1095–1117. New York, Basic Books, 1975
21. Wolpe J: The Practice of Behavior Therapy. New York, Pergamon Press, 1973

Nursing Theory

Judith A. Greene

4

To engage in theorizing means not just to learn by experience but to take thought about what there is to be learned. To speak loosely, lower animals grasp scientific laws but never rise to the level of scientific theory. They learn by *experience, not* from *it, for* from *learning requires symbolic constructions which can provide vicarious experience never actually undergone.*

Abraham Kaplan,
The Conduct of Inquiry, *1964*

An enormous body of literature addresses the subject of nursing theory. These efforts have been directed toward explaining nursing phenomena and delimiting nursing's philosophical, educational, practical, and research boundaries. As a result of these efforts, a wide array of published opinions exists regarding nursing's essence and functions. This diversity is reflected in several conceptual schemes commonly called nursing theories.

Learning Objectives

On completion of this chapter, you should be able to accomplish the following:

1. *Define the term theory.*
2. *Identify three types of theory.*
3. *Discuss the functions of theory.*
4. *Identify types of nursing theory applicable to psychiatric-mental health nursing.*
5. *Analyze selected nursing theories according to type and major conceptual components.*

◆ Theory Defined

A *theory* is a conceptual system consisting of interrelated propositions that describe, explain, and predict selected phenomena. As such, a theory functions to order knowledge about reality. However, no single theory can address all aspects of reality. Rather, a theory orders knowledge about a specific aspect of the real world and suggests ways of further extending and refining that knowledge through scientific research.

All theories are tentative and subject to change or even to obsolescence. The extent to which a theory is verified by scientific research determines its validity and usefulness. When a theory begins to falter under repeated scientific investigations, it is either changed or discarded. Thus, a theory does not represent an absolute truth but rather serves as a tool to increase understanding of the real world.

◆ Types of Theory

Most theories can be classified as deductive, inductive, or analogic. *Deductive theory* consists of a large group of propositional statements based on minimal sensory information developed and interconnected through deductive logic. Because deductive theory is based on minimal sensory information, it may be expected to contain faulty or incorrect theoretical details. It is assumed, however, that these faults will be corrected through scientific research. Examples of deductive theory include psychoanalytic theory, quantum theory, and general systems theory.

Inductive theory, on the other hand, consists of a modest group of summary statements or generalizations based on ample sensory information. Unlike deductive theory, inductive theory maintains a close connection between observation and conceptualization. Consequently, inductive theory uses deductive logic minimally and contains few inferential statements. A well-known inductive theory is Skinner's behavioristic theory.

Analogic theory differs significantly from deductive and inductive theory. An *analogic theory*, more commonly called a model, depicts or explains relationships between things, events, objects, or functions that are basically different yet share similar attributes. Statements of relationships articulated in this way may be based more on imagination than reality, in that analogic theory relies chiefly on "as if" thinking. That is, analogic theory focuses primarily on discerning comparisons, correspondences, parallelisms, or associations that may or may not actually exist. Because of this, hypotheses from analogic theory seldom hold up to scientific investigation. Despite this, analogic theory can be useful in theory construction and scientific research.

Numerous examples of analogic theory exist. Most notable in nursing literature is Roy's adaptation model. When constructing this theory, Roy used Helson's theory of learning and adaptation as a model to organize nursing concepts in a logical pattern. Roy believed not only that the logical pattern of Helson's theory corresponds to the logical sequence of events in nursing practice, but also that some content of Helson's theory applied to nursing.

◆ Functions of Theory

Theory functions not only to organize knowledge, but also to suggest ways of validating and extending knowledge through scientific research. Theory also enables people to predict future events accurately; it is thus a guide to human action. Most important, theory enables individuals to understand phenomena in relation to their unique situations. Through this understanding, individuals may be able not only to predict accurately the outcome of their actions, but also to gain some control over the course of future events.

◆ Nursing Theory

The development of theory, rather than the standardization of roles and procedures, is necessary for the further development of nursing as a profession. Several nurse theorists have made significant contributions toward this goal. Some theorists, such as Peplau, Travelbee, and Orlando, have focused on the interpersonal relationship or interaction between the nurse and the client. Others, such as Roy, Orem, and Johnson, have focused on the behavioral effects of nursing. Still others, such as Neuman and Rogers, have attempted to address the entire field of phenomena associated with nursing from a systems perspective. To a great extent, almost all current nursing theories can be classified as interpersonal, behavioral, or systems-oriented in nature. Some nursing theories, however, reflect mixed characteristics of these types. Nursing theories in each of these classes are useful in psychiatric-mental health nursing and in other nursing specialties. Furthermore, analyzing nursing theories according to classification, theory type, and function assists in their application to psychiatric-mental health nursing practice and research.

◆ Analysis of Selected Nursing Theories

PEPLAU'S THEORY

Hildegard Peplau has been a pioneer in formulating nursing theory. Drawing on the works of Harry S. Sulivan and Rollo May and her own clinical experience, Peplau proposed an *interpersonal theory* applicable to nursing practice in general and to psychiatric-mental health nursing in particular.

Peplau describes the interpersonal aspects of nursing as a process consisting of four phases. The first is the *orientation phase*, in which the nurse and client meet as strangers, exchange social amenities, and then proceed to clarify each other's roles. From this initial phase, the nurse and client enter the *identification phase*, during which the nurse helps the client express feelings and correct or clarify misconceptions based on previous life and health care experiences. Through these transactions, the nurse and client begin to experience each other as unique individuals. As a result, the client experiences acceptance and a high degree of trust in the nurse.

The foundation provided by the first two phases prepares the nurse and client to enter the *exploitation phase*. During this phase, the client begins to derive the full value of the nurse–client relationship. The client begins to test alternative ways of coping with health problems and to formulate goals for the future. As the client becomes more skillful in using the problem-solving process, convalescence begins.

As convalescence progresses, the client and nurse enter the *resolution phase* of the nurse–client relationship. The groundwork for terminating the relationship takes place during the orientation phase. During the resolution phase, however, the nurse and client complete the work associated with terminating the relationship. Ideally, the nurse and client experience termination as a freeing process in which both experience fulfillment; the nurse experiences professional fulfillment, and the client moves toward increased personal maturity.

While working with the client through these phases, the nurse assumes six roles. Initially, the nurse assumes the role of *stranger*, because the nurse and client do not know each other. The tasks of forming trust and acceptance are most prominent at this time.

As the client's needs and limitations are assessed, the nurse assumes the role of *resource expert* in an effort to provide alternative ways of meeting client needs and to assist the client in reducing limitations. Because the client may be incapacitated or immobilized physically and emotionally, the nurse may also need to assume the role of *leader* during the relationship to ensure that client needs are addressed.

Another role often assumed by the nurse is that of *surrogate parent*. Because clients often regress during illness and have dependency needs associated with earlier developmental stages, they often unconsciously view nurses as parent substitutes. As the nurse assumes the role of counselor, the client is assisted to recall past experiences and traumas and to work through these. The nurse may also assume the role of teacher in an attempt to assist the client to learn from present and past experiences and traumas.

Analysis of Peplau's Theory

Peplau's nursing theory can be classified as interpersonal because it focuses primarily on the nurse–client relationship. Although the influence of Sullivan, May, and other theorists is obvious, Peplau's work is considered an inductive theory. This is because it is based predominantly on her observations and clinical experience and is closely attached to observable nursing events. Although this theory is logically developed, it lacks the intricate, formal logic characteristic of deductive theory.

Peplau's theory describes, explains, predicts, and to some extent, permits control of the sequence of events occurring in the nurse–client relationship. It has limited use in short-term, acute care psychiatric nursing settings, in which hospitalizations last only hours or at most a few days, precluding relationship development. Another limitation is that it is applicable only to dyadic nurse–client relationships, not to relationships in which the client is actually a group of individuals—a family or a community. Despite these limitations, Peplau's theory continues to apply to today's nursing scene, especially with respect to long-term psychiatric care in outpatient and home health settings. In these settings, Peplau's work continues to stand the test of time.

OREM'S THEORY

Like Peplau, Dorothea E. Orem has been a pioneer in developing nursing theory. The origins of her theory are not readily recognizable. It appears that the development of her theory was based primarily on her own observations, particularly the self-care behavioral capacities of clients and required nursing care behavior. Orem's theory is considered an inductive theory and is classified as a *behavioral nursing theory.*

Orem's theory is based on the premise that people need a composite of self-care actions to survive. Self-care actions consist of all behaviors performed by people to maintain life, health, and well-being. The capacity of the client and the client's family to perform self-care is called *self-care agency.* Orem states that a need for nursing care exists if the client's self-care demand exceeds the client's self-care agency. Thus, the goal of nursing is to meet the client's *self-care demands* until the client or the client's family is capable of doing so.

Orem's theory describes three types of self-care:

1. Universal self-care behaviors, required to meet physiologic and psychosocial needs
2. Developmental self-care behaviors, required to undergo normal human development
3. Health deviation self-care behaviors, required to meet client needs during health deviations

The classification of self-care behaviors in this manner helps ensure complete assessment of the client's self-care agency.

Although Orem's theory does not specifically incorporate the standard nursing process, three components of the nursing process are easily discernible: assessment, planning, and implementation. Assessment focuses on the client's self-care demand, self-care agency, and self-care deficits. Orem's theory does not specifically address nursing diagnoses derived from analysis of the assessment information. However, a plan is formulated from the information obtained in the assessment, which indicates the nursing approach needed to meet the client's needs, and can be categorized as follows:

1. *Wholly compensatory,* in which the client does not participate behaviorally in self-care
2. *Partially compensatory,* in which the client and nurse participate behaviorally in meeting the client's self-care needs
3. *Educative development,* in which the client meets self-care needs with minimal nursing assistance

To implement the required nursing approach, the nurse uses one of five behaviors: acting or doing for the client, guiding, supporting, providing, and teaching.

The nurse does not evaluate the effects or results of these behaviors, but rather evaluates whether the client still requires nursing care. According to Orem, the need for nursing intervention ceases when either the client or the client's family is able to meet the client's self-care demands.

Analysis of Orem's Theory

Orem's theory consists of a small group of summary statements or generalizations regarding nursing. These statements appear to be based on Orem's observations and analyses of nursing phenomena and are virtually devoid of deductive logic. Consequently, this theory can be typed as an inductive theory. Because Orem's work focuses primarily on behaviors related to self-care, it can also be classified as a behavioral nursing theory.

The strength of Orem's theory lies in its emphasis on clients' capabilities rather than limitations. Orem's theory also explains the necessity of the client's and family's involvement in the nursing process. Furthermore, the theory does not permit the client to be forced into a passive, dependent role.

Orem's theory has two major weaknesses. First, the theory's language is somewhat disorganized and unnecessarily complex and clumsy. For example, the term self-care agency could be rephrased as *self-care capacity.* The second and more important major weakness lies in the theory's failure to address the evaluation of the effects of nursing care behaviors. This failure precludes the use of the theory to guide evaluation research concerning the effectiveness of nursing care. This weakness, however, could be easily eliminated through further development of the theory with regard to nursing diagnosis and criteria for evaluating the results of nursing care behavior.

ROGERS'S THEORY

Martha Rogers, another pioneer in nursing theory development, proposed a theory concerning the nature of humankind from a unique nursing perspective. The theory has close ties to von Bertalanffy's general system theory and to physics. Because Rogers drew extensively on the content and deductive logical form of these two bodies of knowledge, her theory can be typed as analogic and deductive. It can also be classified as a *systems-oriented nursing theory* because of the strong influence of general systems theory.

Rogers's theory is based on four major premises:

1. The human organism is characterized by openness and, as a result, is in continuous mutual interaction with the environment.
2. The human organism is conceptualized as having an energy field that is in constant mutual interaction with the energy fields of the environment and of other human organisms. This dynamic mutual interaction can be perceived as wave patterns or auras.

3. The way in which the energy fields appear is characterized by organized patterns or designs.
4. Human existence is four-dimensional rather than three-dimensional. Four-dimensionality, according to Rogers, is the human being's capacity to transcend conventional concepts of time–space interaction.

Rogers's three principles of homeodynamics rest on the four preceding premises. The first principle of homeodynamics asserts that human life proceeds in one direction along a spiral-like course. Because human organisms are open systems with energy fields capable of continuous, mutual interaction with the environment and each other, organized patterns emerge depicting the mutual interaction of human environmental energy fields along a unidirectional spiral through time and space. The simultaneous mutual interaction of human and environmental energy fields is called *complementarity.*

When complementarity between organisms and their environments encounters interference, the four-dimensional aspect of human existence comes into play. To reduce interference and restore order and complementarity, the person has the capacity to transcend time and space: This transcendence can result in paranormal experiences, such as clairvoyance and other altered states of consciousness. These altered states of consciousness may provide information needed by the person to reduce untoward interference and restore balance and resonance to life. Rogers's theory accounts for these phenomena by suggesting that loops of the person's unidirectional spiral-like trajectory—and their respective energy fields—come temporarily into close proximity, transcending time and space and permitting the occurrence of paranormal phenomena.

The goals of nursing, according to Rogers, are to maintain and promote the maximal health potential of clients, to prevent disease, to formulate nursing diagnoses, and to provide rehabilitative nursing care. From these goals, it is evident that Rogers believed that all people—sick or well, rich or poor, and in all geographic locations—require nursing services. Rogers did not, however, delineate an operational framework for the nursing process in administering these services.

Analysis of Rogers's Theory

Rogers's theory has two major strengths. First, the theory is holistic and takes into account the entire field of phenomena associated with nursing practice. It addresses the psychological, social, environmental, physiological, and physical realms of human existence and attempts to relate them to nursing. Second, the theory addresses the spirituality of human existence by attempting to explain the four-dimensionality of the universe and the occurrence of paranormal experiences. In doing so, Rogers implicitly suggests that further study of these phenomena may eventually change the way psychiatric-mental health nurses and other related professionals regard and treat what are now viewed as mental illnesses. Additionally, by focusing on the nature of human evolution, Rogerian theory has the potential to contribute to psychiatric mental health nursing's understanding of family, group, and community systems.

A major weakness in Rogers's theory lies in the fact that its terminology is overly complex. Additionally, the absence or weakness of logical bridges or transitions between its conceptual components confuses the theory's content. Nevertheless, Rogers's theory has contributed to nursing practice, theory development, and research because it broadens the minds and imaginations of nurses and the field of nursing itself.

As stated previously, Rogers's theory has characteristics of deductive and analogic theory. Rogers used a diagrammatical model of a spiral to depict the life trajectory of the human organism and to illustrate the ways in which energy fields emanate from the individual and the immediate environment; the use of this diagram is one example of the analogic component of her theory. Rogers's use of the logical framework of systems theory and physics laws also reflects the analogic nature of her theory. Because Rogers's theory is organized using deductive logic and is based on minimal observations, her work also may be typed as a deductive theory.

ROY'S THEORY

Callista Roy also has contributed significantly to the formulation of nursing theory. In constructing her theory, Roy used Harry Helson's theory of learning and adaptation to organize nursing concepts in a logical pattern. For this reason, her work can be typed as an analogic theory, and as such, it has been widely used as a conceptual framework for nursing curricula, nursing practice, and nursing research.

According to Roy's theory, the goal of nursing is to promote the client's adaptation in health and illness. This goal is achieved through the nurse's efforts to change, manipulate, or block stress-producing stimuli that may impinge on the client. The theory assumes that this kind of nursing intervention assists the client to cope more effectively through reducing stress.

The concept of *adaptation* in Roy's theory refers to an ongoing process occurring within all living systems. The purpose of the adaptation process is survival, growth, and reproduction. Roy's theory thus assumes that all human beings are adaptive systems and that humans change in response to stimuli. If the change is viewed as positive, one that promotes the person's integrity, then the change can be considered adaptive. If the change does not promote the person's integrity, then the change can be considered maladaptive.

Roy's theory also describes two mechanisms for adapting. The regulator mechanism pertains to physiologic needs and processes. The cognator mechanism refers to perceptual, social, and information-processing functions. These mechanisms are linked loosely to Roy's four modes of adaptation discussed below.

The nursing process used in Roy's theory involves two levels of assessment. The first level includes observation of behaviors related to the four *adaptive modes*: physiologic, self-concept, role function, and interdependence. These four modes represent methods used by the client to adapt. The second level of assessment consists of identifying focal, contextual, and residual stimuli. The *focal stimulus* represents the immediate dominant stimulus affecting the client, such as injury, stress, or illness. *Contextual stimuli* include the environment, the client's family, and all other background factors related to the focal stimulus. *Residual stimuli* consist of the client's previous background, beliefs, attitudes, and traits. These residual stimuli are related to the contextual stimuli and are assumed to also have an effect on the focal stimulus. According to Roy's theory, contextual and residual stimuli are more difficult to assess than the focal stimulus because they are less observable or detectable.

According to Roy's theory, a person's adaptation level is a function of focal, contextual, and residual stimuli. When a person encounters stresses from these stimuli that surpass innate and acquired mechanisms to cope effectively, the person behaves ineffectively, as demonstrated by one or more of the adaptive models. At this point, nursing intervention is required. This emphasis on the client's behavior, stimuli determining the client's behavior, and the nurse intervening in some way to interfere with the stimuli qualifies Roy's theory for classification as a behavioral nursing theory.

Analysis of Roy's Theory

Roy's nursing theory has three major strengths. Of significant importance is the theory's clear language. Second, the theory uses the standard form of the nursing process. Third, it focuses concretely on observable behaviors exhibited by the client that indicate a need for nursing intervention. Moreover, the behaviors used by the nurse to mitigate stimuli impacting on the client can be described in precise, correct terms. This concrete focus on observable behaviors increases the potential for individualized client assessment and care planning.

There are also three major weaknesses to Roy's theory. The first weakness is that the four adaptive modes overlap in meaning and function. For example, each of the four adaptive modes addresses some aspect of psychological and social functioning. For this reason, these modes need to be operationally defined to reduce overlap and redundancy.

The theory's second major weakness is that the nurse's subjective evaluation of what is or is not a positive response to nursing interventions determines what is considered adaptive or maladaptive. Finally, the theory's use of the term *adaptation* can convey a variety of meanings, such as conform, fit, or accommodate. Perhaps, it is implicitly assumed that the term adaptation refers to survival mechanisms studied in evolutionary biology. Nevertheless, objective criteria defining what is or is not adaptive need to be identified to increase the usefulness of this theory.

As stated previously, Roy's theory can be typed as an analogic theory and classified as a behavioral theory. Roy's later versions of her theory assert that it is a systems-oriented theory, but this assertion is debatable. The use of terms such as input, output, and process do not obscure the fact that Roy's theory was modeled from a behavioral theory and thus is a behavioral nursing theory. Of the preceding theories, Roy's adaptation theory is least useful to psychiatric-mental health nursing.

◆ Chapter Summary

This chapter has provided an overview and analysis of the concept of theory, various types and functions of theory, the application of theory to nursing, and selected nursing theories applicable to psychiatric-mental health nursing in particular. This chapter includes the following major points:

1. A theory is a conceptual system consisting of interrelated propositions that describe, explain, and predict selected phenomena.
2. All theories are tentative and subject to change or obsolescence: thus, theories are not absolutely true.
3. The extent to which a theory is verified by scientific research determines its validity and usefulness.
4. Theory can usually be classified as deductive, inductive, or analogic in nature.
5. Theory functions to organize knowledge and to suggest ways of validating and extending knowledge through scientific research.
6. Theory allows prediction of future events and thus is a guide to human action.
7. Many nursing theories can be classified as interpersonal, behavioral, or systems-oriented in nature.
8. Hildegard Peplau, Dorothea Orem, Martha Rogers, and Callista Roy, all pioneers in nursing theory and development, have formulated theories applicable to psychiatric-mental health nursing.

Review Questions

1. Which nursing theory is most often used by psychiatric nurses?
   A. Roy's theory
   B. Rogers's theory
   C. Orem's theory
   D. Peplau's theory
2. Orem's nursing theory is most useful to assess clients in which area of human functioning?
   A. Adaptation
   B. Self-care
   C. Maturation
   D. Homeodynamics
3. Which of the following statements most accurately describes the functions of a theory?
   A. Describes the way reality should be
   B. Serves as a guide to human action
   C. Reports the sequence of past events
   D. Permits control over other people

◆ References

1. Brodbeck M (ed): Readings in the Philosophy of the Social Sciences. New York, Macmillan, 1968
2. Bush H: Models for Nursing. Adv Nurs Sci 1 (2): 13–20, 1979
3. Carboni, JT: The Rogerian Process of Inquiry. Advances in Nursing Science 8(1): 22–37, 1995
4. Ellis R: Characteristics of Significant Theories. Nurs Res 17 (3): 217–222, 1968
5. Fawcett J: Analysis and Evaluation of Nursing Theories. Philadelphia, Davis, 1968
6. Forchuk C, Dorsay JP: Hildegard Peplau Meets Family Systems Nursing: Innovation in Theory-Based Practice. J Adv Nurs 21(1): 110–115, 1995
7. Fitzpatrick J, Whall A, Johnson R, Floyd J: Nursing Models and their Psychiatric-Mental Health Applications. Bowie, MD, Brady Co, 1982
8. Hardy M: Theories: Components, Development, Evaluation. Nurs Res 23 (2): 100–107, 1974
9. Hardy M: Perspectives on Nursing Theory. Adv Nurs Sci 1 (1): 37–48, 1979.
10. Hempel C: Aspects of Scientific Explanation and Other Essays in the Philosophy of Science. New York, Free Press, 1965
11. Johnson D: Development of Theory: A Requisite for Nursing as a Primary Health Profession. Nurs Res 23 (5): 372–377, 1974
12. Kaplan A: The Conduct of Inquiry. New York, Thomas Cromwell, 1964
13. Kuhn T: Structure of Scientific Revolutions. Chicago, University of Chicago Press, 1965
14. McFarlane J: Developing a Theory of Nursing: The Relation of Theory to Practice, Education, and Research. J Adv Nurs 2: 261–270, 1977
15. Nagel E: The Structure of Science. New York, Harcourt, Brace and World, 1961
16. Neuman B: The Neuman Systems Model: Application of Nursing Education and Practice. Norwalk, CT, Appleton-Century-Crofts, 1982
17. Orem D: Nursing: Concepts of Practice, 2d ed. New York, McGraw-Hill, 1980
18. Orlando I: The Dynamic Nurse-Patient Relationship. New York, G.P. Putnam, 1952
19. Peplau H: Interpersonal Relations in Nursing. New York, G.P. Putnam, 1952
20. Peplau H: Interpersonal Constructs for Nursing Practice. Nursing Education Today 7(5): 201–208, 1988
21. Rogers M: Nursing Science: An Introduction to the Theoretical Basis of Nursing. Philadelphia, FA Davis, 1970
22. Rogers M: Nursing: Science of Unitary, Irreducible, Human Beings: Update 1990. In E. Barrett (ed.), Visions of Rogers's Science-Based Nursing. New York, National League for Nursing, 1990
23. Roy C: Adaptation: A Conceptual Framework for Nursing. Nurs Outlook 18 (3): 254–257, 1971
24. Roy C: Adaptation: A Basis for Nursing Practice. Nurs Outlook 19 (4): 254–257, 1971
25. Roy C: Introduction to Nursing: An Adaptation Model. Englewood Cliffs, NJ, Prentice Hall, 1977
26. Suppe F: The Structure of Scientific Theories, 2d ed. Chicago, University of Illinois Press, 1977
27. Sutherland J: A General Systems Philosophy for the Social and Behavioral Sciences. New York, Braziller, 1973
28. Travelbee J: Interpersonal Aspects of Nursing, 2d ed. Philadelphia, FA Davis, 1971
29. Torres G: Theoretical Foundations of Nursing. Norwalk, CT, Appleton-Century-Crofts, 1986
30. von Bertalanffy L: General System Theory. New York, Braziller, 1968

The Therapeutic Relationship

Patriciann Furnari Brady

5

Without deeper reflection one knows from daily life that one exists for other people—first of all for those upon whose smiles and well-being our own happiness is wholly dependent, and then for the many, unknown to us, to whose destinies we are bound by the ties of sympathy. A hundred times every day I remind myself that my inner and outer life are based on the labors of other men, living and dead, and that I must exert myself in order to give in the same measure as I have received and am still receiving.

Albert Einstein,
Ideas and Opinions

Admission to the mental health care system can be a frightening experience. Clients bring with them a variety of thoughts and feelings about mental hospitals. The nurse is the primary individual to meet the care needs of the client. To establish an effective relationship with clients and to meet their needs, the nurse must have an understanding of the nurse–client relationship.

This chapter focuses on the therapeutic relationship—what it is and what it is not, its purpose and phases. The attitude of the nurse and the interventions that facilitate growth are examined as crucial issues affecting the development of the therapeutic relationship.

Learning Objectives

On completion of this chapter, you should be able to accomplish the following:

1. *Define the term therapeutic relationship.*
2. *Differentiate between social, intimate, and therapeutic relationships.*
3. *Describe the characteristics of a therapeutic relationship.*
4. *Identify the anxieties of the nurse and client in a therapeutic relationship.*
5. *Discuss the expectations of the nurse and client in the therapeutic relationship.*
6. *Discuss the impact of the attitude of the nurse-helper on a therapeutic relationship.*
7. *Describe ways in which the nurse facilitates the growth of clients.*

◆ The Dynamics of Relationships

DEFINITION AND PURPOSE OF RELATIONSHIPS

Nursing practice occurs within the relationship of a nurse and a client. A relationship is defined as a state of being related or a state of affinity between two individuals. The nurse and client interact with each other in the health care system, with the goals of assisting the client to use personal resources to meet his or her unique needs. The contributions of each partner in the nurse–client relationship are more important than the individual contribution of either the nurse or the client.[89]

Nursing involves communication: It is a human-to-human event.[12] When clients enter the health care system, they bring with them a preconceived notion of their role and the role of the nurse. The nurse is seen as the provider of care; implicit in this role is meeting the client's psychological needs and facilitating the client's growth. The development of a therapeutic relationship enables the nurse to join in a partnership with the client and to help the client to set goals for solving problems. Nurses who work with clients to identify desired changes empower clients to direct their own treatment and take responsibility for its outcome.

Hildegard Peplau describes nursing as an educative instrument, a maturing force, that aims to produce forward movements of personality in the direction of creative, constructive, and productive personal and community living.[16] Nurses provide the client with the opportunity for an honest and authentic relationship. The care dimension in such a relationship promotes human growth through recognition of the uniqueness of the individual, recognition of the resources within the individual, and provision of an empathetic atmosphere conducive to the client's self-exploration. The focus of caring supports the individual's healing resources.[13] Three categories of nurse behaviors indicate caring:

1. Giving of self
2. Meeting client's needs in a timely manner
3. Providing comfort measures for clients and family members[4]

TYPES OF RELATIONSHIPS

Three possible types of relationships—social, intimate, and therapeutic—can occur between individuals.

Social Relationship

The *social relationship* is the most common kind between individuals in everyday life. Both individuals are equally involved in this relationship and are concerned with meeting their own needs through the relationship. There is no predetermined goal or focus in the relationship, and the continuation of the relationship is not determined at the onset. Platonic friends, work colleagues, and neighbors who help each other out are examples of this kind of relationship.

Intimate Relationship

An *intimate relationship* is a relationship between two individuals committed to one another, caring for and respecting each other. Intimacy is usually exclusive to those involved and implies that they love each other.

According to Erikson, the ability to develop an intimate relationship with an adult of the opposite sex depends on completing developmental tasks.[5] The intimate relationship forms the basis for marriage and other partner-type relationships.

Therapeutic Relationship

In a *therapeutic relationship,* the nurse and client work together toward the goal of assisting the client to regain the inner resources to meet life challenges and facilitate growth. The interaction is purposefully established, maintained, and carried out with the anticipated outcome of helping the client gain new coping and adaptation skills. There are two basic assumptions underlying the therapeutic relationship:

1. The client's difficulties are expressed in the relationship.
2. The previous, learned difficulties of former relationships are amenable to change in this relationship.[9]

Through the nursing process, the nurse establishes a therapeutic relationship to interact effectively with a client. The nursing process can be considered educative and therapeutic when the nurse and client come to know and respect each other as people with similarities and differences who can work together as a team to identify and solve problems.[16] Nurses and clients affect each other; nurses should recognize the effect they have on clients and their clients' effect on them.

Given today's trend toward shortened hospital stays, developing therapeutic relationships poses even more of a challenge for nurses (Box 5-1).

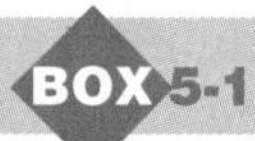

Solution-Focused Therapy

Within the therapeutic relationship, using solution-focused therapy as suggested by Chandler the nurse can assist the client to identify personal strengths and resources to effect change that will lead to a healthy and happier life.

The nurse provides an atmosphere that is conducive to change. This can be accomplished through the development of safety, trust, and empowerment. The nurse assists the client to recognize what inner resources he or she can mobilize to take control of problems. The focus is assisting the client to identify what methods he or she previously used when a change was needed. Through recognition of past accomplishment, change can be seen as possible.

Assisting the client to determine the exact nature of the problem, what needs to occur, and how these changes will be beneficial is the goal of the relationship. Within the client's frame of reference, the client identifies strengths, resources, and attributes needed to make the desired change. The focus becomes the client's actions versus the nurse's actions. The nurse facilitates the client's determination and use of solutions.

As the client begins to generate and implement change, the nurse provides the positive reinforcement. The client is assisted to recognize how these changes have impacted his or her perception of the situation. Assisting the client to assume personal responsibility for the initiation of change empowers the client to believe change can be made, again relieving the feelings of hopelessness and increasing personal competence.

This model permits clients to make and see change in a more rapid manner, and corresponds to the goals of brief treatment and shorter focused hospitalization.

(Source: Chandler, MC, & Mason, WH. Solution-Focused Therapy: An Alternative Approach to Addictions Nursing. Perspectives in Psychiatric Care, 31 (1): *8–13, 1995)*

◆ Dimensions of the Therapeutic Relationship

CONCEPTUAL FRAMEWORK

The nurse–client relationship provides a high degree of validation for clients with emotional problems. Within the nurse–client relationship, the nurse can constantly view clients not only as they are, but also as the people they have the potential to be.[21] As an active member of the treatment team, the nurse has the opportunity to develop a relationship with clients that helps them deal with their fears, symptoms, and interpersonal problems. In a therapeutic relationship, the kinds of interactions in which nurses participate vary from assisting clients with activities of daily living to undertaking individual, group, or family therapy with them.

Psychiatric-mental health nurses have the opportunity to interact with clients across a variety of practice settings and areas. The therapeutic relationship extends from the individual's home to the clinic to the hospital. The therapeutic relationship also extends across a variety of practice areas, including families, schools, community groups, and hospitals. In all these areas, the nurse has the opportunity to develop therapeutic relationships that focus on assisting clients to develop resources to meet their needs.

The nurse recognizes that although not all contacts with clients are therapy sessions, each contact has the potential for being therapeutic, for promoting interpersonal growth, for changing behavior, or for benefitting the client in some way. The therapeutic relationship provides a meaningful context for applying the values of nursing, which include caring, generosity in response to human needs, and courage on behalf of the helpless.[20]

Communication between client and nurse should be carefully planned and implemented so that clients feel protected and accepted and attempt communication with the nurse and others. Through this communication, clients sense the nurse's belief that they have the ability to participate actively in their own care, to effect change, and to function in a healthier manner.

CHARACTERISTICS OF THE THERAPEUTIC RELATIONSHIP

The core of nursing is the relationship between the nurse and the client. This therapeutic relationship is a goal-directed relationship that facilitates the client's development of appropriate coping skills and offers the client the potential to grow. Carl Rogers has described the benefits of a helping relationship in these words: "If I can provide a certain type of a relationship, the other person will discover within himself the capacity to use that relationship for growth and change and personal development will occur."[18]

The client's self-view is affected by the nurse's behavior and attitude. The nurse's effectiveness depends on genuineness, honesty, authenticity, and respect for the client's humanity and dignity. Mentally disturbed clients often misinterpret reality; they lack interpersonal skills and may interpret the nurse's aloofness as rejection. The nurse needs to support the client's constant awareness of verbal and nonverbal behavior. Consistency in approach fosters the development of trust, particularly when the client tests the relationship.

The behavior of clients represents their best adaptation to stress. The nurse must recognize that a change in a client's mood or behavior is a change in the internal situation of that client to which the nurse may not be privy.[19] Unconditional acceptance of the client as a person reinforces the client's sense of worth and dignity. If the client must perform ritualistic behavior, for example, the nurse should plan care to allow time for the client to complete the rituals.

Clients have the right to be involved in their own care. Together the nurse and client determine the goals of the relationship. It falls within the nurse's realm to maintain the therapeutic relationship. To maintain a therapeutic relationship and to provide for the client a safe and therapeutic environment geared toward health, the nurse must stay focused on the client's issues.[17] When the nurse clearly assesses the client's needs and assists the client through the nursing process, the client will move toward emotional health.[17] The nurse's hopefulness and support facilitate the client's development of more adaptive coping skills.

PHASES OF THE THERAPEUTIC RELATIONSHIP

Introductory Phase

The initial or introductory contact between client and nurse can occur in a variety of settings. During the initial contact with the client, the nurse has the opportunity to establish a caring relationship. By acknowledging the client by name and then introducing herself, the nurse communicates interest in the client. Throughout the initial interaction, the nurse may use a variety of techniques to demonstrate acceptance of the client's behavior, establish rapport, and provide an opportunity for the client to establish trust (Case Study 5-1).

During the initial phase of a therapeutic relationship, the nurse focuses on the following:

1. Responding to emergency situations
2. Setting up parameters for nurse–client interactions
3. Explaining the nurse–client interactions
4. Gathering data
5. Helping the client identify problems and plan effective use of community resources and services
6. Reducing client's anxieties

A client may test the nurse's commitment by acting out or missing appointments or meetings. In this phase of the relationship, the client's problems are identified, nursing diagnoses and goals are determined, priorities are set, and plans are formulated to achieve goals.

During the initial interaction, the nurse and client may establish a formal or informal contract to determine the parameters of their relationship. The contract may include such topics as time and place of meetings, evaluating goals, keeping appointments, exploring problems, explaining confidentiality, discussing types of problems to be addressed, and reevaluating expectations at any point in the relationship.

The nurse informs the client when desired goals are beyond the nurse's realm of expertise or the duration of the interaction. Failure of the nurse to share this information with the client in an open and honest manner will interfere with the establishment of trust and the ultimate outcome of the relationship.

In the nurse–client relationship, the nurse exercises a certain amount of power over the client through the use of language and techniques of persuasion, and by assuming control of the agenda.[10] Through the emphasis on a more collaborative and open relationship, these behaviors will not impede the nurse–client relationship.

With the first encounter, the nurse and client in a collaborative relationship begin to identify the client's needs, desires, coping styles, and expectations for the relationship.[1] The nurse will strive to care for the client in such a manner that a sense of trust and confidence

5-1 **Case Study**

Establishing a Therapeutic Relationship With Peter

Peter was brought to the emergency room by the police department after he was found standing on the corner yelling at cars as they drove by. The police stated that it was snowing, there was water flowing in the gutter, and Peter had no shoes on. Peter was wearing slacks, a summer jacket, socks, and no shoes. He appeared frightened and confused.

Barbara asked Peter his name and introduced herself as a primary mental health nurse in the emergency room, who would be caring for Peter this evening. She quickly assessed his physical condition and offered him a blanket and a cup of warm coffee. She explained to Peter that she wanted to help him and questioned what he perceived as his need. He stated someone had run off with his shoes. She told him that she understood it is difficult to be outside when someone takes your shoes. She helped Peter to verbalize his perception of his problem and his needs. Once these initial needs were met, a relationship had been established with Peter, and Barbara completed nursing assessment and planned for further care for Peter.

Questions for Discussion

1. Why were Barbara's initial actions important in establishing a therapeutic relationship with Peter? What did she establish and change through communication with Peter?
2. How might Peter act or react to test Barbara's commitment to the therapeutic relationship?

develops. Therapy begins when the nurse and client progress beyond exchanging information, and the client begins to share subjective content underlying behavior.

Before moving to the next phase of the relationship, the nurse and client should evaluate the initial phase and assess whether the following goals have been met:

1. Security is being established through continued development of trust.
2. The client is assisted to verbalize thoughts and feelings.
3. Areas of inadequate stress adaptation are being identified.
4. Strengths and weaknesses are being identified
5. Goals for the relationship are clearly defined

Middle or Working Phase

In the working phase of the relationship, the client and nurse are actively involved in meeting the goals established during the initial phase of the relationship. During this phase, the client's behavior may fluctuate between dependency and independence as painful aspects of life are faced, and the struggle toward healthy, adaptive behavior begins. The nurse encourages the client to express feelings and attempt new adaptation approaches without danger of punitive treatment, and reinforces effective problem solving.

Nurses need to be aware of the tendency to want to take care of others. Because of this, nursing interventions may be manifested as "overhelping" (going beyond the client's wishes or needs), controlling (asserting authority or assuming control), or narcissistic (needing to find weakness or helplessness in clients).[17]

In this phase of the relationship, the client is likely to feel more secure and openly discusses topics that could not be discussed previously. The client is able to learn new behaviors because the level of anxiety decreases when trust is reinforced through the nurse's acceptance.

Principles of psychiatric rehabilitation may be incorporated in the working phase of the therapeutic relationship, with the aim of increasing the functioning of clients with psychiatric disabilities so that they can be more successful and satisfied with the least amount of ongoing professional intervention necessary.[15]

The therapeutic tasks of the working phase of the nurse–client relationship include the following:

1. Increase the client's awareness and perceptions of the reality of specific personal experiences
2. Develop a realistic self-concept and promote self-confidence
3. Recognize areas of discomfort and verbalize feelings
4. Attempt to make comparisons between the ineffective behavior both within and outside the relationship, and draw conclusions regarding these comparisons
5. Develop a plan of action, implement the plan, and evaluate the results of the plan to alter the client's behavior
6. Assess the client's readiness and provide opportunities for independent functioning

Termination Phase

The termination phase of the therapeutic relationship is bound by the time restrictions established during the initial phase. Time restrictions are often dictated by the place in which the relationship occurs (such as inpatient hospital versus community settings) and the duration of contact with the client (for example, brief hospitalization, long-term hospitalization, or crisis intervention). Regardless of the restrictions placed on the relationship by time or place, the same considerations need to be addressed.

The termination of the relationship may be a traumatic event for the client. The nurse recognizes this imminent loss and helps the client adapt to this stressor.[8] If the client feels rejected and insecure at the time of termination, regression may occur. Recognizing that termination provokes stress, the nurse supports coping behavior and is sensitive to the client's needs. As with other phases of the relationship, however, the nurse must maintain boundaries so that the nurse's own anxieties and wishes do not distort the ability to perceive the client's desires and needs.[17]

Clients' families need to be involved during nurse–client relationships. Families need to be made aware of the client's fluctuating behavior to facilitate the transition out of the therapeutic relationship. Family members need to be informed that improvement in the client's condition is highly variable. They should be told to expect that clients will have periods in which they seem to be worse.[17]

As the termination draws near, the nurse reminds the client of the predetermined duration of the relationship and assists in socialization with others. Tapering contact with the client is a helpful way to encourage independence.The nurse summarizes the client's progress toward attaining goals and freely expresses his or her own feelings regarding the termination. Following are primary tasks for the nurse during termination:

1. Space contacts with the client further apart and begin to decrease the amount of time of each contact
2. Establish a more relaxed, less intense interaction
3. Focus on the future
4. Discourage cues that lead to new areas of exploration
5. Provide necessary referral to others on the health care team[12]

THE THERAPEUTIC RELATIONSHIP AND THE NURSING PROCESS

The various steps of the nursing process can be associated with a therapeutic relationship. During the initial phase of the nurse–client relationship, the nurse and client begin to develop trust. Once the nurse and client have described and clarified this experience, they are able to identify the subjective and objective descriptions of the issues.

During the working phase of the relationship, the nurse and the client assess the data, plan an action, and begin to evaluate the action. Through this process, the nurse trusts the client to generate effective solutions and facilitates the articulation and continued use of these solutions.[13] The relationship ends during the termination phase, when the action has been evaluated as effective.

EXPECTATIONS OF THE NURSE

In a therapeutic relationship, nurses and clients are involved in a stress-producing situation. The openness and honesty inherent in the relationship make both parties vulnerable.

As nurses focus on the caring model instead of the cure model, the focus of the therapeutic relationship changes from therapeutic objectivity to a therapeutic perspective.[13] Therapeutic perspective involves integrating feelings and involvement within a broader framework that is gained from the nurse's knowledge base and experience.[19]

Dealing with the client's dependency needs requires a great deal of skill and self-awareness. The focus of the care is supporting the client's own healing resources.[13] Dependency behavior may elicit in the nurse the feeling of being responsible for the solution to the client's problems. If the nurse does not recognize the client's ability to use inner strengths and resources, the nurse may need to reevaluate the goals of the relationship. It is necessary to determine if the focus of the relationship is the client's needs or the nurse's need to help.

The nurse who strives to understand the client's behavioral needs must be aware of implicit, explicit, rational, irrational, and symbolic patterns. The nurse needs to keep in mind that the client's behavior is his or her best adaptation at the time. Clients' inconsistent behavior can give rise to misinterpretation, confusion, and distress. When the client does not meet the nurse's expectation (eg, when he or she does not appear to be gaining insight into his or her behavior), the nurse may view the relationship as lacking progress. In turn, the client may feel internal stress as a result of trying to please the nurse. The nurse may request assistance from a colleague to provide clinical supervision within the therapeutic relationship. Through the clinical supervision process, the nurse's feelings and concerns can be ventilated as they relate to the educational process of learning about the client–nurse relationship.[6]

The nurse must constantly reevaluate his or her feelings, thoughts, and behaviors within the relationship. The nurse and the client also may need to discuss honestly the course of the relationship. Perhaps the goals of the relationship should be reevaluated. The nurse must be able to tolerate, respect, and redirect the anxiety that accompanies the recognition of possible failure.

EXPECTATIONS OF THE CLIENT

Clients seeking medical or psychiatric treatment expect to gain relief from anxiety.[19] Within the therapeutic relationship, clients are free to verbalize needs and, as the relationship progresses, to verbalize fears and anxieties. The nurse urges clients to evaluate adaptive patterns and the consequences of defensive behaviors. The therapeutic relationship provides clients with the opportunity to test new adaptive skills. As clients receive positive feedback within the relationship and experience growth and increased self-esteem, they are able to relinquish ineffective behavioral patterns. As the relationship approaches termination, the nurse encourages the client to use healthier behaviors in interactions outside the relationship. The goal is independence for the client.

The client's family and friends have expectations of treatment as well. The nurse acknowledges the family unit as a significant part of the treatment process. The nurse must recognize that mental illness sometimes increases the burden and deterioration of relationships between family members; the relationship can be impaired if the family is unaware that many features of the inconsistent behavior are attributable to the illness and situational factors, including the internal state of the client.[193] Therefore, it is imperative that the nurse include the family in the care of the client, which ultimately should lead to the family positively reinforcing the client's attempt to change behavior. The nurse can also empower family and clients by facilitating the development of independent skills in navigating the treatment maze.[22]

◆ Issues in the Therapeutic Relationship

ATTITUDES OF THE NURSE

Self-awareness is an essential skill for the nurse to acquire to be effective in the nurse–client relationship. Attitudes the nurse has developed over the course of a lifetime may determine the nurse's behavior toward the client. To facilitate growth for the client, the nurse must recognize attitudes that may have an influence on the nurse–client relationship.

Mentally ill clients are often viewed by society as hopeless and helpless. This view has been reinforced by the stigma of mental illness associated with the homeless, who are so visible in American society. Such an attitude, whether conscious or unconscious, prevents the nurse from being effective in the nurse–client relationship. This attitude prevents the nurse from encouraging the client toward independence. Feelings of hopelessness are often associated with chronic mental illness.

The nurse must provide hope for the client to lead a productive life. Regardless of the client's present level of adaptation, growth is usually possible. Assisting a client to move from one level of functioning to another is progress, although it may seem minimal to an observer. Through the use of a therapeutic relationship, which could implement the psychiatric rehabilitation process, prognosis for people with long-term mental illness may not be increasing deterioration between episodes, but a gradual improvement over time (see Nursing Care Plan 5-1).

The difference between tolerance and acceptance of behavior is often a misunderstood concept. Tolerance is a passive activity; no action is required by the nurse. Acceptance is an active process that requires recognition of the client's behavior as meeting a need and as the best adaptation at the time. Respecting the human dignity of the individual, hoping for potential growth, and accepting the client's behavior are beginning steps in facilitating growth for the client.

FACILITATING GROWTH

An important objective of the therapeutic relationship is to provide clients with the opportunity to recognize the needs that their behaviors meet and to develop more effective inner resources. The nurse's behavior and approaches give clients feedback about the appropriateness of their behavior. The nurse's behavior must be consistent to provide role modeling. When the nurse makes promises, adequate follow-up must be ensured. Clients may take casual remarks seriously.[2]

The nurse's consistency also provides a secure environment in which clients can deal with problems and develop adaptation skills. When clients perceive inconsistency in the nurse's behavior, they often focus their attention on pleasing the nurse rather than on their personal growth.

To encourage clients to try out new adaptive behaviors, the nurse provides emotional support by helping them pay attention to their feelings, link their feelings to troublesome behaviors, and explore alternative behaviors. The nurse creates a relationship in which clients share decision making and then validate their perceptions of decision outcomes. This offers clients an opportunity to try new behaviors without penalty (ie, they can receive feedback from others and can evaluate the outcome of their behavior) as they develop new adaptation skills that are less destructive than those used previously. During the growth process, the nurse supports and reinforces the healthy aspects of a client's personality, assessing the client's movement toward independence and encouraging assumption of more responsibility.

Nursing Care Plan 5-1

Applying Rehabilitation Principles

Mrs. D, 55 years old, was recently discharged from an inpatient psychiatric facility. She is presently a member of "Heart and Home," which provides apartments for individuals and a meeting place for clients with mental disabilities. She had been a client of the inpatient facility for three years, and has lost the ability to perform specific skills related to shopping, preparing food, and completing laundry, but is able to complete self-care skills such as bathing. Mr. J, a psychiatric-mental health nurse, is providing transitional care for Mrs. D based on the principles of psychiatric rehabilitation.

Nursing Diagnosis

Impaired Home Maintenance Management, related to lack of independent living skills

Outcome

Client will successfully live independently, performing tasks including shopping, cooking, and using appliances.

Intervention	Rationale
Assist client to evaluate her skills and support strengths and reduce deficits in relation to the goal of independent living.	Involves client in own rehabilitation, reinforces self-esteem and desire to learn.
Develop a rehabilitation plan to locate and use resources and teach personal skills.	A structured learning plan provides a framework for potentially new and confusing knowledge.
Facilitate socialization with others in community, including attendance at support groups and recreational activities.	Strengthens client's independence and social functioning.
Teach information about psychotropic medication.	Client knowledge about medication side effects increases compliance.

Evaluation

Note: Client lives independently and functions effectively. After three months of placement in "Heart and Home," Mrs. D was admitted to the inpatient facility for one week. However, she was soon able to return to her apartment and continue developing her skills and resources through her therapeutic relationship with Mr. J.

INTERPERSONAL SKILLS

As Carl Rogers stated, "the degree to which I can create a relationship which facilitates growth of others as a separate person is a measure of the growth I have achieved myself."[18] Nurses must take responsibility for examining their own behavior and making the necessary changes in behaviors when indicated. To function as a healthy role model, nurses must demonstrate sufficient emotional maturity to be able to postpone the satisfaction of their own needs and allow clients' needs to take precedence.[11]

The most basic and important therapeutic tool is the nurse's personality. Many physical, cultural, psychosocial, social, and environmental factors interact to create a unique personality. Nurses who are aware of these factors have increased insight into their own and others' feelings and behaviors. Objectivity and empathy grow out of the nurse's self-awareness, emotional maturity, responsibility, and insight. These tools prevent misinterpretation of the client's needs through interference of the nurse's needs.

CARING

Essential to any therapeutic relationship is the nurse's commitment to caring. The act of caring is one feature that distinguishes nursing from other professions. The nurse wanting to provide a client with a growth-facilitating experience must create an environment reflective of compassion, meaningfulness, tenderness, and love.[5] Providing therapeutic use of self, identifying and responding to the client's needs, and providing basic comfort measures all demonstrate caring.

Distinguishing features of a caring relationship include effective interpersonal communication, expectations for reciprocity, and asymmetry in the relationship.[9] The client's recognition of the nurse's commitment, involvement, and honesty also contribute to a caring relationship.

◆ Chapter Summary

This chapter has presented the dynamics and dimensions of a therapeutic relationship and the issues that arise in such a relationship. It has included the following points:

1. In a therapeutic relationship, the client and nurse participate and work toward the goals of meeting the client's needs and facilitating growth.
2. There are three possible types of relationships: social, intimate, and therapeutic.
3. Therapeutic relationships progress through initial or introductory, middle or working, and termination phases.
4. The core of nursing is the relationship between the nurse and the client.
5. The nurse recognizes that the client's behavior is the best adaptation to stress at the time.
6. The therapeutic relationship provides the client with an opportunity to examine unsuccessfully adaptive (or maladaptive) behaviors and to explore and try out new adaptive skills.
7. The nurse's self-awareness, responsibility, emotional maturity, objectivity, and empathy are powerful tools of intervention.
8. Caring is an essential element of the nurse–client relationship and may be what separates nursing from other professions.

Review Questions

1. Describe the characteristics of a therapeutic relationship.
2. What is the focus of solution-based care as it relates to a therapeutic nurse–client relationship?
3. Describe the tasks that are included in the working phase of a therapeutic relationship.
4. During which phase of a therapeutic relationship does termination begin and why?
5. Describe three ways in which a nurse can facilitate the growth of a client through a therapeutic relationship.

◆ References

1. Arnold E, Boggs K: Interpersonal Relationships: Professional Communication Skill for Nurses. Philadelphia, WB Saunders, 1989
2. Bailey DS, Cooper SD, Bailey DR: Therapeutic Approaches to the Care of the Mentally Ill. Philadelphia, FA Davis, 1984
3. Chandler MC, Mason WH: Solution-Focused Therapy: An Alternative Approach to Addictions Nursing. Perspect Psychiatr Care 31 (1): 8–13, 1995
4. Chipman Y: Caring: Its Meaning and Place in the Practice of Nursing. Journal of Nursing Education 30 (4): 171–175, 1992
5. Erikson EH: Childhood and Society, 2d ed. New York, WW Norton, 1964
6. Farkas-Cameron MM: Clinical Supervision in Psychiatric Nursing: A Self-Actualizing Process. J Psychosoc Nurs 35 (2), 1995
7. Forchuk C: Uniqueness Within the Nurse-Client Relationship. Archives of Psychiatric Nursing 9 (1): 34–39, 1995
8. Forchuk C, Brown B: Establishing a Nurse Client Relationship. Journal of Psychosocial Nursing Mental Health Services 27 (2): 30–34, 1989
9. Gaut DA, Lenninger MM (ed): Caring: The Compassionate Healer. New York, National League for Nursing, 1991
10. Hale JS, Richardson J: Terminating the Nurse-Patient Relationship. Am J Nurs 63 (9): 1116–1119, 1963
11. Hewison A: Nurses' Power in Interaction With Patient. J Adv Nurs 21: 75–82, 1995
12. Lego SM: The One-to-One Patient Relationship. Perspect Psychiatr Care 18 (March/April): 67–88, 1980
13. Montgomery CL, Webster D: Caring, Cursing, and Brief Therapy: A Model for Nurse-Psychotherapy. Archives of Psychiatric Nursing 8 (5): 291–297, 1994
14. O'Toole AW, Welt SR (ed): Interpersonal Relationships in Nursing Practice: Selected Works of Hildegard E. Peplau. New York, Springer-Verlag, 1989
15. Palmer-Erbs V, Anthony W: Incorporating Psychiatric Rehabilitation Principles into Mental Health Nursing: An Opportunity to Develop a Full Partnership among Nurses, Consumers and Families. J Psychosoc Nurs 33 (3): 36–44, 1995
16. Peplau H: Interpersonal Relations in Nursing: A conceptual Frame of Reference for Psychodynamic Nursing. New York, Springer-Verlag, 1991
17. Pillette PC, Berck CB, Archber LC: Therapeutic Management of Helping Boundaries. J Psychosoc Nurs 33 (1): 40–47, 1995
18. Rogers CR: Client Centered Therapy. Boston, Houghton Mifflin, 1952
19. Shafran R, Thordarson DS: Consistency of Behavior: Expected the Unexpected. J Psychosoc Nurs 33 (5): 26–28, 1995
20. Sullivan JL, Deane DM: Caring: Reappropriating Our Tradition. Nursing Forum 29 (2): 5–9, 1994
21. Walker M: Principles of a Therapeutic Milieu: An Overview. Perspect Psychiatr Care 33 (3), 1994
22. Wilson JH, Hobbs H: Therapeutic Partnership. J Psychosoc Nurs 33 (2), 1995

Communication

Julieann Casey Reakes

6

So healthy, sound, clear, and whole.

Alfred, Lord Tennyson

The goal of psychiatric-mental health nursing is to assist the client to live more effectively, learn to solve problems, and recognize when personal coping is ineffective and other resources are needed. Communication is key to achieving this goal.

Nursing has been influenced by a variety of communication theories and has integrated many concepts from these theories into nursing practice. Communication is embedded in the nursing process: It becomes a tool for assessing a client's behavior and an intervention for the nurse to use when developing a therapeutic relationship and a therapeutic setting for client change. It contributes to the accurate development of appropriate nursing diagnoses and subsequent plan. As an intervention, it is a powerful vehicle for helping the client to focus, analyze, and identify problem areas and to facilitate personal development and growth.

Like the nursing process, the communication process includes the components of assessment, problem identification, and the use of specific techniques to facilitate communication with people with specific behaviors or to help appraise client situations.

Learning Objectives

On completion of this chapter, you should be able to accomplish the following:

1. *Define the terms communication and communication process.*
2. *Recognize theories influencing nursing's approach to therapeutic communication.*
3. *Describe the nursing communication model.*
4. *Discuss the interrelationship of components of the communication process.*
5. *Assess the communication needs and problems of clients.*
6. *Explain the nurse's use of listening, attending, and observation skills in the therapeutic communication.*
7. *Identify therapeutic uses of self-disclosure.*
8. *Apply the techniques of therapeutic communication.*
9. *Identify barriers to therapeutic communication.*
10. *List goals for intervening in psychotic communication.*

◆ Communication Theories

THERAPEUTIC COMMUNICATION

Ruesch[13] conceptualized therapeutic communication as building on a meaningful relationship between the client and professional helper. This is a mutual client-centered approach that is powerfully influenced and directed by the professional. Nursing has emphasized the importance of rapport and environmental influences when building a relationship with the client.[13]

FEEDBACK LOOP

The feedback loop and the impact of relationships in communication, acknowledged by Watzlawick and colleagues, have also impacted nursing practice. The nurse who understands a child's withdrawn and anxious behavior as a result of keeping a family secret recognizes the significance of relationships in communication. Feedback as an ongoing sequence of response-stimulus interchange is inherent in many therapeutic communication interventions.[18]

INTERNALIZATION

Birdwhistell recognized that each infant internalizes his or her society's communication systems and that survival depends on the ability to send and receive messages through patterned learning. By the age of 6 weeks, the baby begins to react to vocal stimuli and by 5 months, is responding to phonemes or symbolizations. Through the kinesic and linguistic environmental systems, the infant discovers who he or she is through relationships and societal expectations. Parental directives and responses to behaviors are internalized by the child and influence behavior throughout the life span. Unpredictable behavior in others may be perceived as strange and unfamiliar because it does not fit our system of communication. To understand and accept differences in others, nurses must recognize the influences of gender, culture, and developmental needs on the way various patterns of communication are learned.[4]

TRANSACTIONAL ANALYSIS AND EGO STATES

Berne's[3] theory of communication as a *transactional analysis* process uses the functions of the ego as a way of relating and communicating to promote healthy relationships and behavior. Three *ego states,* parent, adult, and child, evolved from Berne's theory, which is composed of the following: 1) every person was once a child; 2) human beings are capable of reality testing; and 3) adults had parents, in loco or surrogate. Communication patterns reflect these ego states and may facilitate personal growth or contribute to dysfunctional behavior (Box 6-1).

◆ Communication Patterns

Clients are often unaware of their own judgmental (parent) behavior or their rebellious (child) behavior. The nurse can help clients look at their behavior

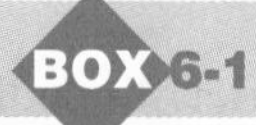

BOX 6-1

Characteristics of Ego States

NEGATIVE CHARACTERISTICS

Critical, demanding, controlling
Adapted, rebellious
Overly compliant

EGO STATE

Parents
Adults
Child

POSITIVE CHARACTERISTICS

Nurturing, facilitative, sympathetic
Problem solver
Reality tester
Spontaneous
Creative

by helping them become aware of communication patterns and the words used in communicating to identify the ego states. Phrases that are evaluative, bossy, judgmental, or critical are usually "parent" communication patterns. Words such as "cool," "not," and "won't" are usually "child" words, communicating a rebellious behavior. Words such as "useful," "practical," and "beneficial" are usually "adult" words. Use of judgmental or rebellious communication behaviors often results in relationship problems. Adult communication patterns that do not communicate rebellion or judgment are more likely to be functional, that is to achieve a desired effect, than parent or child communication patterns.

DYSFUNCTIONAL COMMUNICATION

Several patterns of dysfunctional communication can occur. A *crossed dysfunctional communication* message can occur when messages are addressed to a specific ego state but are not received in that state. An example would be a husband returning home from work and asking, "What's for dinner?" (Message was delivered in an adult ego state.) His wife responds, "I've had a terrible day, and you don't even care what kind of a day I had. You only think of your own needs." (Message was received in a child ego state.)

Another example of a dysfunctional communication pattern is *double messages.* Although it may appear that the communication is an adult-to-adult exchange, the subtle relevant message may be coming from another ego state. An adult message from a mother to an adult daughter may appear to be direct: "I know you're doing the best thing to stay home with the children, but the money we saved for your education may be gone when you want to go back to college." The daughter may receive the ulterior message and on an unconscious level, think, "I'm a bad child. I'll go to school this semester." The daughter's child ego state was hooked by unresolved child problems. This type of situation often results in adult behavior that is controlled and scripted and interferes with the ability to function effectively as an adult.

◆ The Communication Process

Each person manifests his or her unique relationship with the environment in behavior. Behavior can be thought of as a transmission or series of transmissions occurring when the individual interacts with the environment. Communication, the conveyor of these transmissions, is always present and occurring.[19] Even if an individual tried, he or she could never not communicate; the simple lack of verbalization or eye contact communicates something to others.

Communication is a personal, interactive system—a series of ever-changing, ongoing transactions in the environment. Transmissions are simultaneously received (decoded), sent (encoded), and influenced by the total of the experiences and perceptions of the receivers and senders. Through communication and interaction with others, an individual develops a sense of identity and being. Communication is the basis of a person's self-concept and the relationship of this self to another individual, to a group of people, and to the world.

COMMUNICATION SYSTEM

Communication, whether verbal or nonverbal, includes three essential aspects:

1. Transmission of information
2. Meaning of the transmission
3. Behavioral effects of the transmission

The transmission of information is the sending and receiving of messages, or units of information. Through the feedback process, every person in the transaction is affected by the behavior, feelings, attitudes, thoughts, and activities of everyone else involved.

NURSING COMMUNICATION MODEL

Communication models, or graphic representations of various approaches to communication, provide overviews or perspectives about communication. A model of communication compatible with the nursing process is an adaptation of the Wenburg and Wilmot process model of communication (Fig. 6-1).

This model is particularly useful for nursing because it emphasizes the behavioral aspects of the communication process and the internal and external environmental variables that influence the process. Using this model helps the nurse explore the communication process and identify elements pertinent to the communication and nursing processes.

COMPONENTS OF THE COMMUNICATION MODEL

The communication process is composed of the sender, receiver, message, message variables (verbal and nonverbal communication), noise, communication skills, setting, media, feedback, and environment.

Sender

The sender is the encoder, the person who initiates the transmission. This event, the transmission of the message, is verbal and nonverbal.

Receiver

The receiver of the message is the decoder. Encoding and decoding occur simultaneously and are activities of the sender and receiver. The experiences of the sender and receiver influence the transaction.

Message

The message is the unit of information received. A message is made up of many variables that can be verbal or nonverbal.

Message Variables

Message variables are selective verbal and nonverbal stimuli from the internal or external environment that give shape, direction, and focus to the message. Written and spoken language are examples of verbal communication; gestures, facial expressions, and dress are examples of nonverbal communication.

Verbal Communication. Language is the expression of ideas according to society's shared format for sentence structure and grammatical rules. Language is an acquired form of symbolization, a verbal behavior specific to humans.[4]

Although speech is ongoing social behavior, it frequently fails to explain behavior accurately. Speech itself is a complex activity involving the oral, respiratory, auditory, and nervous system components of the body. Structural defects, malfunctioning due to disease, auditory and verbal impairments, sensory deprivation or

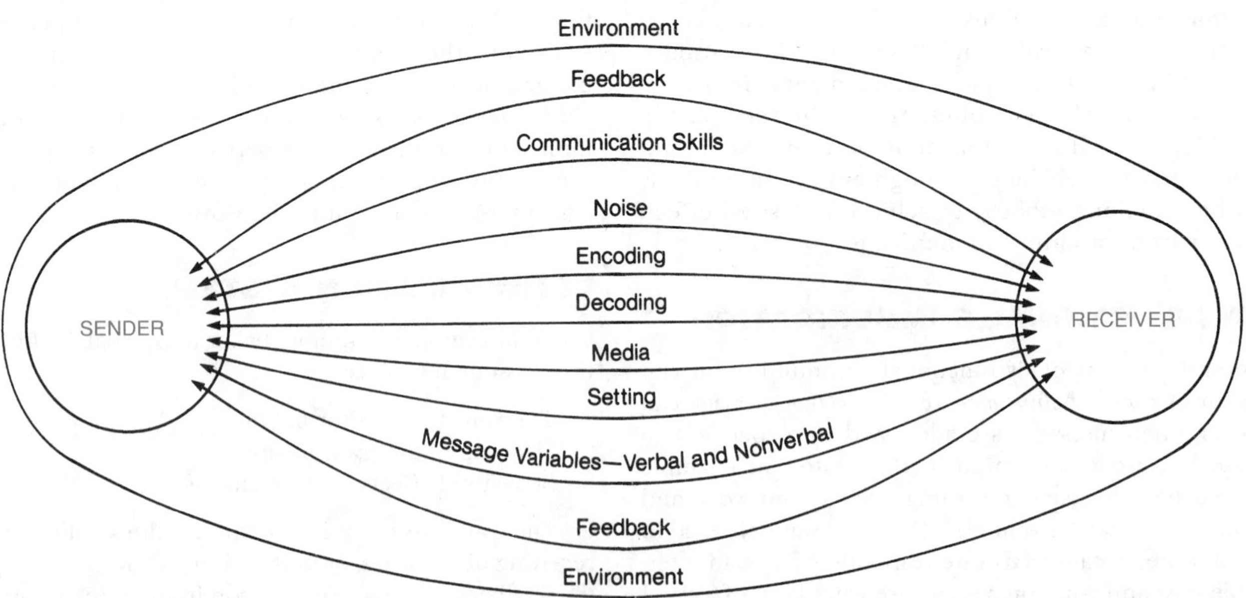

Figure 6-1. Nursing communication model. (Adapted from Wenburg JR and Wilmot WM: The Personal Communication Process. New York: Wiley & Sons, 1973)

overload, and learning disabilities may affect speech and decrease its transmission accuracy.

The following are clinical examples:

- The schizophrenic person is characterized by an inability to abstract and use word symbolization to translate meaning that is reality oriented.
- The stutterer experiences an interruption in the normal rhythm of speech sounds and is impaired in the ability to express his or her relationship with the environment.
- The mentally retarded child may be unable to learn language and is deprived of an expected social behavior.
- The autistic child exemplifies the individual who cannot symbolize with words.

In addition to attending to words and sounds, the nurse recognizes that other factors, such as voice pitch, voice quality (harsh, weak, or strained), and voice amplification (soft or loud), influence the message and are essential components of communication assessment. The choice of words, grammar, and understanding of language also influence the nature of the nurse–client relationship and are therefore included in the assessment.

Nonverbal Communication. Approximately 35% of the meaning of a communication transaction is due to verbal variables; the remaining 65% represents the impact of nonverbal communication. Nonverbal communication may do the following:

1. Contradict verbal behavior
2. Emphasize an emotional tone or mood
3. Complement verbal behavior
4. Control the environment
5. Be the communication of choice

Many nonverbal behaviors are associated with messages. The familiar behaviors of crying, screaming, laughing, moaning, giggling, and sighing are examples of nonverbal communication. Other forms of nonverbal communication include facial expressions, body posture and gait, tone of voice, and gestures.[11]

Use of Space and Territory. The use of space and territory is a form of nonverbal communication. The distance a person maintains from another person or from a group of people is a significant factor in interpersonal activities.

The nurse may observe certain behaviors that indicate that a client's personal space and territory are being invaded. Personal space refers to the space preferred for interactions, whereas social space connotes companionship. Territory implies assigned space, such as a client's room, public room, or a specific seating arrangement. Territory is a designated place that implies ownership or personal possession. Intrusion or violation of someone's space or territory can distract and distort communication.

The concept of distance as a communication variable has been categorized as meeting public, social, and personal needs. The interpersonal aspects of public space involve the greatest distancing of people, whereas intimate personal space involves close contact. Personal (nonintimate) and social space often are reflected in informal gatherings, and interpersonal contact falls between the public and intimate distancing.[11]

The goals and duration of the nurse–client relationship determine the space and distancing involved in the interaction. When designing a therapeutic milieu, the nurse needs to assess the space and territorial needs of all clients.

Noise

Noise refers to sound interferences in the communication system that impair accurate transmission.

Communication Skills

Communication skills include the abilities of the sender and receiver to use message variables to observe, listen, clarify, and validate the meaning of the transmission.

Setting

The setting is the place or location where communication takes place.

Media

Media are the sensory channels that carry the message: hearing, sight, touch, taste, and smell. More than one sensory channel is involved in communication. For instance, a client's verbal message to the nurse for medication to relieve anxiety will be carried through the nurse's auditory channel. The nurse, through the visual channel, sees tears in the client's eyes. The client leans forward and grasps the nurse's hand, emphasizing need through touch.

Feedback

Feedback involves the continuous interpretation of responses of the sender and receiver as messages are simultaneously encoded and decoded. Private variables experienced by the sender and receiver are continually being communicated and therefore influence the transaction. For instance, the receiver may see a sad or depressed expression on the sender's face but decide not to share this perception with the sender, thereby failing to clarify the communication. If the receiver had told the sender of this perception and the sender had explained that the sad expression had nothing to do with the present communication, a positive change might occur, and the facial expression might change to reflect the ongoing transaction.

Environment

The internal and external influences affecting the communication process make up the environment. Contextual cues affect the quality and sometimes the content of communication. Factors in the external environment are seen by everyone but may be perceived differently by each individual. Room temperature, noise levels, smells, and lighting are examples of external environmental factors. Influences in the internal environment are known only to the individual and are not experienced in the same way by others. Feeling tired, experiencing stomach discomfort, and feeling cold are examples of internal environmental factors.

LEVELS OF COMMUNICATION

Communication occurs intrapersonally, interpersonally, in small groups, and in public or large groups. A basic premise of the communication process is that it is intrapersonal in nature; all reactions to communication take place within oneself regardless of the number of people involved in the transaction. In psychiatric-mental health nursing, the main focus of interaction occurs at the interpersonal and group levels. A characteristic of group communication is that the members are interdependent (eg, in social, therapeutic, or task groups). Public communication refers to the public speaking setting in which one person sends a verbal message to a number of receivers.

INTERPERSONAL COMMUNICATION

Interpersonal communication is affected by the participant's sensitivity to his or her own feelings and to the feelings of the other participants. Verbal and nonverbal communication may be spontaneous or calculated to affect the receiver. In therapeutic communication, for example, the nurse communicates to the client by arrangement of the environment, use of space, touch, voice inflection, dress, and so forth. Interpersonal communication is the most direct and pertinent form of communication, because through this transaction, needs are met.

Individuals have interpersonal needs that include knowing that the self is personable, worthy, and able to interact with and use the environment satisfactorily. An individual whose interpersonal needs are not met adequately may be withdrawn, cold, and superficial in relationships. An overly friendly, possessive, and confiding individual also may be giving cues of a less-than-satisfying self-image. A loner, who is shy and passive and a talkative "attention getter" may present behaviors that display feelings of unworthiness.

Submissiveness, lack of confidence, inability to make decisions, domination, and aggressiveness may indicate an inability to use and control the environment.[19] The communication process is a potent approach to assisting others in making adaptive changes to the environment.

Interpersonal Styles of Communication

Three basic interpersonal styles of communicating have been identified as nonassertive or passive, letting others control behavior by not acting in one's own interest; aggressive, which is threatening, blaming, and hostile; and assertive, which is openly expressive, spontaneous, yet considerate of others. Assertiveness training can be useful to professional and nonprofessional people. Table 6-1 provides some examples of assertiveness techniques that can be used by nurses and taught to clients. When using these techniques, assume a relaxed voice tone and body posture, and keep eye contact with the individual.

◆ Therapeutic Communication and the Nursing Process

Client problems may involve various dysfunctional communication patterns. The nurse assesses these client problems as objectively as possible and takes a systematic approach, using listening skills and the nursing process to formulate tentative nursing diagnoses or to identify client problems. The nurse can design the nurse–client interaction during the assessment interview for more than data collection purposes. By creating an environment conducive to communication, the nurse conveys to the client that his or her feelings and needs are important and that the nurse is attuned to them. The ability to communicate in this way is the beginning step toward establishing a therapeutic relationship with the client. By establishing a therapeutic relationship and a therapeutic atmosphere, the nurse can begin to foster change by helping the client to identify and understand his or her own behavior.

COMMUNICATION AND THE ESTABLISHMENT OF THE THERAPEUTIC RELATIONSHIP

The therapeutic relationship as a communication process is applicable to clients throughout the life span and in all settings. It is built on an accurate assessment, spe-

Table 6-1

Assertiveness Techniques

Technique	Example
Using "I" statements	"I feel . . ." "I want . . ."
Restating the message	"I hear you say you care."
Reflecting the other person's feelings without losing your assertive stance	"I know you're frustrated, but this is best for me."
Being neutral; recognizing that the present may not be the optimal time for assertive behavior	"Let's talk about this tonight after dinner."
Accepting responsibility for a mistake	"I did forget to notify you; it was my mistake."
Refocusing	"We're getting off the track. Are you upset?"

cific verbal and nonverbal communication techniques, attending and listening to the client, and intervening appropriately.

Important elements contributing to the establishment of the therapeutic relationship are empathy, attending, observing, and listening. *Empathy* is a communication skill and a behavior. Nursing acknowledges the art of empathy as the inner core of the therapeutic relationship and the infrastructure of therapeutic communication. The use of empathy as a communication skill involves accurate assessment (perception), message delivery (know-how), and assertiveness (timing and focus).

In addition, Egan[7] describes the behaviors of attending, observing, and listening as necessary to the development of a therapeutic relationship. Egan describes *attending* as being with the client in a physical and psychological presence. Specific attending skills include the following:

1. Turning and leaning your face and body to the client
2. Positioning your body to imply an open and natural behavior
3. Maintaining eye contact
4. Assessing one's own nonverbal behavior for nontherapeutic communication messages

Observing and *listening* are crucial elements in enabling the nurse to comprehend nonverbal and verbal messages. The nurse carefully observes the client's nonverbal messages conveyed through body behavior, facial expressions, physiological reactions, skin color, pupil characteristics, and appearance.[7] Simultaneously listening and projecting a neutral presence enhance the nurse's ability to assess the client's verbal messages and vocal behavior.

ASSESSING CONGRUENCE BETWEEN VERBAL AND NONVERBAL COMMUNICATION

There are two levels, content and feeling, to every message. When the content and feeling messages are confused or incongruent, problems occur. A goal of the nurse in a therapeutic relationship is to assess the congruence, or agreement, between the client's verbal and nonverbal communication. The client may not be aware of any disharmony between the two. Consider the following two clinical examples:

1. When interacting with a couple, you observe the husband telling the wife that he is supportive of her being treated for depression but also informing her he has to leave town on business and will not be available for counseling. The husband is giving an incongruent double message to his wife.
2. Although a client has a sad facial expression and tear-filled eyes, he tells the nurse that he feels fine. His nonverbal communication does not agree with his words, and the nurse is alerted to incongruent behavior.

Assessment of the congruence of verbal and nonverbal communication is an integral part of the communication assessment process (Box 6-2).

Barriers to Therapeutic Communication

Various barriers inhibit or interfere with nurse–client communication (Table 6-2). Examples of barriers include lack of planning or inadequate preparation by the nurse during the communication process, which may result in failure to meet the client's identified

BOX 6-2

Communication Assessment Tool

Name ______________________ Age ___ Sex ___ Diagnosis ______________________

I. Sender or receiver impairments
   A. Structural deficit
   B. Sense deficits: hearing, sight, smell, touch, taste
   C. Loss of functions
   D. Disease
   E. Drugs
   F. Other

II. Message variables
   A. Nonverbal communication
      1. Facial expression
      2. Gestures
      3. Body movements
      4. Affect
      5. Tone of voice
      6. Posture
      7. Eye contact
      8. Voice volume, quality pitch
      9. Other
   B. Verbal communication
      1. Content of message
      2. Communication patterns
         a. Blocking
         b. Slow
         c. Rapid
         d. Quiet
         e. Halting
         f. Aphasic
         g. Discontinuous
         h. Excessive
         i. Detailed
         j. Stammering
         k. Circumstantial
         l. Tangential
         m. Long silences
         n. Other

III. Noise

IV. Communication skills
   A. Openness, spontaneity
   B. Use of clarification
   C. Request for feedback
   D. Tolerance of silence
   E. Acceptance of confrontation
   F. Other

V. Setting
   A. Inpatient unit
   B. Community settings
   C. Other

VI. Media

VII. Feedback
   A. Precise
   B. Pertinent
   C. Goal directed
   D. Informative
   E. Solicited
   F. Positive
   G. Negative
   H. Clarified
   I. Opportune

VIII. Environment
   A. External influences
      1. Temperature
      2. Physical arrangement
      3. Lighting
      4. Noise level
      5. Other
   B. Internal influences
      1. Beliefs
      2. Experiences
      3. Thoughts
      4. Attitudes
      5. Other

IX. Cultural influences
   A. Health practices
   B. Religious implications
   C. Language barriers
   D. Food preferences
   E. Other

goals. Precise data collection directs communication assessment. Inadequate data collection or inadequate or inappropriate nursing diagnoses and outcome criteria are significant barriers to facilitative communication.

Nurse–client interaction is built on the development of a trusting relationship. Lack of regard for the other person and being judgmental in an interaction inhibits or is a barrier to therapeutic communication.

Other verbal and nonverbal communication by the nurse may disrupt or end the nurse–client interaction (Table 6-3).

Table 6-2

Barriers to Communication

Category	Barrier
Related to the nursing process	Inadequate data collection Inappropriate nursing diagnosis Inappropriate outcome criteria
Organizational	Lack of planning Inadequate physical environment
Communication	Interrupting Advising False reassurance Belittling Being judgmental Using closed-ended questions Changing the subject Probing Approving Moralizing Social response
Therapeutic use of self	Lack of positive regard Lack of respect Lack of mutual goal setting with client

Table 6-3

Nontherapeutic Communication Techniques

Problem Technique	Definition	Example
Interrupting	Telling the client what he or she is feeling or experiencing and developing his or her ability to understand	Client: "I don't understand my behavior." Nurse: "Well, I think you're denying your feelings on an unconscious level, and this is causing your anxiety."
Approving	Dysfunctional communication; implies that the client must gain your approval and support because you are the expert	Client: "Am I getting better?" Nurse: "You did a good job in group today talking about your relationship with your wife. Keep up the good work."
Moralizing	Passing judgment by using your values as to what is right or wrong	Client: "I use, but I never sold drugs." Nurse: "It's a criminal act to buy drugs, and the user needs to be punished just like the seller."
Social responding	Superficial conversation that is not client centered	Client: "I'm so bored with this place." Nurse: "What book are you reading? What's your favorite television show?"
Belittling	Discounting client's feelings as not being worthwhile	Client: "I feel hopeless most of the time." Nurse: "Look at all the good things in your life—you're fortunate, not hopeless."
Changing the subject	Indicating the nurse is uncomfortable with the communication	Male client: "I feel I've always thought like a female since I was a small child." Nurse: "You played a lot of sports growing up; what was your favorite?"

THERAPEUTIC COMMUNICATION INTERVENTIONS

Communication interventions are an integral part of the nursing process. The following content and examples will provide more depth and refinement in the use of these valuable nursing actions.

Listening

Listening, or focusing on all the behaviors expressed by a client, is the foundation of therapeutic communication. Listening requires energy in a form of concentration that does the following:

1. Minimizes distractions
2. Conveys objectivity
3. Is not evaluative in terms of agreeing or disagreeing with the communicator
4. Focuses on the client's behavior
5. Uses feedback objectively

Listening is an active process that focuses objective, empathic attention on the client. Maintaining eye contact, facilitating close proximity (if not threatening to the client), projecting a relaxed physical orientation and closeness, and speaking in a normal, audible voice are all characteristics of this process.[7]

The nurse attends to physical cues, such as room temperature and physical comfort. The nurse also tries to eliminate noise from the listening environment and tries to discontinue other media channels, such as the telephone, television, or radio, to meet therapeutic listening goals and prevent interruption of the interaction.

Listening to another person requires decoding the content and the feelings expressed in the message. Verbalizations, opinions, thoughts, and impressions make up the content of messages. The feeling portion of a message is the emotional one, which may be described verbally (although this verbal description may or may not be accurate) or nonverbally. A client speaking in a relaxed voice may nevertheless reveal anxiety by nonverbal behaviors, such as chain smoking, clenched hands, tense body posture or movement, and so forth. To individualize approaches to a client, the nurse notes congruence or incongruence between verbal and nonverbal communication and then validates these observations with the client. The anxiety or preoccupation of the nurse or client may be reflected in nonverbal communication that interferes with the therapeutic listening environment.

Observation

The nurse carefully observes for the client's communication of internal influences that may prevent the attentiveness needed for the therapeutic communication process (Box 6-3). The nurse, too, is influenced by internal variables and may be sleepy, hungry, thinking about a meeting with a supervisor, and so on. These kinds of influences can interfere with the nurse–client relationship and should be evaluated and modified, if necessary, to maintain an objective and empathetic environment conducive to the communication process.

Self-disclosure

A major goal of therapeutic communication is to use a planned, systematic approach to foster the client's self-disclosure and enable adaptive changes. In American culture, we learn at an early age to control or conceal our authenticity—we disguise, hide, or deny our feelings. Feelings are expressed in behavior, however, and the client can learn to recognize these inner experiences and express them as adaptively as possible.

Following is a clinical example: A 35-year-old woman was able to identify her promiscuous sexual behavior as a way of dealing with her self-deprecatory feelings resulting from an incestuous relationship with her stepfather during early adolescence. Her suicide attempt at 14 years symbolically ended the relationship, but her sexual behavior during adulthood expressed her continuing rage and low self-esteem. Feelings form the basis of intervention that deals with those feelings realistically.[7]

Cultural Sensitivity. A person's culture influences the expression of feelings; each culture has certain sanctioned verbal and nonverbal channels of expression. Whereas an American may conceal feelings, a member of an Eastern culture may openly and loudly express grief, anger, or joy. Communication is an integral part of the culture of a group, and the nurse must therefore understand how a specific culture uses it. Cultural variables, such as the perception of time, bodily contact, and territorial rights, also influence communication. The communication practices of a culture affect expression of ideas and feelings, decision making, and communication strategies.

Communication Techniques

Therapeutic communication techniques include use of broad openings, clarification, reflection, confrontation, informing, verification, self-disclosure, silence, directing, questioning, and summarizing. (See Boxes 6-4 and 6-5 for examples of applied therapeutic communication techniques.)

The feeling and content components of communication are usually presented simultaneously in a transaction. The client's ability to label feelings and identify whether behavior is adaptive or maladaptive represents therapeutic progress to the psychiatric-mental health nurse. When a feeling has been labeled, the nurse then uses a translating or paraphrasing technique to help the client focus on this feeling, correct misperceptions, and alter the resultant maladaptive or distorted behavior. In this way, clients learn new interpersonal skills and learn to explore their feelings and express them in an adaptive manner.

The content portion of the message is also important because it enables the client to repeat or describe an experience from his or her point of reference. The nurse identifies similarities in themes or concerns of the client and develops an appreciation of the uniqueness of the client's situation. The following are examples of selected therapeutic communication techniques.

Using Broad Openings. Open-ended comments or questions and other broad openings can help the client begin, continue, or focus the expression of communication. Following are guidelines for using broad openings:

1. Wait for the client to finish his or her message.
2. Use phrases such as, "Tell me about what's bothering you." "How are you feeling today?" "What does this mean to you?"
3. Give the client sufficient time to respond.

Advantage: Encourages communication. Helps the client.
Nursing Action: "Tell me what's bothering you. What does this mean? Go on."
Example: Client: "I don't think I can go on anymore."
Nurse: "Tell me what has happened."

Reflecting Feelings. Do the following when reflecting the client's feelings:

1. State your comprehension of the feeling message, using emotional and feeling descriptive words.
2. Use a nonquestioning tone of voice.
3. Wait until the client responds.

Advantage: Helps the client to identify feelings related to a behavior
Nursing Action: State your comprehension of the feeling message, using emotional words and phrases (paraphrase).
Example: Client: "I don't think I can overcome my dependence on my family."
Nurse: "You feel resigned that you can never be independent of your family."

Clarifying Feelings. Do the following when clarifying the client's feelings:

1. Repeat the feeling tone of the message in your own words, or restate an emotional word or phrase used by the client.
2. Use an open, questioning tone of voice that is nondirective and noninterrogating.
3. Wait until the client responds.

Advantage: Helps the client experiençe feelings related to a behavior from a different perspective
Nursing Action: Restate the feeling tone in your own words using emotional words and phrases (paraphrase).
Example: Client: "I feel my family would be better off without me acting so crazy."
Nurse: "You feel your family cannot tolerate your behavior, and you're a liability."

Confronting Feelings. Do the following when confronting the client's feelings:

BOX 6-3

Diagnosing Communication Needs

When analyzing assessment data and formulating nursing diagnoses, the nurse should consider the following factors:

1. The client's use of the communication process:
   - Inability to speak
   - Limited understanding of language
   - Nonassertive communication
   - Distorted decoding
   - Inability to send an accurate message
   - Incongruence of verbal and nonverbal communication
   - Fear of self-expression
2. Etiology of the client's problem:
   - Low self-esteem
   - Feelings of unworthiness and guilt
   - Anxiety about approval of others
   - Inability to express anger or other "*negative*" feelings
3. The client's feelings about his or her communication abilities:
   - Anxiety when talking with authority figures
   - Withdrawal in group communication
   - Continuous talking when interacting in certain situations.

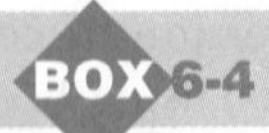

Examining Therapeutic Communication I

Scenario: Harry is a 56-year-old man who is referred to the day hospital following radiation treatment for prostate cancer. His wife died 2 years ago in a car accident. After her death, Harry neglected his printing business, began drinking, and stopped talking to his adult children.

Nurse: Good morning, Harry, I'd like to tell you about the schedule for the day. (Giving information.)

Client: (Silence. No eye contact with nurse.)

Nurse: You look sad. (Making an observation.)

Client: I just want to sit and watch the television. I'm only here because of my children.

Nurse: Your children? (Reflecting content.)

Client: They think I've gotten "crazy" lately.

Nurse: What made them think that, Harry? (Broad opening.)

Client: I don't know, maybe because I took a drink once in a while. I don't know. (Looks irritated.)

Nurse: You seem irritated about their concern for you. (Exploring feelings.)

Client: They don't understand my life was over when I lost their mother. (Becomes teary.)

Nurse: That was a great loss to you when she died. (Verifying perception.)

Client: It was "hell." I've never been able to talk about her—maybe I deserve to be sick.

Nurse: You feel you're being punished for not grieving. (Clarifying feelings.)

Client: Yes. Sometimes I think I've been a coward. (Becomes teary.)

Nursing Diagnosis

Ineffective Individual Coping related to unresolved grief

Criteria for Diagnosis

Unresolved grief
Change in health status
Negative self-concept
Withdrawal from children
Diminished occupational functioning

Outcome Criteria

1. By (identify date), client will express feelings and thoughts about loss of wife and illness.
2. By (identify date), client will decrease negative self-statements and increase use of positive self-statements.
3. By (identify date), client will recognize his drinking as a way of dealing with his feelings.

Communication Intervention (Examples)

Reflect and clarify feelings to encourage expression of feelings.
Reframe negative self-statements.
Use directing to help client to focus.
Attend and listen to client.

1. Describe the emotional message or feelings you are perceiving.
2. Describe the client's ongoing behavior that is influencing your perceptions.
3. Identify the contradictions using a questioning tone of voice.
4. Wait for the client's response.

Advantage: Invites the client to self explore and clarify behavior

Nursing Action: Describe the emotional message and the behavior, identifying contradictions in the client's behavior.

Example: Client: "My husband doesn't care about me. He never comes to visit me."
Nurse: "You refuse to take his calls. I'm confused."

Reflecting Content. Do the following when reflecting the content of the client's communication:

1. State your comprehension of the content message using descriptive or cognitive words.
2. Use a nonquestioning tone of voice.
3. Wait until the client responds.

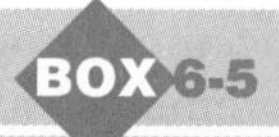

Examining Therapeutic Communication II

Scenario: You are the nurse in an outpatient mental health clinic and see the following client for the first time. Erica is a 34-year-old married housewife who has been persistently depressed since the birth of her third child. Her parents take care of her three children, ages 8 years, 6 years, and 18 months. Erica's husband is a truck driver and works long hours. Erica has difficulty keeping eye contact, is disheveled, and slumps in the chair. Erica tells you that she hasn't any energy, has difficulty sleeping, and "cries over nothing." She has lost 10 lbs this past month.

Dialogue

Nurse: Erica, tell me how you're feeling now. (Using broad openings.)

Client: I can't take care of my children, I'm a poor mother, and I'm ashamed. I feel guilty most of the time because I'm depressed.

Nurse: You feel you're a poor mother because you're depressed. (Reflecting feelings.)

Client: I feel I should "snap out of it." My husband and I can't make decisions. I'm always calling my parents.

Nurse: You're being very hard on yourself. (Clarifying feelings.)

Client: I know, but when I try to make decisions, my parents interfere.

Nurse: Interfere? (Reflecting content.)

Client: Yes. When I want to take the kids for the weekend, they tell me I can't handle them.

Nurse: How does that make you feel? (Clarifying feelings.)

Client: I'm a bad mother. I need their support and approval, but sometimes I think they want to keep me a baby, too.

Nurse: You've always felt like the baby. (Verifying perception.)

Client: Yes. I always ran to them, and my husband and I do the same. Sometimes it's easier than making decisions.

Nursing Diagnosis

Self Esteem Disturbance related to depressive symptoms

Criteria for Diagnosis

Negative self-statements
Physiological and psychological signs of depression
Expressions of guilt and shame

Outcome Criteria

1. By (specific date), client will report a change in depressive mood, discuss fearfulness, and report improved sleeping patterns.
2. By (specific date), client will make one or two decisions and carry through.
3. By (specific date), client will decrease self-deprecatory remarks and verbalize feelings of improved self-concept.

Communication Intervention

1. Clarify and validate to encourage expression of feeling.
2. Give realistic feedback for accomplishments.
3. Reframe negative self-statements.
4. Teach assertiveness skills.
5. Role play using assertive techniques.

Advantage: Implies the nurse is actively listening to obtain an accurate picture

Nursing Action: State your comprehension of the content message, using descriptive or cognitive words.

Example: Client: "I really felt loved by my father when I was in the hospital because of my back pain. It was like old times. He called me his little girl."

Nurse: "You think your father was attentive to you because you were in pain and needed comfort."

Clarifying Content. Do the following when clarifying the content of the client's communication:

1. Repeat your comprehension of the thought or idea in your own words.

2. Repeat a specific word or idea used by the client.
3. Use an open, questioning tone of voice.
4. Wait until the client responds.

Advantage: Acknowledges the client's recollection of the behavior or experience to perceive accurately the behavior or experience

Nursing Action: Repeat your comprehension of the thought or idea in your own words. Repeat a specific word used by the client.

Example: Client: "None of the doctors who examined my back felt I needed surgery. They just told me to deal with the pain."

Nurse: "The doctors didn't see surgery as an option, and you would have to deal with the pain."

Confronting Content. Do the following when confronting the content of the client's communication:

1. Describe the message you are perceiving, using cognitive terms.
2. Describe the mixed-content messages you are perceiving, using the specific cognitive terms of the client.
3. Identify the contraindications using a nonquestioning tone of voice.
4. Wait for the client's response.

Advantage: Invites the client to look at discrepancies in the message being sent

Nursing Action: Describe the mixed message you are perceiving, using cognitive terms.

Example: Client: "I'll never be able to get a job or be able to support myself."

Nurse: "I know you're concerned about your support, but you told me you haven't tried to find a job."

Advantage: Shares with the client the behavior you observe and your awareness

Nursing Action: Describe your perceptions of behavior, using terms similar to what client describes.

Example: Client: "If I didn't have such a traumatic childhood, I could stop drinking."

Nurse: "You feel your inability to stop drinking is still affected by your childhood trauma."

Directing. Do the following when directing the client's interaction:

1. Use nonverbal or succinct, open-ended questioning or declarative statements.
2. Wait for client's response.

Advantage: Encourages client to explore and express thoughts and feelings. Communicates nurse's interest and attentiveness

Nursing Action: Use nonverbal or succinct, open-ended questioning or declarative statements, such as, "You were saying." "Please continue." "Mmmm hmmm."

Example: Client: "I guess I've been treated like the "baby" by the family all my adult life—I can't even take care of my children."

Nurse: "Please go on."

Giving Information. Communicating facts to the client is a common component of intervention. This cognitive, goal-directed function meets an identified objective for the client. Do the following when giving information to the client:

1. State the purpose of the activity, procedure, or situation.
2. Describe the activity, procedure, or situation.
3. Identify the components of the activity, procedure, or situation.

Advantage: Communicates factual information, which increases client trust and mutual goal setting

Nursing Action: State the purpose and describe the action, procedure, or situation to the client in specific terms.

Example: Client: "What's going to happen tomorrow when I have my myelogram?"

Nurse: "You will be taken to radiology at 8:00 AM. The doctor will use a local anesthetic before injecting the dye in your back. The x-rays will be taken with you in various positions. It will take about an hour."

Questioning. Frequently, the nurse uses direct questions or indirect question-like responses during therapeutic communication. A client, however, may become defensive or may intellectualize when asked the "why" of a behavior. Open-ended questions are helpful ways to elicit the how, what, where, and when of the client's behavior. Examples of these responses include questions such as, "Will you elaborate?" "Will you give me an example?" "Am I correct?" The nurse avoids asking questions that require an answer of "yes" or "no" and those that are probing and interrogative during therapeutic communication.

Interviewing

Interviewing is a specific type of guided and limited intercommunication with an identified purpose. An interview is usually conducted to collect a data base for analysis and decision making. The nurse commonly uses structured assessment tools and questionnaires to gather and categorize data (see Chapter 8, Assessment and Nursing Diagnosis).[12] Guidelines for interviewing include the following:

1. Conduct sessions seated in a private, comfortable area with adequate lighting and hearing distance.
2. At the beginning of each session, plan and discuss with the client the length and purpose of the session.
3. Observe, listen, and use facilitative communication techniques.
4. Convey a professional demeanor through dress and manner.
5. Summarize the interaction at the end of the session, and make arrangements with the client for the next session.
6. Positively reinforce the client's attention, effort, and so on.

SELECTED APPLICATION OF THERAPEUTIC COMMUNICATION

Intervening in Crisis Stabilization

Crisis stabilization depends on the therapeutic communication process to help the client regain equilibrium by examining the crisis, correcting distortions, and relieving anxiety. This process also promotes problem solving and strengthens resources and constructive coping behaviors.

Intervening in Psychotic Communication

The nurse does not reinforce a client's psychotic communication. Initial interaction with an individual demonstrating psychotic behavior involves showing interest in and concern for the client. A realistic approach may be to spend time with the client in an activity such as walking (Box 6-6).

The tasks of recognizing feeling messages, decoding content, and clarifying feelings without causing the client to be overstimulated by the interaction are difficult for the psychiatric-mental health nurse. Frequent use of silence may increase the client's anxiety and hallucinatory behavior. Saying, "I can't follow your thinking" or "I'm having trouble understanding your words" to the client who evidences psychotic communication is a way to restore the client to the reality of interpersonal communication.

Listening for any clarifying themes or needs with the psychotic client is difficult and often perplexing for the nurse. The client who needs time to develop a trusting relationship may continue to use psychotic communication and behavior to test the relationship. The nurse continuously evaluates the relationship and the effectiveness of communication with the client. See Chapter 31, Aggressive and Violent Behavior, for further information on communication with a client with psychosis.

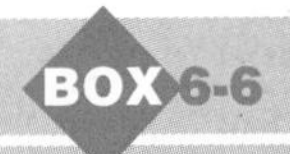

Therapeutic Dialogue: Responding to Psychotic Communication

The following is an example of an interaction between a psychiatric-mental health nurse and a client who is using psychotic communication. The nurse has been meeting and spending time with the client since his admission 1 week ago and has been using various activities within the milieu during their sessions to develop a relationship.

Client: The voices are talking to me again and told me not to go with you on this walk today but to stay in my room and talk to them.

Nurse: Are you confused about whether I want to be with you?

Client: The voices (puts hands to head) are mad at me, and they're saying awful things and using bad words because I'm with you.

Nurse: I look forward to our walks and getting to know you better.

Client: The voices tell me you're just saying that because you want to trick me.

Nurse: I care about you and want to be able to help you. I will be with you every day at this time for the next week.

The nurse was aware of the client's history of abuse by his parents and of spending his adolescence in foster homes. He was diagnosed as schizophrenic and has had repeated admissions to the psychiatric hospital. He has been in a rehabilitation-work program successfully for the past year but became psychotic again when he learned his mother died. Eventually, the nurse and client talked about his feelings of rejection and helplessness. The client was able to return to his rehabilitation-work program and outpatient care.

◆ Chapter Summary

This chapter has explored the purposes, systems, and models of communication. Chapter highlights include the following:

1. The components of the communication process are the sender, receiver, message, message variables, noise, communication skills, setting, media, feedback, and environment.
2. The communication and nursing processes interweave to provide the nurse with a foundation to assist clients' progression toward optimal adaptation.
3. Empathy enables the nurse to view clients in a caring and objective manner and to interact with them in a planned, systematic way.
4. The techniques of therapeutic communication—clarification, reflection, confrontation, verification, self-disclosure, informing, silence, directing, questioning—are the nurse's tools to elicit helpful or facilitative interaction with the client.
5. Barriers to therapeutic communication, such as defending, lack of regard for the other person, and advising, interfere with or inhibit communication between the nurse and client.
6. Therapeutic communication is a powerful tool for the psychiatric-mental health nurse.

Critical Thinking Questions

1. *Cynthia is a 22-year-old woman you are counseling. She married at age 17, has never worked outside the home, and did not finish high school. She tells you her husband is a good provider and father to their young children but does not give her emotional support. He is not affectionate, she says, although she feels he loves her. She says to you: "The strong part of me wants to leave immediately with the children and find someone who will give me emotional security." What are you going to do?*
2. *You are answering the phone on the psychiatric unit when a male voice asks if you care about people. When you inquire about his problem, he tells your life isn't worth living, and he's holding a loaded pistol and is ready to "blow himself away." What are you going to do?*
3. *Debbie, a 42-year-old woman you have been seeing daily, is ready for discharge to an outpatient program. She is diagnosed with borderline personality disorder and was admitted after overdosing on an over-the-counter pain medication. She tells you that you are the best nurse on the unit and is expecting you for lunch at her house the next day. She says, "Now we can be friends because you told me I needed female support." What are you going to do?*

Review Questions

1. The best definition of communication is
   - **A.** the sending and receiving of messages.
   - **B.** the effect of sending verbal messages.
   - **C.** an on-going interactive form of transmitting transactions.
   - **D.** the use of message variables to send information.
2. The foundation of the therapeutic communication process is the nurse's ability to
   - **A.** clarify verbal messages.
   - **B.** listen attentively.
   - **C.** redirect the person's thoughts.
   - **D.** analyze the person's communication.
3. A technique that can help the person begin, continue, or focus on communication is
   - **A.** evaluating the communication intent.
   - **B.** restating the person's message.
   - **C.** giving specific directions.
   - **D.** using broad openings.

◆ References

1. Albert RE: Your Perfect Right: A Guide to Assertive Living, 5th ed. San Obispo, CA, Import, 1986
2. Anvil CA, Silver BW: Therapist Self-disclosure: When Is it Appropriate? Perspect Psychiatr Care 22: 57–61, 1984
3. Berne E: Transactional Analysis in Psychotherapy. New York, Grove, 1961
4. Birdwhistell RL: Kinesics and Context. Philadelphia, University of Pennsylvania Press, 1970
5. Carkhuff RR: The Art of Helping, 6th ed. Amherst, MA, Human Resource Development Press.
6. Coombs A, Avila D, Purkey W (eds): Helping Relationships, Boston, Allyn and Bacon, 1980
7. Egan G: The Skilled Helper, 5th ed. Pacific Grove, CA, Brooks/Cole, 1994
8. Forchuk C, Brown B: Establishing a Nurse-Client Relationship. J Psychosoc Nurs 27(2): 30–34, 1989
9. Kemper B: Therapeutic Listening: Developing the Concept. J Psychosoc Nurs 30 (7): 21–23, 1992
10. Loughlin SN: Symbolism as a Memory Tool in Learning Therapeutic Communication Techniques. Perspect Psychiatr Care 21 (1): 9–17, 1983
11. Pease A: Signals: How to Use Body Language for Power, Success and Love. New York, Bantam Books, 1984
12. Peplau H: Basic Principles of Patient Counseling, 2d ed. Philadelphia, Smith, Kline and French Laboratories, 1964
13. Ruesch J: Therapeutic Communication. New York, WW Norton, 1961
14. Severtsen BM: Therapeutic Communication Demystified. J Nurs Educ 29 (1): 190–192, 1990

15. Stewart J (ed): Bridges Not Walls: A Book About Interpersonal Communication, 5th ed, pp 79–96. New York, McGraw-Hill, 1990
16. Vance B: Human Relationships in Nursing. Provo, UT, Brigham Young University, 1979
17. Wachtel P: Principles of Therapeutic Communication. New York, Gulford Press, 1993
18. Watzlawick P, Beavin J, Jackson J: Pragmatics of Human Communication. New York, WW Norton, 1967
19. Wenburg JR, Wilmot WM: The Personal Communication Process. New York, John Wiley and Sons, 1973
20. Wilson JP: Deciphering Psychotic Communication. Perspect Psychiatr Care 18 (November-December): 254–256, 1979

Biological Bases for Care

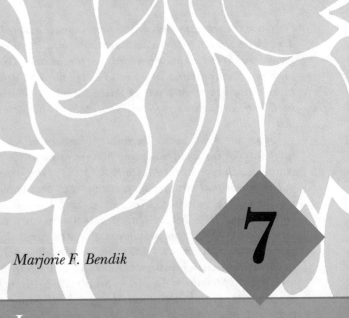

Marjorie F. Bendik

7

It has always seemed astonishing to me that we know vastly more about the first microsecond of the existence of our universe, or about the constituents of any atom, or about the interior of the sun, than we do about the three pounds of tissue inside our own heads. Brain research is truly one of the great frontier areas of science.

D. Allen Bromley, Ph.D.,
Science Advisor to President George Bush and Director, Office of Science and Technology Policy, from **The Decade of the Brain**, *Vol. 2, Issue 1.*

For too many years, mental health professionals adhered to a rigid separation between mental illness and its physiological substrates. This disregard for the ancient Greek ideal of "a sound mind in a sound body" has had disastrous consequences in terms of mistreatment, stigmatization, and care deficits suffered by mentally ill people and their families.

Misinformation about the nature of mental illness is rampant. For instance, according to a recent survey by the National Alliance for the Mentally Ill, 55% of the general public believe that mental illness is caused by poor parenting, and 35% believe it is caused by "sinful behavior." Only a scant 10% believe that mental illness has a biological basis; 45% of the population believe that regardless of the cause, a person can "will away" mental illness. The impact of this misinformation is evidenced by the fact that an estimated 50 million Americans are affected by disorders involving the brain, at an annual cost of $305 billion for treatment and rehabilitation.[7] *According to Dr. Lewis Judd, one in five Americans will have some form of mental illness during their lifetime.*[39]

To address this situation and focus attention on new directions in mental health research, treatment, and rehabilitation, the 101st United States Congress designated the decade beginning January 1, 1990 as the "decade of the brain." The decade of the brain challenges nurses to integrate the biological sciences of genetics, endocrinology, immunology, and neurobiology into the caring concepts of mental health nursing. Moreover, it demands close collaboration among all health professionals to integrate behavioral and biomedical sciences with the goal of achieving a better understanding of mental illness and working toward mental health. To this end, nursing as an applied science must use the expanded knowledge in applying the nursing process.

Learning Objectives

On completion of this chapter, you should be able to accomplish the following:

1. *Discuss the significance of the interrelationships among the nervous, endocrine, and immune systems to psychiatric-mental health nursing.*
2. *Describe several recent advances in genetics relevant to psychiatric-mental health nursing.*
3. *Explain how factors in the physical environment can produce positive or negative effects on mental health.*
4. *Demonstrate holistic nursing principles in creating a care plan for a family with a designated mentally ill member.*
5. *List goals identified collaboratively by families and the psychiatric-mental health team to help a member with mental illness with apparent biological substrates.*

◆ Integration of Mind and Body: Holism

Recent research into the neurological system and mental illness have produced several important findings:

1. Critical relationships exist between environmental stimuli and biological substrates.
2. An abnormality in the structure or function of the brain or the body will affect behavior.
3. Psychosocial stress may physically alter neurochemical pathways, activating depression and physical symptomatology.[31,54]

To help people who have become mentally ill (as manifested by abnormal behaviors, thoughts, and feelings), a psychiatric-mental health nurse must understand the underlying biology of mental illness. To this end, this chapter reviews the pertinent structures of the nervous and neuroendocrine systems and the genetic influences and role of environmental factors in psychopathology.

NERVOUS SYSTEM

Because the anatomy and physiology of the brain and nervous system are enormously complex, this chapter explores only the major components relevant to emotion and behavior, beginning with the brain. The hub of the central nervous system (CNS), the brain generates the thoughts and emotions that make us uniquely human and provides the motivation for all behavior that is not reflexive and autonomic.

Central Nervous System

The CNS is composed of the brain and spinal cord, with associated nerves and end organs that control voluntary acts. Brain structures relevant to psychobiology include the cerebrum, cingulate gyrus and associated structures of the limbic system, corpus callosum, cerebellum, and brain stem, particularly the reticular activating and extrapyramidal systems. Figure 7-1 shows the locations of these structures.

Cerebrum. The *cerebrum* is divided into two hemispheres connected by the *corpus callosum*, which facilitates information exchange between hemispheres. The corpus callosum can also be the location of seizure activation when electrochemical conduction circuits become overloaded. The functions of the two cerebral hemispheres were considered disparate, particularly with respect to producing speech, writing, and understanding language. These functions generally are centered in the left hemisphere, accounting for the typical language-related deficits resulting from a cerebrovascular accident in that area. However, the newer brain-

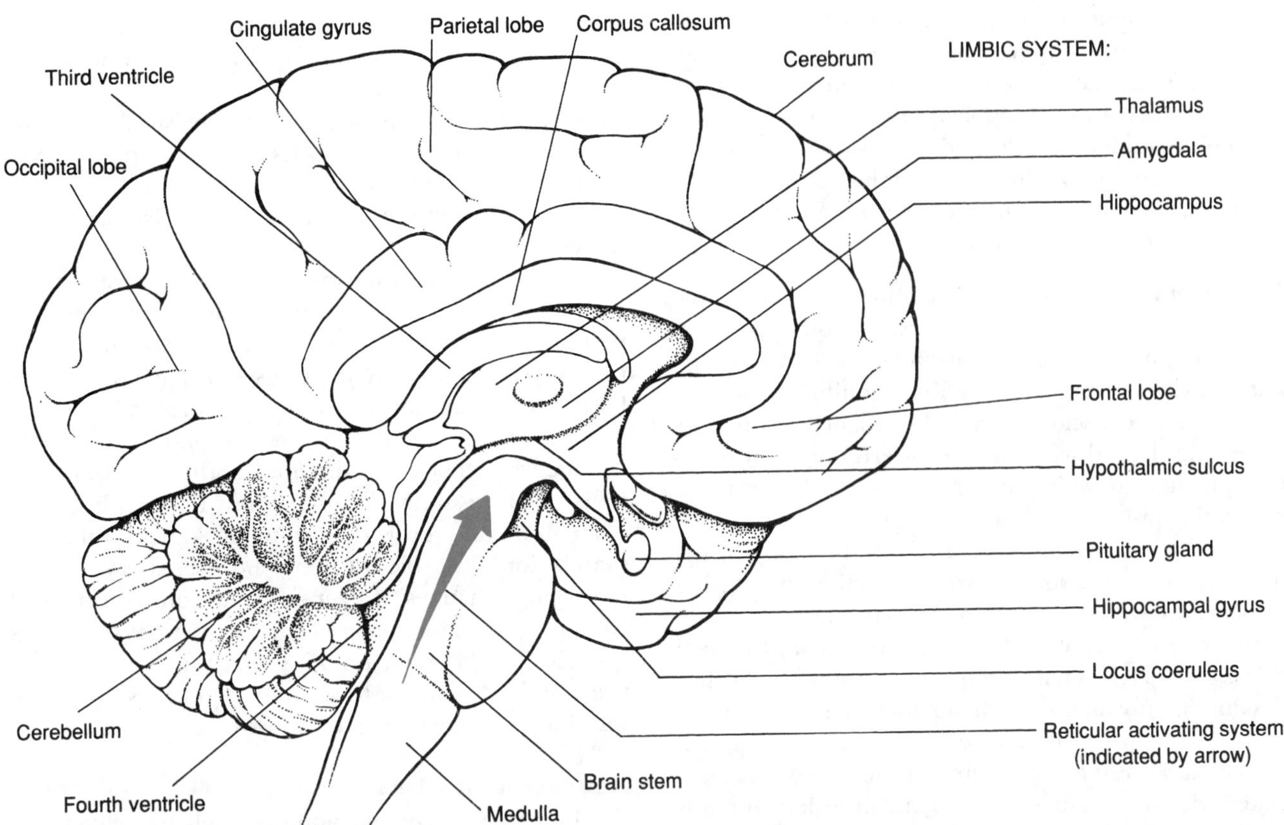

Figure 7-1. The human brain. The temporal lobe, located at the side of the brain, is not shown so that the underlying structures can be displayed.

imaging techniques that view brain activity, such as positron emission tomography (PET) and magnetic resonance imaging (MRI), have uncovered apparent interrelationships between the hemispheres' complex functions.

Each cerebral hemisphere contains four lobes: frontal, parietal, temporal, and occipital. These lobes have distinct functions and some integrated functions. The *frontal lobes* control the organization of thought, moral behavior, and body movement. The left frontal lobe controls right-side body movements; the right frontal lobe controls left-side body movements. The *parietal lobes* interpret sensations and assist in spatial orientation. The *temporal lobes* are dedicated to hearing and memory, the latter in conjunction with the occipital lobe. The temporal lobes are also involved with the limbic system in expressing emotion. The *occipital lobes* contain the structures necessary for visual interpretation; they also coordinate with the temporal lobes' language generation.

Limbic System. Communication between the cerebrum and other areas of the brain is essential to initiating action. Another area, the *limbic system,* arises from the *cingulate gyrus* and encompasses the hippocampus, thalamus, hypothalamus, and amygdala, forming a C-shaped ring above the brain stem. As the seat of emotions, the limbic system plays an important role in behavior: The hippocampus and the amygdala are involved in processing sensations and the emotions associated with memory. Through these structures, emotional arousal through triggering sensations can precipitate the expression of happiness or sadness. The thalamus regulates activity, sensation, and emotion; the hypothalamus is involved in temperature regulation, sexual impulse control, appetite control, endocrine functioning, and impulsive performance, such as excitement, manic behavior, or rage.

A case illustrating the limbic system's involvement in behavior is the famous "Texas tower massacre" of 1966, in which Charles Whitman, a young man in an uncontrollable rage, shot 46 people, killing 16 of them, from a bell tower at the University of Texas in Austin. He was then killed by police. His autopsy revealed a large tumor in the hypothalamic area, causing intense pressure. Although Whitman had complained of intractable headaches, the technology for diagnosing such a tumor was not yet available.

Cerebellum. Lying below the cerebrum, the *cerebellum* is responsible for coordination of movement. Defects in this area related to inhibited transmission of dopamine have been implicated in Parkinson's disease and subcortical dementias, which disrupt smooth, integrated movement. In fact, recent developments in treating these disorders involve intracerebral transplantation of dopamine-producing cells and ablative surgery, which enhances the normal flow of dopamine in the brain by placing a small hole in the globus pallidus or the thalamus to modulate the circuit.[22,47]

Brain Stem. The *brain stem* is significant in psychopathology because of its interactions with the limbic system through the *reticular activating system* (RAS). Originating in the spinal cord, the RAS monitors awareness and states of consciousness. A disturbance in the RAS can cause sleep disruption and interfere with concentration, either of which may precipitate or exacerbate a psychotic episode.

Another brain stem system of psychobiological significance, the *extrapyramidal system*, functions by relaying information from the brain to the spinal nerves. Certain antipsychotic medications may cause extrapyramidal side effects, such as parkinsonism, akathisia, and tardive dyskinesia, in which movements lose their smoothness and become uncontrollable or disjointed.

The *locus coeruleus* is an area in the brain stem associated with stress, anxiety, and panic disorders. It tends to deteriorate with age. This deterioration may lead to decreased anxiety and impulsiveness as a person approaches middle age, causing a mellowing of the intensity of emotions, such as anger. Nurses who have cared for chronically mentally ill or criminally insane clients have observed this phenomenon. The locus ceruleus can also be a factor in depression in later life. Depression may result from failure of the feedback system responsible for suppression of the production of blood cortisol, a stress hormone that is instituted by the activity of the locus ceruleus.[78]

Autonomic Nervous System

Control for the autonomic nervous system (ANS) arises in the hypothalamus, providing for integration with the CNS. The ANS is so named because many of its activities are self-regulating, such as digestion and circulation. However, because the ANS is under the control of the hypothalamus, it also is subject to the influence of the emotions. Thus, the ANS is implicated in certain psychophysiologic disorders, such as heart disease and possibly even breast cancer.[13,25,70] Figure 7-2 shows the locations and functions of important ANS structures.

The ANS has two divisions, the sympathetic and the parasympathetic. The *sympathetic* division, which acts as a unit, includes the chains of ganglia with axons originating in the spinal cord and extending from the ganglia to the viscera. This division also controls secretion of hormones that increase emotional arousal. For instance, the adrenal medulla is a large sympathetic ganglion that secretes epinephrine.

In contrast to the sympathetic division, the *parasympathetic* division restricts its action to one organ at a time. It contains two parts—cranial and sacral—depending on where the nerve fibers arise in the spinal cord.

A final comment on the nervous system structures concerns their neurometamorphosis, or the development of the structural and functional relationships of the nerve cells. Apparently the systems are not strictly bound by the influence of the metamorphic hormones on their development, but they are plastic enough to change with their environment. In other words, heredity is not necessarily destiny; in this there is hope for adaptation and growth in humans. Meanwhile, the search for the role of neurohormonal systems in mediating changes in gene expression continues.[32] Newer research for gene regulators describes sequence-specific DNA-binding proteins that regulate gene expression.[10] Mutants in these gene regulators are implicated in neuropsychological disorders.

Neurotransmitters

The human brain contains approximately 100 billion neurons, or nerve cells, and about the same number of glia (supporting cells). Information passes between neurons through intercellular gaps or synapses through an electrochemical ion exchange involving *neurotransmitters*, which are highly specialized endogenous organic chemicals. Neurotransmitters are synthesized in the cytoplasm of the neuron; for example, tyrosine and dopa combine to form dopamine. This synthesis can be influenced by such factors as diet and drug use. Although many neurotransmitters exist, not all are significant to the study of emotional behavior. Table 7-1 lists the neurotransmitters of particular interest to psychiatric-mental health professionals.

Several psychiatric conditions and personality disorders have been related to neurotransmitter and receptor disorders. Prominent among the former are schizophrenia and mood disorders, such as bipolar psychosis. As for personality disorders, obsessive-compulsive disorder is considered a serotonin-deficit disease; panic disorder has been linked to a deficit in receptor sites for the neurotransmitter gamma-aminobutyric acid (GABA), so GABA's calming effect is not felt within the brain of the panic-stricken person. Panic disorder is strongly familial and is associated with a lactate sensitivity.[89]

Some of the newer imaging techniques, such as emission computerized tomography, PET, or single-photon emission tomography (SPET), now allow researchers to monitor blood flow and the release and tissue concentration of radiolabelled tracers of neuro-

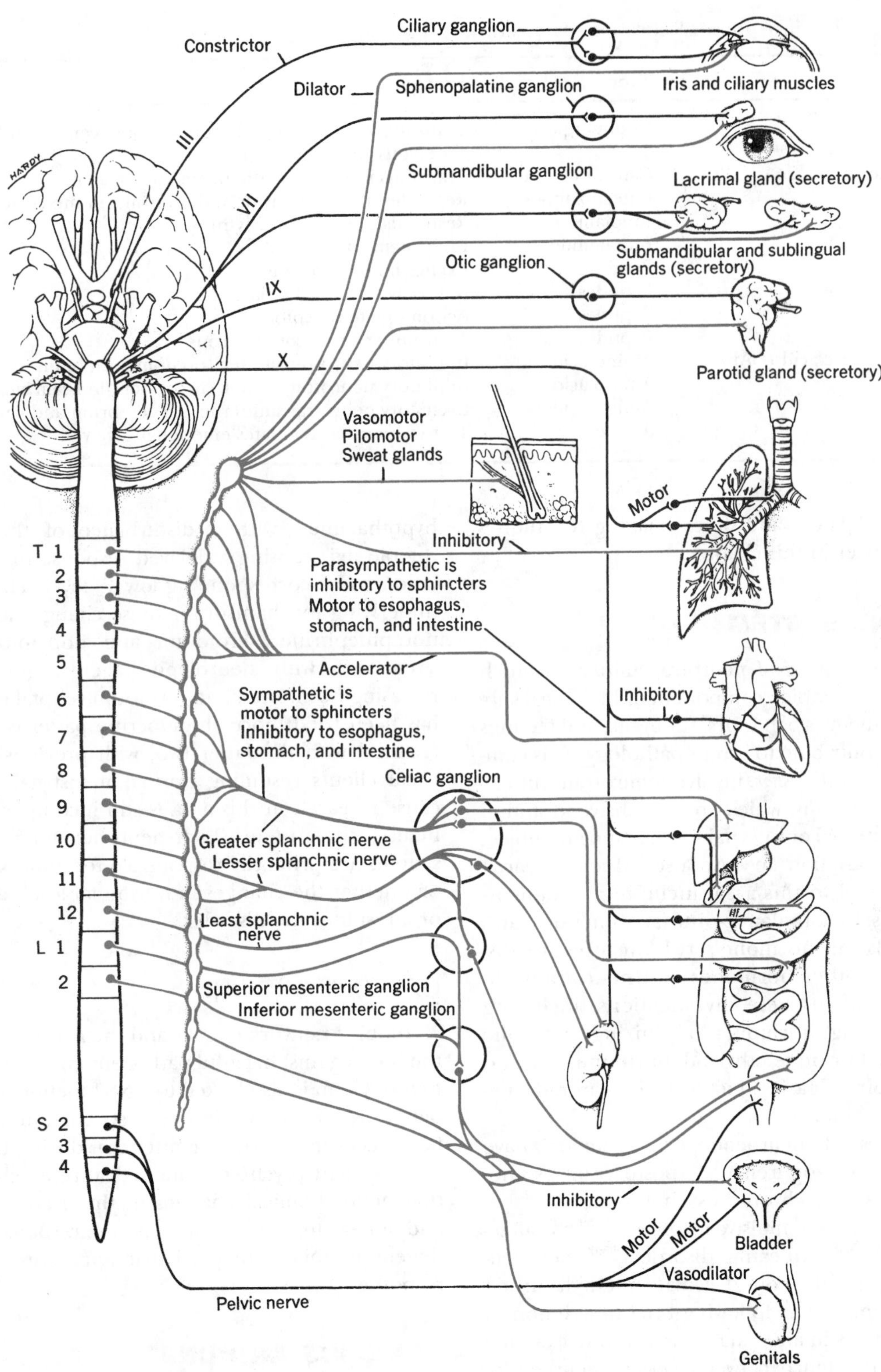

Figure 7-2. The autonomic nervous system. The parasympathetic division (craniosacral fibers) is shown in black; the sympathetic division (thoracolumbar fibers) is shown in color. Note that most organs have a double nerve supply. (In Chaffee EE, Lytle IM: Basic Physiology and Anatomy, 4th ed. Philadelphia, JB Lippincott, 1980)

Table 7-1

Classification and Function of Representative Neurotransmitters

Neurotransmitter	Type	Function
Acetylcholine	Cholinergic	Transmits at nerve–muscle connections (central and autonomic nervous systems)
Norepinephrine	Catecholamine	Transmits in the sympathetic nervous system
Dopamine	Catecholamine	Regulates motor behavior and transmits in the cortex
Melatonin	Indolamine	Responds to circadian rhythms
Serotonin	Indolamine	Brain stem transmitter
Cholecystokinin	Peptide	Excites limbic neurons
Endorphins	Peptides	Naturally produced opiates
Enkephalins	Peptides	Act on opiate receptors
Substance P	Peptide	Transmitter of sensory neurons
Gamma-aminobutyric acid (GABA)	Amino acid	Inhibitory neurotransmitter (predominant brain transmitter)
Glycine	Amino acid	Inhibitory neurotransmitter (prominent in brain stem and cord)
Glutamic acid	Amino acid	Excitatory neurotransmitter in the cerebrum and cerebellum
Histamine	Amine	Transmitter that regulates emotional behavior

transmitters.[37,53] These and other imaging techniques are discussed later in this chapter.

ENDOCRINE SYSTEM

In addition to the role of neurotransmitters, a much larger and more complex component of biological substrates also influences behaviors, thoughts, and feelings and thus may contribute to psychopathology. This component, the *endocrine system*, involves neurotransmitter–endocrine interactions, which are responsive to stimuli arising from external or internal sources and are subject to individual variation in response. Much research has been devoted to this area, including adrenocortical responses, hypothalamic-pituitary functions, and thyroid-stimulating hormone's role in affective disorders.[33] Many other hormones and neurotransmitters are involved in these investigations, including follicle-stimulating hormone, luteinizing hormone (LH), growth hormone, thyroid hormone (T_4 and T_3), thyrotropin-releasing factor (TRF), noradrenaline, and dopamine.

Irregularities of neuroendocrine function have been linked to schizophrenia,[33,46] postpartum psychosis,[74,80] polydipsia in chronic psychotic clients,[6,45,52,75] panic and obsessive-compulsive disorders,[35,39,75,83] affective disorders,[33,35,68] and eating disorders.[55,69] Neuroendocrine function is also considered at fault in disturbed circadian rhythms.[78] The following brief description of endocrine findings in anorexia nervosa is one example of the interdependence between certain neuroendocrine functions and mental disorders.

In the anorectic girl, the circadian pattern of LH secretion is impaired; in the anorectic boy, testosterone levels are reduced. The origin of the problem is in the hypothalamus, with a disturbance of the pituitary-thyroid axis causing a delayed response to TRF stimulation and a corresponding low T_3 level. The apparent underlying mechanism for these changes involves low norepinephrine, serotonin, and dopamine levels.[83] Treatment with neuroleptic agents, gonadotropin-releasing hormones, and serotonin reuptake inhibitors has been tried; normal endocrine patterns have been restored with the latter two, with previously amenorrheal clients resuming normal menstrual cycles. Because research in this area is still incomplete, it is difficult to determine which neurohormonal regulatory systems are primarily responsible for anorexia nervosa or whether the changes in hormonal levels are a cause or a result of the disorder.

IMMUNE SYSTEM

A complex network of cells and their products protects the body against harmful pathogens and toxins; this immune system is also linked to CNS function and thus to behavior. The brain–immune system interaction has been receiving increasing attention during the last decade. Recent psychoimmunological research indicates that neurochemical changes in the brain accompany and appear to mediate the immune response, with endogenous opiates in particular apparently inhibiting response.[24,33,52]

GENETICS AND DNA

Psychobiological research has as a major goal uncovering not only the neuroendocrine substrates of behavior, but also the genetic heritage involved. At the Salk Institute for Biological Studies in La Jolla, California, a human genome project is currently underway to map and isolate all of the genes in the human cell.[20] This project, projected to take 15 years, has intriguing possibilities for understanding and helping people with hereditary physical and mental illnesses. It also raises fears that findings could lead to an increased focus on eugenics and, consequently, increased stigmatization of people who carry undesirable genes. Research on the human genome project is proceeding at a faster than anticipated rate.

To put genome mapping into perspective, DNA resides in the chromosomes, of which there are 46 in each human somatic cell. Half of the chromosomes are inherited from the male parent and half from the female parent. The DNA, two tightly coiled strands of nucleotides, is composed of four bases: cytosine, guanine, adenine, and thymine. Sequences of bases (genes) code for the proteins of life. Humans have an estimated 50,00 to 100,00 genes in each somatic cell nucleus.

Of the many human genes, only about 6,00 are understood from a structural standpoint, and only about 2,600 have been located and mapped on chromosomes. By using restriction enzymes to clip the DNA at specific base sequences, researchers have been able to locate the genes for several transmissible disorders, such as Huntington's disease and muscular dystrophy.

To complicate the picture further, the mitochondria in the cell cytoplasm also contain DNA, which is inherited from the female parent. If this DNA is flawed, it interferes with cellular metabolism. This problem has been implicated in aging changes and in the decreased enzyme activity of Parkinson's disease.[42] To examine these metamorphic and degenerative changes, cell lines can now be cloned and grown indefinitely in vitro.[46] Through restriction enzyme analysis, it is now possible to isolate mutant genes.[73] In the future, it may be possible to regulate gene expression in the brain through cellular surgery and gene transplantation molecular science.[90]

As impressive as these efforts may be, one cannot lose sight of the role that the environment plays in the etiology of certain traits with an apparent genetic component.[74] Genetic inheritance generally accounts for less than half of the phenotypical behavioral disorders and is not restricted to one major gene per disorder; it can involve many small genes at different chromosomal sites.[69] Some important psychogenetic findings are explored in the following section.

HEREDITY AND MENTAL ILLNESS

Mental illness encompasses a broad spectrum of functional and behavioral variations, with four primary aspects:

1. Psychoneurotic behavior, with anxiety states and personality disorders
2. Psychotic behavior, as seen in schizophrenic disorders and psychotic states of mania and depression
3. Psychophysiologic disorders, such as the behavioral malfunctions seen in metabolic imbalance due to drug use, illness, developmental anomaly, or trauma
4. Character disorders, including addictive and sociopathic personalities

Researchers are discovering that many, if not most, of these indications of behavioral dysfunction have precursors in heritage. Moreover, *genetic scapegoating*—attaching stigmas to certain genetic traits—should become less an issue as increasing knowledge reveals that there are no perfectly endowed people.

Genetic Factors in Depression and Mania

Recent exciting discoveries about the role of genetic factors in mood disorder represent new challenges to nursing. These discoveries include linking DNA markers on chromosome 11 to bipolar disorder and increased risk of the disorder in familial descendants.[56,81] A later study has also located a region on chromosome 18, responsible for stress hormone production, that is involved. The research confirms that more than one gene sets the stage for the disorder.[3] About 65% of monozygotic twins have concordance for bipolar disorder. Variance may be accounted for by whether or not the twins shared the same placenta.[16]

However, other biological and environmental factors may impede or contribute to the development of this disorder. These factors include disruptions in circadian and other biological rhythms, altered dietary patterns, the neurobiological nature of stress, and limbic turmoil, such as that caused by seizure activity.[78]

A special case of depression is the one associated with the postpartum period. The syndrome, which can range from the mild "baby blues" through clinical depression to psychosis, may be triggered by the sudden drop in circulating hormones after childbirth.[80] The depression is repetitive, is more prevalent than was commonly believed, is particularly destructive to family relationships, and has a great impact on children in terms of behavior problems, learning difficulties, and affective illness.[67]

Genetic transmission is a possibility, and environmental factors may increase genetic vulnerability.[16,74] When severe postpartum symptoms require clinical treatment, psychiatric nurses have a special opportunity to assist the mother and infant in the attachment process, to provide an opportunity for the mother to rest and regain physical and psychological strength, to help the mother and other family members develop improved coping skills, and to encourage improvement in family relationships. Newer pharmacological treatment, carefully monitored, can alleviate much of the distress of mental illness in the postpartum period, even when mothers are nursing their infants.[94]

Genetic Factors in Schizophrenia

Over the years, from Kallmann's early twin studies to the present day, research into schizophrenia has consistently supported its nature as a familial condition.[2,16,40,51] Dr. David Shore, in his 1989 convention address to the American Psychiatric Nurses' Association in Denver, reiterated that children having one schizophrenic parent have about a 15% chance of developing the disorder, and children with two schizophrenic parents have about a 40% chance, compared with a 2% prevalence in the general population. Concordance in identical twins is 60 times greater than in the general population, but the child of a nonschizophrenic twin is just as likely to develop the condition as the child of a schizophrenic twin.[39] A new study links the likelihood of concordance in twins to their placental status: Twins sharing one placenta were found to be 75% concordant for schizophrenia and other disorders, whereas those with separate placentas and amnions were only 12% concordant.[16] A wide spectrum of schizophrenic illness is present in the inheritance pattern, because schizophrenia is not one distinct entity but several.[17]

Despite the strong heredity connection, it has been difficult to identify a genetic marker for schizophrenia, which has long been recognized as multifactorial and polygenic in transmission.[51] The environmental factors are not strong; a child with a schizophrenic heritage raised by adoptive parents remains at risk according to his or her heritage. Nevertheless, vulnerability is modified by environmental factors to some extent.

Brain imaging techniques show enlarged brain ventricles in some schizophrenic adults. According to Dr. Daniel Weinberger of the National Institute of Mental Health, schizophrenia changes the brain's anatomy, altering its function, especially in communication between the limbic system and the prefrontal cerebral cortex.[92] The significance of ventricular enlargement and increased volume of abnormal white matter seen in computed tomography (CT) and MRI scans is under investigation. Enlarged ventricals are also associated with Alzheimer's disease, but the configuration of the CT scans differs in the two conditions. The pattern of ventricular enlargement in schizophrenia tends to be asymmetric, with more enlargement on the left than on the right, indicating decline in language and communication abilities. In Alzheimer's disease, on the other hand, the pattern of ventricular enlargement is symmetrical, which may indicate a general decline in cognitive functioning.[15] These anomalies are present in affective disorders also but to a lesser degree.[19,21] The effects of ventricular enlargement on surrounding brain tissue are not completely understood.

Meanwhile, neurobiological studies also are proceeding. Findings of one recent study indicated that children whose mothers had influenza in their second trimester of pregnancy were more likely to develop schizophrenia later in life.[1] However, these neurobiological findings often have been identified with other psychiatric conditions, leading to the conclusion that the diagnoses are not correct or are confounded with other disorders (for instance, schizophrenia with an affective disorder or an addictive personality.)[17,26]

Genetic Factors in Dementia

Although schizophrenia usually strikes in youth or young adulthood, some late-life forms that produce dementia develop after age 45. Differential diagnosis is difficult because of the tendency to suspect Alzheimer's disease in older people displaying delirious, demented, or delusional behavior or basic personality changes. Accurate diagnosis hinges on thorough assessment, including careful, continuous nursing observations.[76] Psychoses related to metabolic disorders, drug ingestion, tumors, or depressive or schizophrenic syndromes may be reversed, but there is no effective treatment for the dementias—Alzheimer's disease, Pick's disease, Huntington's chorea, and the dementia seen in the acquired immunodeficiency syndrome (AIDS).

The dementia of AIDS occurs through the entry of the human immunodeficiency virus (HIV) into the brain. This infectious process begins by HIV transportation across the blood–brain barrier, in contaminated monocytes that have ingested the virus. The viruses are thus hidden from the immune system, and the cell vacuoles act as reservoirs of infection. In the brain, the HIV activates an increase in calcium levels, which causes death in neurons.[86]

Grossly similar but somewhat different pictures for the dementias than for other disorders are indicated by MRI. In a recent MRI study, psychotic people showed six times more temporal white matter and four times more frontal and occipital lesions than seen in the normal control subjects. White matter lesions may be linked to psychosis and depression.[21,59,86]

In contrast, MRI in people with Alzheimer's disease (the most common dementia in elderly people) characteristically shows neurofibrillary tangles and enlarged ventricles. These changes indicate damage to the mechanism that screens out excessive stimuli and allows for precise focus, impairing the ability to tolerate multiple stimuli and stress.

Recent neurochemical research into Alzheimer's disease has indicated that the common brain protein amyloid B damages brain cells and causes memory loss in older people in the manner characteristic of

Alzheimer's disease. There seems to be an abnormality in the way that this protein is used by the brain in Alzheimer's disease. The precursor directing the use of amyloid B has been localized to chromosome 21, but it is *not* related to Down syndrome, according to recent information.[39]

Other studies implicate faulty neurotransmitters or defective ribonucleic acid in this process, showing a tendency for the neurotransmitters to diffuse rather than carry through at the synapse.[23] Finally, several investigators have suggested that Alzheimer's disease may be more than one disease or may take more than one form. They cite as evidence genetic studies that have found a familial link in certain Alzheimer's cases but not in others.[58]

The discovery of the gene for Huntington's disease was made in 1993.[94] This situation illustrates some new issues being raised by genetic research. Although the gene can be detected on a genetic probe at a young age, the disease itself does not emerge until middle age. For clients and their families at risk for developing the disease, the decision of whether or not to seek this knowledge may be difficult. As one young client with a family history of Huntington's chorea said to a nurse, "If you were me, would you want to know?" (see Case Study 7-1).

Genetic Factors in Personality, Conduct, and Character Disorders

Genetic research points to a familial predisposition to personality types, addictions, and antisocial behaviors, such as delinquency and crime. Even more common personality factors, such as locus of control, may have a familial basis. For instance, a recent twin study showed that hereditary influences were more important than environmental ones in determining how people felt about the amount of control they felt they had over their own lives and how personally responsible they felt for any misfortunes occurring in their lives. The fact that most participants in the study were older than 50 years points to the persistent influence of heredity despite the various environmental changes that all people experience throughout life.[65]

People have been shown to be at risk for developing certain personality disorders according to family inheritance patterns.[49] Table 7-2 presents data on the incidence of borderline personality disorder and other mental illnesses in relatives of people with borderline personality disorder. Dependent personality disorder and possibly some others may be influenced by hereditary factors. On the other hand, multiple personality disorder is one type of personality disorder with situational antecedents—the most common being severe, persistent child abuse.[8,28]

Of particular interest is the connection between personality disorder and addictive syndromes, such as alcoholism and drug abuse, first identified by Links and colleagues.[49] This connection has been explored in the children of alcoholic parents, many of whom have been diagnosed with major depression, anxiety disorders, or various personality disorders.[87] Subsequent research has pointed to a common genetic marker for these conditions.[12]

Research by Simon Levay of the Salk Institute has focused on homosexuality. Once classified in the Diagnostic and Statistical Manual, second edition, as a "sexual deviation" (pp. 9–10 and 92) and later viewed as a personal lifestyle choice, homosexuality, according to Levay's disputed findings, may have a physiological base. Levay found that in male homosexuals, the anterior hypothalamus apparently contains an unusually small cluster of the cells responsible for sexual behavior. Later, other differences in the brains of heterosexuals and homosexuals were found. Very early research by Kallmann[41] reported virtually 100% concordance for homosexuality in identical twins; until Levay's findings, no anatomical explanation was advanced for the concordance.[4]

Finally, the notion of genetic influences in antisocial behavior is concerned with the influence of many genes interacting with the environment. Researchers at the University of Southern California and the University of California at Irvine, using PET scans, discovered that in people who had murdered or attempted murder, the rates of glucose uptake in the prefrontal cortex areas were significantly lower than those of the control subjects.[71] Findings from this research are a beginning biological look at character disorders. Earlier longitudinal research indicated that biological factors predispose to mild antisocial behavior, even when the person has been raised in a good home environment. In severely antisocial behavior, however, the genetic factors that predispose to antisocial behavior are strongly developed in a poor home environment.[72] Another area of research involves a possible background of childhood or prenatal neurological damage from infection, seizure, or head injury in sexual offenders.

PSYCHOPHYSIOLOGICAL EFFECTS OF ENVIRONMENT

Just as the personality can affect the physiological function (see Chapter 27, Cognitive Disorders), so too can physical abnormalities and traumas affect psychological function. One well-understood example is the psychological effects of physical, psychological, and sexual abuse on children and adolescents. Other important, though less well understood, examples include the psychological effects of toxic substances, illness, accidental injuries and disasters, and seasonal affective disorders on

Case Study

The Client in Genetic Counseling

John G, 20 years old, was the youngest sibling, and the only male, in an affluent family of five children in the town of Huntington, New York. His early childhood memories were of a mother who was unpredictable—kind and loving one moment, cruel and punitive the next. His mother walked and talked only with difficulty. Her clumsy, spastic, twitching movements caused her to drop things on the floor and break them, and she would then become enraged. It was as if she were angry with her own body. John did not remember his father. One of his sisters told him, "Dad got disgusted with Mom's temper and split." His parents were divorced before his mother was diagnosed with "chorea." When John was 8 years old, the housekeeper could no longer contend with his mother's "outbursts," and Mrs. G was admitted to an institution for the mentally ill. She died when he was 16.

John's oldest sister, Mary, was 18 years older than he. Mary took over the family when her mother went to the hospital. Eventually JoAnn and Hester, the two next oldest, married and moved out of the house to start their own families. Mary continued to provide a home for John and Carol, who was 5 years older than John. As time went on, John, then 18, and Carol, then 23, began to notice changes in their older sister that frightened them. Mary, then 36, lost her usual sunny disposition and became forgetful, trembling, morose, and withdrawn. At first they attributed this change to a broken relationship; Mary had intended to marry her long-time fiance in the coming spring. As time went on, Mary did not "snap out of it," and her siblings insisted that she see a physician.

After taking a careful family history and doing some neurological testing, the physician called the family members together and explained the nature of Huntington's disease: It is hereditary, and any child of an affected parent has a 50% chance of developing the disorder. There is no cure or even an effective treatment. With the physician was a clinical nurse specialist in mental health, who also had a master's degree in genetic counseling. The stunned family members were urged to continue meeting with the nurse to have their numerous questions answered: Who else in the family will be stricken and when? How can we protect ourselves? Do men get this disease as often as women? What about our children (from JoAnn and Hester)?

As the counseling sessions unfolded, Carol, then only 25, cried frequently and seemed to see the advent of the disease in every muscle twitch or normal memory lapse. John became very serious and engaged in a flurry of intense productivity. He poured over his college texts with dedication and savored his social life and friends, as if he had to compress living into fewer years than he had anticipated. "Maybe I've got only 10 more Christmases," he said with a laugh. However, he exhibited strong denial: "I won't get this disease because I've always been healthy. I've got to stay healthy to help Mary and Carol and maybe my other sisters as well. After all, I'm the man of the family! I work out every day, and I keep myself in good condition. If I am in charge of myself at all times, I can control my mind, and I won't get it."

When the subject of genetic testing was broached by the counselor, JoAnn and Hester agreed, and both, fortunately, tested negative for the autosomal dominant gene. Carol could not face it. "If they were to say to me, 'Yes, you will get Huntington's disease when you are 30,' what would my life be like? I couldn't live with that!" John was ambivalent "If you were me," he said pathetically to the nurse, "would you want to know?"

Questions for Discussion

1. How did John and Carol's early childhood experiences shape their perceptions of Huntington's disease? Has the treatment picture changed in recent years?
2. What is the history of Huntington's disease? Is it coincidental that the family lives in Huntington, NY?
3. Although Mary was destined to be one of the unfortunate 50% to inherit the disease, what could the breaking of a significant relationship have to do with time of onset?
4. What were the factors that likely prevented the children of the family from learning the true facts about autosomal dominant Huntington's disease earlier?
5. What were the emotions underlying John's statements? Why did he laugh when he talked about "10 more Christmases"?

Table 7-2

Lifetime Prevalence of Disorders in 320 First-Degree Relatives of Borderline Clients

	Prevalence		Risk Periods		
Diagnoses	*N*	*(%)*	*Age (Years)*	*(N)*	Morbid Risk (%)
Schizophrenia	0	(0)	15–45	(218)	0
Schizoaffective					
Depressed	4	(1.3)			
Manic	0	(0)			
Bipolar—mania	8	(2.5)	15–60	(178.5)	4.5
Recurrent unipolar	43	(13.4)	15–70	(161.5)	26.6
Antisocial personality	22	(6.9)	15–40	(229)	9.6
BPD*	35	(10.9)	15–40	(229)	15.3
Alcoholism	48	(15.0)	15–40	(229)	21.0
Drug use	29	(9.4)			
Unspecified psychosis	3	(1.0)			
Other diagnoses	4	(1.3)			

** BPD = borderline personality disorder.*

(Reprinted with permission from Links PS, Steiner M, Huxley G: The Occurrence of Borderline Personality Disorders in the Families of Borderline Patients. J Pers Disorders 2: 17, 1988.)

children and adults. This section discusses recent efforts to sort out the effects of some of these phenomena.

Toxic Substances

The last few years have seen a concentrated effort by the scientific community to categorize the psychophysiological effects of exposure to toxic substances. This effort is largely related to a movement to reduce drug use by pregnant women, because fetal exposure to certain drugs has lasting effects on a child's physical and psychosocial development.[48] The numerous drugs and toxic substances affecting physiology and behavior in people of all ages range from lead, with its well-known effects of exposure,[61] to various prescription and street drugs with widely differing effects (see Chapter 20, Psychopharmacology, and Chapter 33, Substance Abuse and Dependency).

Prescription drugs sometimes have a paradoxical effect on the elderly and on children. In addition, the interactions of multiple prescriptions, especially for the elderly, can be devastating. Such interactions and drug and food interactions may cause confusion, incontinence, delirium, ataxia, and vertigo.[79]

When considering drug interactions, people frequently think of alcohol and its effects but usually do not consider the effects of caffeine in such common substances as coffee, tea, chocolate, colas, and various over-the-counter medications. Overdosing on caffeine produces a syndrome similar to anxiety neurosis. In some people, even moderate amounts of caffeine can precipitate caffeine intoxication, with irritability, sensory disturbances, and depression. Caffeine also may lead to increased consumption of such antagonists as tranquilizers and sedatives, and its diuretic action can dilute the effectiveness of lithium therapy.[38]

The study on the effects of lead ingestion cited previously found that young adults who sustained lead exposure as children still suffer such neurobehavioral impairments as poor hand–eye coordination, decreased reasoning power, and other behavioral deficits tied to CNS dysfunction.[61] Although the effects of lead have been substantiated, the effects of other metals and minerals, such as aluminum, magnesium, iron, and calcium, are under investigation. For instance, aluminum and iron (both of which are commonly present in drinking water) are suspected in interactions that precipitate the neurofibrillary tangles of Alzheimer's disease—namely, displacing the magnesium blocker for calcium and allowing calcium uptake into neurons, which causes cell death.[86]

The effects of mutagenic chemicals on the progeny of exposed men also has been investigated. Mutation has the effect of continuing the transmission of the damaged genes to subsequent generations.[50] Possible transmission of behavioral deficits from men exposed to drugs and other chemicals to their offspring mandates that nurses investigate the drug use and chemical exposure patterns of the father and the mother when assessing psychophysiological effects of exposure on a child.

Illness and Injury

The chapters in Part XI, Mental Health Intervention with the Medical Client, discuss many examples of illness and injury affecting mental health. For instance, diabetes mellitus can cause multi-infarct dementia, and a head injury may cause seizure activity that precipitates panic disorder.

A specific new concern for health professionals in recent years has been the increase in immigration and migration by residents of third world countries who are in search of improved living conditions. These survivors may suffer psychological and physical damage, leading to various neurological and psychiatric problems.[91] Suicide, the ultimate psychiatric emergency, is not uncommon in these survivors. Because health professionals in these people's countries of origin are sometimes participants in a torture routine, establishing a therapeutic relationship with such clients represents a significant challenge for psychiatric-mental health nurses.

Seasonal Affective Disorder

The varying sensitivity of people to different patterns of light exposure, the changing seasons, and the circadian rhythms of their own bodies has received increasing attention during the last decade. Seasonal affective disorder (SAD) is characterized by alternating depressive symptoms in the winter and euphoria in the summer.[60] The etiology of SAD is related to disrupted circadian rhythms due to head injury or failure of the body to adjust to the seasons[84] and to inhibited production of melatonin (a neurotransmitter) due to stress.[56] Treatment often involves timed exposure to a special bright light, which synchronizes circadian rhythms and induces melatonin production.

Application of the Nursing Process

Integration of mind and body is one dimension for the nurse to consider when applying the nursing process; the family as an integrated unit is another. The focus must include the community, because environmental factors greatly influence psychobiosocial health.[44] With the rise of biological determinism, it is important to remember that people are not merely organisms; they have personalities shaped by their interactions and experiences with others. They have psychosocial needs for nurturing and growth as physical and spiritual human beings.[66] This section explores ways to integrate the psychobiological principles into psychiatric-mental health nursing practice.

ASSESSMENT

Assessment represents an ongoing challenge for the psychiatric nurse. The nurse first should obtain an accurate client history, then hold a family conference to explore any possible genetic, environmental, or interactional factors; family history of psychobiological disorders; social support needed and available; and the family's knowledge and use of community resources.[62]

Psychobiological assessment includes an evaluation of anxiety, sexual function, and sleep disturbances and their effects on behavior. The nurse's therapeutic use of self is especially important during this assessment, which touches on topics that many people find sensitive.

For many clients and families, assessment is best conducted during a home visit.[5,34,66] With the emphasis in psychiatric-mental health care shifting from the hospital to the community, home health nursing is becoming an exciting reality in psychiatric-mental health nursing. Home visits provide an excellent opportunity to perform a usual psychobiological assessment while also evaluating the family's socioeconomic and educational level and observing general living conditions, ambience, and hazards. A visit timed to occur at mealtime facilitates the evaluation of dietary patterns. In addition, by being aware of the tenor of the client's home environment, the nurse can observe for triggers and stress buildup that may precipitate undesirable behavior.

The second phase of assessment includes a complete neurological examination. This should include not only tests for common signs of neurological malfunction, such as poor hand–eye coordination, but also some projective tests, such as drawing, to consider how the client perceives himself or herself in particular situations.[9,27]

Finally, the client may be scheduled for diagnostic procedures, such as electroencephalography (EEG), MRI, PET or SPET, or CT. The psychiatric-mental health nurse should be familiar with these tests and their purposes to educate the client and family and allay their anxiety. In brief, the EEG, which maps brain electrical activity, is performed to evaluate Alzheimer's disease, seizure disorder, and emotional arousal in thought disorders, such as schizophrenia.[36] Anatomical detail of brain tissue, such as tumors and the enlarged ventricles and white matter changes in Alzheimer's disease, can be seen on MRI.[85] Using PET scans may help identify specific neurotransmitters related to the actions of drugs, particularly opioids, stimulants, and designer drugs.[43] A variant of PET, SPET uses repeated scans over a short period and can detect certain infections, such as herpes simplex encephalitis. The CT scans show excellent bone detail and are useful for assessing head injuries. Bio-electron activity measure is a specific PET imaging technique to study cognitive functioning.

NURSING DIAGNOSIS

When assessment indicates an underlying physiological cause of a behavioral problem, the nursing diagnoses should reflect the pertinent psychobiological aspects.

For example, an appropriate nursing diagnosis for a client with AIDS might be Impaired Adjustment related to fear of and anxiety about the diagnosis of AIDS, as evidenced by refusing to join group sessions and objection to the medication regimen.

CLIENT OUTCOMES AND GOALS

Nursing process has no value unless it clearly leads to a better outcome for the client and his or her community.[63] Outcome identification conceptualizes the most desirable situation that could ensue from the treatment interventions, given the severity of the client's symptoms, the expectations of society, and the prognosis for the particular diagnosis.[11,39] In the case management focus of today's health care, outcome identification is used to decide whether or not certain resources (eg, reimbursement funds) are appropriate for the particular case. In psychiatric-mental health nursing, the most pragmatic outcome measures usually involve objective measures of functioning, although the client's subjective experience cannot be discounted.[63] For example, outcome identification for a client with paranoid schizophrenia might include criteria that the client no longer exhibits violent behaviors *and* that the client states he or she no longer believes others are plotting against him or her. From a community perspective, accurate outcome identification and effective treatment result in positive relationships and less stigmatization of the mentally ill.

PLANNING

Plans need to include the family and the client, and goals should be agreed on or they will not be achieved. The focus is also on the community, because not all families are able and willing to provide adequate care for mentally ill members, nor is it always in a client's best interest for the family to do so.

Goals for the family of a client with Alzheimer's disease might include the following:

1. Removing all hazardous items from the environment to protect the client from injury
2. Monitoring the forgetful client's diet carefully to ensure adequate nutritional intake
3. Assisting the client with activities of daily living (eg, bathing, dressing, eating) as needed
4. Obtaining counseling help for caregivers to help them develop coping skills for dealing more effectively with the client's difficult behaviors, such as wandering, combativeness, and hiding things
5. Locating community resources for support groups, respite care, and referrals to other psychiatric-mental health professionals

INTERVENTION

Psychobiologically based interventions include newer drugs, biofeedback, soma therapies, hormone treatments, exercise therapy, educational therapy, visual imagery, surgery, and electroconvulsive therapy. Several of these modalities are addressed in other chapters; only examples of innovative strategies are mentioned here.

Promising psychopharmacological research includes how methylfolate (vitamin B_{12}) might enhance recovery from depression and treat schizophrenia,[30] how intramuscular desferrioxamine may slow the clinical progression of Alzheimer's disease,[57] and how understanding the effects of different drugs on cycle length may help prevent recurrence in affective disorders.[82] Newer drugs, such as controlled-release Sinemet, a combination of levodopa and the amino acid inhibitor carbidopa, are used to control the fluctuations in therapeutic L-dopa levels for the treatment of Parkinson's disease.

Educational therapy has a wide range of applications, for example, using an illuminated brain model to teach older children how drugs affect the brain biologically and using communication strategies to enhance the coping abilities of clients affected by Alzheimer's disease.[77] Visual imagery and relaxation therapy have proven effective in various situations and conditions. When undergoing MRI procedures, for example, guided imagery lowers anxiety levels.[88] In substance abuse, endorphin production is stimulated in the brain by relaxation therapy.[18] Other promising and increasingly used interventions include the therapeutic use of humor, music, horticulture, and pets.[14,29,64]

EVALUATION

To keep advancing psychiatric-mental health nursing toward a holistic, theoretically sound art and science, nurses need to evaluate psychobiologically based interventions from an empirical perspective. This is needed to provide evidence supporting the effectiveness of approaches that nurses already know are effective through clinical experience. Horticultural therapy, for example, is not yet supported in the literature, although nurses recognize it as beneficial for some clients. Innovative nursing research in this direction can help psychiatric-mental health nurses achieve their ultimate goal: to understand better the nature of mental illness and more effectively alleviate the pain associated with it.

◆ Chapter Summary

This chapter has presented an overview of the new developments in psychobiology and related them to psychiatric-mental health nursing. Incorporating psychobiological principles will strengthen the body of nursing knowledge and lead to improved quality of psychiatric-mental health nursing care. Chapter highlights include the following:

1. The human person is a holistic entity, with an integration of mind and body so that interference or defect in one aspect affects the function of the other.
2. Understanding mental illness involves a complex effort that delves into the genetic composition and molecular structures of the human organism.
3. Nurses are in a unique position to combine the science of psychobiology with the art of holistic nursing care in assessing and treating many mental illnesses.
4. The timely advent of the decade of the brain presents a challenge for nursing education and an opportunity to expand and advance nursing science through research.

Review Questions

1. One function of the hypothalamus is to
   A. regulate usual activities of the body.
   B. process memory.
   C. control impulsive performance, such as rage.
   D. receive and process sensory input.
2. Characteristic of panic disorder is
   A. the subjective belief that one is having a heart attack.
   B. an excess of the neurotransmitter GABA.
   C. the absence of a familial link.
   D. a feeling of euphoria and manic behavior.
3. In anorexia nervosa, the cause of the disorder is
   A. a change in the hormone levels of the body.
   B. a tumor in the amygdala.
   C. a distorted perception of body image.
   D. difficult to determine because research in the area is incomplete.
4. A psychiatric-mental health challenge that may occur from early discharge of the postpartum client is
   A. lack of the opportunity for parents and newborn to bond.
   B. failure to thrive syndrome in the newborn.
   C. a drop in hormones, leading to postpartum depression.
   D. inability to pharmacologically treat the mother for mental illness in the home setting.
5. Schizophrenic illness
   A. is usually caused by poor parenting or other social problems.
   B. is not one single mental illness entity, but several.
   C. is 100% concordant in identical twins.
   D. shows equilateral brain ventricle enlargement on MRI.
6. Careful nursing observations are necessary for the client exhibiting signs of dementia because
   A. differential diagnosis is difficult, and some forms of dementia are reversible if treated, others are not.
   B. it is possible to arrest Alzheimer's disease in the early stages.
   C. dementia is caused by the HIV virus.
   D. the nurse may want to suggest genetic testing for the family.
7. Studies have shown that
   A. there is a common inheritance pattern in borderline personality disorder and recurrent unipolar depression.
   B. dependent personality disorder and addictive behaviors may be influenced by hereditary factors.
   C. multiple personality disorder may be caused by severe, persistent child abuse.
   D. All of the above are true.
8. The most commonly abused drug on the psychiatric unit is
   A. alcohol.
   B. caffeine.
   C. lithium.
   D. chlorpromazine.
9. In assessing the mental health client's impending discharge to the community, it is *most* important for the interdisciplinary team to
   A. obtain a good family history.
   B. explore the social support and community resources available to the client.
   C. review the current medications the client is receiving.
   D. schedule a series of diagnostic tests.
10. Outcome identification
    A. looks at the most desirable outcome a client could have, given the severity of symptoms and the prognosis expected.
    B. is important to establish because of the case management and reimbursement focus of today's health care scene.
    C. involves objective measures of functioning and the subjective statements and feelings of the client.
    D. All of the above are part of outcome identification.
11. In planning for a client's community living,
    A. the family is always expected to care for the client.
    B. the client is told that he or she will be respon-

sible for his or her own food, clothing, shelter, and medication maintenance.
C. the client and significant other must agree on the goals, or they will not be achieved.
D. community involvement should be minimal.

12. It is most important for psychiatric-community mental health nurses to evaluate their interventions empirically through research because
A. the psychiatric-mental health care team needs documented evidence of successful interventions to help clients.
B. this focus is part of holistic nursing.
C. everyone knows that nursing interventions are effective.
D. it will help the nurse to get published.

◆ References

1. Adams W, Kendall R, Hare E, Munk-Jorgensen P: Epidemiological Evidence that Maternal Influenza Contributes to the Aetiology of Schizophrenia. Br J Psych 163: 522–534, 1993
2. Bender L: Schizophrenic Spectrum Disorders in the Families of Schizophrenic Children. In Fieve RR, Rosenthal D, Brill H (eds): Genetic Research in Psychiatry, pp 125–134. Baltimore, The Johns Hopkins University Press, 1975
3. Berrettini WH: Gene for Manic Depression. Brain Work: the Neuroscience Newsletter 1: 4, 1995
4. Bigelow BV: Minute Brain Cells Tied to Sexuality Are Focus, p A-14. The San Diego Tribune, Friday, August 30, 1991
5. Bloch DA: The Clinical Home Visit. Seminars in Psychiatry 5: 159–165, 1973
6. Boyd MA: Polydipsia in the Chronically Mentally Ill: A Review. Arch Psychiatr Nurs 4: 166–175, 1990
7. Buckwalter KC: The Decade of the Brain and Psychiatric Nursing. Arch Psychiatr Nurs 4: 283, 1990
8. Burgess AW, Hartman CR, Baker T: Memory Presentations of Childhood Sexual Abuse. J Psychosoc Nurs 33 (9): 9–16, 1995
9. Burgess AW, Hartman CR, Howe JW, Shaw ER, McFarland GC: Juvenile Murderers: Assessing Memory Through Crime Scene Drawings. J Psychosoc Nurs 28 (1): 26–34, 1990
10. Chalepakis G, Stoykova A, Wijnholds J, Tremblay P, Gruss P: Pax: Gene Regulators in the Developing Nervous System. J Neurobiology 24: 1367–1384, 1993
11. Cohen C: Poverty and the Course of Schizophrenia: Implications for Research and Policy. Hosp Community Psychiatry 44 (10): 951–956, 1993
12. Comings DE, Muhleman D, Dietz GW Jr, Donlon T: Human Tryptophan Oxygenase Localized to 4q31: Possible Implications for Alcoholism and Other Behavioral Disorders. Genomics 9: 301–308, 1991
13. Cooper CL, Faragher EB: Psychosocial Stress and Breast Cancer: The Inter-Relationship Between Stress Events, Coping Strategies and Personality. Psychosocial Medicine 23: 653–662, 1993
14. Courtright P, Johnson S, Baumgartner MA, Jordan, M, Webster JC: Dinner Music: Does it Affect the Behavior of Psychiatric Inpatients? J Psychosoc Nurs 28(3): 37–40, 1990
15. Crow TJ: The Meaning of the Morphological Changes in the Brain in Schizophrenia. Current Approaches to Psychoses 4: 8–9, 1995
16. Davis JO, Phelps JA, Bracha HS: Prenatal Development of Monozygotic Twins and Concordance for Schizophrenia. Schizophr Bull 21: 357–366, 1995
17. American Psychiatric Association: Diagnostic and Statistical Manual of Mental Disorders, 4th ed. Washington, DC, American Psychiatric Association, 1994
18. Dodge VH: Relaxation Training: A Nursing Intervention for Substance Abusers. Archives of Psychiatric Nursing 5: 99–104, 1991
19. Dupont RM, Jernigan TL, Heindel W, Butters N, Shafer K, Wilson T, Hesselink J, Gillin C: Magnetic Resonance Imaging and Mood Disorders. Arch Gen Psychiatry 52: 747–755, 1995
20. Edelson E: Genome. Popular Science 239 (7): 58–63, 83, 1991
21. Elkis H, Friedman L, Wise A, Meltzer, HY: Meta-analyses of Studies of Ventricular Enlargement and Cortical Sulcal Prominence in Mood Disorders. Arch Gen Psychiatry 52: 735–746, 1995
22. Fazzini E: A Comparison of Neurosurgical Procedures in the Treatment of Parkinson's Disease. The American Parkinson Disease Association Newsletter 1: 4, 1993
23. Finch CE, Morgan DG: RNA and Protein Metabolism in the Aging Brain. Annu Rev Neurosci 13: 75–88, 1990
24. Fisher LA, Brown MR: Central Regulation of Stress Responses: Regulation of the Autonomic Nervous System and Visceral Function by Corticotrophin Releasing Factor-4. Baillieres Clinical Endocrinology of Metabolism 5 (1): 35–50, 1991
25. Friedman M, Rosenman RH: Type A Behavior and Your Heart. New York, Alfred A. Knopf, 1974
26. Garza-Trevino ES, Volkow ND, Cancro R, Contreras S: Neurobiology of Schizophrenic Syndromes. Hosp Community Psychiatry 41: 971–979, 1990
27. Glaister JA: Projective Drawings: Helping Adult Survivors of Childhood Abuse Recognize Boundaries. J Psychosoc Nurs 32 (10): 28–34, 1994
28. Glod CA: Long-Term Consequences of Childhood Physical and Sexual Abuse. Archives of Psychiatric Nursing 7: 163–173, 1993
29. Goddaer J, Abraham IL: Effects of Relaxing Music on Agitation During Meals among Nursing Home Residents with Severe Cognitive Impairment. Archives of Psychiatric Nursing 8: 150–158, 1994
30. Godfrey PSA, Toone BK, Carney MWP, Flynn TG, Bottiglieri T, Laundy M, Chanarin I, Reynolds EH: Enhancement of Recovery from Psychiatric Illness by Methylfolate. The Lancet 336: 392–395, 1990
31. Hammen CL, Burge D, Daley SE, Davilla J, Paley B, Rudolph KD: Interpersonal Attachment Cognitions and Pre-

diction of Symptomatic Responses to Interpersonal Stress. J Abnorm Psychol 104: 436–443, 1995
32. Harris WA: Neurometamorphosis. J Neurobiol 21: 953–957, 1990
33. Hayes A: Psychiatric Nursing: What Does Biology Have to Do with It? Archives of Psychiatric Nursing 9: 216–224, 1995
34. Hellwig K: Psychiatric Home Care Nursing: Managing Patients in the Community Setting. J Psychosoc Nurs 31(12): 21–24, 1993
35. Hollander E, Wong CM: Body Dysmorphic Disorder, Pathological Gambling, and Sexual Compulsions. J Clin Psychiatry 56: 7–12, 1995
36. Hundley J, Sullivan CH, Coburn KL: Computerized EEG: Forming a Mental Image. J Psychosoc Nurs Ment Health Serv 28 (2): 19–23, 1990
37. Jahanshahi M, Jenkins IH, Brown RG, Marsden CD, Passingham RE, Brooks DJ: Self-Initiated Versus Externally Triggered Movements: I. An Investigation Using Measurement of Regional Cerebral Blood Flow with PET and Movement-Related Potentials in Normal and Parkinson's Disease Subjects. Brain 118: 913–933, 1995
38. Jefferson JW: Lithium: The Present and the Future. J Clin Psychiatry 56: 41–48, 1995
39. Judd L: Decade of the Brain and the New Psychiatry. Address given at University of California, San Diego, CA, 1992
40. Kallmann FJ: Heredity in Health and Mental Disorders. New York, Norton, 1953
41. Kallmann FJ: Twin and Sibship Study of Overt Male Homosexuality. Am J Human Genet 4: 136–146, 1952
42. Kiester E Jr: A Bug in the System. Discover 12 (2): 70–76, 1991
43. Kosten TR: Neurobiology of Abused Drugs: Opioids and Stimulants. J Nerv Ment Dis 178: 217–227, 1990
44. Krauss JB: Put the Community Back in Mental Health. Archives of Psychiatric Nursing 5: 1–2, 1991
45. Lapierre E, Berthot BD, Gurvitch M, Rees I, Kirch DG: Polydipsia and Hyponatremia in Psychiatric Patients: Challenge to Creative Nursing Care. Archives of Psychiatric Nursing 4: 87–92, 1990
46. Lendahl U, McKay RD: The Use of Cell Lines in Neurobiology. Trends in Neurosciences 13 (4): 132–137, 1990
47. Lieberman A: Intracerebral Transplantation in Parkinson's Disease. The American Parkinson Disease Association (APDA), pp 1, 4–5, Fall 1990
48. Lindenberg CS, Alexander EM, Gendrop SC, Nencioli M, Williams DG: A Review of the Literature on Cocaine Abuse in Pregnancy. Nursing Research 40: 69–75, 1991
49. Links PS, Steiner M, Huxley G: The Occurrence of Borderline Personality Disorder in the Families of Borderline Patients. J Pers Disorders 2 (1): 14–20, 1988
50. Lowery MC, Au WW, Adams PM, Whorton EB Jr, Legator MS: Male-Mediated Behavioral Abnormalities. Mutation Res 229: 231–239, 1990
51. Malone JA: Schizophrenia Research Update: Implications for Nursing. J Psychosoc Nurs 28 (8): 4–9, 1990
52. May DL: Patient Perceptions of Self-Induced Water Intoxication. Archives of Psychiatric Nursing 9: 295–304, 1995
53. Maziere B, Maziere M: Where Have We Got to with Neuroreceptor Mapping of the Human Brain? Eur J Nuclear Med 16: 817–835, 1990
54. McCain NL, Smith JC: Stress and Coping in the Context of Psychoneuroimmunology: A Holistic Framework for Nursing Practice and Research. Archives of Psychiatric Nursing 8: 221–227, 1994
55. McElroy SL, Keck PE Jr., Phillips KA: Kleptomania, Compulsive Buying, and Binge-Eating Disorder. J Clin Psychiatry 56 (Suppl 4): 14–26, 1995
56. McEnany GW: Psychobiological Indices of Bipolar Mood Disorder: Future Trends in Nursing Care. Archives of Psychiatric Nursing 4: 29–38, 1990
57. McLachlan DRC, Dalton AJ, Kruck TPA, Bell MY, Smith WL, Kalow W, Andrews DF: Intramuscular Desferrioxamine in Patients with Alzheimer's Disease. The Lancet 337: 1304–1308, 1991
58. Mental Disorders and Genetics: Bridging the Gap Between Research and Society. Washington, DC: U.S. Government Printing Office (Stock No. 052-003-01392-4), 1993
59. Miller BL, Lesser IM, Boone KB: Brain Lesions and Cognitive Function in Late-Life Psychosis. Br J Psychiatry 158: 76–82, 1991
60. Morin GD: Seasonal Affective Disorder, the Depression of Winter: A Literature Review and Description From a Nursing Perspective. Archives of Psychiatric Nursing 9: 182–187, 1990
61. Needleman HL, Schell A, Bellinger D, Levitron A, Allred EN: The Long-Term Effects of Exposure to Low Doses of Lead in Childhood. N Engl J Med 322 (2): 83–88, 1990
62. Norbeck JS, Chaftez L, Skodol-Wilson H, Weiss SJ: Social Support Needs of Family Caregivers of Psychiatric Patients from Three Age Groups. Nurs Res 40: 208–213, 1991
63. Olsen DP: Ethical Cautions in the Use of Outcomes for Resource Allocation in the Managed Care Environment of Mental Health. Archives of Psychiatric Nursing 9: 173–178, 1995
64. Pasquali EA: Learning to Laugh: Humor as Therapy. J Psychosoc Nurs Ment Health Serv 28 (3): 31–35, 1990
65. Pedersen NL, Gatz M, Plomin R, Nesselroade JR, McClearn GE: Individual Differences in Locus of Control During the Second Half of the Life Span for Identical and Fraternal Twins Reared Apart and Reared Together. J Gerontol Psychol Sci 44: P100–105, 1989
66. Peplau HE: Some Unresolved Issues in the Era of Biopsychosocial Nursing. J of the American Psychiatric Nurses Association 1: 92–96, 1995
67. Philipps LHC, O'Hara MW: Prospective Study of Postpartum Depression: 4?-Year Follow-Up of Women and Children. J Abnormal Psychol 100: 151–155, 1991
68. Phillips KA, McElroy SL, Hudson JI, Pope HG Jr.: Body Dysmorphic Disorder: An Obsessive-Compulsive Spectrum Disorder, a Form of Affective Spectrum Disorder, or Both? J Clin Psychiatry 56 (Suppl 4): 41–51, 1995
69. Plomin R: The Role of Inheritance in Behavior. Science 248 (4952): 183–188, 1990
70. Powell LH, Shaker LA, Jones BA, Vaccarino LV, Thorensen CE, Ratillo JR: Psychosocial Predictors of Mortality

in 83 Women with Premature Acute Myocardial Infarction. Psychosom Med 55: 426–433, 1993

71. Raine A: Murderers' Brains Found Different. Biol Psychiatry 28: 560–567, 1993
72. Raine A, Mednick SA: Biosocial Longitudinal Research into Antisocial Behavior. Rev Epidemiol Med Social et Sante Publique 37: 515–524, 1989
73. Reilly MM, Adams D, Booth DR, Davis MB, Said G, Laubriat-Bianchin M, Pepys MB, Thomas PK, Harding AE: Transthyretin Gene Analysis in European Patients with Suspected Familial Amyloid Polyneuropathy. Brain 118: 849–856, 1995
74. Reiss D, Plomin R, Hetherington EM: Genetics and Psychiatry: An Unheralded Window on the Environment. Am J Psychiatry 148: 283–291, 1991
75. Ribble DJ, Thelander B: Patients with Disordered Water Balance. J Psychosoc Nurs 32 (10): 35–42, 1994
76. Richards BS: Alzheimer's Disease: A Disabling Neurophysiological Disorder With Complex Nursing Implications. Archives of Psychiatric Nursing 9: 39–42, 1990
77. Richter JM, Roberto KA, Bottenberg DJ: Communicating with Persons with Alzheimer's Disease: Experiences of Family and Formal Caregivers. Archives of Psychiatric Nursing 9: 279–285, 1995
78. Rossen EK, Buschmann MBT: Mental Illness in Late Life: The Neurobiology of Depression. Archives of Psychiatric Nursing 9: 130–136, 1995
79. Schmitz A: Our Other Drug Problem. Health 5 (5): 24, 26, 28, 1991
80. Seeman MV: Schizophrenia in Women and Men. Current Approaches to Psychoses 4: 10–12, 1995
81. Simmons-Alling S: Genetic Implications for Major Affective Disorders. Archives of Psychiatric Nursing 4: 67–71, 1990
82. Solomon DA, Keitner GI, Miller IW, Shea MT, Keller MB: Course of Illness and Maintenance Treatments for Patients with Bipolar Disorder. J Clin Psychiatry 56: 5–13, 1995
83. Stein DJ, Simeon D, Cohen LJ, Hollander E: Trichotillomania and Obsessive-Compulsive Disorder. J Clin Psychiatry 56 (Suppl 4): 28–34, 1995
84. Stuhlmiller CM: The Construction of Disorders. J Psychosoc Nurs 33 (4): 20–23, 1995
85. Sullivan P, Pary R, Telang F, Rifai AH, Zubenko GS: Risk Factors for White Matter Changes Detected by Magnetic Resonance in the Elderly. Stroke 21: 1424–1428, 1990
86. Swanson B, Cronin-Stubbs D, Zeller JM, Kessler HA, Bieliauskas LA: Characterizing the Neuropsychological Functioning of Persons with Human Immunodeficiency Virus Infection, Part I. Acquired Immunodeficiency Syndrome Dementia Complex: A Review. Archives of Psychiatric Nursing 7: 74–81, 1993
87. Tesson BM: Who Are They? Identifying and Treating Adult Children of Alcoholics. J Psychosoc Nurs 28 (9): 16–21, 1990
88. Thompson MB, Coppens NM: The Effects of Guided Imagery on Anxiety Levels and Movement of Clients Undergoing Magnetic Resonance Imaging. Capsules & Comments in Psychiatric Nursing 1: 13, 1994
89. Turner DM: Panic Disorder: A Personal and Nursing Perspective. J Psychosoc Nurs 33 (4): 5–8, 1995
90. vonBernhardi R, Muller KJ: Repair of the Central Nervous System. J Neurobiol 27: 353–366, 1995
91. Warner R: Time Trends in Schizophrenia: Changes in Obstetric Risk Factors with Industrialization. Schizophr Bull 21: 483–500, 1995
92. Weinberger D: Neuroscientist Looks Inside the Brain. Address given at University of Michigan, September 16, 1992
93. Wilke J: From a Survivor. J Psychosoc Nurs 33 (4): 28–37, 1995
94. Wisner KL, Perel JM, Foglia JP: Serum Clomipramine and Metabolite Levels in Four Nursing Mother-Infant Pairs. J Clin Psychiatry 56: 17–20, 1995

The Process of Psychiatric-Mental Health Nursing

II

Assessment and Nursing Diagnosis

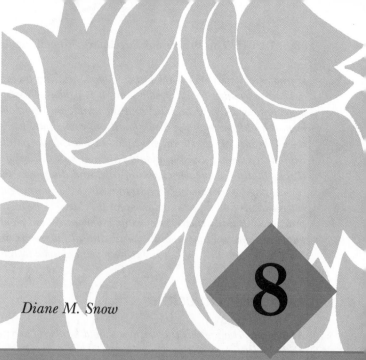

Diane M. Snow

Even as a melody is not composed of tones, nor a verse of words, nor a statue of lines—one must pull and tear to turn a unity into a multiplicity—so it is with the human being I say You. I can abstract from him the color of his hair or the color of his speech in the color of his graciousness; I have to do this again and again; but immediately he is no longer You.

Martin Buber,
I and Thou, *1958*

It has been said and written scores of times, that every woman makes a good nurse. I believe, on the contrary, that the very elements of nursing are all but unknown.

Florence Nightingale,
Notes on Nursing: What It Is and What It Is Not

Psychosocial assessment is the first step of the nursing process used in psychiatric-mental health care. It is a holistic assessment process designed to collect and organize data about the mental health needs of the client, family, or community using sound theoretical and ethical principles. Combining the results with other relevant assessment data culminates in clinical decisions that are the problems, foci of care, and diagnoses, the second stage of the nursing process, that direct the planning of interventions and expected outcomes for the client. If the nurse practices culturally effective communication, interview, observational, and assessment skills, sound clinical judgments are likely to be made to help the client move toward optimal health.

Learning Objectives

At the completion of this chapter, you should be able to accomplish the following:

1. *Define the term psychosocial assessment.*
2. *Distinguish the types and purpose of data and assessment used in clinical situations.*
3. *Describe various tools of psychosocial assessment.*
4. *Discuss the importance of the relationship aspect of the interview in the assessment process.*
5. *Describe the role and expectations of the nurse-interviewer.*
6. *Identify stages and other structural aspects of the interview.*
7. *Apply a focused assessment approach to structure a psychosocial assessment.*
8. *Compare methods of recording assessment data.*
9. *Identify the steps of analysis leading to the nursing diagnosis.*
10. *Formulate a client problem list based on analysis of data into diagnostic hypotheses.*
11. *Define nursing diagnosis within the context of the nursing process, and describe various ways to write diagnoses.*
12. *Explain the use of a taxonomy in writing an accurate nursing diagnosis.*
13. *Explain the use of the five axes of the fourth edition of the Diagnostic and Statistical Manual of Mental Disorders' (DSM-IV) classification of psychiatric diagnoses.*

◆ Assessment

Assessment is defined as gathering, classifying, categorizing, analyzing, and documenting client information about health status; it forms the basis of nursing care planning. Assessment data are derived from data collection, interview, and behavioral observation and validated, when possible, by the client.[2] *Psychosocial assessment* is the term used for assessment of psychological, sociological, developmental, spiritual, and cultural data commonly derived from interviews with a client. Often standardized psychosocial assessment tools are used to provide a basis for treatment decisions and as a baseline for measuring change in behavior or function.

The nurse exercises professional judgment to determine the depth of the assessment of client functioning and to choose the methods of gathering needed data, especially data that include sensitive or emotionally laden topics. Physical assessment data, laboratory data, and relevant chart data are used as part of a holistic assessment. The nurse assesses the client autonomously and collaboratively with other members of the health care team to gather the most comprehensive data base.

TYPES OF DATA

When conducting a thorough assessment of the psychiatric client, it is important to include subjective and objective data. Subjective data include the client's perspective of a situation or series of events, feelings, ideas about oneself, and personal health status in the client's own words.[15] Actual quotes are used to capture the significance of the client's problem or situation that caused him or her to seek help. It is important to accept whatever is reported and then note any inconsistencies or incongruencies that may be explored further.[10]

Objective data include observations, signs, laboratory and chart data,[9] and findings from diagnostic testing and the physical examination.[10] Change in vital signs during detoxification from drugs and alcohol is an example of objective data.

Historical data focus on the past, and current data deal with the present. A lack of historical information may be of significance, for example, when sexual abuse has caused subsequent amnesia for the first several years of a client's life. Current data deal with the present situation. Clients with dementia or delirium may not be able to provide relevant current data. Secondary data sources that support primary sources may be family or friends and chart reviews.

ASSESSMENT IN VARIOUS HEALTH CARE SETTINGS

The setting of a nursing assessment does not necessarily determine the focus of the assessment. A purposeful, comprehensive psychosocial assessment should be conducted in all health care settings; the nurse should collect and analyze information not always identified as problematic for the client at that time. In today's world of managed care health systems and case management, accurate assessments collected in a timely manner are required in home health; outpatient, school-based, and other clinics; homeless programs; and inpatient programs. The goals of prevention and early identification of mental health problems and helping return a mentally ill client to a functional status as quickly as possible necessitate thorough, focused data collection.

TYPES OF ASSESSMENT

The type of assessment used in a particular situation is determined by the nature of the client's history, current problems, and other individual needs. Using a standardized format while maintaining flexibility is important. For example, the nurse approaches a client who is grieving over the loss of a parent differently than a client who presents with severe memory loss and paranoia. Various purposes, goals, objectives, and methods distinguish assessments.

A *comprehensive assessment* includes a complete psychosocial and cultural nursing history, physical examination, and general information about the client. The demands of today's health care delivery services with pressure to decrease length of stay, even in community settings, require a rapid, comprehensive assessment.[2]

A second type of assessment is a *focused assessment*, which includes information concerning a particular problem with subjective and objective data systematically collected and analyzed. This is often done in a crisis situation, such as following a suicide attempt. Analysis involves exploring the nature and intensity of the problem, time and context of the problem, situations that intensify the feelings or problem, associated problems, and the meaning of the problem to the person.

A third type of assessment is a *screening assessment*, in which a specific screening tool or protocol is used to evaluate a particular health problem, such as tardive dyskinesia, in a client on neuroleptic medications. Finally, ongoing assessments are performed on clients to keep the data base and interventions current.[9]

HOLISTIC ASSESSMENT

Based on an understanding of the holistic nature of people, the nurse assesses all aspects of the client's life and experience. This includes spiritual, biological, psychological, social, cultural, cognitive, and behavioral experiences. Even if the client's problems, such as the mood problems of depression, appear to dominate, the nurse gathers assessment data in all areas. Specific potential problem areas that emerge as most significant to the nurse, client, and situation can then be further explored. These may also include physiological complications from the psychiatric problem, such as respiratory distress from heavy cigarette smoking in the schizophrenic client. The nurse should be sensitive to cues, verbal or nonverbal, and to focus questions on these issues rather than waiting for the client to broach the subject directly.[7]

This approach involves broad questions that explore the client's cultural, spiritual, social, cognitive, behavioral, biological, and psychological norms and expectations. Cues and reported data help the nurse and client focus on more specific questions, concerns, and problems.[6]

◆ Special Considerations: Age, Cultural Background, and Physical Health Status

Priorities in the assessment process vary according to client factors that represent special needs, such as age, cultural background, and physical health condition. Briefer assessment tools are used when assessing the elderly client, with greater emphasis placed on observation of the client rather than on information obtained during the interview. Assessment of children requires increased attention to observation of the child's interaction, communication, and play.

The client's sociocultural group also determines priorities in assessment. Client *norms*, or expected behavior and experience in life situations, guide the nurse's assessment, analysis, and diagnosis of client problems and needs. In particular, cultural background may greatly affect a client's responses to questions in the interview, in psychological examinations, or on the mental status examination. Words are used differently in different cultures. Priorities and values differ, and these differences affect clients' answers in areas such as judgment, insight, and general interpretations. Clients from some cultures appear more passive than the nurse might expect yet are within the normal range for their cultures. In general, the nurse must be cautious when deriving conclusions without the benefit of consultation with someone familiar with the client's culture.[5] For the most part, psychological tests and psychiatric rating scales are developed for the white, Anglo-Saxon, Protestant client.

ASSESSMENT TOOLS

The nurse gathers assessment information using various structural approaches and perspectives of inquiry, called *assessment tools*. A comprehensive psychosocial assessment necessitates the use of several tools; many different perspectives are provided by an interdisciplinary mental health team. Within the team, nurses administer some of these assessment tools, interpret the results, formulate a list of client problems and nursing diagnoses, and plan and evaluate nursing interventions. Psychologists administer psychological tests, analyze the test results, and formulate a diagnostic impression from their disciplinary perspective. Other disciplines also use assessment tools to gather essential client data.

HEALTH HISTORY

The client's historical data are collected in a holistic assessment. The depth of the health history is determined by the problem area and the purpose of the assessment. The history's functions are to form a background against which current client functioning may be measured and to gain an understanding of the client's past, present, and potential functioning. Objectives of the history follow:

1. To describe adaptive and maladaptive patterns of behavior
2. To formulate priorities of care
3. To identify client problems and analyze client data in the proper context
4. To consider the client's probable responses to potential therapeutic interventions
5. To analyze the client's perception of the world, health, and illness

The history-taking format chosen by a discipline is generally consistent with its philosophy and approach. A nursing history, for example, focuses on the problems and needs of the client and gathers information to assist in nursing care planning in health and illness adaptation. A *nursing history* form is a vehicle for organizing and recording client information before, during, and after the interview. The sample questions and general categories of examination should be adapted to the client's personality, needs, wishes, and level of communication.[20] Box 8-1 offers a general guide to client assessment, and Box 8-2 provides an example of a nursing assessment of a particular client.

SCREENING AND PSYCHOLOGICAL TESTING

With the changes in health care now focusing on self-regulation or self-management, there is a focus on specific symptom management using formalized testing and evaluation.[17] To provide the necessary detailed assessments to determine the focus of interventions in psychiatric-mental health care, specific symptoms, behaviors, and assets are being identified though circumscribed assessments and formal measurement. Areas that are often appraised with this type of formal testing include depression, anxiety, self-esteem, sleep patterns, and social adjustment.[17] More specialized assessment data may be needed, and the nurse may refer the client for more specialized testing and evaluation.

The nurse may encourage clients to self-monitor and assess their progress through the use of such screening tools as life-stress scales and assertiveness scales.[26] Many self-assessment scales center on clients' wellness and strengths, and help them identify and interpret their own personalities, perceptions, anxieties, coping patterns, and needs. Standardized assessments by the nurse that can be quantified provide for systematic treatment selection and documentation of change.[1] Some that are useful with psychiatric clients include the Brief Psychiatric Rating Scale, which requires a semi-structured interview format; the Symptom Distress Checklist 90-R, which measures subjective distress; the Psychological Well Being Scale, which is appropriate for nonpsychiatric settings; and the Target Complaints Scale, which identifies symptoms the client wants to change.[19]

Screening tools, also called rating instruments, that are used with children have the advantage of helping the child admit to symptoms that are not revealed in the interview. Also, symptoms can be monitored over time through rating instruments. Examples of screening tools used with children include the Children's Depression Rating Scale, which predicts major depression with a score above 40, and the Child Behavior Checklist, which is completed by the parent.[23]

Psychological testing, usually done by a licensed clinical psychologist, is also a structured and systematic process of observing and describing specific behaviors through the use of a numeric or category system.[27] The usefulness of such tests depends on their proper administration and the accurate interpretation of the test results. The significance of psychological test results depends on the degree of agreement of several assessment tools (eg, a battery of psychological tests administered in conjunction with a diagnostic interview and history taking).

The three general categories of psychological tests are projective tests, personality inventories, and intelligence tests.

Projective Tests

The projective test is designed to reveal the structure of the client's mind by focusing on verbalized projections onto ambiguous figures. Projective tests identify patterns of thinking but are not standardized, objective, or predictive of behavior in actual situations.[27]

Personality Inventories

Personality inventories are standardized, objective tests (usually in the form of a questionnaire) that measure attitudes, inhibitions, and action tendencies. The liabilities of personality inventories lie in the limited re-

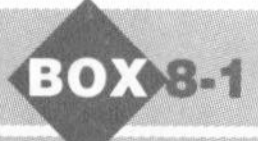

Guide to Client Assessment

Sharon Byers, RN, MSN, CS, Clinical Nurse Specialist, Children and Family Services Department, Minneapolis, MN

DEMOGRAPHIC DATA

Name	Height
Age	Weight
Sex	Date of admission
Marital status	Admitting diagnosis
Religion	

CLIENT'S PERCEPTIONS AND EXPECTATIONS

How does the client define the problem and its cause?
What are the client's expectations of treatment?
What is the length of time the client expects to be involved in treatment?
What are the client's discharge plans?

HISTORY AND EXAMINATION

Sociocultural Data

Occupation
Education
Race, national origin, other cultural data
People living with client
Availability of family or significant others
Client's view of society and world
Recent loss or change in social space, role, habits
Leisure-time activities
Use of tobacco, alcohol, and other drugs

Sexual Data

Is client satisfied with his or her sexual activity and identity?
What is the effect of current problems on sexual functioning?

Medical Data

Allergies
Previous major illnesses, surgeries, and hospitalizations
Medications taken regularly
Review of systems
- Sensory
- Musculoskeletal
- Circulatory
- Integumentary
- Respiratory
- Gastrointestinal
- Urinary
- Reproductive
- Neurological: mental status and thought content and form

continued

BOX 8-1 (Continued)

Spiritual Needs

Religious preference
Spiritual beliefs and practices
Sense of higher power or driving force outside of self

Basic Needs

Dietary preferences, habits, allergies, and restrictions
Rest, sleep, comfort
Personal hygiene
Elimination habits and needs
Psychosocial

General Observation

Appearance
Posture
Gait
Dress
Jewelry, makeup
Facial expression
Behavior
Motor activity
Eye contact
Purposeful or goal-directed actions
Communication
Verbal (rate, pace, flow of speech)
Nonverbal (gestures, body language)
Clarity of communication
Communication of feelings
Communication with family and significant others

SUMMARY

Client functioning and problems
Identified needs and resources
Suggested interventions

sponse choices offered by these tests and the artificial nature of the situation in which the questions are asked. They are normally culturally biased. Nevertheless, these tests are reliable indicators of thought patterns and potential behavior.

Intelligence Tests

Intelligence tests measure intellectual functioning on verbal and nonverbal levels. These tests are standardized according to age but usually do not take into account sociocultural influences on the individual's vocabulary and reasoning. The purpose of administering intelligence tests to a psychiatric-mental health client is to determine the role of intellectual functioning on the development and existence of the problem.

FAMILY ASSESSMENT

The evaluation of family structure, function, and development is a key part of a complete psychosocial evaluation. This information can be used to determine family variables that contribute to the problems of individuals. The response of the individual to family relationships and other factors in the system gives the nurse data that may help to explain the client's signs and symptoms. Overall, the health of the family may be enhanced through careful history taking and observations of communication patterns, rules and roles within the family, how the family adapts to life cycle changes, and the perception of different family members about the problems within the family. The

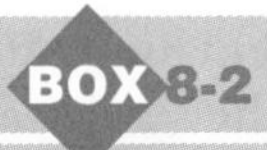

Summary of Nursing Assessment: Mrs. EM

Sharon Byers, RN, MSN, CS, Clinical Nurse Specialist, Children and Family Services Department, Minneapolis, MN

Mrs. EM, a 48-year-old widow, is seen in her apartment by the psychiatric home health nurse following a call requesting services for extreme anxiety and depression. The client has no prior mental health history of treatment but states that she has "always been nervous."

Mrs. EM described the following symptoms: difficulty breathing when getting on a city bus, overwhelming thoughts of being "closed in" when with large groups of people, difficulty sleeping, and reduced appetite. The more dramatic symptoms began 2 months ago, which was about 6 months after her husband's sudden death of a heart attack.

Mrs. EM states she has three children who are supportive and who all live close to her, and several long-time friends with whom she has lost contact since her husband's death. She works in computer software sales and states that her sales have been down for the last 8 months. She is somewhat worried about keeping her job.

Mrs. EM's affect is flat, and her mood seems depressed. She describes obsessive thinking regarding her work, her children, her financial future, and the loss of her husband. She is completely oriented, with memory intact and a good fund of knowledge. She appears capable of appropriate abstract and concrete thought. She reports early morning awakening and frequent crying when alone. She feels "somewhat hopeless" and helpless. She denies suicidal ideation but admits she wishes she were dead "sometimes."

Mrs. EM has no current physical difficulties. She underwent an appendectomy at age 20. A physical examination 3 weeks ago showed that all findings were normal. She reports decreased energy but no physical basis for this symptom.

Mrs. EM was born in Denver, Colorado, the third of six children (three boys and three girls). She states that she had "a pleasant childhood," with no history of mental illness or abuse in her family.

She completed high school and college, receiving a degree in computer science after returning to school when her children were in high school. She married at age 20 and considers her marriage a good one. She did state that her husband took care of all the "household business" and that this responsibility has "overwhelmed" her after his death.

The client appears to be an intelligent, 48-year-old woman in some acute distress, with symptoms of depression and anxiety. Her children are supportive, but she has not developed a good support system outside the family. Her strengths are her intelligence, her past success in her job, and her supportive family. Her liabilities include a lack of an independent approach to the world, a lack of a full support system, and diminished coping with anxiety and grief-produced depression.

DIAGNOSTIC IMPRESSION

Dysfunctional Grieving related to absence of anticipatory grief, evidenced by alterations in concentration and pursuit of tasks

Social Isolation related to depressed mood, evidenced by seeking to be alone and a sad, dull affect

Sleep Pattern Disturbance related to depressed mood, evidenced by early morning awakening and inability to go back to sleep nurse must remain objective and neutral during the interview with the family.

The most common family assessment tool used by psychiatric-mental health nurses is the genogram. In a genogram, a family map is drawn for three generations, and health, culture, religion, mental illness, addiction, and other patterns are assessed. Not only can the nurse use the genogram as a valuable assessment tool, but clients can be taught how to complete the genogram themselves as a therapeutic activity.[12] (see Chapter 17, Families and Family Therapy).

MENTAL STATUS EXAMINATION

The mental status examination (MSE) is an integral tool for assessing objective data in the psychosocial assessment. It includes data about appearance and level of consciousness; motor status and behavior; attitude; intellectual functioning; speech; cognitive status, including attention and concentration; orientation; memory; language and communication; judgment and abstraction; content of thought; affect and mood; and insight. This examination aims to identify psychoneurological status and deviations from the norm. It is particularly useful in identifying cognitive changes, such as memory, orientation, attention, and concentration.

A standardized MSE tool provides a quantifiable measure of function. An example includes the Folstein Mini Mental Status Exam (Box 8-3). These tools are useful in providing data to determine whether dementia or depression are present in an elderly person who is having difficulty with memory. As with all assessment tools, the significance of the results of the MSE can be understood only in relation to the client's history, sociocultural status, and physical condition. The nurse should adapt sample questions and general categories of examination to the client's cultural background, personality, needs, wishes, and level of communication. It is helpful, before beginning the MSE, to reassure the client that these are routine questions. The nurse should not correct a wrong answer unless it may be helpful in testing recall memory during the examination. Box 8-4 outlines various categories and approaches of the MSE.

STRENGTHS AND RESOURCES

Client *strengths* can be reported by the client or assessed by the nurse and validated by the client or family. It is well known that there are healthy parts of any personality; the nurse should always assume a level of competence in the client.[28] Examples of strengths include intelligence, education, support systems, religious or spiritual beliefs, motivation, and physical health.

Assessment of strengths and assets can be used in goal setting and implementation. Most clients will appreciate the validation they receive from identifying these attributes. When the client is unable to participate because of difficulty with thought processes, the nurse can gain this information from the family and from daily observations of the client. For example, a client with suspicious behavior may have high-level intelligence, good physical health, a stable job, and a positive body image. These strengths may be the balancing factors that enable the client to recover from this episode and move quickly along the mental health–mental illness continuum toward a higher level of functioning.

The *resources* available to the client are important to overall coping. These external factors may include social support networks, such as family and friends; financial resources; transportation; community resources; church; or school. The client's history of using potential resources is important when planning nursing interventions to help the client gain access to these resources.

THE INTERVIEW

The most important assessment tool is the interview process. The focused assessment method of structuring the interview ensures that no essential information is overlooked; it also gives clients an opportunity to tell their stories in response to open-ended questions. The interviewer's sensitivity and skill can be developed through training. The crucial element in the psychiatric-mental health interview is the human element—spontaneity, warmth, empathy, and caring. Box 8-5 provides a guide for conducting a client interview.

Conducting the Interview

The *interview* is a purposeful, goal-directed interaction in which the nurse builds an alliance with the client while collecting data for assessment. To foster the development of this alliance, the nurse maintains a nonjudgmental attitude and responds to self-disclosure with honesty, support, and acceptance.[7] The basis for a successful interview is trust, rapport, and respect between the nurse and client.[13] Connecting with the client in this way is a valued aspect of nursing in which the relationship actually becomes an assessment strategy.

The *content,* or factual part, of the interview and the *process,* or relational aspects, are continually observed by the nurse. Clients should be allowed to disclose at their own rate and in whatever manner is comfortable for them. The nurse must attend to the cues that indicate the client's preferences for timing (when to discuss what topic), pacing (how fast or slow to proceed with the data gathering), expectations, and needs. Verbal and nonverbal cues are assessed using knowledge of normal and dysfunctional behaviors.[13] The nurse pro-

(text continues on page 109)

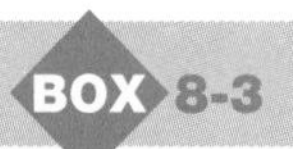

Mini-Mental State Examination

Maximum score 30, Score < 20 suggests significant cognitive impairment.

I. Orientation (Maximum score 10)

Ask "What is today's date?" Then ask specifically for parts omitted; eg, "Can you also tell what season it is?"

Ask "Can you tell me the name of this hospital?"
"What floor are we on?"
"What town (or city) are we in?"
"What county are we in?"
"What state are we in?"

Date (eg, January 21)	1 ____
Year	2 ____
Month	3 ____
Day (eg, Monday)	4 ____
Season	5 ____
Hospital	6 ____
Floor	7 ____
Town	8 ____
County	9 ____
State	10 ____

II. Registration (Maximum score 3)
Ask the subject if you may test his/her memory. Then say "Ball," "Flag," "Tree," clearly and slowly, about one second for each. After you have said all 3 words, ask subject to repeat them. This first repetition determines the score (0–3) but keep saying them (up to 6 trials) until the subject can repeat all 3 words. If he/she does not eventually learn all three, recall cannot be meaningfully tested

"Ball"	11 ____
"Flag"	12 ____
"Tree"	13 ____

Record number of trials ______

III. Attention and calculation (Maximum score 5)
Ask the subject to begin at 100 and count backward by 7. Stop after 5 subtractions (93, 86, 79, 72, 65). Score one point for each number

"93"	14 ____
"86"	15 ____
"79"	16 ____
"72"	17 ____
"65"	18 ____

If the subject cannot or will not perform this task, ask him/her to spell the word "world" backwards (D, L, R, O, W). The score is one point for each correctly placed letter, eg, DLROW = 5, DLORW = 3. Record how the subject spelled "world" backwards: ______________________

OR

Number of correctly placed letters	19 ____

IV. Recall (Maximum score 3)
Ask the subject to recall the three words you previously asked him/her to remember (learned in Registration)

"Ball"	20 ____
"Flag"	21 ____
"Tree"	22 ____

V. Language (Maximum score 9)
Naming: Show the subject a wrist watch and ask "What is this?" Repeat for pencil. Score one point for each item named correctly
Repetition: Ask the subject to repeat, "No ifs, ands, or buts." Score one point for correct repetition
3-Stage Command: Give the subject a piece of blank paper and say, "Take the paper in your right hand, fold it in half and put it on the floor." Score one point for each action performed correctly.
Reading: On a blank piece of paper, print the sentence, "Close your eyes," in letters large enough for the subject to see clearly. Ask subject to read it and do what it says. Score correctly only if he/she actually closes his/her eyes.
Writing: Give the subject a blank piece of paper and ask him/her to write a sentence. It is to be written spontaneously. It must contain a subject and verb and make sense. Correct grammar and punctuation are not necessary.
Copying: On a clean piece of paper, draw intersecting pentagons, each side about an inch, and ask subject to copy it exactly as it is. All 10 angles must be present and two must intersect to score 1 point. Tremor and rotation are ignored

Watch	23 ____
Pencil	24 ____
Repetition	25 ____
Takes in right hand	26 ____
Folds in half	27 ____
Puts on floor	28 ____
Closes eyes	29 ____
Writes sentence	30 ____
Draws pentagons	31 ____

Eg.
Score: Add number of correct responses. In section III include items 14–18 or item 19, not both. (Maximum total score 30)
Rate subject's level of consciousness: ______ (a) coma, (b) stupor, (c) drowsy, (d) alert

Total score ______________

Reprinted with permission from Folstein, M. F., Folstein, F. E., and McHugh, P. R. (1975) Mini-mental state: a practical method for grading the cognitive state of patients for the clinician. Journal of Psychiatric Research 12 189–198.

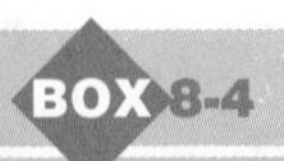

Mental Status Examination

The following general categories should be explored during the mental status examination. Suggestions for pursuing each area are included.

Appearance. General appearance, grooming, motor behavior, mannerisms, posture, gait (Assess through general observations, and record as a general impression.)

Behavior. Speech patterns, tone of voice, use of slang, flow of speech, eye contact, body language, general behavioral responses to others and environment (Assess through general observation; compare findings to the client's usual behavior.)

Orientation. Awareness of reality of person, place, time, situation, relationship with others (Assess through direct questioning.)

Memory. Immediate recall, recent memory, remote memory (Assess through direct questioning.)

Sensorium. Ability to attend and concentrate; perception of stimuli—internal and external (Assess through direct questioning.)

Perceptual processes. Processing of information received through sensorium; includes awareness of self and one's thoughts, reality, and fantasy (Assess by asking questions about delusions, illusions, and hallucinations.)

Mood and affect. Mood—the prevailing emotion displayed; affect—the range of emotion displayed (happy, sad, unchanging); emotion—subjective physiological changes in response to thoughts and perceptions (Assess through observation, and judge the appropriateness of the behavior in relation to the client's usual behavior.)

Intellectual functioning. General fund of knowledge; cognitive abilities, such as the ability to calculate simple arithmetic problems; ability to abstract, or think symbolically and according to categories of association (Assess through direct questioning, such as requesting the client to solve simple math problems or interpret a simple proverb or analogy.)

Thought content. Recurrences of topics of thinking, themes of conversation (Assess by observing what the client discusses spontaneously in conversation.)

Thought processes. Stream of conscious or mental activity, as indicated in speech (Observe for rate, flow, associations made, and ability to pursue a topic logically.)

Insight. Awareness of one's own responsibilities and abilities, especially regarding the current area of concern; ability to analyze problem with objectivity (Ask the client to explain the current problem.)

Judgment. Decision-making abilities, especially regarding delaying gratification for an ultimate gain; style—impulsive, rational, methodological, or trial-and-error (Assess by asking the client what he or she would do in dilemmas requiring important decisions involving personal welfare, such as if he or she inherited a large sum of money or smelled smoke in a theater.

(From Crary WG, Johnson CW: The Mental Status Exam. In Johnson CW, Snibbe JR, Evans LE (eds): Basic Psychopathology: A Programmed Text, pp 50–89. New York, Spectrum, 1975. Also from Margolin C: Assessment of Psychiatric Patients. J Emerg Nurs 6 (July–August): 30–33, 1980.)

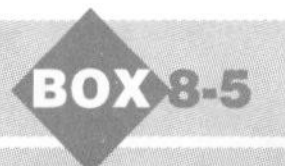

Interview Guide

The following sample questions are intended to aid the nurse in posing appropriate questions during the interview. The nurse relies on overall understanding of the client and the context of the interview to determine specific wording for questions. Remember that open-ended questions will facilitate the interview with higher-functioning clients. However, the more disorganized client may be more comfortable and more cooperative with closed-ended, "yes or no," or short-answer questions. A closed-ended question can introduce a subject as pertinent for the client and be followed by a "tell me about it" question to gain more information.

INTRODUCTORY PHASE

What do you see as the primary problem that brought you here? Why did you decide to seek help at this time? What areas of your life are particularly stressful, and what areas are easy for you now? What kinds of support do you have now? Do you see friends or family regularly? What do they say about the current situation or your coming here? Are finances a problem now? What goals do you have for your life in general and for your experience here? What do you expect from a counselor (or from a hospitalization or treatment experience)? How do you expect us to go about helping you?

WORKING PHASE

Psychological

Have you been having problems thinking clearly lately? How does this problem relate to other problems you've had in the past? Is there a pattern? Is this similar to conflicts with parents in the past? Have there been a lot of changes in your life lately? How do you see yourself now? Has this situation affected your self-esteem?

Social

Are you spending as much time with other people as usual? Are other people responding to you differently now? Have your most significant or intimate relationships changed lately? How do your friends feel about your situation now?

Biological

Have any family members had this kind of problem? Has anyone in your family been hospitalized for a psychiatric illness? Have your eating and sleeping habits changed lately? Have you been feeling unusually sad or happy lately? Have you had unusual experiences that were hard to explain to others? Do your thoughts seem to be moving more slowly or faster than usual? Have there been some thoughts you can't seem to control? How are you feeling physically? Are you feeling pressured by expectations of others? How often (and how much) do you drink alcohol? Do you use any other drugs? Do you have any drug- or alcohol-related problems? What prescription drugs are you on now?

Behavioral

Are there any specific behaviors that always cause you problems? Are there any behaviors you cannot seem to control but would like to stop? Do you feel compelled to do some behaviors you really don't want to do?

How do other people seem to respond to you? Does it seem easy for you to make friends?

Cognitive

Do you tend to fuss at yourself in your head? What kinds of things do you tell yourself about this situation? Are you critical of yourself? What do you think about your ability to get along in this world? How do you think things are going in the world today? Do you feel other people are responsible for your problems today? Does it seem like you act according to your values or other influences?

Cultural

How is your life now different from your parents' lives when you were growing up? Do your family and older friends have trouble understanding you now? How do people from your former culture respond to this sort of problem? How do they explain or make sense of this sort of situation?

Spiritual

Do you believe in a higher power or supreme being? What's your relationship with this being or power like? How does your religion make sense of problems in the world today or of your situation now?

continued

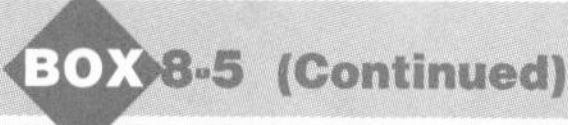
BOX 8-5 (Continued)

MENTAL STATUS EXAM

Orientation

Have you been having trouble realizing where you are or what's around you? Would you tell me where you are now?

Memory

Can you remember what you had for breakfast today? What did you do yesterday? Can you remember what I said my name was? What was the name of the high school from which you graduated.

Sensorium

Do you have trouble concentrating or focusing your thoughts? Can you watch a movie or read a book and follow it through? Do you have trouble keeping up in conversations?

Perceptual

Can you see or hear things that other people do not know are there? Do you have unusual abilities or experiences often now? Are there things you believe that other people say are all wrong? Do you believe people are trying to hurt you? Does it seem easy lately to mistake one thing for another, like a shadow for a man?

Mood and Affect

What has your mood been like lately? Are you more or less emotional than usual?

Intellectual Fund

What is the governor's name? Can you think of one big item in the new lately? Would you please subtract 7 from 100 and keep going with that until I ask you to stop?

What does it mean when people say "Don't cry over spilled milk"?

Thought Content

Are there certain subjects you think about a lot or almost all the time lately?

Thought Processes

Are your thoughts moving more slowly or quickly than usual? Does it seem as if your mind just goes blank lately? Do you have trouble keeping up with your thoughts or understanding your thoughts?

Insight

What do you think the real problem is that resulted in your being here today? How do you make sense of this whole situation now?

Judgment

What would you do if a policeman stopped you for speeding? What would you do if you received a $10,000 check in the mail, just for you to use?

HISTORY

How many brothers and sisters do you have? Where were you born? What were your parents like when you were young? What is your earliest memory? Did you enjoy grade school? How were your grades? Did you play with other children a lot? What was it like at home? What was it like in junior high? What kinds of things did you like to do? Were your grades okay? Did you get into any trouble at school? What were you like in high school? Did you date? How were your grades? Did you use any chemicals? Did you get into trouble a lot? How was it at home? Did you keep your friends from grade school? What did you do after graduation? When was your first significant intimate relationship? When was your first real job? What kinds of jobs have you had? How did you do with your jobs? Have you ever had this sort of problem before? Have you ever had any other emotional problems severe enough to warrant seeking help? Have you had any hospitalization? Do you have contact with family now? Do any family members have a history of psychiatric illness?

TERMINATION PHASE

Are there any other things you would like to tell me that would help me understand you better? Do you have any responses to this interview? Can you tell me what this was like for you? What questions do you have for me?

vides a comfortable environment, uses eye contact, and concentrates on the client's responses with minimal notetaking.[24] The information gathered in a nursing assessment should be treated as confidential.

Skills of the Nurse-Interviewer

A client usually prefers an active, friendly interviewer who verbalizes minimally and uses effective communication techniques.[20] The functions of communication techniques during the interview are to assist the client to make transitions in thinking, to label amorphous experiences, and to gain a clearer understanding of the situation.

The key elements in facilitative communication include active listening and attending skills. *Active listening* concerns the nurse's focused interest in verbal and nonverbal communication, being alert and open without projecting one's own values and ideas on the client, and being empathetic in an active listening response of summarizing what the client is perceived to be saying, reflecting a feeling, and verifying the perception with the client. For example, the nurse might say "It sounds as if you are feeling frustrated and angry about the lack of respect you receive from your teenagers. Is that correct?" The acronym SOLER is used to describe *attending behavior* as sitting squarely, openness, leaning forward, eye contact, and relatively relaxed posture.

Other techniques of facilitative communication are *concreteness* (ie, the interviewer's specificity of communication and persistence in requesting the client to describe feelings and events in specific terms), and *immediacy* (the interviewer's ability to recognize feelings and thoughts of immediate importance to the client and to deal with those issues first).

Experiential and didactic confrontations facilitate authentic relationships. A didactic confrontation occurs when the interviewer objectively offers the client relevant information to correct misinformation. Experiential confrontation involves the nurse's consistently pointing out discrepancies and generalizations in the client's conversation as they occur; this provides firsthand and immediate feedback (see Chapter 6, Communication).[20]

Client Expectations of the Interviewer

Client expectations influence the interview process. The preferred image of the nurse interviewer is that of an expert who is confident in personal and professional roles. The client prefers the professional who conveys warmth and authentic concern while maintaining emotional objectivity. This quality of *emotional objectivity* is the ability to express feelings and responses about the client in a professional and nonjudgmental manner.[4]

The nurse is expected to be competent at starting an interview and keeping the flow of conversation moving. Clients expect the nurse-interviewer to be knowledgeable about human behavior and to interpret *their* behavior, in particular, within the proper context. Clients also expect the interviewer to realize that each client is an expert on himself or herself.[4] Nurses should recognize their powerful position, the client's relative dependency, and the importance of ethics and self-responsibility in accepting the trust of clients. The effects of an interview may be therapeutic or deleterious. A personal and professional code of ethics guides the nurse's actions in the following ways:

1. The nurse does not engage in social, physical, or business contacts with the client.
2. The nurse respects the client's right to confidentiality.
3. The nurse determines when it is necessary to refer a client to another professional.
4. The nurse accepts the role of client advocate and teaches and supports the client regarding mental health care rights.

Finally, the mental health professional is aware that clients seldom fit the ideal image (ie, the energetic, verbal, motivated partner in the interview process). To work effectively with an uncooperative client, the psychiatric-mental health care nurse must find areas of motivation and nurture them (Box 8-6).

Stages of the Interview

Introductory Stage. The *introductory stage* of the interview consists of the client and interviewer introducing themselves, stating their goals and expectations, and discussing the purposes of the interview. During this initial stage, the interviewer scans the client, gathers superficial information about the problem, and makes general observations of the client.

Working Stage. The second stage of the interview is the *middle or working phase.* This stage begins when the client permits a serious pursuit of the problem, to which the interviewer responds with therapeutic skills of problem identification or clarification. During this phase, the nurse-interviewer focuses in depth on the emergence and development of the problem, the extent of disruption caused by the problem, and the client's approaches to the problem thus far. The nurse also assesses the strengths and resources of the client and begins to consider possible intervention strategies.

During the working phase, the nurse and client influence each other; a process of change occurs in both. This is the enactment of the participant-observer role.[14] The middle stage of the interview concludes with an exploration of all potential problems not previously examined.

Termination Stage or Closure. The *termination stage* of the interview begins with a reminder to the client that

BOX 8-6

Motivational Factors and Restraining Forces

SOURCES OF MOTIVATION

To get well
To return home
To feel safe
To find new friends
To stay sober or straight
To solve problems
To have relief from physical pain
To stay in control
To improve a relationship
To decrease medication
To be more productive

RESTRAINING FORCES

Fear of confinement
Loss of freedom
Mistrust
Fear of abandonment
Anxiety
Fear of responsibility
Fear of independence
Fear of reality
Lack of knowledge
Lack of purpose in life
Fear of rejection

the interview will soon be ending. This reminder should be given 5 to 10 minutes before the interview is scheduled to end. The interviewer then reviews and summarizes what has been accomplished and asks the client to add, clarify, or correct information reviewed. The need for follow-up sessions or referrals to other professionals is suggested at that time.

Finally, in recognition of the difficulty clients endure in revealing so much of themselves and their experiences, nurse-interviewers should inform the client that they appreciate the client's cooperation and intrinsic worth. This should consist of a positive and entirely truthful statement that gives clients something that helps them feel better because of the interview.

◆ Nursing Diagnosis

Diagnosing is a cognitive process using skills of critical thinking, problem solving, and analysis. This second step of the nursing process focuses on data analysis so that a nursing diagnosis may be established. The nurse uses theoretical knowledge to cluster data and determine motivational readiness. The resulting problem list is used to formulate the nursing diagnoses. Nursing diagnosis, the formal step of analysis, follows the initial step of assessment and guides the next steps of planning, intervention, and evaluation. A taxonomy is used to organize and categorize the data into appropriate, care-guiding diagnoses. In the interdisciplinary setting of psychiatric nursing, the DSM-IV is an important tool for understanding the signs and symptoms of the psychiatric diagnosis.[3] The manual provides a communication tool for the team to use in understanding a client's problems. Nurses can use this knowledge of the psychiatric diagnosis as a basis for evaluating the client's response to health problems during the analysis phase of the nursing process.

CLUSTERING CUES AND DIAGNOSTIC HYPOTHESIS

After verifying the validity of the cues by confirmation with the client or other reliable sources, the nurse can then group data into units of information or patterns that reflect actual or potential health problems. Data are compared with the client's stated problem and the nurse's initial clinical impression. Examples of patterns at this stage of analysis might be the presence of religious ideation, refusal to eat, refusal to take medication, pacing around the unit, and lack of personal hygiene. The nurse then hypothesizes which nursing diagnosis best represents these cues. Altered Thought Processes and Self Care Deficit are two possible diagnoses.

MOTIVATIONAL READINESS

The nurse cannot assume that the client and family are ready to make any changes in their lives. Patterns of coping develop with time, and it is unrealistic to expect the client to want to change something so familiar that it actually may be more comfortable to continue the behavior than to change it. Even behavior that is self-destructive or obviously harmful to others often will be continued. This can be frustrating for the nurse, who naturally assumes that all people value health and want to improve their own lives. The client, however, may be attempting to survive in a world that he or she perceives as threatening and painful. It is difficult for the client to learn because the focus for behavior is on coping with the pain of living. This involves high levels of anxiety, which narrow the perception of events and cause preoccupation with certain fears. These concerns must be the focus of nursing care until the client feels a degree of safety and security from a trusting, caring nurse–client relationship.

Paradoxically, pain is a powerful motivator. The effort to instill hope by empowering the client to strive for survival and have the will to live is crucial for any type of therapy to be effective. Through analyzing assessment data, the nurse determines potential sources of motivation for the client. Aspects of life that seem important to the client can be sources of power and of an increased sense of personal control and self-esteem. Focusing on helping clients clarify what they want can prevent them from dwelling on their problems.[21]

By accessing sources of motivation, the nurse encourages clients to give up their resistance to changing the forces that impede movement toward wellness. These restraining forces must be identified to reduce them or to change them into motivational factors (see Box 8-5).[18] One approach is to ask outcome-oriented questions, such as "What would having more friends feel like?" Whatever the client's motivation, the nurse needs to recognize it as important to the client and thus to the overall plan of care. If the nurse responds to the request with negative reinforcement or withdrawal, the client's negative self-image and anxiety will be reinforced.

A feeling of powerlessness often prevents a mentally ill client from wanting to change. Clients who do not believe that what they desire is within their control may respond by increasing efforts to control the environment.[25] This may compound the problem, because it is difficult for the client to control most aspects of living. For example, the suspicious client uses projection and blame, the alcoholic client uses denial and rationalization, the depressed client uses self-defeating behavior, and the violent client uses aggression—all in attempts to feel valued. These may be the only ways that clients know to strive for a sense of control. Nursing can play an important role in helping the client tap new sources of power.[25]

PROBLEM LIST

Analysis of the focus of care for the psychiatric-mental health client involves evaluating all the collected information and inferences about problematic behaviors, strengths and resources, and sources of motivation to form a problem list within a holistic nursing framework. Accurate problem identification is necessary for accurate nursing diagnoses. The nurse focuses on the client responses that interfere with the desired quality of life.[10]

Family and related community problems and individual problems should be included in the problem list. The family's level of motivation for change is as important as the client's. The whole family needs support from the nurse, who is often the one health care person with access to the family's concerns. Community resources and other environmental concerns also are important. For instance, the client who lives alone in a rural area with no close neighbors to call on for help has special needs.

Because nurses espouse a philosophy of holism and self-determination, the client's perception and validation of the areas of concern are helpful in formulating a problem list (Box 8-7). Life-threatening problems (eg, suicidal ideation, homicidal ideation, fluid and electrolyte imbalance, threatening hallucinations, and violence) are the exception; the nurse identifies these problem areas from the data, and the problems may or may not be verified by the client.

The nurse must carefully consider the overall context of a client's behaviors, any cultural meaning, and the client's personality before labeling something a problem. Labeling certain areas of concern as problems may not be appropriate if these behaviors are adaptive for the client. The nurse must also consider whether the problem lies within the domain of nursing practice. For example, a low intelligence quotient may be the main reason an adolescent client does not do well in a school program. This is not a problem for the nurse to address. However, the effects of the low score on the client's self-esteem may be a problem that the nurse can address.

NURSING DIAGNOSIS

Determining the nursing diagnoses is the final and most important part of the analysis phase. *Nursing diagnosis* is defined as a statement of the client's response pattern to a health disruption. Tremendous progress has been made in the development of a taxonomy for nursing diagnoses and in assisting nurses to make accurate diagnoses in their clinical practice.

Standard III of The American Nurses Association's (ANA's) *Standards of Psychiatric and Mental Health Nursing Practice,* which guides the practice of psychiatric nursing in any health care setting, states that "the psychiatric-mental health nurse analyzes the assessment data in determining diagnoses."[2] The rationale for this standard is that the "basis for providing psychiatric-mental health nursing care is the recognition and identification of patterns of response to actual or potential psychiatric illnesses and mental health problems" (p 26).[2]

Nursing diagnoses are abstract and broad definitions of phenomena that nurses help clients explore and change if sufficient motivation for change exists. The changes in behaviors or symptoms that initially were clustered to arrive at the diagnoses become the mechanism for evaluation. The goals, predicted and hoped-for changes in behavior, are the outcome criteria for this evaluation.

Making a nursing diagnosis involves informed de-

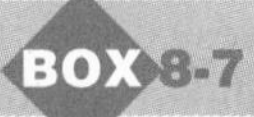

BOX 8-7

Nursing Diagnoses and The Problem List

Each category below represents the first part of a diagnostic statement, and the phrases that follow are examples of problems seen in association with that diagnosis. The second part of the diagnostic statement begins with "related to" and represents, in some way, an etiology of the syndrome described in the first part. The complete diagnosis represents a syndrome that is disruptive to the client's health or adaptation.

Chronic Self Esteem Disturbance
- History of self-injury
- Withdrawn behavior
- Poor hygiene habits
- Ruminations

Ineffective Individual Coping
- Acting out
- Ruminations
- Withdrawn behavior

Altered Thought Processes
- Acting out
- Social isolation
- Restless behavior
- Fear
- Poor social skills

Impaired Social Interaction
- Acting out
- Aggressive behavior
- Limited self-care abilities

Impaired Verbal Communication
- Acting out
- Disorganized speech
- Social isolation

Risk for Injury
- Inability to communicate impending seizure

Note that some problems appear under several diagnostic statements. A phrase listed as a problem in one situation may be listed as a diagnostic syndrome statement in another situation. Making these distinctions carefully and accurately is important when planning nursing interventions. Such decisions must be based on thorough knowledge of the client's problems, of the client as a diagnostic entity, and of the client as a person with a set of behavioral responses.

cision making. Through accurate assessment of the client, family, and community, the nurse collects as much data as possible and clusters the data based on how the pieces fit together. This requires making inferences about the significance of the data to the person and the family. The nurse also uses the results of the nursing history. For example, in the physical dimension, the client may complain of insomnia and early morning awakening, whereas the MSE yields findings of depressed mood and feelings of hopelessness for the affective component. Combining this with a history of a suicide attempt, a series of losses during the last year, and the nurse's theoretical understanding of depression, the behaviors cluster around a sleep pattern disturbance, hopelessness, and a high risk for suicide; these are all areas that nursing can treat. The known causative factors (and there may be several) that confirm the nursing diagnoses are the series of losses and the tendency toward self-destructive behavior. These factors become the focus of nursing intervention by helping the client work through the grieving process and learn more effective coping skills to deal with strong emotions.

TAXONOMY FOR WRITING THE DIAGNOSIS

A taxonomy for nursing diagnoses provides a listing of standardized labels representing health problems and responses to illness and helps build a scientific foundation for the nursing profession.[13] Even when there is no medical diagnosis for a health problem, there can be significant problems for nursing to address. Nursing diagnoses can also emerge from medical diagnoses. For such a list to be valid and reliable, it must be tested by nurses in clinical practice and revised as new diagnoses are determined to be important aspects of practice.

The most recent taxonomy is Nursing Taxonomy I, Revised 1995 to 1996 and endorsed by the North American Nursing Diagnosis Association (NANDA). (See the NANDA list of approved nursing diagnoses on the back endpaper.) In 1994, 19 new nursing diagnoses were approved, including Altered Family Processes: Alcoholism. Some nursing diagnoses are in the developmental stage of validation, while others are still to be identified. An example of one that has not been adequately documented through research is Risk for Relapse. The organizing scheme for NANDA taxonomy, human response patterns, includes the broad patterns of exchanging, communicating, relating, valuing, choosing, moving, perceiving, knowing, and feeling.[13]

The general format for writing a nursing diagnosis that includes all three parts is to begin with the diagnostic label from the NANDA list, followed by the etiology and the defining characteristics (signs and symptoms). A nursing diagnosis should be personalized and descriptive enough to label a client's condition accurately and give direction for intervention. Most NANDA diagnostic labels have definitions that help clarify the titling, and some have an additional qualifying statement that focuses the direction of the concern. For example, Knowledge Deficit may be in the area of medication or treatment, which would be indicated in the label.

The etiology and causative factors (the "related to" clause), the second part of the nursing diagnosis, are specific influencing or contributing factors, such as a series of losses, change in environment, or loss of belief in a higher power. Generally, these factors involve family influences, past experiences, environmental factors, or physically related factors. If the medical diagnosis or an event helps clarify the contributing factor, they can be added as a "secondary to" addition. For example, an etiology for Chronic Low Self Esteem may be related to feelings of worthlessness secondary to a childhood history of sexual abuse and post-traumatic stress disorder.

The signs and symptoms resulting from the medical diagnosis can be the etiological focus but not the medical diagnosis itself. Identified etiological factors should direct the focus of interventions, which are aimed at managing the etiological problems and the health problem.[13] For example, nursing interventions cannot change a client's thought problem if the client is delusional, but it can help the client decrease the anxiety associated with the thought problem, the fear that accompanies the delusion, and the problems with hygiene and safety that may result from the disordered thinking.

The defining characteristics, the third part of the nursing diagnosis, are the subjective and objective clinical cues that are the criteria for the diagnostic label. Accuracy of the label increases if several defining characteristics are present.[9] They can be written as they appear in the NANDA listings, which identify *major* (present 80%–100% of the time) or *minor* (present 50%–79% of the time) defining characteristics. For clarity, it is preferable to use subjective or objective cues from the assessment that specify the client's individual behavior (Table 8-1).

If a diagnosis is written to help prevent a future problem, as in a "risk for" rather than an "actual" diagnosis, then risk factors that verify the diagnosis are listed instead of defining characteristics. They should be risk factors that place the client at a higher risk than the general population.[13] A diagnosis of Risk for Violence: Self-directed or directed at others related to the statements, "I have given up on life, and wish I were dead" and "I won't be around much longer," indicates that there has not been an actual suicidal attempt; however, significant risk factors are present to warrant nursing interventions directed toward safety of the client and prevention of a suicide attempt. It is not necessary to list defining characteristics in a "risk for" diagnosis because the problem does not actually exist. In some clinical situations, the

Table 8-1

Writing the Diagnostic Statement: Incorrect and Correct Examples

Wrong	Right	Rationale
Depression related to loss of spouse	Dysfunctional Grieving related to lack of adequate support secondary to death of spouse, as evidenced by the statement "I have nothing to live for," weepy affect	Depression is a psychiatric diagnosis, not a nursing diagnosis. The complete nursing diagnosis includes an etiology that, in most cases, nursing can change through appropriate interventions. Interventions will focus on development of support. Defining characteristics are usually included from the assessment data ("as evidenced by") to justify the diagnosis from the client's behavior.
Ineffective Individual Coping related to lack of adequate ability to cope	Ineffective Individual Coping related to overuse of denial, rationalization, projection secondary to alcoholism as evidenced by euphoric affect, blaming problems on wife	Etiology ("related to") should not repeat the main idea of the nursing diagnosis.
Sleep Pattern Disturbance related to noise on the unit and lack of adequate supervision	Sleep Pattern Disturbance related to oversensitivity to environmental stimuli	Avoid any statements implying poor nursing judgment or poor staffing that may have legal implications.

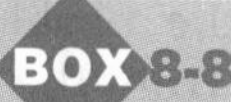

BOX 8-8

Psychiatric Diagnoses Using DSM-IV

Example: Complete psychiatric diagnosis using DMS-IV (for adult)

AXIS I

296.32 Major depression, recurrent, moderate
303.90 Alcohol dependence

AXIS II

301.83 Borderline personality disorder

AXIS III

Obesity
Hypertension

AXIS IV

Problems with primary support group: Family disruption through separation
Economic problems: financial debt

AXIS V

GAF = 50 (current)

Example: Complete psychiatric diagnosis using DSM-IV (for child)

AXIS I

314.01 Attention deficit hyperactivity disorder
296.22 Major depression, single episode, moderate
315.20 Disorder of written expression

AXIS II

V71.09 No diagnosis

AXIS III

None

AXIS IV

Sexual abuse

AXIS V

GAF = 30 (current)

defining characteristics are not written in any nursing diagnosis because the assessment data are readily available.

In certain complex problems, specific clusters of nursing diagnoses are addressed as syndrome diagnoses, such as Rape-Trauma Syndrome and Relocation Stress Syndrome.[9] Wellness nursing diagnoses can also be addressed, especially in community settings where the client is interested in pursuing optimal health. Potential for enhanced parenting may be significant when the outcomes for treatment involve measuring parenting skills. Some psychiatric nurse clinicians are determining clusters of nursing diagnoses, called psychiatric specific nursing syndromes, to fit specific DSM-IV diagnoses.[8]

NURSING DIAGNOSIS AND PSYCHIATRIC DIAGNOSIS

The psychiatric-mental health nurse works closely with other disciplines to arrive at the most appropriate plan of care for the client and family. Physicians and nurse practitioners have the responsibility to make a psychiatric diagnosis when there is sufficient support to determine that a psychiatric problem is present. The taxonomy used to make the psychiatric diagnosis is the DSM-IV of the American Psychiatric Association.[3]

The DSM-IV is a criteria-based diagnostic system that specifies the type, intensity, duration, and effect of the various behaviors and symptoms required for the diagnosis. Guidelines represent the clinical judgments of experts in the field of psychiatry. The nurse assists in this process by sharing important information about the client from the nursing history, mental status assessment, and daily observations. A working knowledge of the DSM-IV is important in maximizing the team effort to help the client. Knowledge of the criteria for deciding on a particular medical diagnosis found in the DSM-IV may help the nurse in making a clinical decision about a nursing diagnosis.

The DSM-IV is a multiaxial system in which the diagnostic criteria are inclusive for each diagnosis. They allow room for individual differences within a pattern of behavior or duration of behavior by including phrases, such as, "at least one of the following" or "for at least 6 months." It is responsive to cultural sensitivities and includes culture-bound syndromes.

Five axes constitute the format for a complete psychiatric diagnosis. A five-digit coding system is used for Axis I and II. Axis I comprises the clinical disorders, such as schizophrenia, bipolar disorder, and substance abuse disorders. A disorder of this nature is usually the main reason the client is seeking help. Axis II is composed of the personality disorders and mental retardation. This axis separates the patterns of lifestyle and coping that have developed from childhood from the more acute manifestation of behavior in the major mental disorders. If the criteria are not met for a personality disorder, then this may be indicated as *deferred* and given a specific code number. A person may have more than one diagnosis on these two axes. Axis III indicates the general medical problems that may be influencing the client's response to the psychiatric problems; for example, asthma, gastric ulcer, or diabetes. Axis IV indicates the psychosocial and environmental problems during the last year, such as economic, housing, primary support group, occupational, educational, social environment, legal involvement, and access to health care services; these are listed as the actual stressors (eg, death of mother). Axis V represents the Global Assessment of Functioning (GAF) currently and during the preceding year; it involves ratings of psychological, social, and occupational functioning on a continuum from mental illness to mental health. On the GAF scale, 81 to 90 means good functioning in all areas, and 1 to 10 means persistent danger of severely hurting self or others, persistent inability to perform minimal personal hygiene, or a serious suicide act with clear expectation of death.[3] Box 8-8 gives examples of the five DSM-IV axes.

Particularly important for nursing directives are Axes IV and V, both of which nurses can use when planning care. If a client has not been functioning well for the last year, for instance, the nursing interventions are individualized so that they are in line with the client's capabilities. In addition, if the stressors have been overwhelming, as in a loss of several family members in a short time, then nursing care is more supportive and less focused on helping the client make major life decisions. Psychiatric nurses are often asked to determine these scorings, another form of nursing judgment.

INTERFACE OF NURSING DIAGNOSIS AND THE DSM-IV

Another helpful way to interface the DSM-IV with nursing is to consider common concerns of clients with certain psychiatric diagnoses. These diagnostic clusters that link with the psychiatric diagnoses include a set of collaborative problems and nursing diagnoses that are predicted to be present with a particular psychiatric diagnosis.[6] The collaborative problem is a potential complication that is monitored or managed frequently, such as seizures with a client in alcohol withdrawal. Even with available diagnostic clusters, each nursing diagnosis should be confirmed or ruled out based on collected data.[6] Also, certain nursing diagnoses (eg, Ineffective Individual Coping and Self Esteem Disturbance) may occur in almost all DSM-IV categories. Thus, it would not be advisable to limit certain nursing diagnoses to particular DSM-IV diagnoses. The danger is a loss of individuality in determining the concerns that are the focus of care for a particular client.

In addition to the advantage of identifying common themes in nursing diagnoses for specific psychiatric diagnoses, there is the added value of including specific age-related nursing diagnoses (ie, child related, adolescent related, young adult related, middle adult related, and older adult related). Another distinction is whether the diagnosis is individual, family, or community focused. Child and adolescent psychiatric nurses especially need family-focused nursing diagnoses, because the philosophy of these specialties is to assist the whole family to make a positive adjustment, which includes changing family and individual patterns of coping. Nurses who work in outpatient settings especially need to make accurate community-focused diagnoses. Box 8-9 identifies several clinically significant nursing diagnoses and collaborative problems that correspond with psychiatric diagnoses. Some or all may apply, and others may reflect the unique variables affecting the client.

DOCUMENTATION

Assessment findings, both initial and ongoing, are documented according to the standards set in each agency and are important as legal references. Most agencies have standard forms to record assessment data. Recording baseline assessment information provides data that may be used for comparison studies on outcome evaluation. Ongoing assessment information is recorded using a variety of formats to monitor the client's progress toward the desired outcomes. Recording formats include block notes with a single entry covering an entire shift, narrative timed notes, and a problem-oriented record. A FOCUSr format, similar to a SOAP or problem-oriented format, addresses repeated or repetitive care in which a particular client problem or nursing diagnosis, change in status, or significant event (eg, use of time out) is addressed using a "data," "action," and "response" format. The FOCUSr format focuses on client concerns and is more positive than the more traditional SOAP format.[10]

Many agencies have progressed to computerized data records where the client records data directly or the staff records data indirectly. Computer prompts alert the staff and client for abnormal findings. Psychiatric home health care is one area where this is taking place so that clients can be monitored between visits. For example, a client who is going through detoxification from alcohol or drugs may have vital signs and other signs and symptoms of withdrawal recorded on a computer and followed by the home health nurse. Ongoing assessment data are available for outcome evalu-

(text continues on page 120)

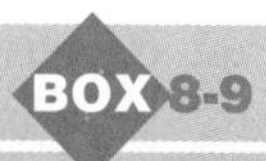

Nursing Diagnoses in Psychiatric-Mental Health Nursing

This chart identifies nursing diagnoses, as specified by the North American Nursing Diagnosis Association (NANDA), that may be associated with selected DSM-IV categories or psychiatric diagnoses. For each DSM diagnosis, the chart presents nursing diagnosis statements using NANDA approved diagnostic labels.

MEDICAL DIAGNOSIS (GENERAL CATEGORY)	POSSIBLE RELATED NURSING DIAGNOSES
Schizophrenia	**Physical**
	Altered Nutrition: Less than body requirements related to mistrust, fear, and disorganized thinking, as evidenced by ritualistic use of food, statement "the food is poisoned," weight loss
	Bathing/Hygiene, Dressing/Grooming Self Care Deficit related to social withdrawal, fear, and confusion, as evidenced by inappropriate dress, statement "the water will kill me"
	Sleep Pattern Disturbance related to environmental distractions, anxiety, and fears, as evidenced by reversed sleep cycles, statement "the hallucinations start at night"
	Altered Nutrition: More than body requirements
	Activity Intolerance
	Sensory Perceptual Alteration
	Psychological/Cognitive
	Ineffective Individual Coping related to poor impulse control, as evidenced by overuse of projection, statement "I spend all my money on Coke and cigarettes"
	Altered Thought Processes related to internal conflict, poor ego boundaries, as evidenced by delusion of being persecuted, difficulty making decisions, poor judgment
	Chronic Low Self Esteem related to repeated feelings of failure, inadequate interpersonal relationships
	Risk for Violence
	Personal Identity Disturbance
	Anxiety
	Impaired Verbal Communication
	Defensive Coping
	Ineffective Family Coping: disabling
	Altered Family Processes
	Noncompliance: clinic aftercare
	Knowledge Deficit: psychotropic medications
	Sociocultural
	Social Isolation related to mistrust of others and fear of closeness, as evidence by statement, "I have no friends," isolation of self
	Altered Role Performance related to feelings of worthlessness and low frustration tolerance, as evidenced by statement, "I keep getting fired from jobs," poor work history
	Impaired Home Maintenance Management related to poor motivation, cognitive disturbance, and lack of family support, as evidenced by cluttered, pest-infested living environment, statement, "I never turn the heat on—it has x-ray radiation"
	Impaired Social Interaction

continued

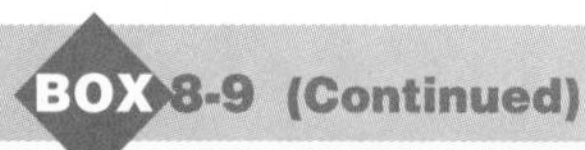

BOX 8-9 (Continued)

	Spiritual Spiritual Distress related to loss of hope, as evidenced by statement, "I can't let anyone see me like this" Hopelessness Powerlessness
Mood Disorders	**Physical** Altered Nutrition: Less or More than body requirements Sleep Pattern Disturbance Bathing/Hygiene and Dressing/Grooming Self Care Deficit Sensory Perceptual Alteration Risk for Injury: lithium toxicity or electroconvulsive therapy Impaired Mobility Constipation **Psychological/Cognitive** Risk for Violence: Self-directed related to history of suicide attempt, giving belongings away, lack of social support system Dysfunctional Grieving related to internalized anger secondary to statement, "I can't go on without him" Self Esteem Disturbance Chronic Low Self Esteem Ineffective Individual Coping Anxiety Altered Thought Processes Impaired Verbal Communication Knowledge Deficit: Medications, depression **Sociocultural** Altered Sexuality Patterns related to high levels of stress, lack of psychic energy, and passivity, as evidenced by statement, "I have no energy" Impaired Social Interaction Altered Family Processes **Spiritual** Hopelessness related to lack of perceived purpose in life, as evidenced by statement "Nothing can be done for me," lack of responsibility for own decisions, extreme apathy Powerlessness
Personality Disorders	**Physical** Risk for Violence: Directed at others related to aggressive acting-out behavior, history of violence **Psychological/Cognitive** Self Esteem Disturbance Anxiety Ineffective Individual Coping Defensive Coping

continued

BOX 8-9 (Continued)

Ineffective Denial
Ineffective Family Coping: Compromised

Sociocultural

Impaired Social Interaction

Spiritual

Powerlessness related to lifestyle of helplessness, as evidenced by manipulative behavior, alternate clinging and distancing behaviors

Substance Related Disorders

Physical

Pain related to withdrawal effects of drugs or alcohol, as evidenced by statement, "Every joint hurts"
Sensory Perceptual Alterations: tactile hallucinations related to withdrawal effects
Risk for Injury
Altered Nutrition: Less than body requirements
Risk for Infection
Risk for Violence: Self-directed or directed at others
Sleep Pattern Disturbance
Self Care Deficit

Psychological/Cognitive

Fear related to loss of substance as coping mechanism, awareness of need for lifestyle changes, as evidenced by facial tension, statement, "I am so scared of the future. I will have to change everything"
Knowledge Deficit related to misconception about drugs, lack of information, as evidenced by request for information about physical effects of cocaine on the body, statement, "No one every told me how hard this detox would be"
Altered Thought Processes related to lack of adequate nutrition, as evidenced by confusion, blackouts, and confabulation
Ineffective Denial related to difficulty accepting lifelong recovery, as evidenced by lack of involvement with peers, negative feedback about 12-step program, statement "I still think I can control my use"
Anxiety
Defensive Coping

Sociocultural

Altered Family Processes: Alcoholism
Altered Role Performance
Risk for Altered Parenting

Spiritual

Spiritual Distress related to conflict between values and behavior, as evidenced by verbalizations of shame and guilt about consequences of drug use

continued

BOX 8-9 (Continued)

Childhood and Adolescent Disorders	**Psychological/Cognitive** Impaired Adjustment related to loss of stability in family, as evidenced by moving from one caretaker to another, failing grades in school, running away from home Personal Identity Disturbance related to lack of development of trust, as evidenced by self-stimulating, ritualistic behaviors Impaired Verbal Communication Risk for Violence: Self-directed or directed at others **Sociocultural** Ineffective Family Coping: Disabling related to rigid roles and rules and enmeshed boundaries, as evidenced by expressions of blame and scape-goating Impaired Social Interaction **Spiritual** Spiritual Distress
Eating Disorders	**Physical** Altered Nutrition: Less or more than body requirements Risk for Fluid Volume Deficit Fluid Volume Deficit Impaired Skin Integrity **Psychological/Cognitive** Altered Thought Processes Body Image Disturbance related to unmet dependency needs, as evidenced by statement, "I have to weigh 75 pounds to have people love me" Self Esteem Disturbance Knowledge Deficit Ineffective Denial **Sociocultural** Altered Family Processes related to lack of ability in family to encourage autonomy, as evidenced by statement, "Our family can't change—my Mom couldn't take it" **Spiritual** Powerlessness
Anxiety Disorders	**Physical** Activity Intolerance related to fears of leaving home secondary to antici-patory anxiety as evidenced by statement, "I can't get out—I may not make it back"

continued

BOX 8-9 (Continued)

	Psychological or Cognitive Anxiety related to perceived loss of feelings of control related to unrealistic fears of dying Self Esteem Disturbance related to feelings of shame and embarrassment Post-Trauma Response Rape-Trauma Syndrome **Sociocultural** Social Isolation related to loss of feeling of safety **Spiritual** Spiritual Distress related to feelings of worthlessness
Dementia and Delirium Disorders	**Physical** Risk of Injury Altered Nutrition **Psychological or Cognitive** Fear related to difficulty with information processing Altered Thought Processes **Sociocultural** Caregiver Role Strain **Spiritual** Hopelessness

ation in which designated indicators evaluate the quality of care.

◆ Chapter Summary

This chapter has discussed the first and second steps of the nursing process, assessment and nursing diagnosis. In these two steps, the nurse assesses the client, analyzes assessment data, looks for clusters of data that fit together in patterns, determines the motivational readiness of the client and family for change, formulates a problem list, and writes the diagnosis. Major points of the chapter include the following:

1. Nursing assessment is the gathering of client data, which are then analyzed in the diagnosis step of the nursing process.
2. Nursing assessment explores the needs, problems, and adaptive resources of the individual and the means by which the nurse may help the client move to a higher level of health.
3. Identification and clarification of the client's problems are major purposes of nursing assessment.
4. Through the holistic approach to assessment, the nurse-interviewer explores client functioning in the psychological, social, biological, behavioral, cognitive, cultural, and spiritual areas of life.
5. A variety of assessment tools should be used to con-

duct a comprehensive assessment of the psychiatric-mental health client.

6. The communication and relationship skills of the nurse constitute the most essential element of the assessment interview.
7. Analysis of the assessment data gathered for a client culminates in the determination of the most important, clearly written, definitive nursing diagnoses.
8. Clients have varying levels of motivation for change and may need help from the nurse to reduce the restraining forces and increase the motivating forces for change; this increases the sense of personal control.
9. The nursing diagnosis is a statement of a client's response pattern to a health disruption and guides the planning and intervention phases of the nursing process.
10. The medical diagnosis is made using the criteria set in DSM-IV. The nurse can use this information in the decisions regarding nursing diagnoses.
11. The DSM-IV is a multiaxial classification system that fosters a holistic approach to the client; it includes specific behavioral criteria for each diagnosis.
12. The current NANDA taxonomy of nursing diagnoses contains useful diagnoses for psychiatric nursing.

Review Questions

1. The DSM-IV contains a multiaxial system for making a psychiatric diagnosis. Which of the following would be an example of an Axis IV diagnosis?
   A. Diabetes and hypertension
   B. Major depressive disorder with psychosis
   C. Mild mental retardation
   D. Economic—loss of job
2. In the nursing diagnosis Risk for Violence: Self-directed or directed at others, the "related to" factors would be
   A. listings of actual risk factors.
   B. behaviors indicating the presence of the problem.
   C. another nursing diagnosis.
   D. the medical diagnosis.
3. A potential complication or collaborative problem for bulimia nervosa might be
   A. major depression.
   B. esophageal bleeding.
   C. loss of social support.
   D. binge cycles.
4. One thing a mental status examination would *not* include is
   A. insight and judgment.
   B. motor behavior and attitude.
   C. history of drug and alcohol use.
   D. hallucinations and delusions.
5. Screening tests that can be scored have the advantage of
   A. a quantitative score that may be diagnostically important.
   B. eliminating the need for a thorough health history.
   C. showing the client the errors in his or her thinking.
   D. providing subjective data for evaluation.
6. How would the nurse complete a psychosocial assessment with a client who was born in another country and could not speak English?
7. Explain nursing diagnosis to someone from a social work background.
8. What are two "risk for" diagnoses for someone with a diagnosis of amphetamine dependency?
9. How do the defining characteristics of the nursing diagnosis influence the goals and interventions?
10. How would the nurse adapt the assessment process for the elderly person and the child?

◆ References

1. Acorn S: Use of the Brief Psychiatric Rating Scale by Nurses. J Psychosoc Nurs Ment Health Serv 31 (5): 9–12, 1993
2. American Nurses Association: Statement on Psychiatric-Mental Health Nursing Practice and Standards of Psychiatric and Mental Health Nursing Practice. Washington, DC, American Nurses Publishing, 1994
3. American Psychiatric Association: Diagnostic and Statistical Manual of Mental Disorders, 4th ed. Washington, DC, American Psychiatric Association, 1995
4. Bernstein L, Bernstein RS, Dana RH: Interviewing: A Guide for Health Professionals, 4th ed. Norwalk, CT, Appleton-Century-Crofts, 1985
5. Boyle JS, Andrews MM: Transcultural Concepts in Nursing Care. Glenview, IL, Scott, Foresman, 1989
6. Carpenito LJ: Handbook of Nursing Diagnosis, 6th ed. Philadelphia, JB Lippincott, 1995
7. Carson VB: Spiritual Dimensions of Nursing Practice. Philadelphia, WB Saunders, 1989
8. Coler MS, Vincent KG: Psychiatric Mental Health Nursing. Albany, NY, Delmar, 1995
9. Collier IC, McCash KE, Bartram JM: Writing Nursing Diagnoses: A Critical Thinking Approach. St. Louis, CV Mosby, 1996
10. Doenges ME, Townsend MC, Moorhouse MF: Psychiatric Care Plans: Guidelines for Planning and Documenting Client Care, 2nd ed. Philadelphia, FA Davis, 1995
11. Dyer JG, Sparks SM, Taylor CM: Psychiatric Nursing Diagnosis. A Comprehensive Manual of Mental Health Care. Springhouse, PA, Springhouse, 1995
12. Fawcett CS: Family Psychiatric Nursing. St. Louis, CV Mosby, 1993

13. Fortinash KM, Holoday-Worret PA: Psychiatric Nursing Care Plans, 2d ed. St. Louis, CV Mosby, 1995
14. Francis G, Munjas B: Manual of Social Psychologic Assessment. Norwalk, CT, Appleton-Century-Crofts, 1976
15. Iyer PW, Taptich BJ, Bernocchi-Lossey D: Nursing Process and Nursing Diagnosis, 3rd ed. Philadelphia, WB Saunders, 1995
16. Kim MJ, McFarland GK, McLane AM: Pocket Guide to Nursing Diagnoses, 6th ed. St. Louis, CV Mosby, 1995
17. McBride AB, Austin JK: Integrating the Behavioral and Biological Sciences. Implications for Practice Education and Research. In McBride AB, Austin JK (eds): Psychiatric Mental Health Nursing. Integrating the Behavioral and Biological Sciences. Philadelphia, WB Saunders, 1996
18. McGovern WN, Rodgers JA: Change Theory. Am J Nurs 86 (May): 566–567, 1986
19. O'Connor FW, Eggert LL: Psychosocial Assessment for Treatment Planning and Evaluation. J Psychosoc Nurs 32: 5, 31–41, 1994
20. Okun BF: Effective Helping: Interviewing and Counseling Techniques, 3d ed. Monterey, CA, Brooks/Cole, 1987
21. Peesuut DJ: Aim Versus Blame: Using an Outcome Specification Model. J Psychosoc Nurs 27 (5): 26–29, 1989
22. Putzier DJ, Padrick KP: Nursing Diagnosis: A Component of Nursing Process and Decision-Making. Top Clin Nurs 5 (Jan): 21–29, 1984
23. Scahill L, Ort SI: Selection and Use of Clinical Rating Instruments in Child Psychiatric Nursing. Journal of Child and Adolescent Psychiatric Nursing 8: 3, 33–41, 1995
24. Shader RI (ed): Manual of Psychiatric Therapeutics, 2d ed. Boston, Little, Brown & Co, 1994
25. Smith FB: Patient Power. Am J Nurs 86 (May): 1260–1262, 1986
26. Sorofman B, Tripp-Raimer T, Lauer G, Martin M: Symptoms of Self-Care. Holistic Nursing Practice 4 (2): 45–55, 1990
27. Talbot J, Hales R, Yudofsky S: Textbook of Psychiatry. Washington, DC, The American Psychiatric Press, 1988
28. Ward M: The Nursing Process. In Krebs MJS, Larson KH: Applied Psychiatric-Mental Health Nursing Standards in Clinical Practice. New York, John Wiley & Sons, 1988

Planning, Intervention, and Evaluation

Kathleen R. Delaney
Donna Lettieri-Marks

9

If the wrong man uses the right means,
the right means work in the wrong way.

Ancient Chinese Proverb

Planning, implementation, and evaluation are the final three phases of the nursing process. Through planning, the nurse prioritizes what needs to be done and how it will be done. The nursing plan sets down the direction, methods, and outcomes for enacting positive change, so the plan is the yardstick for evaluating the client's progress in treatment. The first section of this chapter details the basic principles of planning and some innovations in care planning useful for practicing in managed health care settings.

Once the plan is crafted, the implementation phase of the nursing process begins. Intervening with clients requires nurses to bring the care plan into the current interaction with a client and assess how a suggested approach might apply to the moment. Thus, implementing the nursing care plan requires critical thinking and knowledge of how one translates a strategy into action. Guidelines for learning the implementation process are discussed in the second section of the chapter.

Finally, this chapter discusses how to evaluate the effectiveness of interventions. Beginning practitioners and students usually focus their evaluation efforts on clients' plans of care. However, functioning in new health care arenas demands that even beginning practitioners evaluate the care delivery system, basic outcomes of treatment, and consumer satisfaction with services. The final section explains the evaluation process at the individual and system levels.

Learning Objectives

On completion of this chapter, you should be able to accomplish the following:

1. *Discuss how to organize and use assessment data to formulate a nursing care plan.*
2. *Explain the use of standardized nursing care plans and clinical pathways.*
3. *Describe the critical thinking process that shapes moment-to-moment interventions with clients.*
4. *Understand how to integrate assessment and care plan data with the dynamics of the immediate situation to create therapeutic interactions.*
5. *Explain the relationship of evaluation to the other phases of the nursing process.*
6. *Describe how to evaluate the effectiveness of nursing care interventions and the larger service delivery effort.*

◆ Planning

During planning, the third step of the nursing process, the nurse develops a plan of care that is comprehensive and realistic. Nursing care plans clearly define the goals or outcomes of care and the methods to achieve them.[2] Nursing standards also demand that care plans delineate the responsibilities of interdisciplinary team members, incorporate client education, and include appropriate referrals to ensure continuity of care.[3]

Prior to planning, assessment data have been organized to highlight areas in need of change. The problem areas will have been identified either as foci of care,[27] identified problems,[44] or nursing diagnoses. To begin the planning process, the nurse reviews interview data concerning the client's and family's perspectives on treatment goals, and prioritizes problem areas based on these goals, identified needs, and the clinical problem. Next, the nurse formulates client outcomes applicable to each problem area, and then, as the final step, identifies nursing interventions appropriate to reaching these outcomes. Finally, the nurse estimates a time frame for accomplishing goals and, to ensure continuity of care, begins to anticipate the client's discharge needs. In the following section, these five basic principles of nursing care planning are discussed.

INTEGRATING THE CLIENT PERSPECTIVE: COLLABORATIVE CARE

For a plan of care to be successful, it must incorporate the goals and beliefs of clients and their families. Psychiatric treatment is about change. Change is unlikely unless the client believes that behaviors, thinking, or attitudes should be changed and that such change is possible. Integrating the client's perceptions of problems during the planning process results in outcomes that have a greater potential for success.

To understand how clients define their illness, treatment, and recovery, you must listen to how clients describe their illness experiences.[13] From these descriptions, it is possible to distill how clients define the important aspects of their lives and the critical ways in which illness has affected their self-system.[13] When reviewing client's perceptions, students might ask themselves the following questions:

- What happened in the client's life that prompted him or her to seek treatment?
- What does the client tell himself or herself about why the illness occurred?
- How does the client define getting better?
- How did the client come to think of recovery in this way?
- What does the client believe the treatment team can do to facilitate recovery?

For many years, the family was believed to be either the "cause" or a significant pathological contributor to the client's mental illness.[8] Understanding of the biological bases for mental illness has helped extinguish "parent blaming" and ushered in treatment models focused on promoting the family's involvement in care and expanding their role in facilitating the client's adaptation.[35]

In planning care, nurses should use information from the family to understand better the client's history.[6] Nurses also need to understand the client's social support resources. Critical to planning is integrating knowledge of how the family provides support to the client.[36] Also important is planning for families' support needs, which may arise from the stress of dealing with the client's issues.[43]

PRIORITIZING NEEDS FOR CHANGE

Clients often present with a multitude of needs related to their psychiatric illness. As detailed in the previous chapter, nurses *organize* these needs based on the client's presenting complaint, basic safety issues, current and expectable level of functioning, and social support needs. From this array of issues, nurses must *prioritize* which needs will be addressed in treatment.[17] Nursing Care Plan 9-1 demonstrates how, based on the assessment data, a nurse prioritizes a family's treatment needs.

A client's treatment needs are often prioritized based on safety issues. For example, a client with a diagnosis of schizophrenia is admitted to an inpatient unit experiencing an inability to complete basic activities of daily living, dysphoria, and command hallucinations to attack someone. Basic safety concerns prompt the nurse to prioritize addressing the client's command hallucinations. Once the safety needs of both the client and those in frequent contact with the client are addressed, the nurse then targets interventions to increase the client's competency in activities of daily living.

The context in which treatment will take place also determines how needs and treatments are prioritized. During brief inpatient care, treatments will most likely focus on stabilizing the acute symptoms that required the client to be hospitalized.[44] The goal of brief, focal inpatient treatment is to make the minimal changes necessary so that the client can be referred to less restrictive outpatient treatment.[27] For a client with acute depression, job loss, and marital problems, for example, inpatient work would focus first on the interdisciplinary interventions that initiate therapies for major depression. The team would also develop a discharge plan that addresses the client's support needs and establishes linkages with outpatient sites for continued therapy.

FORMULATING CLIENT OUTCOMES

Client outcomes should logically flow from the nursing diagnoses or collaborative foci of care. Well-formulated client outcomes should be stated in clear behavioral terms.[51] The case study in Nursing Care Plan 9-1 contains several examples of nursing diagnoses and the related client outcomes. Note that the outcomes listed are measurable actions that can be observed by another person. This book contains numerous nursing care plans that supply additional examples of how to formulate client outcomes based on nursing diagnoses or foci of care.

Client outcomes should be realistic and have a good chance of being achieved. To assess if an outcome is realistic, nurses consider the nature of the problem, the efficacy of the treatment approach, the client's contextual resources, and any barriers to treatment.[2] For example, attending therapy at the community health clinic may not be an appropriate outcome for a client with obsessive-compulsive disorder (OCD) if the ritualistic behavior prevents him or her from dressing completely to be able to leave his or her apartment. However, because psychopharmacological medications can help some clients with OCD, a more realistic outcome may be reducing ritualistic behavior through a combination of medication and behavioral plans.

The care plan is a fluid document. Client outcomes should be rethought when evaluation indicates that the outcome is not being achieved. For example, an initial short-term outcome for a client with a history of substance abuse may be for the client to attend an Alcoholics Anonymous meeting in his or her neighborhood. During a home visit, the nurse learns that the client is beginning to break the period of sobriety with "a few drinks." If the client does not attend the meeting after a contracted amount of time and denies the significance of "just having a few drinks," then the short-term outcome for the client might be reformulated to address the client's apparent denial that stands in the way of attending the meeting. Later sections of this chapter will discuss how the evaluation process supports the reformulation of care plans.

DELINEATING THE NURSING APPROACHES

Once the behavioral outcomes are established, the nurse identifies the nursing interventions that will be effective in achieving these outcomes.[18] A wide scope of nursing interventions exists. Box 9-1 delineates categories of nursing intervention listed in the Standards of Psychiatric Mental Health Nursing Practice as appropriate to the basic level psychiatric nurse. Advanced practice interventions, appropriate for the clinical nurse specialist, are geared to activities such as psychotherapy, consultation, and prescriptive authority. When planning care, psychiatric nurses select interventions consistent with their level of practice.[3] However, basic level and advanced practice nurses are required to draw

(text continues on page 128)

Nursing Care Plan 9-1

Planning Care for the P Family

Elizabeth P, a 28-year-old single-parent with two children (a 10-year-old daughter and 7-year-old son), comes to the mental health clinic with vague complaints of "not handling things very well" and "fear of hurting myself."

Elizabeth works at night cleaning buildings, to be at home during the evenings and avoid the child care costs she can ill afford. Divorced and receiving sporadic child support, she had been coping fairly well until recently. She cannot identify any single event or cause for her overwhelmed feelings and certain inability to go on.

Elizabeth reports the children are polite, active, and are doing well in school. Their grades have not changed nor has their behavior altered in any perceptible manner. They both help at home with chores.

During the initial assessment, the nurse learns that Elizabeth's rent has been raised, the children need extensive dental work, and her car requires more repairs than it is worth. Although her family is supportive, especially with the children, she refuses to ask them for any financial help. She does admit to increased difficulty sleeping although she is in bed "almost all the time." She has no plan of how to "hurt herself," just the fear that she may.

A team conference is held to formulate a plan of care. The nurse has contacted the school nurse who verified the children are seemingly doing very well in school. The conference is attended by Elizabeth, the nurse, social worker, pro bono attorney, and psychiatrist.

It is decided during the conference Elizabeth would benefit from antidepressant medication. Hospitalizing her would be best to stabilize her medication, but she has no insurance. Therefore, as case manager, the nurse will coordinate, direct the care plan, and consult with the psychiatrist about medication dosage. The social worker will explore what, if any, options there are for supplemental income while the attorney pursues the child support owed to her. Elizabeth's children will be referred to the county health department clinic for dental care and regular medical care.

During the conference, Elizabeth reveals that she is very fearful of working nights when her children will be in junior and senior high school. She will be referred to vocational rehabilitation for job counseling and possible reeducation.

The nurse will monitor the children by keeping in contact with the school nurse. Elizabeth has been less involved with school activities this year, but she will begin attending PTA meetings once again. Elizabeth will bring the children to therapy on at least one occasion so they can truly be a part of their mother's recovery. Elizabeth will tell her family that she is in therapy, but she is adamant they will not be active participants. "I am not a child," she says.

Because there are many agencies involved in Elizabeth's care, the nurse manager assumes the responsibility of case management. Elizabeth will only have to call her for questions and referral. It is a team goal to keep Elizabeth's involvement with the system minimal so as not to add to her overwhelmed feelings. As she becomes more able once again to cope, these responsibilities will be shifted to her gradually.

After Elizabeth leaves the conference, the team spends a few minutes debriefing. It is crucial that each team member be validated; they are doing what they can with extremely limited resources. The team reinforces that an outcome will be Elizabeth's independence and increased ego strength.

Nursing Diagnosis

Ineffective Individual Coping related to feeling overwhelmed secondary to children's need for dental work, car problems, and rent increase

Outcome

Client will verbalize confidence in ability to handle current problems following provision of situational supports.

Intervention	Rationale
Encourage client to verbalize feelings regarding current situation.	Active listening will enable client to articulate concerns, providing cathartic relief.

continued

Nursing Care Plan 9-1 *(Continued)*

Intervention	Rationale
Assist client to establish priorities for problem solving.	Priority setting by client will help increase client's sense of control and decrease feelings of helplessness.
Encourage client to participate with mental health team's effort to improve her child support payments.	Crisis intervention requires mobilization of resources for assistance of client.
Refer client to agency that will assist in vocational training.	Anticipatory guidance regarding future career planning will increase client's ability to provide for herself and her children.

Evaluation

Client reports adequate coping with current problems.

Nursing Diagnosis

Anxiety related to situational and maturational crises as evidenced by restlessness, insomnia, expressions of not handling things well

Outcome

Client will use specific measures to decrease anxiety.

Intervention	Rationale
Teach client symptoms of anxiety.	Labeling the experiences and feelings described by the client as anxiety will provide reassurance that client is not going crazy.
Encourage client to identify ways she has coped effectively in the past.	Client recognition of past successful coping will increase sense of self-esteem and improve current coping.
Teach other coping skills, such as regular exercise, use of relaxing or enjoyable activities, talking with supportive people.	Healthy coping measures can be learned and will provide client with concrete ways to handle feelings of anxiety.

Evaluation

Client verbalizes that she experiences diminished anxiety.

Nursing Diagnosis

Sleep Pattern Disturbance related to difficulty falling asleep secondary to situational stressors

Outcome

Client will report 6–7 h of uninterrupted sleep daily

Intervention	Rationale
Instruct client to go to bed at same time each night and to wake up at same time each morning.	Regular schedule for sleep-wake pattern will help maintain normal body rhythms.
Teach client information regarding antidepressant medication prescribed by physician.	Antidepressant medication, when taken during the evening, will exert short-term sedative effects, promoting sleep.
Teach client measures to promote sleep, such as elimination of caffeine products in the evening and use of warm bath and warm milk for relaxation.	Simple measures can promote restful sleep patterns.
Instruct client to maintain sleep chart.	The chart assists in monitoring patterns of sleep and will help direct any further intervention.

Evaluation

Client reports adequate amount of restful sleep.

BOX 9-1

Intervention Strategies for Generalist Nurse

Milieu therapy
Psychobiological interventions
Self-care activities
Health promotion and maintenance
Health teaching
Counseling interventions
Problem-solving techniques
Crisis intervention
Stress management
Relaxation techniques
Assertiveness training
Conflict resolution
Behavior modification

Source: ANA (1994) Statement on Psychiatric Mental-Health Nursing Practice and Standards of Psychiatric Mental Health Clinical Nursing Practice. Washington, DC: American Nursing Publishing.

from relevant psychiatric-mental health theory and research for rationales that support nursing interventions. Every intervention should be consistent with its guiding theory, and that theory should provide an explanation for why the intervention should work.[25] For instance, interventions that address the negative thinking of the depressed client are supported by cognitive theory and research that demonstrates that individuals can train themselves to alter negative, automatic thought patterns.[5]

The treatment setting also influences nursing approaches. Today's psychiatric nurse is intervening with clients in community-based treatment, home health care, day hospitals, and sheltered care facilities.[7,23,38] Nurses continue to intervene with clients in acute-care settings, such as psychiatric hospitals, but this traditional nursing role is decreasing with the focus on developing out-of-hospital care. The move to psychiatric community-based care is not new, but the economic force of managed care has accelerated the momentum for clients to be treated outside of hospital settings.[22]

With community-based settings come new treatment modalities, such as assertive case management.[29]Here, the nurse is concerned with stabilizing

Table 9-1

Examples of Standardized Treatment Guidelines

Standard or Guideline	Source	Expected Outcomes
Clinical pathway maps the sequence of the most effective, standard means of care that must occur to move a typical client with a given condition toward desired outcomes within a particular period of time.	Clinical pathways for specific client conditions are developed in treatment settings and often published in specialty nursing journals. Source books that contain examples of clinical pathways are also available.	Expected outcomes of critical events of care are defined. The outcomes for a given time reflect the expected progress of a typical client receiving standard care as defined in the pathway.
Practice guidelines provides specific recommendations for treatment of a particular disorder.	Such guidelines are produced by the Agency for Health Care Policy and Research. The final recommendations for treatment reflect a panel of expert clinicians' synthesis of current clinical knowledge.	The guidelines include some parameters for measuring outcome. Practitioners can also draw applicable outcome criteria from summaries of research included in the guidelines. These summaries document how clinicians have judged the efficacy of particular intervention strategies.
Standard care plan summarizes current nursing practices and interventions for particular clients according to medical or nursing diagnoses. Treatment goals are also defined.	Standardized plans are sometimes written for particular treatment settings, and samples are contained in reference texts.	Expected outcomes are included for each nursing diagnosis and related set of nursing interventions. The outcomes are generally short-term, behaviorally based changes that can be anticipated following interventions.

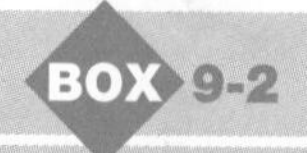

Standardized Nursing Care Plan, Sample 1

Veterans Administration

MEDICAL RECORD	**SUPPLEMENT DEFINED DATA BASE**

SUPPLEMENT TO STANDARD FORMS *(Check one):* ☐ SF 504 ☐ SF 505 ☐ SF 506

SUPPLEMENT TO VAF 10-7978g SERIES *(Check one):* PART ☐ I ☐ II ☐ IV ☐ V

PREPARED BY *(Signature & Title)*	SERVICE	DATE

DATE	NURSING DIAGNOSIS	EXPECTED OUTCOME	NURSING INTERVENTION	EVALUATION SIGNATURE/ DATE
	Sleep Pattern Disturbance related to: a. Anxiety and stress b. Circadian rhythm disturbance (eg, shift work) c. Depression d. Fear e. Inactivity f. Medications as manifested by: a. Difficulty falling asleep b. Difficulty remaining asleep c. Early morning awakening d. Fatigue e. Frequent dozing f. Inability to concentrate g. Irritability	Client will: 1. Identify techniques to induce sleep 2. Fall asleep within 1 h of going to bed 3. Sleep for 90 min 4. Sleep 4–5 h without awakening 5. Sleep through the night 6. Awake feeling refreshed	1. Teach relaxation skills and exercises. 2. Decrease caffeine intake. 3. Adhere to relaxing bedtime ritual. 4. Offer analgesic at least 1 h before bedtime. 5. Discourage napping. 6. Monitor frequency and length of time client is awake at night (night staff).	

Client Identification	Approved by CEB 5/12/88 **SUPPLEMENT** **DEFINED** **DATA BASE** OP-142b [531] MAY 1988

U.S. GOVERNMENT PRINTING OFFICE 1983 381-488/2910

VA FORM
JUL 1982 10-7978g

Table 9-2 Clinical Pathway: Unipolar Depression Without Axis II

The following pathway should be considered a guideline for the management of unipolar depression. It is not intended to be a substitute for clinical judgment. Variation from the pathway depends on the client's condition and the clinical judgment of the health care provider.

Client Name: ______ MR#: ______ Age: ______

Function	Activities	Admission Day (<24 h)	Day 1 (Begins 7 AM)
SAFETY AND CONTAINMENT	Assessment	Client: • Internal control to remain safety (eg, thoughts, agitation, anxiety, impulsivity, alcohol use) • Recent losses • Risk for violence Family: • Perceptions/response to suicide ideation, self-harm • Potential as safety resource • Safety education needs	Reassess client's: • Internal control • Risk for violence • Response to medication Family: • Perceptions/response to SI, self-harm • Safety education needs
	Treatments	• Institute safety interventions • Assess Suicide risk (SR) or close watch (CW) as indicated • Set clear limits regarding specific maladaptive behaviors • Use least restrictive external control for poor impulse control and potential violence (eg, limit-setting, seclusion, to restraints) • Use prn medication	• Institute safety interventions • Verify presence or absence of suicidal or self-harm intent • Adjust SR/CW prn • Identify client and family strengths and resources • Invite client and family to discuss problems related to suicidal and self-harm behaviors • Use least restrictive control prn
	Clinical outcome	• No suicide or self-harm attempts • Decrease in anxiety • Decrease in intensity and immediacy of suicidal impulse • Reports feeling safe • Not violent • Recognizes need for assistance and in controlling thoughts and behavior	• No suicide or self-harm attempts • Decrease in anxiety • Decrease in intensity and immediacy of suicidal impulse • Not violent • Identifies strengths and resources for recovery. Family member(s): • Identifies problem(s) related to suicidal thoughts and behaviors

C. Pitula/RPSLMC

the client's condition by using all available community resources. This approach differs from the hospital-based nurse who may be intervening with a client in crisis using medications and the structure and safety of the hospital milieu.[14] Thus, there may be differences in the approaches nurses delineate when planning to intervene with a client in a community clinic versus a client on an inpatient unit.

When planning interventions for clients, nurses can refer to resource materials, such as standardized care plans, clinical pathways, and universal protocols. Table 9-1 describes each of these clinical tools and how, based on these tools, treatment outcomes are defined.

Standard care plans delineate nursing actions and interventions. They are organized according to the problem areas of a specific diagnostic category or nursing diagnosis. Standardized care plans provide nurses with a documented standard of practice for each diagnostic category.[17] Standardized care plans for a wide range of diagnostic categories are collected in reference texts. Box 9-2 (p. 129) is an example of a portion of a standardized nursing care plan.

Clinical pathways map the work of the treatment team in delivering essential clinical services to clients with a particular condition. The pathway is organized by the clinical functions that identify the important processes of care for a condition.[19] Table 9-2 provides a portion of a clinical pathway developed for unipolar depression.[48]

Physician: ____________________

Day 2	Day 3–4	Day 5
Reassess client's: • Internal control • Risk for violence • Response to medication and side effects	Reassess client's: • Internal control • Risk for violence • Response to medication and side effects Family's: • Response to suicidal thoughts or behavior	Reassess client's: • Internal control • Risk for violence • Response to medication and side effects Family's: • Response to suicidal thoughts or behavior
• Institute safety interventions • Verify presence or absence of suicidal or self-harm intent • Adjust SR/CW prn • Allow off-unit privileges prn • Identify conditions provoking suicidal thoughts or behavior • Use least restrictive control prn	• Institute safety interventions • Verify presence or absence of suicidal or self-harm intent • Adjust CW • Allow off-unit privileges prn • Identify ineffective or harmful clients or family responses to suicidal and self-harm thoughts or behaviors • Alter negative beliefs with new information • Teach family how to protect suicidal client	• Institute safety interventions • Verify presence or absence of suicidal or self-harm intent • Evaluate client and response to teaching new information and how to protect client when suicidal • Communicate evaluation to discharge setting for follow-up
• No suicide or self-harm attempts • Suicidal impulse eliminated • Not violent Family member(s): • Identify problem(s) related to suicidal thoughts and behaviors	• Risk of suicide or self-harm/violence eliminated • Remains safe outside unit supervision • Identifies what provokes suicidal thoughts and behaviors • Identify ineffective and harmful beliefs and responses to suicidal or self-harm thoughts or behaviors	• Client is responsible for own safety • Family is safety resource • Client and family report understanding of ineffective or harmful beliefs and responses • Client and family report ability to perform new responses to suicidal thoughts or behaviors

This pathway details the multidisciplinary plan for clinical interventions and delineates how long they will take and what measurable outcomes can be expected. Clinical pathways demonstrate that a treatment approach that proved to be efficient and cost-effective.[45] This is a type of documentation that third-party payers are increasingly demanding from health care professionals.

Practice guidelines are systematically developed statements that reflect the current state of knowledge about effective and appropriate care for a specific clinical condition.[24] One source of practice guidelines is the Agency for Health Care Policy and Research (AHCRP), which organizes panels of expert clinicians to draw up guidelines for select conditions.[50] This team synthesizes current scientific literature to distill recommendations for assessment and treatment. Guidelines from the AHCRP for the recognition and care of depressed clients were recently published.[16]

DEFINING DEADLINES AND DISCHARGE PLANS

The final step in the planning process is to estimate some time frame for accomplishing outcomes. How deadlines are specified varies. Clinical pathways map interventions on a time line so the time parameters are automatically in place. Most multidisciplinary care plans for inpatient treatment will specify the expected length of stay. Nursing care plans frequently specify time frames by delineating short- and long-term goals. Table 9-3 contains examples of long- and short-term goals and illustrates how they are typically defined.

Time frames are important. They hold professionals accountable for the outcomes they believe treatment will accomplish. Time constraints force professionals to pose the question, "What can be accomplished in this treatment setting in a reasonable, cost-effective length of time?" Once clinicians determine what can be accomplished in treatment in a given time frame, they then ask how these gains can be maintained and what additional issues need to be targeted in subsequent phases of treatment.

Discharge planning or plans for continuity of treatment are an important aspect of the care plan. Discharge planning should begin at the start of treatment.[2] Once the treatment team defines the expected outcomes for their phase of treatment, referrals should begin that target the issues relevant to the continuity of care. Discharge planning ensures that when leaving treatment, a service plan will be in place that matches the intensity of follow-up services with the intensity of the client's needs.

Table 9-3

Long-Term and Short-Term Goals

Changes require goal setting. Goals must be observable and measurable by others. Long-term goals are oriented toward the future, whereas short-term goals are the markers of achievement that one attains along the way toward a goal.
Examples of both types of goals are listed below.

Long-Term Goals	Short-Term Goals
To achieve independence through employment	To graduate from high school or pass equivalency examination
	To graduate from an appropriate vocational or collegiate program
	To apply for and attain a job
To increase ability to cope with stress, as demonstrated by decreased angry outbursts	To seek counseling or self-help group and attend meetings regularly
	To identify one coping strategy and try that coping method for 1 mo
To improve organization and promptness	To organize and list responsibilities of home, work, school, children
	To prepare general schedules based on prioritizing or responsibilities
	To prepare individual daily schedules with daily tasks, appointments
To increase self-esteem by altering body image	To achieve ideal body weight
	To improve body tone through daily exercise
	To assess and redo wardrobe

◆ Intervention

For the beginning student, interactions with clients may be awkward and anxiety-provoking experiences. Although students have been communicating with clients through several clinical practiciums, now an important difference exists. The *therapeutic intent* of words and actions takes center stage. When mentally preparing for a planned interchange with a client, the focus is not on performing a psychomotor skill correctly, but rather on what will be said.

In a typical interaction, the client makes a statement or exhibits a behavior and the student knows that a response is required. The student has read the client's chart and written a care plan. Now this knowledge of the client's history must be combined with what is happening at the moment. As with most new skills, it will require time to master the process of integrating the assessment and care plan data with the dynamics of an immediate situation to create a therapeutic interaction.[49]

Consider as an example the therapeutic principle of empathy. It is not enough to understand the concept of empathy and its use in supporting the client and recognizing the human meaning of illness; face to face with a client who is in distress or facing a stressful recovery, students must use words to forge a mutual understanding of that experience.

The first few attempts at conveying empathy—taking a natural act like talking and adding *intent*—may be rather awkward. Students are aware of the pressure to frame a statement so that the client experiences being understood and responded to. After some practice with the technique, however, using empathy with a client in distress will probably come quite naturally.

The same internalization of principles to frame statements with intent must occur with psychiatric nursing interventions. However, internalizing psychiatric nursing intervention principles is more complicated because the process demands that several considerations remain in focus as the intervention is crafted. The psychiatric nurse's mind must operate like a computer program: first devising a screen that focuses on the possible significance of the present situation, then calling up screens of the assessment data and care plan outcomes, then adding a screen that guides the prioritizing of client needs, and finally matching all this information with an appropriate intervention strategy. The following client vignette illustrates this thinking process.

DETERMINING THE SIGNIFICANCE OF THE PRESENT SITUATION

A student looks across the group room of a day hospital and sees one of her assigned clients, a young man, pacing with a tense look on his face. From previous contacts with the client, the student recognizes that pacing is not a typical behavior. Initially this behavior carries a "meaning" (ie, the client might be in distress). Because the client also appears very agitated, the behavior signals that a crisis might be building.

When a client appears to be in distress and possibly in crisis, an intervention is required. Crisis has the potential to compromise client safety. Clients in crisis may behave in a manner dangerous to themselves or others; therefore, the student's initial response to this behavior should be to approach the client and find out more about the pacing behavior.

CALLING UP THE ASSESSMENT DATA AND CARE PLAN

The student initiates the conversation with a reflective statement, "You're pacing, and have a worried look on your face," and follows it up with an invitation to talk, "What's going on? Is it something we could talk about?" The client responds to this initial probe in the following manner: "I'm just thinking about my life and what a failure I've been and how it really doesn't amount to anything. I feel so nervous inside all the time, and these thoughts keep plaguing me."

The student recalls the assessment data that depicted a client admitted for treatment of major depression. Four days ago, the client began a new trial of antidepressants. The student also knows that negative perceptions and thoughts often accompany depression. The student mentally reviews the client's suicide history and recalls that the client has been troubled with suicidal impulses.

SETTING PRIORITIES

The first priority is always client safety. Based on the current situation and client history, the student asks the client if he is having suicidal thoughts. (Refer to Chapter 42 for more detailed information on conducting a suicide assessment.) The student and client spend some time exploring this issue, and then the student discusses her assessment with the staff. In this case, the client denies suicidal ideation and the physician/nurse team concludes that based on all the available data, special precautions are not necessary. With that critical safety issue resolved, the student mentally turns to the care plan and recalls suggested approaches to the client's anxiety and agitation.

SELECTING THE APPROPRIATE INTERVENTION STRATEGY

The student hopes to use the moment to help the client develop some strategies to cope with anxiety. Based on the care plan, the student might choose between several possible approaches. Box 9-1 lists intervention modalities appropriate for the beginning practitioner. The counseling techniques include problem solving, crisis intervention, stress management, and behavior modification.

A problem-solving approach might focus on reinforcing some thought-stopping techniques the client may have learned in cognitive therapy group. Using a behavioral approach, the student might suggest that when negative thoughts are overwhelming the client should initiate a distracting pleasant activity. The student and the client might compose a list of activities that would be useful in this situation. With a psychoeducational approach, the student would focus on teaching the client about his depression, perhaps discussing how negative thoughts often accompany a depression. A biological approach might point toward the use of antianxiety medication. This book details the conceptual framework for each of these approaches and intervention strategies specific to the major psychopathological disorders.

Which one of these basic approaches nurses use in a moment-to-moment intervention depends on the foci of care, the care plan, and the particulars of the situation. For instance, if it were late in the day and the client were about to travel home, the nurse might talk about behavioral techniques the client could use in the evening hours to cope with negative thoughts. There is no one "right" approach. What is critical is that the student has a clear theoretical rationale for an intervention, and that the intervention is consistent with the assessment and care plan data.[33]

It may appear that a great deal of information must be held in focus as nurses move from planning to intervention. Indeed, the process demands considerable mental energy from the beginning psychiatric nurse. However, as nurses become familiar with integrating information, this type of critical thinking becomes second nature. The challenge for expert psychiatric nurses is never to allow their comfort level with intervening to become so "second nature" that they lose sight of the theoretical rationale for an intervention. Psychiatric nurses should always know what data formed the basis for determining the meaning of behavior and the theoretical rationale for addressing that behavior with a particular intervention.

THE ROLE OF THE NURSE–CLIENT RELATIONSHIP

Central to the practice of psychiatric nursing is using therapeutic communication to forge a relationship with clients.[47] Because principles of the therapeutic relationship are detailed in previous chapters, they are not specifically reviewed here. It should be understood, however, that psychiatric nurses always keep their "third eye" on the relationship, specifically how trust and mutuality are building.[28] In a sense, psychiatric nurses are always involved in the task of cultivating a relationship by communicating empathy, understanding, and interest to clients.[46] These relationship factors are the fabric of every intervention.

INTERVENTION AND THE SUPERVISION PROCESS

When intervening with clients, professionals learn to maintain at least a partial awareness of their own reactions and emotions and question the source of these reactions. This awareness should not interfere with the focus on what the client is communicating. However, this self-awareness is essential so that the nurses's own emotional reactions do not intrude on processing and understanding what the client is communicating. A particular challenge for beginning students is to control their own anxiety often present at initial client interactions.

Students' feelings and reactions that arise when talking with clients should be recalled later in postclinical conferences. Training oneself to recall interactions and the accompanying emotions is at the heart of supervision, a process central to the work of psychiatric nursing.[12] In supervision, psychiatric nurses obtain feedback on interventions and analyze the emotions particular clients generated. This process allows nurses to be objective about their reactions and to decenter emotions. In subsequent interactions, these emotions are less likely to interfere with the moment-to-moment intervention.[53]

◆ Evaluation

Evaluation is the process of determining the value of an intervention or the attainment of a preset treatment goal. Evaluation of practice is essential because of professional accountability and nursing's commitment to clients and families. This commitment to client-centered care demands that nurses continually monitor interventions to determine if they are effective and if they serve the needs of individuals and families.

In health care, evaluation occurs on two levels. First, nurses determine the effectiveness of interventions with particular clients. Here nurses evaluate selected interventions by judging the client's progress toward the outcomes set down in the nursing care plan. On a broader level, nurses also evaluate the effectiveness and efficiency of *care delivery* to populations of clients served in particular agencies and settings.

The evaluation of care delivery is rapidly advancing as an essential element of nursing practice. Even the novice nurse needs to be acquainted with three service-level evaluation methods: process improvement, consumer satisfaction data, and basic standardized outcomes. This section addresses how the evaluation process operates at the client and system level.

EVALUATION IN THE NURSING PROCESS

Evaluation of nursing care is woven into the very fabric of practice. As the fifth step of the nursing process, the evaluation phase of care demands that nurses examine the outcomes of interventions delineated in the nursing care plan.[18] The nursing process is cyclic, so evaluation is the catalyst for modifying the other components of the care plan. The dynamic nature of the nursing process is illustrated in Figure 9-1.

Evaluation of a client's care is twofold: It centers on the changes experienced by the client and the quality or effectiveness of the nursing care itself. For example, the nurse may assess a withdrawn client as disoriented and specify as an outcome of nursing care, "client will verbalize awareness of time and place." Nursing interventions to achieve that goal might include visual cues placed in the client's environment (calendars and clocks) and verbal reinforcement of time and place.

The nurse evaluates the effects of these interventions by observations of the client's behaviors. The nurse may ask the following questions: Is the client present at activities that he or she is suppose to attend? How did the client respond to periodic mental status checks of orientation to time, person, and place? If the client's behavior does not change, the nurse must review and modify the care plan by changing the outcomes or devising new intervention strategies.

This review of the care plan also provides information relevant to the evaluation of nursing care. Was the original assessment of the client complete? Were the client goals realistic, specific, and measurable? Did other nurses who intervened with the client consistently follow the care plan? Were unanticipated complications in the client's response to interventions sufficiently ad-

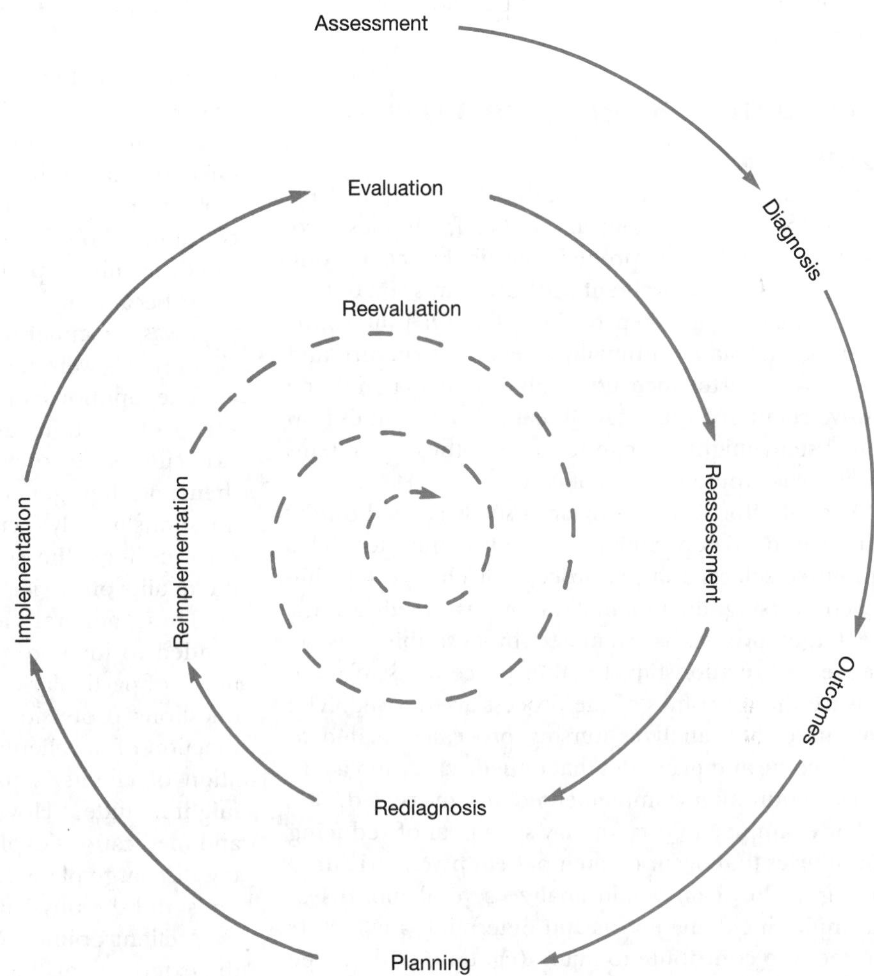

Figure 9-1. The nursing process.

dressed by care plan modifications? Seeking the answers to questions such as these engages nurses in problem solving, which is essential to the evaluation and improvement of nursing care.

For the beginning student, evaluation will most likely focus on the individual client and the extent to which behavioral outcomes are met. The care plan will be focused on relationship-based objectives (eg, establishing consistency and trust) and beginning intervention strategies (eg, problem solving in specific problem areas). Evaluation of these outcomes will be based on behavioral data gathered during your time at the clinical site.

However, as the student progresses through the clinical rotation, the evaluation process and the overall approach to specific clients can be broadened by referring to standardized care plans, clinical pathways, and universal protocols. Box 9-1 differentiates between the design of these clinical tools and how they might be used in practice. Each of these standardized tools has expected outcomes that provide excellent "yardsticks" for evaluating care.

To examine how to use these tools in the evaluation process, consider the clinical pathway presented at the beginning of the chapter. In the pathway, each time period contains specific outcomes of care that the treatment team considers realistic goals of standard care. Each day of treatment holds opportunities to evaluate which outcomes were met. The structure of a clinical pathway usually contains space for documenting variances. In a variance report, the team states why, on any given day, a particular client outcome was not achieved. For example, perhaps by the fourth day, the client is still voicing suicidal ideation. Using a variance note, the staff would chart what factors seem to account for the persistence of the client's suicidal ideation.

In this way, clinical pathways provide the structure for the continual evaluation of care.[45] The final step in the evaluation process is feeding back variance information to improve the interventions or timelines of the pathway. Demonstrating that evaluation data were the basis for modifying a pathway is the backbone of process improvement.

EVALUATION: A BROADER VIEW

Quality Improvement

In process improvement, a health care situation is examined to see how various inputs (staff, supplies, procedures) combine to produce particular client outcomes. Quality improvement (QI) programs aim to take process analysis one step further. The QI philosophy demands that staff continually assess the structure and process of care to uncover variables that may impede positive client outcomes.[4] A QI team also examines how their system might change to correct these problems and improve the outcomes of care.[37]

The QI efforts in nursing are usually carried out by a unit-based or department-based QI committee. This committee selects a target process for change (eg, improved nursing documentation of prn medication). The target process is examined by describing its sequence and relationships to other procedures. Ways to measure the outcomes of the process are derived. The committee then analyzes nursing processes related to this outcome and processes that impede care, and a corrective action plan is implemented and measured.[9]

For example, a QI team may set a goal of reducing staff injuries that occur on an inpatient psychiatric unit. To begin, the team would analyze several months of staff injury incident reports and determine any factors that seem to contribute to injury (eg, time of day, type of client). The QI analysis may conclude that newer, nontrained staff are more likely to be injured. Further exploration of unit procedures may reveal that new staff are not trained in handling potentially dangerous situations until the twice-yearly aggression management class.

The QI team could then set a corrective action plan and a target outcome. The plan might call for the aggression control class to be recorded on a videotape and shown during each new staff member's orientation class. Ideally, a follow-up analysis of incident reports would demonstrate a steep decline in incidents of new staff injury, which supports the use of videotaped instruction.

Since 1987, the Joint Commission on Accreditation of Healthcare Organizations has demanded that units demonstrate that quality assurance programs are grounded in the continual process improvement framework.[30] For a nursing unit, adopting the QI philosophy demands fostering an attitude of problem solving and a commitment to optimizing the treatment system.[5] Students can begin cultivating these attitudes by learning to view the client beyond the individual plan and examining how the system of care operates to meet the needs of the client population.

Consumer Satisfaction

In the 1980s, the health care industry began to embrace management and business strategies to improve care.[20] Of particular influence were the strategies of W. Edwards Deming. Deming[15] believed that the needs of the consumer should determine the nature of services provided. Deming's philosophy took hold in health care. What became increasingly important in treatment settings was consumer satisfaction and the degree to which client needs were identified and satisfied.

The opinions of clients are collected using consumer satisfaction surveys. In these surveys, clients are explicitly asked to evaluate the treatments provided to them and their general satisfaction with services. Survey questions usually focus on satisfaction with the physical surroundings, the competency of treatment staff, and the quality of service.[34]

These general satisfaction categories can be expanded to include questions that identify the unique needs of particular client populations. To develop such questions, professionals ask, "What is critical to the satisfaction of my clients?"[42] Items pertinent to the evaluation of clients' satisfaction with mental health care might include, "How fully were your illness, treatment, and medications explained to you?" "How clearly were the discharge plans explained to you?" "How much interest did the physician take in your problems?"[21]

A client opinion of particular concern to nurses is the extent clients believed treatment was collaborative. In the collaborative treatment framework, clients have opportunities for input into how problems are identified and how the treatment approach is formulated.[10] Opinion questions that tap into this dimension of care might include, "How often did the staff seek your ideas about your problems and your reasons for seeking treatment?"[26] Such items are particularly useful in evaluating nursing's goal of building collaborative treatment plans.

STANDARDIZED OUTCOMES

Evaluation of service delivery demands attention to treatment outcomes. Extreme competition in the marketplace requires psychiatric facilities to demonstrate that treatments are effective and cost-efficient. In the managed care environment, third-party payers are demanding outcome data as a rationale to support services and intervention strategies.[40] A rapidly evolving practice is the use of standardized instruments that measure the basic outcomes of psychiatric care.[31] Standardized instruments are rating scales, checklists, and questions and answer scales that provide an objective and standardized measure of a sample behavior.[39]

The basic outcomes of psychiatric treatment that are important to evaluation include consumer satisfaction, functional status, and symptom stabilization.[11] Consumer satisfaction has been described. Symptom stabilization tools gauge the resolution of symptoms that defined the clinical problem. Typically, clinicians rate the severity of clients' symptoms at the beginning and end of treatment. Instruments, such as the Brief Psychiatric Rating Scale, have been used extensively to rate the impact of treatment on the severity of select symptoms common to the major psychopathological disorders.[1]

Functional status tools assess how the client is functioning at home, at the job, and in life. A popular functional status tool is the Medical Outcomes Study Short Form Health Survey (SF-36).[52] The SF-36 measures health status concepts, such as physical functioning, role limitations, general mental health, vitality, and health perceptions. The SF-36 is completed by the client before and after treatment. It is an efficient way to measure clients' perceptions of their health status and the impact of treatment on these perceptions.

Because psychiatric treatment is a team effort, basic outcomes often reflect the combined effects of the interventions of nurses, physicians, occupational therapists, and social workers. This basic evaluation of treatment does not specifically measure the effects of nursing interventions. However, a basic outcome considered essential to evaluate (ie, functional status) parallels nursing's concern for clients' self-care abilities and quality of life.[41] Thus, some of the basic outcome data will mirror key nursing issues.[32]

Students should investigate the outcome methods being used at their clinical practicum sites. They might examine these data to judge the effectiveness of care being delivered to the client population. If the service unit is not yet collecting basic outcome data, the student might compare the client's functional status (eating, sleeping, ambulation) documented on the admission form with an assessment of clients' self-care abilities exhibited as discharge draws near.

◆ Chapter Summary

Students in psychiatric nursing almost immediately confront the dilemma of what to say to a client: "How do I effectively intervene with the situation that confronts me?" The information presented in this chapter should help with these dilemmas. Principles for devising a psychiatric care plan, moving that plan into action, and then evaluating the effectiveness of the intervention are presented in this chapter. Chapter highlights include the following:

1. During planning, nurses develop a care plan that directs the treatment of the client.
2. Nursing care plans define the goals or outcomes of care and the methods to achieve them.
3. Standardized care plans provide nurses with a documented standard of practice for a client with a particular condition.
4. Implementation requires nurses to combine care plan data with information from what is occurring at the moment, prioritize the client's needs, and then match all this information with an appropriate intervention strategy.
5. Nurses should always know the theoretical rationale that supports addressing a behavior with a particular intervention.
6. Evaluation is the final phase of the nursing process. Here nurses determine the effectiveness of an intervention or the attainment of a preset goal.
7. Evaluation occurs at the client and system level. At the client level, nurses evaluate the outcomes of interventions delineated in the nursing process.
8. Nursing evaluates service delivery systems by participating in quality assurance committees, collecting client satisfaction data, and using standardized instruments to obtain basic treatment outcomes.

Critical Thinking Questions

1. *How does the treatment setting influence how clients' needs are prioritized?*
2. *How do nurses determine if client outcomes are realistic?*
3. *What are some resource materials nurses use to delineate nursing care plans and interventions?*
4. *Explain why the supervision process is critical to the process of intervening with clients in a psychiatric setting.*
5. *How do evaluation data lead to improvements in care planning?*
6. *Why is it important to understand consumers' satisfaction with the care they receive?*

Review Questions

1. All of the following are true regarding the planning stage of the nursing process except which one?
   A. A plan of care should clearly define goals but not address methods to achieve goals.
   B. A plan of care should delineate the responsibilities of interdisciplinary team members.

C. A plan of care should incorporate client education.
D. A plan of care should include appropriate referrals to ensure continuity of care.

2. Mr. D. is a 38-year-old man with major depressive disorder who presents with frequent tearfulness, insomnia, suicidal ideation, few social supports, and estrangement from his family. In organizing treatment needs, the nurse would choose which of the following as the first priority?
A. Mr. D.'s tearfulness and emotional distress
B. Mr. D.'s inability to sleep sufficiently to feel rested in the morning
C. Mr. D.'s active thoughts of trying to kill himself
D. Mr. D.'s lack of ability to develop and maintain sustaining relationships with others

3. The nurse assigned to Mr. D.'s case begins working with him on a regular basis. All are important aspects of intervention with this client except which one?
A. The nurse's interventions must be consistent with the assessment and care plan data.
B. The nurse must keep a "third eye" on the development of trust and mutuality in his or her working relationship with Mr. D.
C. The nurse must follow the "right" approach for a client such as Mr. D. who displays depressive symptoms and suicidal ideation.
D. The nurse must have a clear theoretical rationale for an intervention.

4. When evaluating health care, nurses
A. determine the effectiveness of interventions with particular clients.
B. evaluate the effectiveness and efficiency of care delivery to populations of clients served in particular agencies and settings.
C. use evaluation methods, such as process improvement, customer satisfaction surveys, or basic standardized outcomes.
D. All of the above

◆ References

1. Acorn S: Use of the Brief Psychiatric Rating Scale by Nurses. J Psychosoc Nurs 31 (5): 9–12, 1993
2. Aidroos N: Use and Effectiveness of Psychiatric Nursing Care Plans. J Adv Nurs 16: 177–184, 1991
3. American Nurses Association, American Psychiatric Nurses Association, Association of Child and Adolescent Psychiatric Nurses, Society for Education and Research in Psychiatric Mental Health Nursing: Standards of Psychiatric-Mental Health Clinical Nursing Practice. Washington, DC, American Nurses Publishing, 1994
4. Batalden PB, Nelson EC, Roberts JS: Linking Outcomes Measurement to Continual Improvement. Journal of Quality Improvement 20: 167–180, 1994
5. Beck AT: Cognitive Therapy: Past, Present and Future. Journal of Clinical and Consulting Psychology 61: 194–198, 1993
6. Bernheim KF: Principles of Professional and Family Collaboration. Hosp Community Psychiatry 41: 1353–1357, 1990
7. Blazek LA: Development of a Psychiatric Home Care Program and the Role of the CNS in the Delivery of Care. Clinical Nurse Specialist 7: 164–168, 1993
8. Caplan PJ, Hall-McCorquodale I: Mother-Blaming in Major Clinical Journals. Am J Orthopsychiatry 55: 345–353, 1985
9. Chowanec GD: Continuous Quality Improvement: Conceptual Foundations and Application to Mental Health Care. Hosp Community Psychiatry 45: 789–793, 1994
10. Collins B, Collins T: Parent-Professional Relationships in the Treatment of Seriously Emotionally Disturbed Children and Adolescents. Social Work 35: 522–527, 1990
11. Coyne L: Follow-up Study Methodology: The Menninger Project and a Proposed Ideal Study. In Mirin SM, Gossett JT, Grob MC (eds): Psychiatric Treatment: Advances in Outcome Research, pp 237–253. Washington, DC, American Psychiatric Press, 1991
12. Critchley DL: Nursing's Contributions to a Psychiatric Inpatient Treatment Milieu for Children and Adolescents. In Hendren RL, Berlin IN (eds): Psychiatric Inpatient Care of Children and Adolescents: A Multicultural Approach. New York, John Wiley, 1991
13. Delaney KR: Short-term Hospitalization and the Depressed Patient. In Rogers CA, Ulsafer-Van Lanen J (eds): Nursing Interventions in Depression, pp 37–52. Orlando, Grune & Stratton, 1985
14. Delaney KR: Nursing on Child Psychiatric Milieus: What Nurses Do. Journal of Child and Adolescent Psychiatric and Mental Health Nursing 5 (4): 52–56, 1992
15. Deming WE: Out of the Crisis. Cambridge, Massachusetts Institute of Technology, Center for Advanced Engineering Study, 1986
16. Depression Guideline Panel: Depression in Primary Care, vol 2. Treatment of Major Depression. Clinical Practice Guideline, Number 5. Rockville, MD, US Department of Health and Human Services, Public Health Service, AHCPR Publication No 93-0551, 1993
17. Doenges ME, Townsend MC, Moorhouse MF: Psychiatric Care Plans: Guidelines for Planning and Documenting Client Care. Philadelphia, FA Davis, 1995
18. Duldt BW: Nursing Process: The Science of Nursing in the Curriculum. Nurse Educator 20: 24–30, 1995
19. Dunn J, Rodriguez D, Novak JJ: Promoting Quality Mental Health Care Delivery With Critical Path Care Plans. J Psychosoc Nurs 32 (7): 25–29, 1994
20. Eckert PA: Cost Control Through Quality Improvement: The New Challenge for Psychology. Professional Psychology: Research and Practice 25: 3–8, 1994
21. Elbeck M: Patient Contribution to the Design and Meaning of Patient Satisfaction for Quality Assurance Purposes: The Psychiatric Case. Health Care Management Review 17: 91–95, 1992

22. Freeman MA, Trabin T: Managed Behavioral Healthcare: History, Models, Key Issues and Future Course. Paper prepared for the U.S. Center for Mental Health Services, 1994
23. Francis P, Merwin E, Fox J, Shelton D: Relationship of Clinical Case Management to Hospitalization and Service Delivery for Seriously Mentally Ill Clients. Issues in Mental Health Nursing 16: 257–274, 1995
24. Green E, Katz JM: Practice Guidelines: A Standard Whose Time Has Come. Journal of Nursing Care Quarterly 8: 23–32, 1993
25. Gross D, Fogg L, Conrad B: Designing Interventions in Psychosocial Research. Archives of Psychiatric Nursing 7: 259–264, 1992
26. Hanson JG, Rapp CA: Families' Perceptions of Community Mental Health Programs for Their Relatives With a Severe Mental Illness. Community Ment Health J 28: 181–196, 1992
27. Harper G, Cotten NS: Child and Adolescent Treatment. In Sederer L (ed): Inpatient Psychiatry: Diagnosis and Treatment, pp 320–337. Baltimore, Williams & Wilkins, 1991
28. Heifner C: Positive Connectedness in the Psychiatric Nurse-Patient Relationship. Archives of Psychiatric Nursing 7: 11–15, 1993
29. Hoge MA, Davidson L, Griffith EE, Sledge WH, Howenstine RA: Defining Managed Care in Public-Sector Psychiatry. Hosp Community Psychiatry 45: 1085–1089, 1994
30. Joint Commission on Accreditation of Healthcare Organizations: The Transition for QA to QI: Performance-Based Evaluation of Mental Health Organizations. Oakbrook Terrace, Joint Commission on Accreditation of Healthcare Organizations, 1992
31. Kane RL, Bartlett J, Potthoff S: Building an Empirically Based Outcomes Information System for Managed Mental Health Care. Psychiatric Services 46: 459–461, 1995
32. Kelly KC, Huber DG, Johnson M, McCloskey JC, Maas M: The Medical Outcomes Study: A Nursing Perspective. J Prof Nurs 10: 209–216, 1994
33. Kim HS: Putting Theory Into Practice. J Adv Nurs 18: 1623–1639, 1993
34. Larsen DL, Attkisson CC, Hargreaves WA, Nguyen TD: Assessment of Client/Patient Satisfaction: Development of a General Scale. Evaluation and Program Planning 2: 197–207, 1979
35. Lefley HP: Research Directions for a New Conceptualization of Families. In Lefley HP, Johnson DL (eds): Families as Allies in Treatment of the Mentally Ill: New Directions for Mental Health Professionals, pp 127–135. Washington, DC, American Psychiatric Press, 1990
36. Lefley HP: An Overview of Family-Professional Relationships. In Marsh DT (ed): New Directions in the Psychological Treatment of Serious Mental Illness, pp 166–185. Westport, CT, Praeger Publishers/Greenwood Publishing Group, 1994
37. Marder RJ: The Interface of Clinical Paths and Continuous Quality Improvement. In Spath P (ed): Clinical Paths: Tools for Outcome Management, pp 57–79. Chicago, American Hospital Publications, 1993
38. Mellon SK: Mental Health Clinical Nurse Specialist in Home Care for the 90s. Issues in Mental Health Nursing 15: 229–237, 1994
39. Meyer EC, Gwenyth GH, Rossi JS: Evaluation and Selection of Standardized Psychological Instruments for Research and Clinical Practice. Journal of Child and Adolescent Psychiatric Nursing 8 (3): 24–31, 1995
40. Mirin SM, Namerow MJ: Why Study Treatment Outcome. Hosp Community Psychiatry 42: 1007–1013, 1991
41. Murdaugh C: Quality of Life, Functional Status, Patient Satisfaction. Patient Outcomes Research: Examining the Effectiveness of Nursing Practice. Proceedings of the State of Science Conference. Washingot, DC, NIH publication No 93-3411, 1992
42. Nelson CW: Patient Satisfaction Surveys: An Opportunity for Total Quality Improvement. Hospital and Health Services Administration 35: 409–427, 1990
43. Norbeck JS, Chaftez L, Skodal-Wilson H, Weiss SJ: Social Support Needs of Family Caregivers of Psychiatric Patients From Three Age Groups. Nurs Res 40: 208–213, 1991
44. Nurcombe B: Goal-Directed Treatment Planning and the Principles of Brief Hospitalization. Journal of the American Academy of Child and Adolescent Psychiatry 28: 26–30, 1989
45. Nyberg D, Marschke P: Critical Pathways: Tools for Continuous Quality Improvement. Nursing Administration Quarterly Spring: 62–69, 1993
46. O'Toole A, Welt S: Interpersonal Theory in Nursing Practice: Select Works of Hildegard Peplau. New York, Springer, 1989
47. Peplau H: The Heart of Nursing: Interpersonal Relations. Canadian Nurse 61: 273–275, 1965
48. Pitula CR: Unipolar Depression Without Axis II Clinical Pathway. Manuscript in preparation, 1995
49. Pless BS, Clayton GM: Clarifying the Concept of Critical Thinking in Nursing. J Nurs Educ 32: 425–428, 1993
50. Salive ME, Mayfield JA, Weissman NW: Patient Outcomes Research Teams and the Agency for Health Care Policy and Research. Health Service Research 25: 697–708, 1990
51. Schultz JM, Videbeck SD: Manual of Psychiatric Nursing Care Plans. Philadelphia, JB Lippincott, 1994
52. Ware JE, Sherbourne CD: The MOS 36-Item Short Form Health Survey (SF-36). Medical Care 30: 473–481, 1992
53. Whalley P: Team Approach to Working Through Transference and Countertransference in a Pediatric/Psychiatric Milieu. Issues in Mental Health Nursing 15: 457–469, 1994

Aspects of Care

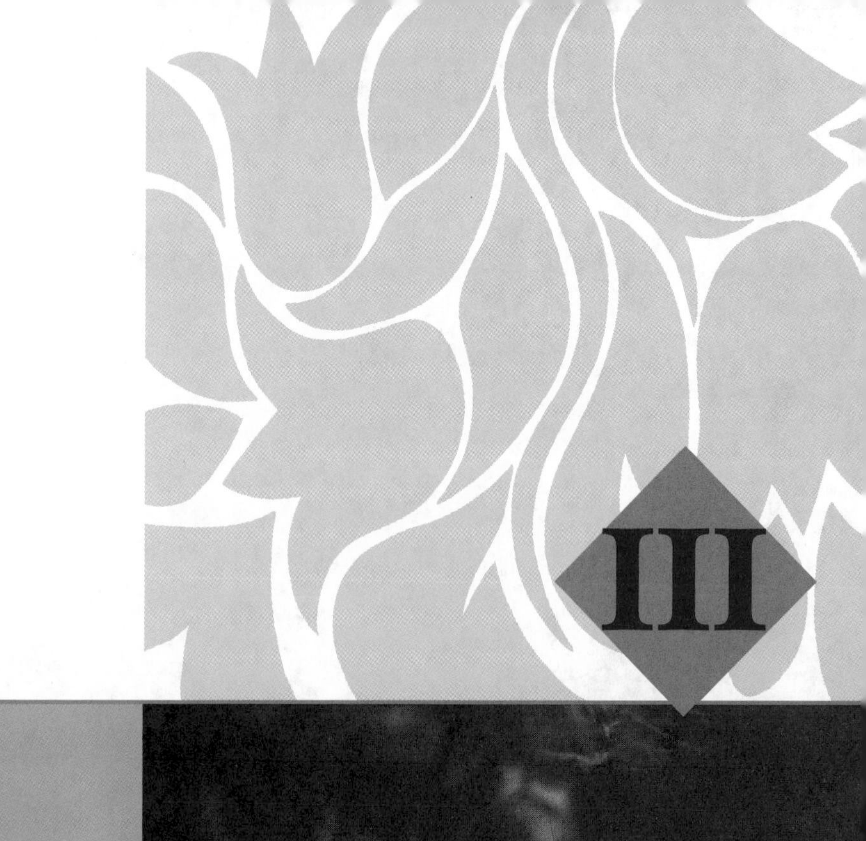

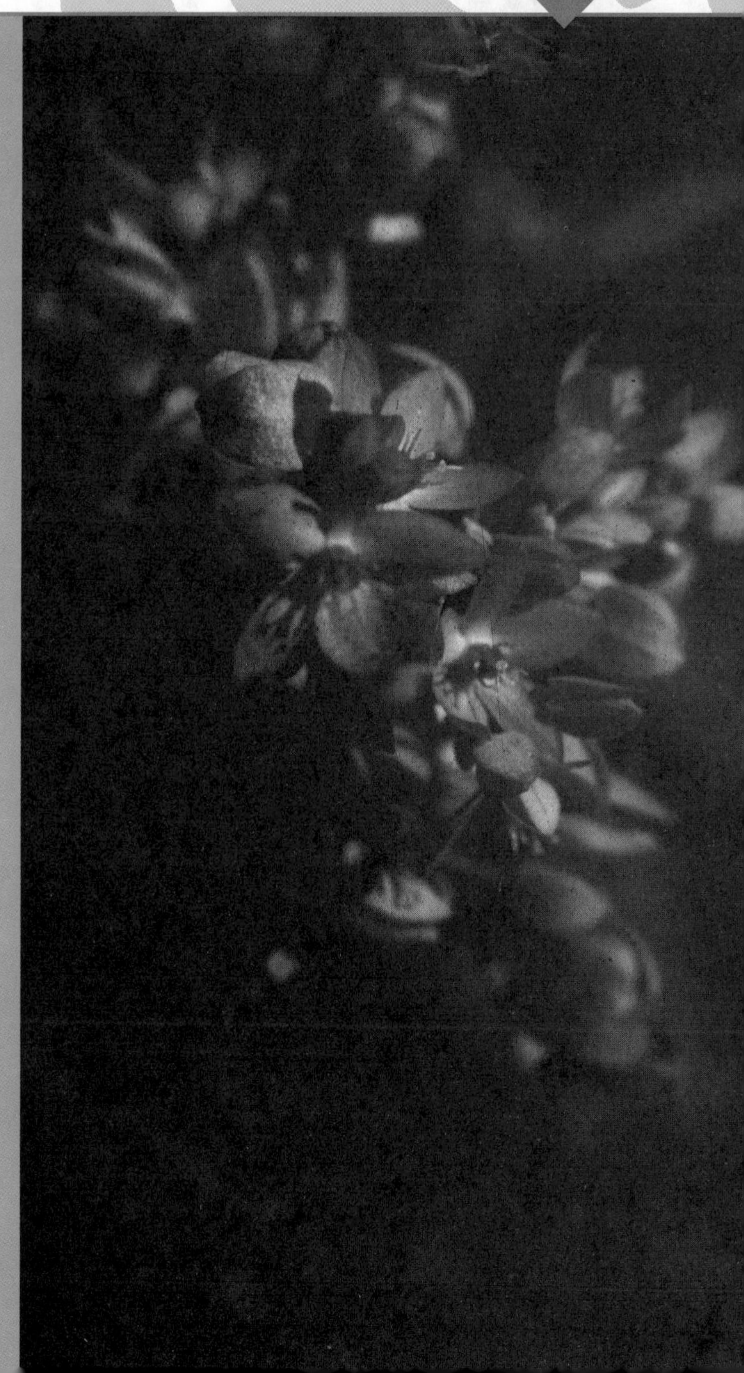

Sociocultural Aspects of Care

Cheryl Taylor
Beverly L. Malone
Kathryn Kavanagh

10

If we are to achieve a richer culture, rich in contrasting values, we must recognize the whole gamut of human potentialities, and so we are a less arbitrary social fabric, one in which each diverse human gift will find a fitting place.

As the diversity of North Americans grows, the need to understand sociocultural aspects of mental health increases. America's cultural diversity challenges psychiatric nurses to recognize complex issues involved in assessing, planning, implementing and evaluating client care. Because culture plays an important role in shaping a person's values, perceptions, beliefs, and behaviors, it is an essential component to understanding mental health. Culture represents the vast structure of behaviors, ideas, attitudes, values, habits, beliefs, customs, languages, rituals, ceremonies, and practices peculiar to a particular group of people and that provides them with a general design for living and with patterns for interpreting reality.[35]

This chapter was written to help the health care provider understand how a person's culture influences behavior in health and illness. The overview of culture focuses on concepts basic to understanding cultural diversity and the nurse's role in designing provision of culturally competent care to clients experiencing mental and emotional stress, and promoting positive mental health.

Learning Objectives

On completion of this chapter, you should be able to accomplish the following:

1. *Describe key concepts essential to understanding culture and mental health.*
2. *Discuss universal characteristics of culture.*
3. *Describe historical, political, societal and cultural contexts of the mental health care delivery system and psychiatric nursing.*
4. *Assess your own heritage, reference group and personal and cultural biases.*
5. *Recognize and discuss feelings, behaviors and personal values that influence your ability to interact with individuals from different cultures in different settings.*
6. *Identify barriers to/of therapeutic communication with culturally different clients.*
7. *Describe skills essential to developing role competence as a psychiatric/mental health care delivery provider.*
8. *Recognize biological variations and the range of social, psychological and spiritual perspectives within ethnic groups and across cultures.*
9. *Discuss criteria for evaluating the effectiveness of culturally competent psychiatric mental health nursing care.*

◆ Universal Characteristics of Culture

Every human being has a cultural dimension that shapes how he or she perceives the world and living in it. In the presence of mental illness or emotional distress in an individual, culture often becomes more evident. Culture is taught and learned from generation to generation. Culture is interactive, adaptive, and satisfying for group needs. Over time, culture represents a systematic blend of the real and the ideal norms or patterns of behavior.

Understanding sociocultural aspects of psychiatric nursing care, approached from a critical thinking perspective, forms a basis for cultural competence. Box 10-1 lists a series of self-assessment questions that nurses ask about their own cultural views and beliefs as a first step to understanding other peoples' culture.

Given that there are hundreds of different cultures, innumerable additional categories of diversity, and as many ways to interpret human experience as there are people, nurses must be reasonable about what it is they should expect themselves to know. It is not possible to know everything that might prove useful in health care, but it is possible to develop and communicate attitudes that express sincere interest, a willingness to learn, and respect for others' views.

Once one begins to assess one's own culture, the next step is in looking beyond to that of other peoples. Consider the following questions:

What is the ethnic/racial profile of the American population?

How culturally diverse is the mental health care delivery system?

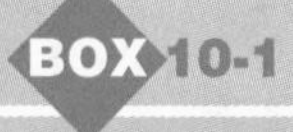

Ask Yourself

1. To what ethnic group, socioeconomic class, and community do I feel a part of or belong? To what extent do I recognize and understand my own racial or ethnic background?
2. What are the values of my ethnic group(s)? What do we generally believe about mental health and mental illness?
3. What are my earliest images of race and color? What are my attitudes toward people who are different from me in appearance or behavior?
4. What have been my personal experiences with other ethnic or racial cultures? What do I know about people from ethnic groups that are different from my own?
5. Sometimes an individual may be a descendent of a variety of racial or ethnic cultures. How do different racial or ethnic cultures come together in my own background?

What are the historical and societal contexts of psychiatric care for clients from diverse cultures?
Are there health issues particular to specific social or cultural groups?
What can be done, personally and professionally, to facilitate positive outcomes for of all social and cultural groups seeking mental health care?

◆ Culture and the Societal/ Historical Context of Psychiatric Nursing

PROVIDERS

Nursing reflects society, and American society is itself in transformation. It is literally changing complexion, "browning" so rapidly that by the middle of the twenty-first century the average resident of the U.S.A. (as defined by census bureau statistics) will trace his or her ancestry to Africa, the Pacific Islands, or the Hispanic or Arab worlds, rather than to European roots.[26] We are diversifying not only by race but ethnicity. Today twenty per cent of people in the U.S.A. speak languages other than English at home.[16] Within fifty years, one out of every five Americans will be Hispanic. Nurses in mental health care settings are in key positions to promote and practice culturally competent care.[34] Camphina-Bacote[6] described a framework for developing cultural competence that delineates practitioner skills on a continuum model (Figure 10-1).

Psychiatric nurses represent approximately 1% of the total 1.8 million nurses employed. Out of 10,567 psychiatric nurses, only 405 (3.8%) have been identified as ethnic minority nurses. Statistics show that psychiatric nursing has fewer providers of color than psychiatry (18.4%), psychology (4.3%), and social work (11.5%).[28] Yet, the leadership exemplified by psychiatric nurses of color has affected not only nursing but the health of the nation (Box 10-2).

CONSUMERS

As a nation, American society has spent the twentieth century learning to hear and attend to the voices of peoples whose views were not previously acknowledged as important. Earlier in this century, when people came from all over the world to the U.S.A, they were expected to become as much a part of the dominant culture as they could. This often meant compromising, even giving up, their original cultures. Language and customs were to conform to norms of American society which, in the realm of health and illness, meant that people were expected to follow the European and American traditions reflected in the health care system. Unmodifiable characteristics, such as race, age and sex, made assimilation more difficult, and often left nonwhites, the very old and very young, and females with significant barriers to full participation in the social mainstream.

The issue of health gaps, whether physical or mental, between the dominant and minority cultures will continue to grow with the changing demographics. Of the 250 million Americans, more that 23% are racially or ethnically different from the dominant culture of European ancestry. Approximately 30 million (11%) are African American, 21 million (8.6%) are Hispanic, and 7.2 million (3%) are Asian Pacific Islanders.[40] In addition to a higher birth rate for Hispanics, this change has been primarily explained by immigrants from Latin American and influxes from the Philippines, China, India and Southeast Asia. By the year 2000, it is predicted that three out of five children will be children of color.[42]

Although these statistics reflect the diversity of America, they do not capture the differences in the

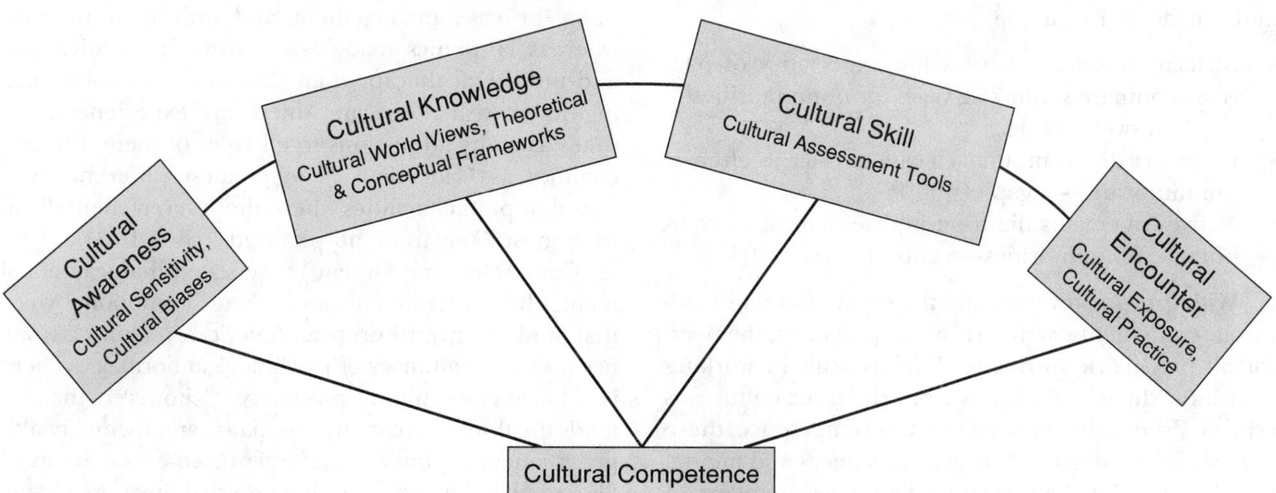

Figure 10-1. A culturally competent model of care. From Camphina-Bacote (1994, p.7) with permission.

BOX 10-2

Culture and the Societal/Historical Context of Psychiatric Nursing

Throughout history, psychiatric nurses of color have made a difference. Their leadership is reflected in psychiatric nurses from Sojourner Truth, who worked with the underground railways to free slaves, and was known as a nurse and counselor, to Hilda Richards, Chancellor at the University of Indiana Northwest.

In 1956, Elizabeth Lipford Kent was the first African American nurse to earn the doctoral degree. Dr. Kent provided administrative guidance to the Lafayette Clinic, a state mental health facility in Detroit, Michigan. Under the leadership of Dr. Ildaura Murillo-Rohde, the Hispanic Nurses Association was established. Through the efforts of Dr. Mary Harper, the ANA Ethnic Minority Fellowship Program was initially conceived and funded by the National Institute of Mental Health (NIMH) in 1974. This outstanding program, which has produced more than 200 doctorally prepared nurses of color, African, Hispanic, Asian and Native American, has continued to be federally funded for more than twenty years under the leadership of dynamic nurses, Drs. Ruth Gordon, Hattie Bessent, and Carla Serlin. During Dr. Hattie Bessent's tenure, Dr. Jeanni Jo, the first Native American nurse earned the doctoral degree. In 1978, Dr. Rhetaugh Dumas, presently vice president of health affairs for the University of Michigan Medical Center, became the first psychiatric nurse and the first African American to serve as Deputy Director of the NIMH. Psychiatric nurses of color have been women and men of extraordinary vision and courage to lead the nursing profession into new arenas of policy making, research and culturally competent clinical service.

health status between the dominant and minority cultures. Infant mortality rates, one of the primary indicators of a nation's health, range from slightly higher rates for Asian Pacific Island groups as compared with those for nonminority infants, to twice as high for African American groups.[33] The health gap is only emphasized when reviewing other major causes of death, such as cancer, AIDS, diabetes, heart disease, homicide, and suicide. For example:[33]

- African Americans have a life expectancy of 69.6 years compared with 75.2 years for nonminorities—a gap of over 5 years.
- Hispanics die from stomach cancer twice as often as nonminorities—a gap of 100%
- Native Americans die from injuries almost twice as often as nonminorities—a gap of nearly 100%

With growing diversity and the small number of culturally competent psychiatric nurse providers, the need for all psychiatric nurses to develop skills in working with individuals and groups from different cultures is critical. Even with increased cultural competence, there is a lack of connection between consumers and mental health care providers. Historically, many members of ethnically and racially diverse populations have avoided the mental health care delivery system. This arose from the fear of being diagnosed or labeled abnormal rather than different. The possibility of misdiagnosis is confirmed in the literature, which consistently reports diagnoses with a high frequency of psychosis and a low frequency of depression in African Americans and other ethnic minorities.[1,39]

African Americans made fewer visits than Caucasians for case management and individual therapy, whereas Hispanics made fewer visits for medications and individual therapy than Caucasians. Despite making fewer visits, African Americans experienced 1.8 times as many admissions to all types of mental health facilities as Caucasians. The greatest difference was found in public facilities where the severely mentally ill were most likely to be hospitalized [39](Box 10-3).

Comas-Diaz and Greene[8] have stated that traditional mental health treatment has been an institutional voice that tends to invest European-American middle-class values with the legitimacy of psychological normalcy. There is a "new cross-cultural psychiatry,"[31] however, that extends the thinking of many psychiatric and mental health practitioners to consider culturally-based explanations of illness and behavior[20]. This is a sign that times are changing. Diversity is increasingly recognized, as is the impor-

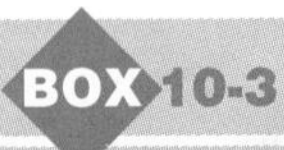

Diagnosis and Race: The Case of Junius Wilson

In 1925, Junius Wilson, a seventeen-year-old black man, was charged with attempted rape in the New Hanover community of Castle Hayne, North Carolina. In court, he was found incompetent to stand trial. The charges were dropped after he arrived at Cherry State Hospital, a state mental institution. However, he was castrated and remained a patient in a locked mental ward for 69 years. In the 1920s, castration was a standard procedure for black males accused of rape. John Badgett, deputy director of the state Division of Mental Health, states that Wilson "has been the victim of social politics that we look back on now and are deeply troubled by." In 1992, after a review of Wilson's medical records, a social worker discovered that Wilson was deaf, not mentally ill. This discovery, with legal assistance, led to the release of Mr. Wilson and compensation by the state for the abuse and years of imprisonment. Mr. Wilson presently lives in a three bedroom house on the grounds of Cherry Hospital. He is enjoying his newly found freedom and speaking in a type of sign language used by blacks years ago, called the Raleigh dialect.

Swofford, S. News and Record, Thursday, December 28, 1995, pp. B1–B2

tance of and right to reference group identity, although these are not always consistently valued. As the century closes, people from diverse backgrounds and orientations increasingly expect, demand and are acknowledged to have a right to opportunities to preserve their varied lifestyles, beliefs, and practices—including those pertaining to health and illness from conception to death. Nursing and other health care disciplines are seriously reconsidering the "one size fits all" approaches that typified health care in the past.

MODES OF CARE

Any attempt to understand the needs of diverse clients begins with finding out from clients, or someone who can truly speak for them, an answer to: "What do you expect (or want) the nurse to do for you?" Intervention might reflect any of the modes of care previously delineated by Leininger for culturally congruent nursing: preservation (that is, maintenance of familiar lifestyles), accommodation or negotiation of some aspect of those, or actual repatterning or restructuring. Nursing's inclination to actively intervene and implement change at times risks wholesale promotion of repatterning of health-related practices that are not harmful or inappropriate, but merely different, and do not require change. This uncritical approach frequently meets with resistance and "noncompliance" by clients who realize that clinicians do not understand (or are not open to learning about) belief and practice orientations that differ from their own (Table 10-1).

A need for cultural maintenance or preservation is demonstrated, for example, when a Native American client expresses a desire to use traditional herbs and to participate in a sweat lodge ceremony to aid in the healing process. The clinician whose attitude communicates sensitivity to, interest in, and even rudimentary knowledge about traditional healing practices has an increased likelihood of learning from the client about the full range of his or her health-related beliefs and behaviors. The client, on the other hand, is more likely to comply with an approach that allows him or her to preserve familiar practices. Since belief can play a major part in healing outcome[32] it follows that every effort should be made to support what clients believe will help—unless there is real evidence that a practice is harmful. This is an area where the difference between stereotype and actual knowledge is readily apparent. Having one's experience discredited or made to seem unimportant is painful.

The second mode of nursing intervention involves assisting clients both to negotiate or adapt to new ways and accommodate old ways.[25] As nurses become sensitive to the complex factors that influence clients' responses to health, illness, treatment, and care, they learn to negotiate. A client who believes his psychiatric problems are punishment for sins he has committed, for example, is more likely to get well and to comply with medication regimes if his spiritual healer (e.g., a priest) is involved with the treatment too.

A third approach to intervention involves culturally acceptable and appropriate care that enables change to new or different behavioral patterns.[25] To be acceptable and congruent, the new standards must be meaningful, satisfying, and beneficial. Changing a person's view of events requires altering the meaning the situation has for that person.[38] However, the need for such restructuring is less common than the need for preservation and negotiation of present beliefs and practices, which involve only partial repatterning.

Beliefs and Practices

Reluctance to seek treatment may involve a different set of cultural beliefs concerning mental health. Each culture has a set of beliefs about the meaning of health and the prevention of illness. Home medicines, prayer

Table 10-1

Concepts Essential to Cultural Competence

Concept	Description or Operational Definition	Verbal Example or Interpretations
Cultural competence	Knowledge based and interpersonal skills that allow health care providers to understand, appreciate, and work effectively with individuals of cultures other than their own	"As a psychiatric nurse in Springfield, Massachusetts, I speak Spanish and work closely with the Puerto Rican People in the community and hospital."
Demographics	Relating to statistical measures of human populations with reference to size and distribution	The Asian population is growing seven times faster than any other minority group.
Difference	The notion that interpretation or meaning is made through contrast and by identifying separateness Differences perceived as an asset or a liability	"I look forward to meeting new people with different ways and views." (asset) "I don't even know her. I don't like the way she looks. Her slanted eyes make me suspicious." (liability)
Enculturation	The process by which an individual learns the expected behaviors of a culture	Marrying a person of another culture and taking on their cultural identity is an example.
Ethnicity	Cultural characteristics, language, religion, perceptions, and values associated with a group	Irish, English, Serbians, West Indians, African-Americans, and Lakota, are examples.
Expectations (client)	Personal anticipated outcome measures of the treatment process	"I want to stop hurting."
Family	A group of people connected by blood, household, or kinship network; the fundamental social unit in society Relationships as the common denominator of all types of families, primary organ of transmission of cultural beliefs and practices	A gang; a traditional group of mother, father, sister and brother; church families are examples.
Generational patterns	Rituals and behaviors transmitted with time and through family tradition	Racial prejudice, domestic abuse, and addiction; "It runs in the family."
Healers	Individuals committed to restoring, renewing, and promoting health on an individual or community level	The medicine man; the midwife; the physician, the clinical nurse specialist; curanderos, and many others are examples.
Interpretation	One's perception or belief about the meaning assigned to an event	"It sounds as if you're saying . . ."
Minor or minority	Smaller, inferior in importance, size, or degree; a smaller segment of a population different from others and often subjected to differential treatment	White students attend school on a historically African American university campus.
Misdiagnosis	Conclusive assignment of label or diagnosis that does not reflect the client's condition	"On the MMPI, the F scale is elevated. This minority male must be paranoid."
Negotiation	Communication designed to reach an agreement when there exists opposing views or goals	"What can I do to arrive at an agreement that will benefit both of us?"
Objectivity	The notion that one can maintain analytical neutrality in approaches to client care	"On a personal basis, I have great difficulty with what you have said. On a professional basis, let's take a look at that. Give me an example of what you mean."
Poverty	Quality or conditions of being poor, experiencing levels of acute deprivation with limited resources to meet basic needs	Parts of the United States of America still have a lot of outside toilets (outhouses).
Preference	To view or give advantage, priority, or privilege to one individual or group over another	Men are much easier to work with than women.

continued

Table 10-1 (Continued)

Concept	Description or Operational Definition	Verbal Example or Interpretations
Prejudice	Negative or hostile attidue toward individuals or groups, based on ignorance, impervious to evidence, and contrary to argument A prejudgment that creates barriers to seeing the facts	A teacher may not expect a student to do well because he or she is a member of "minority" group.
Prescriptive cultural beliefs	Traditional therapeutic culturally bound recommendations for managing illness and health states; cultural *Do's*	Folk practices (eg, wearing a copper bracelet on affected arthritic limb) are examples.
Psyche	The soul, the other self, the second self, living, magnetically combined energy of man with spirit	Examples include spiritual chants, prayers, psychospiritual intervention.
Racism	The process of asserting superiority; racism based on a broad concept referring to racial or physically (biologically) based prejudices and practices exercised against ethnic groups by institutions and individuals in positions of power	Examples include ethnic cleansing; the holocaust; enslavement of African Americans, Jim Crow laws.
Restrictive cultural beliefs	Traditional, culturally bound limitations on behavior; cultural *Don'ts* originally designed to promote health	Women should not take a bath during menstruation.
Stereotype	Accepting generalizations or prevailing assumptions and beliefs about a group of people without regard to their individual differences (seeing individuals as representating a group)	"Black people are dumb, lazy, and violent." "White people all look alike."
Values	A universal feature of all cultures; one's perception of what is important	Values include individualism, groups, unity, consumerism, time, family.
Western medicine	A model of health care delivery based on scientific principles and experimentation to determine cause and effect, understanding disease processes by way of anatomy, physiology, and the mind–body dichotomy	Chemotherapy and surgery are used for cancer treatment.

and rituals often provide cultural solutions to anxiety producing issues, providing a sense of mastery over one's well being.[30] For example, Curanderismo is a type of folk healing sometimes practiced in Mexican-American communities. (Box 10-4)

Many Mexican Americans, like members of other ethnic groups, believe in "folk illnesses." One example is "fright" or "soul loss" (*susto*), which is often associated by members of Hispanic cultures with a sudden start or sneeze.[11] Various conditions thought to result from the "evil eye" (*mal ojo*) are believed to occur unintentionally when, for instance, a nurse fails to touch a child he or she has noticed or examined. Herbal remedies, rubbing, massage and other physical manipulations by *curanderos* (*curanderas,* if they are women) are typical treatments. These might be used with home remedies (such as teas), prayers and trips to religious shrines or charismatic folk healers to alleviate distress.

Some cultural behavior mimics psychopathology. For example, "falling out" is a culture-bound behavior exhibited in some African Americans and Black Caribbeans. Falling out is manifested by sudden collapse and/or paralysis, and the inability to see or speak.[6] The individual is frequently described as caught up in the Spirit, and the behavior is usually associated with a religious experience.

Differences and Commonalities

It is important to realize that the term "Hispanic" actually includes a great deal of cultural variability. The terms Latino and Hispanic refer to generally Spanish ethnicity, language skills, and ancestry, but[37] there is wide variability in levels of acculturation, that is, integration into the mainstream American system.[13] While the average Mexican American was born in the U.S.A. and many members of other Hispanic groups are American by birth, numerous others are immigrants.[29]

Although commonly shared beliefs and practices are often found among members of Hispanic groups, significant differences can also be expected. It is important to avoid stereotyping, since working with fixed ideas about people interferes with understanding who they really are. For instance, the origin of the term "Hispanic" was the US Bureau of the Census, who created

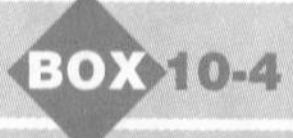

Curanderismo

Juanita Zapata Flint, MS, RN Coordinator/Faculty, El Centro College, Brookhaven College Satellite, Dallas Texas

Curanderismo is the practice of folk healing that evolved from European medical practices of the 15th and 16th centuries and that continues today within the Mexican American community. The Aztecs, Mayas, and other Indian groups left these folk beliefs and curing practices to the Spanish Catholics in Mexico. Curanderismo has persisted as a tradition in the Mexican American culture because of that culture's members' rural background, illiteracy, poverty, and distrust of the modern medical care system.

Curanderas and *curanderos,* or folk healers, are usually women who believe they are endowed with curing powers from God. The healer comes to hold this belief by being involved in the care of a sick person who recovers. Curanderos are sincere in their belief that they were chosen by God and therefore do not usually charge fees for their healing services. They believe that if they expected or demanded payment, their divine gift of healing would be taken away. Recently, however, it has become common for curanderos to develop a fee system, although their charges are minimal.

The diseases treated by the curandera are thought to be due to the will of God or to witchcraft. *Susto,* or fright, is a condition that follows an emotional upset and is characterized by depression, restlessness, loss of strength, and anorexia. If a client suffers from susto, the curanderas are the only ones believed to have the power to perform the necessary healing rituals.

Mal ojo, or evil eye, is thought to be caused by envy, covetous expressions, or attention paid by one person to another. For example, a mother may be told that her child, after making a statement, will cast the spell of mal ojo, and the child will become ill with fever. The person complimenting the child should touch him, thereby breaking the spell of mal ojo.

The belief in mal ojo is widespread. Mexican Americans may take preventive measures, such as wearing amulets, gold earrings, snakes' fangs, garlic, or oil crosses on the head, to deflect the mal ojo.

Mal ojo and susto are only two of the many folk diseases that the nurse might encounter when caring for the Mexican American client. The nurse should not assume that a client who is educated or acculturated does not hold these beliefs in curanderismo.

For example, when I was pregnant with my son, there was a death in the family. I planned on going to the funeral, but when making arrangements with my mother, she told me that I could not go to the funeral due to my pregnancy. It seemed very odd to me that she would say this, because she never seemed to hold much faith in some of the Mexican American cultural beliefs. When discussing this further with my grandmother and mother, they told me that the embalming fluid would be in the air around the body, causing *mal aire,* and this could cause my baby to be born with deformities or make me very ill. They told me that I could possibly miscarry if I came to the funeral. I did go to the funeral, but in respect for their wishes, especially my grandmother's, I sat in the back and did not view the body. (Several months later, I delivered a healthy boy.)

A client's perceptions of health and illness are influenced strongly by cultural beliefs; health care services must acknowledge and understand those cultural beliefs to provide optimal care to Mexican Americans.

References

1. Henderson G: Transcultural Health Care. Menlo Park, CA, Addison-Wesley, 1980
2. Ingham JM: On Mexican Folk Medicine. American Anthropologist, 1970
3. Kiev A: Curanderismo: Mexican-American Folk Psychiatry. New York, Free Press, 1968
4. Madsen W: The Mexican-American of South Texas. New York, Holt, Rinehart, & Winston, 1964
5. Orque SM et al: Ethnic Nursing Care: A Multi-cultural Approach. St. Louis, CV Mosby, 1983
6. Rodriguez J: Mexican Americans: Factors Influencing Health Practices. The Journal of School Health 53 (February): 136–140, 1983
7. Spector RE: Cultural Diversity in Health and Illness, 2d ed. Norwalk, CT, Appleton-Century-Crofts, 1985
8. Swafford-Gonzalez MJ, Gutierrez MG: Ethno-Medical Beliefs and Practices of Mexican Americans. Nurse Prac 8 (November–December): 29–34, 1983

this generic term to identify individuals who identified themselves as being of Spanish origin. But within that generic term, Hispanic, are: Mexican or Mexican American including Chicano; Puerto Rican or Boricua; Cuban or Cuban American; "Other" Spanish or Hispanic, including Central and South Americans; and Latino which is preferred by some Hispanics since it emphasizes Latin America instead of Spanish origins.[9] Interestingly, 63% of the Hispanic population are Mexican Americans with little familial connection to their "Spanish" origins.

Some common influences upon Hispanic American cultural traditions include Catholicism (although increasing numbers of Hispanics are turning to Protestant religions and Pentecostal sects), orientation toward extended family systems (which may include godparents [*compadres*] and other non-biological kin),[14] different concepts of appropriate roles for men and women that are now in flux,[36] a high value of respect for self and others, the priority of spiritual and humanistic over commercial values, relatively clear hierarchy and patriarchy, and fairly common reliance on folk systems of medicine.

Since Hispanic Americans tend to value being listened to and having time spent with them, task-oriented hurrying about is viewed as noncaring. Involvement, loving, and empathy are valued caring behaviors.[26] Spanish American folk medicine, despite some variation with place and group, clearly reflects ancient, humoral roots, as well as Catholic ritual and beliefs about supernatural influences. Many illnesses are "hot" or "cold," so sufferers are treated with medicines and foods of opposite characteristics. These qualities do not refer to temperature but to symbolic properties. Care and treatment regimens can be negotiated with clients within that framework.

◆ Culturally Competent Care

To provide culturally competent care, the nurse must find out from the client and the client's reference group what is considered "normal" and what is "abnormal," both in terms of problem definition and expectations for treatment and care. Culture (including its many expressions as subcultures in the U.S.A.) influences expression, presentation, recognition, labelling, explanations for, and distribution of mental health and mental illness.

Whether or not these are understood, people have reasons for their behavior. They may, for example, refuse to have blood drawn due to a belief that it could be used for sorcery or, as was traditionally believed in some Asian cultures, that blood contains the personality. It does not make sense to risk personality loss with blood donation, or confusion with someone else's as a consequence of transfusion. On the other hand, as unsound as it may be from a biomedical perspective, it does make sense for clients to alter their medication dosage when they believe that the "large" American physicians who prescribe medicines are likely to order too large a dose for someone of smaller stature.[15]

ESSENTIAL CONSIDERATIONS FOR WORKING WITH ANY CULTURE

Since culture is adaptive and interactive, it is important to assess to what degree an individual's traditional views and practices have been modified or replaced with dominant (European-American) cultural values. The dominant culture in the United States is composed of white middle class Protestants of European ancestry. American cultural values stress individualism, reliance on technology, youth and beauty, material comfort, punctuality, and efficient use of time, competition and success through achievement. One example of the above values can be observed with the recent emergence of psychic advisor networks. Psychic advisor networks rely on technology (telephone and television) to access individuals desperate for advice and support. There are multiple networks nationwide that compete with each other, claiming expertise, reasonable rates (advice costs $ per minute) and success stories, all in the name of "entertainment only" which protects them from malpractice claims. Meanwhile, the troubled individual who depends on this service may not receive adequate counseling and may remain apart from the mental health professionals who might help.

Perception of Time

Time takes on different meanings in various cultures. American culture values punctuality, efficiency and conscious efforts to not waste time. Time is a commodity, compartmentalized into appointments and schedules. This approach to communication appears unprofessional and unacceptable in traditional Asian, Hispanic, African American, Native American and other cultures. In their view, ample time should be allotted for clients to explain their situation in detail, and to observe and "size up" the health care professional providing service.[17] In psychiatric nursing, we call it establishing rapport with the client. The key is to recognize alternative cultural views of time and allow the time needed to establish a rapport with the client.

This poses a challenge for the culturally competent nurse. In American society today, "time is money" and time spent relating to others is often not highly valued. Nurses must learn to engage clients in conversation while providing routine care, to advocate for reasonable and client-centered workloads, and to protect valuable nurse-client time together.

Understanding Cultural Patterns

The patterns used by clients to express concern, referred to as "language of distress," vary widely.[18] Although specific socially patterned expectations may or may not be familiar to the provider, knowledge of predictable cultural patterns can be useful for nurses. For example, it is not unusual to encounter clients who deny being depressed, but who complain of headaches, backaches, stomach aches and other physical phenomena prompted (and sometimes consciously associated) with sorrow and suffering. It is beneficial to know that somatic symptoms that express psychological distress occur at high rates, for instance, among clients who are Hispanic[10] or Chinese.[23]

Lack of sensitivity, knowledge and skill (that is, cultural competence) can result in the labelling of people as "noncompliant," "problem clients," or too resistant or defensive to recognize the value of the care being offered or to benefit from treatment. Often the client's ideas about care and caring (and the expression of those), or about priorities, simply differ from those of health care providers. Realizing that perspectives are shaped by values and beliefs (which are, in turn, rooted in orientations to specific cultures, socioeconomic classes, and time periods) allows objective assessment of diverse practices that people use to promote health and cope with illness[21] (Boxes 10-5 and 10-6).

Groups also vary widely in their ideas about appropriate stance, gestures, language, listening styles, and eye contact. Traditional Asian Americans, African Americans, and Native Americans[43] typically consider direct eye contact inappropriate and disrespectful,[20] whereas direct eye contact in American culture is often interpreted as an indicator of self-esteem and assertiveness. Client eye contact is one of the most frequently documented observations noted in clients' psychiatric records. It is important to document clients' appropriate or inappropriate behavior in the context of the clients' cultural norms. Phases such as "poor eye contact" or "good eye contact" should be used with consideration of the context and client's culture.

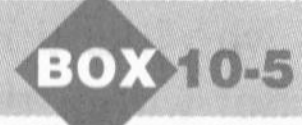

BOX 10-5

Treatment Strategies for Cultural Competence in Mental Health Care Delivery

1. Assess own cultural heritage and behavior patterns.
2. Recognize coexisting belief systems about mental health and illness.
3. Assess client's personal beliefs, concerns, and fears about the illness.
4. Assess and consider family (generational patterns) history.
5. Explain, negotiate, and when indicated, collaborate on a treatment plan that takes into account the client's cultural beliefs. Discuss client expectation of treatment regimen (preserve helpful beliefs or repattern acknowledged harmful beliefs or practices).
6. Recognize informal caregivers as allies in the treatment process.
7. Read documented information about specific cultural groups.
8. Determine if the client is seeking western health care in conjunction with or exclusive of any personal cultural beliefs about mental illness.
9. Collaborate with key informants and others who are adept to interpreting meanings of language and behaviors of specific cultures.
10. Demonstrate patience, a nonjudgmental attitude, and genuine respect for the client no matter what behavior he or she exhibits.

Critical Skills for Culturally Competent Care

Before a psychiatric nurse can provide culturally competent therapeutic care, there is a preparation process. Ideally, psychiatric nurses would acquire these skills in their nursing programs. Battaglia[5] identifies four critical skills:

1. Cross-cultural understanding
2. Intercultural communication
3. Facilitation skills
4. Flexibility

Cross-cultural Understanding. This is the knowledge about how and why individuals of different cultures act the way they do. It may involve studying the relevant culture or identifying a colleague from that culture and learning about the values, norms and mores of the culture. This strategy should not be used in isolation due to the potential fallacy of overgeneralizing that all members of a specific group should be treated the same.

Intercultural Communication. Communication is the crux of cross-cultural psychiatric/mental health nursing. Some differences in communication are readily apparent; others are harder to see, such as differences in degree of openness, self-disclosure, emotional expres-

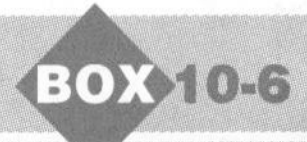

Clinical Considerations for Working With Clients of Asian Ethnic Origin in the Mental Health Setting

1. Do consider the client's level of acculturation.
2. Do assess how the client interprets his or her illness.
3. Do assess the client's concept of the future.
4. Don't be intrusive during the first few sessions. Focus on establishing rapport.
5. Don't misdiagnose submissive women as "psychiatric disorders." Make distinctions between culturally based psychological phenomena and psychiatric disorders.
6. When possible, do pair up same sex client and therapist. Always allow personal space between male and female therapist–client seating arrangements.
7. Do recognize the importance of the family to Asian clients.
8. Do tell your client exactly about prescribed medications, dosage, and side effects. Instruct them not to give their medication to other family members or reduce prescribed medication dosage.
9. Do assess, recognize, and accept the influence of religious beliefs on client's behavior.
10. Do consult with Asian or Asian American practitioners and scholars for advice and recommendations for reading materials, clinical supervision, and staff development.

sion, insight and even talkativeness. Intercultural communication involves the development of listening skills, including deciphering nonverbal behavior and detection of barriers that interfere with communication. The psychiatric mental health nurse should excel in this area unless hindered by intra personal stereotypes and biases that have not been identified.

Communicating across cultures requires testing stereotypes against reality. When cognition and affect are impaired by mental illness, communication can be especially time consuming and complex, although it is no less important. Assumptions must be avoided. Unusual language use may, for example, represent cultural differences rather than thinking or hearing impairments, although those explanations also might be valid. The skilled communicator learns how to identify and bridge differences.[20]

Nearly every "ethnic" category contains parallel variability. There are vast differences among Asian cultures, white ethnic groups, and African American groups. There are also several hundred different Native American and Alaskan Native tribes and nations, some recognized by the federal government and others only at the state or local level.[12] Most Native American populations share a traditional orientation to being in the present (rather than to doing and to the future, which is more typical of European Americans), to cooperation rather than competition, to giving rather than keeping, and to respect for age rather than youth.[1] The traditional Native American life cycle emphasizes rhythmic, natural phenomena; a balance of living, being and working toward shared goals; and acceptance of self development as never completed. On the other hand, many Native Americans are not very traditional and live modern lives indistinguishable from those of many European Americans, or they may combine Native American and other beliefs and practices in any of many different ways.

Differences in communication style may require additional time for the communication that is essential to provision of culturally competent care. Identifying *language* differences between staff and client and among family members will minimize problems that sometimes occur during interviewing (Box 10-7). Determine if the client is fluent in English or any other language. If English is not the client's first language, allow extra time to communicate. Solicit the assistance of a family member, or interpreter but check to see how the client feels about the interpreter selected. Take advantage of the fact that clients may read or write English better than they speak it. Use simple words and avoid professional jargon when speaking to the client. Demonstrate respect for silence as a form of communication. Some cultures (e.g., Navaho) may use silence to show respect. Silence may also be an indicator of endorsement or complicity.

Facilitation Skills. These important skills focus primarily on conflict resolution and the ability to negotiate interactions that may tend to be inconsistent with the value and belief system of an individual or family from another culture.

Flexibility. The quality of flexibility can be described as the ability to embrace change by modifying expectations, readjusting old operating norms and stereotypes and trying on new behavior.

Guidelines for Attaining Cultural Competency

The skills listed in the previous section are critical to the provision of culturally competent care. Malone (1993) recommends the following guidelines for the

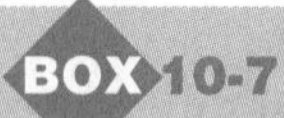

Communication and Culturally Competent Care

Hung Le is a 30-year-old Vietnamese man who reports to the hospital emergency room alone. He presents the following:

- Persistent headaches and generalized fatigue
- Despondent saddened affect
- Disheveled clothing
- Insomnia for 2 weeks
- Anorexia for 3 days
- Downcast eyes when speaking or nodding head to indicate yes or no to interviewer's questions
- Verbally responding in Vietnamese language
- No English spoken

After responding as much as he could to the female staff nurse and female psychiatric resident, Hung Le sat in a noisy waiting area for 40 minutes, looked at his watch, then walked out of the hospital, untreated for his problem. While the English-speaking female staff experienced frustration in communicating with Hung Le, they began planning for culturally competent care by conducting a cultural assessment, beginning with physical cultural variables. Noting no immediate physical concerns, they moved quickly to cultural variables in communication, learning that Mr. Hung spoke French, as do many others from his country of origin. Because a bilingual (French-English) nurse was available, communication was established, and additional information could be obtained about his cultural orientation, mental characteristics, and perception of his current problem. Mr. Hung explained that a fortune teller had predicted his illness, and when symptoms developed, his family avoided letting it be known and treated him with herbs and a special diet. Once Mr. Hung found he could converse comfortably with a culturally competent nurse who accepted him and his situation as he presented it, he began working with the staff toward resolution of the problem.

preparation of students or psychiatric nurse to give culturally competent care[27]:

1. When selecting a school or agency, inquire about the racial and ethnic make-up of the faculty and staff, student or client population, and surrounding community.
2. Seek out learning experiences such as clinical and voluntary community activities that provide exposure to people who are culturally and racially different.
3. Seek out preceptors, mentors, and faculty who are culturally different.
4. Become proficient in another language. Based on the fact that Hispanics are the fastest growing minority population, Spanish may be an appropriate choice as an elective.
5. Study the history, cultural values and mores of the racially and culturally different people in your setting and the community.
6. Attend workshops and participate in learning activities that will increase your knowledge and sensitivity to people from different cultures.
7. Ask an administrator about the institution's short- and long-range plans to increase diversity and the delivery of culturally sensitive care.
8. In clinical postconferences, and during unit meetings, openly discuss cross-cultural issues.
9. Be an active member of your professional organization to use the collective strength of organized groups to support culturally competent care.
10. Practice self-examination of your own value system and that of your family and community of origin. Be specific and replay stereotypes that you have heard during your childhood and present life. Only by facing the reality of one's own views and upbringing can management of prejudices (attitudes) and stereotypes (images) occur.
11. Understand your colleagues,' employers' and fel-

low students' shortcomings in the area of cultural and racial differences. Do not expect everyone to develop the high level of sensitivity, knowledge and skill required of cultural competence, although health care providers should be held accountable for their behavior.

◆ Exploring Client Perspectives

A model designed specifically for psychotherapeutic use is the nurse–client negotiation model. This model acknowledges that discrepancies exist between nurse and client about ideas of health, illness and treatments, and attempts to bridge the gap between the nurse's (scientific) and the client's (popular) perspectives. The major goal of the psychiatric nurse is to explore the client's perspective. Kleinman[23] suggests the following questions as fundamental in determining the client's perspective:

1. What do you think has caused your problem?
2. Why do you think it started when it did?
3. What do think your sickness does to you? How does it work?
4. How severe is your sickness? Will it have a short or long course?
5. What kind of treatment do you think you should receive?
6. What are the most important results you hope to receive from this treatment?
7. What are the chief problems your sickness has caused for you?
8. What do you fear most about your sickness? (or problem?)

These questions are equally appropriate for individuals from the dominant culture. They show respect for what the illness means to the client and respect for the client's involvement in the healing process. A negotiated therapeutic relationship is one in which the client is empowered as a partner in the assessment and resolution of the problem. Kleinman and his colleagues[23] state that the practitioner must move out of an ethnocentric professional framework to recognize clinical reality as constructed by the client's cultural and pluralistic context.

◆ Conclusion

There is an old adage that states, "The cream always rises to the top." This statement implies that one ingredient in a mixture will eventually emerge to be the dominant or most obvious ingredient. In the case of culture and the stress of mental illness, culture is a main ingredient of personality. The greater the amount of stress an individual experiences, the greater the manifestation of their culturally based perceptions, beliefs, and behaviors. In other words, culture, when hidden, eventually rises to the top.

Self-knowledge facilitates personal comfort and understanding of others when caring for culturally diverse clients in a variety of psychiatric/mental health settings. No matter where you are on the cultural competence continuum, ongoing staff development programs are beneficial to improve outcomes of care for culturally diverse psychiatric mental patients. Although diverse cultural groups may have a variety of viewing positions and health care responses to mental illness, an open, honest, and accepting attitude on the part of the nurse can be most effective when providing care.

What you know about yourself is no less important than what you know about others. Recognition of generational patterns within your own culture can assist you to assess and recognize generational patterns in other cultures. The key when working with culturally diverse clients is to develop a balanced contextualized view of the client, family, and community.

◆ Chapter Summary

This chapter emphasizes the importance of nurses' self-knowledge, viewing position, and preparation as culturally competent providers when caring for diverse clients.

1. The more stress an individual experiences, the greater the manifestation of their culturally based perceptions, beliefs and behaviors.
2. A culturally sensitive model of care requires the integration of the individual and the culture while safeguarding the uniqueness of the individual.
3. Knowledge of the typical patterns of other cultures (eg, values, expectations, and behaviors) is useful, for it provides a basis for comparing a given situation with what might be expected.
4. Critical skills for culturally competent care include cross-cultural understanding, intercultural communication, facilitation skills, and flexibility.
5. To provide culturally competent care, the nurse must find out from the client and the client's reference group what is considered "normal" and what is "abnormal," both in terms of problem definition and expectations for treatment and care. It is important to document clients' appropriate or inappropriate behavior in the context of the clients' cultural norms.
6. All cultures have their particular view of communication, space, time and social organization. Differ-

ences in communication style may require additional time to establish the rapport that is essential to provision of culturally competent care.

7. To care competently and confidently requires that we recognize that we are all more alike than we are different and that dealing with differences poses a challenge to psychiatric mental health nurses today.

Critical Thinking Questions

1. *What issues may emerge when working with clients who are culturally different?*
2. *What roles might family play in the mental health treatment of clients?*
3. *How do your personal experiences affect how you think about and feel about clients who have had cultural experiences different from your own?*
4. *What are some experiences that you've had within your lifetime that you consider significant in the way you view a) mental illness? b) clients with diagnosed psychiatric disorders? c) clients who hold viewpoints about mental health treatments that are different from yours?*
5. *What is the most significant action that you could take to increase your ability to provide culturally competent care to clients whose cultural experiences differ from your own?*

Review Questions

1. What is culture?
2. Define and discuss the influence of racial stereotypes on psychiatric nursing and mental health care delivery.
3. Identify significant contributions of psychiatric nurses of color to the nursing profession.
4. What issues may emerge when working with clients who are culturally different?
5. Why is it important to provide culturally competent care to clients?
6. Describe curanderismo.
7. What kinds of roles do healers serve in various cultures?
8. Describe essential assessment parameters for working with diverse clients.
9. What roles might families play in the treatment of clients?

◆ References

1. Adebimpe V: Overview-White Norms in Psychiatric Diagnosis of Black American Patients. American Journal of Psychiatry 138 (3): 279–285, 1981
2. Andrews MM, Boyle JS: Transcultural Nursing. Lippincott-Raven, Philadelphia, PA, 1994
3. Attneave C: American Indian and Alaska Native Families: Emigrants in their own homeland. In McGoldrick M, Pearce JK, Giordano J (eds): Ethnicity and Family Therapy, (pp. 55–83) Guilford Press, New York, NY, 1982
4. Barkauskas: Quick Reference to Cultural Assessment. St. Louis, Mosby Year-Book, Philadelphia, PA, 1994
5. Battaglia B: Skills for Managing multicultural Teams. Cultural Diversity at Work 4 (3):4, 1992
6. Camphina-Bacote J: Psychiatric Mental Health Nursing: A Transcultural Perspective. In Brink,PJ (ed.) Transcultural Nursing: Book of Readings. Eaveland Press, Prospect Heights, IL, 1993
7. Campinha-Bacote J: The Process of Cultural Competence in Health Care: A Culturally Competent Model of Care. Perfect Printing Press, Wyoming, Ohio, 1994
8. Comas-Diaz L, Greene B: Women of Color: Integrating Ethnic and Gender Identities in Psychotherapy. Guilford Press, NY, 1994
9. DeLeon Siantz ML: The Mexican American Migrant Farm Worker: Family Mental Health Issues. Nursing Clinics of North America 29 (1): 65–74, 1994
10. Escobar JJ: Cross-cultural Aspects of the Somatization Trait. Hospital and Community Psychiatry 38 (2): 174–180, 1987
11. Foster GM, Anderson BG: Medical Anthropology. John Wiley and Son, New York, NY, 1978
12. Fleming CM: American Indians and Alaska Natives; Changing Societies Past and Present. In Orlandi, MA (ed), Cultural Competence for Evaluators: A Guide for Alcohol and Other Drug Abuse Prevention Practitioners Working With Ethnic/Racial Communities (pp. 147–171). Office of Substance Abuse Prevention, Division of Community Prevention and Training, Rockville, MD, 1992
13. Garcia J: Yo Soy Mexicano . . . Self-identity and Sociodemographic Correlates. Social Science Quarterly 62 (March): 88–98, 1981
14. Glittenberg J: To the Mountain and Back: The Mysteries of Guatemalan Highland Family Life. Waveland Press, Prospect Heights, IL, 1994
15. Goode EE: The Cultures of Illness. U.S. News and World Report, Feb. 15: 74–76, 1993
16. Grossman D: Enhancing Your "Cultural Competence." American Journal of Nursing, July: 58–62, 1994
17. Hall ET, Whyte WF: Intercultural Communication Guide to Men of Action. In Brink, PJ (ed.) Transcultural Nursing: A Book of Readings. Eaveland Press, Prospect Heights, IL, 1990
18. Helman CG: Culture, Health and Illness. Wright, London, United Kingdom, 1990
19. Henry WA: Beyond the Melting Pot. Time, April 9: 28–29, 1990
20. Kavanagh KH: Transcultural perspectives in mental health. In Andrews & Boyle (eds) Transcultural Concepts in Nursing Care, pp. 253–285, J.B. Lippincott Company, Philadelphia, PA, 1995
21. Kavanagh KH, Kennedy PH: Promoting Cultural Diver-

sity; Strategies for Health Care Professionals. Sage, Newbury Park, CA, 1992

22. Kleinman A: Culture, Illness, and Care: Clinical Lessons From Anthropologic and Cross-cultural Research. Annals of Internal Medicine 88: 251–258, 1978
23. Kleinman A: Rethinking Psychiatry: From Cultural Category to Personal Experience. The Free Press, New York, NY, 1988
24. Kozier B, Erb G, Blais K, Wilkinson J: Ethnicity and Culture; Fundamentals of Nursing, Concepts, Process and Practice, Addison Wesley, Redwood City, CA, 1995
25. Leininger MM: Leininger's Theory of Nursing: Cultural Care Diversity and Universality. Nursing Science Quarterly 1(4): 152–160, 1988
26. Leininger M: Transcultural Interviewing and Health Assessment. In Pedersen, PB, Sartorious N, Marsella AJ (eds), Mental Health Services; The Cross-cultural Context (pp. 109–133). Sage, Beverly Hills, CA, 1984
27. Malone B: Shouldering the Responsibility for Culturally Sensitive and Competent Health Care. NSNA/Imprint: 53–54, 1993
28. Manderscheid, Sonnenschein: 1990
29. McLemore SD: Racial and Ethnic Relations in America, 4th ed. Allyn and Bacon, Boston, MA, 1994
30. Miller M: Culture, Spirituality, and Women's Health. JOGNN: 257–263, 1995
31. Mukherjee S, Skukla S, Woodlke J, Roen A, Olarte S: Misdiagnosis of Schizophrenia in Bipolar Patients; a Multiethnic Comparison. American Journal of Psychiatry 40 (12): 1571–1574, 1983
32. O'Connor BB: Healing Traditions: Alternative Medicine and the Health Professions. University of Pennsylvania Press, Philadelphia, PA, 1995
33. Office of Minority Health, 1985
34. Orlandi M: Cultural Sophistication Framework. In M. Orlandi, R. Weston, & L. Epstein Competence Evaluators (OSAP Cultural Competence Series). DHHS Publication (ADM) 92-1884. Washington, DC: US Government Printing Office, 1952
35. Nobles W: Understanding Human Transformation: The Praxis of Science and Culture. Unpublished paper, 1979
36. Padilla AM, Salgado de Snyder VN: Hispanics; What the Culturally Informed Evaluator Needs to Know. In M.A. Orlandi (Ed.) Cultural Competence for Evaluators: A Guide for Alcohol and Other Drug Abuse Prevention Practitioners Working With Ethnic/Racial Communities, pp. 117–146. Rockville, MD: Office of Substance Abuse Prevention, Division of Community Prevention and Training, 1992
37. Parrillo VN: Strangers to These Shores; Race and Ethnic Relations in the United States. Third Edition. MacMillan, New York, New York, 1990
38. Pesut DJ: The Art, Science, and Techniques of Reframing in Psychiatric Mental Health Nursing. Issues in Mental Health Nursing 12(9): 9–18, 1991
39. Snowden L, Holschuch J: Ethnic Differences in Emergency Psychiatric Care and Hospitalization in a Program for the Severely Mentally Ill. Community Mental Health Journal 28 14): 281–290
40. U.S. Bureau of the Census: Statistical Abstract of the United States: 1990 (110th ed.) Washington, DC, 1990
41. U.S. Department of Health and Human Services: Healthy People 2000. Arlington, VA: CACI Marketing Systems, 1991
42. Waldrop J: You'll Know It's the 21st Century When. . . . American Demographics 12 (12): 22–27, 1990
43. Wood JB: Communicating With Older Adults in Health Care Settings: Cultural and Ethnic Considerations. Educational Gerontology 15: 351–362, 1989

Spiritual Aspects of Care

Evelyn Labun

11

The spirit of the Lord has forsaken Saul, and at times an evil spirit from the Lord would seize him suddenly. His servants said to him, "You see, sir, how an evil spirit from God seizes you; why do you not command your servants here to go and find some man who can play the harp?—then, when an evil spirit from God comes on you, he can play and you will recover." David came to Saul and entered his service; And whenever a spirit from God came upon Saul, David would take his harp and play on it, so that Saul found relief; he recovered and the evil spirit left him alone.

I Samuel 16:14–23.
New English Bible

Spirituality, like the emotions, is a part of every person. It is what makes human beings unique from the rest of nature. A person's spirituality can be a means to growth or may lead to stagnation and regression.

To give effective spiritual care, the nurse needs to understand and feel comfortable with the concept of spirituality as it applies personally and to clients. This chapter addresses the concept of spirituality within the context of mental health care.

Learning Objectives

On completion of this chapter, you should be able to accomplish the following:

1. *Discuss the concept of spirituality.*
2. *Describe, with the use of examples, the expression of spirituality within North American culture.*
3. *Discuss the relationship among religious behavior, spiritual needs, and client behaviors within the mental health and illness context.*
4. *Apply the nursing process for clients with a spiritual need.*
5. *Discuss how the nurse, as a spiritual being, can provide spiritual care.*
6. *Discuss how a group or community setting can be used to provide spiritual care.*

◆ Spirituality

In North America, spirituality has often been associated with religion and religious practices. Religious beliefs and practices are usually an expression of the person's culture and provide an avenue for a person or group to express concern, emotions, and social behavior dealing with spiritual matters. Different churches, denominations, and religious communities develop group and individual ways of expressing their spirituality.

Nurses who are from these communities have a long tradition of acknowledging the spiritual nature of their clients. Along with physical and emotional care, they have recognized the need for spiritual care. A new emphasis on the holistic nature of nursing has led nurses to reexamine their spiritual care in light of a changing pluralistic society. Nurses often ask, "What is spirituality, and how can it be incorporated into nursing practice?"

A starting point in discovering what spirituality involves is to reexamine holistic nursing care. Holistic care has always viewed the client as a total being with physical, sociocultural, and emotional aspects. Each aspect has a clearly defined area for assessment and intervention, even though the areas interrelate and affect the functioning of the total person.

The spiritual aspect of the person is the "inner essence" of the person or the "integrating factor."[26] It integrates the physical, sociocultural, and emotional factors and is the core of the person. The core pervades all of the person's being and makes the person unique. It provides direction, shape, and unique qualities for the person.

Spirituality, however, is more than just the core and integrating factor; it is what causes the person to question the meaning and purpose of life. It creates the desire for relationships with other human beings and the desire to go beyond the self and mere human experience to relationships with what is beyond them. Spirituality has been described as the desire to "touch transcendence."[35] This transcendence might be described as God, a higher power, another world order, or the wonder and mystery of nature around us or beyond our earth.

Positive expressions of spirituality bring out healthy and inspiring qualities in human behavior. Love, hope, faith, trust, and forgiveness are lived out in our relationships with others, with our environment, and with a transcendent God or higher power.[23] Some of these qualities have even been found in people who live in situations where violence is pervasive.[24] Such qualities can be expressed through creative works, such as art, literature, and music, that express love, adoration, awe, or worship. Meaningful work is another avenue of expression.

M. Scott Peck has identified the reality of evil, which may take over a person's spiritual nature and extinguish the existence or possibility of positive or healthy expressions of spirituality.[28] This is not laziness on the part of the person, but rather a distinct movement against the expression of positive human qualities.[27]

Another factor to consider is the person's level of spiritual development. Fowler has identified seven stages of faith development.[16] Box 11-1 outlines these stages. Although Fowler's stages are not directly spiritual in nature, faith development relates to finding life worth living, and so relates to spiritual development.

◆ Expressions of Spirituality

Historically, North American society has expressed its spirituality through religious practices, a sense of mission in humanitarian work, moral and ethical behavior and codes of conduct, and creative works of art. As American society has become more multicultural and pluralistic, other expressions have emerged. Some of these are religious, and some have more secular overtones.[5,12,18] Some are woven into the fabric of cultural beliefs and practices. Cultural factors, spiritual and religious factors, and health beliefs and practices are in-

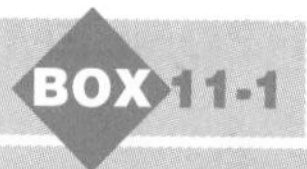

Theory of James Fowler: Faith Development

In the developmental theory contributed by James Fowler, the spiritual identity of humans is essential for holistic care. Fowler's work was influenced by the previous theories of Piaget, Kohlberg, and Erikson. Research was compiled from interviews of people from 4 to 88 years old and from a variety of religious backgrounds, including agnostics and atheists. Fowler explained that "faith is not always religious in its content or context . . . Faith is a person's or group's way of moving into the force field of life. It is our way of finding coherence in and giving meaning to the multiple forces and relationships that make up our lives. Faith is a person's way of seeing him or herself in relation to others against a background of shared meaning and purpose" (p 4). Faith, therefore, is not necessarily religious, but it comprises the reasons one finds life worth living.

Fowler's theory is composed of prestages and six separate stages of faith development. The age when a certain stage exists varies among individuals, but the sequence does not. Equilibrium or the plateau of faith development can occur at any stage, beginning with stage 2.

In the organization of the stages of faith development, Fowler explains a triadic relationship between self, shared causes or values, and others, which is the unifying factor in all stages and is based on trust. During the prestage—called undifferentiated faith—trust, courage, hope, and love compete with threats of abandonment or inconsistencies in the infant's environment. The strength of faith in this stage is based on the relationship with the primary caregiver.

Stage 1, intuitive-projective faith, is most typical of the 3- to 7-year-old child. Children imitate religious gestures and behaviors of others, primarily parents. They follow parental attitudes toward religious or moral beliefs without a thorough understanding of them. Imagination in this stage leads to long-lasting images and feelings that must be questioned and reintegrated in the later stages.

Stage 2, mythical-literal faith, predominates in the school-age child as social interaction increases. Stories represent religious and moral beliefs, and existence of a deity is accepted. Perspectives of others and the concept of reciprocal fairness can be appreciated.

Stage 3, synthetic-conventional faith, is characteristic of many adolescents. As the person experiences increasing demands from work, school, family, and peers, the basis for identity is very complex. An ideology has emerged but has not been closely examined until now. The person begins to question some of the life-guiding values or religious practices in an attempt to stabilize his or her own identity.

Stage 4, individuative-reflective faith, is a crucial stage in which the late adolescent or young adult assumes responsibility for his or her own commitments, beliefs, and attitudes. Many adults do not construct this stage, and at times it does not emerge until they are in their 30s or 40s. Searching for self-identity is no longer defined by the boundaries of faith; compositions of significant others is a primary concern.

Stage 5, conjunctive faith, integrates other viewpoints about faith into one's understanding of truth. One is able to see the paradoxical nature of the reality of his or her own beliefs. Along with this realization, the divisions of faith development among people become apparent.

Stage 6, universalizing faith, involves overcoming paradoxes noted in stage 5 and makes tangible the values of absolute love and justice for mankind. The faith relationship noted in stage 6 is characterized by total trust in the principle of being and the existence of the future, whether derived from the Judeo-Christian image of faith or otherwise.

(From Taylor C, Lillis C, LeMone P: Fundamentals of Nursing: The Art and Science of Nursing Care. Philadelphia, JB Lippincott, 1989 and Fowler JW: Stages of Faith: The Psychology of Human Development and the Quest for Meaning. New York, Harper and Row, 1981)

terconnected.[10] Box 11-2 describes the way various distinct groups in North America express spirituality within society.

Meaning and purpose in living are the central themes in spirituality, especially among the elderly.[34] A study of life experiences in the elderly found that meaningful experiences were those in which the person performs an activity that is perceived as needed by, helpful to, or useful to another person or group. In turn, the person or group receiving the activity also finds it meaningful. The experience is permeated by a sense of positiveness about the self and the activity. In 8 of 11 descriptions in this qualitative study, God, a higher being, or church was described as part of the meaningful experience or as directing or providing the context for the experience.

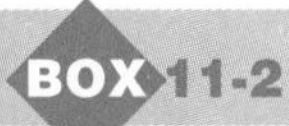

Expressions of Spirituality in North America: The Hmong of Southeast Asia

The Hmong of Southeast Asia are a distinct ethnic group among the thousands of Southeast Asian refugees who arrived in North America during and after the Vietnam conflict. They settled in large numbers in distinct communities in various parts of the continent.

Among the Hmong of Southeast Asia, it is important for the laboring woman to give birth in a place within her husband's family home. The Hmong believe that the souls of infants are easily separated from the body and tend to remain at the place of birth for some time thereafter. The infant must, therefore, be delivered and stay within the family home until the relationship between soul and body is well established.

The child must be cared for within the context of a family group and a familiar place. If nurturing and protection are provided, the child's spirit will become attached to its physical body and then develop into a person. The family's spiritual needs, therefore, are met through cultural practices that express relationships of a spiritual nature, among family members and with members who have died. This practice shows love for the child and expresses a belief about life after death.

(From Labun E: Spiritual Care: An Element in Nursing Care Planning. J Adv Nurs 13: 315, 1988)

◆ Religion and Mental Health

Religious belief and practice are significant avenues for the expression of a person's spirituality that can lead to a deepened sense of reality and purpose and a positive lifestyle. Religion can provide direction and stability in an ever-changing environment.[2,14,19,21]

Although a person's religious beliefs are often a source of strength in times of emotional crisis, in the psychiatric setting, *religiosity*, or the morbid or excessive concern with religion, may reveal a fundamental psychiatric problem.[15] Just as words may be used as a defense against communication, so may religious practice be a negative factor in the person's ability to regain or maintain mental health.

RELIGIOUS OR SPIRITUAL PROBLEMS AND THE DSM-IV

The Diagnostic and Statistical Manual of Mental Disorders recognizes the possibility of a religious or spiritual problem within psychiatric illness.[1] Experiences included under this diagnosis are distressing experiences related to loss or questioning of faith, problems related to conversion or acceptance of a new faith, or questioning of spiritual values, whether they are related to an organized church or religion. Spiritual or religious problems within this diagnosis may also be of a more personal nature not associated with religion or an organized church.

The nurse must assess and make a judgment about whether a particular religious thought or practice will further spiritual health or produce unhealth, facilitate growth and adaptation, or cause stagnation and regression.[9] Three areas to consider when assessing the role of religion in a mentally ill person's problems follow:

1. Is religion a direct cause?
2. Is religion an indirect participating factor?
3. Is religion being used as a symbolic expression of the mentally ill person's feelings and thoughts?[15]

Situations in which religion is a direct cause in mental illness usually focus on God as extremely punitive and demanding.[31] The client may have a history of religious teaching that conflicts with normal biological urges.[4] The client may feel that a relationship with God is no longer possible because of some unforgivable sin. Guilt may pervade the person's consciousness because of sexual urges or the need to feel free from the meaningless or harsh rules of religious beliefs.

USES OF RELIGION

The client in crisis may use religious experience as an explanation for a crumbling hold on reality. In this way, religion may become an indirect participating factor in mental illness. Religion does explain unusual or unfamiliar experiences. Practices and rituals may be used to help the person hold onto reality and provide structure and support. Such practices may be genuine expressions of the person's need and provide support within the crisis situation, or they may be a temporary defense to avoid dealing with self and the mental health issues at hand.[4,15]

Use of religion as a form of symbolic expression in mental illness may provide verbal structure, language, or a reason for the experience. The client might say that God has spoken or that God has visited with a special message. The explanation provides the client with a rationalization for delusions, hallucinations, or bizarre behavior.[4,15]

In some situations, the client may be speaking with the nurse in a conversation that sounds more delusional (unhealthy) than religious. The nurse can proceed to intervene with the delusion while still being sensitive to the underlying spiritual concern.[29] Further explanations about dealing with delusional or hallucinating clients are found in Chapter 30, Schizophrenic Disorders. Remember that "an individual is a spiritual person even when disoriented, confused, emotionally ill, delirious, or cognitively impaired."[7]

Examples of how clients may experience or express their spiritual nature during the course of their mental illness can be seen in the two examples that follow. One client recounts that he found reading Psalm 23 from the Bible a comfort during an acute schizophrenic episode (V.B. Carson, personal communication, June 21, 1995) and helped him have some sense of control over his environment. Another woman who has experienced a number of serious depressions throughout her life says, "Even in my most depressed episodes I have always had a 'song in my heart' because of my relationship with Jesus" (depressed client, personal communication, May, 1994).

Application of the Nursing Process to Spiritual Needs

ASSESSMENT

Assessment of spiritual needs should be approached in the same systematic way that nurses approach assessment in any area.[7] Effective assessment depends on establishing a relationship of mutual trust and respecting the client's beliefs and values. Nursing observations must include the client's environment, feelings, functioning ability, and nursing history data.

An observant nurse will quickly pick up clues from the client's environment—the place where spiritual assessment begins. Religious objects, pictures, greeting cards, or religious programming on radio or television provide information about the client's values and beliefs. The client's relationships with visitors, frequency of visits, and how visits affect the client are also important information.[29] A lack of visitors may indicate that the client is isolated, point to a break in the client's normal relationships, or mean that significant people live far away and can not visit.

A holistic approach to spiritual assessment is necessary to understand more fully the client's spiritual health and to identify spiritual needs. Because spirituality is an integrating factor in a person, it is affected by all physiological and psychological processes, cultural background, environment, and other factors. Thus, all areas of nursing assessment provide important data for developing nursing diagnoses and addressing spiritual needs.

The nurse should begin history taking with questions about the client's view of the primary problem and then move toward more sensitive areas as understanding of the client's condition emerges. Questions directly related to spirituality are generally asked toward the end of the history, at which point the nurse should have a better understanding of the client's condition and will be able to frame questions in a format appropriate to the client's language and in a way that is comfortable for the nurse and client.[13] Box 11-3 provides a guideline for spiritual assessment. Client responses can be used to determine the level of spiritual development using Fowler's stages as a guide.

The initial history taking is merely the beginning of understanding the client's spiritual needs. Spiritual needs arise out of the core of the deepest part of the person's life. Because of the nature of spirituality, the nurse must continue to collect data to ensure a good understanding of the client's needs.

Three general areas need further examination for sensitive spiritual care to occur.[29]

1. Does the client have meaning and purpose in life? This includes hope for the future and faith to believe that life can have meaning.

BOX 11-3

Spiritual Assessment Guide

Ask the client questions about the following:

- Belief in a supreme being or God
- Important personal religious practices
- Any recent changes in beliefs or religious practice
- Whether beliefs or religion offer hope or comfort or cause guilt, shame, fear, or anger
- Whether illness has had an effect on beliefs or religion
- Any creative ways the person uses to express feelings
- What the client find beautiful or appreciates aesthetically

(Adapted from Seifert PC, Beck C: Psychiatric Assessment Tool. In Guzzetta CE, Bunton SD, Prinkey LA, Sherer AP, Seifert PC (eds): Clinical Assessment Tools for Use With Nursing Diagnosis, p 161–178. Toronto, CV Mosby, 1989)

2. Does the person have a means of receiving forgiveness? Can the client deal effectively with guilt?
3. Is the client able to feel loved, valued, and respected by others? Is the client able to trust within relationships, or is there a feeling of alienation and loneliness?
4. Is the client part of a nurturing, caring family or community?

NURSING DIAGNOSIS

Following a careful and ongoing assessment, the nurse establishes the nursing diagnoses. All areas of the assessment provide clues as to the appropriateness of the diagnoses. Further validation by the client should identify incorrect interpretations and avoid ineffective and spiritually damaging care. The data should reflect health-producing and health-inhibiting behaviors.

Spiritual Distress is the North American Nursing Diagnosis Association's accepted nursing diagnosis. It is defined as follows:

> The state in which the individual or group experiences or is at risk of experiencing a disturbance in the belief or value system which provides strength, hope, and meaning to life.[7]

The nurse determines that spiritual distress may result from one or more of the following areas:

- Feelings of guilt
- Inability to practice religious rituals
- Conflict between religious or spiritual beliefs and the prescribed health regimen
- Lack of purpose and meaning in life
- Alienation from God or a higher power
- Lack of forgiveness from self or significant others

Defining characteristics for this diagnosis include a disturbance in the belief system and emotional reactions, such as discouragement, despair, ambivalence about beliefs, a sense of spiritual emptiness, or anger, resentment, and fear about life's meaning, suffering, or death. Further related factors should be identified in the person's pathophysiological condition, such as asking, "Why me?" when diagnosed with cancer; in treatment-related factors, such as chemotherapy or surgery to treat cancer; or in personal or environmental areas, such as anxiety about acceptance by others after removal of a breast.[7]

PLANNING

The main goal in spiritual care is to reduce spiritual distress.[8] Achieving this goal may involve simply strengthening the client's present coping mechanisms or reexamining the client's personal beliefs and values. The client may need to learn to make sense of experiences, to get through a rough time, or to move on.[31] Any goals developed must involve mutual nurse–client planning and further client adaptation and growth. The nurse may need to consult the client's spiritual advisor for help in planning goals and care.

Short-term and long-term goals may be required. For example, for one client, the long-term goal might be to minimize or eliminate spiritual distress, and applicable short-term goals could include assisting clients to mend broken relationships and renew religious practices.

Some clients are in spiritual distress and are unaware of the spiritual nature of their problem (F. Weiss, personal communication, June 22, 1995). After assessment of the client, a spiritually aware nurse may recognize a spiritual problem even though the client does not. The nurse may also recognize areas for spiritual growth that would enhance the client's functioning and promote the client's spiritual health.[3]

Based on the assessment data, the nurse can encourage clients to examine their spiritual needs by saying, "I can see you are hurting. I believe humans are physical, emotional, and spiritual beings. Have you thought of how you are meeting your needs in all these areas?" Within such a context, clients should feel free to talk about their spiritual needs or to explore ways of promoting their spiritual health.

The long-term goal in this situation would be to help clients recognize their spiritual nature and how they may move from spiritual distress to spiritual health. A short-term goal would be to help clients identify spiritual distress as a problem and gain some understanding of their spiritual nature.

INTERVENTION

As the principle provider of spiritual interventions in most health care settings, the nurse must be able to offer hope, inspire faith, and remain open to the client's experiences, needs, and desires. A nurse–client relationship built on trust, caring, commitment, and respect is essential for effective spiritual intervention.

Mentally ill clients may be sensitive to the atmosphere within a nurse–client relationship. Respect for the client may be shown by small acts, such as sharing refreshments during an interview or showing appreciation for an act of kindness or a pleasing personal quality the client displays.

To be effective, intervention also must be appropriate for the client. Factors to consider include the client's ability to think abstractly and understand deeper meanings, the client's level of spiritual development, and the client's goals.[29]

Clients with long-term mental illnesses may begin to

restore spiritual health by reaching out to others and getting a sense of purpose and a reason to live. They may be able to play checkers with others, care for a pet, or play a musical instrument. Some may be able to do volunteer work.

Spiritual growth requires reflection, introspection, and new thoughts and experiences that call old ways into question. Growth often occurs in solitude or in a meaningful relationship with another human being. It may occur while reading about another person's experiences or while recording personal experiences in a journal.[21] Case Study 11-1 illustrates spiritual care in a specific situation.

Spiritual growth may also occur in a supportive, nurturing family; group; or community setting. Examples of supportive communities are 12-step programs, church groups, or weight loss groups. The use of readings, music, rituals, listening, or talking about deep personal concerns sets the stage for the expression of spiritual needs. The development of a community feeling or connectedness between people can provide a feeling of forgiveness, acceptance, growth, and healing. Through meaningful spiritual rituals, the group can experience transcendence and be empowered to look beyond themselves and reach out to others.[11,33] Case Study 11-2 illustrates how spiritual care is provided within a group or community.

The nurse who is sensitive to the client's needs will provide a time and place for private reflection and meaningful sharing. Privacy, a quiet atmosphere, and an aesthetic setting all contribute to these activities. A similarly suitable atmosphere for religious practices and rituals should be provided.

The nurse may be able to suggest suitable religious readings, poetry, music, or art that can speak to the spiritual needs and feelings of the client. Language, music, and art give dignity to suffering and pain.[20,22] The "prayer of the heart" in the Eastern Orthodox Church and the *Zikr* (remembrance) of some Moslem sects are examples of prayers that facilitate meditation and induce a sense of peace.[2]

Another major resource for the nurse is the client's own spiritual advisor or a hospital chaplain. In a multiethnic population, nurses will not be familiar with all the religious traditions and expressions of spirituality within the total population. Some clients with spiritual needs may be more comfortable expressing these to the chaplain.[35] Chaplains are members of the health team with expertise in spiritual matters. The optimum situation occurs when there is dialogue and a spirit of cooperation between the chaplain and nurse.[36]

When working with a delusional client who expresses spiritual questions within a delusional framework, the nurse must make a judgment as to whether the content of the client's conversation is more delusional or spiritual.[29] If the content is more delusional, it is appropriate to respond to the core of the delusion, connecting the belief to the client's feelings. For instance, to the client who says, "I am mightier than Jesus Christ; I am the second son of God," the nurse could respond, "I imagine that saying you are the second son of God makes you feel very important. I wonder if there are times when you feel pretty unimportant."[29] This response reflects on the possible meaning of a delusion and focuses on how the client feels about personal worth and self-esteem. (Further approaches to delusional or hallucinating clients are discussed in Chapter 30, Schizophrenic Disorders.)

EVALUATION

Evaluation, like assessment, is a dynamic and ongoing process. It involves validation and reflection on the meaning of client responses.[25] It requires introspection on the nurse's part as to personal reactions in the light of client behaviors. An evaluation must be based on the reality of the client's situation and the resources available to carry out the plan of care. It must also include evaluation and modification of the care plan in light of new data and understanding of the client situation.

Expected qualities of spiritual health include a sense of inner peace and of meaning in life; an ability to establish warm, loving relationships with other people; and an ability to transcend the self.[8,28]

◆ The Nurse as a Spiritual Being

The nurse's own personal spiritual development is a vital element in providing spiritual care. To understand the client's spirituality, the nurse must do a personal assessment of spirituality.

A study of spiritual care given by nurses found that nurses may respond to spiritual needs at a deep personal level and a broad range of spiritual needs, or they may respond at a more superficial level and more narrow range of needs. Nurses who respond at a deeper level are those with conscious awareness of their own spirituality who have grown personally through a crisis in their lives. They are able to give of themselves at a deep personal level and are particularly sensitive or perceptive to others.[30]

Many nurses agree that spiritual care is important but are fearful and unable to provide this care. Five potential problem areas have been identified:[17]

1. The pluralism in religious and spiritual beliefs within client populations and among nurses leads to

11-1 Case Study

Spiritual Care

Nursing recognizes that spiritual care is an important aspect of client care, yet very little guidance is given to students and nurses on how to help clients with spiritual needs. This scenario illustrates an experience of a nursing student intervening for a client with a spiritual need. The instructor entered a client's room to check on the client and a student, Jane. When she saw the instructor, Jane asked quietly, "Could I speak with you outside?"

They stepped out into the hall, Jane said, "My client thinks he has an evil spirit, and I don't know what to do. I tried to tell him I thought God would forgive him if he prayed and asked for forgiveness, but it didn't seem to do any good." The instructor responded, "Maybe we can help him if we work together."

As Jane and the instructor entered the room, they saw Mr. B, 83 years old, sitting on the side of the bed with his head in his hands and trembling with fear. The instructor sat down on the bed beside him and said, "Mr. B, you told Jane you believe you have an evil spirit. Can you tell us more about that?"

In a low, tremulous voice, the client began to talk about his problem. He said that he believed he had an evil spirit that caused him to begin bleeding again after his surgery and that he hadn't been able to sleep all night because of his fear of death. He felt as though God had rejected him and could no longer hear his prayers. He'd been a Christian for many years and had hosted a small church in his home, but a visit from his pastor yesterday had brought neither comfort nor relief from his fears. He didn't want any further visits; he believed he was doomed.

The instructor put her hand on Mr. B's hand and said that she believed in God too and that she was sure that He loves us all and would not forsake a person who needed Him. She quoted some Bible verses, such as I John 1:9 ("If we confess our sins He is faithful and just to forgive us our sins . . .") and reminded Mr. B that "no matter what we do, God still loves us." The client continued to insist that "The evil spirit won't go away. God can't hear me."

The instructor then offered to pray with Mr. B In prayer, the instructor thanked God for His love and faithfulness and asked that Mr. B be forgiven and receive peace and rest. Following the prayer, Mr. B appeared calmer. The instructor suggested that he repeat the verses to himself should further doubts or fears surface.

Jane and the instructor then helped Mr. B into a comfortable position in bed and left him to rest. Soon after, Jane reported that Mr. B was sleeping peacefully.

Later, Jane and the instructor discussed the incident. The instructor pointed out how the following assessment findings point to a nursing diagnosis of Spiritual Distress.

1. Mr. B had said that although he had been a Christian for many years, God could not hear him anymore.
2. Mr. B believed postsurgical complications were caused by an evil spirit, which required his readmission to hospital.
3. His feeling of rejection and damnation caused him to be very anxious and apathetic.
4. Following a sleepless night, he pleaded for spiritual help.

The nursing actions, carried out within the nurse–client relationship, focused on dealing with Mr. B's fear and helping him restore his faith in God's power and love. Interventions included the following:

1. Sitting down beside him and holding his hand
2. Quoting Bible verses familiar to him and pertinent to his situation
3. Praying with him, thanking God for His love and faithfulness and asking for forgiveness and peace for Mr. B.
4. Encouraging Mr. B to repeat the verses when further fears arose
5. Making him comfortable so he could rest

The instructor helped Jane evaluate the nursing interventions by noting Mr. B's response. He fell asleep within minutes and rested peacefully the rest of the day. Later he stated that he had repeated the verses when fears had arisen and that this had helped reassure and calm him.

Jane stated that she understood the explanation of Mr. B's care but was uncertain about specific interventions. The instructor suggested that she could explore this further by reading a book titled *Spiritual Care: The Nurses Role,* specifically the information on spiritual needs and the use of scripture and prayer.

REFERENCES

Holy Bible, King James Version. Indianapolis, IN, BB Kirkbridge Bible Co., 1957

Kim JJ, McFarlane GK, McLane AM (eds): Pocket Guide to Nursing Diagnosis. Toronto, CV Mosby, 1984

Fish S, Shelly JA: Spiritual Care: The Nurse's Role. Downers Grove, IL, InterVarsity Press, 1978

(Adapted from Labun E: Helping When the Nursing Diagnosis is Spiritual Distress. Venture 2: 5–6, 1987; this experience was recounted by Jean Capes RN, BScN of London, Ontario, Canada)

Case Study

Spiritual Care—A Community of Love and Forgiveness

Mrs. M, 45 years old, was admitted to a psychiatric ward with severe depression. She was unable to sleep, had loss of appetite, and some suicidal thoughts. The center of her problem revolved around her abusive, controlling husband. Although marital therapy had been attempted, her husband remained very angry and unwilling to look at his behavior. At this point, Mrs. M found herself very isolated, had sought counseling, and with the help of her counselor, had initiated divorce proceedings.

Although Mrs. M did not believe in divorce because she saw it as a failure to honor her marriage commitment before God, she could also see how her marriage was affecting her children, 16-year-old Garry and 8-year-old Tammy. Garry was obviously depressed, and Tammy was acting out in school.

In talking with Mrs. M, the nurse identified the nursing diagnosis of spiritual distress. Through her nursing interventions, she helped Mrs. M recognize her anger toward her husband and express it in a letter telling him of her reasons for the divorce. The nurse also talked to Mrs. M about her own personal experience of God as loving and forgiving and helped Mrs. M to accept God's forgiveness by listening to her, reading her scripture about love and forgiveness, and presenting an accepting attitude.

The nurse knew other nurses who were likewise alert to Mrs. M's spiritual distress. Together the nurses provided spiritual care and emotional support for Mrs. M They helped her accept and experience God's forgiveness. They also learned that Mrs. M received regular visits from a group of four to five women from a prayer group within her church. These friends brought cards that spoke of God's forgiveness and love. They brought flowers to lighten her spirits and provide aesthetic beauty as an expression of God's love and thoughtfulness in creation. Mrs. M said that her husband never brought her flowers even though she loved them.

A network of spiritual support for Mrs. M and her children was developed among the nurses and the women in the prayer group. When she was discharged, the prayer group women and their husbands gave her money and moved her and her children into an apartment. Mrs. M continued to feel the support of her prayer group throughout her recovery as she began a new life for herself and her children.

This case is based on a true story recounted by F. Weiss of Lancaster, WI

feelings of inadequacy in knowing how to provide care.

2. Nurses have common fears related to implementation. These fears include not being able to handle a situation, intruding on the client's privacy, or becoming confused or challenged in one's own beliefs.
3. The nurse may lack awareness of a personal spiritual quest. Nurses must ask themselves spiritual questions so that they can become comfortable in providing care.
4. Nurses experience confusion about the difference between spirituality and religious concepts.
5. Nurses are unsure of how to answer questions related to illness, suffering, and aging. Questions that may arise are, "Why am I suffering? How will I face life's losses in aging? How long must I suffer?"

Nurses must begin to deal personally with these questions before they can feel comfortable providing spiritual care.

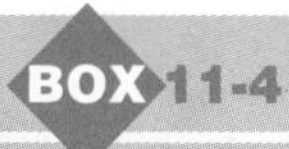

What the Elders Say About Depression: The Nishnawbe of Northwestern Ontario, Canada

One of our investigators interviewed several elders about their perspectives on depression. Although some of the meaning is lost in the translation, her findings are summarized here:

Several words in the Nishnawbe language refer to depression. The actual meanings incorporate the concepts of loneliness and sadness and the implications of the term as used by western medicine.

The elders stated that depression, as they described it, existed in previous times. The hard life and the need to concentrate on survival left little time to dwell on it, so depression was not an obvious phenomenon. One very recognizable cause of depression was shame, and cases were reported in which people died when they were unable to live down a shameful act they had committed. When depression was recognized, an individual family member was assigned to help the person through his or her difficulties.

Several elders elaborated on what they viewed as the roots of depression in Native Canadians today. Their assessments focused mainly on the abandonment of respect for a spiritual way of life in exchange for materialistic things that overwhelm people, preventing them from looking at themselves as they really are.

One elder eloquently stated: "Before the white man came into our world, we had our own way of worshipping the Creator. We had our own church and rituals. When hunting was good, people would gather together to give gratitude. This gave us close contact with the Creator. There were many different rituals depending on the tribe. People would dance in the hills and play drums to give recognition to the Great Spirit. It was like talking to the Creator and living daily with its spirit. Now people have lost this. They can't use these methods and have lost conscious contact with this high power. This goes for white people too. We freeze our lives with all those material things. The more we lose conscious contact with the Creator, the more our consciousness becomes numb. It's like a person going outside. First he would feel the cold, later he would feel very cold, then eventually he freezes. That is what it is like when we stray from the Creator; we freeze our conscious contact and prefer materialistic things. The more distant we are from the Creator, the more complex things are because we have no sense of direction. We don't recognize where life is from."

The elders said that today's parents do not teach this consciousness to the young, show them the mysteries and powers of the universe, or teach them how to improve their knowledge of life to enrich the spiritual part of their life.

Native Canadian spirituality is the maintenance of the contact with one's creator. Meditation, prayer, and symbols are central to it all. God is believed to be in everything, but materialism has caused the loss of conscious contact with God. Each person has his or her own symbols, but the most central symbol in Native Canadian culture is that of the drum, which symbolizes the heart beat. Newborns are close to their mothers, feeling the heart beat even before birth. It is the heart beat that is believed to set the pattern of existence.

The loss of Native Canadian spirituality as a cause for depression goes beyond concepts contained in religious beliefs. It encompasses an entirely different relationship with the world, linked closely with maintaining harmony with nature. The description of the loss of spirituality is remarkably similar to the concepts of normlessness and anomie.

(From Timpson J, McKay S, Kakegamic S, Roundhead D, Cohen C, Matewapit G: Depression in a Native Canadian in Northwestern Ontario: Sadness, Grief or Spiritual Illness? Canada's Mental Health 36 (June/September): 6, 1988; reproduced with permission of the Minister of Supply and Services Canada. 1991)

Spiritual care is provided within the framework of the nurse–client relationship.[32] Even though the nurse may not be able to respond adequately to all of the client's questions, the relationship should bring an atmosphere of mutual sharing and growth. Within this context, the nurse must allow the client to be free to choose and decide on issues, guard against projecting personal beliefs and values on the client, and empathize with clients in their personal struggle.

The nurse must step outside a personal belief system and try to understand the client's values, culture, and beliefs, particularly when they differ from the nurse's own background. Such an approach will enlarge the nurse's understanding of the scope of human spirituality (Box 11-4).

◆ Chapter Summary

This chapter has explored the concept of spirituality from a mental health nursing perspective. This chapter emphasizes the following points:

1. Spirituality is an integrating, core aspect of the whole person. It is the part of the person that searches for meaning, purpose, and relatedness with others. Spiritual qualities of love, faith, hope, and trust are outgrowths of a spiritual nature. These qualities may be extinguished in the presence of evil. Each person's spirituality may be measured on a developmental scale.
2. Historically, North Americans have viewed spirituality as part of religious expression and culture. The diversity of North American culture and the movement away from traditional religions has led to a new examination of spirituality. Meaning and purpose continue to be central to the concept.
3. Religious beliefs and practices may contribute to positive mental health or may be a vehicle for the expression of psychopathology.
4. The nursing process provides a framework for nursing care of the client with spiritual distress.
5. The nurse, as an instrument in providing spiritual care, must develop a personal spiritual identity to be comfortable dealing with the client's spiritual needs. The therapeutic relationship is the context within which appropriate spiritual care is given.
6. Spiritual care that is provided in groups is characterized by a supportive, nurturing community environment guided by reading, music, rituals, and discussions that allow for the expression of spiritual needs. Group members can experience feelings of forgiveness, acceptance, growth, and healing and be empowered to reach out to others.

Critical Thinking Questions

1. *Why do nurses confuse spirituality and religion?*
2. *How are the concepts of spirituality, religion, and culture related?*
3. *Do people from different ethnic groups have the same spirituality? Explain your answer.*

Review Questions

1. Write a working definition of spirituality that reflects your own thinking and experiences. How does it compare with what other writers have said?
2. The nurse is working with a mentally ill client who is experiencing hallucinations. Some of the conversations that the nurse has with the client include discussions about God and Saint Mary. The nurse should recognize that the person
   - A. is using religion to gain power over the environment.
   - B. is inventing stories to rationalize the illness.
   - C. requires an in-depth assessment for the nurse to make judgments about the client's spirituality.
   - D. is expressing a spiritual need in a distorted way.
3. Why is it necessary to use a holistic approach when assessing the client's spiritual health?
4. Assessment of spiritual needs should focus on which of the following areas? Choose the two most correct.
   - A. The church that the client attends
   - B. The things that are most meaningful for the client
   - C. The way the client expresses anger
   - D. The ability of the client to resolve feelings of guilt
5. What is the main goal when a client is diagnosed as having spiritual distress?
   - A. Provide opportunities for confession.
   - B. Remove the client from religious situations.
   - C. Provide individualized approaches that give spiritual support.
   - D. Work on the client's emotional and physical problems first.
6. Explain why spiritual care is often effectively provided in a group or community setting.
7. The role of the chaplain or spiritual advisor in a mental health facility is to
   - A. provide the spiritual care for the nurse.
   - B. provide religious services that nurses are not qualified to give.
   - C. work in collaboration with the nurse by providing spiritual care expertise.

D. respond to requests for consultation on a client's spiritual distress or spiritual needs.

8. Why is it important for the nurse to have an understanding of personal spirituality when caring for clients' spiritual needs?

◆ References

1. American Psychiatric Association: Diagnostic and Statistical Manual of Mental Disorders, 4th ed. Washington, American Psychiatric Association, 1994
2. Baasher T: The Healing Power of Faith. World Health October: 5–7, 1982
3. Bensley RJ: Defining Spiritual Health: A Review of the Literature. Journal of Health Education 22 (September/October): 287–290, 1991
4. Burgess AW: Psychiatric Nursing in the Hospital and the Community, 5th ed. Norwalk, CT, Appleton and Lange, 1990
5. Burnard P: The Spiritual Needs of Atheists and Agnostics. The Professional Nurse 4 (December): 131–132, 1988
6. Burnard P: Discussing Spiritual Issues with Clients. Health Visitor 61 (December): 371–372, 1988
7. Carpenito LJ: Nursing Diagnosis: Application to Clinical Practice, 5th ed. Philadelphia, JB Lippincott, 1995
8. Carson VB: Spiritual Dimensions of Nursing Practice. Toronto, WB Saunders, 1989
9. Clinebell J. Jr: The Mental Health Ministry of the Local Church. Nashville, Abingdon Press, 1972
10. Corrine L, Bailey V, Valentin M, Morantus E, Shirley L: The Unheard Voices of Women: Spiritual Interventions in Maternal-Child Health. MCN 17 (May/June): 141–145, 1992
11. Durkin MB: A Community of Care. Health Progress October: 48–70, 1992
12. Emblen J: Religion and Spirituality Defined According to Current Use in Nursing Literature. Journal of Professional Nursing 8 (January-February): 41–47, 1992
13. Ellis D: Whatever Happened to the Spiritual Dimension? The Canadian Nurse 76 (September): 42–43, 1980
14. Farkas H: Therapeutic Spiritual Experiences. Am J Psychiatry 130 (September): 1045–1046, 1973
15. Field WE, Wilkerson S: Religiosity as a Psychiatric Symptom. Perspect Psychiatr Care 11 (March): 99–105, 1973
16. Fowler J: Stages of Faith. San Francisco, Harper and Row, 1981
17. Granstrom SL: Spiritual Nursing Care for Oncology Patients. Topics in Clinical Nursing Care 7 (April): 39–45, 1985
18. Harrison J: Spirituality and Nursing Practice. Journal of Clinical Nursing 2: 211–217, 1993
19. Harmon Y: The Relationship Between Religiosity and Health, Health Values: Achieving High Level Wellness. 9 (May-June): 23–25, 1985
20. Henderson KJ: Dying, God and Anger. J Psychosoc Nurs 27 (May): 17–21, 1989
21. Horton PC: The Mystical Experience as a Suicide Prevention. Am J Psychiatry 130 (March): 294–296, 1973
22. Lattanzi M, Hale ME: Giving Grief Words: Writing During Bereavement. Omega 15 (January): 45–52, 1984–1985
23. Labun ER: Spiritual Care: An Element in Nursing Care Planning. J Adv Nurs 13: 314–320, 1988
24. Madela EN, Poggenpoel M: The Experience of a Community Characterized by Violence: Implications for Nursing. J Adv Nurs 18: 691–700. 1993
25. Macdonald SM, Sandmaier R, Fainsinger RL: Objective Evaluation of Spiritual Care: A Case Report. Journal of Palliative Care 9 (2): 47–49, 1993
26. Nagai-Jacobson MG, Burkhardt MA: Spirituality: Cornerstone of Holistic Nursing Practice. Holistic Nursing Practice 3 (May): 18–26, 1989
27. Peck MS: People of the Lie: The Hope for Healing Human Evil. New York, Simon and Schuster Press, 1983
28. Peck MS: Further Along The Road Less Traveled: A New Psychology of Love, Traditional Values, and Spiritual Growth. New York, Simon and Schuster Press, 1993
29. Peterson EA, Nelson K: How to Meet Your Clients' Spiritual Needs. J Psychosoc Nurs 25 (May): 34–39, 1987
30. Ross LA: Spiritual Aspects of Nursing. J Adv Nurs 19: 439–447, 1994
31. Simsen B: The Spiritual Dimension. Nursing Times 82 (November 26): 41–42, 1986
32. Slimmer LW: Helping Students to Resolve Conflicts Between Their Religious Beliefs and Psychiatric-Mental Health Treatment Approaches. J Psychosoc Nurs 18 (July): 37–39, 1980
33. Stiles MK: The Shining Stranger: Application of the Phenomenological Method in the Investigation of the Nurse-Family Spiritual Relationship. Cancer Nursing 17 (1): 18–26, 1994
34. Trice LB: Meaningful Life Experience to the Elderly. Image 22 (Winter): 248–251, 1990
35. Widerquist JG: Another View on Spiritual Care. Nurse Educator 16 (March-April): 5, 7, 1991
36. Widerquist J, Davidhizar R: The ministry of nursing. J Adv Nurs 19: 647–652, 1994

Sexuality and Sexual Concerns

Sharon E. Byers
Delia Esparza

12

I am a sexual being. So is she. Together we produce an experience that is exquisite for both of us. She invites me to know her sexually, and I invite her to know me sexually. We share our erotic possibilities in delight and ecstasy. If she wants me and I don't want her, I cannot lie. My body speaks only truth. And I cannot take her unless she gives herself. Her body cannot lie.

Sidney M. Jourard,
The Transparent Self, *1971*

Sexuality is an integral part of the personality, a significant aspect of the functioning of the identity during varied states of wellness. Sexual activity is a form of communication, a method of self-affirmation, a pleasurable form of play, and a reflection of the individual's value system.

This chapter explores the development of sexuality throughout the life span. A humanistic perspective emphasizes the importance of identifying the client's sexual norms and needs and facilitating adaptation accordingly. The chapter describes stages of the human sexual response cycle, traditional and nontraditional methods of sexual expression, and sexual dysfunctions and their treatment approaches. The nurse's role and intervention with clients manifesting sexual problems or concerns are also discussed.

Learning Objectives

On completion of this chapter, you should be able to accomplish the following:

1. *Define the terms sexuality, sensuality, sex role, and gender identity.*
2. *Differentiate between sex derivative, adjunctive, and arbitrary differences.*
3. *Discuss the genetic, hormonal, and psychological influences on sexual development.*
4. *Describe the stages of human sexual response.*
5. *Compare traditional and alternative sexual lifestyles.*
6. *Discuss the client's sexual needs during specific physical or emotional disorders.*
7. *Describe the common sexual problems of men and women who seek sex therapy.*
8. *Describe the treatment approaches for gender identity disorders and paraphilias.*
9. *Apply the nursing process to the care of a client manifesting a sexual problem.*

◆ The Meaning of Sexuality

Sexuality is the expression and experience of the self as a sexual being. It is, therefore, a state of the body and mind and a crucial part of the personality. Sexuality is not limited to overt sexual activity, such as sexual intercourse, but includes solitary activities like studying, walking, and relaxing. Sexuality is a part of every relationship, whether it is primarily a sexual relationship or not.[37]

An important aspect of sexuality is *sensuality,* the expression and experience of self as a sensual being. Sensuality involves experiencing enjoyment through the senses, such as touching a pleasing fabric, listening to good music, or touching the skin of a loved one. Sensuality is a necessary component of fulfilled sexuality. Sensual attraction, however, does not necessarily lead to a wish for sexual activity; it refers merely to pleasure in the company of the other.

One key to unlocking the enjoyment of sexuality and sensuality is through body awareness and acceptance. *Sex roles* are culturally determined patterns associated with male and female social behavior and may be accepted or rejected by the individual. *Gender identity,* or how one chooses to view oneself as a male or female in interaction with others, is an individual and unique expression.

Body appearance holds some limitations for self-direction. The transsexual, for example, rejects his or her physical sexual appearance and prefers to undergo surgery, psychotherapy, and hormone treatments to make a sex change. More common are the problems stemming from men's and women's inabilities to accept their bodies to the fullest extent to enable sexual fulfillment. To gain acceptance, men and women may perceive a need to change their bodies through dieting or exercise. In reality, though, body acceptance ultimately depends on the ability to relax with one's body and to allow physical sensations to be accepted and experienced as they are, without defensively screening out unwanted or perceptually twisting sensations.

People view sexual activity through a paradigm made up of religious values and stereotypical myths. Reality is shaped by choice, assigned sets of meanings, and even anxiety, fear, and lack of knowledge. Religious beliefs and other sets of personal values usually result in classification of sexual activity into one of three categories:

1. Procreational sex, sexual activity for the purpose of conceiving children
2. Relational sex, sexual activity for the purpose of strengthening or fulfilling commitments of a relationship
3. Recreational sex, sexual activity for the purpose of play and personal enjoyment

◆ Sexual Differences

SEX DERIVATIVE DIFFERENCES

The body holds the only inevitabilities of sexuality. These inevitable differences are that men normally are able to impregnate women, and women normally are able to lactate, gestate, and menstruate. Nothing else, including aggressivity, strength, or sex role, has been found to be related strictly to maleness or femaleness. Other differences are relatively arbitrary, some appearing as predispositions created by anatomical differences, such as baldness and the position for urination. These *sex derivative differences* vary from person to person according to familial tendencies, physical makeup, and personality preferences.

SEX ADJUNCTIVE DIFFERENCES

Sex adjunctive differences are seen fairly consistently from culture to culture but are less related to real physical differences than are the sex derivative differences. Examples of sex adjunctive differences are the choice of the man or woman to earn money for the household and the traditional role of the woman in childrearing. These differences are based in part on some physical differences, such as muscle mass and the ability to lactate, but the most important determinants are the preferred roles for men and women in the past. These roles tend to persist due to historic precedence but are now being questioned and challenged frequently by modern male homemakers and career women. Certain sex adjunctive differences may be linked to hormonal or genetic programming in our primate ancestors. For example, one male hormone, androgen, increases physical activity; however, the expression of this activity as physical aggression or dominance is not related to hormonal factors but to individual choice and learning.

SEX ARBITRARY DIFFERENCES

Sex arbitrary differences are purely determined by culture; examples include face painting and genital mutilation. In the Anglo-Saxon cultures, it is acceptable for the female to wear colors on her face called makeup. In other cultures, men wear face paints. In Judeo-Christian cultures, it is common for men to be circumcised as infants. In other cultures, the young girl undergoes similar procedures, such as removing or cutting away a part of the clitoris or the hood of the clitoris. In most of these situations of genital mutilation of infants, the procedure is believed to be painless, despite the infants' cries to the contrary, and is undergone without anesthesia. The procedure is also usually explained as required by hygienic and religious needs.[6]

It is sometimes difficult to understand how arbitrary distinctions come to be viewed as unquestionable and inevitable differences between the sexes. The explanation lies in the fact that our world is shaped by a basic he-schema and she-schema. Our expectations, habits, traditions, mores, customs, norms, and the wielding of power througout history form the basis for these schemata.[15] The interpretations of differences between the sexes are evident from the first days of life, when boys and girls are handled and talked to in measurably different ways.[32] The infant's behavior is also interpreted differently according to sex-related expectations and perceptions.

There are also age-related distinctions regarding sexual differences. For example, in American culture, children are not generally considered to be sexual. Thus, we observe the panic of a mother finding her toddler son fondling his penis or the horror of parents discovering their 13-year-old daughter's birth control pills. The infant's first erection and lubrication occurs soon after birth, indicating the pervasive nature of sexuality. Elderly people also are thought of as asexual by many in the American culture. Two hundred years ago, few people lived long enough to become elderly; we have little precedence on which to form our view of sexuality in the elderly. Our cultural perspective on the sexual needs of the elderly has not progressed as rapidly as the average life span has grown.

NURSES' KNOWLEDGE OF SEXUAL DIFFERENCES

The tasks of the nurse regarding sexuality are fourfold:

1. To be knowledgeable about sexuality and the norms of society
2. To use this knowledge to understand others' behaviors and attitudes that differ in cultural and individual perspectives from one's own
3. To use this understanding to facilitate the client's adaptation and optimal health
4. To be aware of, and comfortable with, one's own sexuality[15]

Adaptation does not mean conforming to others' expectations or norms, but rather responding to the world without losing one's unique qualities. The awareness of personal feelings and others' feelings and attitudes about sexual behavior and differing choices enables the nurse to respond to an encounter based on a sincere understanding of the needs of the client, rather than on emotional taboos or stereotypical beliefs.[27]

◆ Sexual Development

Sexual development occurs in the embryo and continues throughout the life span. A variety of influences (genetic, hormonal, and psychological) have an impact on this development.

GENETIC INFLUENCES

Chromosomes initiate sexual development. *Chromosomes*, found in every cell of the body, are the carriers of genetic programming information. Within the ovum and sperm are the chromosomal offerings of the two parents, which determine the genetic makeup of the child. The male's sperm cell determines the sex of the embryo at conception by adding either an X or a Y chromosome to the X chromosome contained within the ovum. Two X chromosomes result in a female fetus; an X and Y chromosome result in a male fetus.

Sometimes, these groupings of chromosomes occur differently, resulting in such variations as XXY, or *Klinefelter's syndrome.* This extra X chromosome produces a boy who appears normal until adolescence, when decreased production of the male hormone (testosterone) results in small testes, infertility, and a predisposition for a low libido (or sexual interest). Behavior differences may be associated with Klinefelter's syndrome; these include a predisposition to generalized passivity, lack of ambition, and sudden outbursts of aggression. These behavioral and libido differences are reversed with treatments of testosterone, even when undertaken as late as adulthood.[3,21] Apparently, hormonal therapy affects the libido to enable a broader range of behavioral choices.

Turner's syndrome occurs when the second sex chromosome is missing, producing the pattern XO. This syndrome results in short girls without functioning gonads. Until puberty, no problems are noted; however, at the normal age of puberty, the breasts do not develop and there are no menses. The psychological problem associated with this chromosomal variation involves the effect of stigma caused by the differences between this person and the female norm. The absence of hormones during fetal development results in possible deficits in motor coordination, range of affect, and directional sense. The client with Turner's syndrome may have a predisposition to be more complacent and show less initiative than other girls or women of similar age.[14] Hormone therapy results in normal breast development and normal menses in the female with Turner's syndrome, but the short stature does not change, resulting in an adult height of $4^1/_2$ to 5 feet.

The *XYY chromosomal pattern* produces a man with few physical differences from an XY man, except for a slightly taller stature, low sperm count, and some abnormalities of the seminiferous tubules. As children, these boys have a predisposition to appear less socially mature, more impulsive, and less successful in interpersonal relationships than their peers. As men, there is a predisposition to commit crimes but not necessarily of an aggressive nature.[14]

Nursing implications of the diagnosis of one of these chromosomal abnormalities include counseling with the parents and child regarding the effect of the diagnosis on the child's developing self-image. The nurse educates the parents and child about the typical behavioral predispositions and appearance differences associated with the syndrome. The nurse explains that although hormone therapy is a useful means of reducing the difference between the child and the normal boy or girl, it is not a cure for the syndrome. In all cases, hormone therapy can only change superficial differences. Counseling is recommended for intervention in, or prevention of, a crisis in response to the diagnosis as the client and family experience the loss of normal identity. Counseling may also help family members learn to reinforce adaptive behaviors and shape behaviors away from predispositions that may result in maladaptive behaviors.

HORMONAL INFLUENCES

During the first 6 weeks of development, male and female fetuses are anatomically alike. At 6 weeks, primitive gonads are beginning to develop but are not yet differentiated as male or female. Following this time, hormones have the greatest effect on the sexual differentiation of the fetus. At 8 weeks, if testosterone is present in sufficient levels, testes develop from the indistinct gonads. If no testosterone or a less-than-normal amount of testosterone for a boy of this age is secreted by the 12th gestational week, ovaries are formed. Even if the genotype is XY, the absence of testosterone at this time of fetal development causes female differentiation to occur. This would result in an anatomical female who is capable of procreation but who bears an XY genotype.

These sexual differentiations occur in the external genitalia, the internal sex structures, and the delicate nervous pathways and other portions of the brain to create the pattern for further development. The ambiguous gonadal structures develop into uterus, fallopian tube, and vagina in the absence of testosterone. With testosterone and androgen secretion at sufficiently high levels, the same structures become the vas deferens, seminal vesicles, and ejaculatory ducts.

Externally, androgen stimulation results in the urogenital fold joining to form a penis. Without androgen, this fold becomes the labia minora. The hypothalamic-pituitary-gonadal system in the brain responds to androgen by becoming noncyclical. Without androgen, female hormones result in female structures and a cyclical system, with fluctuating hormonal levels producing menses and fertility (Fig. 12- 1).[32]

A variety of hormonal imbalances may affect the development of the fetus so that a genetic girl develops male genitalia or more likely, ambiguous genitalia with a hypertrophied clitoris. A genetic boy could develop internal or atrophied testes, ambiguous genitalia (such as penis and a small vaginal opening), or an atrophied penis. Such variations differ from those seen in chromosomal abnormalities in that the original structures determined by the genotype are sex appropriate, but an improper balance of male and female hormones results in an ambiguous stage of sexual development of the fetus.

Diagnosis and treatment with hormone therapy assist the child with *ambiguous genitalia* to have a normal life and reproduce. Many times, the fetal development

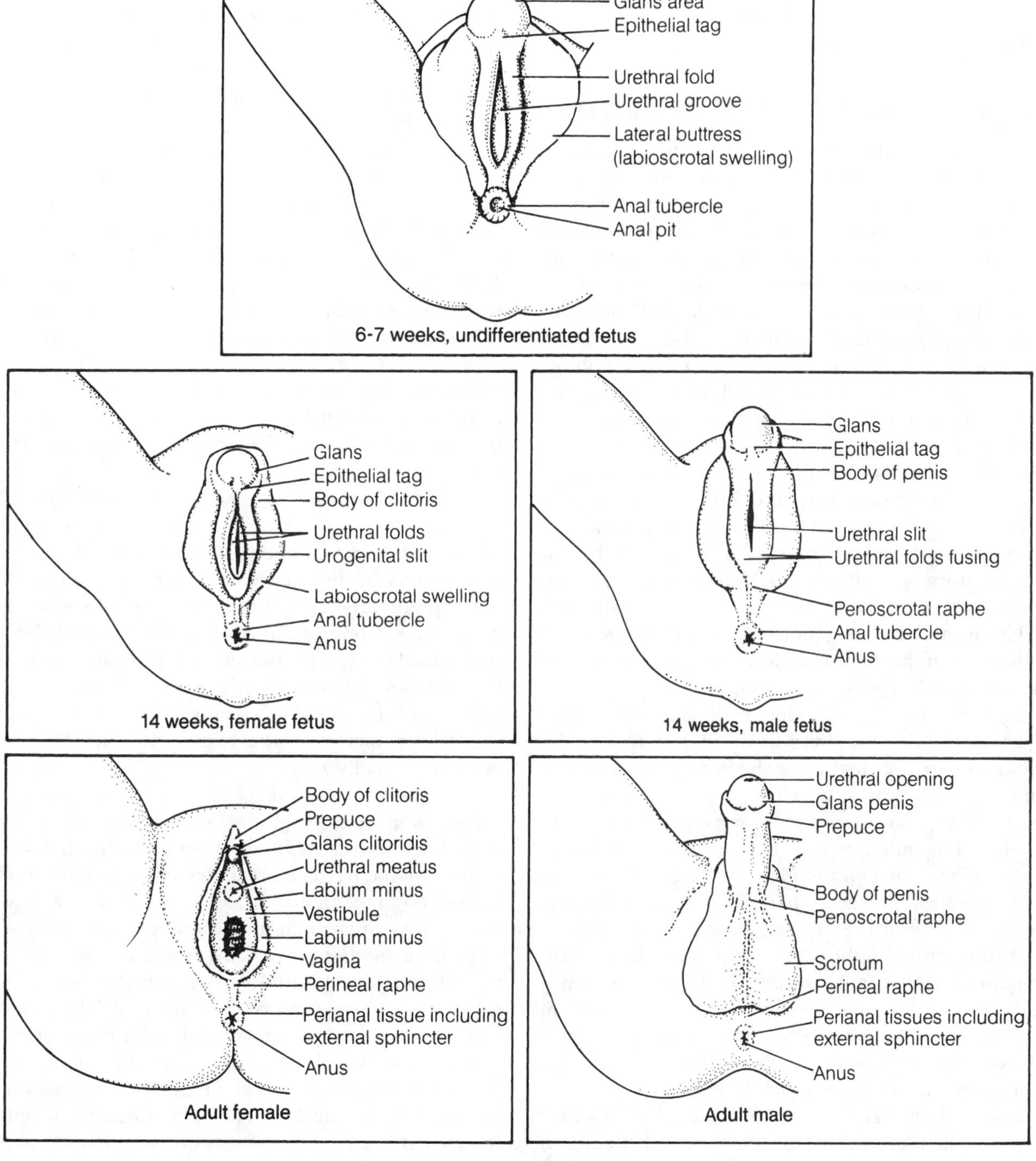

Figure 12-1. Sexual differentiation.

is so different from the genetic structure that the best decision is to raise the child as a child of the sex of the genitalia rather than the genotype. The learned element of sexuality is apparently the most important influence after birth, because these children rarely have problems developing gender identity if they are treated consistently as the sex assigned early in life. Surgery, hormone therapy, and counseling with the parents are crucial elements in a healthy pattern of development. During such procedures, the child is less confused and traumatized if the situation is described as a hormonal imbalance rather than referring to male or female characteristics. Parents will adapt more readily to the birth of a child with ambiguous genitals if the delivery room staff do not refer to the child as either sex, until careful study results in the assignment of the sex of the greatest likelihood of development.[32]

DEVELOPMENT OF GENDER IDENTITY

Many theorists, although accepting the importance of early experience, development, and learning, reject the idea of a fixed identity at a young, seemingly arbitrary age. These theorists believe that a variety of influences develop predispositions (that may or may not be realized) in response to lifelong experience, development, and learning. These theorists believe that maleness and femaleness are not fixed points but exist on a continuum that is open to interpretation and expression according to cultural pressures and preferences. The choices of the individual ultimately become decisive in developing the gender identity in response to the experiences of life. The normally developed boy and girl share most of the same male and female hormones but in differing proportions according to the genetic and hormonal development of the individual. Although they are normally differentiated, the boy and girl are much more alike one another than like less differentiated individuals having genotypes other than XX or XY or than like individuals who developed without the influence of both types of sex hormones.

The first step of gender-identity development occurs as the child becomes aware of the differences of the sexes and perceives that he or she is male or female, as compared with others. This basic recognition of one's sex (whether anatomically clear or assigned due to anatomical ambiguity) is called *sexual identity*.[32] Sexual identity allows the child to interpret clearly the behaviors of others as behavior appropriate for a boy or girl and as different or the same as the sex of the child.

During early childhood, the child forms bonds with male and female significant people. How these bonds are formed affects how the child will prefer to develop his or her sexual identity. Parents and other important adults are role models and teachers about how men and women act and relate with each other.

Gender identity refers to how the child feels about his or her sexual identity, that is, how the child decides to interpret his or her sexual identity for himself or herself. The development of *gender role* refers to how the child's gender identity will be expressed socially in behavior with others of the same and opposite sex.

Children tend to prejudge themselves and others regarding sexual orientation and identity based on information and attitudes mimicked from parental behavior because they have little real experience on which to base their own behavior. Often, this results in rigid distinctions of gender roles. On the other hand, if children are told about sexuality, differences and similarities between the sexes, and sexual behavior between the sexes before puberty, they develop a more matter-of-fact approach to sex. Later they are able to make important decisions about their own behavior based on information rather than on emotions, stereotypes, or expectations of others.

During early childhood, fantasies also play an important role in the child's developing gender identity. These fantasies include images of ultimate self-satisfaction and feelings of self-fulfillment. Children's fantasies do not tend to be as structured or realistic as those of adults. These fantasy associations are formed according to feelings of pleasure and are instrumental in the development of the child's system of symbols pertaining to self. These symbols are uncensored by the expectations of society and loved ones and are therefore truly creative events of the child. This system of symbols and fantasies takes on an erotic quality when the child reaches puberty.[32]

These fantasies guide the choice of *sexual object*, that is, the individual's choice of an object for sexual expression. For most people, symbols and fantasies are abstractions during childhood, but in adolescence, they develop into an image of the ideal man or woman. For others, the system of abstractions persists, and the adult's sexual interest is invested in objects, events, or particular types of people; this is termed *paraphilias*. The fantasies of the child before puberty probably correlate with later choices of sexual expression when he or she becomes sexually active.[32]

The preadolescent years are an important period in the development of gender identity because, during these years, the child experiences his or her first bond of an adult nature. The preadolescent usually forms this intense bond or friendship with a peer of the same sex, although he or she may have a strong case of hero worship of an older person. This sensitive preadolescent period enables the child to begin to shed childhood values and interests and replace them with those of the adult world. The intense preadolescent relationship is not unlike a love relationship. It is usually not one sided like the crushes of earlier childhood but may be just as fantasy oriented and romantically obsessive, whether the romantic element is covert or overt. These intense relationships sometimes become sexual, resulting in an early homosexual or heterosexual experience. This does not, however, indicate the lifelong sexual object choice of the preadolescent. Nevertheless, the resolution and success of this bond creates early perceptions about roles in a sexual relationship.

During the adolescent phase of development, the adolescent expresses his or her perceptions of roles through sexual interest in another. Although sexual object choice is usually determined during adolescence, this choice can, and frequently does, change in adult years. The way in which early romantic relationships develop and satisfy the adolescent's needs and desires greatly affects future behavior in relationships.

Gay and lesbian adolescents have a doubly hard time developing healthy sexual identities. In addition to the normal identity problems of the teenage years, gay adolescents who are afraid of their homosexuality (internalized homophobia) are found to have a higher incidence of teenage acting out, such as drug and alcohol use, promiscuity, and suicidal ideation. Sensitive and helpful responses from health professionals can make a big difference.[34,35]

Life experience and opportunities and increasing self-awareness influence gender identity, gender role, and sexual object choice throughout the adult years. The early and middle adult years focus on sexually solidifying a long-term relationship and procreating. In middle age and later maturity, the focus turns again to the self and to personal fulfillment. In older age, sexual activity becomes symbolic of the continuation of social abilities and the reaffirmation of the self.

◆ Sexual Expression

Sexual object choice determines sexual expression. This choice is formed by an internal fantasy image of the ideal other. Dating behaviors are attempts to find this perfect other and develop a relationship rich in personal satisfaction. The success or failure of early adolescent relationships depends greatly on how well the fantasy actually fits the person. As people mature, their fantasies change. The ideal person image usually is altered by learning more about the needs, desires, and behaviors of others. A more mature person may be successful in falling in love because the fantasy may be more realized.[32] If the individual's fantasy is of an object, as in the paraphilias, he or she may still develop feelings of concern, affection, and erotic interest in another person in response to experience.

The state of "being in love" means deep involvement with and devotion to another person. In this state, sexual activity is undertaken according to perceived mutual needs and desires, which are expressed nonverbally during acts of lovemaking. The ability to send and receive these nonverbal cues accurately is necessary in sexual relationships. Also, people usually engage in sexual activity in a state of abandonment, in which each partner abandons his or her body to the pleasure of the other and becomes totally immersed in delighting the body of the other.

Being in love obviously is not the sole motivation for sexual activity. Sometimes, people are unable to integrate their images of an ideal relationship partner and an ideal sexual partner. They then find themselves in a relationship with one person with whom they are in love but deeply sexually attracted to another person. Some people do not like the man or woman with whom they enjoy the most intense sexual pleasure. Some men and women, perhaps due to conflicting feelings about sexual activity, believe that they can only experience sexual abandonment with someone they do not like or respect. It is probably true that relationships endure when they contain the potential for both sexual and personal pleasure for both parties.

HUMAN SEXUAL RESPONSE

The research of Masters and Johnson developed physiological information about the *human sexual response cycle.* They identified four phases of the cycle and labeled them excitement, plateau, orgasm, and resolution. Kaplan's work suggested renaming these desire, excitement, and orgasm for better understanding of the physiological process.[20] More subjectively experimental or psychological approaches suggest a preexcitement or transitional phase during which the partners are psychologically receptive to erotic stimuli.

The body cycles through natural phases of activation that lead to increased sexual receptivity.[20] The following discussions are based on Kaplan's system. The phases are discussed as specific and consistent. In fact, individuals may experience these phases in variations of these descriptions, according to individual differences and a variety of relationship, health, and environmental influences.

Desire

This phase involves the activation of areas of the brain to produce sexual appetite or drive; it does not include actual changes in the genital organs. This may include genital sensations or may be experienced as a feeling of restlessness, "sexiness," or just interest and openness to sex. The exact way in which the neural system of the brain creates these sensations is not clearly understood. It is assumed that these neural pathways are connected with pleasure and pain centers of the brain. This would explain the pleasurable, euphoric feeling people have when engaging in sex and the absence of sexual desire when a person is in pain. The *desire* phase seems to be controlled by the individual's perception of the environment, personal preferences and attractions to other people, and the absence of inhibitory influences. Sexual desire will exist and build only in the absence of inhibitory forces, such as fear, anxiety, discomfort, mental preoccupation (eg, worry), a higher level need (eg, hunger), or an intense emotion (eg, anger). However, forces that are inhibitory in some people, such as pain or anger, may create a higher base level of excitement and actually increase sexual arousal in people who do not perceive these sensations as frightening or aversive. Although we do not understand this mechanism, it is another example of the highly individualistic nature of the sexual experience.

Excitement

The next phase, *excitement*, is brought on by the psychological stimulation of the desire phase, such as fantasy or romantic communication. Physiological stimulation, such as touching, kissing, fondling, licking, or biting erotic parts of the body, produces the genital changes of the excitement phase. The areas on the body that are particularly sensitive to erotic stimulation are called erogenous zones. These zones differ among individuals but generally include the neck, mouth, breasts, inner thighs, and genital areas. The anus and navel are also erogenous areas for some people.

The petting and fondling activities of the excitement phase of the sexual response cycle are called *foreplay*. The caring, nurturing, and attentive behaviors between the sexual partners communicate concern and appreciation for each other's needs, desires, and sexual nature. Young men and women of various ages sometimes reach orgasm in response to intense foreplay alone. Nevertheless, this phase of sexual activity is the one most frequently omitted, especially if the couple perceives sex as relational or procreational rather than recreational.

This phase in the female begins with lubrication, expansion of the clitoris, and nipple erection. There is a generalized tensing of muscles throughout the body and increased heart rate, respirations, blood pressure, and motor restlessness. A fine rash or "sex flush" may appear over the abdomen and chest.

In men, this phase begins with erection of the penis, elevation of the testes, erection of the nipples, and sometimes a sex flush. Heart rate, respiratory rate, blood pressure, and motor restlessness increase in men as in women.

In women, vaginal vasocongestion results in a reduction of the opening of the vagina and the development of a swollen and tensing area called the orgasmic platform in the lower third of the vagina and the labia minora. The clitoris retracts from the normal position. Breasts enlarge through areolar engorgement. The sex flush, generalized muscle tension, rising heart rate, blood pressure, and respiratory rate continue.

In men, there is an increase in size of the coronal area of the glans penis. The testes continue to increase in size and elevate. The sex flush and motor restlessness increase. Heart rate, blood pressure, and respiratory rate rise.

Orgasm

The next phase of sexual response is called *orgasm*. In women, orgasm consists of three to 15 strong, rhythmic contractions of the orgasmic platform of the vagina. These may be followed by spastic contractions. During this phase, the vagina remains enlarged, and the uterus contracts irregularly. There is generalized muscle spasm and loss of voluntary muscle control throughout the body. Hyperventilation, blood pressure, heart rate, and sex flush reach peak. The rectal sphincter may contract, and the urinary meatus may dilate.

In men, the orgasm phase consists of emission and ejaculation and is characterized by ejaculatory contractions along the entire length of the penis, three or four expulsive contractions, then several contractions of less intensity. Response patterns of muscles, rectal sphincter, heart rate, blood pressure, and respiratory rate are the same as those seen in women during this phase.

The Kaplan model does not include the stage of *resolution* included in the Masters and Johnson model, because resolution is not actually a part of sexual response. However, it is helpful to examine this return of the body to normal state following orgasm.

In the female, resolution is marked by the return of the orgasmic platform to its normal size and position. The clitoris returns to normal size and position in 5 to 30 minutes. Breasts return to their normal size. Sex flush and muscle tension disappear as heart rate, blood pressure, and respiratory rate return to normal. In many women, lubrication recurs during the resolution phase, indicating an ability to reach orgasm again if stimulated.

In the man, the resolution phase involves a similar return of the genitalia to their normal sizes and positions but also includes a refractory period, during which time ejaculation cannot occur. This refractory period varies widely in length among individuals, and it changes throughout the life span. During the resolution phase, the penis reduces in size about 50% almost immediately after orgasm. The remaining enlargement of the penis disappears more slowly, sometimes over 2 hours. Similarly, vasocongestion of the scrotum and testes reduces by 50% rapidly, then continues to resolve over a longer period of time. Sex flush, nipple erection, muscle tension, heart rate, blood pressure, and respiratory rate all normalize fairly quickly during this phase.

These phases have many variations according to the individual's health state, energy level, and environment. For example, decreased lubrication or erection may have nothing to do with decreased desire. Orgasm may not be reached, yet both partners may have experienced a fulfilling sexual encounter. The subjective experience often does not match the physiological event, especially in women. Women frequently have long or slowly increasing plateau phases. Some women may even lose excitement during this phase yet feel fulfilled. All of these variations are normal, and it is important that clients understand them as normal. For example, some people experience orgasm as a release but not as the intensely pleasurable or euphoric experience that other people do. Neither orgasm is "better," nor do the differences reflect any significant physiological or psychological differences. An individual's sexual response is based on more than just physiological factors and is affected greatly by attitudes about sexual activity and the relationship and by many other less obvious factors.[24]

METHODS OF EXPERIENCING ORGASM

Orgasm may be reached through a variety of techniques. *Masturbation* refers to the self-stimulation of erogenous areas to the point of orgasm. In men, masturbation is usually performed by gripping the shaft of the penis and moving the hand up and down. Vibrators are also commonly used in masturbation, by rubbing the moving area of the machine over and around the penis. Women masturbate by either directly or indirectly stimulating the clitoris, rubbing over or around the clitoris, or inserting an object into the vagina to simulate the action of the penis in intercourse.

Cunnilingus is oral-genital stimulation performed on a woman. *Fellatio* is oral-genital stimulation performed on a man. Many men and women prefer this method of reaching orgasm over other methods. Lips, tongue, and teeth are used to stimulate the clitoris and vagina in cunnilingus and the penis in fellatio. Sucking, licking, nibbling, and blowing activities are used in this method of sexual stimulation.

Sexual intercourse, or *coitus,* is penetration of the vagina by the penis. Coitus is performed in a variety of positions. Face to face with the woman above and face to face in side-lying positions allow more control by the woman and usually result in less depth of vaginal penetration than many other positions for intercourse. The face-to-face with the man above position facilitates deeper penetration, especially if the woman has her legs over the shoulders of the man. This position does not facilitate as much ejaculatory control by the man. The rear-entry position allows deeper penetration and manual clitoral stimulation. Seated and standing positions offer varying degrees of control for either partner, depending in the positon of each partner, and they tend to decrease the depth of penetration.[3,21]

Anal intercourse is common among male homosexuals and also occurs in heterosexuals. A lubricant is necessary because the anus does not have the natural lubrication of the vagina. Anal intercourse is very stimulating to the penis because the anal opening is tight. The penis inserted into the anus stimulates the clitoris or penis of the receiving partner indirectly and is psychologically erotic for many people. For others, anal intercourse does not produce erotic sensations and may result in pain. Some women and men are excited by the partner stimulating the anus with a finger during intercourse. The finger or penis inserted into the anus should be washed before insertion into the vagina to avoid infecting the vagina with the normal bacteria of the rectum.

Other activities for reaching orgasm include penetrating the vagina or anus with the hand, vibrator, or other object, simulating actions of the penis. The hand and fingers create widely different sensations than does the penis or other penis-shaped objects and offer variations for heterosexual and homosexual couples. In addition, the penis, scrotum, clitoris, and vagina may be stimulated by the hand or other body part of the partner to result in orgasm.

TRADITIONAL LIFESTYLES OF SEXUAL EXPRESSION

In the current, dominant society of the country, many men and women engage in some sexual activity before marriage. Although this is counter to the teachings of most American religions, this practice does allow the adolescent to survey sexual attractions and erotic relationships before making a lifetime choice of marriage.[32] In addition, masturbation is common among adolescents and may help the adolescent and young adult develop sexual responsiveness and range of sexual preference.[32] Dating extends through the high school years, and the time of marriage generally depends on career choices. Many men and women choose to establish themselves in a profession or other career before marriage; however, subcultural and individual values, goals, and norms help determine the time of marriage. Committed relationships are now commonly formed as partnerships in the true sense of the word, with marriage contracts defining the shared responsibilities and the obligations of both partners.

With the current increase in sexually transmitted diseases, sexual activity is generally initiated with a great deal of thought and consideration. *"Safer sex"* involves avoiding unprotected sex with an unscreened partner and using a glove, finger cot, dental dam, or condom when exploring anal or vaginal areas and stimulating the penis. Kissing and hugging are generally safe, though French kissing may pose a hazard in some individuals. The general rule is to avoid contact with blood, feces, vaginal secretions, or semen. See Box 12-1 for a more detailed list of safer sex guidelines.

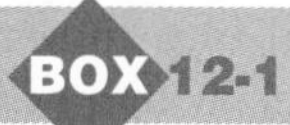

Safer Sex Options for Physical Intimacy

Safe sex guidelines are being taught by nurses and other health care professionals to clients and community groups in a variety of health care settings. Below are some safer sex guidelines you may wish to share with your clients:

SAFE

Massage
Hugging
Body rubbing
Dry kissing
Masturbation
Hand-to-genital touching (hand job) or mutual masturbation
Erotic books and movies
All sexual activities, when both partners are monogamous, trustworthy, and known by testing to be free of HIV

POSSIBLY SAFE

Wet kissing with no broken skin, cracked lips, or damaged mouth tissue
Vaginal or rectal intercourse using latex or synthetic condom correctly
Oral sex on a man using latex or synthetic condom
Oral sex on a woman using a latex or synthetic barrier such as a female condom, dental dam, or modified male condom, especially if she does not have her period or a vaginal infection with discharge
All sexual activities, when both partners are in a long-term monogamous relationship and trust each other

UNSAFE IN THE ABSENCE OF HIV TESTING AND TRUST AND MONOGAMY

Any vaginal or rectal intercourse without a latex or synthetic condom
Oral sex on a man without a latex or synthetic condom
Oral sex on a woman without a latex or synthetic barrier such as a female condom, dental dam, or modified male condom, especially if she is having her period or has a vaginal infection with discharge
Semen in the mouth
Oral-anal contact
Sharing sex toys or douching equipment
Blood contact of any kind, including menstrual blood, or any sex that causes tissue damage or bleeding

(Reprinted with permission from Contraceptive Technology, 16th edition, Hatcher et al. Irvington Publishers, 1994)

CULTURAL DIFFERENCES IN SEXUAL EXPRESSION

Sexual expression is inextricably bound with numerous intrapersonal and extrapersonal factors, including cultural ones. Cultural groupings include not only racial and ethnic cultures, but also the culture of the family of origin, the culture of the organized religion or spiritual philosophy, the culture of a particular region of the country, and the culture of the discipline (nursing). These cultural influences are visible in our values, beliefs, and behaviors, including sexual expression. For example, psychiatric nurses are bound by the American Nurses Association's Standards of Nursing Practice not to engage in sexual behavior with clients.

Because values and beliefs form views regarding sexual expression, the nurse needs to be aware of his or her own views and learn about the views of the client populations with whom he or she works. In general, sexual expression that occurs between two consenting adults, is not harmful (physically or psychologically) to either party, does not involve any form of force or coercion, and occurs in private is thought to be within the range of acceptable sexual expression. Sexual behaviors that violate these parameters, such as pedophilia, incest, or voyeurism, are not acceptable because they violate the will of others and may fall into the category of criminal behavior (eg, incest, pedophilia).

Also, not everyone agrees on what types of sexual expression are harmful to the parties involved. For example, American society tends to view prostitution as a criminal activity despite the fact that many believe that prostitution meets the parameters noted previously. However, among the many complaints about prostitution is the belief that this activity is at a minimum psychologically demeaning and may include physically destructive or dangerous practices by the parties involved. Interestingly, society tends to punish the one who sells the sexual behaviors and not the buyer of these behaviors as evidenced by the fact that prostitutes are prosecuted and their customers are frequently let go free.

Within the increasingly culturally diverse American society, many variations regarding sexual expression exist. Nurses should expect to encounter these variations. Further, the nurse's response to these variations should include a willingness to learn about others' ways and to be responsive to the client's sexual concerns. These attitudes are inherent in the efforts to treat the client with respect and dignity.

Research in the area of cultural differences in sexual expression is sparse. Many previously largely homogeneous groups are becoming increasingly diverse due to political and economic changes resulting in the influx of other cultural norms. Some general guidelines, however, can help the nurse know what to expect regarding clients' cultural values.

Within the Hispanic communities of the United States, research suggests that Hispanics are more reticient to discuss issues of sexuality.[1] In one study of Spanish-speaking sex offenders, researchers found that programmatic adjustments were necessary because of their subjects' difficulty discussing sexuality in a group setting, their reluctance to criticize other members in the group, and their adherence to rules of etiquette or politeness toward the therapist in which discussion of sexual matters is a breach of etiquette.[7]

Studies of Hispanic adolescents and young adults suggest that sexuality remains a sensitive issue among the young, and their views of sexual roles and behaviors tend to be more traditional.[10,23,31] However, sex education,[29] peer pressure and achievement orientation, and parental attitudes[13] have been found to influence sexual behavior in Hispanic adolescents.

Within African American communities in the United States, sexuality is also a sensitive and private concern. For example, a study of racial differences in social support and mental health in men with HIV infection found that African American men were less likely to be open about their sexuality to their primary social support network than white men.[30] Another study of African American teenage girls and women (ages 15–45) found that these women perceived that the African American community continues to value traditional sexual roles that permit men to have sexual freedom but censure women for the same activities.[12] Additionally, one study that examined the interaction between African (strong independent women and reciprocity between spouses) and American (European-derived American heritage of sexuality as a male status symbol and of male control of women's lives) gender-role ideologies suggests that these conflicting ideologies contribute to other stresses of African American families regarding gender role behaviors.[38]

In the case of immigrants to the United States, the most likely predictors of "Americanized" sexual attitudes seem to be the length of time the client has been in the American culture, the education of the client, and the client's parents' education level.[1] Between African Americans and whites in this country, gender is a more significant variable than race in predicting sexual attitudes.[38] Religious attitudes have a strong influence on sexual attitudes and sexual behavior in some cultures. For example, premarital sexual behavior in African American women has been shown to be related to religious involvement.[5] Sex role attitudes seem to predict attitudes about sexual behavior as well. Cultures that value equality between the sexes also reflect more liberal notions about sexual freedom and tend to be more open to discussing sexuality. In cultures that value a strictly patriarchal household, such as the Laotian Hmong people and Iranians before the Islamic revolution, there is clear double standard, with men accepted as sexually promiscuous and inclined toward extramarital sexual relationships and women expected to be virgins before marriage and to remain monogamous throughout marriage.[21] Such beliefs, however, sometimes are changed when these people move to a more sexually permissive country and are enculturated in that country.

The nurse must develop trust with the client and then interview the client to uncover his or her sexual norms and values. Nursing intervention must be based on an understanding of the client's cultural context for sexual values, norms, and behaviors.

Much more research regarding sex role ideologies within the numerous diverse cultural groups is necessary to understand and care for clients better. However, this lack of knowledge is no excuse for nurses to remain poorly informed about the sexual behaviors and needs of the populations with which they work. Nurses pledge (by ethical code and by standards of practice) to assess and respond to the health care (including sexual health care) needs of their clients. Nurses, therefore, need to perform careful assessments that include discussions of cultural factors that may contribute to differences in the client's expression of his or her sexuality.

ALTERNATIVE SEXUAL LIFESTYLES

Homosexuality and Bisexuality

For about 2% to 4% of the population, the sexual object choice is a member of the same sex.[22] Preferring a member of the same sex as a sexual partner is called *homosexuality;* male homosexuals are sometimes referred to as gay men, whereas female homosexuals are known as lesbians. The incidence of homosexuality varies geographically; in some major cities, for example, the percentage of male homosexuals may be as high as 14%.[22]

Bisexuality refers to an equal or almost equal preference for either sex. Some bisexuals, however, do not feel fulfilled with a solitary (or monogamous) relationship with a member of either sex but prefer to be involved in equally intense and meaningful relationships with a man and a woman. Approximately 7% to 9% of the general population can be identified as bisexual, which includes those who refer to themselves as bisexual if they have ever had a sexual experience of any kind with a person of the same sex, even if they generally prefer and are engaged in a heterosexual relationship.[22] As with homosexuality, bisexuality is not uniformly distributed in the population; the percentages are likely to be highest in urban areas.

These sexual identities are due not only to predisposition for sexual activities, but also to a perceived preference for sharing emotional intimacy with either a man or a woman and with the man or woman chosen for a sexual relationship. The development of homosexual or bisexual orientation is not well understood. Research suggests that as with heterosexuals, numerous biological, genetic, social, and environment factors play a role in the development of a person's sexual preference. Animal studies, for example, suggest that sexual object choice and sexual behavior can be influenced by the presence or absence of fetal androgenic substances. Genetic studies of male homosexuality suggest that familial constellations contribute to the development of male homosexuality. However, other studies have found little correlation between family constellations or parental characteristics and adult homosexuality. Much remains to be understood about homosexual and bisexual preferences. Most of the research to date has focused on male homosexuals with little attention to lesbians or bisexuals.[19]

Gay men, lesbians, and bisexuals are sometimes collectively called gays. Transsexual and transgender individuals are sometimes included in this category as well. In most areas of the country, a united force of gay, lesbian, and bisexual people is working through political means for elimination of discrimination. There is really no such thing as a typical gay or lesbian person, just as a typical heterosexual person exists only statistically. The mannerisms and preferences of dress that are seen as associated with gay people are sometimes exaggerated in response to stigmatization from the heterosexual world.

The sexual behavior of gay people varies as much as the sexual behavior of heterosexuals. Sexual dysfunction or pedophila is no more prevalent among gay men, lesbians, and bisexuals than among heterosexual groups. Promiscuity is no more common among homosexuals than heterosexuals. Gay and lesbian people do tend to enter a greater number of sexual relationships, perhaps because there are fewer societal supports for long-term relationships among gay people. Nevertheless, their relationships tend to last for 2 to 3 years and tend to be monogamous. For many homosexual people, the gay or lesbian bar provides one of the few places where it is acceptable to meet with and talk to other homosexuals. The heterosexual or "straight" world, on the other hand, has a variety of places within which heterosexuals can display affection for each other and be considered socially acceptable.

In recent years, community centers, organizations, and publications devoted to gay, lesbian, and bisexual activities and concerns have emerged. Gay and lesbian concerns have also become more visible in mainstream movies and television sitcoms. Community celebrities, such as politicians, actors, and activists, are more open about their sexual orientations. Despite these forward strides, many individuals still hold values and beliefs that are discriminatory toward homosexuals. Gay men and lesbians continue to be stigmatized and persecuted by laws denying them equal rights and opportunities as those available to heterosexuals (ie, service in the military, legal recognition of marriages, and antidiscrimination laws for work and housing).

Nursing care for people with homosexual or bisexual preferences should include completing a thorough nursing assessment (Box 12-2), displaying sensitivity regarding various lifestyle concerns in a predominantly heterosexual society (ie, homophobia, disclosing or not

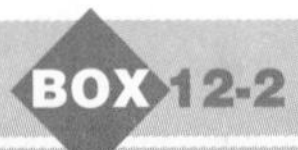

Sexual Assessment of Homosexual or Bisexual Clients

1. Do you consider yourself homosexual or bisexual? How long have you been "out" to yourself about your orientation? Do you wish to have, or have you had, any actual same-sex sexual experiences?
2. What are your thoughts or feelings about your orientation? If you have positive feelings about being homosexual or bisexual, how do you feel you developed this outlook? If you have negative feelings about being homosexual or bisexual, how do you cope with these feelings? Do you feel you have accepted your homosexuality?
3. Are you very "out" in your life (at work or school)? Of your family and friends who know, how do they feel about your orientation?
4. Whom do you consider as your support system? Do they know you are homosexual or bisexual? Do you have homosexual or bisexual friends? Has being "out" or "closeted" about your orientation caused any problems in your family, place of work, church, or social relationships? How do you deal with these problems?
5. Do you have a lover or life partner? Do you and your partner have any unresolved issues that need to be addressed? How has the issue of acquired immunodeficiency syndrome and other sexually transmitted diseases affected your sex life and relationship? Do your family and friends know the nature of your relationship? Are they supportive?

(Adapted from Smith BS: Nursing Care Challenges: Homosexual Psychiatric Patients. J Psychosoc Nurs 30 (12): 15–21, 1992)

disclosing a homosexual or bisexual orientation), including the homosexual's life partner or significant other in the treatment plan, and being knowledgeable about specific community resources.[36]

Nurses should also be prepared to discuss and respond to questions regarding sexuality from their gay clients. For example, the nurse may need to provide education on "safer sex" practices (see Box 12-1) or be knowledgeable about when a gay man may resume having anal sex following a hemorrhoidectomy. Issues regarding AIDS, such as loss of family, friends, or a partner to this terminal disease, may also be part of addressing the gay or lesbian client's health care needs (see Chapter 48, The Client on the Human Immunodeficiency Virus Spectrum).

VARIATIONS IN SEXUAL EXPRESSION DUE TO PHYSICAL OR MENTAL CONDITIONS

The Client's Sexual Needs

Illness, disability, hospitalization, and surgery are frequent factors in the disruption of the self-concept, including the sexual identity and gender identity. The client may demonstrate these disruptions as withdrawal from the family, anger toward the hospital or clinic staff, and deterioration of normal practices of hygiene and dress. Sometimes, hospitalized clients respond to crises by making obscene or sexually suggestive remarks or gestures toward nursing personnel. Although this behavior cannot be reinforced by the nurse, the response should not be one of anger. The nurse first clarifies the nature of the nurse–client relationship and then clearly states that the nurse is interested in maintaining this therapeutic, nonsocial relationship. If the client is persistent, the nurse repeats the limits of the relationship and that violation of these limits will not be tolerated. Often, the client accepts the more clearly defined relationship and perhaps indicates a need for a closer relationship with staff on a therapeutic level. Illness and hospitalization weaken most normal coping mechanisms of clients and remove them from significant relationships, thereby creating a need for intimacy on some level with staff members. This need is met by understanding nursing staff responding with emotional warmth and support within a professional relationship.

Many nurses are bothered by the client who masturbates. Perhaps one reason for this lack of tolerance and empathy is a mistaken belief that seriously ill people do not have sexual needs and desires. The nurse should provide for privacy and respect this privacy by knocking on the door before entering, keeping the curtain drawn around the client's bed unless requested otherwise, and so forth. If the nurse finds a client masturbating, he or she should apologize for the invasion and provide the necessary privacy. It is important to convey respect and appreciation for the client's needs and individual values. Similarly, a client may need sexual activity with his or her sexual partner while hospitalized. The nurse should be sensitive to cues of these needs and should respond by providing privacy.

Whenever the client's sexual values and expression differ from those of the nurse, the nurse should be alert to any tendency to act out biases on the client. Instead, the professional nurse must be able to empathize with the client's sexual concerns and difficulties. This empathy is essential for truly therapeutic interactions between the nurse and the client.

Changes in Sexual Abilities

Certain physical and mental conditions affect one's ability to perform sexually and create a threatening crisis for the client's self-esteem. The nurse needs to be aware of such conditions and encourage the client to verbalize feelings and frustrations. Often, if the usual mode of sexual expression is not possible, an alternative method could be successful in meeting the client's sexual and relationship needs. For example, the quadriplegic client can participate in sexual intercourse if she or he is comfortable taking on a new role, perhaps a more passive one. A man who has lost the ability to achieve and maintain an erection may undergo a relatively simple procedure to have a penile implant placed surgically that enables erection, although not ejaculation. Many times, the client will feel satisfied with the ability to please his or her partner sexually, even if orgasm as formerly experienced is impossible (Case Study 12-1).

Many surgical treatments and diseases can result in impotence in men or decreased sexual excitement in women. These include perineal prostatectomies, sometimes ileostomies and colostomies, and in some cases, diabetes. These problems may be caused by psychological or physiological changes. The client may require referral for more tests or therapy to discern the nature of the problem. A man with physiological erectile dysfunction might be encouraged to try activities other than intercourse for sexual fulfillment. A penile implant may be preferred by some men. Male or female clients might be assisted to find greatr sexual pleasure by trying more foreplay, increased patience on the part of the client and partner, and improved communication about thoughts and feelings in response to sexual activity.

Some women experience a loss of libido following bilateral oophorectomies and difficulty reaching orgasm following abdominal surgeries to create colostomy or ileostomy. Both partners must understand the physiological causes of these reactions and openly communicate their responses. These are also good suggestions for clients who may have sexual changes due to diabetes mellitus. This disease may cause orgasmic dysfunction in women and retrograde ejaculation in men (which would prevent conception).[21] Some women experience dyspareunia, or pain with sexual intercourse, following hysterectomies and radiation treatments for uterine or cervical cancer. Coital positions providing the woman with more control in directing the penis and preventing deep penetration may restore sexual satisfaction in the relationship.

Elderly people experience changes in sexual abilities that they sometimes perceive as an inability to engage in sexual activity. The elderly person should be counseled regarding the normalcy of changes, such as a longer refractory period in the man, less firmness of the male erection, a longer time required to achieve erection and reach orgasm, and occasional incidents of inability to achieve erection. Many men adapt to such changes by trying alternative sexual activities, such as having the partner stimulate the penis manually before

Case Study

A Client With Spinal Cord Injury

Ms. K, 36 years old, suffered a spinal cord injury in a motor vehicle accident, leaving her paralyzed from the waist down. Recently divorced, she had been dating two men, one of whom she was "strongly attracted to." During her stay in a rehabilitation center, Ms. K talked with the nurse about her body image and fear of never being able to have a "real" sexual relationship again.

The nurse listened to Ms. K's concerns and acknowledged her grief and fears. She then discussed various sexual activities that possibly could be fulfilling to both Ms. K and a partner. The nurse addressed Ms. K's body image concerns, emphasizing that although the injury had confined her to a wheelchair, it had not otherwise altered her appearance. The nurse encouraged Ms. K to look in the mirror more often, to develop a more realistic and positive attitude, and to share her concerns with a support group. The nurse also gave Ms. K copies of journal articles and book excerpts about sexual activity after spinal cord injury.

Later, Ms. K shared her concerns and this information with her support group. She received much positive feedback from group members for bringing up a subject of concern to them all. As a result, she began to feel reassured that she could rebuild a new, positive body image for herself and enjoy active sexual expression.

Questions for Discussion

1. What would you say to Ms. K to enhance her body image?
2. How did Ms. K show that she was adapting well?
3. How would you react if Ms. K came to you with questions about sexual activity in which she was engaging?

attempting coitus and oral sex if erection cannot be achieved fully enough to engage in coitus. Women tend to experience a loss of lubrication and some dyspareunia with the normal physical changes of aging. Engaging in sexual activities other than coitus, trying new coital positions, or using a water-soluble lubricant may allow the elderly woman to enjoy a full sex life.[3]

The Effects of Drugs

Some drugs affect libido and sexual abilities. When possible, the drug should be discontinued, and a drug without this side effect should be administered. If this is not possible, the nurse should explain the cause of the problem to the client and encourage the alteration of sexual activity as necessary. One such alteration might be the adoption of new coital positions or longer periods of foreplay before attempting coitus. Again, it is necessary that the client's sexual partner know the reason for the client's changing sexual abilities. Alcohol affects sexual interest and abilities in many men and women, but these changes are reversed when the alcohol use is curbed or stopped. On the other hand, chronic alcohol or drug use may affect the relationship to an extent that it interferes with normal sexual activity. Couple therapy or counseling may be needed to help restore open communication between the partners.

Some drugs are used in the treatment of sexual dysfunction, paraphilias, and gender identity disorders. For example, antianxiety medications are sometimes used with clients whose anxiety and tension interfere with their ability to engage in sexual relations. Fluoxetine (Prozac), tricyclic antidepressants, haloperidol (Haldol), lorazepam (Ativan), thioridazine (Mellaril), and the monoamine oxidase inhibitors have been used to prolong sexual activity in men suffering from premature ejaculation.[19] Clients who engage in paraphilic behavior, especially those whose behavior endangers the safety of others (pedophiles, violent sadists), may be treated with drugs that reduce their sexual desire, arousal, and paraphilic fantasies. Cyproterone acetate (Androcur) and medroxyprogesterone acetate (Provera) reduce testosterone levels, which results in decreased levels of deviant sexual behavior.[19] Additionally, sertraline (Zoloft) and fluoxetine (Prozac) have been useful in reducing depressive symptoms in paraphilics and decreasing some paraphilic behaviors.[4,17,18]

Clients with gender identity disorders frequently want to take hormones to produce the physical sexual characteristics of the gender with which they identify. Clients should be discouraged from taking hormones without a doctor's supervision and from purchasing black market hormones and quack "feminization pills." In male-to-female transsexuals (MTFs), the effects of estrogen include less frequent erections, sterility, breast enlargement, decreased testicular volume, and more rounded body contours. Side effects include hypertension, hyperglycemia, hepatic dysfunction, and thromboembolic phenomena. Female-to-male transsexuals (FTMs) who take androgens will experience an increase in sex drive, clitoral tingling and enlargement, amenorrhea, and deepening of the voice (over several months). With weight lifting exercise, increased muscle mass will develop. Some changes in hair distribution of the face and body may occur, including development of frontal balding. Side effects include thromboembolic phenomena, hepatic dysfunction, and elevations in cholesterol and triglycerides.[19]

Sexual Behavior During Psychoses

The schizophrenic client may evidence bizarre sexual habits during psychotic episodes. These are usually part of the client's delusional system and probably do not represent covert sexual desires.[16] The client with manic behavior often exhibits increased sexual interest along with the loss of usual inhibitions. This results in a period of sexual promiscuity and flirtatious behavior. The depressed client may experience a loss of sexual interest and ability during the acutely depressive period. Family members, friends, and sexual partners of these clients must be informed of the causes of erratic behavior and understand that the behavior may never recur during healthier periods. The client should be protected by limit setting; punishment or chastisement will not change the inappropriate behavior.

Posttraumatic Stress Disorder

Many women and some men unfortunately have been victims of rape, incest, or other forms of sexual assault. The result of these traumatic events is often lifelong emotional trauma. Many victims of sexual abuse and assault develop psychological problems that prevent them from being vulnerable and thus accepting love or from being strong with another and thus creating equal relationships.

Victims of sexual abuse or assault may have distorted body images or unusual anxiety and fear about sexual behavior or sexual touch. All of the common sexual problems listed in this chapter could potentially have been caused by traumatic sexual events in some period of the client's life. The nurse must ask clients if they have experienced such trauma and help them explore thoughts and feelings about this if they are willing and able to do so. Psychotherapy may be advisable for clients who have experienced sexual trauma (Box 12-3).

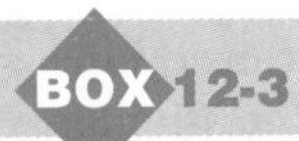

BOX 12-3

Therapeutic Dialogue Regarding Sexual Concerns

Ms. K., 35 years old, was seen for her yearly pelvic examination. The nurse had the following interview with the client:

Nurse: Have you ever had any unwanted sexual contact or experience?

Ms. K.: Well, not as an adult. When I was about 7 years old, my uncle lived with my mother and me for awhile. He used to make me touch him. (Client looks embarrassed and she looks down at her feet.)

Nurse: I am so sorry. That must have been a very difficult experience for you.

Ms. K.: (Client becomes tearful.) I was so scared and ashamed. I never told anyone.

Nurse: (Brings client tissues and sits quietly allowing the client to cry and collect herself.) That is a heavy secret to carry around with you all these years.

Ms. K.: (Client nods head in agreement.)

Nurse: Do you feel ready to continue our interview or would you like a few minutes to collect yourself?

Ms. K.: I'm OK. I guess this stuff still bothers me. Sometimes I dream about it. The idea of sex is ugly to me. I avoid men. I have never dated because the idea of being with a man makes me feel nervous and anxious. The thought of being with a man makes me want to run far away.

Nurse: I agree with you that the sexual abuse you experienced as a little girl is still bothering you and has affected the way you feel about sex and relationships with men. These problems are frequently reported by women sexually abused as children. You should know that these are problems that can be treated. Would you like the names of some therapists who treat this problem?

Ms. K.: Yes, I would. I think it's time for me to work on this problem.

◆ Sexual Disorders and Gender Identity Disorders

The Diagnostic and Statistical Manual of Mental Disorders (fourth edition) lists three categories of sexual disorders. These categories are the sexual dysfunctions, the gender identity disorders, and the paraphilias.

SEXUAL DYSFUNCTION DISORDERS

Sexual Dysfunctions are those disorders that involve the disturbance of the sexual response cycle. These disorders are listed in Box 12-4. There are few systematic epidemiological data regarding the prevalence of these various sexual dysfunctions, and these show extremely wide variability, probably reflecting differences in assessment methods, definitions used, and characteristics of sample populations.[8]

Desire Disorders

Hypoactive sexual desire disorder is characterized by persistently or recurrently deficient or absent sexual fantasies and desire for sexual activity. Low sexual desire may be global and encompass all forms of sexual expression or may be situational and limited to one person or to a specific sexual activity (eg, intercourse but not masturbation). These people do not initiate sexual activity and only engage in it reluctantly when it is initiated by the partner. Hypoactive sexual desire is frequently associated with problems of sexual arousal or with orgasm difficulties. Also, depressive disorders are associated with low sexual desire. Some studies have found increased levels of serum testosterone in men complaining of this problem. Because of lack of normative age- or gender-related data on frequency of sexual desire, the diagnosis must rely on clincal judgment that takes into account factors such as age and the context of the person's life. Treatment targets individual and contributing causal factors that are related to the hypoactive sexual disorder, such as childhood sexual abuse, hormonal imbalances, depression, and other sexual disorders.[8]

Sexual aversion disorder is characterized by persistent or recurrent extreme aversion to, and avoidance of, all (or almost all) genital sexual contact with a sexual partner. The aversion to genital contact may be focused on a particular aspect of sexual experience (genital secretions, vaginal penetration) or may be generalized to all sexual stimuli, including kissing and touching. When confronted with a sexual situation, some individuals with severe sexual aversion disorder may experience panic attacks with extreme anxiety, feelings of terror, faintness, nausea, palpitations, dizziness, and breathing difficulties.

Individuals may avoid sexual situations or potential sexual partners by covert strategies: going to sleep early, traveling, neglecting personal appearance, using substances, and being overinvolved in work, social, or family activities. Treatment focuses on the anxiety symptoms, such as the dynamic issues that may be related to the sexual aversion (eg, sexual abuse or other related trauma).[8]

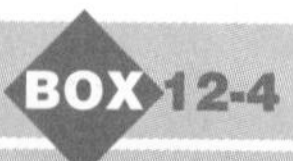

DSM-IV Diagnoses of Sexual Dysfunctions

The following specifiers apply to all primary sexual dysfunctions:

Lifelong Type/Acquired Type
Generalized Type/Situational Type
Due to Psychological Factors/Due to Combined Factors

SEXUAL DESIRE DISORDERS

Hypoactive Sexual Desire Disorder
Sexual Aversion Disorder

SEXUAL AROUSAL DISORDERS

Female Sexual Arousal Disorder
Male Erectile Disorder

ORGASMIC DISORDERS

Female Orgasmic Disorder
Male Orgasmic Disorder
Premature Ejaculation

SEXUAL PAIN DISORDERS

Dyspareunia (Not Due to General Medical Condition)
Vaginismus (Not Due to a General Medical Condition)

SEXUAL DYSFUNCTION DUE TO A GENERAL MEDICAL CONDITION

Female Hypoactive Sexual Desire Disorder Due to . . .*
Male Hypoactive Sexual Desire Disorder Due to . . .*
Male Erectile Disorder Due to . . .*
Female Dyspareunia Due to . . .*
Male Dyspareunia Due to . . .*
Other Female Sexual Dysfunction Due to . . .*
Other Male Sexual Dysfunction Due to . . .*
—— Substance-Induced Sexual Dysfunction**

Arousal Disorders

Female sexual arousal disorder is characterized by a persistent or recurrent inability to attain, or to maintain until completion of the sexual activity, an adequate lubrication-swelling response of sexual excitement. In women, the arousal response includes vasocongestion in the pelvis, vaginal lubrication and expansion, and swelling of the external genitalia. *Male erectile disorder* is characterized by a persistent or recurrent inability to attain, or to maintain until completion of the sexual activity, an adequate erection. There are different patterns of erectile dysfunction. Some individuals report the inability to obtain any erection from the outset of the sexual experience. Others will complain of first experiencing an adequate erection and then losing tumescence when attempting penetration. Still others report that they have an erection that is sufficiently firm for penetration, but they lose tumescence before or during thrusting.[8]

Male and female sexual arousal disorders may be due to psychological factors, such as depression, anxiety, psychological trauma, or medical conditions, including reduction of estrogen or testosterone levels, atrophic vaginitis, diabetes mellitus, radiotherapy of the pelvis, multiple sclerosis, renal faliure, or spinal cord injury. These difficulties may also be related to the side effects of antihypertensive medications, antidepressants, neuroleptics, and substance abuse. Treatment targets the related causative factors.[8]

Orgasmic Disorders

Female orgasmic disorder and *male orgasmic disorder* are characterized by a persistent or recurrent delay in, or absence of, orgasm following a normal sexual excitement phase. Premature ejaculation is characterized by a persistent or recurrent onset of orgasm and ejeculation with minimal sexual stimulation before, on, or shortly after penetration and before the person wishes it. Men and women exhibit a wide variability in the type or intensity of stimulation that triggers orgasm. These diagnoses should take into account the person's age, life circumstances, and the adequacy of intensity and duration of the sexual stimulation, as these disorders may be due to psychological and or medical conditions. Treatment focuses on the related causative factors.[8]

Dyspareunia (not due to a general medical condition) is characterized by genital pain that is associated with sexual intercourse in either a man or woman. Although it is most commonly experienced during coitus, it may also occur before or after intercourse. The intensity of symptoms may range from mild discomfort to sharp pain. *Vaginismus* (not due to a general medical condition) is characterized by the recurrent or persistent involuntary spasm of the musculature of the outer third of the vagina that interferes with sexual intercourse. The physical obstruction due to muscle contraction usually prevents coitus. These conditions tend to be chronic unless treated (Table 12-1).[8,25]

Paraphilias

Paraphilias are recurrent and intense sexually arousing fantasies, sexual urges, or behaviors lasting at least 6 months that generally involve nonhuman objects, the

Table 12-1

Common Sexual Problems and Suggested "Homework"

Sexual Difficulty	Exercise or Homework Suggested	Intended Goal of Homework
Female orgasmic dysfunction	Sensate focus (first nongenital, then genital)	Reduces pressure to "perform," increases awareness of sensual pleasure; teaches partners about preferred areas and methods of nongenital and genital touch; teaches woman to avoid spectator role
	Masturbation or use of vibrators	Teaches woman how to pleasure herself; teaches her how to achieve orgasm; teaches her more about her genitals; sensitizes her to sexual stimulation
	Education and psychotherapy	Explores attitudes about self, sexuality, sexual behavior; increases partner's understanding
Low sexual desire	Medical examination	Rules out hormonal imbalance
	Facilitative communication, psychotherapy, and education	Explores attitudes about self, partner, relationship, and sexuality; increases partner's understanding
Erectile dysfunction	Sensate focus	Reduces perception of pressure to "perform" sexually, teaches to avoid spectator role in sexual activity
	Facilitative communication and psychotherapy	Explores attitudes and feelings about self, partner, relationship, and sexual behavior; increases partner's understanding
	Medical examination	Rules out organic cause
Rapid ejaculation	Squeeze technique	Educates about level of sexual arousal
		Teaches inhibition of ejaculation, control of cycle for maximum satisfaction
Vaginismus	Relaxation exercises	Decreases anxiety about penetration and sexual intercourse
	Graduated dilators	Increases vaginal tolerance of and relaxation with insertion of penis
	Facilitative communication and counseling	Explores attitudes and feelings about self, partner, relationship, and sexual behavior; increases partner's understanding of situation

suffering or humiliation of oneself or one's partner, or children or other nonconsenting people. For some individuals, paraphiliac fantasies or stimuli are necessary for erotic arousal and are always included in sexual activity. In other cases, the paraphiliac preferences occur only episodically (eg, during period of stress). The behavior, sexual urges, or fantasies cause clinically significant distress or impairment in social, occupational, or other important areas of functioning.[8]

The paraphilias are described in Box 12-5. Some clients experience psychological distress about paraphilias. Other clients' paraphilias may only be fulfilled through commiting crimes, such as molesting children, "flashing" exhibitionism, or making obscene phone calls (scatalogia). However, some clients with paraphiliac interests may not be distressed by them, but may view them as an interesting part of their personal sexuality and seek to fulfil them with similarly interested adult partners. These clients may be active with their partners or visit specialized prostitutes; may read books, magazines, and Internet information about their paraphilias; or may participate in paraphiliac subcultures. Some clients may attend support groups that encourage responsible behavior. Frequently, involvement in treatment is not voluntary but rather the consequence of criminal prosecution (court-ordered treatment).

Problems can occur when one partner, who is comfortable with a paraphilia, tries to pressure an uninterested spouse to participate or is rejected by the uninterested spouse. An example of this is when a husband asks his wife to aid him with cross-dressing, and the wife is not comfortable or pleased with his cross-dressed sexuality and persona or with his activities in cross-dressing subculture.

Estimates regarding the prevalence of paraphilic behavior in the general population are not available. However, although paraphilias are rarely diagnosed in general clinical facilities, the large commercial market in paraphiliac pornography and paraphernalia and the presence of support groups suggest that its prevalence in the community is high. The most common presenting problems in clinics that specialize in the treatment of paraphilias are pedophilia, voyeurism, and exhibitionism. Approximately one-half of the individuals with

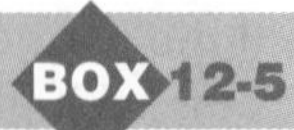

DSM-IV Definitions of Paraphilias

Exhibitionism—exposure of one's genitals
Fetishism—the use of nonliving objects such as female undergarments
Frotteurism—touching and rubbing against a nonconsenting person
Pedophilia—sexual activity with a prepubescent child
Sexual Masochism—real, not simulated, humiliation; being beaten, bound, or otherwise made to suffer
Sexual Sadism—real, not simulated, acts that inflict psychological or physical suffering of the victim sexual partner
Transvestic Fetishism
Voyeurism—observing an unsuspecting person who is naked in the process of disrobing or engaging in sexual activity
Paraphilia Not Otherwise Specified

paraphilias seen clinically are married, and, except for sexual masochism, where the ratio is estimated to be 20 males for each female, the other paraphilias are almost never diagnosed in females, although some cases have been reported.[8]

Treatment for paraphilic disorders that distress the client or lead to criminal behavior is often difficult. Some methods to treat these disorders include the use of drugs (cyproterone acetate or medroxyprogesterone) that reduce sexual desire, satiation (a boredom technique in which the sex offender uses his most erotic fantasies postorgasm in a boring, repetitive manner to extinguish the erotic quality of his fantasies), signaled punishment (combining aversion therapy with biofeedback of one's erections to deviant stimuli), and treatments aimed at the paraphiliac's deficits (eg, deficits in arousal to adult partners, deficits in assertive skills, and treatment to reduce distorted cognitions regarding their paraphilic behavior). For example, a child molester may describe his 4-year-old victim as seductive because the child invited him to join in her play or ran around the house in her panties.[19] These and other personality deficits are treated using a variety of treatment modalities and approaches.

GENDER IDENTITY DISORDERS

Gender identity disorders (Box 12-6) are characterized by strong and persistent cross-gender identification accompanied by persistent discomfort with one's assigned sex. No recent epidemiological studies provide data on the prevalence of gender identity disorder. Data from smaller countries in Europe with access to total population statistics and referrals suggest that roughly 1 per 30,000 adult men and 1 per 100,000 adult women seek sex-reassignment surgery. In child clinic samples, approximately five boys for each girl are referred with this disorder. In adult clinic samples, men outnumber women by about two or three times.[8]

In children, disturbance is manifested by four (or more) of the following:

1. Repeatedly stated desire to be, or insistence that he or she is, the other sex
2. In boys, preference for cross-dressing or simulating female attire; in girls, insistence on wearing only stereotypical masculine clothing
3. A strong and persistent preference for cross-sex roles in make-believe play or persistent fantasies of being the other sex
4. Intense desire to participate in the stereotypical games and pastimes of the other sex

In adolescents and adults, the disturbance is manifested by symptoms such as a stated desire to be the other sex, frequent passing as the other sex, desire to live or be treated as the other sex, or the conviction that he or she has the typical feelings and reactions of the other sex.[8]

In addition, these individuals experience a persistent discomfort with his or her sex or sense of inappropriateness in the gender role of that sex. In children, this aspect of the disturbance is manifested by any of the following: Boys may assert that their penis or testes are disgusting or will disappear or that it would be better not to have a penis. They may avoid rough-and-tumble play and reject male stereotypical toys, games, and activities. Girls may reject urinating in a sitting position, assert that they have or will grow a penis, or assert that they do not want to grow breasts or menstruate. They may show marked aversion toward normative feminine clothing.[8]

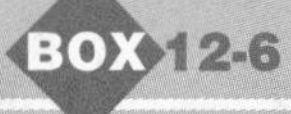

DSM-IV Diagnoses of Gender Identity Disorders

Gender Identity Disorder
  in Children
  in Adolescents or Adults
Gender Identity Disorder NOS
Sexual Disorder NOS

In adolescents and adults, this discomfort with the biological sex is manifested by symptoms such as preoccupation with changing primary and secondary sex characteristics to fit the desired sex (eg, request for hormones, surgery, or other procedures to alter sexual characteristics) or the belief that he or she was born the wrong sex.[8]

Treatments available for those suffering with gender identity disorders include hormone treatment, sex reassignment surgery (SRS), and psychotherapy. Surgical techniques for the creation of a vaginal barrel or a penis are limited, expensive, and may have unpleasant side effects. At least 35% of clients complain of inadequate vaginal depth in the years following SRS, and as many as 30% regret having undergone SRS.[19] In MTFs whose hormone treatments did not produce great breast enlargement, surgical breast implants may be an option. Due to expense and lack of sophisticated surgeries, many FTM transsexuals undergo a double mastectomy with cosmetic chest resculpting, without attempting to create a penis.

As described in the previous section on drugs, hormonal treatment in MTFs results in less frequent erections, more rounded bodily contours, decreased testicular volume, and a limited but pleasing breast enlargement. In FTMs, testosterone produces an increased sexual drive, amenorrhea, and hoarseness. If weight lifting is undertaken, a pronounced increase in muscle mass may occur. Also some increase in the amount and coarseness of facial and body hair may occur, as may frontal balding.[19]

Psychotherapy for adult clients focuses on assisting them to find a workable, comfortable sexual identity. Clients often find it difficult to find partners who accept them as they are and consequently suffer from depression, anxiety, or other disorders related to their lack of an intimate connection to another person.[19] Support groups of other transsexuals and newsletters and magazines for transsexuals may alleviate distress and loneliness, providing friends, correspondence, and a safe space for clients to explore their gender identities.

Application of the Nursing Process to Sexual Problems

ASSESSMENT

The first step of the nursing process, assessment, includes reviewing the client's record for a clearer understanding of all aspects of the sexual problem. A sex history is obtained in which the client's earliest sexual experiences are described, along with how the client first learned about sex. The nurse compiles data that clarify the client's feelings and attitudes about sex. The assessment process also focuses on the sexual relationship, exploring such issues as what sex roles and gender roles are taken by each partner, how well the partner's attitudes agree with those of the client, how each partner percieves the needs of self and the other, how sexual needs and preferences are expressed in the relationship, and whether each partner gives equal consideration to the needs of the other. The nurse also may wish to investigate the past relationships of the client and partner to explore how these earlier relationships have affected the client. This information facilitates a clarification of the problems and assists the nurse in identifying educational deficits and other needs.

The nurse gathers the sexual history and explores sexual problem areas through the interview process. The nurse must maintain a relaxed, but respectful, matter-of-fact attitude through this interview. Data gathering should progress gradually from easier, more comfortable material to more difficult material by means of focused and open-ended questions. When introducing potentially uncomfortable material, the nurse should first make an accepting statement that assumes the client has has a full range of experience in this area. An example is "When did you start masturbating?" rather than "Do you masterbate?" Another example is, "Men sometimes are unable to have an erection even when they really want to have intercourse; what is that like for you?" rather than "Do you have difficulty achieving an erection sometimes?" Also be sure to use words familiar and comfortable to the client. For example, if the client uses the word lovemaking instead of intercourse, the nurse uses this word also (Box 12-7).[2]

The interview includes questions about when and how the client learned about sex, current attitudes about sex, how the current health problem influences his or her sexual attitudes or behavior, and questions about current sexual habits and functioning. The interview also should gather information about self-image, body image, and sexual image. These refer to the client's feelings and thoughts about his or her body, the self in general, gender identity, sexual object choice, and sexual behavior and attitudes. Other areas to explore include history of sexual trauma, rape, or sexual abuse or harassment. It is also helpful to understand how the client's family of origin dealt with sexuality and nonsexual touching and affection. Is the client comfortable with nonsexual touch and friendly hugs? Especially important in the assessment is information about the client's current sexual relationship. Important areas for exploration include how needs are communicated, how satisfied the client is with the frequency and quality of the sexual relationship, and what the client assumes his or her partner's answers to these questions are. Box 12-8 gives an example of a therapeutic dialogue that assesses the client's sexual concerns.[2]

The nurse must include cultural data in the assessment process. Identifying religious and ethnic influ-

BOX 12-7

Discussing Sexuality With A Client

1. Sexual concerns are often not voiced by clients unless the nurse indicates this is an area she feels comfortable addressing. Therefore, asking clients if they have any concerns about their sexual relations with others is the nurse's responsibility.
2. All clients (men and women) should also be asked about unwanted sexual experiences. Between 20% to 25% of women in the United States will be raped during their lifetime. As many as 75% of women will experience some type of unwanted sexual experience during their lifetime. Estimates of rape of men are lower (10%–14%); however, this may be due to the fact that men are less likely to report sexual abuse or assault. Do not ask if a client has been raped. The use of the term "rape" is often limiting, suggesting to clients that you are only interested in past rape experiences. They may not reveal other unwanted sexual experiences that they do not consider to be rape. Every unwanted sexual experience has the potential to be injurious to the wellness of the survivor of that experience.
3. Present an open and accepting attitude whenever discussing sexual matters with the client. Many clients will not discuss these matters if they feel they are being judged negatively or fear that you will be embarrassed or uncomfortable by what they might say. If you are uncomfortable (eg, nervous, giggly, embarrassed) discussing sexual concerns, practice these discussions using hypothetical situations with peers or friends until you feel comfortable discussing sexual matters. Being able to help clients with their sexual concerns is a skill that every nurse should possess.
4. Discussion of sensitive matters, such as childhood sexual abuse, sexual dysfunction, or sexual assault, requires time and empathy from the nurse. This content will not emerge if the client feels rushed. Also, clients frequently express intense feelings related to their sexual experiences or concerns (eg, anxiety, sadness, shame, guilt, anger). The nurse has a role in supporting the expression of these feelings, validating them, and helping the client seek further assistance with these feelings if necessary.

ences on the client's perceptions of sexuality assists the nurse in understanding the client's responses and determining realistic treatment approaches. If the client has rejected his or her culture of origin and adopted another lifestyle or subculture, the culture of origin still may have a covert influence on behavior and responses. If the client's lifestyle is nontraditional, the nurse may suggest ways the client can respond to discrimination, either by controlling exposure in society or by locating a support group and alternative system of approval.

NURSING DIAGNOSIS

After gathering the assesment data most pertinent to the client's sexual problem or concern, the nurse formulates a nursing diagnosis. This second step of the nursing process involves synthesizing information about the client's sexual health, needs, problems, knowledge level, and satisfaction to help lead the nurse develop a more precise plan of care. Possible nursing diagnoses include the following:

1. Sexual Dysfunction related to lack of sexual fulfillment, as evidenced by vaginismus
2. Altered Sexuality Patterns related to socially unacceptable sexual practices, as evidenced by exhibitionism
3. Rape-Trauma Syndrome related to fears associated with violence, as evidenced by panic in sexual encounters
4. Sexual Dysfunction related to knowledge deficit about safer sex, as evidenced by unsafe sexual practices

PLANNING

Treatment approaches are planned following the data gathering and analysis processes. These approaches may be suggested by the nurse or other health care professionals, based on an understanding of the cultural and religious preferences that influence the client's sexuality and sexual activity. The nurse ascertains the client's acceptance of the suggested interventions and explains the process involved. In most situations, both sexual partners must accept and understand the therapy program. The couple, not one or the other partner, is the client in sex therapy. The client (ie, the couple) works with the nurse through the planning process.

INTERVENTION

The attitudes held by health care providers can make the occurrences of sexual problems more difficult or less difficult for the client and family to address and overcome. During the early recovery period, the nurse

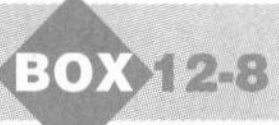

Therapeutic Dialogue

ASSESSING THE CLIENT'S SEXUAL CONCERNS

Client: I don't know what she likes. She said last week that our sex life was no good; what am I doing wrong?

Therapist: Well, maybe nothing. We'll see. Did you have an argument last week?

Client: Yeah. She said she's tired of me going out with my friends every Friday night and she thinks I drink too much.

Therapist: Is she usually critical of your habits like that?

Client: No. This is the first time she's ever criticized me. We've been married 3 years!

Therapist: Do you think you might drink too much sometimes?

Client: Well, yeah. But she never used to care.

Therapist: Maybe she's just now getting to a point that she has to say what she doesn't like. So, one thing is going out with friends every Friday night and one thing is drinking too much. So, what do you make of her comment about your sex life?

Client: I don't know. Unless it's that she doesn't like it when we have sex when I'm drinking.

Therapist: You think that might be it?

Client: Well, sometimes she acts that way.

Therapist: I think it's time the two of you really talked, maybe in here if not at home. And give each of you a chance to say what's bothering you.

Client: Okay. I guess you're right. I'll talk to her about coming in here.

Therapist: And one more thing. Do you ask her what she likes sexually?

Client: Well, no, I mean, she's always just liked it.

Therapist: Well, maybe it's time you both told the other what you like and what you want.

DISCUSSION

This couple is entering a new phase of intimacy in which each partner is more aware of his and her needs and wants. There has been a lack of communication in several areas, confused with the sexual issues, which requires exploration of each problem, open discussion, and assertiveness about each person's needs and wants.

or other staff member who works with the client who underwent injury or surgery resulting in a change in body function and image must convey an attitude of acceptance of the ostomy, the amputation stump, or the paralyzed limbs. Nurses must be sensitive to cues that a concern exists and support the client's attempts to discuss the problem or fear. The nurse must be aware of the sexul needs of the hospitalized client, the elderly client, and the client's sexual partners.

The nurse also must facilitate the family's understanding of the client's condition. This may be done by suggesting a family meeting, during which the nurse supports the client in talking with the family or sexual partner. The nurse may wish to suggest a private meeting between the client and the sexual partner or the family. The nurse helps the client prepare for such a meeting by talking about the problems that need to be discussed and perhaps by role playing a situation of talking with the family member about a sensitive topic. The nurse also may decide to talk with family members about changes and needs of the client, with the client's permission, to make future discussions easier for him or her. Clear communication is an essential element in the relationship between client and family or sexual partner.

Nurses often are uncomfortable with topics of sexuality and discuss such topics with clinical detachment. This may be harmful to the client struggling with the issue of how to continue as a sexual being while hospitalized or chronically ill. American society tends to consider physically and mentally ill people as asexual or to attribute their sexual activities to their illness states. This is detrimental to the self-image of the client. The nurse can facilitate a change by being comfortable with sexual topics, open to discussing concerns and answering questions, and respectful of client's sexual choices.[6,10]

The nurse's role in the intervention process is frequently one of clarifying communication.[11] The nurse encourages expression of feelings by both partners, eliciting feedback, separating thought and feeling, and helping the client learn other means of clear, open communication. The nurse often suggests activities for the couple to try to encourage the development of new sexual patterns. Often, the nurse acts as a teacher, clarifying vague information for the client and giving new information about sex positions or habits. The nurse might help a partner explore why he or she has some preference or fear based on historical or cultural information.

Nurses are effective in interventions if they are knowledgeable and sensitive to their own and the client's sexual attitudes and concerns and if they are comfortable with their own sexual choices and with discussing the client's choices. Many sexual issues can be resolved through effective nursing intervention and may not require formal sex therapy.[10]

Sex Therapy

Sex therapy is a particular approach to sex counseling practiced by masters-level clinicians with additional training in this therapeutic specialty. While the nurse generalist is in a position to assess the client's sexual concerns and is prepared to educate the client regarding normal sexual functioning, he or she is generally not prepared to provide sex therapy.

Sex therapy was first formalized by Masters and Johnson in the 1950s as an outgrowth of their research on human sexuality. Their model of treatment was based on the idea that most sexual dysfunctions were the result of lack of sexual knowledge and negative attitudes toward sexuality. The Masters and Johnson approach involves two therapists (a man and woman) who gather a comprehensive sexual history on the couple seeking treatment and then following a review of their sexual difficulties with the couple, provide sexual education and step-by-step instructions regarding sexual behavior. The Masters and Johnson model also provides supportive psychotherapy to the couple as necessary.[26]

One sexual exercise developed by Masters and Johnson is the *sensate focus* exercise in which the partners take turns instructing each other in specific ways of pleasuring each other without engaging in coitus. These exercises teach the couple many lessons, including increased comfort with their bodies and themselves and increased communication and cooperation with each other sexually.[26]

In the 1960s and 1970s, Helen Singer Kaplan developed her model for treatment of sexual disorders. Her model integrates psychodynamic behavioral principles into conjoint therapy. In addition to specific sexual homework, she makes use of psychodynamic insights, dream interpretations, and gestalt and transactional techniques. The Kaplan model uses only one therapist and tailors the sexual homework to the dynamics at work in the couple's relationship. Thus, a less assertive spouse may be instructed to act as the initiator of sexual activity and be given instructions to be more active during the couple's sexual encounters. The Kaplan model, like the Masters and Johnson model, emphasizes communication between the partners; however, it also focuses on exploration of the relationship and emotional concerns and then works with the relationship dynamics as they present in the sexual disorder of the couple.[20]

Today, sex therapy is offered using a variety of modalities; however, the principles of the Masters and Johnson and the Kaplan models are commonly used in many treatment programs. Sex therapy for couples involves carefully assessing a couple's sexual difficulties, then clarifying each member's perceptions of the other and of sexual activities in general. The therapist facilitates communication between the two partners and their acceptance of each other's feelings and attitudes.[2]

The approach of sex therapy is that sex is to be enjoyed and must not be viewed as an obligation of a relationship. The therapist may suggest certain exercises for the couple, most of which focus the couple on the sensual pleasures of touching and foreplay and deemphasize the demand aspects of sexual activity. One such exercise is a sense awareness activity during which the partners are not to attempt any activity to achieve orgasm but spend time relaxing and enjoying the physical closeness of the other. This exercise also encourages immediate involvement and discourages dissociation or the spectator role.

The couple may also be taught new coital positions or different sexual activities that may better suit the needs of both partners. Other types of exercise assist a partner to maintain more control during the sexual activity and to help him or her overcome fear or anxiety about sexual behavior. The *squeeze technique* is an exer-

Nursing Care Plan 12-1

The Client With A Sexual Dysfunction

Mr. C is a 25-year-old single man who was admitted to the inpatient psychiatric unit with a diagnosis of major depression. During her initial interview with Mr. C, the nurse learned that he had problems with premature ejaculation and had stopped dating because of his inability to control this problem. He expressed feelings of humiliation and embarrassment and of inadequacy as a man. He also related that approximately 1 year ago, his fiance had broken their engagement. He became tearful saying he still loves her but has "nothing to offer her."

Nursing Diagnosis

Self-esteem Disturbance: humiliation and inadequacy related to depression and feelings of sexual inadequacy

Outcome

Client will report increased self-esteem and self-confidence.

Intervention	Rationale
Encourage client to explore feelings about self and identify realistic strengths and resources	Exploration and discussion of issues promote a more realistic image of self.

Evaluation

Client's statements and behavior indicate an improved level of self-esteem.

Nursing Diagnosis

Ineffective Individual Coping and guilt related to unresolved grief

Outcome

Client reports decreased feelings of guilt associated with loss of the relationship.

Intervention	Rationale
Encourage expression of feelings, especially guilt, associated with loss of relationship	Engaging client in discussing loss conveys that these feelings are a normal part of the grieving process.
Explore with client his fears associated with loss	Exploring fears provides a means for identifying potential coping mechanisms

Evaluation

Client verbalizes feelings and fears associated with the loss and displays grieving behaviors.

Nursing Diagnosis

Impaired Social Interaction: cessation of dating related to depression, grief, and sexual dysfunction

Outcome

Client will work through feelings of depression, grief, and fear and resume dating behavior.

Intervention	Rationale
Encourage client to participate in activities with others	Participating in activities with others increases client's social interactions
Discuss with client the consequences of various behaviors exhibited in relationships	Discussing the events of social interaction helps client recognize the effects of interpersonal behavior and learn more satisfying ways to relate to others

Evaluation

Client interacts socially with others and resumes dating.

cise suggested to help a man delay ejaculation during coitus to promote a mutually more pleasurable experience for the couple. This technique involves the man's partner stimulating the penis to near-orgasm, then firmly squeezing the head of the penis with the thumb and two fingers until the man's urge to ejaculate has subsided. This may be done during coitus also, if a female partner is on top of the man and can remove the penis from the vagina when her partner informs her of his impending orgasmic inevitability.[32]

Sex therapy is composed of four general modes of treatment: simple counseling, couples therapy, individual therapy, and group therapy. Simple counseling is an ideal format for the nurse and may be done individually or with the couple or group. This includes education, specific suggestions (such as exercises or new positions), permission and reassurance, and facilitative communication. Couples therapy involves more in-depth exploration and intervention and is most often done by a sex therapist. This includes making "homework" assignments for exercises, then observing and responding to the couple's responses to the homework. Resentments and anxieties surface and are discussed during therapy. Obstacles to completion of assignments are observed and modified through the therapy process. Individual therapy proceeds in a similar manner but with increased focus on individual emotional blocks and self-exploration homework through the use of a mirror, masturbation, and relaxation and imagery exercises. Group therapy involves discussion of problems and concerns, homework for individual or couple exploration, and group support and reassurance.

EVALUATION

Nursing interventions are evaluated by follow-up sessions in which the nurse explores whether the client accepted or tried the suggested interventions. Evaluation also includes determining whether the suggested activities or positions were realistic for the client's situation. In some cases, the client may not want to change or may not be ready to try something new. The nurse assesses the client's progress and suggests new activities, if appropriate. The nurse may decide to refer the client to someone else (perhaps someone with a perspective more consistent with the client's) or to a clinician with more experience or greater training in sex therapy (see Nursing Care Plan 12-1, p. 194).

◆ Chapter Summary

This chapter has discussed the development of sexuality as an integral part of the personality. Some of the chapter's major points include the following:

1. The sexual nature of the personality affects the emotional, spiritual, and psychological natures of the self; indeed, they are not separate natures but integral parts of the personality, the self.
2. Sexual development is influenced by genetic and hormonal factors and by the development of gender identity.
3. The human sexual response cycle consists of three phases: desire, excitement, and orgasm.
4. Sexual expression, whether in traditional or alternative lifestyles, is a reflection of various intra- and extrapersonal factors, including cultural influences.
5. Clients who undergo injury or surgery resulting in a changed body image often suffer a blow to their sexual identity.
6. Nursing interventions with clients whose physical or mental disorders interfere with their sexual abilities include client and family teaching, support, and counseling.
7. Sex therapy may be the treatment of choice for certain common sexual problems: erectile dysfunction, rapid ejaculation, vaginismus, and orgasmic dysfunction.
8. Many different interventions, including behavioral, surgical, educational, and pharmacological methods, are used to treat paraphilias and gender identity disorders.
9. The steps of the nursing process are applied to clients with sexual problems.
10. Research in the areas of sexuality and sexual issues demonstrates the need for more information and openness when working with clients.

Critical Thinking Questions

1. *Why is the issue of sexuality an essential part of every nursing assessment?*
2. *How does your sexuality reflect your environment, family and spiritual values, and societal norms?*
3. *What would your sexuality be like if you belonged to a different cultural group or if you had a different sexual orientation? How would your sexuality have been influenced by these differences?*
4. *What are some of the potential sexual implications for the following health problems: hypertension, heart disease, menopause, chronic alcohol or drug abuse, diabetes, and depression?*
5. *Review the American Nurses Association's Standards of Nursing Care. What does this document say about addressing the client's sexual concerns? What does it say about the nurse's sexual behavior toward the client?*

Review Questions

1. Which of the following statements is not true?
   - **A.** Sex-related differences vary from person to person according to familial tendencies, physical makeup, and personality preferences.
   - **B.** Certain sex adjunctive differences may be linked to hormonal or genetic programming in our primate ancestors.
   - **C.** Sex arbitrary differences are determined by culture, not for any biological reason.
   - **D.** Sexuality is not a part of every relationship.
2. Which of the following statements is true about the XYY chromosomal pattern?
   - **A.** The XYY chromosomal pattern is called Klein-felter's syndrome.
   - **B.** Men with this chromosomal pattern have a predisposition to commit crimes.
   - **C.** The XYY chromosomal pattern predisposes the individual to passivity, lack of ambition, and sudden outbursts of aggression.
   - **D.** The XYY chromosomal pattern is called Turner's syndrome.
3. Cultural influences are inextricably bound with sexual expression. Which one of the following statements is not true?
   - **A.** Cultural groupings include the culture of the family of origin and the culture of one's spirituality or chosen profession or occupation.
   - **B.** The nurse should be aware of his or her own cultural influences, beliefs, and values to avoid imposing them on the client.
   - **C.** Sexuality is expressed in the same way across cultures.
   - **D.** The nurse should be responsive to the client's sexual concerns and be willing to learn about the client's sexuality.
4. The origin of sexual orientation preference in human beings is not well understood. Which of the following statements regarding sexual orientation is not true?
   - **A.** Research suggests that biological, genetic, social, and environmental factors play a role in the development of sexual orientation.
   - **B.** Most sexual orientation research has been done on lesbians.
   - **C.** There really is no such thing as a typical gay or lesbian person.
   - **D.** Nursing assessment of a gay or lesbian client should include a discussion of pertinent life-style issues and stresses.
5. Describe a comprehensive sexual assessment of the client.
6. Describe how drugs may be used to treat certain sexual dysfunctions or paraphilic disorders.
7. What are the basic principles of sex therapy for couples?

◆ References

1. Abramson PK: Parental Attitudes About Sexual Education—Cross Cultural Differences and Covariate Controls. Arch Sex Behav 12 (5): 381–397, 1983
2. Andrews S: Coping With the Sexaul Health Interview. J Nurs Midwifery 33 (6): 269–273, 1988
3. Bell N: Sexuality: Promoting Fulfillment. Nursing Times 58 (6): 35–37, 1989
4. Bradford JM, Pawlak A: Double-Blind Placebo Crossover Study of Cyproterone Acetate in the Treatment of the Paraphilias. Arch Sex Behav 22 (5): 383–402, 1993
5. Brown SV: Premarital Sexual Permissiveness Among Black Asolescent Females. Soc Psychol Q 48 (4): 381–387, 1985
6. Brown Y, Calder B, Rae D: Female Circumcision. Canadian Nurse 85 (4): 19–22, 1989
7. Cullen K, Travin S: Assessment and Treatment of Spanish-Speaking Sex Offenders: Special Considerations. Psychiatr Q 61 (4): 223–236, 1990
8. American Psychiatric Association: Diagnostic and Statistical Manual of Mental Disorders, 4th ed. Washington, DC, 1994
9. Durchame S, Gill KM: Sexual Values, Training, and Professional Roles. J Head Trauma Rehab 5 (2): 38–45, 1990
10. Ford K, Norris A: Methodological Considerations for Survey Research on Sexual Beahvior: Urban African American and Hispanic Youth. J Sex Res 28 (4): 539–555, 1991
11. Frank D: Attributions About Sexual Experiences. Clin Nurs Spec 4 (1): 17–20, 1990
12. Fullilove MT, Fullilove RE, Haynes K, Gross S: Black Women and AIDS Prevention: A View Towards Understanding the Gender Rules. J Sex Res 27 (1): 47–64, 1990
13. Gibson JW, Kempf J: Attitudinal Predictors of Sexual Activity in Hispanic Adolescent Females. J Adol Res 5 (4): 414–430, 1990
14. Greydanus DE: Adolescent Sexuality and Gynecology. Philadelphia, Lea & Febiger, 1990
15. Hoskins CN: Activation: A Predictor of Need Fullfillment in Couples. Res Nurs Health 12 (6): 365–372, 1989
16. Jacobs P, Bobek SC: Sexual Needs of the Schizophrenic Client. Perspect Psychiatr Care 27 (1): 15–20, 1991
17. Kafka MP: Sertraline Pharmacotherapy for Paraphilias and Paraphilia-Related Disorders: An Open Trial. Annals Clin Psych 6 (3): 189–195, 1994
18. Kafka MP, Prentky R: Flouxetine Treatment of Non-paraphilic Sexual Addictions and Paraphilias in Men. J Clin Psychiatry 53 (10): 351–358, 1992
19. Kaplan HI, Sadock BJ (eds): Comprehensive Textbook of Psychiatry/V. Baltimore, Williams & Wilkins, 1989
20. Kaplan HS: Disorders of Sexual Desire and Other New Concepts and Techniques in Sex Therapy. New York, Simon & Schuster, 1979
21. Katzin L: Chronic Illness and Sexuality. Am J Nurs 90 (1): 55–59, 1990

22. Laumann EO, Gagnon, JH, Michael RT, Michaels S: The Social Organization of Sexuality: Sexual Practices in the United States. Chicago, University of Chicago Press, 1994
23. Lefley HP, Scott CS, Llabre MH, Hicks D: Cultural Beliefs About Rape and Victims Response in Three Ethnic Groups. Am J Orthopsychiatry 63 (4): 623–632, 1993
24. McKenzie F: Sexuality After Total Pelvic Externation. Nursing Times 84 (20): 27–30, 1988
25. Manley G: Treatment and Recovery For Sexual Addicts. Nurs Pract 16 (6): 34–41, 1990
26. Masters WH, Johnson VE: Human Sexual Inadequacy. Boston, Little Brown, & Co, 1970
27. Medler T, Medler J: Nursing Management of Sexuality Issues. J Head Trauma Rehab 5 (2): 46–51, 1990
28. Meredith W, Rowe G: Changes in Lao Hmong Mental Attitudes After Immigrating to the United States. J Compar Fam Stud 17 (1): 117–125, 1986
29. Moran JR, Corley MD: Sources of Sexual Information and Sexual Attitudes and Behaviors of Anglo and Hispanic Adolescent Males. Adolescence 26 (104): 857–864, 1991
30. Ostrow DG, Whitaker RE, Frasier K, Cohen C: Racial Differences in Social Support and Mental Health in Men With HIV Infections: A Pilot Study. AIDS Care 3 (1): 55–62, 1991
31. Padilla AM, Baird TL: Mexican-American Adolescent Sexuality and Sexual Knowledge: An Exploratory Study. Hispanic Journal of Behavioral Sciences 13 (1): 95–104, 1991
32. Poorman S: Human Sexuality and the Nursing Process. Norwalk, CT, Appleton & Lange, 1988
33. Roo VVP, Roo VN: Sex Role Attitudes: A Comparison of Sex Race Groups. Sex Roles 12 (9): 939–953, 1985
34. Roo VVP, Roo VN: Sex Role attitudes Across Two Cultures: United States and India. Sex Roles 13 (11–12): 607–624, 1985
35. Schneider SG, Farkeraw NL, Kruks GN: Suicidal Behavior in Adolescent and Young Adult Men. Suicide and Life-Threatening Behavior 19 (4): 389–391, 1989
36. Smith GB: Nursing Care Challenges: Homosexual Psychiatric Patients. J Pschosoc Nurs 30 (12): 15–21, 1992
37. Thomas B: Asexual Patients. Nursing Times 85 (33): 49–50, 1989
38. Ucho LG: Culture and Violence: The Interaction of Africa and America. Sex Roles 31 (3–4): 185–204, 1994

Grief and Loss

Katherine T. Pritchett
Patricia M. Lucas

13

I walked a mile with Pleasure,
She chatted all the way,
But left me none the wiser
For all she had to say.
I walked a mile with Sorrow,
And ne'er a word said she,
But, oh, the things I learned from her
When Sorrow walked with me!

The Westminster Press, *Philadelphia, 1565*

Birth, loss, and death are unique experiences common to all individuals. Grief is one of the most universal human responses to loss. Nurses frequently encounter clients who are experiencing loss in a wide variety of settings. To intervene appropriately, the nurse must be able to recognize grief and understand the significance of loss.

This chapter discusses the theoretical viewpoints of grief and loss. The meaning of loss to the client, family, and health care provider is explored. The nursing process is used as the framework for assisting the nurse in assessing, planning, and implementing care for the client experiencing grief and loss.

Learning Objectives

On completion of this chapter, you should be able to accomplish the following:

1. *Discuss theoretical perspectives on grief and loss.*
2. *Describe grieving as it relates to special circumstances, such as death of a child and sudden death.*
3. *Discuss the meaning of loss to the client, client's family, and health care providers.*
4. *Apply the nursing process to a client and family who are experiencing grief and loss.*
5. *Formulate a comprehensive nursing care plan for the client and family experiencing grief and loss.*

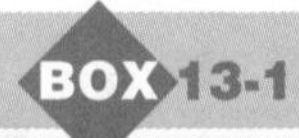

Somatic and Psychological Symptoms of Normal Grief

1. Somatic distress
   - Feeling of tightness in the throat
   - Choking sensation and shortness of breath
   - Sighing
   - Empty feeling in abdomen
   - Fatigue or lack of strength
   - Intense subjective distress described as tension or mental pain
2. Preoccupation with image of the deceased
   - Has a sense of unreality
   - Has a feeling of emotional distance
   - Imagines the presence of the deceased one
   - Believes these feelings indicate approaching insanity
3. Guilt feelings
   - Searches for evidence of negligence for preventing the death
4. Hostile reactions
   - Loss of warmth in interactions with others
   - Tendency to respond with irritability and anger
   - Not wanting to be bothered by friends and relatives
5. Loss of usual patterns of conduct
   - Restlessness
   - Continually searching for something to do
   - Inability to initiate and maintain organized patterns of activity

(Modified from Lindemann E: Symptomatology and Management of Acute Grief. Am J of Psychiatry 101: 141–143, 1944.)

◆ Perspectives on Grief and Loss

THEORETICAL VIEWPOINTS: GRIEVING PROCESS

Grief is a universal response to a loss encountered by all ages and cultures. The concept of grief was first explored by Freud in 1917. He described the normal emotion of grief and its expression in mourning. Grief resolution as described by Freud is a painful process not easily completed.[14]

Lindemann (1944) saw grief as a natural response to loss and described common characteristics of acute grief that occur within 6 to 8 weeks following a loss. He used the term *grief work* to describe steps taken toward grief resolution.[28] These symptoms are listed in Box 13-1.

In 1969, Elisabeth Kübler-Ross presented a framework for understanding the process of dying. Her extensive case study investigations with the terminally ill, their families, and professional staff have profoundly affected how society views death and dying.

Kübler-Ross identified five stages of dying experienced by clients and loved ones:

1. *Denial*—"No, not me." Denial is a necessary mechanism to protect the person from the impact of awareness of inevitable death.
2. *Anger*—"Why me?" The initial stage of denial is followed by felt and expressed anger. The dying person's anger is directed at self, God, and others.
3. *Bargaining*—"Yes, me, but . . ." The anticipation of the losses through death brings about a time of bargaining. Through this bargaining, the person attempts to postpone or reverse death. The client may pray for more time to complete important goals in life. During this time, promises are made to alter lifestyle, go to church more often, or give to charity; the client usually promises something in exchange for life.
4. *Depression*—"Yes, me." When the full effect of the diagnosis is felt, and the loss can no longer be delayed, the client moves into the stage of depression.

This depression is a therapeutic state that aids the client to detach from life and living and thereby accept death. The depression involved in death and dying is different from the pathological depression seen in the process of life. Pathological depression must be treated and its cause determined; in the process of dying, depression is a necessary stage of growth rather than a regression.

5. *Acceptance*—"My time is very close now, and it's all right." This stage occurs when the bereaved person comprehends the reality of the ensuing loss and feels at peace about the outcome.

In her research, Kübler-Ross found that not all individuals sequentially progress through the five stages, nor does everyone experience all five stages.[24,25]

Important insights into the process of dying were noted in Glaser and Strauss's long-term sociological study of dying. They postulated that dying clients and their families, friends, and professional staff may be at different levels of awareness of the dying process. The levels include the following:

1. *Closed awareness,* or "keeping the secret," when clients are not aware that they are dying but the family and professional staff are
2. *Suspicion awareness,* involving a suspicion that death may occur but without sufficient information to verify it
3. *Mutual pretense awareness,* in which all people involved in the situation are aware of the active dying process but maintain a ritual of pretense
4. *Open awareness,* when all involved in the situation are aware of the active dying process and demonstrate their awareness in actions, communication, and taking care of unfinished business[13]

Colin Murray Parkes, in his classic research with widows and widowers, has identified four phases of the grief process:

1. *Shock and disbelief.* The numbness that occurs in this first stage protects the bereaved from overwhelming pain. Only specific details can be recalled concerning spontaneous decisions.
2. *Expressions of the emotions of grief.* After the numbness subsides, the bereaved person experiences intense yearning and loneliness for the deceased. Symptoms of acute grief are also present, along with feelings of guilt and anger.
3. *Disorganization.* Emptiness, apathy, and depression occur during this stage of mourning.
4. *Recovery.* Recovery from the loss is a gradual process in which the survivors attach meaning to the loss and begin to develop new relationships. The pain of the loss is never completely gone; the memory of the deceased is not erased, but a readjustment to life is made.[14]

Engel (1964) integrated the theories of grief and grieving with practical nursing applications.[9,11] Benoliel, a frequently cited nurse-author on the concept of grief, describes grief as a total human response to the loss of a significant relationship. The grieving individual must incorporate the changes created by loss into a new definition of reality.[5]

Recent research findings have described grief as a pervasive, highly individualized dynamic process with a strong normative component. This contemporary view of the grief concept as dynamic removes the rigid phases or stages of the classic grief process.[9,22] The limits of normal grieving behaviors are defined by social and cultural parameters.[29] When grief work has been successfully accomplished, two primary outcomes are evident: 1) the establishment of a new reality and 2) the development of a new identity.[9]

BEREAVEMENT

There is much ambiguity relating to the definitions of bereavement, mourning, and grief. Some authors use the terms interchangeably.[20] Other authors note distinctions in the terms. *Bereavement* is the feelings, thoughts, and responses that occur following a loss. *Mourning* is the process of detachment from the loss. It involves the grief work necessary for resolution.

Some grieving individuals have symptoms characteristic of a major depressive episode (ie, feelings of sadness, insomnia, poor appetite, weight loss).[1] The normalcy of these symptoms varies from one culture to another. Symptoms not characteristic of a normal grief reaction differentiate bereavement from a major depressive episode. The Diagnostic and Statistical Manual of Mental Disorders, fourth edition, lists these symptoms as follows:

1. Guilt about things other than actions taken or not taken by the survivor at the time of death
2. Thoughts of death other than the survivor feeling that he or she would be better off dead or should have died with the deceased person
3. Morbid preoccupation with worthlessness
4. Marked psychomotor retardation
5. Prolonged and marked functional impairment
6. Hallucinatory experiences other than thinking that he or she hears the voice of, or transiently sees the image of, the deceased person[1]

◆ Grieving and Special Circumstances

DEATH OF A CHILD

The death of a child, regardless of age, is one of the most traumatic losses a parent can experience. The loss is unique due to the complex issues involved in the parent–child relationship. The parent must deal with the loss of self in addition to the loss of the child. The child's death robs the hopes, dreams, and expectations for the future that the parent has invested in the child.[6,35]

In viewing the family's grief following the death of a child, attention must be given to the grieving siblings. Although children demonstrate grief differently than do adults, their grief work is similar. Children may have somatic complaints and exhibit behavioral acting out as a response to their sadness and fears about death. These behaviors and complaints may also be an effort to illicit the attention their grieving parents are unable to give. Children may find it difficult to live up to the parent's idealized image of the deceased child. The death of a child may also cause a conflict in the marriage relationship. Couples often grieve differently, and these differences bring discord to their relationship.[31]

Perinatal loss, whether by miscarriage, stillbirth, or death in the neonatal period, is a great tragedy for the parents. Pregnancy is viewed as an emotional crisis because of the major changes that occur in physical and psychological equilibrium. The crisis of pregnancy is normally resolved in the birth of the child. A pregnancy that results in a perinatal loss creates an additional crisis. A bereaved mother must resolve the crisis of perinatal loss in addition to the crisis of pregnancy.

Perinatal death is a narcissistic loss for the mother. Such a loss can be described as losing part of oneself, which can be more difficult to mourn than the loss of a separate person. The mother identifies with the growing fetus throughout the pregnancy. Thus, the mother perceives perinatal death as a threat to her own developing maternal self-worth. During the pregnancy, a woman fantasizes about the personality traits and particular characteristics of her child-to-be. The loss of the fetus means the end of a real life and a fantasy. The fantasies of the child-to-be make the loss of the real child even greater. According to Leon, "what has been lost is not a child one did not know so much as fantasies of one who will never be."[27]

To appreciate the depth of the perinatal grief response, one must understand the concepts of attachment and detachment during the mourning process. Klaus and Kennell describe the attachment process as a series of steps through which parents progress during pregnancy and birth: planning, confirming, and accepting the pregnancy; feeling fetal movement and accepting the fetus as an individual; giving birth; and hearing, seeing, touching, holding, and caring for the newborn. Many of the steps occur before the birth. Because bonding has already begun, parents can experience an acute grief reaction at birth. The concept of detachment is also an important part of the mourning process. This phase of the process involves "letting go."[3,23]

The expression of grief and the process of mourning following the death of an infant are similar to the normal grief stages identified by Kübler-Ross.[24] Searching and yearning and disorientation have been added as specific to stages of perinatal grieving.[7,26]

SUDDEN DEATH

Much work has been done with the survivors of victims of sudden or unexpected deaths. Sudden death produces greater emotional turmoil and shock in survivors than does a gradual, expected death. Survivors do not have time to engage in anticipatory grief. The most disturbing and unbalancing feature of a sudden death is its unexpectedness.

Many times interpersonal circumstances at the time of death, such as emotional stress, anger, or hurt, may evoke severe guilt feelings in the survivors. Immediate reactions are usually severe and include disbelief, guilt, fear, remorse, and despair. Many families feel guilt for not having been able to do something special or extra for the deceased. For example, families who experience the sudden death of a child may have recurring memories of the death experience and may grieve forever over the missed options or developmental achievements that would have occurred.[22]

◆ Meaning of Loss to the Client

The dying person is faced not only with physical and social losses from the disease itself but with the ultimate loss of personal existence.[4] It is almost impossible to be truly prepared for death, because we cannot imagine ourself as nonexistent. Although fear of death is a part of the human experience, we often find that older people seem less fearful than younger people, and consequently they are more often concerned about the deaths of loved ones, friends, and pets. A person with a lengthy terminal illness may even welcome death as a release from pain. A client's religious belief or philosophical orientation may alter acceptance of death and the dying process. The acceptance of death as an inevitable and individual process may begin early in life for one person, whereas for another, this realization may not be reached until the physical signs and deterioration of aging are experienced. Some people attempt to deny death to the very end of their lives.

A dying person may have fears related to the loneliness and isolation they may feel in the institutional setting. The client's isolation is potentiated by such nonverbal gestures as dimming lights and drawing blinds and verbal gestures of whispering and giving stereotypical answers to the client's questions. Despite increasing public and professional attention to the subject of death and dying, dying still remains a lonely and isolated event in which the client often feels "dehumanized, impersonalized, and mechanized"[24] (Box 13-2).

To understand the meaning of loss to the dying client, spiritual needs should be considered. Included in these needs are 1) a search for meaning, 2) a need for love and hope, and 3) a sense of forgiveness. The dying person must feel that his or her life and approaching death have purpose and meaning. In reviewing their life, the dying person must have a sense of forgiveness for guilt experienced from unmet self-expectations. The dying person needs to feel unconditional love from all those around him or her—family, friends, and professional caregivers—even when the person is unresponsive to the love offered. Hope is an integral part of human existence. "If a patient stops expressing hope, it is usually a sign of imminent death."[24] Hope fluctuates throughout the dying process because the perception of reality changes as life changes.[8,10] The process of dying places the client in a dependent position called the "sick role." By accepting the sick role, clients lose control over the environment, decision making, and familiar and secure social roles. These losses and the change in role expectations place clients in a vulnerable position, and may make them feel at the mercy of the professional staff. Previously determined advanced directives assure the client that his or her wishes will be protected (Box 13-3).

Hospice provides an alternative treatment plan for the adult or pediatric client with a life-limiting medical problem. The services are often directed by the client's own personal physician and provided through a hospice

BOX 13-2

Therapeutic Dialogue: Living With a Terminal Illness

Dave is a 16-year-old diagnosed with terminal bone cancer. In the last year, he has undergone two surgeries and chemotherapy. This interview took place at a recreational center where Dave spends time with his friends. Dave was expecting the interviewer and was aware of the topic of the interview.

Nurse: Hi, Dave. I'm Dr. M.

Client: Yeah, hi. I've been expecting you. Let's go sit under the tree by the courts.

Nurse: You look like you're having fun.

Client: Yep, it's about time. I was letting myself die too long until I finally got a little smarts and I said to myself, this death thing you've been just going down, down. You've got to LIVE! You know you can make the decision to die, like my doctor said, just give up, lay there and finally die.

Nurse: Did that happen to you?

Client: Oh yeah, for a long time all I did was stay in bed in my room . . . didn't do a thing.

Nurse: Just stayed alone. Did you experience anger?

Dave: Yep, when I was laying there I used to think over and over again, why me, why me . . . why did I get picked out for cancer? It seemed like I just finally said to myself, "Dave, you're just gonna have to die or live—not live just like I was—you're gonna have to really LIVE!! I just can't do everything I used to do before. So I went back to my regular school and did most of what I used to. Most of my friends knew I was going to die—and it was hard—nobody would say anything at first and they didn't invite me to do all the things we used to. But it got better—I guess they just forgot about me dying.

Nurse: That was difficult.

Client: Yep, for a while it made me more scared, but now it's okay.

Nurse: You might have to have more surgery.

Client: That's what they wanted, but after my last surgery when I finally woke up, I said to myself, "No way am I ever going to go back for any more. My mom said that I had the choice, and I don't want to go through all that pain any more for nothing. I know that they can't cure it, and that's okay. It hurts my mom, but she understands.

DISCUSSION

One of the greatest stressors experienced by the dying client is the isolation from family and friends. Sometimes this occurs when significant others avoid conversations dealing with the client's feelings about illness and impending death. Nurses and other health care professionals can fill this need for openness and truthfulness by accepting the client's expressions. The nurse listens to, acknowledges, and refrains from making judgments about these expressions.

The person with a terminal illness faces multiple real losses. Interpersonal or social support should not have to be one of these losses when health care providers intervene therapeutically.

BOX 13-3

Texas Directive

Directive made this ________ day of ________, 19____.
I, ______________, being of sound mind, willfully and voluntarily make known my desire that my life shall not be artificially prolonged under the circumstances set forth in this directive.

1. If at any time I should have an incurable or irreversible condition caused by injury, disease, or illness certified to be a terminal condition by two physicians, and if the application of life-sustaining procedures would serve only to artificially postpone the moment of my death, and if my attending physician determines that my death is imminent or will result within a relatively short time without the application of life-sustaining procedures, I direct that those procedures be withheld or withdrawn, and that I be permitted to die naturally.
2. In the absence of my ability to give directions regarding the use of those life-sustaining procedures, it is my intention that this directive be honored by my family and physicians as the final expression of my legal right to refuse medical or surgical treatment and accept the consequences of that refusal.
3. If I have been diagnosed as pregnant and that diagnosis is known to my physician, this directive has no effect during my pregnancy.
4. This directive is in effect until it is revoked.
5. I understand the full import of this directive, and I am emotionally and mentally competent to make this directive.
6. I understand that I may revoke this directive at any time.

____

DECLARANT

I am not related to the declarant by blood or marriage. I would not be entitled to any portion of the declarant's estate on the declarant's death. I am not the attending physician of the declarant or an employee of the attending physician. I am not a patient in the health care facility in which the declarant is a patient. I have no claim against any portion of the declarant's estate on the declarant's death. Furthermore, if I am an employee of a health care facility in which the declarant is a patient, I am not involved in providing direct patient care to the declarant and am not directly involved in the financial affairs of the health care facility.

____

WITNESS — Print Name

____

Address and Telephone Number

____

WITNESS — Print Name

____

Address and Telephone Number

This directive complies with the Natural Death Act, Tex. Stat. Ann. Ch.672 (1977, amend. 1989).

care system. Medicaid, Medicare, and most private insurance payers will cover services rendered through a hospice plan. The type and extent of the service are monitored by these agencies.

The client and family benefit from the multidisciplinary approach of the hospice program. The purpose of these programs is to improve the quality of life for clients and to assist them in dealing with the significance of a life-limiting illness. When the focus of treatment changes from cure to palliative, the services of a hospice program can help make a client's life as comfortable and fulfilling as is possible. This palliative treatment concentrates on comfort and quality of life, not on cure.

The hospice program can be used by clients who want to stay at home and benefit from services provided to them by hospice caregivers. The client whose care is provided within a nursing home may also use the services of a hospice program. An inpatient facility is associated with most hospice programs designed to treat acute problems and return the client to his or her home setting. Examples of services that may be available to the client or family through a hospice program include medications; equipment; supplies; nursing care; personal care with bathing, dressing, and feeding; housekeeping assistance; emotional counseling; chaplain support; social work support; bereavement counseling; financial counseling; physical therapy; physician support; and volunteer support.

◆ Meaning of Loss to Family Members and Loved Ones

THE EXPERIENCE OF LOSS

The loss of a loved one is experienced not only through death, but also through lengthy illness, divorce, and separation. Each new loss requires adjustment to the specific life circumstance. All losses, including the loss of a loved one through death, involve a loss of part of the self; therefore, the experience is unique for each person. A family's adaptation to a terminal illness is affected by ethnicity and religious beliefs. The experience of terminal illness may also make demands of social and financial resources requiring major lifestyle changes.[4] Communication difficulties may arise within the family. Conspiracy of silence occurs when no one is willing to discuss the family member's impending death.[18]

The loss of a sibling is a traumatic event in the life of a child. Children tend to manifest grief through various emotions, somatic symptoms, and acting-out behavior.[18] Common problems frequently experienced by bereaved children include school difficulties, physical symptoms, health fears, and sleep disturbances. Studies further denote that grieving siblings demonstrate more behavior problems than the normal population. The most frequent behavior observed in grieving children centered on their demands for attention. A recent study on grief behaviors in bereaved siblings suggests that girls demonstrate more internalizing depressive behaviors, whereas boys' behaviors were of the hyperactive, externalizing type.[30]

The age and developmental level of a child delineate their grief response. Children younger than 2 years can understand the concept of separation but not death. Between 2 and 5 years, the child views death as a temporary rather than real event. Children between 6 and 10 years begin to understand the reality of death. By adolescence, the child's concept of death compares to that of an adult.[31] Investigators note that youth begin to use religion as an important means of coping.[2] The teenager impacted by a sibling's death must incorporate this traumatic loss into normal developmental losses of adolescence.[15] Health professionals working with the bereaved adolescent must consider the complex family dynamics inherent in the mourning process.[19]

ANTICIPATORY GRIEF

According to Lindemann, anticipatory grief is the progression through the phases of grief prior to the death of a loved one. This process may be beneficial to the mourner by buffering the impact of sudden death, but the process could be adversely affected if the anticipatory grief was done too effectively, and the death did not occur.[28] Rando (1986) proposed that anticipatory grief is not simply postdeath grief begun early. The anticipatory grieving done prior to the death cannot be merely deducted from the total grief work necessary for resolution. Within anticipatory grieving, there is a delicate balance among the conflicting demands of holding onto, letting go of, and drawing closer to the dying client.[41] Although anticipatory grief work may be a positive experience in the adjustment of the survivors by allowing them gradually to let go of their loved one, it may be difficult for the dying person to cope with the loss of emotional support by their family.

Another issue of anticipatory grief occurs when the loved one's actual death and funeral are confronted. Historically, funeral rites have functioned as ceremonies to provide emotional support to the survivors and to strengthen familial, friendship, and community bonds. When anticipatory grief has helped the survivors separate from the dying client, their expected mourning behaviors are minimized. They may be criticized for this less intense grief response.

THE MOURNING PROCESS

Dying people and their families may move through the stages of dying identified by Kübler-Ross—denial, anger, bargaining, depression, and acceptance—although not necessarily at the same time or at the same pace. Successful mourning brings comfort when the family or friends attain a sense of peace or acceptance with the death. To grieve is to allow expression of the sorrow and other feelings but not to use these feelings as an excuse to avoid the gift of life that the mourners still possess.

In the process of grieving, the deep feelings of ambivalence—love, anger, and guilt toward the lost loved one—are the emotions seen in major depression. Although these emotions of the grieving person are, in varying degrees, identical to those of major depressions, they differ in origin and process. The grief process is healthy, necessary, and growth producing, whereas major depressions are personality structure-oriented and growth-blocking processes.

The length of the grieving reaction and the final adjustment made to a new social environment depend on the success of what is called the *grief work,* that is, freedom from the bondage of the deceased, reorientation to the environment in which the deceased is no longer present, and establishment of new relationships. Some people resist accepting the discomfort and distress of mourning. They may choose to avoid the intense pain connected with the grief experience and expression of the feelings associated with grieving. The avoidance or disruption of normal grieving may be the prelude to a morbid grief reaction. This morbid reaction may be reflected in physiological and behavioral responses, ranging from psychosomatic conditions, such as asthma, ulcerative colitis, and rheumatoid arthritis, to antisocial behavior and even psychosis.[28]

When dealing with a bereaved person, certain factors can aid in understanding and predicting reactions and facilitating the helping relationship. The factors can be grouped to include the following:

1. Type of relationship lost
2. Nature of the death
3. Characteristics of the survivor
4. Social and cultural milieu
5. Nature of the support group[29]

◆ Meaning of Loss to Health Care Professionals

To care effectively for dying clients, the health care professional must accept and recognize his or her own mortality and examine the personal meaning of death. Even when these steps have been accomplished, death is still difficult to view, and the accompanying feelings are painful.

A recent research study was done to determine methods nurses use to assist them in their grief work. From the results, it was noted that the informal network of peer group support was most important in helping nurses grieve effectively. The nurses also indicated that a formal support group, in addition to increased grief resolution training, would be helpful.[39] The stress related to prolonged contact with the dying client or family should be a focus during the actual time of care and after death.[18] Collegial and supporting relationships among health care providers are important to the provision of emotional and physical care for the terminally ill client and family.[4]

Nurses also profit from using stress-reducing strategies. Examples of such strategies include maintaining good health habits, regular exercise, and diversional activities. Another technique that some nurses have found helpful in reducing stress and resolving grief is the concept of shared ritual experiences.[17] These caregivers must learn to focus on the positive aspects of their unique roles. Remembering the positive responses from families can increase self-esteem and job satisfaction. Hospice nurses use a care, rather than cure, framework to achieve satisfaction in their work.[40] The use of a scrapbook of letters to clients who have died in which the caregiver shares thoughts and feelings relating to the significance of the client's life is another way of preserving memories and facilitating grief resolution.[31]

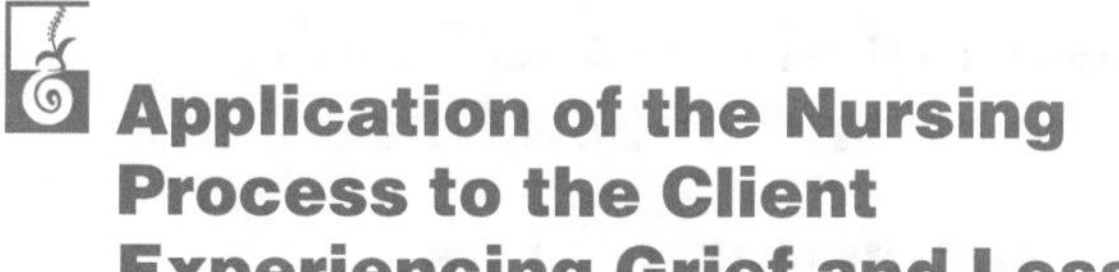

Application of the Nursing Process to the Client Experiencing Grief and Loss

ASSESSMENT

Assessment of the Dying Client and Family

Effective nursing care of clients and family experiencing grief and loss requires an ongoing collection of data oriented toward understanding the strengths and limitations of the dying person and his or her family. Key assessment areas include the following:

- Client and family goals and expectations
- Client and family awareness of terminal diagnosis
- Stage of death and dying
- Availability of support systems for client and family
- Client perception of unfinished business that needs to be completed
- Referral needs for financial, emotional, or legal problems
- Coping skills of client and family

- Perceptions of client and family relationships with health care providers
- High-risk family members prone to adaptation problems during and following illness (eg, children)[4]

Assessment of the Client With a Perinatal Loss

After a perinatal loss, grief expressions typically follow the stages of grief and mourning identified by Lindemann and Kübler-Ross.[24,28] During the period of disbelief and denial, parents have difficulty concentrating and making decisions. Mood swings and emotional turmoil also may be observed. Common somatic manifestations include dizziness, pallor, perspiration, palpitations, and aching arms.[38]

As the reality of the perinatal death is felt, behaviors of the next phase begin to appear. Anger and guilt predominate among the feelings of confusion, anxiety, and sadness. Authors have referred to this phase as a period of *yearning and searching.* In the phase of *disorientation* occurring several months after the loss, disorganization, despair, and depression can be noted. Feelings of loneliness and emptiness intensify, and there is a preoccupation with the deceased infant.[26] During the acceptance or resolution phase, the preoccupation with the loss begins to subside, and reorganization of life begins. Lindemann believed that the normal acute grief response would be resolved within 4 to 6 weeks. Current belief is that the normal acute grief response may take up to 12 weeks, with resolution of grief extending over 1 to 2 years.

Pathological grief may manifest itself in several possible ways. There may be an absence of grief or a delay in reaction to loss in the first 2 weeks. A prolonged or a distorted grief reaction may also signal pathological bereavement. Other possible indicators may be anxiety symptoms, unrealistic idealization of the fetus, and a desire to have a replacement child.

The following risk factors have been linked to increased incidence of pathological grieving:

1. A reported crisis during the pregnancy (eg, death of a loved one, marital conflict)
2. Perceived or experienced lack of emotional support from husband or family
3. Seeing but not holding the baby
4. Conception of another pregnancy within 5 to 6 months of the perinatal death
5. A surviving twin
6. History of emotional disorders (eg, depressive reaction)
7. Intense ambivalent feelings about the pregnancy
8. Strong cultural view of the mothering role[16,26]

The nurse also needs to be aware of individual differences in the process of grieving among mother, father, siblings, and other family members. Fathers follow the same grief response as do mothers; however, a man may feel a need to be strong for the sake of his wife and not add to her grief. Fathers may feel angry and cheated at the loss of the father role. The difference between the mother's and father's progress through the stages of grief may be related to the mother's prenatal emotional attachment to the baby. This difference has been termed *incongruent grieving.*[33] Confusion and resentment may result if partners equate the length of time spent grieving to the intensity of the loss. Siblings may experience guilt feelings about the death of a new baby—especially young children, who may have perceived the pregnancy as a rival. It is not uncommon for young children to wish for a new baby to go away. Thus, they may feel responsible for the death of the new baby. Young children's distorted concepts of illness and death may cause them to have fears related to the possible death of their parents.[31,38] Grandparents may also feel the intensity of grief and mourning of the perinatal loss. They grieve for the grandchild they will never have and for the suffering that their own child is experiencing.

NURSING DIAGNOSIS

When caring for a client and family experiencing grief and loss, the nurse analyzes assessment data gathered to determine actual and potential problems and formulates appropriate nursing diagnoses. Examples of nursing diagnoses for the grieving client and family follow:

1. Anticipatory Grieving related to
   - Perceived potential loss of significant other
   - Perceived sense of loss accompanying fetal or neonatal death or birth of a newborn with a defect or disorder
2. Dysfunctional Grieving related to
   - Absence of anticipatory grief
   - Chronic terminal illness
   - Lack of resolution of previous grieving response
3. Self Esteem Disturbance related to the grieving process
4. Spiritual Distress (distress of the human spirit) related to
   - Separation from religious and cultural affiliation
   - Perinatal loss and grieving process
5. Social Isolation related to
   - Inadequate personal resources
   - Withdrawal following death of an infant or child
6. Anxiety related to
   - Failing or deteriorating physiological condition
   - Knowledge deficit about perinatal loss
   - Diagnosis, tests, therapies, and prognosis

PLANNING

Grieving is the natural response to loss. Inherent in goal setting for a client and family experiencing grief and loss is the promotion and protection of individual self-esteem and self-worth throughout all the phases of the mourning process. Also significant in planning are goals to assist the client and family to resolve grief, accept the reality of the loss, and resume normal activities and relationships. Physiological needs of the client and family experiencing grief and loss must also be met. In goal planning with bereaved individuals, it is important to keep in mind that their preoccupation with thoughts of the deceased may interfere with their participation and understanding. A thorough plan of care involves collaboration with members of the multidisciplinary team, family members, significant others, and community resources (Case Studies 13-1 and 13-2).

INTERVENTION

Caregivers must initiate intervention strategies for the client and family experiencing grief and loss. Interventions should be designed to help the client and family cope with the immediate significance of loss, facilitate the process of detachment, and help make this experience an opportunity for growth (Nursing Care Plan 13-1).

Facilitating Understanding of the Mourning Process

The client and family experiencing grief and loss need to be made aware of the normal process involved in the stages of grief. Initially, people have difficulty determining their own needs and lack the initiative or energy to search out the needed helping service. After the initial loss, mourners experience loneliness and a need to speak about the deceased. Those who have experienced anticipatory grief appear to have less severe grief reactions.

In addition, professionals must recognize the typical behaviors seen in a healthy response to the death of a significant other. Grief may be manifested in tears, overwhelming feelings of loss, desire to withdraw, imagined guilt about omissions, and physical symptoms, such as anorexia, headache, and dizziness. Health care professionals must accept grief-related behaviors, which help survivors reorganize and resume productive, functional living. These behavioral expressions loosen the ties to the deceased and allow the survivors to form new ties. It is particularly helpful for survivors to understand that the emotions they are experiencing are common and that the deep hurting does come to an end.

The grieving process does not necessarily take place only after the death of a loved one. During a long illness, family members and significant others may actively move through the stages of mourning and may "let go." In this way, they accept the person's death before death actually occurs. Therefore, when death does occur, the survivors may express, through verbal and nonverbal behavior, a sense of relief and peaceful acceptance.

Perinatal loss presents a special challenge in mourning. Differences exist depending on the gestational age at the time of loss. For example, with a first-trimester miscarriage, the pregnant woman perceives the fetus as part of herself and thus mourns self-loss rather than loss of a separate being. The loss of the parent role must also be considered. In a stillbirth or early neonatal death, there often is a lack of anticipatory grieving; the suddenness of the loss precludes preparation for grieving. With the birth of a preterm infant or a baby with a congenital defect, parents must mourn the loss of their expected perfect child.[32] The grieving couple mourn not only the child that they have lost, but also the child that never will be. Interventions should assess the couple's progress through the mourning process and facilitate their understanding of this process. Information on grief response should include normal behaviors, common somatic discomforts, realistic expectations, and time parameters for grieving. The nurse needs to realize that even after perinatal death has been mourned and there is a return to normal living patterns, the mother or couple may continue to grieve on birth dates and other dates that signify hoped-for expectations of the lost child. If incongruent grieving occurs, the nurse needs to encourage open communication between family members.

Providing Information

Clients and family members want to be kept informed about what is happening. Without appropriate information, clients and families cannot take an active part in decisions regarding their care. The nurse's role in working with clients and families experiencing grief and loss is one of liaison between the client, family, physician, hospital, and community. The nurse also assumes the vital role of clarifier, explainer, and interpreter of symptoms, communications, agency rules, and expectations.

Communicating With Sensitivity

The nurse's role is of primary importance in creating a therapeutic environment in which the grieving client and family feel comfortable in expressing loss. Through verbal and nonverbal communication, the nurse can help bereaved individuals integrate the loss into their lives. Statements that acknowledge the loss (for example, "I'm so sorry about your loss; it must be so difficult

(text continues on page 212)

Case Study

The Client Who Has Experienced a Perinatal Loss

Joan N. Yanda, M.S.N., R.N., ACCE, Staff Nurse, Labor and Delivery, Columbia Medical Center, Plano, Texas; consultant, RTS Bereavement Services, La Crosse, Wisconsin.

Bob and Sue have been married 6 years. They met in high school and still live in the same town where they grew up. Bob is a policeman, and Sue is a receptionist. They have a 4-year-old son, Kevin. Sue is 38 weeks' gestation.

Sue calls her physician because she has not felt her baby move in 24 hours. Sue and Bob arrive in the labor and delivery department for a sonogram. There are no fetal heart tones. There is no fetal heartbeat on the sonogram. The doctor tells Bob and Sue that their baby has died. Bob is confused and asks if something can be done—a cesarean—something! The doctor explains that nothing can be done.

Labor is induced. During labor, Bob and Sue are quiet, but show no tears. After 8 hours of labor, Sue delivers an 8 lb, 2 oz girl with blond hair. The delivery room is very quiet. Bob looks away as the infant is born. The nurse weighs the infant and wraps her in warm blankets. She asks if they would like to see the infant. They say no. In a private recovery room, Sue and Bob sob uncontrollably in each other's arms. The nurse takes pictures of the infant. She asks the parents if they would like to see the picture and tells them that their daughter looks as if she is sleeping. They agree to see the picture and then ask to see the baby. Through tears, the mother sees that the little girl has her family's nose and her husband's chin. The nurse asks what name they had chosen for her—it was "Jennifer." The chaplain visits and answers questions about funeral options. The father holds his daughter. The parents unwrap the infant, counting fingers and toes. The nurse leaves them alone between vital signs and lochia checks. The father requests pictures of the three of them, saying, "It is the only chance we will get." This picture is taken and added to the memory packet, which contains a lock of hair, footprints, birth certificate, bracelet, and crib card. The packet is given to the parents. After recovery, the mother is transferred to a gynecology floor, where she stays overnight. The nursing staff makes time to allow the mother and father to verbalize their feelings about their daughter, Jennifer. The parents are given a book about grieving for support after discharge. The social worker provides information and the phone number of a parent support group. Sue is discharged to home the next day.

Questions for Discussion

1. Discuss the different types of crises involved in the obstetrical situation.
2. Identify the symptoms and behaviors of the grieving process that can be observed in the bereaved couple.
3. Discuss behaviors that may indicate potential problems occurring in the mourning process.
4. List nursing interventions that facilitated the concept of attachment and detachment.

Case Study

The Client and Family Experiencing Grief and Loss

Mama Lillie, as her family called her, was 97 years old. She had lived most of her life within a 10-mile area. She had been widowed for 30 years. Only she and her 84-year-old sister remained of the six siblings. Her own family of four children had become much larger—12 grandchildren (1 deceased), 22 great-grandchildren, and 5 great-great-grandchildren. She had worked very hard all of her life. When her husband had a cerebral aneurysm and could not work, they moved to her parents' farm, and she carefully rationed their small earnings to provide for their family. She later worked in a hat factory to provide income for herself, her husband, and her mother. They moved in with her mother after Mama Lillie's father died.

At the age of 72, she retired. She was known far and wide for her cooking, quilting, and love of family. Her strength had always been her reliance, but age was beginning to take its toll. Her hearing was diminishing, her spryness decreasing, and her heart weakening, but her love of family endured it all. At 94 years old, she moved from her home of 42 years into a retirement home. She graciously gave her possessions to family members. She rallied in her new home. She had friends to talk to, games of 42 to play, trips with the group to the beauty shop, church services coming to her. When cooking became difficult, Meals on Wheels supplemented. When frequent health care monitoring was needed, a visiting nurse met the needs. The declines were becoming more obvious now, and her physical needs were more than her new home could provide. Her decision, though a difficult one, was made. She would go into a nursing home. She wanted to continue to be her own person and definitely not to be a burden. The episodes of congestive heart failure came more frequently, and her 97-year-old heart was getting tired—still her eyes twinkled as family visits, calls, and letters came.

The last episode was emotionally taxing. Already weakened from the previous illness, her strength was gone. She told her daughter-in-law that God had called her home, and she was ready. During the days to follow, most of her large family were at her bedside. She did not talk much but was aware of those present. No one wanted to admit that this was probably goodbye. In the last few hours of her life, the medications no longer effective, her children, daughter-in-law, and sister encircled her bed and were beside her when she died. Time and the losses it creates had taken their toll, but Mama Lillie's legend would live on through her family.

Questions for Discussion

1. Discuss the types of losses noted within this situation.
2. What impact did these losses make on the outcome?
3. Explore community resources that were used.
4. What potential outcomes do you see for this family after Mama Lillie's death?
5. Compare these outcomes with those from a sudden unexpected death of a family member.

Nursing Care Plan 13-1

Grief After A Sudden Death

While away on a business trip, 46-year-old Mr. V is killed in a motor vehicle accident. His 42-year-old wife and 2 sons, ages 16 and 18, are in a state of shock. Through the wake and funeral Mrs. V remains stonefaced and silent. She speaks little, never cries, and refuses the food offered by family and friends. One month later she confides to her sister, "How could he do this to me? Was I that terrible of a wife?"

Nursing Diagnosis

Dysfunctional Grieving, related to failure to grieve at time of loss and lack of resolution of grief response

Outcome

Client will acknowledge awareness of loss and communicate feelings and thoughts about loss.

Intervention	Rationale
Acknowledge client grief through empathetic interaction and explain that anger, guilt, and distress are normal grief reactions.	Validating feelings promotes normalization of her experience and gradual acceptance of reality.
Establish rapport by spending time with client and by actively listening to her concerns.	Nonjudgmental listening promotes development of a therapeutic relationship.
Encourage use of support groups.	Sharing feelings with others decreases sense of isolation and loneliness after a loss.

Evaluation

Client discusses her feelings of grief and uses support groups, family, and friends as supports.

Nursing Diagnosis

Self-esteem Disturbance related to the grieving process

Outcome

Client will verbalize positive self-worth, identify her own and sons' strengths, and plan for their future.

Interventions	Rationale
Use open-ended questions to encourage verbalization of feelings of anger, guilt, depression of all family members.	Loss is frequently associated with feelings of anger toward and guilt about the deceased, and clients must learn to express these normal feelings without shame.
Approach client and sons in warm, nonjudgmental manner.	This approach encourages acceptance of self as worthy individual.
Encourage and support decision-making.	Appropriate decision-making reinforces sense of competency.
Encourage open communication of family members.	Sharing and acknowledging feelings decreases loneliness, isolation, and sense of abandonment.
Assist with referrals to support groups, such as Widow to Widow program and Widowed Persons Service of AARP.	Self-help groups provide additional support beyond family members who are often also struggling with personal grief.

Evaluation

Client reports improved sense of self-worth, open and honest communication with sons and other family and friends, and use of support services.

for you to be here alone") convey the nurse's concern and empathy and may assist individuals in their grief expression. The bereaved person may have difficulty communicating because of the intensity of the grief. The nurse must not push the client to communicate but should allow the client to communicate when ready. This is an appropriate time for the nurse to listen, touch, and simply to be present (Box 13-4). Nurses should not try to hide their own feelings to protect families. It is okay if the nurse cries. People will long remember sincere expressions of empathy.

Communication with the dying client should involve active listening and a minimum of idle chatter. Many times, all that is needed is a mutual silence in which the nurse is comfortable. During active listening, the nurse carries on the ongoing assessment of the client's feelings

BOX 13-4

Losing a Baby

Reverend Renee Gaston Hoke, Associate Minister, First Christian Church, Duncanville, Texas

Few events in my life have affected my attitudes and emotions as profoundly as the loss of a baby—babies in our case, since my husband Greg and I lost twins at birth almost 10 years ago. I remember those first few days in the hospital vividly even today, and I remember clearly the care I received from the hospital staff.

My pregnancy had been normal in every way, so our loss was first and foremost a complete surprise. For several days, my primary emotions were disbelief and a great, dark, emptiness. It would be weeks and months before I wrestled with deeper spiritual needs and emotions connected with our loss. For those first few days, I felt only numb . . . and very, very empty.

The first hours were a fog of physical pain and exhaustion. I was moved to the last room on the maternity hallway, but I could clearly hear crying babies being carried to their waiting mothers. I could only guess what it must be like for those mothers to nurse their new babies.

These were normal, happy sounds. I could hear them very clearly because my own room was so quiet. When Greg was not visiting, I turned off the television and stared silently out the window into the winter sky. There were no calls or visits from my friends or relatives yet—most of our friends had not yet heard the news, and our immediate relatives were making plane reservations to attend the funeral. Two or three days later, Greg and I were surrounded by more love and nurturing than we could have dreamed possible. But those first few days were silent.

Who became the only living, breathing humans in my world during those empty days? The nurses—making their rounds, taking my temperature, delivering meals or medication. I remember that most of them entered and left my room uttering only the few words necessary to do their jobs. They performed their tasks in seconds, almost as if they were timed for efficiency. I felt contagious. Soon the door would close and I would hear them move down the hall to the next room, where they would chat comfortably with the next patient.

I understand now how they must have felt in my presence. I was the abnormality—the woman *without* a baby. If they stopped to chat with me, would I burst into tears? Would I blame them for my loss? Would I ask them to explain how something so terrible could happen?

Far from it! I was not in search of answers yet. In fact, I wasn't even sure of the questions. What I needed most was a friendly voice to talk with me about the weather or a new recipe, to distract me from my loss and remind me that normal, ordinary life continues no matter what.

A nurse can be a wonderful, comforting distraction for a grieving patient. As she or he bustles around your room, taking your pulse or straightening your bed, you are transported back to your childhood and the tender loving care that mom or grandmother lavished on you. How special you feel to have someone near whose only thought is for your well-being! How nice to feel the touch of a hand or hear a kind word!

I do remember one nurse who knew just what I needed in the midst of my ordeal. She cared for me in recovery, when my pain was still more physical than emotional. As she fluffed my pillow and brushed back my hair, I thanked her.

"You're welcome," she answered softly, and then she paused. "This just isn't fair, is it?"

That was all I needed. A voice, a human being who cared. The burning spiritual and philosophical questions could wait until another day. For now, what I wanted was ordinary sights and sounds to remind me that life goes on . . . regardless. For a while, thanks to those kind words, the emptiness was more bearable.

and coping abilities. The dying client may express concern about specific problems or business that must be completed before reaching any sense of peace or acceptance. Together with the nurse or other health care provider, the client can then make appropriate plans.

Communicating With Parents Who Have Experienced Perinatal Loss

Nurses should be careful to avoid stereotypical statements, such as "I know how you must be feeling," "You're young; you can have other babies," "It must be God's will; it must be for the best," and "You were just barely pregnant; it's fortunate that you really didn't get to know this baby." These statements negate the mother's feelings and interfere with the process of attachment and detachment needed for normal grief resolution.

Supporting Meaningfulness

Frequently, the dying client's world is filled with loneliness, isolation, and feelings of rejection. This triad is the source of feelings of meaninglessness in an existence that holds no purposeful actions or goal attainment activity. Alleviation of pain, the lessening of discomfort, and positive give-and-take relationships support the dying client during the remainder of life. During the dying process, the presence of at least one significant other—at times, the nurse—is necessary for open sharing and expression of feelings. Given the opportunity and appropriate milieu, dying clients tend to be frank and direct in expressing their feelings and thoughts.

The exploration of feelings may be appropriate at any time in the dying process. It is too global to assume that certain feelings are occurring because the client is dying. Examining expressed feelings opens the way for sharing deeper or more submerged ones. The search for meaning that many dying clients undertake is an introspective process examining not only the meaning of death, but also the meaning of life. Clients may reaffirm their earlier philosophical or religious orientations or may make major changes in religious or philosophical beliefs. The value of accomplishments, achievements, and relationships is examined. Relationships with family members and significant others may take on increased importance and immediacy. When all the pieces begin to fit together and some order has been put to life and death, dying can become a meaningful growth experience (Box 13-5).

The act of leave-taking or saying goodbye may be possible when the dying client feels a sense of order to life and death. The nurse's role in this stage is one of support to the dying client, family members, and significant others.

Providing for Human Comfort and Support

Individuals experiencing grief and loss often feel isolated, abandoned, or undesirable when staff are hesitant to become involved in physical and emotional care. Nurturing is important to feelings of self-worth and self-esteem. When providing for the client's physical care, the nurse should carry out activities with gentleness and concern. In implementing care, the nurse acknowledges the client's cultural and religious values.

Maintaining Autonomy

Ill or dying clients find themselves in a situation of extreme dependency. A balance between autonomy and dependency must be maintained as long as clients are able to remain involved. Areas of involvement, including aspects of self-care and decision making, allow the client a degree of personal power and control. A client may be totally dependent for physical care yet maintain autonomy through decision making. This is an important aspect in a health approach, rather than an illness approach, to the dying client. Offering personal control means allowing the client a voice in the care decisions. The nurse provides the client with the basic rights of all clients, including that of informed consent and the alternative of saying "no" to those things that intimately affect the client.

As with any behavior, extremes on the autonomy-dependence continuum may exist. Clients who are basically dependent may react by exhibiting dictating, controlling behaviors toward health care professionals and family. A more intense look at the client may reveal a frightened and lonely person whose greatest fear is that of abandonment. This dynamic of behavior has probably existed throughout the client's life with family members and significant others and probably will not change during this aspect of life.

If the client's behavior represents a major change in behavior, the nurse demonstrates quiet acceptance, gentle limit setting, and trust through reliable and predictable administration of nursing care. Listening, role modeling, and open communication with loved ones are necessary to maintain a balance of integrity and support a continued interaction with the dying client. The nurse facilitates family interactions and provides a place for the expression of feelings.

Encouraging Reality of Loss

Through history, death rituals have helped bereaved individuals cope with the reality of loss. The health professional encourages the bereaved individual to express grief verbally and nonverbally. Active involvement in a self-help group enables the bereaved person to integrate the loss and validate grief feelings and experiences.[12,21]

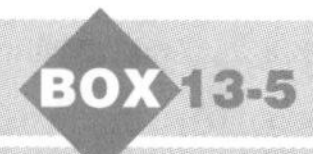

Personal Reflections on Death

Felicitas Alfaro, RN, MEd, Instructor of Nursing, El Centro College, Dallas, Texas

When I stop to analyze or reflect on the major events of my life, I necessarily have to think about the significant losses that I have experienced and the tremendous impact they had on me and my development.

Six to seven hours after I was born, my mother died. When I was 2 weeks old, my oldest sister and my father brought me home to a family of two sisters and nine brothers ranging in age from 2 to 25 years. They all played a role in raising me, as did my aunts and even a friendly neighbor or two.

I grew up hearing, "That's the baby of the family—poor thing—you know her mother died when she was born." Often, I was introduced as "This is my baby sister—the one that was born when my mother died." There was no malice here, just fact; however, for many years, I felt guilty. I used to think that if I'd never been born, then my mother would have never died and my brothers and sisters would have had a mother. It was not until I was in college that I was truly able to verbalize this and work it through, to realize that I had no control over my being born or over my mother's life or death.

When I was 8 years old, my oldest brother died of cancer at the age of 33. He had struggled for 7 years. The last few months of his life were the most uncomfortable. A couple of my older brothers and my oldest sister helped his wife with his care. He died at home—surrounded by those who loved him most. I remember it being Valentine's day because his daughters and I were comparing our Valentine's day cards. As an adult looking back, I am struck by the vivid memories of my brother's colostomy, his pneumonectomy scar, the whispers and the crying at home when the doctor pronounced him dead—and the Valentine's day cards.

By the time I graduated from high school, one of my paternal aunts, who had taught me to sew and embroider, was found to have metastatic bronchopulmonary carcinoma. Because she had no children, she and my uncle moved in with my other aunt. My sister, cousins, and I took turns helping with her care until she died—again, very peacefully at home.

My father died a couple of months later of a massive heart attack. It was new year's day afternoon, and we were getting ready to go to Mass. I remember him walking by my room and out the back door where he collapsed after looking out one last time. I ran to him, sat him up, and held him in my arms. He died there, but I didn't realize it because I had never seen anyone actually die. A neighbor helped me bring him into the house to his bed. I called my brother, who is a mortician, to come quickly. He arrived within minutes. He knew my daddy was dead, but he also knew that I still thought he was alive. Daddy was pronounced "D.O.A." I could not cry, just as I was not able to look at him in his coffin. After the shock wore off, all I felt was anger. I was very angry at God—I could not and did not want to understand. Then I was very depressed.

The depression was what drove me to see the doctor I had had as a child. He was Hispanic, and he knew my family well. He was very sensitive and gentle with me and helped me to realize that I had to get out of the "poor me's" and get on with living. I became a volunteer in the clinics at the county hospital, and that experience led me to become a nurse—the one thing I had sworn I would never be.

Since then, I have lost all my aunts and uncles and several very close and dear friends and a sister-in-law who died suddenly and tragically. I have to think of all that uncalled-for guilt of a child who did not understand. I reflect on the years when anger would surface and then subside. I'm glad that it is finally resolved. I'm thankful for all the love and support from my family and friends, the love and support that I believe is a reflection of God's love and support. It is the enduring love, the steadfast love, the patient love, and quiet love of those around us that keeps us going.

The interesting thing is that even after many years, I still cry, and I still miss them. The feelings never go away—the changes in understanding and the tears are different—but the feelings never go away. I'm sure some of you can understand what I am saying.

> Those who living fill the smallest space, in death have often left the greatest void. —W.S. Landor, "Geri"

The encouragement and support by the health care team of the parent's decision to see, touch, or hold the infant after death is important. This private time when the parents can say goodbye to their infant helps make their loss real. Assisting the parents to plan funeral arrangements is another way of allowing the baby's existence and death to become real. Concrete reminders of the baby's birth and death can be provided by the

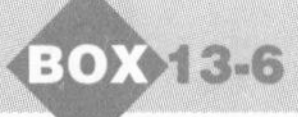

Grief Support Program

Joan N. Yanda, M.S.N., R.N., ACCE, Staff Nurse, Labor and Delivery, Columbia Medical Center, Plano, Texas; Consultant, RTS Bereavement Services, LaCrosse, Wisconsin

At Columbia Medical Center in Plano, Texas, for the past 6 years, we have had a multidisciplinary perinatal loss support program called Healing Matters for parents and familes who lose infants through ectopic pregnancy, miscarriage, stillbirth, and neonatal death.

The perinatal loss support team is composed of the physician, nurse, social worker, and chaplain. The nurse caring for the grieving family is a gatekeeper to coordinate all supportive efforts with two cardinal rules in effect: 1) he or she cannot provide support alone, and 2) he or she cannot be finished by the end of her shift. The goal for each family is to meet them at the point of their need and help them move through the grief experience without incurring additional pain. At the first interaction, the nurse begins to counsel the parents about their plan of care and options: labor experience; seeing and holding the baby; taking pictures, clothed and unclothed; gathering mementos; funeral and burial options; baptism or blessing; dressing the baby; and siblings and other family members seeing and holding the baby.

Many parents say that the most important thing they did was to see and hold their baby—"One must say hello to say goodbye." The parents have a limited time to parent this baby. The next most important thing is to have pictures—35 mm can be focused better and provide a background that makes treasured pictures. Polaroids fade with time. A memory packet is gathered. It contains a lock of hair (if parents grant permission), footprints, identification bracelet, tape measure, clothing—anything that was actually used with the baby. If the parents refuse either the pictures or the packet, it is filed and kept indefinitely. Parents almost always change their minds.

The parents are given a choice to recover in a medical-surgical unit or in women's services. At any time during the labor and before or after the death in the neonatal unit, the chaplain and social worker may see the couple to assist in gathering mementos. The chaplain facilitates the grieving process, provides spiritual comfort, and explains the funeralization process, which is compatible with the beliefs of the family. The social worker provides information on the grieving process and community resources (eg, support groups and follow up after discharge). The physician continues his or her relationship with the couple by offering sympathy and answers to "why" whenever possible so future pregnancies may be realized. Grief literature appropriate to the loss is given before discharge, available in English and Spanish. The nurse will provide follow up for 1 year, following the loss through phone calls, especially at 1 week, 3 to 4 months, estimated date of delivery, the anniversary of the birth or death, and holiday times.

At the Medical Center, we have two support groups. One group is for perinatal loss, and one group is for any other loss of spouse, siblings, parents, and children. The format is similar, with a guest speaker for the first 20 to 30 minutes on general topics of grief, followed by small-group discussion where each participant may share as much as they desire of their story. These are self-help groups with people reaching out to people who share a common tragic experience as each tries to come to terms with grief and learn how to live without their loved one.

In addition, we train interested staff from all disciplines to be grief counselors, role models, and resources for other staff members who are not as comfortable with death. Based on the RTS Bereavement Service's counselor training, three 8-hour days on perinatal loss are provided to discuss personal feelings about death, grief theory, current research on grief, theoretical framework of caring, care of the caregiver, what parents tell us they appreciate and remember, what to say and what not to say, telephone counseling, ethnic differences in grief expression, funeralization process, picture taking, and support following discharge. These counselors share consistently that working with grieving families integrates the art and science of nursing and provides the most meaningful experiences of their professional practice.

bereavement team. Examples of articles confirming the reality of death include photographs, identification bracelets, footprints, and documentation of the baby's weight and length. Parents should also be encouraged to name their baby. If the infant has an anomaly, the nurse should prepare the parents for what they will see. If the parents do not view the baby because of the anomaly, their fantasized picture of the child may be more frightening than is actually true. Miscarriages present a unique difficulty for the parents in that there can be no keepsakes of the baby. This lack of tangible keepsakes can create an unreal event for the grieving parents.[3,26,34,36,37]

Planning for the Future

Bereaved individuals must be aware that friends and even family members may respond in well-meaning but nontherapeutic ways. Anticipatory guidance from the bereavement team may allow them to respond to these difficult situations more effectively. Written information concerning available resources (eg, support groups, helpful literature) should be provided, because individuals initially may be unable to hear due to the intense grief and preoccupation with the loss. Follow-up counseling to answer families' questions about the medical condition or the events surrounding the death is important. In the perinatal situation, this counseling also can explore the possibilities of future pregnancies. Parents usually are advised to wait 6 months or more before another pregnancy to avoid the replacement child syndrome; the new baby should not be thought of as a replacement for the infant who died. Follow-up visits also can be a time to assess for any signs of pathological grief. If symptoms are present, appropriate referral for psychotherapy should be made. An example of one hospital's approach to perinatal loss intervention is provided in Box 13-6.

EVALUATION

Evaluating the effectiveness of interventions relating to grief and loss requires an ongoing assessment throughout each of the stages of the mourning process. Specific observations should be made to determine whether desired client outcomes have been achieved. Evaluation of the resolution depends on the strength of follow-up interventions. Further clinical research also is needed to distinguish early symptomatology of pathological grief responses.

◆ Nurse's Feelings and Attitudes

Involvement in the physical and emotional care of a family experiencing loss causes a grief response in the nurse similar to that in bereaved individuals. Dealing with grief and loss is exhausting work for health professionals. To avoid emotional burnout, strategies such as group sessions to receive information and emotional support are necessary for team members. The strength of intervention strategies is contingent on the emotional well-being of the staff and their commitment to the value of the program.

◆ Chapter Summary

This chapter has explored the topic of grief and loss and their effect on the client and family experiencing grief and loss. Chapter highlights are as follows:

1. Grief, a universal human response, affects all ages and cultures. Ambiguity exists among researchers as to operational definitions of grief, bereavement, and mourning.
2. Contemporary grief research has a less restrictive view of the time involved for grief resolution than did the classic grief research.
3. Phases of the grieving process differ among theoretical perspectives, but the grief work that is necessary for resolution is inherent.
4. The death of a child of any age is a traumatic and devastating loss for a parent and family.
5. Sudden, unexpected death does not allow time for survivors to engage in anticipatory grief.
6. The dying person is faced with physical and social losses in addition to the ultimate loss of personal existence.
7. Hospice provides an alternative treatment plan for the adult or pediatric client with a life-limiting medical problem.
8. Family and friends of the dying person experience feelings of loss and anticipatory grief in preparation for the individual's death.
9. Health care providers also go through the grieving process when dealing with clients experiencing loss and must have adequate available support and encouragement.
10. Assessment of a client and family experiencing grief and loss may include normal symptoms and behaviors of grief and indicators of potential pathological bereavement.
11. Goals and outcome criteria are formulated for the client and family to help them accomplish the mourning process.
12. Intervention strategies are designed to assist the client and family in the resolution of grief and the acceptance of the loss.
13. Evaluation of the specific interventions determines whether projected client outcomes have been achieved.

Review Questions

1. Differentiate among the concepts of grief, mourning, and bereavement.
2. Differentiate the concept of palliative care from a medical cure concept.
3. At what age does a child's concept of death most resemble that of an adult?
   A. Adolescent
   B. School age
   C. Toddler
   D. Preschool
4. A child younger than 2 years would view death as
   A. separation.
   B. reality.
   C. personal.
   D. abstract.
5. List stages of death and dying according to Kübler-Ross.
6. Which of the following symptoms would not be included in Lindemann's symptomatology of acute grief?
   A. Choking sensation
   B. Restlessness
   C. Feelings of guilt
   D. Increased interactions with others
7. Identify the main difference between contemporary and classic research on the concept of grief.
8. Give examples of interventions appropriate to include in a perinatal loss support program.

◆ References

1. American Psychiatric Association: Diagnostic and Statistical Manual of Mental Disorders, 4th ed, rev. Washington, DC, American Psychiatric Association, 1994
2. Balk DE: Sibling Death, Adolescent Bereavement, and Religion. Death Studies 15: 1–20, 1991
3. Beckey RD, et al: Development of a Perinatal Grief Checklist. J Obstet Gynecol Neonatal Nurs (May-June): 194–199, 1985
4. Benoliel JQ: Loss and Terminal Illness. Nurs Clin North Am 20 (June): 439–448, 1985
5. Benoliel JQ: Definitions of Grief [Letter to the Editor]. Res Nurs Health 15 (4): 319–320, 1992
6. Braun MJ, Berg DH: Meaning Reconstruction in the Experience of Parental Bereavement. Death Studies 18 (March-April): 105–129, 1994
7. Brost L, Kenney JW: Pregnancy After Perinatal Loss: Parental Reactions and Nursing Interventions. J Obstet Gynecol Neonatal Nurs 21 (November-December): 457–463, 1992
8. Conrad NL: Spiritual Support for the Dying. Nurs Clin North Am 20 (June): 415–426, 1985
9. Cowles KV, Rodgers, BL: The Concept of Grief: A Foundation for Nursing Research and Practice. Research in Nursing and Health 14: 119–127, 1991
10. Dubru M, Vogelpohl R: When Hope Dies—So Might the Patient. Am J Nurs 80: 2046–2049, 1980
11. Engel GL: Grief and Grieving. Am J Nurs 64 (9): 93–98, 1964
12. Gifford BJ, Cleary BB: Supporting the Bereaved. Am J Nurs (February): 49–55, 1990
13. Glaser BG, Strauss AL: Awareness of Dying. Chicago, Aldine Publishing, 1965
14. Glick I, Weiss R, Parkes C: The First Year of Bereavement. New York, John Wiley and Sons, 1974
15. Grogan LB: Grief of an Adolescent When a Sibling Dies. MCN 15 (January-February): 21–24, 1990
16. Hall RCW, Beresford TP: Grief Following Spontaneous Abortion. Psychiatr Clin North Am 10 (September): 405–419, 1987
17. Hammer M, et al: A Ritual of Remembrance. MCN 17 (November-December): 311–313, 1992
18. Heiney SP, Hasan L, Price K: Developing and Implementing a Bereavement Program for a Children's Hospital. Journal of Pediatric Nursing 8 (December): 385–391, 1993
19. Hogan NS, Balk DE: Adolescent Reactions to Sibling Death: Perceptions of Mothers, Fathers and Teenagers. Nurs Res 39 (2): 103–106, 1990
20. Jacob SR: An Analysis of the Concept of Grief. J Adv Nurs 18 (November): 1787-1794, 1993
21. Joffrion L, Douglas D: Grief Resolution: Facilitating Self-Transcendence in the Bereaved. J Psychosoc Nurs 32 (3): 13–19, 1994
22. Kachoyeanos MK, Selder FE: Life Transitions of Parents at the Unexpected Death of a School-Age and Older Child. Journal of Pediatric Nursing 8 (February): 41–49, 1993
23. Klaus M, Kennell J: Maternal-Infant Bonding. St. Louis, CV Mosby, 1982
24. Kübler-Ross E: On Death and Dying. New York, Macmillan, 1969
25. Kübler-Ross E: Death—The Final Stage of Growth. Englewood Cliffs, NJ, Prentice Hall, 1975
26. Lake M, et al: The Role of a Grief Support Team Following Stillbirth. Am J Obstet Gynecol 146 (August): 877–881, 1983
27. Leon IG: Psychodynamics of Perinatal Loss. Psychiatry 49 (November): 312–324, 1986
28. Lindemann E: Symptomatology and Management of Acute Grief. Am J Psychiatry 101 (September): 141–148, 1944
29. Martocchio BC: Grief and Bereavement Healing Through Hurt. Nurs Clin North Am 20 (June): 327–339, 1985
30. McCown DE, Davies B: Patterns of Grief in Young Children Following the Death of a Sibling. Death Studies 19: 41–53, 1995
31. McIntier TM: Nursing the Family When a Child Dies. RN (February): 50–55, 1995
32. Pederson DR, et al: Maternal Emotional Responses to Preterm Birth. Am J Orthopsychiatry 57 (January): 15–21, 1987

33. Peppers LG, Krapp RJ: Motherhood and Mourning. New York, Praeger, 1980
34. Primeau MR, Lamb JM: When a Baby Dies: Rights of the Baby and Parents. J Obstet Gynecol Neonatal Nurs 24 (3): 206–208, 1995
35. Rando TA: Bereaved Parents: Particular Difficulties, Unique Factors, and Treatment Issues. Social Work 30 (January-February): 19–23, 1985
36. Rappaport C: Helping Parents When Their Newborn Infants Die: Social Work Implications. Soc Work Health Care 6 (Spring): 57–67, 1981
37. Ryan PF, Cote-Arsenault D, Sugarman LL: Facilitating Care After Perinatal Loss: A Comprehensive Checklist. J Obstet Gynecol Neonatal Nurs (September-October): 385–389, 1991
38. Sahu S: Coping with Perinatal Death. J Reprod Med 26 (March): 129–132, 1981
39. Spencer L: How Do Nurses Deal With Their Own Grief When a Patient Dies on an Intensive Care Unit and What Help Can be Given to Enable Them to Overcome Their Grief Effectively? J Adv Nurs 19: 1141–1150, 1994
40. Sumner L, Hurula J: Making the Most of Each Moment. Nursing 93 (August): 50–55, 1993
41. Walker RJ, et al: Anticipatory Grief and Alzheimer's Disease: Strategies for Intervention. J Gerontological Social Work 22 (March-April): 21–39, 1994

IV

Intervention Modes

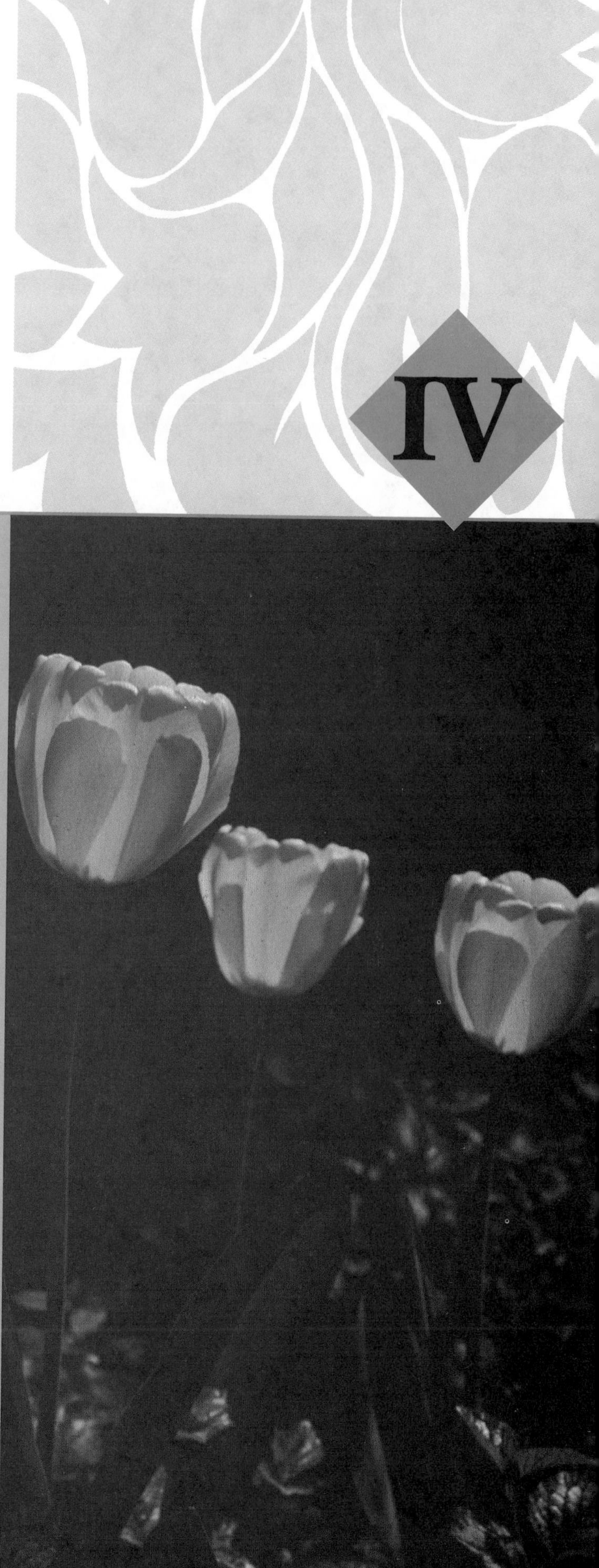

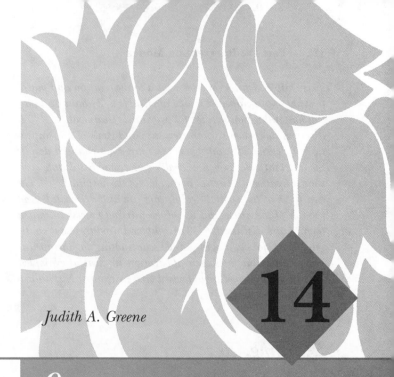

Milieu Therapy

Judith A. Greene

14

Once from a big, big building
When I was small, small
The queer folk in the windows
Would smile at me and call.
And in the hard wee gardens
Such pleasant men would hoe:
"Sir, may we touch the little girl's hair!"
It was so red, you know.
They cut me coloured asters
With shears so sharp and neat,
They brought me grapes and plums and pears
And pretty cakes to eat.
And out of all the windows,
No matter where we went,
The merriest eyes would follow me
And make me compliment.
There were a thousand windows,
All latticed up and down.
And up to all the windows,
When we went back to town,
The queer folk put their faces,
As gentle as could be;
"Come again, little girl!" they called, and I
Called back, "You come see me!"

Edna St. Vincent Millay,
"A Visit to the Asylum"

This chapter defines concepts related to the creation and maintenance of a therapeutic milieu applicable to 24-hour and partial hospitalization settings for psychiatric treatment.[6,13,17,18] *It describes components, characteristics, and goals of a therapeutic milieu and illustrates how these have not changed despite the fact that today's mental health care economics dictate ever-shorter treatment processes in and out of the hospital.*[4,11,15] *The functions of the mental health team are also delineated, and the role of the nurse and use of the nursing process in milieu therapy are discussed.*[7,16] *The chapter introduces some basic guidelines for managing and coordinating a therapeutic milieu and illustrates their application in clinical examples, reflecting the current trend toward brief psychiatric hospitalization and treatment.*

Learning Objectives

On completion of this chapter, you should be able to accomplish the following:

1. *Discuss concepts related to the creation and maintenance of a therapeutic milieu.*
2. *Identify the components, characteristics, and goals of a therapeutic milieu.*
3. *Describe the functions and humanistic attributes of a mental health team.*
4. *Discuss the nurse's role and functions within the therapeutic milieu.*
5. *Discuss challenges confronting nurses in providing milieu therapy in short-term hospital-based psychiatric treatment processes.*
6. *Apply general guidelines for facilitating a therapeutic milieu in a 24-hour or partial hospital setting.*

◆ Therapeutic Milieu Defined and Described

The term milieu is a French word meaning "middle place." In the English language, milieu means environment or setting. As used in psychiatric-mental health nursing, milieu refers to the people and all other social and physical factors in the environment with which the client interacts.[3,6]

Historically, milieu therapy referred to a 24-hour therapeutic experience lasting several days or even weeks. As a result of shrinking financial resources for mental health care, milieu therapy is provided in 24-hour and partial (less than 24 hours and usually 4 to 6 hours per day) hospitalization settings. This trend has challenged nurses and other mental health professionals to adapt milieu therapy approaches to brief or partial hospitalization treatments to ensure quality psychiatric care without diluting the effectiveness of this therapeutic modality.[4]

In either of these cases, a therapeutic milieu is an environment designed to provide a secure retreat for individuals whose capacities for coping with reality have deteriorated. As such, the therapeutic milieu affords them opportunities to acquire adaptive coping skills. Offering secure, comfortable physical facilities and providing recreational, occupational, social, psychiatric, medical, and nursing therapies, the therapeutic milieu can do the following:

1. Shelter clients physically from perceived painful, terrifying stressors
2. Protect clients physically from discharges of their own and others' maladaptive behaviors
3. Support the physiological existence of clients
4. Provide pleasant, attractive sensory stimulation[1]
5. Teach clients and their families about adaptive coping strategies

To accomplish these goals, the therapeutic milieu must consist of caring, concerned, intelligent health care providers who can work together effectively as a mental health team. Psychiatric-mental health nurses and other mental health and medical personnel working together create a therapeutic milieu—a healing environment.

CHARACTERISTICS OF A THERAPEUTIC MILIEU

The overall goal of the mental health team is to maintain and create a therapeutic milieu characterized by the following elements:

1. Individualized treatment plans
2. Self-governance
3. Progressive levels of responsibility
4. Variety of meaningful activities
5. Links with the client's family and significant others
6. Links with the community
7. Effective interaction among mental health team members
8. Humanistic mental health team members

Individualized Treatment Plans

A therapeutic milieu is tailored to the client's individualized needs as much as possible without infringing on the needs and rights of other clients and mental health team members. Nevertheless, to provide organization and predictability within the environment, a definite structure, schedule, overall guidelines, and social controls are set forth.

Self-Governance

To assist clients to develop self-responsibility and appropriate interdependence with peers, a therapeutic milieu must provide some formal mechanism whereby clients participate in decision making regarding milieu issues. Such a mechanism might include structured community meetings and client–team committee meetings held at regularly scheduled intervals. Involving clients in milieu issues enables them to exert a positive therapeutic influence on the environment and on each other.[10]

Progressive Levels of Responsibility

In a therapeutic milieu, clients are expected to assume a responsible role in maintaining the environment. A client's degree of responsibility should be commensurate with his or her capabilities at any point during the treatment process. Matching expected responsibilities with capabilities promotes feelings of self-responsibility in the client.

Various approaches can assist a client in becoming self-responsible. One approach is to use a level system designating what the client must do to earn a specific set of privileges (Table 14-1). This approach is a form of behavior modification in that it rewards and reinforces responsible behavior. Assigning a level to a client is primarily the responsibility of the mental health team; however, comments from clients during community meetings about their peers' readiness for a level change are taken into consideration when making level assignments. Using a level system based on behavior modification is most appropriate with adolescents and much less so with adults.

A Variety of Meaningful Activities

To encourage proactive social behavior and adaptive coping skills, a therapeutic milieu should provide each client with an individualized activity schedule. Such activities may include structured exercise classes, jogging, weight lifting, interpersonal skills training (eg, assertiveness training, listening and communication skills), leisure skills classes, and work and occupational therapies.[12]

Table 14-1

Progressive Levels of Responsibility According to Self-Care Capacity

Classification Level	Characteristics of a Client Assigned to This Level	Requirements for Progression to the Next Higher Level
Severely limited self-care capacity	• Displays injurious behavior • Disoriented to time, place, and person • Unable to function in group therapy • Exhibits poor personal hygiene	• No longer exhibits severely limited self-care capacity
Level I	• Does not display dangerous behavior • Knows the current date, time, and place • Attends at least one therapeutic group daily • Attempts to maintain good personal hygiene and grooming	• States the names of the primary nurse, physician, and at least three other mental health personnel • Attends at least three assigned activities
Level II	• Successfully completes requirements for progression to this level and consistently maintains this level of performance	• Attends all therapeutic activities • Participates actively in community meetings and serves on at least one client committee • Develops a self-directed behavior plan to change or resolve a personal problem • Knows the names of all of his or her medications and the times they are due • Participates in a family session
Level III	• Successfully completes requirements for progression to this level and consistently maintains this level of performance	• Takes an active role in assisting other clients to gain level changes • Demonstrates willingness to serve as an officer on the client committee • Assumes leadership role in the community, acts as a positive role model, and ensures that other clients are prompt in their attendance of regularly scheduled activities and group meetings • Initiates with the mental health team discussions concerning discharge planning

Links With the Client's Family and Significant Others

Besides providing respite, a therapeutic milieu also should provide opportunities for the client to reenter the mainstream of family life at his or her own pace. This may be accomplished in several ways. One way is through family education programs. Led by a mental health professional—preferably a psychiatric-mental health nurse clinical specialist—family education programs aim to help family members and significant others understand the client's problems and learn how they can contribute to the client's recovery. Family assessment and brief family therapy may help a client and family members identify maladaptive relationship patterns. With 24-hour psychiatric hospitalization, visitation programs for family members and significant others can be incorporated into the overall therapeutic milieu by involving them in selected milieu activities, such as interpersonal skills classes, mental health classes, family group therapy, and psychotropic medication classes.

In partial hospitalization psychiatric settings, family members and significant others may participate in education programs instructing them how to provide appropriate home care for the client. Home care issues, such as recognition of signs and symptoms indicating exacerbation of the client's psychiatric illness, administration of psychotropic medications in the home, and provision of a facilitative home environment to assist the client's recovery, are often taught in partial hospitalization family education programs. Additionally, guidelines to assist clients and their families to select an appropriate psychiatric home care service may be addressed.

Links With the Community

Activities outside the structured milieu, such as attending support groups, such as Alcoholics Anonymous, Emotions Anonymous, and Overeaters Anonymous, and others, link clients with community life. Participating in these activities with mental health team members can help a client develop the social skills and confidence needed to reenter the community. Such activities also can provide the client with opportunities to acquire or rekindle enjoyable leisure-time interests. Establishing such links with the community demonstrates to the client that he or she can once again be an active participant in the world.[12]

Effective Interaction Among Mental Health Team Members

Interpersonal conflict occurs periodically in any group, including a mental health team. Consequently, team members must be able to resolve interpersonal conflicts effectively and promptly. If they cannot do so, the effectiveness of the therapeutic milieu may decline to the point at which clients are placed in jeopardy. When mental health team members can engage in effective conflict resolution, they are more apt to trust each other and act and interact as a team and not as "lone therapists."[17] Further, mental health team members who can resolve interpersonal conflicts are effective role models for clients.

Humanistic Mental Health Team Members

For a therapeutic milieu program to be effective, mental health team members need to possess high degrees of the following attributes:

1. Optimistic attitudes toward people in general
2. Ability to inspire hopefulness in clients and their families and team members
3. Creativity in working toward more effective ways of involving clients in their own recovery processes
4. Lack of fear or prejudice when confronted with people exhibiting unconventional, bizarre, or aberrant behaviors
5. Willingness to maintain frequent daily personal contact with clients
6. Ability to set limits on personal behavior and the behavior of others in a nonpunitive manner
7. Willingness to share control and decision making with team members and clients
8. Belief that controls and limits should be provided by therapeutic relationships with clients to the greatest extent possible rather than by physical or chemical restraints[17]
9. Ability to provide effective mental health education to clients and their families and home caregivers

◆ Facilitating a Therapeutic Milieu

COMPONENTS OF A THERAPEUTIC MILIEU

Comfortable, secure physical facilities; a qualified mental health team; and an effective therapeutic milieu program are the essential components of a therapeutic milieu. In other words, the total milieu, not just one component or mental health member, is the therapeutic agent. The total milieu acting as the primary therapeutic agent—milieu therapy—is a group therapy approach that uses a total living experience (recreational, occupational, psychosocial, psychiatric, nursing, medical therapies, and mental health team–client relationships) to accomplish therapeutic objectives.[9,12]

These therapeutic objectives in the broadest sense include assisting clients to do the following:

1. Correct or redefine perceptions of stressors
2. Correct maladaptive coping behavioral patterns
3. Develop adaptive coping behavioral patterns
4. Acquire interpersonal and stress-management skills to conduct themselves more effectively and strengthen or correct their coping strategies
5. Generalize what they learn about themselves, other people, and adaptive coping behavior to a variety of social contexts

Developing and maintaining a therapeutic milieu that helps clients achieve these objectives require management of the environment and coordination of the mental health team's collaborative efforts.

As a microcosm of society, a therapeutic milieu should match the client's cultural background. The absence of such a match can create even greater cognitive dissonance or inner conflict within the client. For example, it would be more destructive than helpful to recommend a milieu therapy program reflecting the religious values of the Christian faith to a devout Orthodox Jew. Therefore, before recommending milieu therapy, mental health team members must ascertain that the therapeutic milieu is to some extent compatible with the client's cultural background. Similarly, a therapeutic milieu needs to reflect to a great extent the socioeconomic values held by its clients and mental health team members, especially in light of the current high cost of psychiatric treatment.

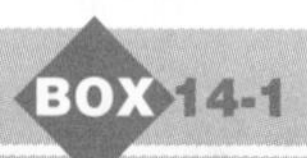

Managing and Coordinating the Therapeutic Milieu: Nursing Responsibilities

Direct Client Care

- Manage the day-to-day care of clients.
- Assist in contributing to the formulation and implementation of individualized client treatment plans—assessment, diagnosis, planning, implementation, and evaluation, including plans for discharge and reentry into the community.

Indirect Client Care

- Maintain ongoing communication with other mental health team members.
- Enforce rules, policies, and regulations of the therapeutic milieu.
- Maintain cooperative, supportive working relationships with other mental health team members.
- Schedule, assign, manage, and evaluate clinical work.
- Conduct quality improvement studies to improve client care and the effectiveness of the therapeutic milieu.

◆ Nursing in the Therapeutic Milieu

Traditionally, psychiatric-mental health nurses have assumed responsibility for managing and coordinating milieu activities. Viewing clients from a holistic rather than fragmented perspective enables nurses to fulfill these responsibilities. Unlike many other mental health team members, nurses possess the knowledge and skills to help clients meet their physiological, psychological, psychosocial, and spiritual needs. Further, because nurses maintain almost continual contact with clients in 24-hour and partial hospitalization psychiatric settings, they have more opportunities to assume management and coordination responsibilities to ensure continuity of care (Box 14-1).

To manage and coordinate a therapeutic milieu effectively, nurses use the nursing process to assess clients within the therapeutic milieu, to plan and implement client and milieu strategies, and to evaluate client and milieu outcomes. More specifically, nurses assess the physiological and psychological status of each client within the milieu. Making these assessments continually enables nurses to play a major role in individualizing each client's treatment plan and activity schedule. Assessing the influence of the milieu on each client and the influence of each client on the milieu is another important aspect of the nursing role in the therapeutic milieu. Such assessments are invaluable in assisting the mental health team as a whole to understand the group dynamics of the milieu and to select and implement appropriate milieu strategies and activities.[8] Other ways in which nurses contribute to the management and coordination of the therapeutic milieu include the following:

1. Physical and safety care
2. Medication administration and education
3. Psychosocial care
4. Mental health education
5. Health education

Physical and Safety Care

To meet a client's physical care needs, the nurse must assess the client's ability to perform activities of daily living (ADLs)—eating, eliminating, ambulating, bath-

Nursing Care Plan 14-1

Providing Physical Care in the Therapeutic Milieu

Nursing Diagnosis

Altered Nutrition: Less than body requirements related to client's refusal to eat secondary to belief that food is poisioned

Outcome

Client will eat at least 75% of each meal and cease stating his belief that food is poisoned.

Intervention	Rationale
Point out to client that all trays are filled from the same food containers	This presents reality without arguing about client's delusion.
Provide client with food from unopened containers, such as yogurt, microwavable foods, closed milk or juice containers.	Until client's paranoid feelings decrease, allowing him or her to open own containers and fix microwavable foods will ensure adequate nutrition.
Unobtrusively observe client's intake and output; weigh all clients every 5 days.	Monitoring intake and weight provides means to evaluate adequacy of nutrition.

Evaluation

Client gains one pound per week and stops talking about the food being poisoned.

Nursing Diagnosis

Sleep Pattern Disturbance related to paranoid thoughts and possible anxiety

Outcome

Client will sleep 4 to 5 consecutive hours without waking for three consecutive nights and without use of hypnotic drugs.

Intervention	Rationale
Provide a restful, quiet environment and relaxation therapy before bedtime.	Decreased stimuli promotes relaxation.
Encourage warm bath before bedtime.	A warm bath promotes relaxation and decreases tension.
Provide bedtime snack high in amino acid L-tryptophan, such as milk or cheese, unless client is taking a monoamine oxidase (MAO) inhibitor.	This promotes sedation and relaxation. Antidepressants of the MAO type when taken with certain foods containing tyramine, such as cheese, can cause hypertensive crisis.
Allow quiet activities if client has unsuccessfully tried to sleep.	Activity will decrease restlessness and help divert client's attention from difficulty falling asleep. When drowsiness returns, client can again attempt sleep.

Evaluation

Client sleeps 4–5 consecutive hours at night and reports relief from insomnia.

continued

Nursing Care Plan 14-1 (Continued)

Nursing Diagnosis

Bathing/Hygiene Self Care Deficit related to low self-esteem and anergia

Outcome

Client will bathe and wear clean clothes each day, brush teeth twice daily, comb hair and shave daily.

Intervention	Rationale
Gently confront client regarding hygiene and self-care behaviors.	Presenting reality and identifying the problem is the first step in promoting change.
Offer kind, consistent encouragement to client in attempts to become more independent in self-care.	This validates the idea that the client is capable of performing independent self-care activities.
Guide the client verbally and nonverbally with gradual withdrawal of assistance until client becomes independent in self-care.	This guidance structures and motivates depressed, anergic clients to perform self-care.
Positively reinforce signs of progress in hygiene and self-care.	Commenting on client's efforts at self-care helps reinforce the continuation of that behavior.

Evaluation

Client bathes, brushes teeth, wears clean clothing daily, and has no body odor.

ing, dressing, and so forth. This allows the nurse to plan and implement, directly or indirectly, an individualized treatment plan designed to reinforce or promote the client's independence in performing ADLs (Nursing Care Plan 14-1). Assessing the client's physical status for signs of physical illness or adverse reactions to psychotropic medications or activity schedules constitutes another important nursing function. Additionally, in a therapeutic milieu designed for chemically dependent clients, the nurse must assess clients' physiological reactions to detoxification from addictive agents.

To meet safety care needs, the nurse assesses the extent to which the client displays self-destructive or other-destructive behaviors.[5] A client with destructive tendencies requires surveillance, usually in a 24-hour hospitalization setting. Surveillance usually consists of unobtrusively observing the client at least every 15 minutes until destructive tendencies are no longer evident.[8] The nurse also must ensure that the physical environment is safe for a client with such tendencies.

Frequently, clients with destructive tendencies are treated in psychiatric partial hospitalization programs. In this setting, the mental health team uses the behavioral approach of forming a safety contract to help the client refrain from acting out his or her violent tendencies. Additionally, violence-prone clients may form a safety contract with their peers during community meetings to enhance their commitment to remain safe in the therapeutic milieu and after returning to their own homes.

To ensure client safety, the nurse and other mental health team members should conduct periodic safety checks of the entire milieu. These checks include not only community areas within the milieu, but also the surrounding external areas. These safety checks must, however, be conducted in a manner that does not violate clients' rights.

Adequate staffing with psychiatric-mental health nurses and other mental health professionals also is necessary to ensure safe care in 24-hour and partial hospitalization programs providing milieu therapy. As a rule, a ratio of one registered nurse to five clients helps guarantee safe care on a 24-hour basis.[18] Additionally, at least one activity therapist should be available 12 hours a day to help implement the activity schedule, and at least two paraprofessionals or mental health workers should be continuously available to help ensure client safety.

In partial hospitalization programs, clients are usually less acutely impaired. In such settings, a ratio of at least one registered nurse to 10 clients is considered sufficient to provide a safe milieu. Additionally, at least one activity therapist and two paraprofessionals or mental health workers should be available to help implement milieu therapy.

Medication Administration and Education

In the therapeutic milieu, as in other hospital settings, nurses manage medication administration. Certain administration methods, however, differ significantly from those used in other hospital settings. For example, in the therapeutic milieu, nurses often are expected to gain the client's informed consent before administering psychotropic medications. This process involves explaining in general terms the desired and undesired effects of the psychotropic drug to be administered and the dose, frequency, time, and route of administration. The client is encouraged to ask questions about any aspect of medication administration and may decline to take the prescribed drug.

Approaching medication administration in this manner shows respect for the client and provides a realistic point for beginning medication education. More important, this approach is more likely to encourage clients' compliance with prescribed medication regimens because it allows clients to participate actively in this important aspect of treatment.

Another way medication administration differs in the therapeutic milieu is that the client commonly is expected to approach the nurse for medication at specific times and places. In some progressive settings, a capable client may be given responsibility for self-administering medications under the nurse's supervision. For example, a responsible client may be given a 24-hour supply of medication to take independently in the milieu setting. Successful completion of this assignment would thereby demonstrate the client's readiness to assume self-care with regard to medication administration and for discharge from the therapeutic milieu. Whatever the method used, however, the goal is to assist the client to assume responsibility for taking his or her own medication to avert recurrence of psychiatric symptoms and rehospitalization. Nurses can assist clients to reach this goal by providing a caring and humane approach to medication administration and education.

Psychosocial Care

Providing psychosocial care consumes the greatest proportion of nursing time and effort in a therapeutic environment. To provide such care, the nurse engages in various helping behaviors. One helping behavior involves reducing stressors within the milieu that the client perceives as psychonoxious, such as loud voices, violent television programs or video games, unsightly visual stimuli, unpleasant odors, and crowded spaces. Reducing the frequency and intensity of perceptual stressors may be helpful.

Encouraging the client to identify his or her problems and conflicts, to attempt to understand them, and to experiment with new ways of handling problems and conflicts constitutes another form of psychosocial care offered by the nurse in the therapeutic milieu. The nurse may use informal group interventions, such as community meetings and structured or unstructured group therapy sessions.

Conducting brief on-the-spot reality therapy with clients to help them deal with problems arising in the therapeutic milieu is another important aspect of the nursing role. Periodically, the nurse may need to engage in limit setting to help the client deal with behaviors destructive to self, others, or the environment (Box 14-2). Other important nursing actions include helping the client use time productively for leisure and work, involving a withdrawn client in the milieu, encouraging a client with low self-esteem to value himself or herself, and serving as a role model by demonstrating interpersonal effectiveness in relating to clients and other mental health team members.[8]

The nurse also may provide brief on-the-spot individual therapy. A client in a therapeutic milieu may have one or more such therapy sessions daily with the nurse assigned to his or her care. This therapy aims to assist the client in the following:

1. Clarifying and correcting perceptions of current stressors
2. Identifying thoughts and feelings evoked by stressors
3. Examining how thoughts and feelings influence behavior
4. Evaluating the extent to which coping behaviors are adaptive or effective
5. Identifying alternative adaptive coping strategies in the therapeutic milieu
6. Test identified alternative coping strategies in the therapeutic milieu

By working with a client in this manner, the nurse can help increase the client's self-awareness, thereby enabling the client to acquire the adaptive coping skills needed to reenter family and community life as soon as possible.

The nurse also may work with clients in small therapeutic groups on a daily basis to assist them in gaining self-awareness about how they affect and are affected by others.[9] Group therapy can give clients the opportunity to develop and refine their social skills and more importantly, to learn to trust others and view themselves as trustworthy. This form of psychosocial care can help a client learn adaptive roles and behaviors that can be

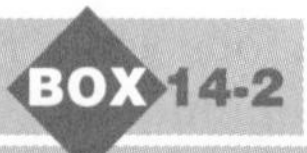

Providing Psychosocial Care: Limit Setting on Maladaptive Group Behavior

Situation: A group of clients conspired to receive extra privileges by requesting them from various mental health team members; they then attempted to pit team members against each other by repeating different versions of staff responses.

Problem: Dysfunctional group behavior as evidenced by conspiratorial manipulative behaviors

Outcome: Clients will become more functional as a group as evidenced by honest, open interactions.

INTERVENTION	RATIONALE
Initiate a mental health team meeting to discuss the problem, and arrive at a team decision regarding milieu strategy.	Effective milieu therapy requires team discussion, identification of problems, and determination of a therapeutic team approach to client behavior.
Initiate a community meeting to share the mental health team's assessment of the problem.	The mental health team role models effective group behavior as a cohesive work group.
Inform group that each client will be assigned to one specific team member and that seeking extra privileges from other team members will not be allowed.	This provides boundaries and guidelines for client and staff behavior.
Confront a client every time he or she attempts to revert to former behavior pattern.	This confrontation allows clients to become more self-aware regarding individual contributions to group behavior.

Evaluation: Client group does not engage in conspiratorial manipulative behaviors.

generalized to group situations outside the therapeutic milieu.

Mental Health Education

The nurse commonly provides client and family teaching centering around psychotropic medications or coping strategies for psychiatric illness. Effective teaching can increase a client's understanding of treatment plans and thereby improve compliance. Mental health education also focuses on interpersonal effectiveness (eg, assertiveness training, communication, problem solving, and parenting skills), which can help clients relate to others in the milieu more effectively and help them prepare for return to family, friends, and community on a full-time basis. Similarly, involving family members in such classes assists them to cope with and adapt effectively to the client's changed behavior.

Another area of mental health teaching offered by nurses and other mental health team members deals with stress management. In the therapeutic milieu, this focuses on helping the client learn to cope with stress through physical exercise, relaxation therapy, and enjoyable leisure pursuits. Engaging in these activities not only fosters a sense of well-being, but also cultivates self-confidence, self-control, and increased self-esteem. Added benefits of physical exercise include improved body image, weight loss, and increased muscle tone, poise, and balance. In some instances, these activities also promote positive social interactions among clients.

Relaxation therapy, another useful method of coping with stress, can involve progressive muscle relaxation, visual imagery, soothing auditory experiences, and massage. This therapy is especially helpful for clients with psychiatric disorders characterized by maladaptive anxiety, such as chemical dependency, anxiety and stress-related disorders, and depressive reactions.

The nurse can teach relaxation therapy techniques in individual or group sessions. Usually, the nurse first demonstrates the technique and then coaches clients in their use. Audio or video training cassettes help teach these techniques and allow clients to practice them as needed.

Health Education

Besides mental health education, the nurse also provides client teaching regarding physical health problems. A client may be at risk for various physical health problems, such as hypertension, obesity, hypercholesteremia, diabetes, and other stress-related physical illnesses, due to the self-neglect associated with chemical dependence, depression, and other psychiatric disorders. Health principles helpful in preventing and controlling these illnesses can be presented in a combination of lectures and discussion groups. Another area of health education focuses on preventing sexually transmitted diseases, especially HIV infection, which is particularly important for chemically dependent clients. Various teaching aids can help the nurse present this information in an objective, informative, nonthreatening manner.

Other Nursing Considerations in the Therapeutic Milieu

Depending on the organizational structure of the milieu, the nurse may be responsible for developing individualized nursing care plans rather than contributing assessment data to an overall interdisciplinary or multidisciplinary treatment plan. In either case, however, the nurse must function within the context of the total mental health team to manage and coordinate milieu activities in an effective, harmonious manner. Failure to do so can result in clients pitting mental health team members against one another, thereby sabotaging the therapeutic milieu's effectiveness.

Similarly, the nurse who makes clinical assignments for nursing and other personnel must remain cognizant of the overall purposes of the therapeutic milieu program, clients' needs, and the needs and capabilities of personnel. As much as possible, nursing and other personnel should be in recovery from their own emotional or mental health problems. Often, this means that mental health professionals and paraprofessionals must be actively involved in their own therapeutic process. Active involvement in a therapeutic process and clinical supervision can help psychiatric-mental health nurses and other mental health personnel increase the effectiveness of their interactions with clients.

Although it would be ideal for all members of the mental health team to work effectively with all clients, such an expectation is unrealistic. Nurses and other mental health personnel are human and subject to all the life stressors and strains affecting clients. For this reason, nurses may find the following guidelines useful in implementing their role in the therapeutic milieu:

1. Cultivate self-awareness through self-evaluation and evaluation by supervisors and peers.
2. Relate objectively to the emotionality of clients, team members, and the therapeutic milieu's social climate without becoming overly involved or taking sides.
3. Be sensitive to the needs of all people concerned yet sensible enough to recognize personal limits in attempting to address the needs of others.
4. Communicate clearly and do not hesitate to seek clarification of others' communications while recognizing the inevitability of miscommunication.
5. Always expect the unexpected despite the best efforts and plans.
6. Be clear at all times regarding one's own values, principles, and beliefs regarding what is and is not clinically appropriate for adequate client care to ensure one's own survival in the current mental health care system.

◆ Chapter Summary

This chapter has described the components of a therapeutic milieu, applicable to 24-hour and partial hospitalization settings, and discussed how the total milieu acts as the primary therapeutic agent. Additionally, this chapter has delineated nursing functions important in creating and maintaining a therapeutic milieu. The following information has been discussed:

1. From a stress-adaptation framework, a client may require milieu therapy in a 24-hour or partial hospital psychiatric setting as a result of decreased ability to cope with and adapt to life stressors.
2. The therapeutic milieu provides a temporary, safe haven from life stressors while offering a client opportunities to acquire adaptive coping behaviors; that is, the therapeutic milieu affords asylum in the truest sense of the word while extending an invitation to the client to return to the mainstream of living and being in the world.
3. Essential characteristics of a therapeutic milieu include individualized treatment plans; links with the client's family, significant others, and community; effective relationships among members of the mental health team; and humanistic attributes of mental health team members.
4. Milieu therapy is a group therapy approach that uses the client's living experience as the primary therapeutic agent.
5. Nurses have traditionally assumed responsibility for managing and coordinating therapeutic milieu activities.
6. One important nursing function of the therapeutic milieu is teaching clients about mental health and other health concerns (eg, information about psychotropic medications, psychiatric disorders, interpersonal and communication skills, stress management, relaxation therapy, sexually transmitted diseases, and stress-related physical disorders).
7. Due to decreasing financial resources for mental health care, nurses are challenged to provide safe, quality care in the therapeutic milieu.
8. Nurses in the therapeutic milieu must communicate

the following message by their every action and word: "Come join us in the world. You are welcome here."

Review Questions

1. Which of the following statements best describes the purpose of milieu therapy?
   A. Provides primarily a group approach to family therapy
   B. Provides protection for people with ineffective coping
   C. Provides individual therapy primarily in a group setting
   D. Provides a facilitative environment in a home setting
2. Which of the following characteristics would be most helpful in a milieu therapy treatment team member?
   A. Acts alone without conferring with team members
   B. Administers chemical restraints initially to protect clients
   C. Acknowledges the need to share control and decision making
   D. Actively practices personal involvement with clients
3. Which of the following statements best reflects the concept of personal responsibility in a therapeutic milieu?
   A. Self-governance by clients promotes adverse treatment outcomes.
   B. Self-governance by clients promotes staff negligence and conflict.
   C. Self-governance by clients promotes appropriate interdependence with others.
   D. Self-governance by clients is contraindicated in most hospitals.

◆ References

1. Arieti S: Interpretation of Schizophrenia, 2d ed. New York, Basic Books, 1974
2. Bulechek G, McCloskey J: Nursing Intervention. Philadelphia, WB Saunders, 1985
3. Carleton E, Jonson J: A Therapeutic Milieu for Borderline Patients. In Mereness D (ed): Psychiatric Nursing, vol 1, 2d ed, pp 288–293. Dubuque, IA, WC Brown, 1971
4. Delaney K, Ulsafer-Van Lin J, Pitula CR, Johnson ME: Seven Days and Counting: How Inpatient Nurses Might Adjust Their Practice to Brief Hospitalization. J Psychosoc Nurs Ment Health Serv 33 (8): 36–40, 1995
5. Duffy D: Out of the Shadows: A Study of the Special Observation of Suicidal Psychiatric In-Patients. J Adv Nurs 21 (5): 944–950, 1995
6. Gunderson J, Will D, Mosher L (eds): Principles and Practice of Milieu Therapy. New York, Jason Aronson, 1983
7. Holmes MJ: Psychiatric Mental Health Nursing. In Arieti S (ed): American Handbook of Psychiatry, vol 5, 2d ed, pp 652–665. New York, Basic Books, 1975
8. Jacobs A, Brotz C, Gamel N: Critical Behaviors in Psychiatric-Mental Health Nursing, vol 2. Palo Alto, CA, American Institutes for Research, 1973
9. Janosik E, Phipps L: Life Cycle Group Work in Nursing. Monterey, CA, Wadsworth Health Sciences Division, 1982
10. Kahn EM: The Patient-Staff Community Meeting: Old Tools, New Rules. J Psychosoc Nurs Ment Health Serv 32 (8): 23–26, 48–49, 1994
11. LeCuyer EA: Milieu Therapy for Short Stay Units: A Transformed Practice Theory. Archives of Psychiatric Nursing 6: 108–116, 1992
12. Linn L: Occupational Therapy and Other Therapeutic Activities. In Kaplan H, Freeman A, Saddock B (eds): Comprehensive Textbook of Psychiatry III, vol 2, 3d ed, pp 2382–2390. Baltimore, Williams & Wilkins, 1980
13. Luker R (ed): Partial Hospitalization. New York, Plenum Press, 1979
14. Mason WH, Breen RY, Whipple WR: Solution-Focused Therapy and Inpatient Psychiatric Nursing. J Psychosoc Nurs Ment Health Serv 32 (10): 46–49, 1994
15. Murray R, Baier M: Use of Therapeutic Milieu in a Community Setting. J Psychosoc Nurs Ment Health Serv 3 (10): 11–16, 1993
16. O'Toole A: Psychiatric Nursing. In Kaplan H, Freeman A, Saddock B (eds): Comprehensive Textbook of Psychiatry III, vol 2, 3d ed, pp 3001–3004. Baltimore, Williams & Wilkins, 1980
17. Robbins L: The Hospital as a Therapeutic Community. In Kaplan H, Freeman A, Saddock B (eds): Comprehensive Textbook of Psychiatry III, vol 3, 3d ed, pp 2362–2368. Baltimore, Williams & Wilkins, 1980
18. Walker M: Principles of a Therapeutic Milieu: An Overview. Perspect Psychiatr Care 30 (3): 5–8, 1994

Individual Psychotherapy

Jeanneane Lewis Cline
Joy Randolph Davidson

15

Carpe diem, lads. Seize the day!

Why do I stand up here? I stand upon my desk to remind myself that we must constantly look at things in a different way!

You see—the world looks very different from up here. You don't believe me? Come see for yourselves. Come on; come on!

Just when you think you know *something, you have to look at it in another way. Even though it may seem* silly *or* wrong! *You must try!*

Now when you read, don't just consider what the author thinks, consider what you think. *You must strive to find your own voice. The longer you wait to begin, the less likely you are to find it at all!*

Break out! Don't just walk off the edge like lemmings! Look around you! There! There you go! Dare. . . Dare to strike out and find new ground!

John Keating, English Professor played by Robin Williams in "Dead Poets Society," A Peter Weir film

Psychotherapy is a method of facilitating change in a person's feelings, attitudes, and behaviors. For most of us, this is both intriguing and disturbing. The idea that major changes can be brought about by talking with another person seems almost like magic; it brings out hopes and fears in everyone.

Aeschylus, the father of medicine, had a name for what is now called psychotherapy. He called it the use of iatroi logoi, *or "healing words." As Plato put it, through Socrates, "It may be that the art of rhetoric follows the same methods as does the art of medicine. . . . In both cases you must analyze a nature, in the one that of the body, in the other that of the soul." Even Jesus can be seen as practicing psychotherapy with the use of metaphoric stories and the curing of both the body and the soul. Anton Mesmer, trained in medicine and theology with a method described as* magnetism, *soon discovered that he was able to induce the state of hypnosis himself and did not need the magnets. Initially, Sigmund Freud used electrotherapy, then hypnosis, and finally perfected the ceremonial, or therapeutic, conversation, earning him the title of father of psychoanalysis.*[72,73] *Carl Jung, his star pupil, broke from him and developed a theory of psychotherapy that incorporates symbols (a symbol is the "best expression obtainable . . . for something that is essentially unknown"), the collective unconscious, and mandalas (mostly designs with circles, crosses, and four quadrants).*[34,41]

People hope for more happiness and less pain, yet they fear changes in themselves and in the people they love. How will change, no matter how desirable, affect important relationships? What does it mean in terms of time, effort, and responsibility for the individual? What will the person have to do in therapy, and how can the habits and feelings of a lifetime be altered?

This chapter discusses how people can change in the therapeutic process, achieve their hopes and dreams, and increase their strengths. Emphasis is placed on the origins of therapy, the evolution of therapeutic techniques, and the qualities that a therapist—and a psychiatric nurse— need to have to facilitate change. Certain commonly used terms are defined and discussed in relation to the specific meanings and concepts they convey about the nature of human behavior and the therapeutic process.

Although psychotherapy is based largely on Freudian theory, it is now viewed as a mixed, continually changing and improving discipline with contributions from many areas: general systems theory, social work, nursing, medicine, and cybernetics. Therapy, defined as change and growth, is an open-ended process that continues throughout a person's life. New ways of perceiving, relating, and being are learned as life situations change and the individual reaches new developmental levels, experiencing traumas and successes.

Learning Objectives

On completion of this chapter, you should be able to accomplish the following:

1. *Discuss the purposes of individual psychotherapy.*
2. *Contrast social and therapeutic relationships.*
3. *Discuss the qualities of an effective therapist.*
4. *Compare client and therapist expectations of therapy.*
5. *Discuss various concepts of psychotherapy.*
6. *Discuss current trends in psychotherapy.*

◆ Historical Discussion of Psychotherapy

Psychotherapy is the use of techniques that facilitate or allow people to modify their feelings, attitudes, and behaviors. In therapy, two people come together in an encounter that is specifically designed for the purposes of relieving emotional pain, treating mental illness, and facilitating change and growth. In a therapy situation, one person is designated as the therapist (the facilitating or helping person), and the other is called the client (the person seeking help). The dialogue between them is focused on issues of great importance to the client. Most people who choose to enter therapy have a strongly perceived need to understand themselves, to make some kind of change in themselves, or to get relief from pain (psychosocial, emotional, or physical). Often, more than one of these factors motivates the client to enter therapy.[59]

Therapy has also been described as "peeling off the crust of self-deceit and stripping the ego of its defenses in order to uncover the core self."[69] The therapist uses both verbal and nonverbal communication to build a relationship with the client. The basic concept of therapy involves understanding of the self, understanding of others and being understood by others, and choosing to make changes, achieve relatedness, and relieve emotional pain.

Psychotherapy may be a treatment choice for a variety of reasons: to treat an emotional disorder, to deal with problems in people who would not be described as emotionally ill, to gain insight and self-knowledge, and to train people in the helping professions. Other motivations for therapy are reducing stress or anxiety, working through crises or traumas, and treating medical problems, especially psychosomatic and terminal illness.

Specificity of purpose of the interaction, identification of the roles of the therapist and client, and use of primarily verbal communication mark the differences between psychotherapy and other human relationships. Additionally, nonverbal techniques are critical in therapy and include silence, body language, facial expression, and respect for personal space.[66]

Nursing is most likely to meet the needs of affordable, accessible, and accountable mental health service. In the caring—rather than curing—relationship, one maintains therapeutic perspective rather than therapeutic objectivity. Although objectivity requires distance from feelings, a therapeutic perspective integrates involvement or interaction and feelings. When distance is needed, it is from the pathology, not the person. The good facilitator is attendant to the process, does not control, lets clients move at their own pace, and integrates softness with toughness, intuition with logic, and assertiveness with compliance (Box 15-1 and 15-2).[55,65]

LEVELS OF PSYCHOTHERAPY

The abilities, needs, and motivation of the client and the resources available help determine the level of psychotherapy in which the client participates. These levels of therapy are classified generally as supportive, re-educative, and reconstructive.

Supportive Therapy

Supportive therapy allows the client to express feelings, explore alternatives, and make decisions in a safe, caring relationship. It may be needed briefly, for a period of months, or intermittently for years. In supportive therapy, there is no plan to introduce new methods of coping; instead, the therapist reinforces the client's existing coping mechanisms.

Re-educative Therapy

Re-educative therapy involves new ways of perceiving and behaving. The client explores alternatives in a planned, systematic way, which may require more time (10–25 sessions for 3–4 months or 40–50 sessions for 6–24 months). Crisis therapy, the term for the briefest of interventions, may be only one to four sessions. Clients enter into a contract that specifies goals or desired changes in feelings and behavior. Changing a behavior may change the way clients perceive themselves, or, conversely, changing feelings may change the behavior. Talking about alternative ways of coping opens up new options that the client may decide to try. Examples of re-educative therapy include short-term, brief, solution oriented, reality, cognitive restructuring, and behavior modification. Today the majority of therapy is in this general category.[47,48]

Reconstructive Therapy

Reconstructive therapy, typically involving deep psychotherapy or psychoanalysis, was pioneered by Freud, Jung, and others. It may require 2 to 5 years of therapy or more and delves into all aspects of the client's life. Emotional and cognitive restructuring of the self takes place. Positive outcomes include greater understanding of self and others, more emotional freedom, development of potential abilities, and heightened capacity for love and work.[2,3,26] The hallmarks of Freud's theory of psychoanalysis are transference and resistance, and the hallmarks of psychotherapy, as developed by Jung, are the collective unconscious, archetypes, and individuation.[29,41]

STAGES OF PSYCHOTHERAPY

The three previous levels of psychotherapy each contain some element of the following stages.

Introductory Stage

In the *introductory stage,* the client and therapist meet and begin to work together. This stage usually involves taking a history of the client's life, including any medical problems and current medications. If the client is a referral, the therapist may already have the information. Many physical illnesses resemble emotional problems or the reverse. Referrals or consultations may be indicated at this time to understand the problem better.

The exploration of the client's background and problems will include any precipitating factors or events that led the client to seek help. Clients are asked to discuss their perceptions of their challenges or problems, needs, or expectations and their desired outcome of the therapy sessions.

During the introductory stage, the therapist forms some preliminary ideas about the client's needs. Together, client and therapist discuss issues such as the length of time therapy will require, meeting dates, location, fees, and so forth. The current popularity of health maintenance organizations (HMOs), with their focus on cost-effectiveness, may influence this process. The number of sessions, fees, and copayments may be predetermined by a client's HMO. This includes set fees, percentage fees, and copay fees; time limitations of only three sessions at a time up to 50 per year (generally with a much lower fee, 20%–30% of a basic rate); and lifetime dollar maximums.[47,81]

The client and therapist also begin to form some ideas about each other regarding personality and compatibility—whether there is mutual respect and liking and whether they can work together effectively. The ability to work together and to be invested emotionally in the task of therapy is known as the *treatment alliance.*

The introductory phase in the past may have lasted from a few weeks to up to 2 or more years, especially in a situation with an extremely withdrawn, defended, or psychotic person. For the majority of managed care clients today, the introductory stage will usually be one to three sessions, because the whole process may be only 6, 10, or 20 sessions. With justification, the therapist usually is able to get additional sessions authorized. The goal of this first stage of therapy is to establish a degree of trust that will allow clients to give up their defenses so they can enter into the second, or working, stage of treatment.

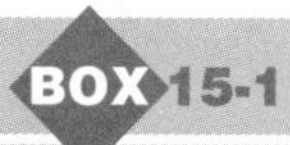

Students and Psychiatric Nursing

Nursing students sometimes work with psychiatric-mental health clients on a one-to-one basis in inpatient and outpatient settings. The students usually function as members of the treatment team and participate in carrying out a plan of care.

Members of the treatment team have input in planning and implementing client goals and regularly provide feedback on client and team interaction. Within this setting, the nursing instructor acts as a resource person and supervisor to the student. Together, the treatment team and instructor provide direction, support, and role modeling for the student.

The central element of therapy is the ongoing process that involves the client, the student, and the staff. The term *process* means the experience of self-discovery, understanding, practicing, exploring, and relating to others. This process extends to everyone involved and in a truly therapeutic setting, leads to growth and self-actualization as defined and desired by the client.

Students have a great deal to contribute to clients because they bring interest, concern, and caring to the clinical setting. Clients respond to this and often feel less threatened by students than they do by the professional staff.

Problems may arise because of the students' vulnerability and tendency to become overinvolved with a client. Both of these tendencies are also related to the students' therapeutic qualities. Without empathy and concern, little therapy could occur. Nurses, or any therapists, have the responsibility of separation of personal needs from the client's needs. Therapists must be aware of their own individual, personal needs before discerning those of the client.[59]

One method to help nursing students recognize and integrate their feelings is the use of critical thinking using a weekly journal of anecdotal notes of significant events during the clinical experience. The writings are to discuss the event, identify the feelings, reflect on the experience, and share the impact the event had in their lives.[45] Critical thinking activity is an involvement in the present and a reflective process (see Box 15-2).

As the clinical experience progresses, students often realize that they and their family and friends are not very different from the client. There is a common humanity, and most human problems are similar. Students begin to question long-held values and beliefs and to wonder just how healthy they are. The students' personal problems often become more visible.

Overidentification with the client seems to be related to this awareness that we are not very different from each other. As an increased self-awareness, recognition of similarities, and empathy occur, the student may develop very intense emotional ties with the client. Students must learn to recognize when their emotional responses are becoming focused on themselves rather than on the client. This may be evidenced through disclosing family matters, expressing their own fears, and sharing other personal information.[59]

Students need to realize that their feelings and concerns are not wrong, bad, right, or good and that all feelings about client–staff interactions do need to be shared with the nursing instructor or staff. This openness will keep the student–client relationship in a therapeutic framework and will help students relieve their own anxiety. It is important to be congruent—matching verbalizations with facial expressions, voice tones, body language—and demonstrate positive respect and regard with the client. A staff member who has these qualities is able to bring out feelings in the client, and the student experiences a therapeutic environment in action.[59,60]

A large part of the anxiety many students feel stems from the fear of harming the client. They often express this fear as, "What if I say the wrong thing?" "Do you think I said the right thing?" The student's fear or anxiety, therefore, relates to the student and the client. Students must recognize that they do not have the power to destroy the client, even thought they can elicit anger. A student may want or need to work further on personal problems and may be referred for counseling. A need for counseling is not to be considered a weakness but rather an opportunity for change. Working out one's own problems or challenges allows for personal and professional growth.

BOX 15-1 (Continued)

The cornerstone of the nurse–client relationship is the helping process. Knowing when to help and when to refrain from helping is the fulcrum that supports this therapeutic, yet delicate, relationship. Empowerment and advocacy remain central concepts for nursing; the art of accurate empathy is a prerequisite for contemporary mental health care.[59]

Psychiatric nursing education for the future is moving from the identification of roles and functions in the 1950s to the 1960s, from the focus on psychosocial aspects of practice in the 1970s to the 1980s, to the increasing complexity of the biopsychosocial phenomena that differentiate between mental health and mental illness in the 1990s.[60] It is also moving to community, self-responsibility, and critical thinking skills beyond 2000.

Working Stage

In the *working stage* of therapy, the client is able to become more trusting, to disclose, and to begin exploring with the therapist the thoughts, feelings, and behaviors that lead to the pain or problems. Again, in the past, this exploration may have taken months or years to complete. Today, the whole process may be completed in 20 sessions. Increased trust allows the client to experience greater recall and insight and to express previously repressed feelings. As the client understands and functions more effectively, the last stage of working through is reached.

Working-Through Stage

In the final stage of therapy, the *working-through stage,* the client achieves a higher level of understanding of the self and relationships with others and begins to try out new ways of perceiving, thinking, feeling, and behaving. As the client interacts with others and uses newly acquired coping skills, changes are reflected in external behaviors and in interactions with others. The client may need a great deal of support and encouragement during this stage and may rework emotional material more than one time. Although clients do become more autonomous and ready to live their own lives, termination of therapy is viewed as a kind of separation and loss, and the client may experience grief.[27,64]

ISSUES OF CLIENT AND THERAPIST

During individual psychotherapy, clients explore issues of such an intimate and personal nature that they can be discussed only with a person they consider trustworthy. Trust is a necessary condition for growth and change.

Many of us have experienced a trauma and then a change in our own lives; it probably happened because someone was therapeutic at a time of need. Looking back, we remember a grandparent, parent, friend, or teacher or minister who had a profound effect on our lives. Somehow, the presence, compassion, or example of that person helped us to understand, feel better, or make a needed change. Some quality in that person met our own need to find new meaning or direction in life.

Our own change and growth may have resulted from a love that made no demands and set no conditions. We may have responded to another's acceptance and ability to see worth in another human being. Perhaps it was the integrity of mind and spirit that made it safe to confide in that person. We say of such people, "He always loved me and believed in me." "She understands me and was always there when I needed her." "She is solid as a rock."

The qualities that are so powerful in our personal lives are also the qualities that are effective in therapy. In therapy, there are two people, the client and the therapist. The client is in conflict, in a process of growth and change, and is experiencing enough pain or discomfort to cause awareness of a need for help. Another

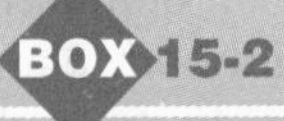

Critical Thinking Process

Some questions to ask yourself when using critical thinking include the following:

- What is occurring? (Describe the event.)
- What is my response?
- What are my feelings?
- What are the choices of action?
- What are the steps involved in the decision-making process?
- What choice did I make?
- What did I do?
- What is the significance of this event for me?

person, the therapist, has the essential qualities to provide that help. One of the goals of therapy is to learn to relate more effectively to others and to meet more of our needs and their needs.

Most people have families, friends, or someone available in times of need. Even the poorest and most lonely have some available resources, such as volunteers or public health systems. Why, then, might it be necessary for someone to go to a therapist to get help? Why can't all people achieve the same results simply by talking to those who are important in their lives?

For many people, the realities of living and relating to others have been difficult and painful. Some may have grown up in a family that was conflicted, chaotic, or dysfunctional to a greater extent than most families (most families have some dysfunction).[14] Perhaps family members were locked in constricting roles, had hidden agendas, used unclear communication patterns, or were responsible for incidents of physical, emotional, sexual, or spiritual abuse. Ways of relating and expressing feelings may have been distorted, causing painful, unproductive encounters with the people most important to the client as a child; these people were not able to understand or give the child what was needed.

Early ways of relating and early experiences are carried from the past into the present. Often faulty or unproductive ways of relating are modified by other experiences and other relationships. The processes of relearning and emotional repair may be seen as children enter school and form friendships; adolescence is also a time of major reworking and relearning. Therapy is designed to provide emotional relearning experiences in a safe relationship.

Initially, clients relate to the therapist and behave in the same way as with the other significant people in their lives. The patterns of client relationship behaviors become evident as the process of therapy continues. In classical psychotherapy, a great deal of emphasis is placed on the client's memories of childhood relationships and events. In present and future oriented therapies, the emphasis is on the client's feelings and behavior in current relationships. In both kinds of therapy, distortions in thinking and interpersonal relationships are identified and become the foci of therapy.[27]

Selecting a Therapist

When faced with a challenge, the client may consult any helping person; usually a therapist is chosen because of his or her objectivity. The therapist is not related to or involved with the client outside of the therapy situation. This is one of the therapist's important ethical responsibilities. The therapist should not engage in a social relationship—and never in a sexual relationship—with a client. If this occurs, it is an abuse of the therapist's power, and the relationship becomes nontherapeutic and detrimental to the client. Even after completion of the counseling contract, the therapist should not engage in a social relationship with the client; if additional counseling were needed, the relationship could not return to a therapeutic one.

With care and caution, people may consult friends or those who are already known to them for therapy. The therapist then is mandated to discuss the need for objectivity with the client, and if there is conflict, refer the client to another therapist. On occasion, a friend or acquaintance may be able to be both objective and therapeutic.

Therapists provide a different perspective for clients and give them the opportunity to discover alternative ways of perceiving, thinking, feeling, and behaving. Clients may be locked into one mode of being, but the therapist is not limited by the client's special set of circumstances.

The therapist also brings specialized knowledge to the relationship with the client in the areas of human behavior and therapeutic relationships, and possibly a nursing, social work, psychology, medicine, counseling, or ministry background.

Having the qualifications of empathy, objectivity, perspective, and specialized knowledge, the therapist observes ethical standards and operates outside the framework of the client's daily life and within the context of goals jointly designed by the client and therapist for the client's benefit (see Nursing Care Plan 15-1).

Competencies of the Therapist

Carl Rogers identified some qualities that promote a therapeutic relationship.[61] He believed that therapists' attitudes provide "necessary and sufficient conditions" for therapeutic change. These attitudes are congruence, unconditional positive regard, and accurate empathetic understanding.

Congruence, or genuineness, means that the feelings, thoughts, and behaviors of a person are consistent. To be congruent, therapists need to understand themselves, be aware of their feelings, and be free of deceit or misleading behaviors. This does not imply that the therapist expresses or acts on every thought or feeling, but with awareness, he or she makes a deliberate decision to interact—to speak, move, or touch—with the client.

Clients are often incongruent and unaware that their feelings, thoughts, and accompanying behaviors do not fit. They may express feelings and ideas that do not match what is really being felt or thought (ie, smile when talking about a loss). Congruence in feedback from the therapist allows clients to become more aware of their true feelings and thoughts and to feel free and safe enough to express them, however tentatively. Satir

Nursing Care Plan 15-1

Therapy for an Individual

30-year-old James has just learned that he is HIV-positive. He delayed acknowledging possible symptoms, and seeking medical tests, for four months. Now that his HIV-+ status is confirmed, he is afraid that his parents and brother will reject him for his homosexuality and for being HIV-+. His sister is aware of his homosexuality, and supports his lifestyle. James's affect is notably depressed. He communicates in brief, flat sentences, saying that he feels worthless and is afraid "everyone will abandon me."

Nursing Diagnosis:

Anxiety, related to anticipated family response to client's illness and sexual orientation

Outcome:

Client will verbalize reduced anxiety after planning method of communicating with family.

Nursing Interventions	Rationale
Assist client in role-playing discussions with family, in four different ways, leading to four different outcomes.	Supports client in gaining realistic perspective on family responses.
Encourage client to contact sister by telephone.	Contact with a supportive relative will reinforce client's feeling he "belongs" in family.
Provide positive reinforcement for client choices.	Nonjudgmental therapeutic relationship will increase client self-esteem.

Evaluation

Client reports decreased anxiety and honest communication with family.

Nursing Diagnosis:

Loneliness, related to fear of rejection

Outcome:

Client will communicate feelings currently internalized and reestablish social interactions.

Nursing Interventions	Rationale
Encourage client to use "I" statements to express feelings and thoughts.	"I" statements increase acceptance from others and resolution of fears and emotions.
Encourage client to discuss feelings in group therapy and with support group.	Provides opportunity for support and relationships from social sources.

Evaluation

Client reports decreased feelings of loneliness with group interaction.

and colleagues[62] note that verbal expression is the part of awareness that indicates past, present, or future; affect is nonverbal expression originating in the right hemisphere of the brain that always reflects the present. Therefore, discrepancies and conflicting messages can occur, especially when discussing the past.[5]

Unconditional positive regard involves being able to feel absolute acceptance for the client but not necessarily the client's behaviors. This attitude allows the client to increase self-acceptance and self-worth and to move toward the realization of self-potential. It is well known that expectations influence outcomes; therefore, the solution-oriented therapist maintains presuppositions that empower the client. These assumptions focus on client strengths, enhancing client–therapist cooperation, and helping create positive self-fulfilling prophecies for the client.[57]

Accurate empathetic understanding involves feeling and experiencing with the client "almost as if" the therapist were having those feelings and experiences. This empathy allows the client to become more aware of feelings and to feel validated. Someone, the client realizes, has heard what he or she is trying to express, and understands.

According to Milton Erickson,[36,68] therapeutic intervention requires a combination of observation, creativity, flexibility, practice, and a willingness to take risks. Being a master of observation, one of the tools considered most essential, Erickson took and used whatever the client brought into the session: attitudes, interests, emotions, symptoms, or worries. He considered observation skills more valuable than the learning of any one theoretical model. An effective therapist must be able to detect the slightest nuance in the client's flow of words that might betray the feelings well hidden beneath the words.

Erickson had the ability to be "totally present," and his observation skills were so acute that he could almost immediately speak and act out of a similarly patterned reality. It is important to speak the client's language because no two people understand the same sentence the same way. With one client who was in a mental hospital for 5 years and had communicated almost entirely in a meaningless "word salad," Erickson studied transcripts until he could improvise a similar word pattern. Each time he interacted with this client, he responded with the same intonation and number of words and phrases. Eventually, although unable to give up nonsense words entirely, the client began to use understandable words. Creativity is involved when whatever the client presents is transformed or redirected into a therapeutic response.

The role of the therapist is to facilitate change and promote growth and development. Therapy is not a matter of giving to or doing for someone; rather, it is a way of reaching and freeing the client's own energies and potentials.

EXPECTATIONS OF THE CLIENT

The energies and potentials of the client are powerful. The great emotional energy invested in wishes, hopes, and dreams provides keys to understanding what motivates people to go into therapy. To understand themselves or to change behavior in even small ways, people must have a strongly perceived need to change, a hope that change is possible, and at least some belief that someone can help them. These feelings must be strong enough to cause the client to risk self-disclosure and to continue in therapy even when it is painful and embarrassing.

Sometimes clients expect the therapist to solve all of their problems—to "make things all right." This may not be a conscious thought; however, the wish to be loved and cared for, like a cherished child in a loving home, is a very human desire and probably one that everyone has had at one time or another. The therapist makes it clear from the beginning that therapy is a joint effort in which the challenges or problems, the alternatives, and the choice to change belong to the client. Facilitating, rather than helping or doing for the client, will promote the autonomy and growth that therapy is designed to accomplish.

EXPECTATIONS OF THE THERAPIST

The major expectation of the therapist is that clients will be as open and honest in discussing the situation as they are consciously able to be. This is part of the *therapeutic contract.*

Other therapist expectations include keeping appointments on time and being paid for services. Therapists will arrange a method for the client to contact them in case of need, let clients know in advance when holidays and vacations are scheduled, and arrange for another therapist to provide care when needed.

Usually, the therapist will use a collaborative approach in planning therapy, identifying challenges or problems, and setting goals. In the past, this may have taken several sessions; however, today it is usually accomplished in the first session, with the caveat that goals may change or new ones may evolve as therapy continues. Therapy uses verbal and nonverbal (movement, music, song, and writing) techniques.

Physical acting-out of loving or hostile feelings between client and therapist is inappropriate and will be clarified with the client if any confusion or misunderstanding is present. The inappropriate feelings or behaviors will be identified and discussed in the format of the treatment plan with the client rather than as a rebuke (ie, "let's discuss your understanding of the agreement or plan").[59]

The therapist has an obligation to protect clients who are suicidal or likely to harm another person. In this situation, it may be necessary to hospitalize a client. Taking steps to protect clients is often reassuring to them, even though they may be angry and protest. Hospitalization can supply the needed external control at a time when a client feels, acts, or threatens to act out of control. Being or feeling out of control is frightening for the clients and the people around them.

Sometimes people use threats of suicide to get their needs met, albeit inappropriately, or to manipulate others. The nurse must realize that even when the client threatens suicide for these reasons, the possibility of suicide is real. This kind of behavior also provides fertile ground for exploring the client's need to manipulate others and the feelings that have lead to this behavior.

The therapist may expect to feel pleasure from facilitating growth and change and from understanding more about human behavior. The therapeutic relationship is always maintained within the ethical standards of a professional person working with a client to meet the client's needs. Personal and social needs of the therapist are met outside the therapeutic relationship through his or her own family, friends, other professionals, and the community.

How client challenges or problems are defined and what kind of therapy is used depend to a great extent on the therapist's orientations. The therapist has formed a theoretical framework of values, beliefs, and concepts from education and life experiences. The following discussion focuses on how some of the concepts used in individual therapy developed.

◆ Origins and Development of Psychotherapy

A tremendous amount of information is available about human behavior. Some of it is old and some new. Contributions to the study of human behavior have come from medicine, psychiatry, nursing, sociology, psychology, and biology. A particularly interesting area has been that of ethology, the study of animal behavior in relation to habitat. Studies of animal behavior have inspired much of the current research on human behavior. Such seemingly diverse areas as Harlow's[35] work with monkeys and studies of imprinting in animals have helped researchers to understand humans. Studies of social behavior have also broadened the conceptions of how people develop and relate to each other.[30,66] Many of the original ideas of Freud and his colleagues about individuals and therapy are still in use; many other theories have been developed and modified as new information and new perspectives become available.

Theories, concepts, and hypotheses (ideas that try to explain how or why something occurs) are formed within the context of a historical period. They arise in a given culture out of the general level of knowledge of that time, and as the culture changes, the theories change. Improved research techniques provide additional and more accurate information. By understanding behavior, we may be able to predict it and perhaps make desired changes.

Therapists shape their beliefs and values out of their own experiences within the larger cultural framework. For example, a person who had difficulty forming a warm, close realtionship with parents during infancy might grow up to form or believe in a theory that interpersonal difficulties during infancy may cause or contribute to mental illness. Research on infant attachment, in fact, tends to support this belief.[1,11-13] Self-understanding helps the therapist to understand others.

In therapy, both the client and therapist are engaged in trying to discover solutions and sometimes in trying to understand and form ideas about what led to the current challenges or problems. Exploring the client's beliefs and values is helpful (Case Study 15-1).

FREUD'S THEORIES

Sigmund Freud (1856–1939)[2,3,29,63] certainly was affected by his culture and the state of knowledge at that time. His genius lay in his ability to transcend culture and from his observations of his clients, develop ideas that are still influential in therapy.

Freud studied in Vienna, then the world center for medical education, and could be described as a middle-class, Jewish, professional man who had access to the knowledge of his day. A tremendous amount of work was being done in all the sciences during the Victorian era and the first part of the 20th century. Application of the scientific method, the use of the microscope and telescope, and the new theory of evolution opened up new areas of investigation.

A neurologist, Freud was interested in applying the scientific method to his work. At that time, people in the sciences were engaged in describing, classifying, and labeling their discoveries; mental illness and the workings of the mind could also be studied, described, labeled, and classified. Originating in this way, the medical model proclaimed that mental illness is a disease manifested by symptoms. This was a radical idea and represented a significant change from older ideas that mental illness was caused by sin or constitutional inferiority.

Freud became convinced that the mind was a major

Case Study

Solution-Focused Therapy and Reframing of Thoughts to Decrease Anxiety

Mrs. M is a 53-year-old married woman who reports having "panic attacks" about every 2 weeks for the last 6 months. She states that her husband leaves town for 3 days at a time every other week with his new job. She relates that she becomes dizzy, has a pounding in her chest, and is afraid to leave the house. She will talk with her husband on the telephone, but that does not help the "bad feelings" that she has inside. These "bad feelings" have grown to the point where she experiences them as her husband begins packing for his business trips and they expand into "full-blown panic" after he is gone. This is Mrs. M's first time seeking therapy. She says she does not want her husband to quit his job, and that is why she is here today.

As she interacts with the therapist, she talks about the strong marriage of her parents and the security she felt as a child. It seems that her parents both died recently. Her father was hit by a drunk driver and was killed immediately. When her mother heard this news, she had a massive heart attack and died 1 week later. Mrs. M has been married 30 years and feels she has a good, stable marriage. Her husband has always worked during their marriage but recently received a promotion to a position that requires regular travel out of the city.

"I came to see you because my family doctor recommended you," she said during her first interview with the therapist. When asked more about her feelings, she stated, "I feel like my world is ending. I'm afraid that my husband will die."

The therapist used reframing as they talked about fear of abandonment as related to the deaths of her parents. They identified and reframed her expectations about the separation occurring with the out-of-town travel. Mrs. M was helped to see that most travel is safe and people do return and that she was generalizing the situation. Additionally, the bad feelings were reframed into feelings of loneliness and missing her husband. These feelings were then "normalized" as expected with the changes in the job. Mrs. M was able to accept this and integrate these feelings into her experience of her husband's business travel.

Questions for Discussion

1. Explain Mrs. M's perception of her situation. Are these consistent with the situation?
2. How else might her uncontrollable feelings have been handled?
3. What strengths and skills does Mrs. M. have?
4. In what ways would you help her identify her goals?
5. What measures would you use to include her husband in therapy?

factor in mental illness when he observed that clients suffering from amnesia or from hysterical paralysis became symptom free under hypnosis. Clients were able to remember or were able to use the previously paralyzed body part, thereby demonstrating that the illness was not an organic impairment but a functional one. This distinction is still used in health care. Organic illness can be demonstrated by alterations in the anatomy or physiology of the body, yet in functional illness, an organic cause for the alteration cannot be demonstrated. With improved diagnostic studies, such as positron emission tomography, magnetic resonance imaging, and the thyroid function test, these classifications may change.

Freud observed that when talking about their lives and experiences, clients often remembered previously forgotten experiences. Talking allowed them to express some of the painful thoughts and feelings attached to those experiences. Sometimes, their physical or emotional distress was relieved, and they became free of symptoms. Laing[44] later described this same phenomenon, saying that once the catastrophic experience is relived and reintegrated, its "original spell evaporates." Freud began to try to understand and account for these experiences. In time, he called this work *analysis* or *psychoanalysis,* a study of the workings of the mind. From his experiences with clients and his self-analysis, Freud formed major concepts about mental functioning.

PSYCHOTHERAPY CONCEPTS

Insight

A person is said to gain *insight* when he or she becomes consciously aware of the old, painful, angry, or socially unacceptable thoughts or feelings that have been repressed. *Intellectual insight* is an understanding of the origins and consequences of a symptom or behavior. *Emotional insight* involves understanding and re-experiencing the painful, frightening, or angry feelings that are associated with a symptom or behavior. This re-experiencing, also called *catharsis,* frees a person's fixed emotions and allows for emotional growth.

Repression

The concept of repression is central to Freudian theory. Through repression, feelings, thoughts, and experiences that are too painful or threatening to a person are pushed into the unconscious part of the mind. *Unconscious* literally means not available to consciousness. Repression is an unconscious phenomenon; that is, a person does not purposely try to forget the events or ongoing situations that threaten the ego integrity (ie, the person's self-image or safety). Sometimes there is partial repression; for example, knowledge of a situation may be in a person's awareness, but the feelings about the situation are repressed.

Exerting powerful influences on people, repressed knowledge and feelings come out in all kinds of ways. "Freudian slips," or slips of the tongue, may occur; sometimes a word or a phrase that seems funny or inappropriate in the context of a sentence makes good sense in expressing the person's real feelings. Items, appointments, and so forth may be broken, forgotten, or otherwise damaged.

Dreams also provide a way of releasing repressed thoughts and feelings. Recurring dreams may have been present for a long time and may represent the client's attempt to solve a problem. It is common for people to have vivid dreams or to remember more dreams when anxious or excited. Paradoxically, therapy represents a form of stress that causes anxiety and an emotionally secure situation. The security offered by the therapist allows for weakening of repressions and access to emotionally important material that may be disguised in dreams.

Originally, therapists attempted to analyze both manifest and latent dream content because they believed that a specific kind of dream had a special meaning. Now therapists believe that the most productive use of dream material comes from clients' discussions of their thoughts and feelings and of what the dreams mean to them.

Free Association

Free association is the free expression of thoughts and feelings as they come to mind. This method encourages the lowering of the client's defenses. It is the primary method of treatment in psychoanalysis and in much of psychotherapy.

Resistance

Resistance means that the client resists receiving information or recalling feelings. It often occurs as *blocking,* which is when the client "blanks out" and is unable to finish a thought or idea. The client may suddenly change the subject without any cue or obvious reason to do so. Blocking involves repression of painful knowledge and feelings and resistance to recalling and understanding the thought.

Techniques such as having the client lie on a couch and face away from the therapist are used in psychoanalysis to avoid influencing what the client says. It is a way of trying to decrease resistance. Using accepting, nonjudgmental, therapeutic attitudes also decreases resistance, especially when allowing the client to express any and all thoughts and feelings.[2] In the newer models of therapy, eye contact is important.

Maslow[51] helps us to understand resistance through his assertion that people have both a need to know and a fear of knowing. Knowing and understanding imply action and change. The therapist supports the client's need to know. This support is needed because the knowledge that has been repressed is literally unthinkable. In this way, therapy represents both threat and opportunity.

Everyone has secrets—things they are reluctant to reveal out of fear of disapproval, rejection, anger, withdrawal of affection, or even abandonment. With unconscious material, the fear that drives or mediates the repression is so strong that it is experienced as a threat to the person's existence—a fear of total rejection, abandonment, or loss of existence, or intolerable feelings of worthlessness and self-loathing.

Infants and small children depend completely on significant adults, parents, or caregivers for survival in both a physical and an emotional sense. Lack of love, disapproval, or an inability to accept and love the child unconditionally is a threat to that child's survival.

Sometimes a family will place adult burdens of emotional responsibility on a child and expect that child to meet the dependency needs of the parents. Each family also has standards of behavior for children that include which feelings may be expressed and how they may be expressed. If a child learns that it is not safe to express pain, anger, love, tenderness, and vulnerability, then repression is the price the child pays for surviving in that family. The effects of that repression may include shame and guilt (see Chapter 22, Children).

Miller[54] feels that traditional psychoanalysis does not allow for the voice of the abused child because the child was not allowed to feel but perhaps was told how to feel. According to Miller, Freud's focus on client fantasies only banished the fears and did not permit working through. Many well-documented studies indicate that 50% to 60% of inpatients, 40% to 60% of outpatients, and 70% of all psychiatric emergency room clients report childhood physical or sexual abuse; this suggests that prolonged, severe childhood abuse may play an underestimated role in the development of many psychopathologies currently related to biological factors, intrapsychic conflicts, or other family-of-origin issues.[80]

Reworking

Through *play* and *reworking*, children learn other ways of behaving as they grow and develop. Family members, peers, and people outside the immediate family model different ways of feeling and behaving. Adolescents especially rework earlier developmental stages and modify earlier feelings, beliefs, and attitudes.

To a great extent, this *emotional relearning* is what happens in psychotherapy. This relearning or reworking is mainly of the nonfunctional, usually negative messages that were introjected or internalized throughout childhood. Jeffers[39] refers to these messages as the "chatterbox," a broken record or noise in the head. Early therapists believed that the personality was fairly rigid and could only be modified slightly. Now therapists believe that there is far more plasticity and potential for change, even in middle or old age.

Transference

Transference, a major tool or technique, is a powerful force in psychotherapy. In therapy, when clients are deeply involved with their feelings and experiences, they can transfer feelings and attitudes held toward significant others onto the therapist. The term *significant others* is applied to the people who have profound importance in the client's life. Clients are often almost as concerned with the feelings and needs of their significant others as they are with their own feelings and needs. There are usually different sets of feelings and attitudes for each person—mother, father, brother, sister, or lover. Clients often react toward the therapist in the same ways they react—or have reacted in the past—toward these important people in their lives, yet this time clients receive different responses.

The sex of the therapist does not seem to make much difference, but the appearance and behaviors of the therapist may trigger transference. The transference may be positive or negative; in either case, the therapist becomes all good or all bad. As the client first gets in touch with feelings of pain, anger, and hurt, a positive transference may become negative. As the client begins to establish trust with the therapist and work through the hurt and anger, the negative transference may become positive.

With transference, the client realizes as therapy continues that the therapist is not like the significant others. The processes of projection and transference allow both the client and the therapist to understand the feelings, attitudes, and behaviors that the client has learned. An important part of this emotional relearning is the client's realization that other people do not possess the stereotyped or punitive reactions that have been present in past relationships. Clients also realize how transference and projections contribute to and feed into current relationships and maintain faulty, incongruent, and inappropriate perceptions and behaviors. The experience of being valued and understood allows the client to have new perceptions and form new perspectives.[27]

Countertransference

In *countertransference*, the therapist transfers his or her feelings for significant others onto the client. Usually, something about the client (appearance, tone of voice, mannerisms, or behavior) will trigger countertransference. An unusual like or dislike of the client is a clue to the therapist to analyze the reaction. If not detected, countertransference can cause problems. Therapists should be open to comments that staff members may make about "spending too much time with the client," "giving the client special privileges," or "having a lot of concern." Therapists will often consult a colleague or request supervision to deal with the client affectively in a way that is therapeutic and beneficial for both (Table 15-1).[63]

Ambivalence

Ambivalence is the experience of two strong, opposing feelings or wishes toward the same object or person and results in conflict when these approach and avoidance tendencies are both present. Dollard and coworkers[21] were able to create ambivalence in laboratory rats by giving them an electric shock while they were eating.

Table 15-1

Issues and Responses of Therapeutic Nursing

Issue	Response
Nurse self-disclosure—therapeutic on a limted basis; progress inhibited by overuse	Limit personal information to simple facts; may be a reality check for client.
Confidentiality—the basis of trust; sharing important information modified with adolescents and children	Clarify record keeping and sharing information with treatment team. Discuss legal requirements of duty to warn and duty to protect.
Transference—unconscious transference of feelings toward therapist from significant, childhood relationships	Assist with identification of possible meanings of positive or negative transference responses.
Countertransference—limits nurse's ability to be therapeutic with client	Increase awareness of specific feelings toward client (ie, anger, sympathy).
Resistance—delays working on issues and making changes in coping responses or skills	Identify and discuss meaning to client; it will resolve itself at right time.
Insight—helps client understand disease process and interpersonal relationships and facilitates treatment outcome	Encourage expression of feelings about client situation and condition. Assist client to become aware of feelings and then aware of the meaning of the feelings and behaviors.

The strong drive or need (hunger) caused approach to the food, and recall of the painful shock caused strong avoidance tendencies; thus, confusion and useless back and forth activity resulted.

In human beings, the opposite feelings or needs are often love-hate, love-fear, or need-fear. Anger usually results when strong drives or needs are frustrated and not allowed an appropriate expression. Another outcome of this frustration may be what is called learned helplessness, which some believe to be a major component of depression.[56]

Ambivalence causes a great deal of conflict, which gives rise to the varied reactions of doubt, indecision, inertia, fickleness, and inconsistency.[29] It may also manifest as extreme anxiety, panic, or frozen immobility. To different degrees, ambivalence is present for everyone; feelings toward people vary with the amount of closeness of the relationship and with different situations. A small child expresses these feelings directly by saying "I hate you" when frustrated and a few minutes later saying "I love you" with equal intensity. Both feelings are real at the time, and the older child comes to realize that anger and love can coexist.

In a functional family, children are taught to own their feelings and to label them correctly. The family meets the child's need for love and security and socializes the child by teaching him or her how to meet needs in socially acceptable ways. Parents who cannot allow a child to separate and become autonomous contribute to ambivalence about dependence-independence and love-hate issues. If being dependent means being loved and being independent means being emotionally abandoned, a tremendous amount of conflict and anger will be generated within the child.

Parents who have difficulty allowing feelings of anger, aggression, or sexuality may react to the child's expression of these feelings in such a punitive way that these feelings are repressed. In this culture, girls are often taught to repress angry, aggressive, and sexual feelings and boys to repress feelings of love, tenderness, and dependency. There are indications that this is changing, and people are being encouraged to integrate both male and female characteristics within themselves.[56] By repressing strong feelings, emotional development of the repressed feelings is inhibited, as is the appropriate expression of the opposite feelings.

Ambiguity

Ambiguity describes the experience of uncertainty. One measure of emotional competence is how well a person is able to tolerate living with a degree of uncertainty. An element common to many people in therapy is difficulty tolerating ambiguity, generally indicating a strong need for certainty and stability. Many people would like to live in a reasonably predictable environment and feel that they have some control over their lives. Children who live in chaotic or deprived environments or never experience stability will be at risk in the world. Often as adults, they will cling to very rigid ideals to feel secure.

Tolerating ambiguity means that a person is able to perceive the world and other people in a way that allows for variations and shades of meaning and includes being able to have different feelings about a person or situation. Even though it may seem easier or safer to live in a world where things could be categorized as good or bad, there would be fewer possibilities and experiences would not be as rich in meaning.

Object Constancy

The feeling of security or stability is known as *object constancy* or *object permanence.* It is a general feeling that people are reliable and that the world is a pretty good place.

Object constancy comes about partly as the result of a secure maternal–infant attachment.[1,11-13,49] A secure maternal–infant attachment has survival value for the infant and for the human species. It is manifested in the infant's maintenance of proximity to the mother in times of stress and by exploration away from the safe haven in times of security.

Maternal qualities that foster attachment are sensitivity to the infant's needs, warmth, and nurturance. The infant both initiates and limits interaction with the mother or primary caregiver through eye contact or vocal cues (eg, crying, cooing). The mother cues in to the baby's signals, then mirrors and selectively emphasizes a behavior; for example, the first faint twitch of the baby's lips is identified as a smile and then positively reinforced by mirroring that behavior.

Accurate, empathetic mirroring reinforces desired social behaviors. The sensitive mother is aware that her baby is tired when eye contact is ended, the signal to end interaction. Soon after birth, the parents identify the baby's cries as indicating hunger, pain, or a need for attention. This awareness of the infant's behavior ensures that his or her needs will be met. Studies indicate that babies seem to be genetically programmed to prefer the human face. Babies quickly learn to recognize and prefer the mother or primary caregiver. After about 7 months, babies begin to discriminate and prefer mother, father, and known people to strangers and are anxious with strangers. Distinctions made between self and others and between known people and strange people are precursors of a clear sense of self and identity.

As the babies become more mobile, they begin the gradual processes of separation and individualization. For very young children, for example, the fun of peek-a-boo and hide-and-seek lies in discovering that people do exist even though they are not seen for a little while. As babies become toddlers, they can be observed to play happily for a while, go to another room, come back to the caregiver, and then return to play, discovering that the parent exists even when in another room. The ability to say "no" and to control bowel and bladder functions also reinforces autonomy and emphasizes the distinction between what is "I" and "mine" and what is "you" and "yours."

As these processes of identification, separation, and autonomy occur, there is a corresponding internalization of the feelings, attitudes, and behaviors of the parents and significant others. This internalization is known as *introjection.* The infant incorporates aspects of significant others as part of the self. This internal representation of others then supplies the object constancy. Throughout their lives, people continue to carry a realistic conception of those they love that remains constant and will persist even after the loved ones have died.

Acting In

Acting in is the kind of resistance that circumvents therapy through blocking, forgetting, changing the subject, or trying to elicit the therapist's approval or disapproval while trying to recall or express feelings. Consciously, the client is earnestly trying to express everything as it comes to mind, as requested.

Acting Out

In *acting out,* the client substitutes some kind of action for feeling or thinking. As painful memories, feelings, and thoughts begin to reach awareness, a kind of reflex substitution of action occurs, and the feelings are not allowed to reach consciousness.

The behaviors seen in acting out are learned and often become a defensive pattern. Common defenses are the use of alcohol or drugs, getting involved in fights, running away, or compulsive or promiscuous sexual activity. Even ordinary activities like work or exercise may be used or overused as defenses.

Sometimes while in therapy, a client will get divorced, married, form new friendships, move, or change jobs as a shortcut to getting support or their dependency needs met. This is another way of avoiding the more difficult task of becoming aware of feelings and understanding the self. The therapist may ask the client to sign an agreement or contract to postpone major lifestyle changes during therapy until less vulnerability and better self-understanding exist.

Interpretation

Interpretation appears very exciting in movies in which the analyst arrives at a brilliant interpretation of the client's problem, and the client says, "Aha! That explains everything!" Actually the important aspect of interpretation is the client's own explanation and understanding of the feelings and behaviors. A therapist may make beautiful formulations of the client's problems and their origins and causes, but this is not helpful unless the client arrives at self-understanding. The client's insight is the therapeutic element.

Sometimes the therapist will offer a tentative explanation or ask whether it is possible that a particular feeling or experience is connected to another. Questions such as this are best asked infrequently. With respect for the client's anxiety and need for defenses, even a cautious and accurate comment may arouse a good deal of anxiety, anger, or denial. Interpretations of this kind are useful when clients are ready to deal with the aspect of themselves that lies just below the surface.

Working Through

Working through comes in the later phase of therapy. At this point, the client has reached a fairly good understanding of the feelings and patterns of behavior that have caused distress. Having more emotional energy available, the client is able to perceive more of the world and to form new perspectives.

Working through means that the client's insights are discussed and reworked over a period of time. The long repressed pain, guilt, anger, shame, grief, or sadness must be expressed—not just once but many times—to be owned and integrated into the self. Often there are periods of regression, discouragement, or acting out.

Part of the process of working through is the knowledge that therapy will end, and the relationship that has been of great importance will gradually become less important and also end.

Translating

Translating insight and understanding into new behaviors is the final aspect of working through. Discussion is not enough; practicing new behaviors is highly reinforcing. As the client feels less angry, vulnerable, or frightened, there is more freedom to practice the new behaviors. Feelings are often more vivid and more consciously experienced. This in turn allows the client to become more autonomous, more aware of options, and better able to live with tensions, ambivalence, and ambiguity.

As the process of emotional re-education or the development of new behaviors is internalized, the emotions become more congruent, and a greater choice of behaviors is available. Psychotherapy is a process of being—a process of learning, tuning out the nonuseful, and adapting to changes.

◆ Current Psychotherapeutic Theories

The current psychotherapeutic theories are generally present and future oriented and focus on solutions, changes, and outcomes, rather than the "problem," in a collaborative atmosphere that empowers and recognizes client strengths. The therapist does not need to know about the past, except for successes, and changes are expected. Even though requiring a shorter length of time, the newer theories do not mean that less skill or training is needed (Table 15-2).

SOLUTION-FOCUSED THERAPY

In *solution-focused therapy*, the emphasis is not on the cause of the problem or what is continuing the problem, but on the belief that all individuals or families have the resources and are capable of solving their problems. It is a collaborative model with the therapist as a facilitator, rather than an all-knowing expert, and the final solutions are constructed by clients who know themselves and their situation better than the therapist.

Solution-focused therapy is particularly efficient because it focuses on clear, realistic goals; uses tasks; and develops client cooperation and efficacy. The emphasis is on "change talk" to build the expectation of change. It is action and future oriented and requires an extreme sensitivity to and awareness of client strengths to empower the client.

Walter and Peller[76] have defined 12 assumptions for a solution-focused approach. They were guided by the works of Insoo Kim Berg, Steve de Shazer, Milton Erickson, William O'Hanlon, and Michelle Weiner-Davis. These assumptions are used to guide decisions about therapy with clients, as differentiated from merely following a technique or procedure.[10,19,20,28,57,68,78] Solution-focused therapy has also been successful with children (Box 15-3).[43]

With decreased inpatient lengths of stay (ie, from 16 to 10 to 5 days or less), problem-solving interventions that require reasoning skills are not suitable for the more severely mentally ill client population. Simple, brief, solution-focused interventions are more effective when using what the clients bring with them to facilitate the clients' meeting their needs in such a way that they can make satisfactory lives for themselves. It is important to emphasize that the client possesses competence by saying, "Tell me how you dealt with a similar situation in the past." "I'm impressed with how you . . ." "You really do know how to. . . ." When working with feelings, the therapist can say, "When you are not feeling depressed, what will you be feeling instead?" It is important to use the client's words without rephrasing them.[52,75]

Table 15-2

Psychotherapeutic Theories (Selected)

Theorists (Selected)	Therapeutic Process	Role of Client and Therapist
Psychoanalytic (Sigmund Freud, Carl Jung, Milton Erickson, Erick Fromm, Frieda Fromm-Reichmann)	Explore unresolved early developmental conflicts and intrapsychic feelings, thoughts, and experiences that interfere with living a full life.	Client verbalizes all thoughts, dreams. Therapist is remote; he or she encourages and interprets thoughts in terms of conflict, transference, and resistance.
Behavioral (Ivan Pavlov, B.F. Skinner)	This educational process is based on the assumption that behaviors or responses are learned and may be relearned; positive or productive behaviors are reinforced.	Client selects and practices new behaviors. Therapist determines technique (relaxation therapy, assertiveness training, desensitization techniques).
Brief, solution focused (Insoo Berg, Steve de Shazer, William O'Hanlon, Michelle Weiner-Davis)	This cognitive process is based on solutions, past successes and exceptions, rather than causes; it has a present and future focus.	Client participates in development, evaluation, modification of plan. Therapist helps explore alternative behaviors.
Interpersonal (Hildegard Peplau, Harry Stack Sullivan)	Based on interactions between client and therapist in a safe setting, participant observations and reactions of the client and therapist are used.	Client shares anxieties, feelings. Therapist develops close empathic relationship that is used as a corrective interpersonal experience.
Existential (Victor Frankl, William Glasser, Fritz Perls, Carl Rogers)	Emphasis is on the courage to diverge, consider, survive a severe change in life. Client is encouraged to accept self and assume control of own behavior.	Client shares meaningful experiences, takes responsibility for behavior. Therapist helps clarify reality, recognize value of self, explore feelings.
Communication (Eric Berne, Richard Bandler, John Grinder)	Unclear communication causes behavior disruptions, incongruence in verbal and nonverbal messages.	Client looks at communication patterns and works at clarifying own and validating others' messages. Therapist identifies patterns and helps improve communication.
Cognitive (Aaron Beck, Albert Ellis, Mara Palazzoli)	Emphasis is on restructuring thought processes (the way people think about themselves) by changing the words that are used.	Client identifies distortions, learns more realistic responses. Therapist suggests new views of life, different behaviors, and responses.

Reframing, a key concept, is taking information or beliefs and putting them in a different perspective. For example, chances for success are greater for the client seen as cautious rather than paranoid, unhappy rather than depressed, needing to learn a new skill rather than having low self-esteem, beginning to do the same task differently.[4,16,19,71]

Huber[38] defines equilibrium therapy as a reframing or rebalancing that can increase alternatives and new beliefs, define a different reality, and let people experience themselves differently. The change in the meaning of behaviors is illustrated by being able to see the glass that is half full or half empty as half full and half empty. Things can both stay the same and change: "It seems that you are very angry about ______, and you are seeing a therapist as a way to resolve some of these feelings."

The concept of reframing can work for nurses who have reached an impasse in their search for professional growth. In this time of decreased staffing, it is easy for the psychiatric nurse to stay behind the wall, work on the chart, and spend very little time with the client. One study exploring this situation identified this behavior of nurses but did not identify any reason for it.[60] If psychiatric nurses are unhappy, desire a change, and believe that they have power, they can reframe their environment and role, using the solution-focused model. Nurses may be given this opportunity, or they may have to take the initiative and ask for its development.

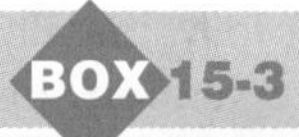

Assumptions and Steps in Using Solution-Focused Therapy

I. Investigate strengths—Use clients' talents to develop rapport and hope; believe that clients are cooperative and do work on solutions.
   a. How do you spend your days?
   b. What do you do well?
   c. What else do you do well?
   d. What are your hobbies or interests?

II. Problem construction—Use client language to construct solvable problems as clients are the experts and determine what to work on in therapy.
   a. What brings you here?
   b. What could I help you with?
   c. When clients say they want to know why they are having a "problem," say, "Would it be enough if the problem were to disappear, and you never understood why you had it?"
   d. What is the problem not about?
   e. What is the most important situation to which a solution must be found?

III. Investigation of solutions—The client is to leave with some sense of being able to handle the problem; taking one step at a time leads to greater changes.
   a. Usually between the time an appointment is made and the first session, people notice that things are already better.
   b. How did you get that to happen?
   What needs to happen for you to keep doing what worked? c.

IV. Exceptions—Nothing "always" happens. Exceptions to the situation, created by therapist and client, can then be used to create solutions.
   a. There are two kinds of exceptions:
      1) Deliberate—a conscious effort is made to do something different.
      2) Spontaneous—Nobody knows how it happened. This is a clue worthy of further investigation.
   b. What was different when you expected the problem to happen and it did not?
   c. What was different about times when the problem did not happen?

V. Goal investigation—Focusing on a positive solution and the future leads to a change in the desired direction; changing the meaning affects future interactions with involved others.
   a. Miracle question: "Suppose you go home tonight and while everyone is asleep, there is a miracle and the problems are resolved."
   b. How would you know the next day? What would be different?
   c. How would your spouse, child, parent, friend know?
   d. Who would be the first to notice?
   e. What would they do or say?

VI. Goals or tasks may be assigned.

Using the theory itself is suggested when teaching this approach to nursing staff. Questions to ask nursing staff include, "What do you think about the health care system today?" "What is already working for you?" "Does your nursing care (behavior) reflect what you know?"[78] Again, the focus is on what is simple and easy, knowing that often just the reframing of an idea, rather than the problem, results in changed feelings, actions, and behaviors (see Case Study 15-1).

COGNITIVE THERAPY

The client has the key to understanding and solving a psychological disturbance within the scope of his or her own awareness. For Beck, *cognitive therapy* suggests that the individual's problems are derived from certain distortions of reality based on erroneous premises and assumptions that originated in defective learning during the cognitive developmental phase. The goal of therapy is to help clients "unravel" their distorted thinking, to normalize rather than pathologize events ("Yes, it is expected that you would be upset," not horrified), and to learn alternative, more realistic ways to respond to their experiences. Because reality is a product of personal meanings that individuals create, it is important to teach people to hear themselves.[5-7,53] Cade and O'Hanlon[16] maintain that people are much more likely to be persuaded by self-generated arguments and counterarguments than by information received from others.

After experiencing the horror of World War II concentration camps, Frankl[25] developed logotherapy. Logotherapy is defined as the "will to meaning" (of life) in this world rather than within the psyche. This meaning is unique and specific to each person in that it must and can only be fulfilled by that person. "The last of the human freedoms" is the ability to "choose one's attitude in a given set of circumstances" (ie, how I describe it, how I feel about it, what it means to me).[25]

The goal of logotherapy is to counteract the anticipatory anxiety of phobias and fears by prescribing an excess of the unwanted behavior, a concept known as *paradoxical intention.* Paradoxical techniques, which are not easy to construct, are interventions in which the therapist seemingly promotes the continuation or worsening of the problem rather than its removal. Paradoxically, the therapist's directive to continue or worsen the problem can actually work to solve the problem.[58,68] For example, the person having trouble going to sleep is told not to try to fall asleep and to stay awake as long as possible, which is soon followed by sleep. To the man who stutters, the advice is, "You are going out this weekend and show people what a good stutterer you are, and you are going to fail in this, just as you have failed in previous years to speak properly." This works!

Palazzoli, from Milan, Italy, initially was known for the unique paradoxical intervention of "prescribing the symptom." According to this technique, therapists would argue against a change in behavior and explain to clients that "the most troublesome symptom was ultimately in the service of the family."[58] Palazzoli's treatment team achieved particular success with anorectic and schizophrenic children (clients) by using the *invariant prescription,* a fixed sequence of unusual directives that was used with every family. One of these directives requires parents to disappear without forewarning, have no contact with their children or anybody else in the extended family, and increase the time from a few hours to a whole weekend. Success is attributed to interruption of the counterproductive family triangulation patterns that existed in multiple areas of their lives.

Several studies indicate that cognitive therapy is effective in a number of different disorders. One study on the use of cognitive retraining with 16 clients with schizophrenia indicated some improved performance on the training tasks but no change in the basic deficits of information processing as measured by attention.[9] A study of 64 clients with panic disorders showed that 82% of those receiving cognitive therapy and 68% of those receiving relaxation training were classified as treatment responders; only 36% of the control group responded.[8]

Burns and coworkers'[15] cognitive-behavioral study with 115 depressed clients unexpectedly found that low-level depressions may have a stronger association with interpersonal problems than other forms of depression, such as major depressive episodes. Cognitive therapy seems to help depressed people by changing their views of life from pessimistic to optimistic and decreases subsequent relapses after the period of initial treatment has been completed. Although it is not clear that verbal behavior is a cause for change, there is a high probability that it produces stimuli that lead to different behaviors.[74,79]

Cognitive therapies also are now well established as a component for the treatment of a wide range of child behavior problems. A great deal of evidence suggests that deficits and distortions in cognitive processes play a role in disorders of affect and behavior in children and adults.[50,70] With only brief training for the therapists, a study in Great Britain indicated that cognitive therapy was more likely to be effective with chronically anxious clients than psychodynamic psychotherapy.[23] Salzinger[63] has expressed concern about the length of time a client will be able to maintain behavior changes that are accomplished by changing the thinking and automatic thoughts that lead to nonproductive, stereotypical behavior. However, clients can alter their self-instruction with enough variability to respond to additional changes in their lives.

RATIONAL-EMOTIVE THERAPY

Rational-emotive therapy (RET), designed by Ellis, encourages flexibility, minimizes emotional disturbance through rational thinking, and allows individuals to separate the emotionality from the illogical, inconsistent, and unworkable values with which they have indoctrinated themselves. Two primary beliefs included are global negative self-evaluations and low frustration tolerance or discomfort disturbance. Even though RET has grown and changed since it was first developed in 1958, it still includes the interrelatedness of cognitive, emotive, and behavioral processes; the importance of cognition in psychological problems; a humanistic view of the self; and the futility and danger of negative self-rating. "Dogmatic" beliefs are called "preferences", a change in wording that decreases intensity and increases options.[22,33]

A general format for RET is, "It would be nice if Jane would . . . ; maybe I can influence her to . . . , but that does not mean that she should not continue to. . . ."

Catastrophizing, a term applied to exaggerated thoughts, is when a hypothesis is equated with a fact (ie, a wart means cancer; a boyfriend or girlfriend arriving late for a date means he or she wants to end the relationship). "Irrational beliefs" in RET are comparable to "automatic thoughts" in cognitive therapy.[8] Using RET changes the way some experiences are reported; there is less reported anxiety and depression and hopefully less actual anxiety and depression.[32]

Rational-emotive therapy works for many different clinical situations, especially addictions and depressions,[7] psychoeducative programs with children, and self-help situations for lay people (especially for chemical addictions). Research is being done regarding the use of RET for migraine headaches[40]; however, it is difficult to pin down exactly what it includes as a therapeutic system. Even with mixed reviews in the literature about the effectiveness of RET, it is one of the most viable and widely used of the cognitive-behavior therapies (Box 15-4).[24,32,33]

BOX 15-4

Steps in Using Rational-Emotive Therapy

1. Identifying problem-causing situation or statement
2. Altering the usual irrational beliefs about the situation through repeated challenges to the thoughts and words
3. Changing the words and behavior
4. Changing philosophy with the following beliefs:
    a. I create my own psychological disturbances.
    b. I can significantly change these disturbances.
    c. Emotional and behavior disturbances come from irrational beliefs.
    d. I can discriminate between rational and irrational beliefs.
    e. I dispute the irrational ones through logical, scientific reasoning.
    f. I am working toward internalizing new, rational beliefs.

TREATING DUAL DIAGNOSIS: CONCURRENT CHEMICAL DEPENDENCY AND PSYCHIATRIC DISORDER

The *dual diagnosis* of chemical dependency and psychiatric disorder is common: Approximately 50% to 80% of people in drug treatment programs have psychiatric difficulties; 50% of psychiatric emergency room visits also have a substance abuse component; and 60% to 80% of people in psychiatric inpatient programs and 30% to 40% of people in psychiatric outpatient programs have a substance abuse disorder.[48] Nearly all the psychiatric syndromes can be precipitated by the use of an addictive substance.[18]

For centuries, alcoholism was seen as a "weakness." There has been an increasing belief in the disease concept for the last 100 years. Today genetic markers have been identified that indicate that some people have a predisposition to develop an addiction because of altered processes in the metabolism of alcohol.

Along with the current biological information, there is also a psychodynamic perspective that focuses on understanding addictions as adaptive attempts to repair self-regulatory deficiencies (the ability to maintain abstinence) and to alleviate emotional suffering. The idea of alleviating emotional suffering was included in Freud's idea of regressive infantile autoeroticism (masturbation) that was first experienced as pleasure and then as unpleasure; this is the cycle of most addictions. A second view is that unconscious aggression and sadism are important factors in developing an addiction; the addiction is seen as a coping mechanism that is primarily defensive.[48]

People often are motivated to escape from aversive self-awareness through the artificial means of drugs or alcohol and by decreasing attention and focus to sensory stimuli through cognitive narrowing. Shutting out painful self-awareness improves the mood and health problems that were being intentionally inhibited. Seemingly against the will, being stressed, anxious, or depressed leads to an increase in the behaviors people are trying to eliminate (eg, food, alcohol, self-injury). Development of skills to cope with negative emotional states, especially threats to self-esteem, may be the single most important factor in successful treatment of addictions.[37]

Szapocznik pioneered one-person family therapy when there was only one willing participant, the identified client. With the drug-abusing adolescent, this form of therapy was more effective in symptom reduction and improved overall family functioning; the results continued for 6 to 12 months after therapy ended. A later study indicated that the families deteriorated even though the adolescents improved.[46]

Managed care organizations are demanding integrated programs that address chemical dependency and mental health issues. Clients with secondary substance abuse disorders may be using alcohol and drugs to medicate psychiatric symptoms; the chemically dependent client also may have a severe depression related to the toxic effects of alcohol on the brain and hopelessness from repeated failures to stop drinking or using drugs. For the dual recovery client, an effective treatment program could be designed with the use of the biopsychosocial assessment grid, which integrates the physical, psychological, and social symptoms of chemical dependency with mental disorders, personality disorders, and situational life problems. The cognitive behavioral and brief therapy models are particular useful in these situations.[31]

◆ Future Considerations

The America of today has become diverse in the varieties of cultures represented. Therefore, it is imperative that psychiatric nursing of the future be culturally cognizant of all the people, open to the different lifestyles, and ready to understand and accept various health-related beliefs.

All methods of psychotherapy are effective with any given individual part of the time. Therefore, the skill (or serendipity) is to match the client with a therapist able to use the method most effective for that individual. Regardless of the conceptual base, the value of the psychotherapeutic process is determined by the client.

◆ Chapter Summary

This chapter has discussed how feelings, attitudes and behaviors are changed through individual psychotherapy. Some of the important points discussed in the chapter are as follows:

1. People choose to participate in a therapeutic process to facilitate changes, resolve interpersonal issues, and develop self-understanding.
2. The level of psychotherapy—supportive, re-educative, and reconstructive, will depend on the degree of severity and the discomfort level of the client.
3. As individual psychotherapy develops, the client and therapist will discuss some historical information, current challenges, past successes, feelings, needs, and goals.
4. Because of their objectivity, perspective, and specialized knowledge, therapists generally can be more effective than family or friends in facilitating the client's work with challenges and growth.
5. The client and therapist need to communicate clearly their expectations of each other and of the therapeutic process.
6. The important concepts of psychotherapy, insight, repression, resistance, transference, and reworking are explored and applied to client involvement in various methods of individual psychotherapy.
7. Current issues in individual therapy include solution-focused therapy, cognitive therapy, rational emotive therapy, dual diagnosis, and economic concerns.

Review Questions

Erica Brown is experiencing difficulty after the loss of her fiance in an automobile accident involving an intoxicated driver. She is having trouble sleeping and concentrating on her work and frequently argues with her family, especially her father, who "drinks too much."

1. Erica has an appointment with a nurse who has first suggested that
   - **A.** her family is insensitive to her needs and should come in for joint therapy.
   - **B.** a change in diet will be helpful in increasing sleep time.
   - **C.** responsibilities of client and therapist be outlined, goals determined, possible approaches and solutions discussed and evaluated, and a suggested time frame for therapy identified.
   - **D.** methods to increase concentration be practiced.
2. Erica is very pleased with the progress of the sessions and invites the therapist to attend a play with her. The therapist responds:
   - **A.** "That is very thoughtful of you, and I have been wanting to see that play; what time does it start?"
   - **B.** "I already have plans for that date, but thank you."

C. "My spouse would get upset if I attended that play with you."
D. "Thank you for the invitation. Our relationship is defined as therapeutic and can only be effective when we attend to the 'business of therapy' rather than social activities."

3. Erica's therapist was able to identify specific body movements with different feelings and provide feedback immediately; this is an example of the following therapist:
   A. Carl Rogers and congruence
   B. Milton Erickson and total presence
   C. Carl Jung and the meaning of symbols
   D. Sigmund Freud and dream interpretation
4. Erica initially told the therapist that she had come because she knew the therapist would solve all her problems. The therapist's best response is:
   A. "I have been successful in helping people in the past."
   B. "You will be able to solve all your problems better than I can."
   C. "We will also need to have your family come in for a joint session."
   D. "This will be a joint effort, coupled with your courage and honesty."
5. Late for her third appointment with no explanation, Erica came in, sat off center in the chair, and angrily said to the therapist, "That shirt looks like something my father would wear!" This is an example of
   A. acting out and transference.
   B. countertransference and interpretation.
   C. ambiguity and acting out.
   D. translating and working through.
6. Erica and her therapist were able to resolve her issues by defining her beliefs about responsibility, identifying the irrational parts, and believing that she could make changes. This is an example of
   A. cognitive therapy.
   B. rational-emotive therapy.
   C. critical thinking therapy.
   D. solution-focused therapy.

◆ References

1. Ainsworth MD, Blehar MD, Waters E, Wass S: Patterns of Attachment: Assessed in the Strange Situation and Home. Hillsdale, NJ, Lawrence Erlbaum, 1978
2. Arieti S: Handbook of Psychiatry, vol. V, 2d ed. New York, Wiley & Sons, 1975
3. Arieti S, Chrzanowsk G: New Dimensions in Psychiatry: A World View. New York, Wiley & Sons, 1975
4. Bandler R, Grinder J: The Structure of Magic I. Palo Alto, Science and Behavior Books, 1975
5. Beck AT: Cognitive Therapy and the Emotional Disorders. New York, Penguin Books, International Universities Press, 1979
6. Beck AT: Cognitive Therapy: Past, Present, and Future. J Consult Clin Psychol 61 (2): 194–198, 1993
7. Beck AT, Wright FD, Newman CF, Liese BS: Cognitive Therapy of Substance Abuse. New York, The Guiford Press, 1993
8. Beck JG, Stanley MA, Baldwin LE, Deagle EA III, Averill PM: Comparison of Cognitive Therapy and Relaxation Training for Panic Disorder. J Consult Clin Psychol 62 (4): 818–826, 1994
9. Benedict RH, Harris AI, Markow T, McCormick JA, et al: Effects of Attention Training on Information Processing in Schizophrenia. Schizophr Bull 20 (3): 537–546, 1994
10. Berg IK: Solution-Focused Approach to Family Based Services. Milwaukee, Brief Family Therapy Center, 1990
11. Bowlby J: Attachment, vol. I. New York, Basic Books, 1969
12. Bowlby J: Separation, Anxiety and Anger, vol. II. New York, Basic Books, 1973
13. Bowlby J: Loss, Sadness and Depression, vol. III. New York, Basic Books, 1980
14. Bradshaw J: The Family A Revolutionary Way of Self-Discovery. Deerfield Beach, Health Communications, 1988
15. Burns DD, Sayers SL, Moras K: Intimate Relationships and Depression: Is There a Causal Connection? J Consult Clin Psychol 62 (5): 1033–1043, 1994
16. Cade B, O'Hanlon WH: A Brief Guide to Brief Therapy. New York, WW Norton, 1993
17. Christensen AP, Oei TP: The Efficacy of Cognitive Behavior Therapy in Treating Premenstrual Dysphoric Changes. J Affective Disord 33 (1): 57–63, 1995
18. Dackis CA, Gold MS: Psychopathology Resulting from Substance Abuse. In Gold MS, Caby ARE (eds): Dual Diagnosis in Substance Abuse, pp. 205-220. New York, Marcel Decker, 1991
19. DeShazer S: Keys to Solution in Brief Therapy. New York, WW Norton, 1985
20. DeShazer S: Words Were Originally Magic. New York, WW Norton, 1994
21. Dollard J, Doob LW, Miller N, Mowrer OH, Sears R: Frustration and Aggression. New Haven, Yale University Press, 1939
22. Dryden W, Bond FW: Reason and Emotion in Psychotherapy: Albert Ellis. Br J Psychiatry 165 (1): 131–135, 1994
23. Durham RC, Murphy T, Allan T, Richard K, et al: Cognitive Therapy, Analytic Psychotherapy and Anxiety Management Training for Generalised Anxiety Disorder. Br J Psychiatry 165 (3): 315–323, 1994
24. Ellis A: Reflections on Rational-Emotive Therapy. J Consult Clin Psychol 61 (2): 199–201, 1993
25. Frankl VE: Man's Search for Meaning An Introduction to Logotherapy. New York, Washington Square Press, 1969
26. Fromm E: Greatness and Limitations of Freud's Thought. New York, Meridan, Penquin, 1980
27. Fromm-Reichmann F: Principles of Intensive Psychotherapy. Chicago, University of Chicago Press, 1950

28. Furman B, Ahola T: Solution Talk Hosting Therapeutic Conversations. New York, WW Norton, 1992
29. Glover E: Freud or Jung, Forward by Anderson JW. Evanston, Northwestern University Press, 1991 (London, Allen & Unwin, c1950)
30. Goffman I: Behavior in Public Places. New York, The Free Press, 1963
31. Gorski TT: Trend Watch. Treatment Today 7 (3): 40–41, 1995
32. Gossette RL, O'Brien RM: The Efficacy of Rational Emotive Therapy in Adults: Clinical Fact or Psychometric Artifact? J Behav Ther Exp Psychiatry 23 (1): 9–24, 1992
33. Haaga Da, Davison GC: An Appraisal of Rational-Emotive Therapy. J Consult Clin Psychol 61 (2): 215–220, 1993
34. Hannah G: Jung: His Life and Work. Boston, Shambhala, 1991
35. Harlow HF, Zimmerman RR: Affectional Response in the Infant Monkey. Science 130: 421–432, 1959
36. Haven RA: The Wisdom of Milton Erickson, vol. II. New York, Irvington Publishers, 1992
37. Heatherton TF, Renn RJ: Stress and the Disinhibition of Behavior. Mind/Body Medicine 1 (2): 72–81, 1995
38. Huber, CH: Encompassing Individual and Family Treatment: Equilibrium Therapy. Family Counseling 2 (1): 1–15, 1994
39. Jeffers S: Feel the Fear and Do it Any Way: New York, Fawcett Columbine, 1987
40. Johnson NB: Rational-Emotive Therapy in the Management of Migraine Headache. J Am Acad Nurse Pract 6 (5): 201–206, 1994
41. Jung CG: Memories, Dreams, Reflections. Recorded and edited by Jaffe A, Revised Edition. New York, Random House, 1965
42. Kirkby RJ: Changes in Premenstrual Symptoms and Irrational Thinking Following Cognitive-Behavioral Coping Skills Training. J Consult Clin Psychol 62 (5): 1026–1032, 1994
43. Klar H, Coleman WL: Brief Solution-Focused Strategies for Behavioral Pediatrics. Pediatr Clin North Am 42 (1): 131–141, 1995
44. Laing RD: The Voice of Experience. New York, Pantheon Books, 1982
45. Landeen J, Bryne C, Brown B: Exploiting the Lived Experiences of Psychiatric Nursing Students Through Self-reflective Journals. J Adv Nurs 21 (5): 878–885, 1995
46. Leitch C: A Clinician's Researcher: Jose Szapocznik. The Family Therapy Networker 17 (5): 77–82, 1993
47. Lerner: The Assault on Psychotherapy. The Family Therapy Networker 19 (5): 44–48, 1995
48. Lowinson JH, Ruiz P, Millman RB, Langrod JG (eds): Substance Abuse: A Comprehensive Textbook. Baltimore, Williams & Wilkins, 1992
49. Mahler MS, Bergman A, Pine F: The Psychological Birth of the Human Infant. New York, Basic Books, 1975
50. Mahoney J: Introduction to Special Section: Cognitive Therapies. J Consult Clin Psychol 61 (2): 187–193, 1993
51. Maslow AH: The Need to Know and The Fear of Knowing. J Gen Psychol 68: 111–124, 1963
52. Mason WH, Breen RY, Whipple WR: Solution-Focused Therapy and Inpatient Psychiatric Nursing. J Psychosoc Nurs Ment Health Serv 32 (1): 46–49, 1994
53. Meichenbaum D: Changing Conceptions of Cognitive Behavior Modification: Retrospect and Prospect. J Consult Clin Psychol 61 (2): 202–204, 1993
54. Miller A: The Drama of the Gifted Child. New York, Basic Books, 1979
55. Montgomery CL, Webster D: Caring, Curing, and Brief Therapy: A Model for Nurse-Psychotherpay. Arch Psych Nursing 8 (5): 291–297, 1994
56. Nerin WF: Family Reconstruction Long Day's Journey into Light. New York, WW Norton, 1986
57. O'Hanlon WH, Weiner-Davis M: In Search of Solutions. New York, WW Norton, 1989
58. Palazzoli MS, Boscolo L, Cecchin G, Prata G: Paradox and Counterparadox. New York, Jason Aronson, 1978
59. Pilette PC, Berck CB, Achber LC: Therapeutic Management of Helping Boundaries. J Psychosoc Nurs 33 (1): 40–47, 1995
60. Porter S: The Determinants of Psychiatric Nursing Practice: A Comparison of Sociological Perspectives. J Adv Nurs 18: 1559–1566, 1993
61. Rogers C: On Becoming A Person. Boston, Houghton-Mifflin, 1961
62. Satir V, Banmen J, Gerber J, Gomori M: The Satir Model, Family Therapy and Beyond. Palo Alto, Science and Behavior Books, 1991
63. Salzinger K: Cognitive Therapy: A Misunderstanding of BF Skinner. J Behav Ther Exp Psychiatry 23 (1): 3–8, 1992
64. Saul LJ: The Childhood Emotional Pattern and Psychodynamic therapy. New York, Van Norstrand, 1980
65. Schaef AW: Beyond Therapy, Beyond Science. San Francisco, Harper Collins, 1992
66. Scheflen AE, Scheflen A: Body Language and Social Order. Englewood Cliffs, NJ, Prentice Hall, 1972
67. Scott J: Cognitive Therapy. Br J Psychiatry 165 (1): 126–130, 1994
68. Simon RS: One on One: Conversations with the Shapers of Family Therapy. Washington DC, New York, The Family Therapy Network and Guilford Press, 1992
69. Sines D: The Arrogance of Power: A Reflection on Contemporary Mental Health Nursing Practice. J Adv Nurs 20 (5): 894–903, 1994
70. Spence SH: Cognitive Therapy with Children and Adolescents: From Theory to Practice. J Child Psychol Psychiatry 35 (7): 1191–1228, 1994
71. Stiles WB, Shapiro DA: Verbal Exchange Structure of Brief Psychodynamic-Interpersonal and Cognitive-Behavioral Psychotherapy. J Consult Clin Psychol 63 (1): 15–27, 1995
72. Szasz T: The Myth of Mental Illness. New York, Harper & Row, 1974
73. Szasz T: The Myth of Psychotherapy: Mental Healing as Religion, Rhetoric, and Repression. Syracuse, Syracuse University Press, 1988
74. Teasdale JD, Segal Z, Williams JM: How Does Cognitive Therapy Prevent Depressive Relapse and Why Should At-

tentional Control (Mindfulness) Training Help? Behav Res Ther 33 (1): 25–39, 1995

75. Tuyn LK: Solution-Oriented Therapy and Rogerian Nursing Science: An Integrated Approach. Arch Psych Nurs 6 (2): 83–89, 1992
76. Walter JL, Peller JE: Becoming Solution-Focused in Brief Therapy. New York, Brunner/Mazel, 1992
77. Weber RL, Costikyan N, Fales H, Morgan S: An Observation and Group Dynamics Model for Teaching Psychoanalytic Psychotherapy. Academic Psychiatry 19 (1): 12–21, 1995
78. Webster DC, Vaughn K, Marinez R: Introducing Solution-Focused Approaches to Staff in Inpatient Psychiatric Settings. Arch Psychiatr Nurs 8 (4): 254–261, 1994
79. Weissman MM: Psychotherapy in the Maintenance Treatment of Depression. Br J Psychiatry Suppl 26: 42–50, 1994
80. Wylie MS: The Shadow of Doubt. The Family Therapy Networker 17 (5): 18–29, 1993
81. Wylie MS: The New Visionaries. The Family Therapy Networker 19 (5): 20–29, 1995
82. Yapko MD: The Seductions of Memory. The Family Therapy Networker 17 (5): 31–37, 1993

Groups and Group Therapy

Barbara G. Tunley-Crenshaw

16

No man is an island, entire of itself; every man is a piece of the continent, a part of the main; . . . any man's death diminishes me, because I am involved in mankind; and therefore never send to know for whom the bell tolls; it tolls for thee.

John Donne, **Devotions** ***XVII***

We live and work in groups: Each of us is born into a family, we attend school with groups of our peers, enter into friendship and work-related groups, and establish our own groups of family or significant others. In psychiatric-mental health and other areas of health care, nurses interact with groups of students, faculty, professional colleagues, clients, and the client's family. An understanding of group dynamics and their application is essential to effective functioning in our personal and professional lives.

The family may be defined as the individual's primary group. The characteristics of this primary group influence how the individual is socialized into future groups and how various roles within groups are adopted. This chapter discusses group process, dynamics, theory, norms, roles, decision making, and outcomes. It examines various types of groups and the advantages and disadvantages of group therapy. An overview of theoretical frameworks for group therapy is presented, including a discussion of Rogerian, gestalt, transactional analysis (TA), and T (training) groups. The chapter focuses on nursing intervention through the media of group process therapy.

Learning Objectives

On completion of this chapter, you should be able to accomplish the following:

1. *Identify the characteristics of a group.*
2. *Explain group norms and how they are developed and enforced.*
3. *Compare styles of group leadership and their effects on group members' functioning.*
4. *Describe the process of structuring a group.*
5. *Define three major categories of group roles.*
6. *Discuss the purposes, advantages, and disadvantages of group therapy.*
7. *Discuss the therapeutic factors of group therapy.*
8. *Compare the various types of therapy and self-help or growth groups.*
9. *Describe the stages of group development.*
10. *Apply therapeutic interventions to groups of clients.*
11. *Identify process communication in group behavior.*

◆ Group Process

WHAT IS A GROUP?

A group is three or more people with related goals. These goals are influenced by many factors—intrapersonal and interpersonal needs, the physical environment, and the unique interaction of the group.

The physical environment is one factor that affects group development. For example, the physical environment or climate in some countries is so severe that the survival of the individual depends on relationships with other individuals. The individuals form relationship bonds that develop into groups. These groups develop structures, characteristics, and roles. The further creation of systems and subsystems leads to the development of more complex societies that display certain characteristics called *culture.*

CHARACTERISTICS OF GROUPS

The following are characteristics of groups:

1. Size of the group
2. Homogeneity or heterogeneity of group members
3. Stability of the group
4. Degree of cohesiveness, or bonding power, between members
5. Climate of the group (eg, warm, friendly, cold, aloof)
6. Conformity to group norms
7. Degree of agreement with the leader's and the group's norms
8. Ability to deal with members' infractions
9. Goal-directedness and task orientation of the group's work

TYPES OF GROUPS

Groups may be primary or secondary, formal or informal. Members of *primary groups* have face-to-face contact. They have boundaries, norms, and explicit and implicit interdependent roles. An example of a primary group is a family.

Secondary groups are usually larger and more impersonal than primary groups. Members of secondary groups do not have the relationship bonds or emotional ties of members of a primary group. An example of a secondary group is a political party or a business.

A *formal group* has structure and authority. Authority in a formal group usually emanates from above and interaction in the group is usually limited. A faculty meeting is an example of a formal group. *Informal groups* provide much of a person's education and contribute greatly to his or her cultural values. The members of an informal group do not depend on each other, such as in friendship groups and hobby groups.

GROUP NORMS

A *group norm* is the development, over time, of a pattern of interaction within a group to which certain behavioral expectations are attached. Group norms affect the scope and functioning of a group. Norms also help to structure role expectations and provide sanctions, taboos, and reference power to the group.

To explain group norms, consider the example of a

nursing team meeting designed to discuss client care planning and communication among the nursing staff. A role expectation norm is that the team leader will chair the meeting. A membership norm is that the members will be on time and will possibly sit in certain places. There may be a *formalized norm* called an agenda of the meeting, which states that communication among nursing staff members will occur before the discussion to plan client care. Other group norms may be universal with regard to the task role of one member, such as the role of the secretary who records the minutes of the meeting. Group members who present their clients' history and assessment accurately, clearly, and with organization receive sanction. A group taboo is to fall asleep and snore while another member is talking. When a group member falls asleep and snores during meetings, especially if this occurs numerous times, the member is viewed as a deviant. A deviant may eventually be isolated by the group. Members neither speak nor listen to him or her when he or she speaks. They may physically isolate the deviant by not sitting next to him or her. Therefore, punishment, formal or informal, is meted out to the deviant along with criticism.

Norms exert a controlling element over groups by setting the boundaries of group activities. To promote the growth and stimulation of group members, groups must learn to change their norms when they no longer function for the group. A group is more creative if each member becomes a so-called change agent for norms no longer needed (Nursing Care Plan 16-1).

GROUP LEADERSHIP

To become an effective group leader, the nurse must understand the concepts of leadership and their accompanying forces, scope, and limitations. The three concepts of power, influence, and authority have an impact on leadership. *Power* is the perceived ability to control appropriate reward, therefore lending *influence* to the leader. The nurse leader gains *authority* through influence, power, and knowledge or expertise. The leader also understands that there are effective ways of using authority and decides to what extent he or she will expand or limit this authority.

The effective leader also decides to what extent the authority will be autocratic (centralized) or democratic (decentralized). The leader reaches this decision, in part, according to the type of group. For example, the leader may relinquish authority readily in a training group. The purpose of the T group (or training group) is to improve the group members' ability to communicate or relate to others in the group. The members, however, generally possess a certain degree of knowledge and experience in relating to others and are therefore capable of imparting their skills to other group members.

In groups where members are likely to exhibit high degrees of personality disorganization and faulty communication and interpersonal skills, the leader may exercise centralized authority. In other types of therapy groups, such as gestalt groups, which deal with the here and now and whose members are generally healthy, the distribution of power within the group may depend on the age and emotional maturity of the group members.

Styles of Group Leadership

Leadership styles are influenced by several factors, including the philosophy of treatment; personality of the leader; traits, characteristics, and purpose of the group; and degree of mental, emotional, or cognitive impairment of the group members.

The nurse group leader alters the style of group leadership according to the demands of the therapeutic situation. The three basic styles of group leadership are autocratic, democratic, and laissez-faire.

An *autocratic* leader is one who exercises significant authority and control over group members; rarely, if ever, seeks or uses input from the group; and does not encourage participation or interaction from the group.

In some circumstances, such as in emergencies, the autocratic style of leadership may be the most effective; it conserves time and energy and dictates roles and responsibilities to members. On the other hand, constant use of an autocratic leadership style may cause hostility, scapegoating behavior, dependence on the leader, and limitation of growth potential for group members.

The *democratic* style of leadership encourages group interaction and participation in group problem solving and decision making. A democratic group leader values the input and feedback of each group member, seeks spontaneous and honest interaction among members of the group, and creates an atmosphere in which members are rewarded for their contributions. The group's opinions are solicited, and the group's work is tailored to their common goals. A group with a democratic leadership style may require more time and effort than an autocratic group to accomplish its goals; however, the group's efforts are more productive and cohesive and instill in members a sense of participation in decision making.

In a *laissez-faire* style of leadership, group members are free to operate as they choose. This style of group leadership may be effective if the members are highly knowledgeable, task oriented, and motivated. On the other hand, the laissez-faire approach is time consuming and often inefficient in the accomplishment of group tasks.

(text continues on page 263)

Nursing Care Plan 16-1

Interventions in Group Process and Group Therapy

Group Problem

Fear of authority, resulting in timid, hostile, aggressive, or withdrawn behavior

Outcome

Group members will deal with authority directly and openly.

Intervention	Rationale
Use nonverbal and verbal communication techniques; listen to and encourage the client to share and explore feelings.	The nurse-therapist functions as a role model of healthy communication.
Reassure the client that the nurse-therapist will not respond punitively to the expression of feelings.	An initial task of the group is to deal with and work through authority issues to facilitate the group's progress.
Respond in an understanding manner when the client expresses feelings (even when they are hostile).	Acceptance of feelings allows group members to acknowledge and own their feelings.

Evaluation

Group members discuss their views and feelings about authority.

Group Problem

Initial anxiety in a group, displayed by silence, fidgeting, nervous movement, and selective hearing

Outcome

Group members' anxiety will be lessened so they can function more effectively in a group.

Intervention	Rationale
Give "strokes" for positive interaction. Help the client establish a role in the group, one related to the client's skills.	Reinforcing group members' interaction increases their continuing interaction and promotes the development of group roles.
Share with the client that discomfort in the initial stage of group development is not uncommon. Meet the client's dependency needs.	Reassurance and meeting group members' dependency needs allows them to feel safe in the group.

Evaluation

Group members respond to leader and other members in a productive manner.

Group Problem

Hidden agenda

Outcome

Group members will express communication and act openly.

Intervention	Rationale
Identify the souce of individual and group anxiety causing the hidden agenda.	Hidden agendas sabotage the group's progress, create anxiety in members, and may cause members to form subgroups or leave the group.
Explore the hidden agenda with the group and its meaning and effect on the group's functioning.	

continued

Nursing Care Plan 16-1 *(Continued)*

Evaluation

Group members express their feelings about the issues being discussed.

Nursing Diagnosis of Group Problem

Subgrouping

Outcome

Unproductive subgroups will be eliminated.

Intervention	Rationale
Establish clarifying goals and purpose of the group (thereby lessening the group's anxiety and aiding in elimination of subgroups).	Clarification allows group members to establish their group roles that aid in problem-solving.
Direct subgroup interest toward the goals of the group, thereby lessening subgroup preoccupation with outside themes.	A sense of belonging to the group increases members' participation and furthers their comfort in role-taking.

Evaluation

Members discuss content related to group topics in the group.

Group Problem

Deviant behavior

Outcome

Members' deviant behavior will be modified.

Intervention

Identify deviant behavior and discuss it with the client.

Identify sources of discomfort in the environment that affect the client.

Explore with the client whether or not he or she identifies the behavior as deviant.

Help members of the group identify deviant behavior.

Help the client explore how this behavior affects his or her relationship in the group.

Use group pressure to help the deviate member change or conform to group norms.

Help the group identify which behavior is destructive and which might foster group growth.

Rationale

Dealing directly with deviant behavior helps the group learn effective ways to problem-solve.

The leader explores the deviant behavior first with the client and then with the group as a whole to prevent its interference with group process.

Evaluation

Group members take on task roles and building and maintenance roles, and less individual roles in the group.

Group Problem

Overdependency

Outcome

Members will demonstrate appropriate independence in accomplishing the group's task.

continued

Nursing Care Plan 16-1 *(Continued)*

Intervention	Rationale
Provide a leadership void to make the client more independent.	Overdependency prevents the group from exploring and problem-solving.
Explore the client's feelings about dependency and how it affects the group's growth.	Giving the client an independent role in the group allows the client to explore, achieve, and receive reinforcement.
Share specific techniques with the client, such as a list of the group's tasks, and request that the client volunteer for the job for which he or she is most suited.	

Evaluation

Group members function comfortably and effectively in an independent fashion; group does not disintegrate in leader's absence.

Group Problem

Resistance to therapy (*eg,* grunting, moaning, staring into space, overresponding to situations, changing the subject, absence from group

Outcome

Members will demonstrate increased acceptance of, and participation in, therapy.

Intervention	Rationale
Explore resistance behavior with client.	Some degree of resistance is common in every group.
Confront the client with his or her actions and behavior, using an understanding approach.	To promote individual and group progress, resistance must be confronted.

Evaluation

Members will discuss problems and feelings in place of acting out.

Group Problem

Termination of the group, resulting in increased anxiety and self-defeating behavior

Outcome

Members will accept group termination and learn from termination experience.

Intervention	Rationale
Help the client identify what he or she has accomplished while a member of the group.	Learning process in the group depends on the ability to express feelings and evaluate members' achievements at termination.
Help the client work through feelings of loss during termination (*i.e.,* feelings of anger, depression, euphoria, rejection).	
Help the client express both positive and negative feelings about the group and evaluate the group experience realistically.	
Plan a termination activity that allows expression of group members' feelings.	
Lessen intensity of group interaction as group nears termination.	

Evaluation

Members explore achievements accomplished in the group and feelings related to termination.

Decision Making

Decision making is a necessary component of leadership, power, influence, authority, and delegation of authority. In formal groups, specific guidelines determine which decisions will be made by the leader and which decisions will be decentralized, that is, delegated to group members.

The ability to make effective decisions depends on the group's knowledge of the subject, its ability to choose appropriate methods to solve problems, its ability to test and evaluate problem solving and decision making after a decision has been put to the test, and its maturity and ability to reverse or modify a decision that has proven to be unwise, unfair, or otherwise unacceptable.

Decisions may be made by consensus, majority vote, or minority decision. In a *consensus,* all members of the group agree on a decision. Although consensus may prove to be time consuming and costly, especially in a large group, it gives more satisfaction to the total group. The democratic leader uses consensus whenever possible. *Majority vote* is a form of decision making in which the issue is decided by the larger number of group members. This method is often used by democratic leadership when it is not possible to reach a consensus. A *minority decision* may be formulated by a self-delegated subgroup or a group appointed as a subcommittee to explore the situation in greater depth and reach a decision.

Structuring the Group

The group leader is instrumental in establishing and maintaining cohesiveness in the group. The leader also selects and orients new group members in beginning and continuing groups. An effective leader ensures that the structuring process for the group defines group norms, clarifies expectations, sets standards for group performance, and maintains cohesiveness as new members are introduced into the group. The leader discusses some of these issues with new members before introducing them to the group. An example of such a discussion follows.

> Leader: Jane, welcome. I am Ms. C., the group leader. I always meet with new members to share with them the goals and expectations of the group. (pause) The group will have eight members, including you. We will meet from 1 to 2 PM each day in the blue room. Members will enter and leave the group as their behavior and needs change. (pause)
>
> Jane: What are we expected to do?
>
> Leader: Group members are expected to share their problems and their feelings about those problems with other members of the group.
>
> Jane: Is that all?
>
> Leader: No. It is also my expectation that group members will discover techniques of problem solving through exploring these problems and feelings and that eventually, when members learn to relate more effectively to each other, they will transfer these newly acquired skills to other relationships.
>
> Jane: That sounds difficult and frightening.
>
> Leader: Changing and growing have a certain amount of pain.

The leader structures the group by determining its size, homogeneity of group members, and leadership style. The group's purpose and goals define its scope, limitation, and desired accomplishments. The group leader's responsibilities to members include ensuring the psychological safety of group members, establishing and maintaining group norms, role modeling relationship skills, and commenting on group process. To receive gratification from group membership, members must participate by introspecting, self-disclosing, nurturing others, expressing feelings, and contributing to the maintenance of the group.

ROLES IN GROUPS

The functions of group leaders and members are interdependent. Member roles can enhance the effectiveness of a group leader and vice versa. Roles observed in groups are categorized as group task roles, group building and maintenance roles, and individual roles.

Group task roles identify group problems and select methods to solve those problems. Problem solving helps the group to reach its goal or mission. Some examples of group task roles include the initiator-contributor, who suggests or proposes to the group new ideas or different ways of regarding the group problem or goal; the information seeker, who asks for clarification; the information giver, who offers facts or generalizations that are considered authoritative or who shares personal experiences in relation to the group problems; the coordinator, who shows or clarifies how ideas can work; the orienter, who keeps the group on target by defining where the group is in relation to its goal; and the recorder, who is the group's memory and writes down productive discussion and group decisions.

Group building and maintenance roles are oriented toward the functioning of the group as a whole. They alter or maintain the group's way of working to strengthen, regulate, and perpetuate the group. Some examples of group building and maintenance roles include the encourager, who given acceptance to the contributions of others; the harmonizer, who reconciles differences between group members; the gatekeeper, who facilitates the contributions of others, thereby keeping communication open by encouraging remarks about these contributions; the group observer, who notes what is occurring in the group and feeds it back to the group with an evaluation or interpretation of the group's procedure; and the follower, who goes along with the ideas of other members, assuming more of an audience role.

Individual roles are those that meet only the needs of the group member, not of the group. They hamper rather than enhance group functioning. They support individual needs and goals not group needs and goals. Some examples of individual roles include the aggressor, who deflates the status of individual and group accomplishment; the blocker, who resists progress by arguing or disagreeing beyond reason; the recognition seeker, who calls attention to himself or herself through boasting and pointing out achievements; the play person, who horses around, demonstrating lack of involvement; and the dominator, who asserts authority and superiority in manipulating the group or certain members of the group.

All of these roles are observed in group behavior. Individually oriented behavior, which often grows out of anxiety, distracts from and temporarily stymies the group and its progress, whereas task, maintenance, and building roles promote group growth and productivity.

◆ Group Therapy

PURPOSES

One of the purposes of group psychotherapy is to intervene in mentally disordered behavior, thinking, and feeling. Group therapy offers multiple stimuli to reveal, examine, and resolve distortions in interpersonal relationships. The purpose of a group is related to its goals and expected outcomes. For example, a training group's purpose is to help members improve their present styles of relating to others. An individual needing to develop or heighten these skills would join a training group instead of a psychotherapy group.

ADVANTAGES AND DISADVANTAGES

Group therapy as a form of treatment for psychiatric-mental health clients has advantages and disadvantages. The advantages of group therapy include the following:

1. A greater number of clients can be treated in group therapy, making the method cost-effective.
2. Members profit by hearing other members discuss their problems. This discussion decreases members' feelings of isolation, alienation, and uniqueness, which encourages them to share feelings and problems.
3. Group therapy provides an opportunity for clients to explore their specific styles of communication in a safe atmosphere where they can receive feedback and undergo change.
4. Members learn multiple ways of solving a problem from other group members, and group exploration may help them discover new ways of solving a problem.
5. Members learn about the functional roles of individuals in a group. Sometimes a member shares the responsibility as the cotherapist. Members become culture carriers.
6. The group provides for its members' understanding, confrontation, and identification with more than one individual. The member gains a reference group.

There are also disadvantages of group therapy:

1. An individual's privacy may be violated, for example, when a conversation shared within the group is repeated outside of the group. This behavior obstructs confidentiality and hampers complete and honest participation in a group.
2. Clients may experience difficulty in exposing themselves to a group or believe that they lack the skills to communicate effectively in a group. Some clients may use these factors as resistance; others may be reluctant to expose themselves to the group because they do not want to change.
3. Group therapy is not a helpful form of therapy if the therapist conducts the group as if it is individual therapy. Such a therapist may see dynamics and group processes as incidental or antagonistic to the therapeutic process. The effective group leader must be skilled in techniques and interventions that foster group interaction and shape group behavior and growth.

THERAPEUTIC FACTORS OF GROUP THERAPY

Various authors, such as R. Corseni, B. Rosenberg, and most recently, I.D. Yalom, have researched and described the therapeutic factors in group therapy. Yalom describes 11 therapeutic factors of group therapy:

1. Instillation of hope
2. Universality
3. Imparting of information
4. Altruism
5. Corrective recapitulation of the primary family group
6. Development of socializing techniques
7. Imitative behavior
8. Interpersonal learning
9. Group cohesiveness
10. Catharsis
11. Existential factors[40]

Instillation of hope helps the client maintain faith in the therapeutic modality. The client is optimistic and believes that he or she will get better. Instillation of hope is important in pretherapy and can be correlated with a positive therapy outcome. Inpatient groups have selected the instillation of hope as a therapeutic factor effecting outcome more so than outpatient groups.[24] Therapists may enhance this process by bringing attention to the progress of group members.[40]

Universality prevents the client from feeling unique and different. Within the group, the client begins to feel less isolated and more like other people. This feeling is strengthened by the client's learning that others in the group have similar problems, thoughts, and feelings. Universality limits the fears that clients have about being alone in having unacceptable thoughts, impulses, and fantasies. Group therapy provides more opportunity for universality and consensual validation than individual therapy.[40]

Imparting of information is the use of information in a planned, structured manner, such as didactic instruction given in a lecture format. These lectures may be accompanied by audiovisual and other teaching aids. The topic of the didactic presentation is clear.[40]

Altruism is the process of clients aiding or helping each other. The act of giving to others becomes therapeutic for the giver by increasing his or her self-esteem.[40]

Corrective recapitulation of the primary family group means that the client is influenced in therapy group by his or her history. Initially in group therapy, clients usually perceive the behavior of other members as being like their siblings' and the behavior of the leader (or therapist) as being like their parents'. When neither the members nor the leader respond as siblings or parents have in the past, clients begin to gain insight into their own behavior. Examples of these refocused problems are authority, rivalry, intimacy, competition, hostility, love, and others. Early conflicts with parents and siblings, and even conflicts with peers and teachers, are relived and corrected.[40]

Development of socializing techniques occurs in group therapy. Social skills are related to interpersonal success in American society. Feedback and role playing of social events are two techniques used in group therapy to develop social skills. It is expected that clients will terminate their group therapy experience with greater social skills than they previously had. Clients with regressed behavior may learn elementary social skills, such as not belching during group, whereas clients in higher functioning groups may learn to respond to feedback about styles of communication, such as rushing one's words, repeating oneself, and interrupting other members when they are speaking. Through feedback in the group, maladaptive social behavior is lessened, and the client becomes more acceptable to members of his or her therapy group and to other associates.[40]

Imitative behavior is a powerful therapeutic tool through which a group member identifies with the healthier aspects of the other members and the leader. Imitating the behavior of an assertive group member or leader, for example, demonstrates growth. In groups, the imitative process is more diverse than in individual therapy. Clients also benefit by observing the therapy of other clients with a similar problem. This is often called "spectator therapy" and usually has a more important role in the initial stages of the group.[40]

Interpersonal learning results from therapy groups because the groups are, in effect, microcosms of society. Learning from a therapy group can be transferred to other groups. The client learns to profit from the therapeutic use of anxiety. When anxiety is minimized, the client relates more openly and learns to trust, expose, give of self, expect from others, test reality, and experience growth. Interpersonal relationships in group therapy are therapeutic when parataxic distortions, as described by Harry Stack Sullivan, are modified through consensual validation in a group. Correction of interpersonal distortions is the goal. There are more opportunities to work through distortions in a group, which is related to transference with group members not only with a single therapist.[40]

Group cohesiveness relates to bonding or solidarity, the feeling of "we" instead of "I." Cohesiveness is demonstrated through group attendance and the ability of the group to communicate positive and negative expressions to each other without the group disintegrating. In cohesive groups, members try hard to impress one another, are accepting of each other, and enter and leave the group with minimal disruption of the process. There is a protection of group norms and low tolerance of members who deviate from the norms. The client's role in a cohesive group greatly influences his or her self-esteem. Cohesive groups produce positive client outcomes.[40]

Catharsis is the expression of feelings, especially those that involve deep emotions. Expression of feelings is a particularly important therapeutic factor. Catharsis is effective in group therapy when it is followed by insight and cognitive learning.[40]

Existential factors emphasize the present quality, content, subjective awareness, freedom of choice, and state of being. They are important in boundary situations as clients work through impending death and inevitable developmental life experiences, such as retirement and aging, that is, things that "are." Existential factors, such as responsibility, capriciousness of existence, and recognition of mortality, are factors with therapeutic value that are explored in group therapy.[23,40]

Interdependence of Therapeutic Factors

Therapeutic factors are interdependent; they do not operate separately. Different factors are more functional and helpful to group process at different stages of the group. Although the same therapeutic factors operate in all types of therapy groups, their emphasis and importance vary according to the type of group.

Every therapy group emphasizes various therapeutic factors according to the group's purpose and goals. Group therapists focus on the process of interpersonal learning and change.[40]

NURSES AND GROUP PROCESS AND THERAPY

Historically, nurses have used groups and group process in hospitals and other health care settings. As nursing progressed from functional assignments to the team approach, many studies were undertaken to discover ways to enhance the team's tasks and maintenance roles. Nurses have collaborated with colleagues in examining group theory, group dynamics, and group functioning in various health care delivery systems. Psychiatric-mental health nurses have specifically explored the use of groups as a teaching method, a therapeutic tool with clients, and a form of peer group supervision.

Nurse educators use group seminars as part of the teaching-learning process to enable nursing students to participate in groups, learn group roles, and learn the function and dynamics of the student-participant role. Instructors delegate a certain amount of authority to the nursing students yet serve as democratic leaders who structure the course and define expectations of the class. This experiential learning sparks an exciting way to learn group theory, enabling students to transfer their knowledge of, and experience in, group dynamics to other arenas of therapy, such as milieu, client groups, and supervision groups. Often these seminars are prerequisites for advanced courses in group therapy in graduate nursing programs.

In the past, psychiatric-mental health nurses learned group therapist and cotherapist roles and responsibilities. Dr. Hildegard Peplau, an early authority on psychiatric nursing specialist programs, augmented nurses' involvement in group therapy through what is known as experiential learning. Nurses developed increasing skill in the techniques of group therapy; psychiatric nursing clinical specialists became highly skilled in group intervention.

The mental health revolution, sponsored by President John F. Kennedy, demanded that greater numbers of health professionals administer formal and informal group therapy in community mental health centers. Responding to this need, psychiatric-mental health nurses and particularly psychiatric clinical nurse specialists have become more active in group leader roles in the therapeutic communities, outpatient settings, and private therapy. They also have become more active as liaison psychiatric nursing consultants in general hospital settings.

Psychiatric-mental health nurses participate as leaders or coleaders in many formal and informal group therapies, including revitalization, resocialization, reeducation, supportive therapy, insight, psychoanalytic therapy, TA, family therapy, couple therapy, adolescent therapy, T groups, and prevention groups in the community.

TYPES OF THERAPY GROUPS

Growth Groups and Psychotherapeutic Groups

In the past 3 decades, numerous forms of growth groups, including self-help groups and group counseling, have developed. Factors that determine the maximal therapeutic benefit of a growth or therapy group include the following:

1. Extent of personality disorganization of the participant
2. Effect of personality disorganization on interpersonal functioning, as a family member, provider, productive citizen
3. Degree of functional ability and role success or failure of the participant
4. The participant's ability to harness impulses in stressful group situations
5. The member's purpose or goals in joining a group, both articulated goals and hidden agendas
6. The participant's ability to share and support others in problem-solving tasks
7. The participant's ability to use the material produced in a group to solve problems in his or her own situation

Leaders of psychotherapeutic and self-help groups have different functions. The leader of the psychotherapy group assumes more responsibility for the group than does a leader of a self-help group. In the psychotherapy group, the members or clients may have limiting maladaptive to severe emotional disorders. The members may be referred to the group from individual therapy, where they were seen in an initial crisis state but later are able to tolerate the group setting. Clients in a therapy group do not become the therapist, and the therapist never assumes the client's role in the group. The leader also provides more support for members of a therapy group who may have less tolerance for stress.

In a growth or self-help group, such as a T group, the leader and members have attainted a certain degree of emotional stability, and there is not a great discrepancy between their functioning by the end of the growth group experience. The group initially uses the leader to provide guidance and clarification. However, toward the end of the group experience, the leader becomes a part of the group, and several leadership functions may be performed by the group members. In a growth group, the members may receive less support from the leader while dealing with their anxiety, but there is conflict resolution by the end of the group.

Psychoanalytic Group Psychotherapy

In a psychoanalytic group, the therapist holds a prominent position. Each client in the group has a relationship with the therapist. Group communication is focused on the three levels of unconscious, semiconscious, and conscious material. The group focuses on interpretation of dreams, free association, and other latent content produced in the group. The therapist turns these experiences into conscious, healthy learning experiences for the client. This process is accomplished by transference to the therapist and multitransference to group members.

Transactional Analysis

The three ego states of the individual—the parent, child, and adult—are examined in TA groups. A goal of TA groups is that individuals in the group will communicate from the proper ego state for the situation and the responses of others, thereby lessening conflict and promoting mature relationships.

Rational-Emotive Therapy

Based on the theory of Albert Ellis that human beings, although subject to powerful biological and social forces, still have the capacity for being rational, rational-emotive group therapy aims to maximize a person's rational thinking. People, says Ellis, tend to overgeneralize situations when they are anxious. If they do not use thinking and reasoning at this point, they become irrational. The therapist designs activities to rid the members of the group of their irrational ideas.

Rogerian Group Therapy

In a Rogerian group, the therapist's goal is to help the members express their feelings toward one another during group sessions. The therapist's role is one of encouraging this expression of feelings, clarifying these feelings with clients, and accepting clients and their feelings nonjudgmentally. Through this process, the client learns to accept his or her own feelings, a first step toward self-acceptance. The client gains positive self-regard through the relationship with the therapist. Inherent in Rogerian theory is the belief that change and growth can take place at any age.

Gestalt Therapy

Fritz S. Perls pioneered the techniques of gestalt therapy. Gestalt theory emphasizes the here and now, that is, self-expression, self-exploration, and self-awareness in the present. Clients and therapist focus on everyday problems and try to solve them. The individual becomes aware of the total self and the surrounding world; awareness of the problem renders the person capable of change. The leader's role in gestalt therapy groups is to help members express their feelings and grow from their experiences.

Interpersonal Group Therapy

Interpersonal theory development is attributed to Harry Stack Sullivan, who also worked extensively with Peplau to introduce interpersonal theory into nursing. Anxiety is the focus of interpersonal therapy—how individuals develop anxiety and how they resolve it. Anxiety has the potential to hamper, distort, or enhance relationships between individuals. Interpersonal group therapists explore the members' anxiety and stress and their effects on the individual.

It is believed that anxiety arises from interpersonal relationships and is reduced or relieved through interpersonal support. One of the main goals of interpersonal group therapy is to promote the individual's comfort with others in the group, which then transfers to other relationships.

Psychodrama Groups

Psychodrama in the United States has its origin, implementation, and direction in the work of Jacob L. Moreno. He promoted this method of group therapy with individuals, small groups, and large groups. He even tried to help the citizens of America resolve their guilt about John F. Kennedy's assassination through sociodrama.

Psychodrama can be used as a form of group psychotherapy that explores the truth through dramatic methods. During psychodrama, the subject (or client) produces a topic to be explored. The director (or therapist) directs the subject through role playing of scenes related to the topic and incorporates the use of auxiliary egos (or therapeutic aides) in the action. The audience experiences the feelings and identifies with the action on the stage. A catharsis occurs for the subject and for the audience.

Bion Method

Also termed the Travistock conference, the Bion method emphasizes experiential learning that is translatable into action in work and community life. The group provides a setting in which experience can be studied and partially understood as it occurs. The group examines transactions, boundaries, the function of leadership, and attitudes toward authority.

Marathon Groups

The term marathon group refers to the amount of concentrated time the participants spend together as a group. Marathon groups are similar to each other, not by virtue of the leader's theoretical orientations or techniques, but because each is a single uninterrupted session. These sessions may last from 12 hours to 2, 3, or more days, allowing short periods away from the group for sleeping and eating. These groups have a clearly stated goal of personal change or growth of the participants.

Encounter Groups

The purpose of an encounter group is personal change, often as a result of deeply felt experiences. The differences between marathon and encounter groups are minimal, and the theoretical orientations of group leaders are diverse. Examples of themes of encounter groups are "The Challenge of Change, Danger, and Fulfillment"; "Closeness: Can It Hurt?"; and "Marriage: How to Survive It."

T Groups

The T group is the oldest and best known therapeutic method coming out of the sensitivity training group movement. The first T group conference was held in Bethel, Maine, in 1946. The goal of each T group conference is to verify experimentally the T group method. This involves the study of group norms, roles, communication distortions, and the effects of authority on behavior patterns, personality, and coping mechanisms. Group members receive feedback by exposing themselves to others in the group, and they experiment with new and more productive behavior.

Other sensitivity groups may have similar objectives, such as interpersonal skill groups, discussion groups, self-analytical groups, and process groups. All of these groups focus on the growth process of the individual through the help of the leader and the group.

Community Support Groups

Numerous support groups have emerged under the category of community mental health psychiatry. Some were founded to lend continued or added support to previously hospitalized psychiatric clients. Other groups have been formed as a result of the needs of individuals in the community. Self-help groups have been developed by lay people to address specific needs shared by group members. Community support groups, of which there are more than 500 examples, may be classified in various ways (Table 16-1).

The main purpose of community support groups is to provide identification, clarification, understanding, role-modeling, feelings of togetherness, and group cohesion. They help prevent the individual from feeling lonely and isolated. Some groups evolve into educational models that enhance communication, self-image, body image, problem solving, decision making, and growth processes.

Most community support groups help their members decrease levels of stress and increase levels of self-acceptance. With the help of the group, the member is better able to deal with the problems that he or she brought to the group. The outcome of this process is rewarding; the member develops new or more effective patterns of behavior.

Although community support groups have structures similar to those of other groups, they may be larger than therapy groups. Leadership in community support groups may be shared among the members; that is, *leadership as a process.* Senior members are expected to provide direction and structure and help establish norms.

NURSING GROUPS IN THE 1990s

Reassessing the need for change in individuals, groups, and environments has led nurses to seek alternative ways to improve communication. Economics and nurses' expanded collaborative and cooperative practice have encouraged nursing toward innovation in group work. Because computer networks are interactive media, computer groups have been established to diminish the problems of distance, time, and need for speedy feedback.[31]

Economics has also fostered short-lived crisis groups with a solution-focused framework. It has encouraged the use of more "open-open" groups (members can enter or leave the group at any time), which also provides a richer medium of information that can lead to problem solving.

In nursing education, the use of groups has increased in the form of study groups, special project groups, and testing groups. The following is an example of Front Range Community College nursing program, which formed student groups to help their students learn about groups and group theory. With increased challenges, the nursing faculty formed additional groups with the following objectives:

1. Initiate brain storming among the members to enhance critical thinking
2. Foster "bonding" of group members
3. Help students increase their survival skills
4. Help students learn conflict resolution and assertiveness and become change agents
5. Practice collaboration in the student role to apply

Table 16-1

Community Support Groups

Type of Group	Support Offered	Examples of Groups
Community support groups for victims of violence	Individuals and families who have been physically or emotionally abused.	Safe house, rape trauma, battered children
Birth anomaly support groups	Individuals and families with birth defects and congenital anomalies	Down syndrome, cerebral palsy
Acquired diseases support groups	Individuals and families coping with, and adjusting to, diseases originating after birth that are not inherited or innate	Leukemia, acquired immunodeficiency syndrome, Diabetes
Chronic illness support groups	Individuals and families in which there is an illness of long-term duration, slow progression, and often little change in the symptomatology	Chronic obstructive pulmonary disease, cancer, arthritis
Developmental adjustment groups	Individuals and families with physical or emotional development that deviates from the norm	Autistic children, cretinism, runaway teens
Grief education and resolution groups	Individuals and families with physical and emotional loss	Loss due to death of a significant person, sudden infant death syndrome
Interracial and biracial support groups	Individuals and families of interracial siblings, children, spouses, parents, and neighborhoods	Asian American families; greater Park Hill Neighborhood Association
Self-help and improvement support groups	Perspectives on behavior and attitude change	Assertiveness, Weight Watchers, Alcoholics Anonymous
Family structure support groups	Individuals and families of nontraditional (non-nuclear) family structure	Step-parenting, Parents without Partners, Lucky Mother's Club
Work-related support groups	Workers who experience job-related stress	Burnout groups, Friday evening groups

this process on the job after graduation and thus prevent unhealthy competition

6. Build self-esteem
7. Learn how to teach clients and families by teaching each other
8. Learn decision making and the responsibility that accompanies this process
9. Foster achievement of peers, for example, an "A" student helping students with lower grades

Study groups developed their own operational rules and norms. They established tolerance, limit setting, and group problem solving. Student group members learned group dynamics and how to reach out for help through the group. Groups sponsored individual growth through imitative behavior. Students learned about the change process by developing these skills in their groups and discovered that diversity of group members fosters strength.

Evaluation of these nursing student groups revealed that the experience was positive. Members gained knowledge about group functioning through their participation and expressed individual growth. Identified problems were group meeting times that conflicted with family schedule and finding a mutually convenient meeting time for all group members.

STAGES OF GROUP DEVELOPMENT

Initial Stage

The initial stage of group development is likely to involve superficial, rather than open and trusting, communication. The members are becoming acquainted with each other and are searching for similarity between themselves and other group members. Members may be unclear about the purposes or goals of the group. A certain amount of structuring of group norms, roles, and responsibilities takes place (Table 16-2).

Working Stage

During the working stage of group development, the real work of the group is accomplished. Because members are already familiar with each other, the group leader, and the group's rules, they are free to approach and attempt to solve their problems. Conflict and cooperation surface during the group's work.

Characteristics of a Mature Group. The mature group demonstrates its maturity through such positive characteristics as empathy, effective communication skills, and a definite, inclusive group culture. Its characteristics are described in detail in Table 16-2. Even if a group

Table 16-2

Stages of Group Development

Stage	Characteristics
Initial	1. Works on getting acquainted with group leader and members 2. Depends on the leader for direction 3. Searches for meaning and purpose of the group 4. Restricts content and communication style 5. Searches for similarity among members 6. Gives advice
Working	1. Solves selected problems of working together 2. Conflicts between members or between members and leader 3. Works on issues of dominance, control, and power within group 4. Cooperates to accomplish the group's work
Mature	1. Develops workable norms and a group culture 2. Resolves conflict when it occurs; conflict arises due to issues of importance, not emotional issues 3. Evaluates own work and individuals assume responsibility for their work 4. Accepts each others' differences without placing value judgments on them 5. Sanctions role assignment by members of the group 6. Discusses topics and makes decisions by means of rational behavior, such as sharing information and open discussion 7. Provides a feeling of "we" for the leader and members 8. Demonstrates cohesion 9. Validates itself; has a group image
Termination	1. Evaluating and summarizing the group experience 2. Exploring positive and negative feelings about the group experience

reaches a mature stage in its development, its members can regress as individuals. This change may be precipitated by the addition of a new group member or members, loss of a member, or a group problem that introduces stress. All of these can cause some degree of return to an earlier stage of functioning. The more serious the disturbance, the greater the potential regression. The more experience the group has in applying problem-solving skills, the more able it is to be resilient in the face of difficulties and return to its former stage of mature functioning. If the group "image" is one of a "problem solver," this also facilitates group functioning. Leadership is also important in sustaining the group and returning it to a mature level of functioning after crisis or change.

Termination Stage

During termination, the group evaluates the experience and explores members' feelings about it and the impending separation. The termination of the group may be an opportunity for group members who have difficulty saying goodbye to learn to deal more realistically and comfortably with this normal part of human experience, separation.

◆ Group Communication and Nursing Intervention

THERAPEUTIC INTERVENTIONS WITH GROUPS

The use of therapeutic communication techniques with groups requires that nurses possess considerable preparation and skill in group work. Examples of these communication techniques are described in Table 16-3.

LATENT AND MANIFEST COMMUNICATION

Groups use latent and manifest communication. *Latent content* is content that is not discussed, occurs on a feeling level, and is seldom verbalized, such as hidden agendas. *Manifest content* involves spoken words (Fig. 16-1). Groups are most effective when their latent and manifest content are similar. The further apart these levels of communication are, the more communication problems are experienced by the group.

Table 16-3

Examples of Group Communication Techniques

Technique	Description	Example
Approval	Condoning or encouraging an attitude, feeling, or action	Frank: "I decided to move to a new apartment." Nurse: "You made a wise decision."
Acceptance	An attitude or a relationship that recognizes an individual's worth without implying approval of behaviors or personal affection	Marty: "Nurse, I was angry at you for not cancelling the session." Nurse: "It's all right for you to get angry at me, Marty."
Clarification	Restatement of the substance of what the client has said	Abel: "I feel hopeless, no way out." Nurse: "You feel you have no way out?"
Exploration	A shift from considering one aspect of a situation to considering another	Frank: "My son decided to leave the business." Nurse: "Tell me how that came about."
Identification	Delineating specific factors for the purposes of understanding or clarifying	Frank: "I often do favors for others, like my father did. He said it is rewarding, and makes us better people." Nurse: "Sounds like you had respect for your father's opinions and judgment."
Interpretation	Finding or explaining the meaning or significance of the information	Mr. B.: "All this talking is really a pain in the neck." Nurse: "Mr. B., you seem annoyed at all the talking," or Abel: "I feel hopeless, no way out." Nurse: "You sound suicidal."
Information giving	Stating facts about a problem	Marty: "All the staff write notes in the charts after the group meeting and put their own interpretation on what we say, don't they?" Nurse: "I can only speak for myself. I write notes in the chart, but I try hard not to misinterpret what members state in the group."
Encouraging expression of feelings or ideas	Indicating in some way that it is permissible or desirable to talk about feelings or ideas	Mr. W.: "It takes me 10 or 15 minutes to get oriented in the morning and then I'm all right." Nurse: "Are there others who feel this way?" Ms. S. "I always get up to eat and have some coffee. Then I feel more like facing others."
Reassurance	Offering the client confidence about a favorable outcome through suggestion, persuasive arguments, or comparing similar situations	Frank: "I was afraid to move at first." Nurse: "Frank, we are always here to listen to your fears and try and help you work them out."
Support	Giving comfort, approval, or acceptance	Marty: "My busted arm has played heck with me. Getting anything for it has been a federal case. And I'm not one who shows pain easily." Nurse: "This must be pretty infuriating." Marty: "Well, it really bugs me."
Intervention	An action that directs or influences the client's behavior	Nurse: "Frank, you've been silent, inattentive, and haven't shared with the group since your weekend pass. Will you tell us what is going on with you?" Frank: "I had a horrible weekend. I don't know how to share what happened, but I'll try."
Understanding	Indicating verbally or nonverbally that the feelings being communicated by the client are comprehended	Marty: "Nurse, I feel frightened about discharge." Nurse: "I can understand your feeling frightened. Leaving the hospital is not always easy."
Reflection	Repeating to clients what they said; mirroring their statement	Mr. B.: "All this talking is really a pain in the neck." Nurse: "This talking is a pain in the neck."
Listening	Concentration on the client's communication without interruption	Nurse listens and attends to client.
Teaching	Helping the client learn specifics in relation to events and behavior	Abel (to the nurse): "You were irritated at me, weren't you, but we were able to talk about it and work it out." Nurse: "Yes, we did. I was irritated because I felt you were not listening, and we did talk about it."

continued

Table 16-3 (Continued)

Technique	Description	Example
Silence	The use of no verbal or spoken words	Nurse is silent while attending to client.
Structuring	Shaping the content of the group meeting	Frank: "I'm going home soon." Mrs. C.: "Really?" Nurse: "Maybe you would like to talk about it?
Limit setting	Deciding how far group members and the group may go before the therapist ceases or restricts to a point the behavior, activity, or verbal expression of members	Marty: "I feel we need to cancel our therapy session next week because the next day is a holiday and we need a long weekend to travel." Nurse: "Holiday weekends are difficult; however, we will not cancel our group session."

A group may not solve its problems readily, due to the interference of latent content. Hidden agendas hinder group communication. For example, if a group member feels that he or she would be punished if he or she verbalized an opinion in the group, especially if it disagrees with the leader, his or her latent communication would influence overt behavior and interfere with group growth.

CONTENT AND PROCESS COMMUNICATION

Content and process are other ways of observing group communication. When observing the group's discussion, what is being said is the *content.* How the group is handling its communication is *process.* Who talks to whom, what is said, and what is left unspoken are examples of process.

Examples of content and process communication follow:

Content	Process
1. Discussing how a mother does not take care of her children may mean . . .	the leader or therapist is not meeting the dependency needs of the group.
2. Talking about the fighting of sisters and brothers at home may mean . . .	there is a lot of conflict and fighting in the therapy group.

TRANSFERENCE AND COUNTERTRANSFERENCE

Transference occurs when a client attributes characteristics and behavior of a family member or significant other to the therapist, thereby responding to the therapist in a certain manner. The clarification of this distortion with the client helps to create a therapeutic process of learning. *Countertransference* occurs when the therapist responds in a negative manner to the client's transference, further complicating communication.

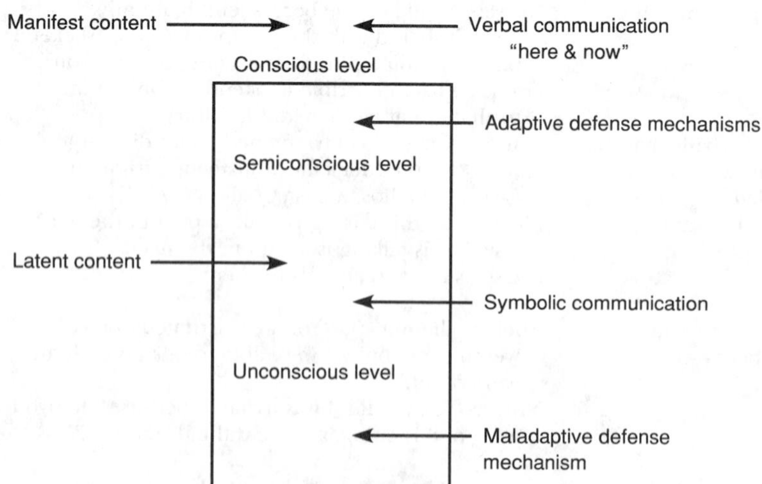

Figure 16-1. Communication diagram: "The group mind."

THEMES

The group leader observes for *themes* in the group's communication that relate one group session to another and then explores the meanings of these themes. Through therapeutic communication, the leader may help the group uncover and solve the problem. Group functioning is also evaluated by observing changes in members' behavior, such as their ability to apply these new techniques to solving future problems. Box 16-1 illustrates how communication themes are used.

Higher functioning groups or those with less overt psychopathological symptomatology will work through problems with minimal hidden agendas and symbolic language. The therapist can encourage the group to deal with here and now material and can manage anxiety more readily than in a group that communicates on a symbolic level. The cotherapist in Box 16-1 listened for latent and manifest content to identify the group theme and used techniques of communication to help the group solve the problem.

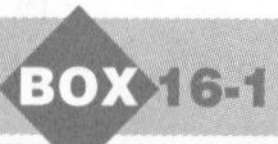

Therapeutic Dialogue: A Group Case

Theme: The group theme is authority, or more pointedly, transference. Our therapist is punitive to the group, like our mothers, if we disagree.

Countertransference

Therapist I, Mrs. A (angry): You are rebellious and won't listen to reason. I am particularly angry at Marty because she started this . . .

Resistance

Three-fourths of the group did not attend the next meeting.

Interpretation

Therapist II, Mr. B (at a later session): Marty, when you stated we were like your mother, it sounded as if you were angry.

Acceptance

Marty: Yes, and afraid.

Exploration

Therapist I, Mrs. A: Marty, I wonder if you felt that your weekend pass being canceled was related to you disagreeing with me in group?

Acknowledgement

Marty: Yes.

Consensual validation

Group: You know, Mrs. A, we all thought that.

◆ Chapter Summary

This chapter has discussed group process and theory and their application to therapeutic needs. Some of the major foci of the chapter have included the following:

1. A group is three or more people with related goals.
2. Groups vary according to their size, homogeneity of membership, climate, norms, and goal directedness.
3. Group norms are the patterns of interaction that develop within a group.
4. A group leader designs the group's structure, style of leadership, and decision-making policies.
5. Roles in groups are task building and maintenance and individual roles.
6. The advantages of group therapy include its effectiveness and efficiency in time and cost.
7. Nurses participate as leaders and coleaders in multiple formal and informal groups.
8. Most therapeutic group experiences can be categorized as psychotherapy or growth groups.
9. The three stages of group development are the initial, working, and termination stages.
10. Nurses and other group leaders use a variety of therapeutic interventions with groups; they identify and explore latent versus manifest communication and process versus content communication.
11. There are at least 11 therapeutic factors observed in group therapy.

Critical Thinking Questions

1. *List the stages of a group and a characteristic of each stage.*
2. *Discuss six characteristics of a mature group.*
3. *Explain how a client in a therapy group becomes a culture carrier.*
4. *State six advantages of group therapy.*
5. *Discuss five therapeutic factors observed in group therapy.*
6. *Give an example of how a leader can affect the initial stage of a group.*

Review Questions

1. Identify the stages of a group.
   - A. In the initial stage, most of the goals of the group are developed.
   - B. Initial stage, working stage, mature stage, disruptive stage

C. In the initial stage, evaluation of the group's work is done.
D. Initial stage, working stage, mature stage, and termination stage

2. Characteristics of a mature group are
   A. criticism of group members at most of the group sessions.
   B. the group making very few decisions.
   C. the group remaining very dependent on the group leader.
   D. the group demonstrating cohesion and problem solving.
3. An explanation or description of a primary group may be as follows:
   A. Primary groups have distant contact.
   B. Primary groups have face-to-face contact, boundaries, and group norms.
   C. Primary groups are usually larger and more impersonal than secondary groups.
   D. Most group members have never belonged to a primary group.
4. Group norms
   A. do not influence role expectations in the group.
   B. influence patterns of interaction and behavioral expectations in the group.
   C. are developed over a short period of time.
   D. are not connected to sanctions, taboos, or the reference power of the group.
5. Group roles are usually described in three major categories:
   A. Group building and maintenance roles, group task roles, and individual roles
   B. Group harmonizer as an example of a the task role
   C. Disruption roles, complaining roles, and harmonizing roles
   D. Initial roles, developmental roles, and mature roles
6. Therapeutic factors of group therapy as stated by I.D. Yalom include
   A. attending all therapy sessions,
   B. instillation of hope and altruism.
   C. discussing in detail all thoughts and feelings.
   D. not trusting other group members.
7. Advantages of a group are
   A. learning multiple ways of problem solving.
   B. that clients can be treated more economically.
   C. that clients always feel comfortable and supported.
   D. that therapists need less education to facilitate group therapy.
8. Styles of group leadership can be described as
   A. punitive and forgiving.
   B. democratic, socialist, and despotic.
   C. counter-transferring.
   D. autocratic, democratic, and laissez-faire.

◆ References

1. Agazarian Y: Contemporary Theories of Group Psychotherapy: A Systems Approach to the Group-as-a-Whole. Int J Group Psychother 42: 177–204, 1992
2. Alonzo A: Training for Group Psychotherapy, Group Therapy and Clinical Practice, pp 521–532. Washington, DC, American Psychiatric Press, 1993
3. Aveline M: Principles of Leadership in Brief Training Groups for Mental Health Professionals. Int J Group Psychother 43: 102–120, 1993
4. Bloch S, Crouch E: Therapeutic Factors: Intrapersonal and Interpersonal Mechanisms, Handbook of Group Psychotherapy. New York, Wiley, 1994
5. Butheil T, Gablard G: The Concepts of Boundaries in Clinical Practice: Theoretical and Risk-Management Dimensions. Am J Psychiatry 150: 188–196, 1993
6. Dies R: Group Psychotherapies in Modern Psychotherapies: Theory and Practice. New York, Guilford Publications, 1993
7. Evans M, et al: A Triage Model of Psychotherapeutic Group Intervention. Archives of Psychiatric Nursing 7 (4): 244–248, 1993
8. Franko D: The Use of a Group Meal in the Brief Group Therapy of Bulimia Nervosa. Int J Group Psychother 43: 237–242, 1993
9. Gilbert C: Twenty Years: A Great Beginning . . . Including Commentary by Pothier, P. Journal of Child and Adolescent Psychiatric Mental Health Nursing 5 (4): 41–51, 1992
10. Goldman BM, et al: Young Children of Alcoholics: A Group Treatment Model. Soc Work Health Care 16 (3): 53–65, 1992
11. Goodman G, Jacob M: The Self-Help, Mutual-Support Group, Handbook of Group Psychotherapy. New York, Wiley, 1994
12. Hardy J, Lewis C: Bridging the Gap Between Long and Short Term Therapy: A Viable Model. Group 16: 5–17, 1992
13. Hooking P: Utilizing Roger's Theory of Self-Concept in Mental Health Nursing. J Adv Nurs 18 (6): 980–984, 1993
14. Horvath A, Gaston L, Luborsky L: The Therapeutic Alliance and its Measures in Dynamic Psychotherapy Research. New York, Basic Books, 1993
15. Kaul T, Bednor R: Experimental Group Research: Can the Cannon Fire. In Handbook for Psychotherapy and Behavior Change: An Empirical Analysis, 4th ed. New York, Wiley, 201–203, 1994
16. Kimmel LH: The Concept of Elastic Boundaries Applied to Group Therapy With Veterans Over 60 Years Old. Archives of Psychiatric Nursing 5 (2): 91–98, 1991
17. Koss M: Sharing: Research on Brief Therapy in Handbook of Psychotherapy and Behavioral Change: An Empirical Analysis, 4th ed, pp 664–700. New York, Wiley, 1994

18. Lambert M, Bergin A: The Effectiveness of Psychotherapy in Handbook of Psychotherapy and Behavioral Change: An Empirical Analysis, 4th ed, pp 143–189. New York, Wiley, 1994
19. Lieberman M: Self-Help Groups. Comprehensive Group Psychotherapy 300–301, 1993
20. MacKenzie K: Time-Limited Theory and Technique in Group Therapy in Clinical Practice. Washington, DC, American Psychiatric Press, 1993
21. MacKenzie R, Tschusche V: Relatedness, Group Work and Outcome in Long-Term Inpatient Psychotherapy Groups. Journal of Psychotherapy Practice and Research 2: 147–156, 1993
22. McCallum M, Piper W, Mortin H: Affect and Outcome in Short-Term Group Therapy for Loss. Int J Group Psychother 43: 303–319, 1993
23. McDougall GJ: Existential Psychotherapy With Older Adults, Journal of the American Psychiatric Nurses Association I (1): 16–20, 1995
24. McLeod J, Ryan A: Therapeutic Factors Experienced by Members of An Outpatient Therapy Group for Older Women. British Journal of Guidance and Counseling 21: 64–72, 1993
25. Miller CR: Group Therapy for Women: Benefits of Ethnocultural Diversity. Journal of Women's Health Fall (3): 189–191, 1992
26. Moreno J: Group Therapy for Eating Disorder. In Fuhriman A, Burlingame, G (eds): Handbook of Group Psychotherapy. New York, Wiley, 1994
27. Mueller A, Ladewig P, Falco J: The Use of Group Process in Developing Nursing Articulation Models. Nurse Educator 18 (1): 29–32, 1993
28. Munich R: Varieties of Learning in an Experiential Group. Int J Group Psychother 43: 345–361, 1993
29. Pearlman IR: Group Psychotherapy With the Elderly. J Psychosoc Nurs Mental Health Serv 31 (7): 7–10, 32–33, 1993
30. Pollack LE: Content Analysis of Groups for Inpatients With Bipolar Disorder. Applied Nursing Research 6 (1): 19–27, 1993
31. Ripich S, Moore S, Brennan P: A New Nursing Medium: Computer Network For Group Intervention. J Psychosoc Nurs 30 (7): 15–19, 1992
32. Ronaldson S, et al: Validation Therapy: A Communication Link With the Confused Older Person. Australian Nursing Journal 21 (10): 19–21, 1992
33. Schodler M: Brief Group Therapy with Adult Survivors of Incest, in Focal Group Therapy, pp 292–322. Oakland, CA, New Harbinger Publication, 1992
34. Shrivers B, et al: The Clinical Nurse Specialist as Brief Psychotherapist. Perspect Psychiatr Care 28 (4): 15–18, 1992
35. Wallace B, Nosko A: Working With Shame in the Group Treatment of Male Batterers. Int J Group Psychother 43: 45–61, 1993
36. Wheeler I, O'Malley K, Waldo Mad Murphey J: Participants' Perception of Therapeutic Factors in Groups for Incest Survivors. Journal for Specialists in Group Work 17: 89–95, 1992
37. Wifley D, Agras S, et al: Group Cognitive-Behavioral Therapy and Group Interpersonal Psychotherapy for the Nonpurging Bulimic: A Controlled Comparison. J Consult Clin Psychol 61: 296–305, 1994
38. Wilson WH, Vaccaro JV, Kahn EM, et al: Group Treatment Assignment for Outpatients with Schizophrenia: Integrating Recent Clinical and Research Findings . . . Including Commentary. Community Ment Health J 28 (6): 539–560, 1992
39. Worthington C: An Examination of Factors Influencing the Diagnosis and Treatment of Black Patients in the Mental Health System (review). Archives of Psychiatric Nursing 6 (3): 195–204, 1993
40. Yalom ID: The Theory and Practice of Group Psychotherapy, 4th ed. New York, Basic Books, 1995

Families and Family Therapy

Christina R. Hogarth
Susan Mace Weeks

17

. . . And what of Marriage, Master?
You shall be together when the white wings of death scatter your days.
Ay, you shall be together even in the silent memory of God.
But let there be spaces in your togetherness,
And let the winds of the heavens dance between you.
Love one another, but make not a bond of love:
Let it rather be a moving sea between the shores of your souls.
. . . Sing and dance together and be joyous, but let each one of you be alone,
Even as the strings of a lute are alone though they quiver with the same music.
Speak to us of children . . .
. . . They are the sons and daughters of Life's longing for itself.
They come through you but not from you.
And though they are with you yet they belong not to you.
You may give them your love but not your thoughts.
You may house their bodies but not their souls,
For their souls dwell in the house of tomorrow, which you cannot visit, not even in your dreams.
You may strive to be like them, but seek not to make them like you:
For life goes not backward nor tarries with yesterday.
You are the bows from which your children as living arrows are sent forth.

Kahlil Gibran,
The Prophet, *1923*

Fairy tales, television, and the wedding industry would have us believe that marriage is finding a prince or princess and living happily ever after. In recent years, however, "happily ever after" has given way to unprecedented rises in divorce, intrafamilial abuse, substance abuse, adolescent suicide, crime, teenage pregnancy, and heavy reliance on social welfare and mental health services. Many families have lost hope and control over their own destinies, while others have organized to avoid becoming one of these alarming statistics.

For many years, nurses, sociologists, anthropologists, psychiatrists, psychologists, and social workers have explored the structure and form of the family. Families have been studied in relation to their developmental stages, structure and function, communication patterns, and dynamics as a living system. More recently, attention has been focused on varying types of families and the different settings in which families encounter mental health care professionals. Nursing literature is also increasing the focus on effective nursing interventions for family systems and ways to measure the outcomes of these interventions. The ability of families to adapt to stress and change while continuing to provide an atmosphere of care has become a central theme of family-focused care.

This chapter presents major theories of family functioning, with emphasis on the family systems approach. Stressors and changes that may impact families are addressed and analyzed through the use of the nursing process.

Learning Objectives

On completion of this chapter, you should be able to accomplish the following:

1. *Define the term family.*
2. *Describe the theoretical approaches to the study of family: developmental theory, structure and function analysis, communication theory, and systems theory.*
3. *Identify the characteristics of living systems.*
4. *Discuss family variables that are instrumental in producing competent individuals.*
5. *Discuss historical, developmental, role-related, and environmental stressors affecting families.*
6. *Apply the nursing process to healthy and dysfunctional families.*
7. *Describe characteristics and skills essential to psychiatric-mental health nurses who work with troubled or dysfunctional families.*

◆ Family Theories

DEFINING THE FAMILY

The *family* is the basic unit of society, composed of two or more individuals who come together to share common beliefs and values. The bonding factor of a family is that of commitment. The individuals within the family may be related by marriage, blood, adoption, mutual consent, or economic necessity.

The family ideally interacts in ways that allow the attainment of common goals, such as the maintenance of a household, socialization, companionship, rearing of children, and providing care to impaired family members. A family attempts to provide for the needs of its members, including physiological needs, safety needs, belongingness and love needs, esteem needs, and the need for self-actualization.[26] Martha Craft defines the family as, "a social context of two or more people characterized by mutual attachment, caring, long-term commitment, and responsibility to provide individual growth, supportive relationships, health of members and of the unit, and maintenance of the organization and system during constant individual, family, and societal change."[10]

The form or structure of an individual family may vary greatly. In addition to the traditional nuclear family, families may be composed of people not related by blood or marriage living together as a family group, single-parent families, and extended family groupings. Although the form and structure of the family continue to change, the family persists as the most important force in providing stability for individuals, groups, and cultures.

The importance of family structure and function within society has made the family the focus of much analysis. Various disciplines have studied the family from differing theoretical perspectives, including developmental stages, structure and function analysis, communication theory, and systems theory. Psychiatric-mental health nurses do not have the benefit of a single well-tested theory to guide their interventions with families. However, many nursing theories can be easily applied to psychiatric nursing interventions with families. Two theories that are useful in family interventions and that blend well together are Hildegard Peplau's interpersonal psychodynamic theory[31] and the family systems nursing theory of Wright and Leahey.[43] Both theories focus on interpersonal relationships and view nursing in an interactive manner.[14] Other family theories with application to psychiatric nursing are discussed below.

DEVELOPMENTAL STAGES OF FAMILIES

Development refers to an orderly evolution of events moving from simple to complex. Human development has been studied extensively in all spheres of human experience, including biological, psychological (ie, cognitive and emotional), social, and spiritual realms. The family is a group of people in varying stages of development and a family group in a stage of development.

Duvall has described the basic tasks and development stages of families. The eight basic tasks of families follow:

1. Physical maintenance
2. Allocation of resources—meeting family needs and apportioning goods, facilities, space, authority
3. Division of labor
4. Socialization of family members
5. Reproduction; recruitment and release of family members
6. Maintenance of order
7. Placement of members into society
8. Maintenance of motivation and morale—encouragement and affection, meeting personal and family crises, refining a philosophy of life and sense of family loyalty through rituals[11]

Duvall identified the eight stages of family development as follows:

1. Beginning families (married couple)
2. Early childbearing families (oldest child up to 30 months)
3. Families with preschool children (oldest child 2–5 years)
4. Families with school children (oldest child 6–13 years)
5. Families with teenagers (oldest child 13–20 years)
6. Launching center families (children leaving home)
7. Families of middle years (empty nest through retirement)
8. Family in retirement and old age (retirement to death of both spouses)[11]

Stevenson has identified four stages of family development based on the length of the couple's relationship:

1. Emerging family (stage I)
2. Crystallizing family (stage II)
3. Integrating family (stage III)
4. Actualizing family (stage IV)[37]

The *emerging family* stage encompasses the first 7 to 10 years of the relationship. The couple is initiating work and career paths, and children often enter the family during this stage. Both developments—career and children—are stressful events, as are the beginning stages of the relationship. By the end of this stage, basic patterns of family life are established.

The *crystallizing family* stage, extending from 10 to 25 years of cohabitation, usually is calm until children reach adolescence. There also is considerable contact between children and parents before the children are launched from the family. The adults continue to grow and begin to participate in community life.

The *integrating family* stage lasts from about the 25th year of the relationship until the 40th. Usually, the children are young adults by this time, and the couple or adults who lead the family renew and enhance their relationship. Although work roles continue to be important, humanistic tendencies appear, and leisure is significant to the couple during this stage. The grown children may need to make adjustments to aging parents.

The *actualizing family* stage encompasses the period after about 40 years of living together. The couple continues to develop, or if one partner dies, the remaining partner grieves and continues to grow. Family members deal with aging, chronic illness, dying parents, and death.

STRUCTURE AND FUNCTION OF FAMILIES

The structure, or organization, of the family includes the type of family (ie, nuclear or extended) and the value systems that dictate the roles, communication patterns, and power distribution within the family. The value system includes basic beliefs about mankind, nature, the supernatural, time, and family relationships. Value systems tend to cluster by socioeconomic status or ethnic group.

Families with low incomes, for example, tend to have a present-time orientation and view themselves as subjugated to the environment and the supernatural or fate. Due to severe economic difficulties, family relationships tend to be disrupted by desertion of spouses and early emancipation of children. Families cope, however, by taking in other extended family members' children and often by the grandmother's provision of direct assistance to family members. Power usually is authoritarian or not exerted.

Middle-income families tend to espouse the Protestant work ethic prevalent in this country. This ethic dictates the importance of work and planning for the future and the belief that humans are somewhat inherently evil but changeable through hard work. Financial stability and success are viewed as rewards for hard work. Family relationships center around the nuclear family, with socialization among work-related or neighborhood friendships. Power is more egalitarian in middle-income families than in low-income families, but it becomes more male-dominated as the economic level of the family rises. Middle-income families see themselves as able to control and work for mastery over the environment.

These statements are broad generalizations of social values and do not account for cultural differences. Many ethnic groups, for example, place great importance on extended family relationships, rather than on the individualism valued by middle-income Americans.

Functions of the family may include procreation and socialization of children, maintenance of a household, affection, health and illness care, adapting to change within and from outside the family, and providing necessities for family members.

FAMILY COMMUNICATION THEORY

The family communication theory was developed in the 1950s by researchers at the Mental Research Institute in Palo Alto, California. Jackson, Watzlawick, Haley, Beaven, and Satir contributed to a theory of family dynamics in schizophrenia and double-bind communication; this theory has since been disproved as more was learned about the biological aspects of schizophrenia. They also pioneered efforts in family therapy.[32,40]

These researchers and practitioners found that children learn and develop by responding to verbal and nonverbal communication. A child's interpretation of himself or herself and the environment depends on messages received from parents. The messages are powerful because the child depends on the parents for survival.

Communication, says Satir, is the way members "work out to make meaning with one another." In nurturing families, communication is congruent, "direct, clear, specific, and honest," and family members have positive feelings about themselves. Rules (norms for how members should think and act) are "flexible, human, appropriate, and subject to change," and links to society (the ways family members relate to the community) are "open and hopeful." Satir views families as people making factories, with the parents as engineers or architects of the family.[32] Communication, self-worth, rules, and links to society are assessed by observing interactions among family members. Communication is the focus of intervention in the family.

FAMILY SYSTEMS THEORY

Family systems theory developed during the 1950s on the East and West coasts. The West Coast group of Jackson, Haley, and associates in Palo Alto explored the notions of communications theory (ie, cybernetics and feedback loops) and homeostasis applied to the family with a schizophrenic member.[4] In Washington, DC, Bowen based his family systems concepts on a biological system model.[8] In Philadelphia, Minuchin used the systems model in research with families exhibiting psychosomatic disorders.[27] More recently, in Dallas, Lewis and Beavers explored disturbed and healthy families from a systems viewpoint.[5,25]

A *system* is a whole that consists of more than the sum of its parts. Although a system can be divided into subsystems, the subsystems are not representative pieces of the whole. Human beings are complex organisms who respond, grow, and change in the context of relationships with others and in response to the environment. To study family research, theory, and therapy, one must understand the basic characteristics of living systems.

Characteristics of Living Systems

Limits are imaginary lines drawn to define the areas into which one should not intrude. These *boundaries* pertain to the system as a whole and to subsystems within it. Boundaries exist between people, between subsystems, and between the family system and the environment. The family's values, style, and self-worth determine the permeability of the boundaries to outside influences, such as the media, friends, school, and church. Boundaries may be clearly defined but open to change and input, so poorly defined that confusion and chaos exist, or so rigid that little input can permeate.

Negentropy is a tendency toward openness to the environment, both inside and outside the family. Living, open systems tend to increase in complexity with time, a phenomenon known as *differentiation*. An example of differentiation is human growth and development. The child grows from a dependent infant to a child with concrete thinking and a short attention span who feels safe at home, and then to a young adult with abstract thinking and a lengthy attention span capable of living independently in a complex environment. *Entropy* is the tendency of a system to be closed to the environment. A person who remains closed to feedback from others tends to develop distorted and peculiar perceptions, thoughts, and feelings.

Time is important to families. Systems change with the passage of time, as people age, and as children are born and leave home. *Stresses* and strains impinge on and occur within family systems. Stress is normal and inevitable as change occurs. Adolescence is an example of a common developmental stressor. *Conflict* often results from stress and change and is a normal and common phenomenon. A family's ability to manage change and conflict is termed *adaptation*. Adaptation may range from failure to adapt, to mere survival, to growing and changing into a more highly differentiated system.

It is useful to view families on a continuum from negentropic to entropic, or from more growth oriented to less growth oriented. Families that are mostly negentropic, or more open and growth oriented, produce the most personally and interpersonally capable people. In contrast, families that are more entropic, or less open and growth oriented, produce less capable people who often come to the attention of health care workers, mental health care providers, educators, and law enforcement personnel.

Producing Competent People

Beavers described eight critical variables for producing competent people.[5] Optimal families have an *open system orientation,* which assumes that an individual needs a group from which he or she derives satisfaction and personal definition. Optimal families also believe that life is complex, with experience flowing not from a single cause but from multiple factors.

Optimal families have *permeable boundaries.* The family views the world outside of itself positively, uses input from society and the environment to enrich its members' lives, and discards input it does not value. The boundaries between subsystems within the family, such as the subsystems of parents and children, permit privacy and aloneness but allow for the inclusion of others.

The optimal family experiences *contextual clarity.* Verbal and nonverbal communication are congruent and clear, and generational lines are clear with a strong parental coalition. In these families, developmental issues are resolved appropriately.

Power in optimal families is shared and flows from the parental couple, an egalitarian partnership involving complementary role behaviors. Roles are not shared but complement one another. For instance, one partner may be more aggressive and the other more supportive. These complementary roles may exist without sexual stereotyping but often follow the prevalent social patterns of the time. Gender does not define overt power in optimal families. People in these families do not lose their power by becoming close and intimate. Children do not assume parental responsibilities, and parents are able to use authoritarian approaches if needed.

Optimal families encourage *autonomy.* They consciously believe that children are being prepared to leave the family and live interdependently and progressively encourage independent thinking and behaviors. Each member's views are respected, and members claim responsibility for and communicate clearly their thoughts, feelings, and actions. People from optimal families possess a high degree of initiative and performance.

The *affective tone* in optimal families is caring, warm, empathic, and hopeful. Members ask about and attend to feelings; they are involved with one another. Conflict, which is inevitable, is confronted and resolved. The family members believe that they are able to survive difficult or unpleasant situations and occurrences. Their management or resolution of conflict strengthens their relationships and increases their confidence in the relationships.[1]

Negotiation and task performance are accomplished with input from all members and attention to the developmental capabilities of children. No one is excluded. Parents lead the negotiations, typically in family meetings.

The optimal family has *transcendent values,* a belief system that tolerates and transcends the pain of loss and change. This belief system may be based in part on conventional religious beliefs but usually is an intrinsic belief that love is a worthwhile risk even though the loved one may be lost. The family has an altruistic bent toward society. Children, of course, cannot conceptualize these notions until they near adulthood. Nevertheless, mature parents set the tone for the family with their own abilities to transcend the inevitability of loss, death, and change.

Change

The concept of change is central in the family systems theory. Western, particularly American, views about marriage and family are influenced by fairy tales and the media, wherein the hero and heroine find each other and live happily ever after. The couple soon finds, however, that living happily ever after is indeed a fairy tale. They discover that their lives and the environment are constantly changing. If children enter the family, change and conflict are inherent. Every system works to maintain homeostasis, that is, some kind of stability that provides a balance between what is valued and desired and the changes that impinge on and disrupt that homeostasis. Change causes stress within the system.

◆ Stressors and Their Impact on Families

HISTORICAL VIEW OF FAMILIES

During this century, immense social and technological change has occurred in the United States. Following the sacrifices and pain of World War I, the great depression, and World War II, families settled into a conservative nuclear family pattern. The wife-mother often stayed home as the primary parent to the children, while the husband-father developed his career and was the primary source of financial income for the family. In greater numbers, families moved away from the city to suburban areas as a sign of increasing affluence. The adults of the 1950s were children of the depression who feared economic deprivation and wanted to spare their children the pain of poverty.

During the 1960s, tremendous social change occurred. Youth rebellion against a materialistic society and the United States' increasing involvement in Vietnam disrupted the long-accepted values of patriotism and the work ethic. Humanitarian social values became prevalent. Minority groups in the United States insisted on their rights to participate in the affluent life of middle-income America. Their insistence took place through political influence, passive tactics (eg, civil disobedience), or violence. The rights of the individual became paramount in education, health care, hiring practices, housing, and business opportunities.

The 1970s brought the women's movement and emphasis on self-awareness and fulfillment. Divorce rates skyrocketed, and the family's typical configuration of homemaker-mother, breadwinner-father, and children was threatened. Individual freedom was important. Inflation was rampant. By the end of the 1970s, the dual-earner family was the predominant family form, and half of the mothers in the work force had preschool children.[7,45] Violent crime, sexual promiscuity, adolescent pregnancy, substance abuse, mental health problems, and suicide became almost epidemic. The emergence of ultraconservative groups, such as the Moral Majority, and increased membership in conservative churches signaled a swing of the pendulum toward more traditional values.[44]

In the 1980s and into the 1990s, families continued to experienced severe strain. The trends of the previous decade persisted, resulting in serious decline for the well-being of children. Children of all socioeconomic classes were increasingly affected. Problems of poverty, divorce, out-of-wedlock births, absentee parents, latchkey kids, violence, and drugs were no longer confined to the lower socioeconomic classes.[21]

According to the National Commission on the Role of the School and the Community in Improving Adolescent Health, "never before has one generation of children been less healthy, less cared for, or less prepared for life than their parents were at the same age."[28] The House Select Committee on Children, Youth, and Families stated that childhood is now "far more precarious and less safe for millions of America's children."[35]

In the mid-1990s, we now see families as systems that are characterized by change.[22] Regardless of the nature of the changes, whether life stage changes, changes in roles and family structure, or societal changes, change is a constant force impacting family systems. A major focus of professionals interfacing with families is that of empowering the family to deal in an optimal manner with the numerous changes they will encounter.

DEVELOPMENTAL STRESSORS

Besides developing as a unit in the context of historical events, the family undergoes changes related to the growth and development of its members. The birth of the first child, whether planned or unplanned, is a significant stressor. The physiological and emotional changes of pregnancy test the couple's ability to support one another. Lifestyle changes related to nausea or fatigue also may be difficult for the couple. Childbirth is now usually a shared experience for the couple and often a peak experience in their lives. However, the demanding infant soon commands a central position in the family by requiring a great deal of energy, time, and emotional investment. The couple must learn to meet the baby's needs without neglecting their own, a task that persists through childhood and adolescence.

The adolescent period is a highly stressful time for families. The teenager's ambivalence about dependence versus independence and resultant limit testing are frightening and frustrating for parents. Finding a balance between giving the adolescent freedom to grow and learn versus protecting him or her from harmful experiences until sound judgment is developed requires much time, energy, thought, and sensitivity. Open communication must be centered on the teenager's thoughts and feelings regarding important issues, such as money, rules, school achievement, sex, love, career choice, and friends. Parents need to set appropriate, fair limits with consequences for the breaking of rules. On the other hand, every aspect of the adolescent's life should not be subjected to scrutiny, probing, and checking. Trust should be established through childhood and early adolescence, and opportunities for role taking, examining moral-ethical issues, and developing good judgment should be provided *with* the child.

The middle years present two major crises: the midlife crisis and dealing with aging parents. The crisis of midlife begins when the middle-aged person confronts the fact of mortality, often triggered by the appearance of wrinkles or competition from younger people at work. The middle-aged person accepts limitations and hopes for success and comes to terms with accomplishments in life thus far, including work, family relationships, sexuality, and hopes for children. This is a painful time and often coincides with the presence of teenagers in the family. Moreover, the decision to care for elderly parents may leave the middle-ager responsible for two generations, a considerable burden.[37]

The older adult must cope with the loss of work, friends, spouse, and often economic resources. Looking back on life, the older adult concludes that it has been a meaningful experience with which he or she is satisfied or that it has not been meaningful. A conclusion of lack of meaning may lead to despair.

ROLES AND CHANGE WITHIN FAMILIES

Role development and change cause considerable challenges for families. Since the late 1970s, the predominant family structure has been the *dual-earner family*. Often there are children in the dual-earner family. Providing physical and emotional care for children, maintaining the household, participating in children's activities, providing transportation for children, and maintaining and developing the self and the relationship with a spouse dictate a full, interesting life or a frustrating, exhausting one. Women in these families typically experience more role strain and feel more overwhelmed by their responsibilities than do men in these families.[18]

The skyrocketing divorce rate profoundly affects the families involved. The self-esteem of the involved spouses often suffers a severe blow. The children may become angry and confused and are often forced to choose the parent with whom they will live. Because of their stage of development, they may feel self-blame for the breakup of the marriage. Most families cannot adequately recover from divorce without counseling. The counseling is often prompted by the mother-wife's stress or by the children's acting-out behavior. Serious economic setbacks occur when one household becomes two households with the same income. Women usually earn less money than their male counterparts and are more likely than men to receive custody of the children. Child support payments often are not paid regularly. Children of divorce may undergo moves to new schools, loss of friends and activities, and loss of the parent who does not have custody (Box 17-1).

Other families experience change through the loss of a family member through death or desertion. Economic conditions in these families vary according to socioeconomic class, whether the lost member was a breadwinner or the sole breadwinner, and whether the death was due to catastrophic illness.

The *single-parent* family is often at risk because of its limited financial resources and the parent's limited time and energy. Moreover, the absent parent's role modeling is not available for the children. Twenty-four percent of all households in the United States are headed by a single parent; 88% of these are headed by women.[19] Single-parent families are much more likely to experience economic strain than are two-parent families.

An increase in remarriages has resulted in more *blended* families. Putting two families together, particularly if children are involved, takes time and patience. Adoptive families of an older child also experience role change. This change requires considerable patience and love for the child, who has often been in a succession of foster homes.

A dramatic rise in teenage pregnancy has resulted in increasing numbers of *teenage parents.* Adolescent parents have not reached adulthood themselves yet have the responsibility for a baby, for which they are emotionally and financially ill equipped. In addition, the adolescent mother and her infant also experience physiological risk.

ENVIRONMENTAL INFLUENCES ON THE FAMILY

Although descriptions of the family often refer to "middle-class" families, a variety of cultures are represented in the United States. Effective family assessment and intervention require an awareness and understanding of family members' ethnic backgrounds and the skills needed to provide culturally competent care.[23] Different cultures have different definitions of family, varying family life cycles, and variations in attitudes of family solutions. They often seek care from their culture's folk health systems rather than seeking care from the professional systems of the dominant culture.[9]

Poverty is an overwhelming obstacle for many families. The struggle to obtain food, clothing, and shelter, often substandard and far from the American dream, occupies the family's time and energy and depletes its dignity. Frustration is high, and desertion and violence are common. Reliance on public assistance may be seen as demeaning and limiting individual initiative. A low socioeconomic status is the most significant risk factor for children demonstrating behavior problems.[38]

Television and other media have been significant influences on families during the last 40 years. The media has been blamed for contributing to unprecedented materialism, increase in violent crime among young people, irresponsible sexual behavior, sapping of creative thinking, undesirable dietary practices, and lack of communication between family members. In one survey, eighth-grade students reported watching 21.4 hours of television per week and spending only 5.6 hours per week on homework. Sixty-three percent of the students said their parents "rarely or never" limited television watching time.[2]

The changing *values* of society have an impact on schools. Schools, in turn, impact on the families of their students. Schools at all levels have been concerned with students' rights and with providing curricula for the development of the whole self. Some critics have claimed that this concern has resulted in a decline in college entrance examination scores and serious discipline problems, particularly in high schools. Some schools are responding by raising academic standards and adopting stricter disciplinary policies. At the same time, however, schools are challenged by a lack of parent involvement in school.

The rise in violent crime and in the incidence of *family violence* is staggering. Suspected child abuse and neglect reports have increased more than 10% per year, rising from 669,000 in 1976 to 2,163,000 in 1987.[13] One in 10 American women are abused by intimate partners.[34] Many of the previously discussed changes and stressors that impact families contribute to family violence.

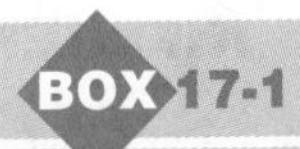

How Children Adapt to Divorce

In addition to the already strenuous developmental tasks of childhood and adolescence, children of divorce must master six more psychological tasks, according to Judith Wallerstein, who has conducted a longitudinal study of children of divorce. This study has produced some sobering data. The process of recovery from divorce is a lengthy one, lasting through late adolescence or early adulthood. Even when the psychological tasks of coping with divorce are mastered, the child of divorce experiences "some residue of sadness, of anger and of anxiety about the potential unreliability of relationships." The tasks of coping with divorce include the following:

Task I, *acknowledging the reality of the marital rupture,* is usually completed within 1 year; however, it is usually accompanied initially by considerable regression. Younger children have more difficulty with this task because of their inability to conceptualize time, space, and the nature of relationships.

Task II, *disengaging from parental conflict and distress and resuming customary pursuits,* is also usually completed by the child within 1 to 2 years of the divorce. In the year following the divorce or separation, the child often has difficulty learning and has other school problems. Some children become involved in sexual activity or stealing. All children must distance themselves from their upset parents and overcome their own depression and anxiety. After the initial upset, most children resume their usual activities.

Task III, the *resolution of loss,* takes many years. In addition to grieving the multiple losses that the divorce precipitates, the child strives to recover from an overwhelming sense of rejection. This sense of rejection is diminished by frequent, reliable visiting arrangements and by the development of a relationship with the noncustodial parent.

Task IV, *resolving anger and blame,* also takes many years to accomplish. Usually in late adolescence, the child begins to understand the parents and the reasons for the divorce. Typically, the child forgives the parents and perhaps himself or herself.

Task V, *accepting the permanence of divorce,* is a gradual process during which the child wishes intensely for and fantasizes about the restoration of the family. It is not uncommon for mature adults to continue to wish for and fantasize about the reconciliation of their parents.

Task VI, *achieving realistic hope regarding relationships,* is a normal task of adolescence, but for the child of divorce, it is complicated by fears of rejection and failure based on earlier experience.

Clearly, the child of divorce faces a dilemma—to learn to trust in his or her own lovability, capacity to love, self-worth, and in the reliability of relationships. Findings from a 10-year follow-up of 38 youngsters now 16 to 18 years old, whose parents divorced during the children's early latency, suggest that separation from families and the transition into young adulthood are burdened by fear of disappointment in love relationships, lowered expectations, and a sense of powerlessness. A need for the father, especially among boys, appears to burgeon at middle and late adolescence.

(From Wallerstein JS: Children of Divorce: Report of a Ten Year Follow-up of Early Latency Age Children. Am J Orthopsychiatry 57 [April]: 199–211, 1987.)

The presence of *chronic illness* or *disability* in a family member taxes physical and emotional energy, time, and economic resources of the ill or disabled person and other family members. *Alcoholism* and other *chemical dependencies* are major stressors for families. The National Council on Alcoholism and Drug Dependence reports that 43% of American adults have been exposed to alcoholism in their own families.[29] There is increasing evidence that this disease is genetically transmitted and mediated by environmental factors. Families of alcoholics are often characterized by intense conflict, shame, lack of trust, denial, and physical illness. Family members take on roles that help to stabilize this distressed family but ultimately result in increased problems for the family and enable the deterioration of the alcoholic and the family (Table 17–1).

Although the stressors that have been presented are significant and prevalent, a critical variable in whether the family survives and produces capable people is the parents' self-esteem. The family can tolerate and cope with a great deal of stress if parents feel satisfied with themselves and their relationship. Low parental self-esteem is a major stressor to any family. Therefore, family nursing interventions are often targeted toward the parents as individuals and the parenting partnership.

Application of the Nursing Process to the Family

ASSESSMENT

Nursing assessment of families has often focused on illness. However, a perspective of assessing families related to wellness rather than illness is more appropriate for nursing's goal of health promotion.[20] The assessment framework presented here incorporates variables that affect the development of competent people with the addition of a category related to health (Boxes 17-2 and 17-3).

People are continually subjected to stress and change; how a person manages stress and change determines relative wellness. The ability to adapt and grow stems directly from an individual's experiences in family life. Nurses who assess families will examine data regarding the family's structural, functional, developmental, and communicational patterns. This information allows the nurse to assess the family member's adaptation or "fit."[12] Families' levels of adaptation fall on a continuum from optimal to midrange to severely disturbed.[5] Families also may be described as nurturing or troubled.[32]

Optimal Families

As described previously, the *optimal family* has little physical illness and usually practices high-level health care, including excellent nutrition and abstinence or near abstinence from substances with the potential for abuse, such as alcohol and drugs. The family also participates in regular exercise and recreation, avoids dangerous activities, and demonstrates concern for the environment. In short, the optimal family is the ideal family. Most families function in the adequate and midrange area, and a smaller proportion of families function in the troubled range.

Adequate Families

Adequate families produce people who do not have mental health problems. The adequate family maintains an open systems orientation; the family is flexible

Table 17-1

Roles and Dynamics of an Alcoholic Family

Role	Motivating Feeling	Identifying Symptoms	Payoff: For Individual	Payoff: For Family	Possible Price
Dependent	Shame	Chemical use	Relief of pain	None	Addiction
Enabler	Anger	Powerlessness	Importance; self-righteousness	Responsibility	Illness; "martyrdom"
Hero	Inadequacy; guilt	Overachievement	Attention (positive)	Self-worth	Compulsive drive
Scapegoat	Hurt	Delinquency	Attention (negative)	Focus away from dependent	Self-destruction; addiction
Lost child	Loneliness	Solitariness; shyness	Escape	Relief	Social isolation
Mascot	Fear	Clowning; hyperactivity	Attention (amused)	Fun	Immaturity; emotional illness

(Wegschieder S: Another Chance: Help and Hope for the Alcoholic Family, Palo Alto, CA, Science and Behavior Books, 1981).

BOX 17-2

Characteristics of Optimal Families

1. *Open-system orientation*
   Multiple causation of events
   Need for each other and other people
2. *Boundaries*
   Touching
   Interaction between family members
   Allocation of space in household
   Links to society
3. *Contextual clarity*
   Developmental issues resolved
   Clear generational lines
   Strong parental coalition
   Communication; clear, direct, honest, specific, congruent
4. *Power*
   Flows from parental coalition
   Delegated to children appropriate to age
   Clear role definition
   Not sex-defined
   Rules
5. *Encouragement of autonomy*
   Differentness accepted
6. *Affective issues*
   Warmth and caring
   Empathy
   Feelings attended to
   Amount of conflict
   Resolution of conflict
   Self-esteem of members high
7. *Negotiation and task performance*
   Input from all members
   Led by parents
   Little conflict
8. *Transcendent values*
   Expect loss
   Recover from and prepare for loss
   Hopeful
   Altruistic
9. *Health measures*
   Healthy diet
   Free of drugs and chemicals
   Regular exercise and recreation
   Concern for the environment
   Abstinence from dangerous activities
   Family history of health

and open, does not believe causation of events is linear, and expresses need for each other and other people. The intrasystem boundaries are clearly defined but open. Members of the family respect each other's privacy, but there is considerable face-to-face interaction and touching.

The family's links to society are numerous and viewed positively. Societal links are likely to include work, school, church, friends, extended family, family physician, and community service organizations. The family is not likely to have connections with social welfare agencies. Contextual clarity is present, and developmental issues are resolved appropriately according to the ages of the children. The parents provide strong leadership and maintain their relationship as a couple. Communication is clear, direct, honest, specific, and congruent.

In adequate families, power flows from the parents, who use authoritarian measures when necessary. Parents delegate responsibility to children as deemed appropriate for their age and stage of development. Roles are clear; that is, family members know and agree on their functions and performance of activities. Family members understand and generally respect family rules. Power and authority are not ascribed by sex but rather by the individual characteristics and abilities of each family member. Achievement of an egalitarian relationship necessitates commitment and perseverance. Both of the adult partners may sacrifice some aspect of self-realization to meet the children's needs in an adequate or optimal manner.

Adequate families promote autonomy by encouraging children and adults to try new activities and express their ideas, even when those ideas diverge from the family's values. Family members are valued for their differences and their similarities with others. Idiosyncracies are tolerated with good humor.

The affective tone is warm and caring. Members are empathic, often at early ages, and consider and ask about others' feelings. Although there is more conflict in the adequate family than in the optimal family, it is resolved without loss of self-esteem. Self-esteem is high in these families; however, because of extra responsibility and higher demands from the family, the mother may experience more stress, loneliness, or depression than other family members.

Negotiation and task performance are accomplished with considerable ease but not as easily as in optimal families. Decisions often are reached at family meetings; parents lead the discussions and have the final say in decisions. Some conflict about household work exists, and the mother is likely to assume a dispro-

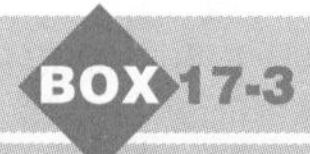

Family Assessment Guidelines

1. *Open-system orientation*
   What do you believe are the reasons for the difficulty?
   What do you think the solution is?
2. *Boundaries*
   (Notice who touches whom, who talks to whom, presence of eye contact.)
   (Notice whether the touching is parental, kind, loving, seductive, rought, or violent.)
   Where does everyone sleep?
   Do you all have time alone?
   How do you get along with your child's teacher, scout leader, and other significant people in your child's life?
   How do you like your child's friends?
   Are you in touch with your child's friends' parents?
3. *Contextual clarity*
   Who's in charge in this family?
   Who gets along best with whom?
   Who does what around the house?
   (Notice whether parents agree on what is happening.)
   (Notice whether there is unusual closeness between child and opposite-sex parent.)
   (Is communication clear, honest, specific; do members make "I statements" or blaming "you statements"?)
   (Can the interviewer get an answer to a question? Can family members get an answer?)
   (Can the interviewer follow the family conversation?)
   (Are verbal and nonverbal communications congruent?)
   How much is your television turned on?
4. *Power*
   (Do the parents set the tone for the interview, set limits on children's behaviors? Are the limits reasonable, not just talk or punitive?)
   (Does one person control the group by talking or distracting?)
   (Does everyone talk or at least seem involved?)
   Tell me your rules.
   What happens if they are broken?
   What are everyone's jobs at home?
5. *Encouragement of autonomy*
   If you (wife) like to stay home and read and you (husband) like to go to parties, how do you deal with these different desires?
   (Are members stereotyped as "the angel," "the wild one," "just like his Uncle so and so," and so on?)
   What kinds of things are you (a child) interested in
   How are you different from your sister?
6. *Affective issues*
   (Can the interviewer feel warmth and caring, or does the interviewer feel uncomfortable, fearful?)
   What do you think your child is feeling? What are you feeling as you listen to your child?
   (Notice whether family members seem ashamed or embarrassed.)
   (Are conflicts resolved?)
   What do you do when you get angry?
7. *Negotiating and task performances*
   Do you argue about household chores?
   (Can the family solve a problem with parents having final say in the issue?)
   Do you have meetings?
8. *Transcendent values*
   (Do family members believe that problems can be solved?)
   What do you think and feel about your child going to camp, getting married, and so on?
   What do you (parents) do for fun?
   (Do family members accept that life is complicated, difficult, joyous, routine?)
   In what kinds of community activities are you involved?
   (Do family members laugh at themselves, have a sense of humor?)
9. *Health measures*
   When and where do you eat meals?
   Do you eat one meal each day together?
   What kinds of things do you eat?
   How often do you have a drink?
   Does anyone take medications?
   Tell me how you have fun.
   Do you participate in sports or other exercise?
   What do you do to relax?
   What illnesses have family members had (grandparents, aunts, uncles)? Any suicide, mental illness, drug or alcohol addictions in the family?

portionate share of the work. Nevertheless, the adequate family usually can work out ways to prevent overload of one person. Family members are competent in all areas and excel in some areas. There is no significant deviance in performance in school or work or in relationships with others.

Transcendent values include a hopeful, positive outlook; the expectation and preparation for loss of children, retirement, and so forth; and altruism toward neighbors. These families also practice adequate health measures and do not suffer significant health problems.

Midrange Families

Midrange families produce people with mental health problems. The "identified client" in the family is likely to be behaviorally disordered or demonstrate a personality disorder. Family members may also have physical illnesses. Although family members are reasonably effective, they are restricted. An open-system orientation is absent in these families; family members need others but under certain conditions. The family tends to believe that there are causes for events, but they are not sure what they are. They continuously strive to find answers and do well.

Boundaries remain fairly clear, although when under pressure, the family will solidify its boundaries and turn inward (ie, keep the trouble inside) or lose its boundaries and spill into the environment. Interaction between family members (intrasystem interaction) is restricted. Links to society are present, but they disrupt when the family is under unusual pressure. Families who tend to externalize trouble (ie, push it into the environment) have contact with law enforcement agencies.

Midrange families also have difficulty with contextual clarity. Developmental issues are not resolved adequately or appropriately. Parental coalition is present but weak, and other coalitions develop that undermine the effectiveness of the parents. Communication in these families is generally clear but expressed with fear, guilt, or anger.

Power is the central difficulty in midrange families. The family confuses love and power. Midrange families often believe that caring means controlling the life of another and through overt or covert coercion, applying a system of "oughts" and "shoulds." The "shoulds" are often sex-stereotyped. The parents believe in doing the "right" thing and are constantly struggling for control of the children through discipline, money, and so forth. Children become powerful by manipulating the parents, not by learning to assume power and responsibility. Family roles are defined by sex or by other beliefs about the family member, such as "she's so good and never causes any trouble" or "he's the athletic one." The family behaves as if someone is judging the goodness or badness of the family's actions, thoughts, and feelings.

Encouragement of autonomy is not found in midrange families. On the contrary, children are expected to adhere to the family's norms. The constant power struggles and repression of feelings and ideas within the family drain the family members' creativity. Children tend to stay in the parental home well into adulthood or leave home very early in a kind of pseudoautonomy.

The affective issues that characterize midrange families are depression, anxiety, and anger. The enormous resultant conflict may be overtly expressed in angry exchanges or repressed through submission to the "oughts" and "shoulds." As a result, members display little empathy, much conflict over rules and norms, considerable frustration, and caring that is controlling rather than growth producing. The self-esteem of the family members is low, and the identified client has very low self-esteem.

Negotiation and task performance are accomplished by coercion, because the parental team cannot agree on who does what. These families do not hold family meetings. Nevertheless, the work of the family is accomplished.

Transcendent values of hope and altruism are lacking. The family eventually accepts change and loss but with a great deal of pain, anger, and frustration. They look toward the future as if to say, "What difficulty will present itself?" Martyrdom is not an unusual stance for members of these families.

Health problems in midrange families include excessive use of alcohol, prescription tranquilizers, and other drugs for relief of the pain of daily living. The stressful existence of midrange families produces some psychophysiological illnesses, such as headaches, ulcers, and obesity. Because the family is concerned with doing the "right" thing, they meet their basic health needs.

The family attempts recreation and exercise, but the conflict that surfaces during the planning of events reduces their pleasure. In some families, the presence of a great deal of anger leads to dangerous activities, such as hitting, driving at excessive speeds, and running away. The midrange family is too preoccupied with daily events to explore health promotion and wellness activities.

Troubled Families

Families functioning on the more dysfunctional end of the family health continuum tend to produce people who exhibit disorders of conduct, personality, or addiction. *Troubled families* display qualities opposite to those of optimal families' characteristics. The family tends to be very rigid or disordered, rather than open and flexible.

Boundary issues in troubled families are problematic. The family system boundary is rigid with minimal links to society. The links are tentative and mistrustful, and input from the larger society is limited. Troubled families may also have diffuse boundaries, with family business tending to spill over into the environment. Interpersonal boundaries are also diffused, resulting in global response to input. Distancing between people is prevalent.

Contextual clarity is blurred in troubled families. Due to a weak parental coalition, cross-generational clinging occurs, and developmental issues remain unresolved. The parents deal with their pain of disappointment in each other by reaching across generational boundaries for comfort or control of the situation. Often this cross-generational clinging takes the form of a triangle; for example, mother and son form a coalition against father. Often, covert or overt incestuous behavior occurs. The child who is "triangled" is usually the symptom bearer in the family. This child (or young adult) responds to these pressures with mental disorder, physical illness, or delinquent behavior.

Communication is not clear, congruent, specific, direct, nor honest. Because family members have low self-esteem, they fear rejection from others and are embarrassed about this fear. To cover up their fear of rejection, members of troubled families tend to use four patterns of communication described by Satir:

1. Placating, or doing anything to prevent others from getting angry
2. Blaming, or attempting to look strong and reject first
3. Computing, or treating others as if they were insignificant by using big words
4. Distracting, or eliminating the possibility of rejection by changing the subject or talking in a "crazy" way[32]

Another characteristic of communication in troubled families is the lack of congruence between verbal and nonverbal communication, for example, smiling when talking in an angry tone of voice. *Double-bind communication* occurs when an incongruent message is sent that includes a direction to do something with a nonverbal message to do the opposite. Furthermore, the receiver of the message is not permitted to comment on it. For example, a father says to his child in angry tone of voice, "Come here and let me hug you. You know Daddy loves you." The child answers, "You sound mad." The father responds, "I don't know what you're talking about." The child is then faced with the dilemma of determining to which communication he or she should respond. A child faced with continuous double-bind communication is unable to determine the true meaning of statements or identify and name normal feelings. As the child's ability to test reality becomes impaired, he or she may invent a language and peculiar explanations for events. In some troubled families, anger is communicated through hitting and other forms of assault.

Another communication difficulty found in troubled families, *disqualifying,* occurs when an individual fails to attend to another's message by silence, ignoring, or changing the subject. Evasiveness in communication is also common in these families.

Power is diffuse and does not flow from the parents. Autonomy is discouraged rather than encouraged. In fact, the troubled family does not tolerate differences. Paradoxically, the family tends to view one of its members as "different" and the cause of its trouble; this process is called *scapegoating.*

The affective tone in troubled families with diffuse boundaries tends to be exaggerated. Members react inappropriately to threats or to one member's difficulties. In families with rigid boundaries, the affective tone is restricted, depressed, and despairing. There is a lack of empathy, and great distance exists between members. Undue attention (confusing, smothering, or rejecting) is paid to one member. Self-esteem in troubled families is low, and hate, inability to respond empathetically to others, loneliness, and hopelessness predominate.

Negotiation is not accomplished, and performance of tasks varies widely. Conflict may be a constant, overt, and unresolved presence in families with diffuse boundaries. This conflict is denied, not discussed, and unresolved in families with rigid boundaries. Transcendent values are absent. The inability of troubled families to tolerate loss or differences leads to a cynical, hopeless outlook rather than an altruistic, hopeful one. The stresses of unhappy family life often produce serious physical illness, usually in one member.

NURSING DIAGNOSIS

The nurse can formulate nursing diagnoses to address a family's functioning or adaptive abilities. The following nursing diagnoses are appropriate descriptions for altered or ineffective family interactions:

1. Altered Family Processes
2. Ineffective Family Coping: Compromised
3. Ineffective Family Coping: Disabling
4. Family Coping: Potential for Growth[30]

These nursing diagnoses assist the psychiatric-mental health nurse in planning interventions for the family whose less-than-optimal coping methods or responses to stress, crisis, or change prevent it from attaining its goals. Often the nurse uses family-focused nursing diagnoses in addition to individual-centered diagnoses, especially when working with child, adolescent, and chemically dependent clients. Incorporating family diagnoses may be appropriate during the application of the nursing process for any client exhibiting emotional or behavioral problems.

PLANNING

Optimal and adequate families are not likely to present themselves for assistance in traditional mental health care settings. These families may interact with mental health professionals through church activities, Parent-Teacher Association meetings, community functions, adult education centers, and other such events. They educate themselves through newspapers, magazines, books, and select television programs. Therefore, the nurse must plan to reach optimal and adequate families in nontraditional health care settings, such as preventive and health maintenance programs. Family members may be enriched in four areas: enhancement of existing strengths, anticipatory guidance, parent education, and holistic health measures.

Enhancing existing strengths may be as simple as a word of praise or as complex as a series of structured, goal-directed activities. Providing encouragement and praise for the successful performance of parental functions develops trust and increases self-esteem. Anticipatory guidance refers to teaching parents and families what to expect next, particularly in terms of developmental events and crises. Childbirth education and classes on adolescence or aging parents are examples of anticipatory guidance. Family nursing programs are also being used in tertiary care settings.[39] These education programs may be formal or informal.[17]

Midrange families are likely to use mental health facilities and interact with nurses in community health settings. The midrange family with school-age children is likely to come in contact with the school nurse. These families benefit from enhancement of strengths and parenting programs. The nurse may help the family with problem solving, conflict management, and education about normal growth and development, especially as it relates to their present difficulties. The nurse may also make referrals to family therapy if problem solving and education approaches fail to relieve problems.

Troubled families often receive family therapy through therapists in private practice, community mental health centers, or psychiatric inpatient units. Networking the family with other social service agencies is often essential, particularly if economic problems exist, if protection for one or more members is needed, or if the legal system is involved. The responsible nurse, therapist, social worker, or other health care professional seeks sources of support for the family and assists them in arranging for these services. These services may include churches, social welfare agencies, emergency supply pantry services, Red Cross, voluntary agencies, hospices, and community health services.

The planning of nursing care for families involves matching nursing interventions to specific domains of family functioning. Such domains may be cognitive, affective, or behavioral.[42]

INTERVENTION

Nursing interventions with families may include family support, maintenance of family process, promotion of family integrity, family involvement, family mobilization, caregiver support, family therapy, sibling support, and parent education.[10] To be effective in intervening with families, the psychiatric-mental health nurse must first develop necessary characteristics and skills.

Characteristics and Skills of the Nurse

To work effectively with families, the nurse must possess self-awareness, empathy, therapeutic communication skills, and knowledge of family theory. The nurse expands understanding of family life through formal education, self-directed learning, observation, and supervised practice.

Self-awareness is crucial to an understanding of the behaviors of others. One must be able to identify and "own" one's thoughts, feelings, and biases before understanding others' feelings and behaviors. The psychiatric-mental health nurse pursues personal growth as part of ongoing education. Nurses must also become aware of their own family dynamics, roles, and values so that they will not confuse or compare their own family style with others and impose their style on others.

Another crucial characteristic is *empathy*. The nurse interacts and intervenes with families experiencing varying problems and strengths. The nurse must be able to experience the family's trouble from their perspective and then step back to analyze and intervene. Empathy is essential to building trust.

Therapeutic communication skills also are essential. The nurse is a role model of clear, open, direct, honest, and congruent communication and clarifies the family's unclear communication. The nurse who works effectively with families possesses certain knowledge about families, which includes the beliefs that families are functioning as well as they are able, that no one is to blame, that parents want very much to do a good job, and that people behave in nonproductive ways because they are in pain. The nurse, empathizing with the family's pain, works from the position of their strengths; he or she assists them, primarily through communication skills, to learn that the problem is a family problem and that there are more satisfying ways to live as a family and as people.

Skillful use of the nursing process, particularly defining the problem accurately, leads to a more productive plan with successful outcomes. So-called *noncompliance* often results from failure of the nurse or other health care provider to discover important underlying issues that result in nonresolution of the problem. Knowledge of various *teaching* strategies, an understanding of *learning* principles, and the ability to make adequate *referrals* for other services are important. The nurse actively assists the family through the steps to ensure entry into the desired system. Box 17-4 lists some self-help groups and resources for families.

An important activity that nurses have always performed, *case management,* ensures that families with a severely mentally ill member receive assistance in obtaining help for all problems. Case managers also provide crisis intervention. Nurses with psychiatric experience and adequate educational background perform well as case managers. The role of a nurse case manager with mentally ill clients is expanding with the current economic incentives toward limited mental health care. These limitations promote new, creative approaches to meeting the needs of families.

Collaboration is working with others as equals toward a common goal. The nurse is a peer on the mental health team and strives to provide the best service to clients by using the contributions of other disciplines in the interest of the family. Nurses also are *consultants* on family health in the community by serving on advisory boards, committees, and school boards and by communicating with legislators and candidates about the needs of families.

The development of *personal coping* skills is essential to the well-being of the nurse who works with families. The intensive nature of family health nursing, especially psychiatric-mental health nursing, necessitates that the nurse obtain sufficient rest, exercise, relaxation, and nurturance and support from colleagues, friends, and significant others. Adequate *clinical supervision* from an experienced clinician promotes objectivity, continued professional growth, and support of the nurse.

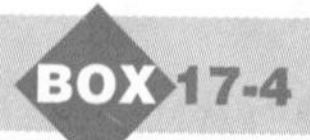

Support Groups and Resources for Families

There are many support groups and resources available to troubled families. People who are interested in them should consult their local libraries, telephone directories, or mental health centers for the groups in their area or contact the group's national office. A partial listing follows.

Al-Anon/Alateen
Al-Anon Family Group Headquarters, Inc.
PO Box 862
Midtown Station New York, NY 10018-0862
1-800-344-2666

Alcoholics Anonymous
PO Box 459
Grand Central Station
New York, NY 10163-0371
(212) 686-1100

Families Anonymous
PO Box 528
Van Nuys, CA 91408
(818) 989-7841

Mothers Against Drunk Driving (MADD)
511 E. John Carpenter Freeway, Suite 700
Irving, TX 75062-8187
(214) 744-6233

Narcotics Anonymous
N.A. World Service Office, Inc.
PO Box 622
Sun Valley, CA 91352

National Alliance for the Mentally Ill (NAMI)
2101 Wilson Boulevard, Suite 302
Arlington, VA 22201
(703) 524-7600

Parents Anonymous
7120 Franklin Avenue
Los Angeles, CA 90046

Parents Without Partners
7910 Woodmont Avenue
Bethesda, MD 20814

Toughlove
1-800-333-1069

Psychoeducation for Families

Families with a seriously mentally ill member require extensive teaching about the illness. Families of mentally ill people are now a highly visible political entity represented through the National Alliance for the Mentally Ill, both nationally and in local chapters. Families in this group are sensitive to any potential or actual blaming by professionals, and they consider traditional family therapy countertherapeutic because of the blame it places on the family members of mentally ill individuals. Comprehensive care for the families of mentally ill clients includes preventive, restorative, and palliative nursing care.[3] Nurses and other mental health professionals must always provide concrete, specific information on the etiology, symptoms, and prognosis of the illness and information about medications, how to manage disorders behaviorally, and how to access and manage the mental health system.[15] They must also provide empathic support for a family dealing with a catastrophic, chronic illness. The family may agree to family therapy after trust is established.

Family Therapy

Family therapy is conducted by clinicians of various disciplines, including nurse therapists who have undergone formal training in family therapy during graduate or postgraduate education. *Family therapy* is a specific intervention mode based on the premise that the member with the presenting symptoms signals the presence of pain in the whole family. This pain may arise from the disappointment of the marital partners with each other. Their unhappiness, anger, and hurt are expressed overtly or covertly in a number of ways, such as triangling, scapegoating, psychophysiological illness, mental illness, and substance abuse. Whatever the presenting diagnosis, the therapist works to assist the family to identify and express their thoughts and feelings, define family roles and rules, try new and more productive styles of relating, and restore strength to the parental coalition. Although family therapy is most often conducted with the members of the nuclear family, other variations include extended family therapy and multiple family therapy.[6]

Family History. Family therapy begins by exploring the family's history, starting with the parents' relationship. This strategy starts the process of focusing on the couple as leaders of the family and takes the pressure off the identified client. During the history taking, each person in the family is identified and recognized in chronological order, thereby acknowledging each member's uniqueness and defining their roles. History taking may also include a three-generational map of family structure and relationships (Box 17-5).[36] This map is called a genogram. As the therapist draws the map, he or she questions the family about significant events and identifies family roles. This nonthreatening technique may be useful in diagnosing the family's problems and for helping the family members understand that their present structure, roles, values, and entire system evolved from the past. It is an excellent approach for nurse-therapists and other psychiatric-mental health professionals who work with dysfunctional families.

Communication Techniques in Family Therapy. Family therapy may be initiated by asking the family to talk together about the trouble and then monitoring the conversation.[1] The therapist intervenes in the family's conversation by clarifying; interpreting double-level, double-bind, and nonverbal communication; and assisting members to identify their own thoughts, feelings, and actions and to communicate them clearly and congruently to others. The therapist deals with anger by talking about it openly and nonjudgmentally, interpreting anger as hurt, handling emotionally loaded issues through moving from least to most emotionally loaded material, and tying feelings to the facts. The therapist uses humor and empathy, points out positive aspects of the individuals, never blames anyone, and assumes good will even when it is expressed poorly.[33]

Experiential Activities. Other therapeutic techniques available to the nurse-therapist and family include homework assignments, paradoxical injunction, and sculpting. Homework assignments might require family members to engage in one recreational activity together during the next week, eat one-third of their meals together, or verbally reinforce each family member once each day. Paradoxical injunctions are instructions to perform the opposite of what is intended, also called the therapeutic bind.[24] Sculpting is a technique wherein the family enacts an experience without words, then "freezes." The sculpture expresses the feeling tone without word games and is a powerful device for assisting families to understand their relationships. The therapist may instruct a particular member to arrange the sculpture as he or she would like it to be, thereby initiating change with action.[16] Other interventions might include story telling, respite planning, and interventive questions (questions designed to promote change).[42]

EVALUATION

Successful outcomes of work with families can be measured by comparing family functioning with the assessment criteria described previously. Successful outcomes may include more optimal levels of biological, emotional, or spiritual functioning.[10] The family who functions optimally has an open systems orientation, clear boundaries, positive links to society, contextual clarity with clear and congruent communication, a strong parental coalition, appropriate power distribution, autonomous people, a warm and caring affective tone with high self-esteem of members, efficient negotiation and task performance, and transcendent values of hope and altruism. As Satir says, "Family therapy is terminated when everyone in the family can use the first person singular followed by an active verb and ending with a direct object."[33] At that point, family members are free to express feelings and thoughts without fear of losing self-esteem. Case Study 17-1 and Nursing Care Plan 17-1 outline a specific family situation and goals and interventions for family care.

◆ Chapter Summary

This chapter provides an overview of family theories, stressors that impact families, and nursing process application to families. Chapter highlights include the following:

(text continues on page 296)

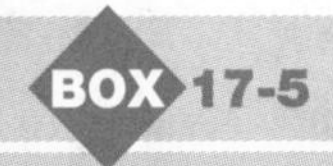

Preparing a Genogram

GENERAL INSTRUCTIONS

1. Divide the paper sideways into three levels.
2. Begin in the middle, with husband on left.
3. Males are in squares; females are in circles.
4. Place birth dates below symbol, prefaced by a "b."
5. Place death dates below symbol, prefaced by a "d."
6. Place marriage date, preceded by "m" on the paired solid line. Separation = "s." Divorce = "d."
7. Adoption date is "a."
8. For first generation (the grandparents), indicate the sibling structure by "oldest of _____" or "youngest of _____" and so forth.
9. Indicate occupation and ethnicity of the first generation along with symbols.
10. Indicate the occupation of the middle generation.
11. Indicate the school year or occupation of the third generation (children of major couple).

NOTATIONS

1. Solid paired line indicates marriage.
2. Broken paired line indicates nonmarriage relationship.
3. Solid vertical line indicates children of the couple.

SAMPLE

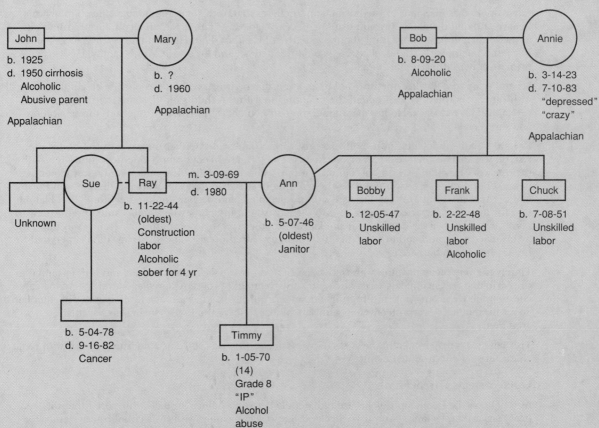

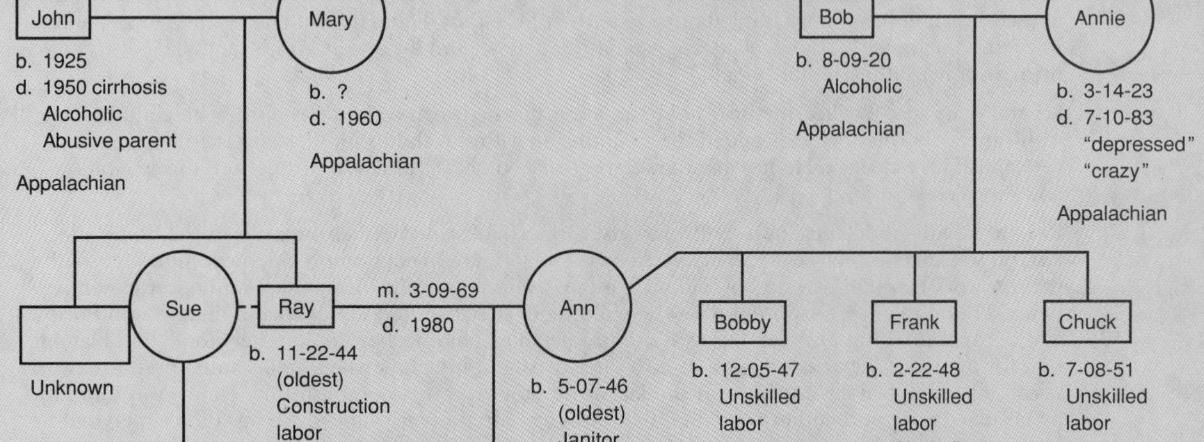

(Adapted from Smoyak S: Family Systems: Use of Genograms as an Assessment Tool. In Clements IW, Buchanan DM (eds): Family Therapy: A Nursing Perspective. New York, John Wiley & Sons, 1982.)

Nursing Care Plan 17-1

The M Family

Assessment

Fourteen-year-old Timmy called the adolescent inpatient facility saying he wanted to "get off drugs and alcohol" and that he could not get along with his parents. An appointment was made with him and his family. Timmy and his mother, Ann, came for several appointments. When outpatient family therapy failed to assist the family, and the potential for violence increased, inpatient admission was arranged.

Timmy is the only child of Ann and Ray M. They were divorced years ago and are now getting back together. The couple have known each other from childhood. Ann is a small, obese, woman who wore the soiled jacket from her janitor's uniform on every occasion that the therapist saw her. Ann talks continuously in a low voice and tells her "story" at every opportunity, whether or not it is relevant. Ann is a high-school graduate. She is one female of four siblings of an alcoholic father and a "mental case" mother. Two brothers are alcoholics. She describes her childhood as working very hard at keeping house, studying, and later working as a nurse's aide at an early age. She was, and remains, ashamed of her family or origin and is angry and ashamed that her son, whom she had hoped would be President of the United States, has been drinking for 2 years, cursing, skipping school, and generally not meeting her expectations.

Ray is angry that his son is in the hospital and believes that, with some reasonable rules, Timmy can behave and quit drinking. Ray quit drinking 4 years ago. Ray's father was an alcoholic and physically abused him and his siblings until about age 6; then his father died. His mother was ineffectual, and Ray left home in early adolescence. He was befriended by, and lived with, Ann's family. He learned to drink with her father and brothers.

Several years ago, Ray became involved in an affair during which a child was born. The child became ill with cancer and died. He has ended the relationship with the child's mother and is attempting to reestablish his marriage. He has maintained regular contact with his son throughout the separation and divorce.

Ray has a sixth-grade education. Both parents work two jobs and neither parent is in the home after 4 P.M. on weekdays or before 4 P.M. on weekends. The jobs are needed to provide necessities, but both parents work extra, in part, to buy Timmy a moped, computerized video games, and other expensive items. They do this so he will not have the childhoods they had. Ray also works so that he won't drink and because he cannot tolerate his wife's unpredictable behavior: her "telling her story" and blaming him for his affair. Ray tried to leave or end the assessment interview when he became upset. Ann works because it raises her self-esteem, and she knows no other way to accomplish this. Timmy was cared for by his maternal grandmother, who died 6 months ago after a year's illness. He was then supervised by his alcoholic grandfather.

Timmy is a very pleasant youth who is working hard on his goals in the program and is determined to stop drinking and maintain sobriety. He finds the treatment program's privilege level system logical and helpful. He is outgoing and friendly but angers quickly. He has average intelligence. He complains about his mother's overprotectiveness and says he has to leave the house during his parents' arguments.

This family has deficits in all nine areas of assessment and is described as a midrange family with some characteristics of a troubled family.

Open Systems Orientation

Ann believes the family's problems are unilaterally her son's failure. Initially, Ray stated that the problems are Ann's fault, but quickly decided that placing Timmy with his alcoholic grandfather for care, buying him too many things, and failing to set rules with logical consequences are errors. Timmy believes that being with his alcoholic grandfather and his parent's fighting are the problems. All family members imply or express a need for others in their lives.

Boundaries

No touching was noted during the assessment interview. Interaction occurs between parent and child with very little between parents. Ann has very few relationships outside the family.

continued

Nursing Care Plan 17-1 (Continued)

Contextual Clarity

The parental coalition is absent. Ann uses her son, rather than her husband, for companionship and support. Ray behaves in a parental role but is unavailable to both his wife and Timmy because of his long work hours and his inability to negotiate with his wife. The parents use blaming patterns of communication and communicate with each other through their child. Only Ray is able to make "I statements."

Power

Ray and Timmy are essentially powerless. Although Ann is very passive superficially, she manipulates her family by not communicating in any other way than "telling the story," thereby inducing guilt and frustration. Her manipulations are a result of her very low self-esteem, shame, and loneliness. Role definitions are based on each individual's perception. Ann's role with her husband is that of a punitive parent; with her son, she assumes a peer role and expects her son to behave like an adult. Ray has a parental role but no husband role. Timmy wishes he were treated like an adolescent son, which his father does but his mother does not. Apparently, his grandmother fulfilled the role of parent for Timmy, but this was offset by the grandfather's treating Timmy as a peer.

Ann and Ray have different sets of expectations that are not clearly defined. Ann expects Timmy to stay at home at all times and bring his friends to their home; however, she does not approve of his friends. When Ray directs Timmy to perform a household chore without consulting Ann, she then tells Timmy not to do it. Timmy, in turn, becomes angry and confused, leaves the house, and drinks.

Encouragement of Autonomy

Although family members identify differences in each other, they are unable to accept them and they hold distorted, unrealistic, and unexpressed expectations of each other.

Affective Issues

Although this family had intense, painful conflicts, the very intensity indicates their concern about losing each other. Both parents care deeply for their son, who reciprocates the feeling. The parents were seriously hurt by their experiences in their families of origin and in their experience with each other. The family earnestly desires to be together as a family but has been unable to negotiate the changes needed. Self-esteem is low in all three members of the family with Timmy having the highest levels.

Negotiation and Task Performance

This family is unable to negotiate.

Transcendent Values

This family is in a great deal of pain and not hopeful because Timmy's drinking has upset their hopes for him to have a better life than the parents had.

Health Measures

Although the family has a regular dinner daily, other meals are irregular and unplanned. Timmy abuses alcohol and marijuana. Ann is obese. Ray has regular recreation with his friends, but Ann and Timmy do not. There is no family recreation at all. Ann's and Timmy's recreation together is watching soap operas.

Although there are deficits in all nine assessment areas, several major themes emerge as appropriate areas for nursing intervention. These are expressed as nursing diagnoses. Because the parental coalition is the critical factor in family functioning, the therapy is directed toward the couple.

continued

Nursing Care Plan 17-1 (Continued)

Nursing Diagnosis

Ineffective Family Coping: compromised, related to unclear boundaries between parents and child and conflictual communication patterns

Outcome

Family members will communicate needs and feelings clearly and negotiate limits and expectations of one another.

Intervention	Rationale
Role model clear, effective communication for family members, eg, use of "I" statements, rather than blaming.	Learning of new, more effective means of communication can take place through role modeling.
Help parents identify acceptable expectations of son's behavior and rules with natural consequences.	Parents must agree on acceptable behavioral norms before expecting compliance with rules; natural consequences are powerful modifiers of behavior.

Evaluation

Communication among family members improves and parents provide son with reasonable expectations of, and natural consequences for, his behavior.

Nursing Diagnosis

Ineffective Individual Coping related to alcohol abuse

Outcome

Timmy will achieve and maintain sobriety from drug and alcohol abuse.

Intervention	Rationale
Involve client and family in addiction recovery program.	Addiction treatment is accomplished through 12-step programs and the participation of all family members.
Help Timmy develop and follow an aftercare program.	Maintaining sobriety requires adherence to an aftercare program.
Teach parents to use positive parenting skills.	Parenting skill development results in improved child and parent functioning.

Evaluation

Timmy remains free of drugs and alcohol.

1. A family is a culturally produced social system composed of two or more people in a primary group.
2. The developmental level of a family's adult members or oldest child may be an index of family development.
3. According to the family systems theory, the whole (the family) is more than the sum of its parts (the members of the family).
4. Living systems possess clear but open boundaries, negentropy, differentiation, and adaptation.
5. Successful families produce competent people through mature leadership of parents.
6. Historical, developmental, role-related, and environmental stressors influence families.
7. Assessment of families includes examination of the family's open systems orientation, boundaries, contextual clarity, power, encouragement of autonomy, affective tone, negotiation and task performance, transcendent values, and health.
8. Goals for families may include enhancement of ex-

isting strengths, anticipatory guidance, parenting education, and holistic health measures.

9. Nurses working with families need to possess self-understanding, empathy, therapeutic communication skills, and knowledge of family theory.
10. The family therapist helps family members identify and express their thoughts and feelings, define family roles and rules, try more productive styles of relating, and restore strength to the parental coalition.

Critical Thinking Questions

1. *Think about a client family with which you have worked. Apply the family nursing process described in the chapter to this family.*
2. *Identify three assumptions you have made about families in the past that you now believe may not be factual.*
3. *List changes you might want to make in your nursing practice as a result of challenging the assumptions you identified in question 2.*
4. *Review the interventions listed in the nursing care plan in this chapter. What changes might you make in these interventions if you were the nurse intervening with this family.*
5. *Based on the evaluation outcomes listed in the nursing care plan, suggest revisions you would make to the plan of care for continuing nursing intervention with this family.*

Review Questions

1. Define the term family.
2. Name four theories used to understand families.
3. Identify at least one family stressor from each of the following categories: historical, developmental, role development and change, and environmental.
4. List the four types of families that nurses may assess.
5. Name two nursing diagnoses that may be applied to families.
6. List three interventions that may be used by nurses intervening with families.

◆ References

1. Andrews E: The Emotionally Disturbed Family. New York, Jason Aaronson, 1977
2. Bacon KH: Many Educators View Involved Parents as Key to Children's Success in School. Wall Street Journal July 30, 1990
3. Basolo-Kunzer M: Caring for Families of Psychiatric Patients. Nurs Clin North Am 29 (1): 73–79, 1994
4. Bateson G, Jackson D, Haley J, Weakland J: Toward a Theory of Schizophrenia. In Jackson DD (ed): Communication, Family, and Marriage. Palo Alto, CA, Science & Behavior Books, 1968
5. Beavers WR: Psychotherapy and Growth: A Family Systems Perspective. New York, Brunner/Mazel, 1977
6. Bender PJ: Multiple Family Therapy for Adolescents: A Case Illustration. Journal of Child and Adolescent Psychiatric and Mental Health Nursing 5 (1): 27–31, 1992
7. Bohen HH, Viveros-Long A: Balancing Jobs and Family Life. Philadelphia, Temple University Press, 1981
8. Bowen M: Family Therapy in Clinical Practice. New York, Jason Aaronson, 1978
9. Campinha-Bacote J: Transcultural Psychiatric Nursing: Diagnostic and Treatment Issues. J Psychosoc Nurs 32 (8): 41–46, 1994
10. Craft MJ, Willadsen JA: Interventions Related to Family. Nurs Clin North Am 27 (2): 517–540, 1992
11. Duvall E: Family Development, 4th ed. Philadelphia, JB Lippincott, 1971
12. Dzurec LC: Assessing Fit: A Key Indicator of Family Health. J Nurse Midwifery 40 (3): 277–289, 1995
13. Finkelhor D: The Main Problem Is Still Underreporting, not Overreporting. In Gelles RJ, Loseke DR (eds): Current Controversies on Family Violence. Newbury Park, CA, Sage, 1993
14. Forchuk C, Dorsay JP: Hildegard Peplau Meets Family Systems Nursing: Innovation in Theory-Based Practice. J Adv Nurs 21: 110–115, 1995
15. Fowler L: Family Psychoeducation: Chronic Psychiatrically Ill Caribbean Patients. J Psychosoc Nurs 30 (3): 27–32, 1992
16. Fowler J, Rigby P: Sculpting With People: An Educational Experience. Nurse Education Today 14 (5): 400–405, 1994
17. Gordon T: Parent Effectiveness Training. New York, PH Wyden, 1970
18. Hall WA: Comparison of Experience of Women and Men in Dual-Earner Families Following the Birth of Their First Infant. Image: Journal of Nursing Scholarship 24 (1): 33–38, 1992
19. Hanson SMH: Healthy Single Parent Families. In Whall Al, Fawcett J (eds): Family Theory Development: State of the Science and Art. Philadelphia, FA Davis, 1991
20. Hartrick G, Lindsey AE, Hills M: Family Nursing Assessment: Meeting the Challenge of Health Promotion. J Adv Nurs 20: 85–91, 1994
21. Hewlett SA: When the Bough Breaks: The Cost of Neglecting Our Children. New York, Basic Books, 1991
22. Kavanagh KH: Family: Is There Anything More Diverse? Pediatric Nursing 20 (4): 423–426, 1994
23. Kuo CL, Kavanagh KH: Chinese Perspectives on Culture and Mental Health. Issues in Mental Health Nursing 15: 551–567, 1994
24. Lantz JE: Family and Marital Therapy. New York, Appleton-Century-Crofts, 1978

25. Lewis JM, Beavers WR, Gossett JT, Phillips VA: No Single Thread: Psychological Health in Family Systems. New York, Brunner/Mazel, 1976
26. Maslow AH: Motivation and Personality. New York, Harper & Row, 1954
27. Minuchin S: Families and Family Therapy. Cambridge, Harvard University Press, 1974
28. National Commission on the Role of the School and Community in Improving Adolescent Health: Code Blue: Uniting for Healthier Youth. Washington DC, National Association of State Boards of Education and the American Medical Association, 1990
29. National Council on Alcoholism and Drug Dependence. The Alcoholism Report 20 (3): 3, 1991
30. North American Nursing Diagnosis Association: Nursing Diagnosis: Definitions and clarification 1994–1995. Proceedings of the Eleventh National Conference, April, 1994
31. Peplau HE: Interpersonal Relations in Nursing. New York, GP Putnam's Sons, 1952
32. Satir V: Peoplemaking. Palo Alto, CA, Science and Behavior Books, 1972
33. Satir V: Conjoint Family Therapy. Palo Alto, CA, Science and Behavior Books, 1983
34. Sampselle C: Violence Against Women. New York, Hemksphere, 1992
35. Schuckit MA: Biological Vulnerability to Alcoholism. J Consult Clin Psychol 55 (3): 301–309, 1987
36. Smoyak S: Family Systems: Use of Genograms as an Assessment Tool. In Clements IW, Buchanan DM (eds): Family Therapy: A Nursing Perspective. New York, John Wiley & Sons, 1982
37. Stevenson J: Issues and Crises During Middlescence. New York, Appleton-Century-Crofts, 1977
38. Verhulst FC, Koot HM: Child Psychiatric Epidemiology: Concepts, Methods, and Findings. Newbury Park, CA, Sage, 1992
39. Vosburgh D, Simpson P: Linking Family Theory and Practice: A Family Nursing Program. IMAGE: Journal of Nursing Scholarship 25 (3): 231–235, 1993
40. Watzlawick P, Beaven J, Jackson D: Pragmatics of Human Communication. New York, Norton, 1967
41. Wegschieder S: Another Chance: Help and Hope for the Alcoholic Family. Palo Alto, CA, Science and Behavior Books, 1981
42. Wright LM, Leahey M: Calgary Family Intervention Model: One Way to Think About Change. Journal of Marital and Family Therapy 20 (4): 381–395, 1994
43. Wright L, Leahey M: Nurses and Families: A Guide to Family Assessment and Intervention, 2d ed. Philadelphia, FA Davis, 1994
44. Yankelovich D: Stepchildren of the Moral Majority. Psychology Today November: 5–10, 1981
45. Yankelovich, Skelly and White, Inc: Family Health in an Era of Stress: The General Mills American Family Report, 1978—1979. Minneapolis, General Mills, 1979

Behavioral Approaches

Juliann Casey Reakes

18

We are controlled by the world in which we live, and part of that world has been and will be constructed by men. The question is this: are we to be controlled by accident, by tyrants, or by ourselves in effective cultural design?

B.F. Skinner,
Freedom and the Control of Men, *1955*

This chapter discusses principles of behavior therapy, strategies of learning theory, and the application of these principles and strategies in assisting clients to replace maladaptive behavior with adaptive behavior.

Behavior therapy has proven to be a practical, efficient, and parsimonious way of helping clients and families to change behavior by applying learning theories. Behavior therapy is the essence of behaviorism, a philosophical approach to life and a psychological discipline built on a precise scientific orientation to the problems of humans and other living organisms. Behaviorism represents reality and thus views behavior outside the expanded social norm as maladaptive and not as a symptom of disease, a form of deviance, or a deficit. In behavior therapy, the cause of maladaptive behavior is not a relevant issue, because the focus is on assisting clients to adapt objectively to the real world by learning ways to change responses to the internal and external environments.

The components of the nursing process and behavior analysis and application are similar. Assessment, nursing diagnosis, planning, intervention, and evaluation by means of specific outcome criteria are inherent in both methodologies. The goals of nursing and behavior therapy are also parallel—to help people deal more effectively with reality.

Learning Objectives

On completion of this chapter, you should be able to accomplish the following:

1. *Define terms specific to behavior therapy.*
2. *Apply principles of behavior therapy to nursing practice and client problems.*
3. *Discuss the goals of behavioral therapeutic approaches.*
4. *Differentiate among classical conditioning, operant conditioning, cognitive therapy, and other forms of behavior modification.*
5. *Discuss the use of various forms of behavioral intervention.*
6. *Apply the steps of the nursing process to the process involved in behavior therapy.*

◆ Principles of Behavior Therapy

The term behavior refers to the overt and covert responses an individual makes to internal and external environmental stimulation. These responses include feelings, cognitions, verbalizations, activities, and biological parameters. Behavior modification techniques and cognitive interventions provide diverse approaches for dealing with maladaptive behavior through behavior therapy. Maladaptive behavior may be learned or may result from the failure to learn adaptive behavior.

The approach to behavior therapy is similar to the nursing process. Assessment, specific description of the identified behavior, accurate problem identification, and goal setting are the steps in designing a behavioral therapy program. Overt responses or behaviors are measurable; mediating processes or cognitions, such as thoughts, feelings, and attitudes provide subjective data to assess, diagnose, and intervene in the client's behavior (Box 18-1).

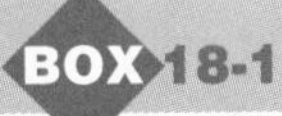

18-1

Describing Adaptive and Maladaptive Behavior

Following are examples of maladaptive behavior:

1. Continually talking about feelings of worthlessness and guilt
2. Reporting voices from the television telling client to hurt self
3. Bingeing on 10 to 12 slices of pizza, a quart of ice cream, and 2 dozen cookies, followed by forced vomiting 3 times a week
4. Continuing to abuse alcohol after completing a detoxification and rehabilitation program
5. Denying physically abusing children even with an eyewitness account
6. Continuing to support a husband who refuses to work
7. Pacing the room continually while wringing hands
8. Stating that he or she cannot leave the house alone without feeling acute fear

These behaviors increase tension and illness, maintain negative patterns, and show profound fear of change.

In contrast, examples of adaptive behavior include the following:

1. Participates in relaxation exercises daily
2. Uses assertive techniques with family members
3. Exercises for 30 minutes 3 times a week
4. Attends daily Alcoholics Anonymous meetings
5. Keeps a journal to record feelings when angry and frustrated
6. Complies with medication treatment
7. Identifies cognitive distortions
8. Initiates conversation with group members

These behaviors provide release of tension, promote physical and mental health, and show acceptance and successful use of positive change.

◆ Types of Behavior Approaches

Behavior therapy includes classical conditioning, operant (instrumental) conditioning, modeling and observational learning, and cognitive processing.[19,31,34]

CLASSICAL CONDITIONING

In Pavlovian learning, an *unconditioned stimulus,* such as food, elicits an *unconditioned response,* for example, salivation, in a hungry dog. When a *conditioned stimulus,* like a bell, is paired with the food, over time the conditioned stimulus results in salivation in the dog, a *conditioned response.* The unconditioned stimulus is a reinforcer for the conditioned stimulus and the conditioned response. This type of learning is affected by events that occur before the behavior. The preceding events elicit a certain response. The unconditioned stimulus may be rewarding or pleasant (eg, a smile from the nurse) or unpleasant noxious, painful, or aversive (eg, a drug that induces nausea). Aversive therapy has been used to treat alcoholism by pairing the drinking of alcohol with a nausea-producing drug.

There are many examples of classical conditioning in health care. Fear of injections may be conditioned by the nurse's white uniform or by the sight of the needle or syringe. The nurse's uniform, an unconditioned stimulus, may elicit discomfort or fear, the unconditioned response. The needle may be a conditioned stimulus and fear a conditioned response.

More than one stimulus not originally associated with a response may reinforce learning by binding a response to a series of stimuli. By the process of chaining, more than one unconditioned stimulus may become a conditioned stimulus, and higher order conditioning, or learning, can result. For example, a child receives a toy at the doctor's office when she responds favorably to examination and treatment. The office nurse verbally praises the child and hands her a toy while giving her a hug or a pat on the back. At the same time, the child's mother tells her the reward is a stop at a restaurant for a special treat because she was such "a good girl." The toy is a primary reinforcer for the child's behavior in the doctor's office; the praise, pleasant touching, and the treat are successive reinforcers.

Many emotional responses, such as an unfounded fear of objects, may become conditioned responses due to higher order conditioning, despite the fact that there may have been no direct association with the feared object. Words, which can be symbols of experiences or events, may become conditioned stimuli that trigger respondent behavior or that signal dangerous or feared situations.[31,35]

The classic example of respondent conditioning is the work of psychologist John B. Watson and nurse Rosalee Rayner of Johns Hopkins Hospital. Albert, an 11-month-old boy, was conditioned by noise associated with a white rat to fear white furry objects. This illustrates the behavioristic view that phobias are conditioned fears learned when a stimulus is paired with a feared object or event.[37]

Joseph Wolpe built on the theory of classical conditioning to demonstrate clinically that learned anxiety may be inhibited by another behavorial response. When behavioral responses, such as muscle relaxation, assertive responses, and sexual arousal responses, occur in the presence of cues that originally triggered anxiety, anxiety is lessened. These responses eventually become associated with the cues and weaken the anxiety response. Wolpe called this counter-conditioning process *reciprocal inhibition.* For example, the person who experiences unsatisfactory job interviews and becomes anxious may become conditioned to employment situations because of encounters with similar cues and stimuli. The anxiety evoked may cause the person to avoid job situations.

Learning to deal assertively with this situation in the presence of these cues can reduce anxiety. Assertive responses, sexual responses, and muscle relaxation are associated with the parasympathetic nervous system; increased activity of this system decreases anxiety responses associated with the sympathetic nervous system, such as dilated pupils, increased blood pressure and heart rate, and increased blood supply to voluntary muscles. Systematic desensitization based on reciprocal inhibition theory has been effective with a broad group of client problems, including phobias, obsessive-compulsive disorders, sexual disorders, psychosomatic disorders, and alcoholism.[41]

OPERANT CONDITIONING

B.F. Skinner and a colleague introduced a specific type of behavior therapy, *operant conditioning,* in 1954. Operant or instrumental behavior (such as eating or writing) refers to activity strengthened or weakened by its consequences (such as weight loss or weight gain). Operant behavior is under the control of the individual, who can use behavior to change or modify the environment and is influenced by a reinforcer. A *reinforcer* is anything that increases the probability of a response.

In operant conditioning, reinforcement strengthens a wide range of behaviors, as the client learns to duplicate certain responses. The criteria for reinforcement are that the reinforcer meet a need and be goal directed. Food, for example, may not always elicit an adaptive behavior if hunger is not a priority need. A positive reinforcer, or *reward,* strengthens a behavior; removal of a negative reinforcer strengthens or facilitates adaptive behavior when the client is able to evade or avoid the harmful reinforcer.

Positive and negative reinforcers are specifically defined with regard to previous impact on the behavior to be changed. Punishment is not a negative reinforcer because it is designed to eliminate a behavior, whereas true negative reinforcement produces adaptive behavior. Punishment often suppresses the maladaptive behavior but does not eliminate it from the client's behavioral pattern. If not offered a specific alternative, the individual may respond with a behavior that is more maladaptive than the original behavior. Regressive behavior or generalization to other situations may also occur if an alternative behavior is not available. For example, a child may be scolded for eating too much junk food at home and may, therefore, learn to eat junk food at fast-food stands. Children often become enuretic when punished, whereas adults may resort to overeating, drinking alcoholic beverages, or retaliating with aggressive behavior toward spouse or children.[36]

Operant conditioning has been successfully used with many clinical and behavioral problems that have not responded to other treatments.

Operant Control of Verbal Behavior

According to Skinner, verbal behavior is also under operant control and like other operant conditioning, is influenced by its outcome. Verbal behavior influences personal interaction and is maintained by social behavior. It translates other behavior into word symbols. As in any translation, the interpretation is subjective. When reinforced and under similar contingencies, words become maintained as behavior patterns. As an example, psychotic verbal behavior may be eliminated by positively reinforcing rational verbal behavior with special privileges.[36]

Generalization

Adaptive behavior specific to one situation may occur in similar situations because of a phenomenon called *generalization*. For example, rational verbal behavior learned in client–health team interactions may generalize to client–family and client–friend relationships.

Discrimination

Discrimination refers to a specific response occurring in a situation. The client who is positively reinforced for completing an activity task and ignored when the task is not completed and who then consistently completes assigned work is making a differential or a discriminating response.

Extinction

Extinction involves withholding reinforcers to reduce the probability of the response. For instance, if staff ignore a client's attention-seeking behavior and positively reinforce group-participating behavior, the first behavior may be extinguished by an increase in the response to the second.

Prompting and Fading

Prompting and fading refer to creating conditions that facilitate or accentuate the reinforcer. *Prompting* is a cuing process; *fading* is a gradual reduction of this process. Carefully enunciating a word for an aphasic client learning to identify objects again after a stroke may be eliminated or faded as soon as the client begins to name the object without cuing by the nurse.

The following example illustrates the application of fading and prompting. A program was initiated to emphasize the need for client compliance with a prescribed daily program. The client was instructed to notify a staff member hourly when completing an activity. The staff member prompted the client to check the schedule and reinforced the client's actions with praise when the task was completed. After a 3-day compliance with this plan, the hourly check was expanded to 2 hours for another 3-day period, to 4 hours for the next 3 days, and so forth until the schedule was checked only once a day.

Shaping

Shaping refers to patterning a group of actions by continued reinforcement of responses essential to the desired target behavior. For instance, a neat, clean physical appearance is targeted as the priority behavior to be achieved by a client. When the client is consistently rewarded with verbal praise and attention from the health team when hair is combed, teeth are brushed, and nails are trimmed and clean, the overall target behavior—a neat, clean physical appearance—is often achieved.

Reinforcers

The choice and timing of reinforcers are important for adaptive change. When the response or operant conditioning occurs and is recognized as bringing about a desired action or modification in the environment, the client has discovered a potent tool for change. *Social reinforcers* may include praise, attention, touch, or interest. *Material reinforcers* may include food, prizes, redeemable tokens, or money. *Activity reinforcers* may include watching television; attending plays, movies, or dances; playing cards; or shopping.

The psychiatric-mental health team may observe a client modifying a favorable response other than the target behavior. An unplanned event may become a reinforcer. For example, smiling associated with verbal praise (the primary reinforcer) may strengthen the target behavior when used alone. Withdrawing a reinforcer to bring about a desired behavior is an excellent intervention in many client management situations. For instance, sending a disruptive client to a time-out area may increase a targeted behavior.

Chance Reinforcement

Chance reinforcement also may strengthen maladaptive behavior. For example, a nurse who immediately spoon feeds a client refusing to eat—even though extra cigarettes might be given to him for eating without help—may be unknowingly reinforcing the noneating behavior.

Secondary Reinforcement

Secondary reinforcers or conditioned responses are as influential in changing behavior as are primary reinforcers. They also may be interchangeable. For example, participation with others by playing bingo, the primary reinforcer, may become a secondary reinforcer for increasing verbal communication. This is an application of the *Premack principle,* which states that a high-probability behavior can reinforce a low-probability response. To illustrate, a client who likes to watch television may be allowed to watch his or her favorite program if he or she attends an occupational therapy activity. An anorectic client may be rewarded for weight gain by being permitted to participate in desired activities.[25]

Reinforcement Schedules

Reinforcement may be continuous or may occur at fixed or varying intervals. Designing a reinforcement schedule for a specific client requires careful planning. All staff involved in the client's 24-hour care must follow the schedule according to the protocol.

Reinforcement schedules may be of three types:

1. Continuous: Every expected response is reinforced.
2. Intermittent: Every expected response is not reinforced; only selected responses are reinforced.
   a. Fixed ratio: Every certain response is reinforced, such as the third, eighth, or tenth response.
   b. Variable ratio: The responses being reinforced are changed at certain times; at first, the third response may be reinforced, and the next day the sixth response may be reinforced.
3. At intervals: Variable or fixed ratios are defined by the time between reinforcement.[34]

MODELING AND OBSERVATIONAL LEARNING

Cognitive Processing

Cognitive processing therapies recognize that thinking processes are involved in the experience of psychological distress. These approaches try to correct distorted thinking patterns and recognize that beliefs, attitudes, and assumptions underlie faulty thinking patterns. Emotions and behavior that are activated by faulty thinking result in maladaptive behavior patterns. Perception of life events is filtered by stereotyped views based on these irrational thoughts; thus, reality is distorted.

Beck identified the cognitive triad of the depressed person—a negative view of self, the world, and the future. The resulting feelings of hopelessness are responses to the faulty thinking processes that reinforce feelings of low self-esteem and the inability to cope with depressive symptoms.[6,7]

The goal of cognitive therapy is to decrease subjective distress and increase productive, rewarding behavior. Clients who benefit from this approach are able to learn the association of counterproductive beliefs, distorted thinking, self-defeating feelings and behaviors, and logical fallacies. These illogical ideations include the following:

1. Personalization: taking responsibility for an event or situation that is not under one's control
2. All-or-nothing thinking: seeing things in black-and-white categories; unrealistic self-expectations
3. "Awfulizing" or minimizing: exaggerating or minimizing an event, a situation, or one's own qualities
4. Overgeneralization: basing behavior on a single negative event or situation, resulting in self-defeating patterns of behavior; often involves labeling or mislabeling
5. Selective negativism: preoccupation with a negative issue or happening, which blots out any productive logical thinking
6. Making assumptions: mind reading or fortune telling without logical, objective data to support conclusions
7. Words such as *want, ought,* and *should,* which convey rigidity, unrealistic expectations, and perfectionism; all-or-nothing thinking reinforced
8. Negating positive thoughts: rejecting positive experiences and maintaining negative beliefs
9. Emotional reasoning: basing decisions and self-evaluation on negative thinking[9]

The main focus of cognitive restructuring is logical thinking to evaluate situations by recognizing the criteria that emphasize irrational and distorted thoughts and neutralizing the situation so that rational thought is initiated.

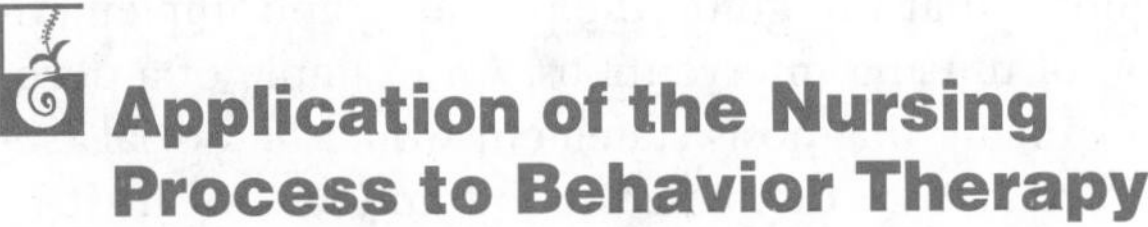

Application of the Nursing Process to Behavior Therapy

ASSESSMENT

Collection of Data

The first step in the nursing process and the application of behavioral principles, assessment involves collecting objective and subjective data. Objective data can be measured, observed, or validated. Subjective data reflect the client's feelings, perceptions, and verbalization (self-talk) about any problems.

Information about the client's problem may be obtained from the following sources:

1. Nursing history
2. Systems review
3. Physical examination findings
4. Psychosocial, cultural, and mental status findings, including developmental data, demographic data, and the duration, frequency, and extent of the presenting problem
5. Description of the behavior and situation before and after the problem
6. Consequences of the problem behavior
7. Client resources: likes, dislikes, support systems, and interests
8. Client expectations and motivations

The nurse may identify problem areas that the client does not recognize but that influence the presenting problem. For example, the nurse may perceive that a client has poor verbal communication skills, which may be directly related to the presenting problem of feeling anxious in situations with strangers.

Careful listening and observation during the interview, examinations, and testing contribute valuable information in identifying the following:

1. The problem behavior
2. The situations in which the behavior occurs
3. The consequences of the behavior
4. The parameters of the problem
5. The client's perception of the problem

Problem Identification

The behavior or target problem must be clearly identified (Box 18-2).

NURSING DIAGNOSIS

In this second step of the nursing process, the nurse examines the assessment data and formulates nursing diagnoses that will guide the planning and implementation of nursing interventions. An example of a pertinent nursing diagnosis statement would be Social Isolation related to depressed mood and lack of trust in others, as evidenced by sad, dull affect; uncommunicative behavior; preoccupation with own thoughts; and absence of supportive significant others. Each part of this diagnosis provides the nurse and other mental health team members with information on specific client behaviors to be modified by behavioral techniques.

PLANNING

Planning of behavioral interventions is a cooperative effort among psychiatric-mental health team members. Objectivity is a necessary component of planning behavioral methods; subjectivity affects the evaluation of the client's behavioral progress and treatment planning.

Planning involves *goal setting,* in which treatment goals are identified based on the assessment and analysis of client behavior. Possible goals could include the following:

1. Provide a safe physical environment.
2. Increase a defined behavioral performance.
3. Promote self-care and independence.
4. Implement competent, individualized care.
5. Select learning methods.

A client treatment plan typically would incorporate the following elements:

1. Client's name
2. Purpose of the behavior modification program
3. Goals of the program
4. Place where the behavior occurs
5. Target behavior
6. Reinforcement schedule
7. Staff objectives (eg, how to record behavior, reinforcement protocol)
8. Time the behavior is to be observed or is to occur
9. Data-collection methods

INTERVENTION

The fourth step of the nursing process, intervention, involves compliance with reinforcement schedules, manipulation of the environment, and other treatment activities, some of which are described in the following sections.

Self-management Programs

Nurses have directed self-management programs with clients motivated for behavior change in the areas of weight control and smoking control. Self-management programs follow the same format as other modification programs; observing and recording one's own behavior are additional reinforcers.

Contracting

Behavioral contracting, an agreement with a client for a specific behavior, is often used in self-control programs. A contract may be oral or written. If written, the contract identifies behavior or other criteria and is dated and signed by the nurse and client.

Therapeutic Dialogue: Identifying the Problem

The following dialogue between the nurse and client illustrates the importance of the client identifying the problem. A female high school teacher and part-time bookkeeper, age 44 years, works 60 hours a week. She is depressed and has irritable bowel syndrome.

Nurse: You've talked about a lot of losses in your life.

Client: I thought I had resolved the issues with my divorce 5 years ago, but recent conflict with my 22-year-old son has made me angry about it all again.

Nurse: Tell me about the conflict.

Client: I asked my son to try and find his own place since I remarried a year ago. He's been with us, not helping with the bills, and being dependent.

Nurse: Go on.

Client: He finally left, but he went to his father's and told him and his sisters I kicked him out. (Begins to cry.)

Nurse: It's hard for you to talk about.

Client: When my first husband asked for a divorce out of the blue, I was shocked. The children took sides; my daughters went with their father, and my son stayed with me. My daughters blamed me for their father's dissatisfaction with our marriage.

Nurse: What were your feelings when this happened?

Client: Depressed, angry, and I guess I felt abandoned.

Nurse: Abandoned?

Client: As I look back, I had this same feeling as a child. I felt my parents didn't care about me, and when my marriage broke up (crying, head down), I covered it up with my anger.

Nurse: (Puts arm around client's shoulders.) You're feeling those same feelings now.

Client: I guess that feeling has always been there, stronger than the anger and depression that I was dealing with.

Nurse: (Silence . . . but holds client's hand.)

Client: I've never really dealt with my growing up. I just ran away and got married. When that "blew up" on me, and I pushed those old feelings away.

Nurse: As painful as it may be, resolving this issue may make some connections for you.

Discussion

The client is beginning to identify her irrational belief on emotional reasoning. Because she felt angry and depressed, she blamed her divorce and the conflict of her children rather than her deeper feelings of abandonment and fear, resulting in self-defeating behaviors.

Other Behavioral Activities

Positive or negative reinforcement of behavior, *prompting* (cues), *fading* (removing cues), extinction (ignoring a behavior), *time out,* and *revoking privileges* may be included in the nursing plan. Teaching the client to *discriminate* (make a certain response) or *generalize* (apply a response to other situations) also may be goals of a treatment plan. *Overcorrection* (another behavior is added to one that the client is repeating in an acceptable way) or *simple correction* (a repeat of the acceptable behavior) may be useful.

Narrative Interventions

Narrative interventions can help clients clearly identify the problem that they perceive as disrupting their life and reinforcing dysfunctional behaviors. Often the problem is distorted or disguised. This may occur because the client erroneously perceives as the problem issues that are really effects of the problem. The client's interpretation of the problem continues to cloud the real problem. Connecting events, cues, or behavioral patterns can help the client externalize the problem as objective fact. When clients recognize that it is not the problem—but the misinterpretation of its effects—that causes them difficulty in their lives, self-blame or blaming others is reduced. In addition, motivation to seek solutions or to reframe the problem increases options, alternatives, and awareness that the problem and its effects can be controlled. Increasing self-management and finding new meanings in lived experiences neutralize the power of misperceived problems and their effects.

Narrative interventions enable a client to become the story teller, the principal actor in his or her life's scenarios. Through oral or written narrations, clients recognize their resistance and correctly identify their real problems. Narrative interventions include writing autobiographies, letters, projections of how problems will be solved, or stories that symbolize the client's experiences. Audiotaping can be substituted for clients who are not able to express themselves in writing.

> A 52-year-old woman who experienced chronic depression for a number of years recognized after writing her autobiography that her three failed marriages were due to her rescuing behaviors. When the men she married became more independent, her relationship with them deteriorated. Eventually she was able to recognize that her own needs were not being met, which contributed to her low self-esteem and self-defeating behaviors.[40]

Journaling is a specific way to help clients become aware of their experiences, thoughts, and feelings. Journaling provides a record for clients to review and use for self-discovery. This can also result in clients' finding new meanings, examining values, and clarifying relationships.

Teaching clients to describe their behavior and record their observations increases self-awareness through feedback and reflection. Examples of journaling include writing about conflicts (such as feelings or choices), strengths, weakness, changes, and self-affirmations. Particularly powerful is expressing emotions in writing, a constructive way to deal with feelings.

Assignments for clients may include recording thoughts and feelings about themselves, interests, relationships, specific situations, creative ideas, memories, and goals for the future. Clients should be instructed to note the date and time in their entries and leave room to add material when they review their journaling.

> A client who used journaling to record her thoughts and feelings on days that represented special events in her life, such as birthdays, anniversaries of losses, and holidays, identified that she had been displacing her anger onto her husband. She had not resolved her feelings about her father and brother who had died accidently and the recent death of her grandfather.[10]

Cognitive Therapies

Through cognitive therapies, the client learns to change behavior and decrease subjective distress by initiating relaxation exercises, thought stopping, visualization activities, modeling, facilitative self-talk, and self-modeling techniques. Cognitive therapy emphasizes identifying alternative creative and logical thinking to offset distorted thinking. Assertiveness training, an integral part of this approach, teaches the importance and rights of the self.

Homework assignments are fundamental to this approach, helping clients learn to monitor their own behavior. Homework assignments may take the form of monitoring and recording dysfunctional thinking, prescribing activities to alter environmental variables, and countering distorted cognitions. Other valuable tools include writing an autobiography and composing letters (not necessarily to be sent), in which a conflicting issue is explored and feelings expressed. To counter resistance and help the client perceive the reality of a situation, it may be helpful to prescribe activities that emphasize specific situational events and other characteristics that reinforce distortions.[26]

The nurse can use various approaches to teach a client to monitor feelings and thoughts. When preoccupation with these dysfunctional thoughts overwhelms the client, teaching thought-stopping techniques may be helpful. A slow increase in activities often increases the client's efficiency and can be a positive reinforcement to show progress.

Reframing or shifting illogical labeling helps the client use a problem-solving and positive approach that facilitates the countering technique. The client also can use self-talk and visualization techniques to dissipate the anxiety that comes from irrational thinking. Countering techniques include the following:

1. Decreasing subjective distress (calm oneself, visualize a pleasant scene, use relaxation techniques)
2. Using thought stopping (say the word *stop*; see a red stop light; clap hands; snap a rubber band on wrist)
3. Allowing oneself to become neutral (rid the self of distractions, distorted thoughts, preoccupations)
4. Visualizing a mental white screen
5. Visualizing self countering own distorted thinking

The following two scenarios illustrate the use of countering techniques:

A 40-year-old engineer loses his job of 15 years. He has a son starting college in the fall, two school-age children, and a wife whom he supports financially. His interpretation is, "I'm a failure, and I'll never get another job; my family will be in need."

Countering techniques might include the following:

1. "I've been thinking of changing jobs, because that one's no longer a challenge."
2. "I turned down two jobs a few years ago and was told to call when I was ready to change jobs."
3. "My company has lost a lot of money recently, and its change in philosophy disturbs me."
4. "My wife and I have been unhappy with our current lifestyle."

A 30-year-old man who has been taking alprazolam (Xanax) for a number of months because of panic attacks decreases his medication at the order of his doctor.

His interpretation when he begins to feel anxious is to think that his panic attacks are beginning again.

Countering techniques might include the following:

1. "These feelings are normal because I'm decreasing this medication."
2. "I've been under stress lately because of a business deal, and these feelings could be due to this situation."
3. "I want to come off all medication and know that the other techniques I've learned will help."
4. "I've been keeping long hours at work and only sleeping a few hours each night. I'm overworked."

Box 18-3 gives an example of an automatic thought record.

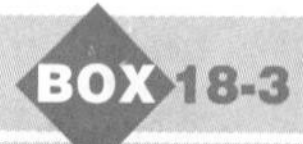

Automatic Thought Record

Situation: The client is an anxious, depressed 32-year-old divorced man. His 7-year-old daughter lives with her mother in another state. His business failed and he filed bankruptcy 1 year ago. He has quit three jobs within the last 6 months.

Automatic thought: I will never be able to have my daughter visit me or keep a job.
- Belief in thought (scale 0–10): 9
- Emotion (scale 0–10): Anxiety, feelings of worthlessness—9
- Evidence for thought:
  - Business failed
  - Quit three jobs within the last 6 months
  - No savings
- Evidence against thought:
  - Business successful for 10 years; business failed when shopping center where shop was located deteriorated.
  - Daughter visited every holiday and for 1 month last summer.
  - Client had purchased airline ticket for daughter's next trip before bankruptcy.
  - Client quit jobs because they were in outdoor settings, which aggravated his asthma.
- Errors in thinking:
  - Emotional reasoning
  - Personalization
  - Negating the positive
- Realistic view of thought based on evidence: "I need to identify career plans that will build on my strengths. I will take time and sacrifice to become financially stable."
- Rerated thought (0–10): 6
- Rerated emotion (0–10): 6
- Summary: Client recognized cognitive distortion and was able to reframe thought.

Rational-Emotive Therapy. One form of cognitive therapy, *rational-emotive therapy* (RET), is based on the premise that an individual's behavior is controlled by values and beliefs. Many people evaluate their behavior based on illogical and irrational beliefs and assumptions. Following are examples of such false assumptions:

1. A person should be loved and approved by all.
2. A person should be competent and talented and prove herself or himself.
3. A person has little control over life, and pressures make one feel angry, hostile, and depressed.
4. Dangerous and threatening situations should be feared.
5. Past experiences are the most important influence on present behavior.
6. Dependence on stronger individuals or a supernatural power is necessary for living.

7. Understanding the world is necessary for a happy life.
8. Performing well and being liked are necessary to feel adequate as a person.
9. Being depressed, angry, or anxious is giving in to situations or feelings that should be faced.
10. Beliefs of society and authority figures should not be questioned; if they are, punishment will follow.[15]

The following example illustrates the RET model, which is diagrammed in Figure 18-1.

A 42-year-old engineer admitted to the hospital reports severe anxiety, diarrhea, a pounding feeling in his chest, difficulty breathing, insomnia, a sensation of suffocation, and difficulty swallowing. His behavioral pattern occurred after his 17-year-old daughter told him and his wife that she was pregnant and wanted an abortion (Fig. 18-1**A**).

The client told the nurse that he is "no good" and a "harsh disciplinarian," that his wife and children do not love him, that he is to blame for his daughter's problems, and that he is worthless (Fig. 18-1**B**).

This father is experiencing anxiety, guilt, depression, and anger (Fig. 18-1**C**). The nurse focuses with the client on his self-talk, or assumptions, and the validity of these beliefs (Fig. 18-1**D**). The client is helped to discriminate between information that is rational and logical and information that is distorted, demanding, and negative. The nurse and the client focus on his feelings of worthlessness and blame.

The client realized his thinking was illogical, and that it would not be catastrophic if his family did not love him. The client was able to think rationally and realize that he was not responsible for his daughter's behavior. He also realized that he quickly assumed responsibility for all family problems, which excluded his family from responsibility (Fig. 18-1**E**).

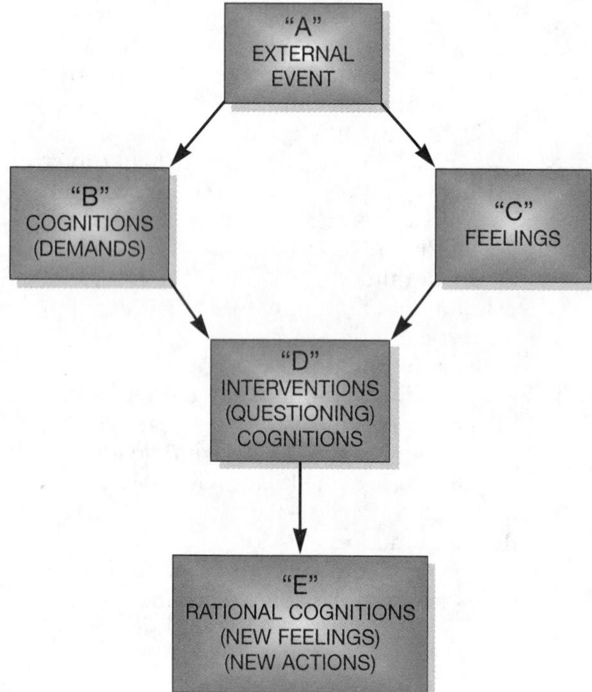

Figure 18-1. The rational-emotive therapy model. Rational-emotive therapy uses the model above to illustrate a therapeutic approach to faulty assumptions or beliefs.

A. External event
B. Cognitions (self demands) associated with A
C. Feelings and emotions associated with A
D. Interventions that modify B
   Questioning self demands
E. Rational cognitions
   New feelings
   New actions

(Adapted from Ellis and Dryden: The Practice of Rational-Emotive Therapy. Springer Pub. Co. 1987)

In RET, cognitive methods involve the client and nurse in approaches that apply learning principles to question illogical thinking and to increase the client's problem-solving ability, social skills, and assertiveness. Box 18-4 demonstrates the application of several RET techniques. Self-assessment, self-monitoring, behavior reversal, role playing, modeling, visual imagery, thought stopping, and interventions with operant and respondent conditioning are included in this diversified approach to meeting clients' needs.[6,10,15]

When using RET to treat individuals with depressive behaviors, success has been proven. The depressed person typically interprets cues and data illogically, thereby deprecating affirmative information and enlarging negative data. Based on the assumption that people are depressed because of inadequate social skills, lack of positive social reinforcement, and negative environmental events, the emphasis is on increasing the client's social skills through assertiveness training, assessing events that may reinforce negative feelings, setting goals, and rehearsing new social skills.

Thought Stopping. *Thought stopping,* developed by Wolpe, also has been successful in treating individuals with depressive disorders. Irrational, brooding, and anxiety-provoking behaviors are inhibited by a specific therapeutic approach. For example, by shouting the word *stop* after expressing an illogical behavior, a client realizes he or she can control his or her own thoughts. Another approach to thought stopping is to request the client to substitute a positive thought for a negative, distorted thought.

Thought stopping reportedly is useful in treating obsessive-compulsive disorders. The word *stop* initiated by the therapist is often followed by an oversized stimulus, such as a loud noise or by the client's loudly echoing the word *stop.* The troublesome thought is interrupted or blocked by counter-conditioning principles.[8]

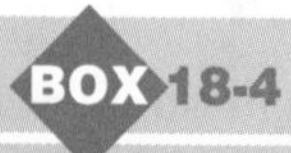

Applying Rational-Emotive Therapy

Mr. F, 58 year old retired salesman with major depression and suicidal ideation, is attending a day treatment program. His depression began two years ago at the time of his retirement. His 28-year-old son, who had been living at home and complying with medication for treatment of schizophrenia, left home, stopped taking his medication and has been living as a "homeless person." Mr. F tells the nurse he was a "bad father," never did anything with his son, and is to blame for the son's present homeless lifestyle. Mr. F's relationship with his wife has become strained with little or no communication (see Fig 18-1A).

This man is experiencing depression, guilt, anxiety, and anger (see Fig 18-1C). The nurse focuses with the client on his self-talk, and the validity of the demands he perceives (see Fig 18-1B). Mr F is helped to discriminate between information that is rational and logical and information that is distorted and negative. He is able to connect his feelings of worthlessness and self-blame with the unrealistic self-demands and distorted thoughts (see Fig 18-1D). Eventually, Mr. F realized that he was not responsible for his son's behavior. He acknowledged his need to take responsibility for his wife and son, by assuming responsibility for his son's illness related to his absences from home and lack of involvement with his son (see Fig 18-1E). After he shared his feelings with his wife, communication between them improved.

Modeling

Learning through another's performance, even if the behavior is not practiced or rewarded, is a principle of social learning theory. *Modeling,* or imitation, is a method of behavior change in which a client learns vicariously by observing others' behavior or by verbal descriptions of a desired behavior, which is a cue for initiating new responses.

Aggressive and nonaggressive behavior may be demonstrated by modeling techniques. In one study, children who watched aggressive actions by real-life models on film and by cartoon characters displayed more aggressive behavior than children exposed to nonaggressive behavior or children in a control group. Modeling strategies also have been effective in reducing children's fears. Brief filmed experiences showing a child overcoming fear in certain situations—such as visiting a dentist's or physician's office or interacting with a feared animal—were shown to children who then rehearsed their own responses to the feared situation.[4]

Imagery

Imagery is an adaptable therapeutic approach used to facilitate positive self-talk. Mental pictures under the control of and initiated by the client may correct faulty cognitions. The client pictures past significant memories and present events; combined with relaxation therapy and role-playing, this can increase the client's awareness of situational events and other variables resulting in maladaptive behavior.

Behavior Rehearsal

In *behavior rehearsal* (or role playing), used in conjunction with modeling, the client rehearses new responses to problem situations after learning new adaptive responses portrayed through modeling. The nurse's specific attention to detail reinforces characteristics of assertive behavior, such as eye contact, clear and audible vocal tone, posture, and gait.

Behavior rehearsal often is useful in group settings for teaching social skills and for meeting specific therapy goals. Sharing simulated situations and modeling approaches provide opportunities for participation by the group members.[18]

Assertiveness Training

Role playing is the most commonly used technique in *assertiveness training,* which deconditions anxiety arising from interpersonal relationships. An interfering emotional process free of anxiety, assertive behavior is expressive, spontaneous, goal-directed, and self-enhancing.[1]

Assertiveness training increases self-esteem and confidence, teaches ways to accept criticism and make it productive, teaches effective coping mechanisms for stress, and teaches the effectiveness of positive self-talk (Box 18-5). In their early years, people often are punished for expressing their authentic selves. As nonassertive behavior is rewarded, people become unassertive about their rights as human beings. Poor role models, lack of opportunity, and cultural differences discourage assertiveness.

Problem Solving

Behavioral goals include increasing adaptive behavior and learning problem prevention and problem solving. *Problem solving* involves the following phases:

1. A general approach to the problem
2. A specific definition of the problem and its parameters
3. Generation of possible solutions and implications
4. Selection of a solution
5. Testing and evaluation of the solution

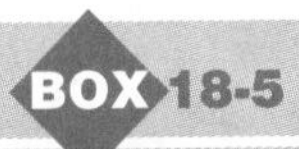

Assertive Techniques

Evaluate the situation, then do the following:

Identify the legitimate rights and responsibilities of the people involved.
Identify the short- and long-term consequences.
Determine how you will behave.

1. Express your own views, using "I" statements.
2. Maintain eye contact.
3. Assume a relaxed posture.
4. Use humor when appropriate.
5. Keep your nonverbal behavior congruent with verbal behavior.
6. Listen and wait for other people to respond.
7. Use reflecting and clarifying techniques.
8. Recognize your right to repeat assertive statements.
9. Acknowledge criticisms.
10. Use a firm, but empathetic, voice tone.

Other assertive techniques include the following:

- Recognize other person's feelings.
- Repeat assertive message calmly.
- Compromise.
- Stay neutral if conflict is escalating.

Counter nonproductive, illogical thoughts by reversing these irrational thoughts. Acknowledge that these are illogical thoughts and that subsequent negative and maladaptive feelings evolve from these thoughts. Use thought-stopping techniques to initiate the countering procedure. When countering, be creative but logical.

1. Are your expectations unrealistic?
2. Are your thoughts aligned with cognitive distortions?
3. Do you have objective data to support these thoughts?
4. Do you acknowledge the "shoulds," "oughts," and "musts" that support maladaptive behavior?

A lack of problem-solving skills is often associated with distorted cognitive processing and interpersonal problems. In conjunction with other cognitive therapy methods, the client is taught to identify the situational and personal aspects of the problem that may inhibit the problem-solving process.[19,31]

Progressive Muscle Relaxation

Muscle relaxation is a potent treatment strategy for dealing with psychophysiological distress and chronic sleeplessness. Anxiety lessens when muscles relax. More than 40 years ago, Edmund Jacobson recognized that muscle relaxation was a therapeutic tool for stress-related problems. After studying the physiological and psychological effects of muscle relaxation, he comfortably positioned clients and taught them to tense and relax the main muscle groups of their bodies. He then shared the monitoring information with the clients, who eventually were able to use only passive activity to relax.

Wolpe demonstrated that progressive muscle relaxation, combined with mental pictures (images) of a feared situation or increased association with the feared object in graduated increments, could desensitize phobic clients. Muscle relaxation is physiologically incompatible with the anxiety-evoking response.[41]

The following guidelines are suggested for using relaxation therapy:

1. Keep the environment as quiet as possible, and request that the client sit comfortably in a chair or lie down to facilitate muscle relaxation.
2. Tell the client that this technique may help reduce tension and anxiety. Encourage the client to close the eyes and let thoughts focus on pleasant, quiet scenes, as he or she tenses and relaxes various muscle groups.
3. Demonstrate the technique, and emphasize that muscles should not be strained but should be tensed to about 75% of their potential. In some client situations, a doctor's order and a careful physical assessment may be necessary to reduce the risk of any complications of this procedure. Use a ratio of a 5- to 10-second cycle of tension followed by a 20-second cycle of no tension.
4. Instruct the client in a quiet, calm way to tense the hands by making a fist and then relaxing. You may suggest that the client "let go" and become very relaxed and comfortable. Tell the client to tense and relax the biceps, triceps, shoulder, neck, mouth, tongue, eyes, back, midsection, thighs, stomach, calves, feet, and toes in the same manner.
5. Teach the client to breathe in a deep, relaxing way and "let it all out" as the final relaxation technique. Overdoing the breathing exercise may cause hyperventilation.[19]

EVALUATION

Objectives of behavioral change are stated in specific performance terms or in terms of detailed, precise, and measurable outcome criteria. Although careful monitoring is necessary to validate the desired behavioral outcome, evaluation is more simplified than it is in client situations with highly subjective descriptions of behavior.

During assessment, behavior is measured over time until a clear response is identified. An intervention is then applied and the behavior measured again for a specific period. If there is a change in behavior, the intervention is removed to validate that the intervention was responsible for the change. This technique is called the *reversal technique.*

Multiple baseline recording is another technique for assessing and evaluating interventions. Through this technique, several behaviors are measured over time, and an intervention is applied to one of these behaviors until a change in the behavior is noted. Little or no change may occur in the other behaviors. The intervention is then applied to one of the other behaviors to determine if a change occurs.[34]

The importance of evaluation cannot be overemphasized, because the effect of interventions may be unique to one targeted behavior or may influence other behaviors. Continually revising treatment plans as necessary and recognizing needed modifications help individualize care for psychiatric-mental health clients.

◆ Chapter Summary

The nursing process and behavior therapy are concerned with predicting behavior and providing accurate interventions for client problems. This chapter has included the following major points:

1. Following a complete assessment, including health history, physical and mental status examinations, laboratory tests, and client and family interviews, objective observation of the maladaptive behavior for a period of time is essential for accurate behavioral assessment.
2. The health team documents the observation period and the frequency of the behavior.
3. Specificity, a key factor in behavioral analysis, results from objective systematic approaches to client problems.
4. Descriptions of adaptive and maladaptive behavior and behavioral outcomes must be detailed to allow precise measurement and evaluation.
5. Behavioral interventions, including behavioral contracting, cognitive therapy, modeling, imagery, assertiveness training, and progressive muscle relaxation, are powerful approaches to dealing with clients' problems and needs.

Review Questions

1. The main goal of cognitive therapy is to
   A. emphasize contrasting.
   B. identify positive affirmation.
   C. correct faulty thinking.
   D. teach problem solving.
2. Reframing is an important intervention in cognitive therapy and relates to
   A. using thought therapy to decrease distress.
   B. looking at an event or situation from a different perspective.
   C. relaxation exercises to decrease anxiety.
   D. self-management in decreasing distress.
3. Behaviorists believe that maladaptive behavior is
   A. learned.
   B. genetically linked.
   C. due to a conflict.
   D. the result of trauma.
4. Operant conditioning is behavior that is
   A. specific to one situation.
   B. due to chance.
   C. strengthened or weakened by consequences.
   D. built on cues.
5. Social reinforcers include
   A. money, candy, tokens.
   B. praise, attention, touch.
   C. dancing, watching television, playing games.
   D. All of the above
6. When clarifying the content portion of a message, it is important to
   A. focus on the thought or idea being communicated.
   B. focus on the feeling tone of the message.
   C. focus on the thought and feeling tone of the message.
   D. address the problem using your own interpretation.
7. All of the following are therapeutic communication techniques except which one?
   A. Verifying
   B. Directing
   C. Summarizing
   D. Changing the subject

◆ References

1. Alberti RE, Emmons ML: Your Perfect Right, 2d ed. San Luis Obispo, CA, Impact, 1974
2. Alladin A: Cognitive Hypnotherapy With Depression. Journal of Cognitive Psychotherapy 8 (4): 275–288, 1994
3. Anderson-Malico R: Anger Management Using Cognitive Group Therapy. Perspect Psychiatr Care 30 (3): 17–20, 1994

4. Bandura A: Social Learning Therapy. Englewood Cliffs, NJ, Prentice-Hall, 1977
5. Baucom D, Epstein N: Cognitive-Behavioral Marital Therapy. New York, Brunner/Marel, 1990
6. Beck AT: Cognitive Therapy and the Emotional Disorders. New York, International Universities Press, 1978
7. Beck AT, Rush AJ, Shaw BF, Emery G: Cognitive Therapy of Depression. New York, The Guilford Press, 1987
8. Burns DD: Ten Days to Self-Esteem. New York, William Morrow, 1993
9. Burns DD: The Feeling Good Handbook. New York, A Plume Book, 1990
10. Carr JB: Communicating With Myself: A Journal. Dubuque, IA, Wm. C. Brown Publishers, 1984
11. Coon D: Cognitive-Behavioral Intervention With Avoidant Personality. A single case study. Journal of Cognitive Psycho Therapy 8 (3): 243–253, 1994
12. Crane DR: Introduction to Behavioral Family Therapy for Families With Young Children. Journal of Family Therapy 17 (2): 229–241, 1995
13. Demarest AP: The Personal Script as a Unit of Analysis for the Study of Personality. Journal of Personality 63 (3): 560–592, 1995
14. Duncan B, Salovey A, Rusk G: A Client-Directed Approach to Therapy. New York, The Guilford Press, 1992
15. Ellis A, Dryden W: The Practice of Rational Emotive Therapy (RET). New York, Springer, 1987
16. Ellis A, Dryden W: Rational Emotive Therapy. An excellent Counseling Therapy for NPs. Nurse Practitioner 12 (7): 16–37, 1987
17. Emery G: Own Your Own Life. New York, Penguin Books, 1982
18. Freeman A, Simon KM, Beutler LE, Arkowitz H: Comprehensive Handbook of Cognitive Therapy. New York, Plenum Press, 1989
19. Goldfriend MR, Davison G: Clinical Behavior Therapy. New York, Holt, Rinehart & Winston, 1976
20. Greenberg LS, Safran JD: Emotion in Psychotherapy. New York, The Guilford Press, 1987
21. Jacobson E: Progressive Relaxation. Chicago, University of Chicago Press, 1938
22. Johnson HM: How Do I Love Me? 2d ed. Salem, WI, Sheffield Publishing, 1986
23. Lavallee L, Campbell JD: Impact of Personal Goals on Self-Regulation Processes Elicited by Daily Negative Events. Journal of Personality and Social Psychology 69 (2): 341–352, 1995
24. Lynn SJ, Gaske JP: Contemporary Psychotherapies Models and Methods. Columbus, OH, Charles E. Merrill, 1985
25. McMorrow MJ, Cullinan D, Epstein MH: The Use of the Premack Principle to Motivate Patient Activity Attendance. Perspect Psychiatr Care 16 (January-February): 14–18, 1978
26. McMullin RE: Handbook of Cognitive Therapy Techniques. New York, WW Norton, 1986
27. Meichenbaum D: Cognitive-Behavioral Therapies. In Lynn SJ, Garske J (eds): Contemporary Psycho Therapies Models and Methods, pp 261–283. Columbus, OH, Charles E. Merrill, 1985
28. Owen SV, Fullerton ML: Would it Make a Difference? A Discussion Group in a Behaviorally Oriented Inpatient Eating Disorder Program. J Psychosoc Nurs Ment Health Serv 33 (11): 35–40, 1995
29. Smith G, Schivekel AI: Using a Cognitive-Behavioral Family Model in Conjunction With System and Behavioral Family Therapy Models. The American Journal of Family Therapy 23 (3): 203–212, 1995
30. Perry S, Frances A, Clarkin J: A DSM-III Casebook of Differential Therapeutics. New York, Brunner/Mazel, 1985
31. Price RH, Lynn SJ: Abnormal Pschology. Chicago, IL, The Dorsey Press, 1986
32. Reeder DM: Cognitive Therapy of Anger Management: Theoretical and Practical Considerations. Archives of Psychiatric Nursing 5 (3): 147–150, 1991
33. Rimm D, Cummingham HM: Behavior Therapies. In Lynn SJ, Garske J (eds): Contemporary Psycho Therapies Models and Methods, pp 221–250. Columbus, OH, Charles E. Merrill, 1985
34. Rimm DC, Masters JC: Behavior Therapy: Techniques and Empirical Findings. New York, Academic Press, 1974
35. Schwartz A: The Behavior Therapies. New York, The Free Press, 1982
36. Skinner BF: About Behaviorism. New York, Vintage Books, 1976
37. Watson JB, Rayner G: Conditioned Emotional Reactions. J Exp Psychol 3: 1–14, 1920
38. Webster DC: Solution-Focused Approaches in Psychiatric/Mental Health Nursing. Perspect Psychiatr Care 26 (4): 17–21, 1990
39. Weiss JC: Cognitive Therapy and Life Review Therapy. Theoretical and Therapeutic Implications for Mental Health Counseling 17 (2): 157–172, 1995
40. White M, Epston D: Narrative Means to Therapeutic Ends. New York, WW Norton, 1990
41. Wolpe J: The Practice of Behavior Therapy, 2ed. New York, Pergamon Press, 1973
42. Young JE: Cognitive Therapy for Personality Disorders. Sarasota, FL, Professional Resource Exchange, 1990
43. Zerhusen JD, Boyle K, Warner W: Out of the Darkness: Group Cognitive Therapy for Depressed Elderly. J Psychosoc Nurs 29 (9): 16–21, 1991

Alternative Therapies

Jeanneane Lewis Cline

19

A New Metaphor For Reality:
"The Whole Ball of String"
This ball of string represents reality-with-a-capital R.
It is immense.
It is made up of many, many strands . . . all interwoven, knotted, diving deep into the center, hanging out as loose ends at the surface.
Reality is complex and bigger than we are.
There are many ways to approach and approximate reality.
Every string captures an aspect of reality,
but no strand captures all of it.

Claire Monod Cassidy, 1994

Some people believe that in western medicine, the chief block to understanding and healing human beings is an overemphasis on technique, a tendency to view the client as an object to be analyzed, calculated, and managed. The alternative to this is an existential approach to healing, based on the view that understanding the client as an individual provides the basis for applying specific techniques. The task of psychotherapists is to understand the client "as a being and as being in their own world."[74]

This chapter presents a selected history and overview of alternative therapies as they pertain to psychiatric and psychological conditions. It includes a limited overview of how alternative therapies may pertain to the psychiatric considerations of selected medical conditions. Topics include spirituality, crystal healing, yoga, acupuncture, therapeutic touch (TT), movement therapies, art therapy, light therapy, massage, psychonutrition, and the development and implementation of these concepts for psychiatric nursing.

This chapter is not meant to teach the nurse how to apply alternative therapies, even though some of them, such as TT, are easy to learn. Expertise in alternative therapies requires study and apprenticeship, even professional accreditation.[55,56] *Instead, this chapter is designed to provide information to motivate the reader to seek additional information on alternative therapies and their relevance to psychiatric nursing.*

Nurses must be aware that many clients seek alternative therapies because of fear, mistrust, cultural differences, and a desire for a more holistic mind-body-spirit approach to care.[51,58,96] *Among clients who are reluctant to take pharmaceuticals, there is an increased interest in psychoneuronutritional therapy, herbal medication, homeopathic remedies, and mechanical aids, such as light boxes, for seasonal affective disorder (SAD).*[7,12,21,87,99]

Learning Objectives

On completion of this chapter, you should be able to accomplish the following:

1. *Define alternative therapies.*
2. *Discuss three concepts of alternative therapy.*
3. *Apply alternative therapies in nursing care.*
4. *Describe the usefulness of spiritual healing, therapeutic touch, acupuncture, imagery, movement, relaxation, or humor in the care of clients with mental illness and addiction.*
5. *Discuss other alternative therapies: herbal treatments, massage therapy, art therapy, light therapy, healing with crystals, and psychoneuronutritional medicine.*

◆ Alternative Therapies

Alternative Medicine, the broad domain of complementary and alternative medicine (CAM) encompasses all health systems, modalities, and practices other than those intrinsic to the politically dominant health system of a particular society or culture. CAM includes all practices and ideas self-defined by their users as preventing or treating illness or promoting health and well-being.[46]

The last part of this statement, "all practices and ideas self-defined by their users as preventing or treating illness or promoting health and well-being," immediately elicits many questions. What are these other modalities and practices? How do they work? Are they safe? Will they hurt? Can they be used with other methods? Can the practitioners be trusted? How much will they cost? Are they compatible with my beliefs? What are the client's responsibilities?

Many alternative health care practitioners believe that the client must be self-aware to be involved in the healing process. Awareness of how people view their personal situation, what they believe, and what they expect to happen is the base for understanding their perception of reality. Perception influences all the choices people make regarding their actions, including those that have an impact on self-healing.[14,31,44,85] It may be necessary to ask a client to reexamine some aspect of his or her lifestyle that may be out of balance rather than diseased. In many cases, nurses must consciously put their own beliefs aside and focus on understanding what a client is experiencing; this is similar to the process used to help a client explore hallucinations.

USE OF ALTERNATIVE THERAPIES

The last decade has seen an increasing focus on alternative therapies. More than 22 million (8.8%) Americans[58,79,86,96] use alternative rather than allopathic methods, or a combination, for health care, and spend more for out-of-pocket alternative services than for out-of-pocket allopathic or hospital services. Americans spend $26 billion per year for questionable medical therapies and an additional $10 billion per year on health "quackery."[34] Insurance companies do not pay for most alternative health care services, yet these services are inexpensive and available to many.[39] Meanwhile, approximately 75% of visits to the doctor are for illnesses that will ultimately get better by themselves or for disorders related to lifestyles filled with anxiety and stress.[14,96]

The Office of Unconventional Medicine of the National Institutes of Health (NIH) was created in June 1992 with a $2 million budget. By October 1992, the name was changed to the Office of Alternative Medicine (OAM), and the budget was increased to $7.5 million for 1996. Goals for the OAM are to gain recognition, inclusion, and reimbursement for the services.[79] An additional focus is research on many of the existing methods and treatments. A comprehensive reference book,

Alternative Medicine: Expanding Medical Horizons, A Report to the NIH on Alternative Medical Systems and Practices (also known as the Chantilly Report) was prepared for NIH in 1992. Internet sites, primarily established in academic centers include Paracelsus @teleport.com; wellnesslist @wellness mart.com; and altmed-res@virginia.edu.[105] Table 19-1 provides a sample of alternative therapies.

Some nurses may be uncomfortable when a client expresses his or her preference for alternative therapy over conventional medical and psychiatric treatment. This preference should be respected and valued as a part of that individual's belief system (Case Study 19-1). When appropriate, it is important to help clients identify *effective* alternative health care for their needs in the current health care environment. As an example of the efficacy of alternative therapies, a family practice group in Arizona established a clinic that provides services representative of 21 alternative health care methods. Their practice has since experienced a decrease in emergency room visits, hospitalizations, and overall costs. These findings support the belief that alternative methods can be less dangerous and more effective than standard therapy.[78] Additionally, more than 80 companies, including many Fortune 500 companies, are using alternative interventions, such as 15-minute massage sessions twice a week during lunch break, acupuncture for smoking, arts as a creativity enhancer, and "Lunch and Laughs" for relief of stress.[66]

LEGAL ISSUES

Licensing laws for alternative healing practices are specific to each state. For example, some states license massage and reflexology therapists; some permit the skills to be practiced by licensed physical therapists, chiropractors, or unlicensed individuals; and some require physician supervision.[8]

Herbal remedies have been in a "regulatory gray zone" in the United States for a long time. The Euro-

Table 19-1

Sample of Alternative Therapies

Model	Practitioner	Treatment	Goal
Allopathic	Physician, nurse, rehabilitationist	Medical, surgical, specific for diagnosis	Treat, restore function, obtain knowledge
Curanderismo	Curandera(o) herbalista, espiritista	Ritual incantations, suggestion, chanting, incense	Restore balance, practice religion in context of illness, assist recovery, preserve traditions
Chinese herbal medicine	Physician, herbalist shaman, masseur	Acupuncture, herbs, diet, massage, increase of qi flow, use of moxibustion at focused qi points	Relieve pain or tension, promote harmony in body and environment
Yoga	Practitioner, physical therapist	Breathing control, body positions (asanas), movement of body's internal energy	Purify body, relieve tension, promote peace
Native American	Shaman with benevolent spirits	Herbs, chanting, trance, sand painting, use of therapeutic communication through metaphor and ritual	Practice healing religion in context of illness
Homeopathy	Certified homeopath	"Likes cure like" with infinitesimal doses of herbs, minerals	Assist recovery, influence development of vaccines
Flower essences	Homeopath, herbalist, self-administered	Spiritual or metaphysical qualities of flowers and herbs in extracts to alleviate psychological spiritual problems	Rebalance physical, emotional, spiritual, and mental aspects
Therapeutic touch, acupuncture, shiatsu, reflexology, massage	Practitioner, nurse, massage therapist	Pressure, touch and patterning to change energy flow in body	Rebalance energy fields; improve mental state
Dance-movement therapy	Dance therapist	Facilitating movement, expressing feelings, providing growth experiences	Restore function in family, society
Crystal and color therapy	Practitioner, shaman, self-administered	Meditation based on crystals and colors	Rebalance energy fields

19-1 **Case Study**

Respecting the Client's Belief System

A 28-year-old woman of Asian background had been on the psychiatric unit for three days and was not participating in the program. The husband was asked to sit in with the nurse for additional information. The nurse suspected that the family was uncomfortable with the male physician and the direct questions of the group therapists. The discussion was directed mainly with the husband, who validated these concerns. After changing to a female physician and providing information to the staff about using less threatening questions and not requesting eye contact, the woman began to attend the scheduled activities.

Questions for Discussion

1. Considering the woman's culture, how would you sensitively inquire about the family's beliefs about and use of healing practices?
2. If the client and her husband wished to use traditional (non-Western) healing methods, how would you incorporate them into her plan of care?

pean phytomedicine (*phyto* means plant) market tops $3 billion in Germany. Phytomedicine tops $6 billion in the United States. The Food and Drug Administration (FDA) has not acted on a 1992 request to allow "old drug" status to European phytomedicines for over-the-counter sales. Current FDA regulations require them to be approved as new drugs, which is costly.[41,105] The American College of Apothecaries, primarily composed of pharmacists who compound medications, established a Committee for Alternative Medicine in 1995.

Alternative medicine may be viewed as less credible than traditional western approaches because of nonadherence to approved scientific models and methodologies and limited control and governance of the practitioner.[39] To establish accountability, some attempts have been made to generalize the undocumented and unsubstantiated claims of a particular therapy. Claims that a therapy is applicable to all people with a particular condition, irrespective of the stage of the disease, specific demographics, and other forms of individual variability, may undermine the perceived value of alternative therapies.[34]

◆ Spirituality and Alternative Therapies

Spirituality has always been a component of healing in many cultures and is making a reappearance in the United States. Nightingale wrote that spirituality is intrinsic to human nature and is the deepest and most potent resource for healing. She believed that science is necessary for the development of a mature concept of God. Believing that the "Laws of science are the thoughts of God," she did not see a conflict between science and spirituality.[73]

Spirituality, sometimes used interchangeably with religion, refers to a sense of meaning and purpose in life and a source of love and relatedness. The definition of spirituality differs from that of religion. Religion may be defined as an "adherence to beliefs and practices of an organized institution." Spirituality may be defined as a "transcended relationship between the person and a Higher Being."[69] Spiritual healing may be defined as "direct influence of one or more people upon another living system without using known physical means of intervention," "treating the soul injured by sin," or "deliverance from adverse effects of demons or spirits."[5] Spiritual support may be defined as "the perceived, personally supportive components of an individual's relationship with God."[65]

A review of 2,348 articles in four leading psychiatric journals from 1979 to 1982 showed that only 59, fewer than 2.5% of the articles, included any type of quantified religious variable. Only one article used a state-of-the-art approach to measuring religious factors, and some even view religious variables as pathological.[60] The Diagnostic and Statistical Manual of Mental Disorders, third edition revised (DSM-IIIR), referred to spirituality and religion as Religious or Spiritual Problem (V62.61) within another diagnosis. In contrast, the 1994 DSM-IV (V62.89) acknowledges for the first time that religious and spiritual issues can be the sole focus of psychiatric treatment.

Recent studies have found positive relationships between spirituality and mental health. People reporting mystical experiences scored lower on psychopathology scales and higher on measures of psychological well-being than the control group. Mystical experiences were reported by 30% to 40% of the population, suggesting that this is normal rather than pathological.[69] Another study reports that 48% of the sample, especially those with little social support, stated that spirituality was central to coping with their serious mental illnesses. Spirituality helped the individuals feel cared for, comforted, and socially supported and gave them a sense of belonging to a community.[101]

Twelve-step programs, such as Alcoholics Anonymous, include the concept of spirituality with a reference to God in five of the 12 steps and do not believe that recovery is possible without the help of a *higher power.* Some theorists and clinicians suggest that addictions are essentially spiritual crises, not mental disorders.[69]

Spiritual factors associated with health include patience, hope, forgiveness, grace, meditation, fellowship, and prayer. How does prayer heal? Healing may come through faith, belief, or a surrender to God that then increases one's receptivity to a supernatural force. One becomes receptive to healing prayer through self-preparation (eg, fasting); from the love, caring, and healing belief of the healer or intermediator; and through cooperation of faith and physical aids (eg, medication), stimulating the body forces and inspiring them to do the work God made them to do.[64,94] Dossey believes that *not* to use prayer is analogous to withholding a treatment.[26]

Healing prayer may have an immediate effect, or it may require many sessions. MacNutt believes all people have the potential for invoking healing prayer; Krieger also believes all can learn TT.[55,56,71] Some people seem to have the power to pray for certain things and not others; others pray for generalized improvement, the "highest good," or the best possible outcome because something else may need to be accomplished before the specific condition heals. In a review of more than 100 studies, the majority demonstrated that prayer brought about significant changes.[26,50,54,71] Many studies blind the participants to the true nature of the experimental protocol and the fact that a healing study is being conducted to control for suggestion, expectation of healing, and the placebo effect.

A group in a community setting, designed and led by nurses, facilitated people telling about their dreams as a means to gain spiritual awareness. For the first time, group members were able to talk about what was of great importance in their lives.[23] Nurses have the capacity to include spirituality selectively when caring for the client.

ILLNESS CAUSATION THEORIES

Hay has proposed the theory of *metaphysical* causation of disease, asserting that words and thoughts have power to create and maintain experiences and that life experiences do "mirror our beliefs." A change in thinking can bring about a change in the experience or condition. This theory of disease, which applies to physical and mental illness, reflects similar theories to those behind cognitive and solution-oriented therapies. Hay believes that for every unwanted physical condition, there is a need to be fulfilled, and one must go beyond the physical expression to the mental cause behind it. For example, constipation could indicate a belief in limitation, an unwillingness to let something go because of a fear that there will be no replacement, or the need to hold on to a painful memory. Willpower and discipline will not bring about changes; one must work on the "willingness to release" the need for cigarettes, excess weight, cancer, or depression. She suggests that "incurable" only means that a condition cannot be cured by "outer" methods and that one must go within the self to effect healing.[42]

These concepts support the nurse's use of talk therapy and the positive outcome of people who restate or reframe their thoughts and change the words. The belief that healing mechanisms can be activated at the mental level reinforces the impact of people's words on belief and sensory systems

SHAMANISM

For thousands of years, shamans, the earliest healers, have been responding to a primal drive; their intense spiritual experiences begin with an initiatory crisis of affliction that leads to enlightenment and the power to heal. The modern doctor and the priest have descended from shamanic traditions. Shamans are expected to transform and heal themselves, learn from their own illness experiences, and access altered states of consciousness (ASC) for the benefit of those seeking healing. Shamans are the most psychologically healthy members and leaders of their community and are the healers and spiritual leaders.[1,27] The shaman or therapist is sensitive to the listener's immediate needs, often uses story telling, and models the skills of the "hero."[61]

Changing how people see things and expanding on their inner positive qualities are fundamental shamanic arts.[20,58] Ritual work has a direct therapeutic effect on the client by creating vivid healing images and inducing ASCs that are conducive to self-healing. Physical disease is believed to be an externalized image of thought[2] or to arise from an imbalance in one's relationship with the spirit world.[3,27] Rhythmic auditory stimuli, such as drums or chants, help the shaman to determine the proper balancing actions by engaging in profound dialogue with the imaginal realms.[27,114]

Shamanic Healing Rituals

Shamans and native healers share four basic concepts of healing with contemporary health care:

1. A shared world view that makes diagnosis possible in each culture

2. Qualities that appear to facilitate the client's recovery
3. Positive expectations of the client to assist the healing process
4. The ability to impart a sense of mastery that empowers the client[57]

Shamanic healers use spiritual insight gained from transcendental meditation to produce ceremonies that change clients' perceptions of their illnesses. Although the foundations of shamanism differ from those of western medicine, both traditions provide experiences that convince clients that specific procedures alleviate illness.[75] Myths, symbols, and rituals also can be effective interventions for pain.

One example of a shamanic healing ritual comes from the Tamang tradition. The kara puja ritual of playing drums and singing sacred stories is a successful means of treating "soul loss and spirit possession," other terms for variations of dissociative and somatoform disorders (ie, conversion reaction). The ritual alters the client's relationship with the spiritual cosmos and affects significant interpersonal relationships. The family is included in the ritual to reestablish unity. The inability of a person to fulfill social responsibilities is viewed as an impending spiritual death.[83]

Today, Native American shamans are likely to designate those physical conditions (ie, tuberculosis and malaria) that are best treated by the allopathic physician. [114] One Native American man explained his criminal behavior as episodic ghost possession. After traditional exorcism failed to help, a western diagnosis of dissociative state with paranoid schizophrenia was made. The client underwent remission during neuroleptic treatment, despite previous evidence of possession. Neuroleptics may relieve symptoms of exorcism-resistant possession.[40]

Clinical Application and Nursing

The nurse can encourage the use of traditional rituals in the psychiatric unit; in the receptive client, such rituals may help unclutter the mind and allow the client to visualize healing images, practice healing chants, and convey healing messages to self.[3] Rituals may consist of music, storytelling, and movements. The Native American will respond to storytelling or metaphors rather than the more direct information that Americans value. Using the phrase "remember when" lets a person begin to attain an ASC and begin to consider changes or reframe thoughts. Metaphors use figurative language to suggest a likeness of one idea used in place of another and provide a strong image with a feeling tone that is powerful in communicating meaning. Using metaphors requires practice; however, the nurse can listen for the client's metaphors and assist with clarification. To integrate treatment better with Native American, Asian, Southeast Asian, Chinese, Japanese, or Pacific Island clients, the nurse must explore their cultural traditions of medication, charms or amulets, dietary practices, and religious beliefs. The nurse can then consider how to maximize the supplementary use of shamans or healers if the client so desires.

◆ Chakras and Energy Fields

CHAKRAS

Chakras are part of the practice of Ayurveda, Chinese, and New Age medicine and yoga meditation. Clients involved in these belief systems or practices may refer to chakras with varying levels of self-awareness. Chakras are centers in the body located in the pelvis, abdomen, chest, neck, and head that are energy conduits or foci to specific organs and emotional states. For example, the heart chakra, situated near the heart in the chest area, affects the heart and lungs and emotions and affection. Both TT and acupuncture involve direct or indirect manipulation of the chakras and energy fields. The practice of crystal healing also relies on chakras. See Figure 19-1 for a representation of each chakra.

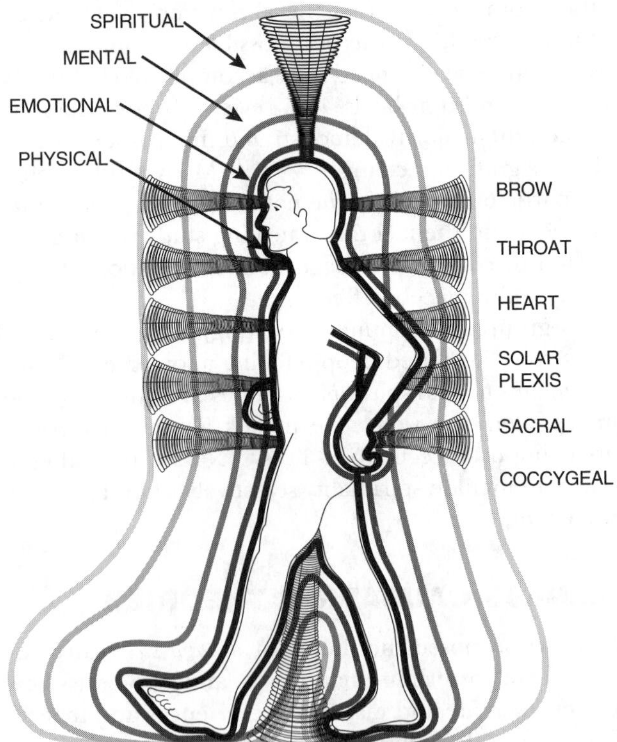

Figure 19-1. The chakras in relation to the layers of the energy field. (Reprinted with permission from Janet L. Mentgen, Program Administrator, Healing Touch.)

The systems of Egypt, Japan, and Tibet teach that the center of the body is the solar plexus or abdomen. Other modern alternative healing theorists propose that the center is the heart chakra. When operating from this chakra, the practitioner will always come from "unconditional love" and do no harm,[49] a concept important to the nurse. Clients who are aware of chakras may somatize specific mental distresses in chakra areas.

ENERGY FIELDS

Chakras can be thought of as transformers; they transform various universal energies into energy that is usable by humans for different body functions. In energy field theory, the chakras may be a mechanism that interrelates the physical body, acupuncture meridians, and the "etheric bodies" formed by human energy fields. Each chakra has a specific function in each of the energy fields. The four sequential energy fields that envelop the body in layers are as follows:

1. The *etheric* or vital field is most associated with energy-balancing work by practitioners; it is about 2 inches out from the skin.
2. The *aura* or emotional field holds the affective and feeling energy.
3. The *causal* or mental field embodies thinking patterns and visual imagery.
4. The *astral* or intuitive field relates to the spiritual dimension and is about 12 inches out from the body.[26,45,49,56,62]

These fields reflect mental and physical illness by distortion and change in "feel" and color.

THERAPEUTIC TOUCH

Therapeutic touch is a method of modifying a client's energy field. It was pioneered and developed by Delores Krieger and Dora Kunz. Therapeutic touch has been taught to more than 72 thousand people since 1975, in more than 80 American universities and in more than 70 foreign countries, especially in schools of nursing. In part, the practice of TT is derived from ancient concepts of "energy transfer," the "inner healer," and the "laying on of hands" (although the TT practitioner does not actually touch the client). This nonintrusive practice is still a matter of controversy, even though enough current, supportive data indicate that TT is effective in promoting healing.

Role of Therapeutic Touch Healers

Practitioners or healers and work with the person's energy field, or aura, to consciously direct an energy exchange. The practitioner is a conduit to focus universal energy—also described as love, spirit of a god, or white light—on the client. Using his or her own healthy energy field as a support system, the practitioner provides the "scaffolding" to guide the repatterning of the client's weakened and disrupted flow. The goal of support is to stimulate the immunological system so that the clients can heal themselves.

Use of Therapeutic Touch

Each therapeutic touch session consists of four steps: centering, assessment, treatment, and evaluation. The sessions generally last 1 to 2 minutes for neonates and 20 minutes for adults.[55,56,59,70,72] Although most reported studies of TT examine its use in medical conditions,[109,110] TT has been used with depression, fatigue, and lethargy. It has also been shown to alleviate some of the symptoms of acquired immunodeficiency syndrome, which is caused by the human immunodeficiency virus (HIV). Therapeutic touch has positively affected hyperkinetic children, catatonic adults, and people with bipolar disorder. It has shown no impact on schizophrenia.[56]

One study explored various psychological and immunological effects of TT on bereaved clients and practitioners. Although affect of clients improved, results varied considerably between the two practitioners in the study. The practitioner with greater experience who administered 50 to 60 treatments per month had better outcomes than the practitioner who administered 10 treatments per month,[84] again reinforcing the value of experience and expertise for the nurse (Table 19-2).

◆ Acupuncture

In our era of "high-tech" medicine, many Americans are turning to acupuncture, a centuries-old form of therapy, to deal with chronic pain and the physical effects of mental stress. There are 9,000 to 10,000 practicing acupuncturists, including 3,000 physicians, in the United States today.[86]

PROCEDURE AND EFFECTS

Acupuncture stimulates or sedates selected points along channels or meridian lines going from the head to the feet to treat the desired region of the body. During treatment, tiny 1- to 2-inch needles are inserted at selected acupuncture points on the 12 major meridians or eight auxiliary tracts. There are up to 1,000 interconnected acupuncture points. The needles are twirled clockwise or counter-clockwise to evoke, intensify, or change the needle tip's polarity and cause a change in condition. Disposable acu-

Table 19-2

Simplified Steps of Therapeutic Touch

1. Centering—This initial act of centering your consciousness quiets the chattering "monkey brain" and focuses attention on inner responses to receive information.
2. Assessing—Sensitize the hands; with open hands 2–3 inches from the body begin to scan from the head down. Repeat on the opposite side of the body (front or back). Be aware of differences you may feel.
3. Treatment—This involves the conscious, deliberate engagement of the healer with intentionality and compassionate interest in helping others, and a willingness of the healee to change. Use hands to unruffle, rebalance, facilitate, mobilize congestion, dampen, and synchronize energy flow.
4. Evaluation—When cues are no longer present or the client has had enough, reassess the field for balance. Treatment is completed.

puncture needles should be used to avoid any risk of HIV or other infections.[3,4]

ACUPUNCTURE THEORIES

Why is acupuncture effective? One theory proposes that because the needle is a metal conductor with opposite polarities at the tip and handle, manipulation of the needle impacts the energy flow in the body.

Another theory is that acupuncture stimulates the production of enkephalins and endorphins, the body's natural pain relievers. These morphine-like substances are similar to the chemical morphine yet have no addictive properties.

The traditional philosophical theory proposes that the body and its organ systems are under the influence of two opposing forces, known as yin (the negative, dark, cold, female) and yang (the positive, light, hot, male) and that the interaction of these two forces creates *ch'i*, or *qi*, life energy. The acupuncturist believes that imbalances in *qi* are the cause of disease processes.[4,98] The skill of working with *qi* to regulate the body and thus affect the mind is sometimes referred to as Qi gong.[91] Qi gong, acupuncture, and the use of herbs are the three pillars of Chinese medicine.

Critics believe that acupuncture is little more than an "elaborate triggering" of the placebo effect. However, one characteristic of the placebo effect is that its efficacy decreases with time, whereas acupuncture's benefits have a cumulative effect. None of the many theories alone explains the multiple analgesic, anti-inflammatory, sedative, or regenerative effects of acupuncture.[4,99]

Some insurers and Medicaid programs cover acupuncture. Half of the states have licensing agencies.

Clinical Application and Nursing Considerations

Acupuncture has been used successfully to provide pain relief and treat drug addiction, headaches, nerve and muscular disorders, and allergies.[4] It is also used for mental imbalances, particularly stress. The psychiatric nurse can support clients in the mental health setting who prefer acupuncture alone or in combination with a traditional program by assisting with the decision-making process and validating their choice. Education of the staff will help in decreasing anxiety and acceptance of this treatment format.

◆ Healing With Crystals

Healing work with stones and gems dates back thousands of years in Native America, South America, Africa, Europe, Egypt, and India. Healing with crystals became popular again in North America and Europe during the 1980s. As discussed previously, each chakra has an energy field and a corresponding color or colors. In crystal healing, clear quartz crystals or gemstones of corresponding colors are applied to chakras to heal physical, emotional, or mental maladies associated with those chakras. Specific colors and gemstones have specific purposes, assigned by their traditional and spiritual associations. For example, heart chakra colors are rose and green and healing gem stones include rose quartz, green aventurine, green jade, tourmaline, and rhodochrosite. These gem stones are used to treat broken hearts, thymus or immune system weakness, circulation, infections, loneliness, self-image, trust, and recovery from abusive childhoods or relationships.

Crystals may be set on a table, put on the client's body in various places, or laid out in a sacred space pattern. The "laying on of stones" is believed to activate a particular energy that releases emotional, mental, or spiritual blocks to well-being. When the healing is accomplished, the gemstones have absorbed negative energy and let their positive energy "clear" the chakra area. Some feel energized, and others feel relaxed.[99] Crystals may be worn, carried in a pocket, or set on a chakra area of the body.

Stone healing practitioners are not licensed. Healing with stones is usually a form of self-medication in clients with strong spiritual beliefs. When healing with stones is important to the client, nurses can communicate acceptance of the practice, help the client acquire stones and crystals, and provide for safe care of these items. As with other alternative methods and the mind-body-spirit beliefs, combining crystal healing practice with traditional means may be more acceptable, and therefore more beneficial, for the client.

◆ Yoga

Often called "mindfulness meditation," yoga is a gentle and powerful form of body meditation that cultivates musculoskeletal strength, flexibility, and balance and inner stillness. In one method, the mindfulness is a stillness that allows the individual to focus on thoughts, sensations, or physical discomfort. Participants practice this mindfulness by attending to breathing and various physical sensations while lifting, stretching, and balancing in a wide range of physical postures and moving slowly between them with concentration. Yoga invokes physiological changes of the relaxation response and is a means of escaping the mental activities that often cause suffering.[14] It was widely practiced in the United States during the 1960s and remains popular today, specifically as a means of relieving stress.

◆ Imagery

Imagery is an ancient healing technique and a cognitive tool to facilitate communication between perception, emotion, and body changes. Imagery decreases pain and stress, alters the course of disease, engenders a feeling of control, and improves one's outlook on life.[100]

USE OF IMAGERY

Imagery is applicable in mental health when resistance to change is a treatment concern. Using imagery dialogue, the client is asked to image or personalize the feeling of being ambivalent about change; if the client is willing, he or she then invites the "feeling" to emerge for conversation and exploration to understand more about what is occurring. In the process, the client tends to disidentify with the struggle and see the "feeling" as something that also has needs, fears, concerns, and wants. Ultimately the client can befriend, accept, and then negotiate with the feeling. Resistance may also appear in the image in the form of an immovable, unchanging object, such as a huge black mountain. In this situation, the therapist suggests that the person walk around to see the other side, usually a very different perspective presenting different solutions.[89]

Clinical Application and Nursing Considerations

Symbolic imagery seems to be more powerful than concrete images.[24] Imagery is a means of consciously involving the mind in a situation in which it unwittingly may have been playing a role. The goal of imagery is to help people recognize that by being responsible for their own reactions, they can learn to respond differently and gain a sense of control over themselves and their lives.[67,95] Assisting people with using imagery and descriptions is similar to facilitating problem solving with different ideas and words, a psychiatric nursing skill. The nurse can help the client relax and provide some initial cues for starting imagery work. Case Study 19-2 includes the use of imagery.

◆ Movement and Relaxation

Frederick M. Alexander (1869–1955) developed a technique involving breathing and gentle posture changes designed to increase the awareness of the self and rectify the lack of balance and coordination in everyday activities. Based on the mind-body-spirit concept, feelings and thoughts that occur with habitual, distorted movements lead to tension that, in turn, leads to sickness and pain. His process of "reeducation," rather than therapy, includes awareness and "letting go" of excessive, unconsciously held tension in the body. Inhibiting habitual responses to stimuli frees the body to develop different reactions to stimuli by conscious, de-

Case Study

The Use of Imagery

A 45-year-old man with bipolar disorder was readmitted because of inconsistency with medication use and many problems in his life. He was a commercial artist whose wife and grown children had become disillusioned, disgusted, and disappointed. The nurse asked him to describe his illness. He stated that it was like a roller coaster attached to a comet that traveled from fluffy pink, golden clouds to huge gray, rolling thunderheads. Wanting to reestablish contact with his family, he was willing to begin to reconsider his bipolar condition through the use of imagery. The nurse did not discuss medication, and when the client was sensing more control and less interference from staff, he asked for information about medication.

Questions for Discussion

1. Using imagery, how would you coach a person to maximize his 5 senses and move toward a new vision of his condition?
2. What steps would the person take to experience the realization of his new vision?

liberate direction. His theory is, "If you stop doing the wrong thing, the right thing will happen automatically."[96]

With similar beliefs and techniques, Jacobson developed a progressive relaxation technique that includes relaxing the eyes to avoid reviewing visual impressions of negative experiences and focusing on specific muscle groups. The overall effect is a decreased tension in muscle groups and an energy conservation.[47]

Moshe Feldenkrais also believed that a correction or change of body movements is the best means of improving self-image and performance. An increased awareness of body parts and their relationship to each other leads to a "harmony rule" with activities, abilities, and passions for an improved vitality of life. Particular emphasis is placed on working with the back—the "spine of your personality." When the back is impaired, the ability to say "no" to the world is also impaired. To be happy, sad, angry, or express any feeling requires certain body postures. The following components of self-image are present in every action of the body:

1. Movement—temporal (time) and spatial changes
2. Sensation—the senses plus kinesthetics, which include pain, orientation in space, passage of time, and rhythm
3. Feeling—self-respect or its lack and the emotions
4. Thinking—the intellect[6,31]

The Hendricks, a husband and wife team, believe that talk therapy keeps discussions at the level of concepts and does not allow a person to experience the feelings and reconnect the mind and body. The Hendricks' work with clients includes awareness of breathing, movements, and tension patterns to decrease fragmentation and increase aliveness, well-being, and creativity. Rather than giving an interpretation of an action or gesture, the therapist may request that the client magnify the action, saying for example, "Make that gesture a little bigger," rather than "Stop that!"as the family usually says. The gesture might be an eye twitch that signifies sadness or a hand straying to the belly, which often indicates fear. The therapist uses nonjudgmental inquiry. The client is helped to reclaim feelings associated with an action through comments such as, "that feeling reminds you of. . . ."[44] This reinforces the need for nursing to focus on observation skills, feelings, and communication.

DANCE AND MOVEMENT THERAPY

The discipline of dance or movement therapy is a more formalized means of using the body and various movements in therapeutic activity. Every emotion has its expression in the postural model of the body (motion), and changes are connected with expressive attitudes. The therapists are accomplished dancers who incorporate psychological theory into an "interactive process" with individuals or groups. Clients of all ages and many diagnoses, even with catatonia, are included. Dance therapy began with several distinct foci:

- Marian Chase with a Freudian psychoanalytic base in the early 1940s on the East Coast
- Mary Whitehouse with a Jungian spiritual-myth base in the 1960s on the West Coast
- A complex system of movement observation, analysis, and notation brought to the United States by Rudolf Laban and Irmgard Bartenieff from Germany in 1936

Labananalysis, originated for dance, was adapted for dance or movement therapy and includes, for example, the elements of the following:

1. Notation, quantitative aspects of body movements: time and number of movements
2. Effort/shape, qualitative aspects: fast or slow, light or heavy, direct or indirect
3. Space/harmony, body's relationship to space: up or down, side to side, back and forth

Dance therapy starts with the client or mover letting the movement happen; the therapist then reflects, encourages, and responds to the client's movements. Dance therapy is the experience of the mover or client, the witness or therapist, and the relationship between them.[18] Like all forms of psychotherapy, dance therapy is involved with the diagnosis and treatment of emotional dysfunction because the emotions are the bridge between the *psyche* and the *soma*.

Clinical Application and Nursing Considerations

The nurse must recall that movement is a means of communication and can often facilitate verbalization in the mute, resistant client. Effective questions include, "Of what is this condition (not illness) an expression?" "In what ways are the body and the psyche colluding with this condition?" These questions imply that the client can change things, as opposed to questions such as "What did you do to bring this on yourself?"

Heber, a nurse, designed a movement program for psychiatric clients, excluding the psychotic and suicidal, that demonstrated improved affect, decreased muscle tension, and an overall sense of "feeling good." The data were based on more than 350 clients, 18 to 60 years old, with anxiety, tension, depression, and low self-esteem; they attended 30-minute movement therapy sessions on 6 consecutive days.[43] Nurses not trained in movement therapy can use directed and undirected movement which, in its unskilled clumsiness, gives clients permission to try something different and may even be the cause of laughter.

VOICE AND MOVEMENT THERAPY

Less common than dance therapy is voice movement therapy. Newham developed voice movement therapy from the notion that in preverbal cultures, singing was a means to release emotional energy and express psychological excitation generated from life experiences. After analyzing breathing, sounds, and movements, the therapist massages and manipulates the client's body, gives instructions for ways of moving, and suggests changes in moods and images that the client may have unconsciously allowed to infiltrate and affect the voice quality. The changes release vocal functions from social and psychophysical constrictions.[80]

◆ Humor

Humor comes from the Latin *umor* meaning liquid or fluid; in the Middle Ages, it referred to an energy that affects particular body fluids and emotional states, determining health and disposition. Today's definition of humor is a quality of perception that enables us to experience joy even when faced with adversity. Humor involves the whole brain, integrates and balances activity in both hemispheres, shifts internal chemistry, enhances perceptual flexibility, and renews spiritual energy. Laughter appears to be the perfect antidote for stress.[113] The Greeks used comedians to help heal the sick, and the Ojibwa Native Americans have "clown-doctors." Guffawing for 20 seconds gives the heart the same workout as 3 minutes of hard rowing.[53]

In one hospital program, 70 humorous movies were shown to a group of chronic schizophrenic clients for 3 months. Compared with a control group that viewed assorted movies, the treatment group showed a decrease in verbal and motor aggression, were more supportive of each other, and improved relationships with staff. However, because of the clients' regressed state, the improvements did not carry over into social relationships outside the program.[32,33]

Goodheart has used therapeutic laughter for more than 20 years. Techniques such as having the client wear a red clown nose and say "tee-hee" when describing a problem stimulate humor and laughter and change the client's and others' perspective of the situation (Box 19-1). Painful emotions are red flags telling us we need to act; if we do not act, the emotions may emerge later in different disguises. Laughter causes a shift in attitudes, body language, and emotions. People who laugh then think more clearly and carefully and enjoy their lives more.[35]

An Example of the Effect of Changing One's Perspective

1. Place a flattened hand, fingers together, up to the face with the palm just touching the nose and observe what you see—not much.
2. Now move the hand in the same position out about 12 inches and observe what you see and whether you laughed.
3. Move the hand in the same position to the end of the outstretched arm and observe what you see.

The first position gives a very limited vision.
The second position gives a broader view, and the hand looks somewhat smaller.
In the third position, the hand, identified as the problem, looks even smaller and a larger context with more alternatives comes into view.

Finding humor in nursing activities can lift the spirit's energy level and help nurses replenish themselves from "compassion fatigue." Although there may be a risk in poor timing, nurses can focus on the laughing *with* and not *at* people.[53] Use of the distance-perception activity (see Box 19-1) is helpful with clients when words get in the way.

◆ Massage

The American Association for Massage Therapy increased from 1,500 members in 1983 to 22,000 in 1995, and the accredited schools increased from 12 to 60 in the same time.[66] Massage therapies include Rolfing (a technique developed by Ida Rolf, a biochemist, that uses deep, vigorous massage), Reichian therapy (developed by Wilhelm Reich, with the goal of working on the body's "armor"), and Trager therapy (designed to provide relief from tensions through passive, gentle movement of the head, neck, shoulders, and legs).[96]

Body-related therapies are often the lay person's first exposure to a body-mind maintenance concept of health. Massage has a time-honored place as the art and science of muscle relaxation and stress reduction. Healing touch, which requires less specific anatomical knowledge and includes awareness of energy fields, may be integrated into body therapies and often facilitates a quicker response. The nurse can help the client by using body therapies as an adjunct to traditional psychotherapy. When mental blocks are encountered in psychotherapy, from childhood trauma for example, body therapy may be a means of release, followed by continuation with the original therapist.[45]

◆ Art Therapy

Art therapy is a frequently used therapeutic specialty. Clients and program directors who have difficulty accepting TT or meditation are often more open to art therapy because of its long and successful history. Art as therapy uses painting, sculpture, or drawing to assist clients to express inner stories in a psychotherapeutic way that frees emotions and heals the psyche. It focuses on the power of the creative process to heal without analysis. It also provides therapists and care providers with information about the client and enables them to support changes.

Art therapy is particularly useful with children and adolescents because it provides a safe expression of pain. It facilitates emotional expression and release; images of pain and darkness are brought to light and changed into images of love, lightness, and control. Art therapy may be used in diagnosis and treatment.[92] The nurse, although not an art therapist, can offer clients this means of self-expression. Interpretation is allowed and encouraged only by the client; the nurse's responses must be objective, as are behavioral observations. For example, statements such as "I see blue and green," "That line is jagged," "There is an empty space," "Tell me about the picture,"or "Explain what this means to you" would be appropriate. It may be necessary to use positive statements to encourage the client who is having difficulty complying with art therapy because of shyness or self-perceived "lack of talent."

◆ Light Therapy

Since the second century, natural light has been known to be a general contributor to health. Seasonal rhythms are affected by neuronal pathways that transmit light from the eye to the hypothalamus and then to the pineal gland to suppress nocturnal melatonin (synthesized from serotonin) secretion. Several studies have associated seasonal variations, such as fewer daylight hours and decreased sunlight in the winter, with altered mood and physical functioning.

Light therapy has been effective with depression, especially SAD; delayed sleep phase syndrome; premenstrual symptoms; bulimia; drug addiction; and alcohol withdrawal. The best times to administer light therapy are before noon and after 2 PM. Light therapy may be initiated at any convenient time of the day for intervals of 10 to 15 minutes, with 90 minutes the maximum practical amount. It may consist of simply sitting or walking in full sunlight, spending time underneath full-spectrum light bulbs, or using "light boxes" designed to provide intense, full-spectrum light while the client does daily activities. Consistency is important in light therapy; it works well in conjunction with meditation or administration of serotonin uptake inhibitors.[7]

Photostimulation produces as much as an 85% improvement in SAD. Unlike classic depression, SAD is generally characterized by oversleeping, overeating, craving carbohydrates, and weight gain in the winter.[87] The nurse should evaluate depressed clients for possible symptoms of SAD, which will influence treatment and education for aftercare.

◆ Psychoneuronutritional Medicine

Nutritional therapy is one of the most commonly self-administered alternative healing methods. It may take the form of specific diets, such as the macrobiotic diet, or nutritional supplements, often more varied and obscure than simple multivitamins from the drugstore. Many naturopaths, homeopaths, and physicians in holistic practice make extensive use of nutritional therapy. Certification of nutritional therapists varies from state to state.

Nutritional therapy is based on the clinical relationship between psychology, neurochemistry, and nutrition. Bland developed a multidisciplinary field of psychoneuronutritional medicine to treat problems ranging from behavior disorders in children to cognitive or emotional disorders in adults. For example, serotonin is derived from the essential amino acid tryptophan; decreased tryptophan decreases the pain threshold, so foods rich in tryptophan may be recommended for some clients. Other clients might benefit from an increased intake of the B-complex nutrient folic acid, which is involved in the conversion of phenylalanine to dopamine, a neurotransmitter.[12]

Use of herbal remedies and extracts is increasing in popularity today. Herbs were used for healing in Egypt in 2300 BCE, by the Hebrews in 1500 BCE, and in Greece in 506 BCE, where the primary healers were women. Hildegard of Bingen (1098–1179), an abbess, wrote medical books for natural healing and herb use of 213 plants and 55 trees, plus mineral and animal-derived remedies. Herbs are more the basis of the Chinese healing system than is acupuncture. The tradition of Chinese herbals and herb healing goes back to 400 BCE; there are almost 6,000 entries in the modern Chinese herbal pharmacopoeia.[99]

One herbal remedy system, the Bach flower remedies—formulated in the mid-1900s by Edward Bach—focuses specifically on mental disorders as perceived by the client. This system coordinates 38 herbal extracts with states of mental distress, including codependency, posttraumatic stress disorder, depression of several sorts, and lack of motivation.

The current increased interest in herbal and nutritional remedies appears to be based on the high costs of, and disillusionment with, modern medicine and the myth that plant remedies are "naturally" superior to drugs.[104] Another myth is that herbs and nutritional supplements do not produce side effects; this is not true. Very high doses of vitamin A and vitamin C can cause dermatological, visual, and digestive problems; excessive mineral supplements can cause rashes; and certain popular herbs, such as goldenseal (produces diarrhea) and ma huang (accelerates heart rate) can produce negative side effects.

Clients interested in nutritional and herbal therapy for psychiatric disorders should be encouraged to consult with a physician who specializes in nutrition, or with a nutritionist. If this is not possible, they should be encouraged to explore nutritional and herbal remedies with reasonable caution and to avoid unsubstantiated fads. Poor eating habits can affect mood and alertness, especially in active people; clients who are taking nutritional remedies should consume a healthy, regular diet to obtain their full effect.

◆ Nursing Paradigm

Watson discusses a change in nursing's caring–health paradigm that has moved beyond the industrial, mechanistic, and interactionistic models for humanity and science to one of caring. Caring has been linked to healing as part of nursing and described as a sacred art that honors the sacredness and unity of all life.[106] Nightingale states, "Nature alone cures . . . and what nursing has to do . . . is to put the client in the best condition for nature to act upon him."[81] Likewise, as the nurse cares for others, it is imperative that a balanced self-care lifestyle be role modeled with the methods discussed previously—awareness, focus, imagery, relaxation, and patience.[107] Teaching occurs best through the modeling of behaviors.

> Imagine that each scientific discipline has, so to speak, caught hold of the end of one of these many strands hanging off the whole. As different disciplines run up individual strands doing research, they do indeed approach closer to Reality. However, each single strand does not make up Reality, and even if one discipline followed its strand successfully through all its twists and turns, it could never encompass the *whole ball of string.* At the intersections and knots, people of different backgrounds have the opportunity to work together to unravel mysteries.[17]

◆ Chapter Summary

With the increasing diversity of people living in the United States, psychiatric nurses must begin to approach "healing" and "nursing" with a cross-cultural focus. An awareness that truly hears, sees, and clarifies the client's words and movements in collaborative treatment planning is imperative. The Office of Alternative Medicine has been established by the government to ensure accurate knowledge through research, proficiency of practitioners, and adequate funding. This chapter has highlighted the following points:

1. Alternative therapies, originated in many cultures thousands of years ago, include beliefs about touch, eye contact, gender roles, and family and community relationships.
2. Alternative therapies that rely on healers, family involvement, and more natural substances, such as herbs, vitamins, nutrients, and noninvasive therapies, can be a more cost-effective approach to health.
3. Even though the major focus of alternative therapy has been on medical conditions, the client with psychiatric disorders also may be helped with these methods.
4. Spiritual concepts and belief in an invisible and powerful higher force permeate most healing practices of East and West. It is the client's faith in these beliefs that has the most impact.
5. Therapeutic touch, developed by nursing, is based on the concepts of acupuncture, chakras, and energy fields.
6. Psychoneuronutrition, herbal medicine, and homeopathy are fields involved in health care today.
7. Imagery, movement therapy, humor, massage, relaxation techniques, yoga, art therapy, music therapy, and light therapy are treatment modes that may be incorporated into traditional nursing care.
8. Work with energy fields, therapeutic touch, and imagery is rapidly increasing and being accepted by the public and may be incorporated into psychiatric care.
9. The practitioner may be a shaman, healer, doctor, medicine person, curandero, therapist, or nurse.
10. Nursing has the ability and opportunity to increase awareness of cross-cultural issues and alternative therapies, as well as to realistically implement the knowledge and practices both in assessment and in provision of mental health care.

Review Questions

1. Often misunderstood and feared by some in traditional health care, alternative therapy is defined as
   A. a method of care and healing that applies the best possible techniques to maintain health.
   B. a method that focuses on the individuality of the client within the family.
   C. health systems whose practices are defined by the users as being preventive and promoting well-being.
   D. stating that information is more important than one's belief in a health care system.
2. Concepts involved with alternative health care include
   A. legal issues of practitioner licensure, medication (herbal) regulation, and scientific methodologies of concern.
   B. spirituality.
   C. cultural influence and beliefs.
   D. stress in industry, family relationships, and individual lifestyles.
   E. all of the above.
3. Alternative therapies are to be included in a new psychiatric program in a midsize city. Nursing care will incorporate
   A. a client class on acupuncture conducted by the nurse therapist.
   B. the extended family in treatment planning.
   C. client interview about health beliefs and practices.
   D. art therapy for all clients.
4. Therapeutic touch, acupuncture, movement, relaxation, and humor may be used as conjunctive treatments with mental illness and addictions because
   A. they are cost-effective.
   B. there is documentation that these therapies have a positive impact on mental health and addictions.
   C. these health care methods are easily learned and applied by nurses.
   D. it is easier for clients to use imagery than traditional talk therapy.
5. Though useful, the alternative therapies of art therapy, light therapy, and psychonutritional medicine
   A. are readily accepted by the majority of people seeking psychiatric care.
   B. have been used for centuries by famous people.
   C. can increase the nurse's risk of malpractice.
   D. may have limited use on the treatment unit if not sanctioned by program directors and health insurance companies.

◆ References

1. Achterberg J: Imagery in Healing, Shamanism and Modern Medicine. Boston, Shambhala, 1985
2. Achterberg J: Woman as Healer. Boston, Shambhala, 1991
3. Achterberg J, Dossey B, Kolkmeier L: Rituals of Healing Using Imagery for Health and Wellness. New York, Bantam, 1994
4. Acupuncture: An Ancient Therapy Edges Into Mainstream. Lifetime Health Letter, University of Texas, Houston, 7(5): 3–8, 1995
5. Aldridge D: Is there Evidence for Spiritual Healing? Advances: The Journal of Mind-Body Health 9(4): 4–21, 1993
6. Alon R: Mindful Spontaneity Moving in Time With Nature: The Feldenkrais Method. Bridport, Dorset, England, 1990 (Distributed by Avery Publishing Group, Garden City, NY)
7. Avery DH, Bolte MA, Dager SR, Wilson LG, Weyer M, Cox GB, Bunner DL: Dawn Stimulation Treatment of Winter Depression: A Controlled Study. Am J Psychiatry 150(1): 113–117, 1993
8. Beck RL: An Overview of State Alternative Healing Practices Law. Alternative Therapies in Health & Medicine 2(1): 31–35, 1996
9. Benor DJ, Benor R: Spiritual Healing, Assuming the Spiritual is Real. Advances: The Journal of Mind-Body Health 9(4): 22–30, 1993
10. Benson H: Commentary: Placebo Effect and Remembered Wellness. Mind/Body Medicine 1(4): 44–45, 1995
11. Berland W: Unexpected Cancer Recovery: Why Patients Believe They Survive. Advances: The Journal of Mind-Body Health 11(4): 5–19, 1995
12. Bland J: Psychoneuro-Nutritional Medicine: An Advanced Paradigm. Altern Therap in Health and Medi 2: 22–27, 1995
13. Bolletino RL, LeShan L: Cancer Patients and "Marathon" Psychotherapy: A New Model. Advances: The Journal of Mind-Body Health 11(4): 19–35, 1995
14. Borysenko J: Minding the Body, Mending the Mind. New York, Bantam Books, 1987
15. Brennan R: The Alexander Technique. Rockport, MA, Element Books, 1991
16. Campinha-Bacote J: Transcultural Psychiatric Nursing: Diagnostic and Treatment Issues. J Psychosoc Nurs 32(8): 41–46, 1994
17. Cassidy CM: Unraveling the Ball of String: Reality, Paradigms, and the Study of Alternative Medicine. Advances: The Journal of Mind-Body Health 10(1): 5–31, 1994
18. Chodorow J: Dance Therapy and Depth Psychology: The Moving Imagination. New York, Routledge, 1991
19. Cousins N: Anatomy of An Illness. New York, WW Norton & Co, 1979
20. Courtney J: Memories, Part III: Reality IS, Atlantis Imagery Newsletter 3:6, 1995
21. Davidson J, Gaylord S: Meeting of Minds in Psychiatry and Homeopathy. An Example in Social Phobia. Altern Thera in Heal & Medi 1(3): 36–43, 1995

22. Dein S: The Management of Illness by a Filipino Psychic Surgeon: A Western Physician's Impression. Soc Sci Med 34(4): 461–464, 1992
23. Dombeck MT: Dream Telling: A Means of Spiritual Awareness. Holistic Nursing Practice 9(2): 37–47, 1995
24. Dossey B: Using Imagery to Help Your Patient Heal. AJN: Nurse Practitioner Extra 95(6): 41–46, 1995
25. Dossey L: Space, Time, and Medicine. Boulder, Co, Shambhala, 1982
26. Dossey L: Healing Words, San Francisco, Harper Collins, 1993
27. Dossey L: Whatever Happened to Healers? Altern Thera in Health and Medic 1(5): 6–13, 1995
28. Dossey L: In Praise of Unhappiness. Altern Ther in Health and Medic 2(1): 7–10, 1996
29. Emery M: Intuition Workbook. Englewood Cliffs, NJ, Prentice Hall, 1994
30. Fawzy FI: Immune Effects of a Short-Term Intervention for Cancer Patients. Advances: The Journal of Mind-Body Health 10(14): 32–33, 1994
31. Feldenkrais M: Awareness Through Movement. New York, Harper & Row, 1972
32. Gelkopf M, Kneitler S, Sigal M: Laughter in a Psychiatric Ward: Somatic, Emotion, Social & Clinical Influence on Schizophrenic Patients. J Nerv Ment Dis 181(5): 283–289, 1993
33. Gelkopf M, Sigal M, Kramer R: Therapeutic Use of Humor to Improve Social Support in An Institutionalized Schizophrenic Inpatient Community. J Soc Psychol 134(2): 175–182, 1994
34. Gellert G: Global Explanations and the Credibility Problem of Alternative Medicine. Advances: The Journal of Mind-Body Health 10(4): 60–67, 1994
35. Goodheart A: Laughter Therapy. Santa Barbara, Less Stress Press, 1994
36. Gordon R: Your Healing Hands: The Polarity Experience. Mill Valley, CA, Orenda Unity Press, 1978
37. Greenfield SM: Spirits and Spiritual Therapy in Southern Brazil: A Case Study of an Innovative, Syncretic Healing Group. Culture, Medicine, and Psychiatry 16(1): 23–51, 1992
38. Grossman D, Taylor R: Cultural Diversity on the Unit. Am J Nurs 95: 64–67, 1995
39. Gruman JC: Should Alternative Medicine Stay Alternative? Advances: The Journal of Mind-Body Health 11:(4): 65–69, 1995
40. Hale AS, Pinninti NR: Exorcism-Resistant Ghost Possession Treated With Clopenthixol [available in Europe]. Br J Psychiatry 165(3): 386–388, 1994
41. Harris ML: Office of Alternative Medicine: Still Under Construction. Vegetarian Times 102: 65–71, 1994
42. Hay LL: Heal Your Body. Santa Monica, CA, Hay House, 1982, 1984
43. Heber L: Dance Movement: A Therapeutic Program for Psychiatric Clients. Perspect Psychiatr Care 29(2): 22–29, 1993
44. Hendricks G, Hendricks K: At the Speed of Life: A New Approach to Personal Change Through Body-Centered Therapy. New York, Bantam, 1993
45. Hower-Kramer D: Healing Touch A Resource for Health Care Professionals. Albany, Delmar Publishing, 1996
46. Hufford DJ: Whose Culture, Whose Body, Whose Healing? Altern Therapies in Heal & Med 1(5): 94–95, 1995
47. Jacobson E: You Must Relax, 5th ed. New York, McGraw-Hill, 1978
48. Jones D, Churchill JE: Archetypal Healing. American Journal of Palliative Care 11(1): 26–33, 1994
49. Joy BW: Joy's Way: A Map for the Transformational Journey. Los Angeles, JPTarcher, 1979
50. Karagulla S: Breakthrough to Creativity, Your Higher Sense Perception. Santa Monica, DeVorss, 1967
51. Kim MT: Cultural Influences on Depression in Korean Americans. J Psychosoc Nurs 33: 2, 13–18, 1995
52. Kim S, Rew L: Ethnic Identity, Role Integration, Quality of Life, and Depression in Korean-American Women. Archives of Psychiatric Nursing 8: 348–356, 1994
53. Klein A: The Healing Power of Humor. Los Angeles, Tracher, 1989
54. Koenig HG: The Relationship Between Judeo-Christian Religion & Mental-Health Among Middle-Aged and Older Adults. Advances: The Journal of Mind-Body Health 9: 4, 33–49, 1993
55. Krieger D: Therapeutic Touch: How to Use Your Hands to Help or to Heal. New York, Prentice-Hall, 1979
56. Krieger D:Accepting Your Power to Heal. Santa Fe, Bear & Company, 1993
57. Krippner S: Some Contributions of Native Healers to Knowledge About the Healing Process. Int J Psychosom 40: 1–4, 96–99, 1993
58. Krippner S: A Cross-Cultural Comparison of Four Healing Models. Altern Therap in Health and Medi 1(1): 21–29, 1995
59. Kunz D: Compassion, Rootedness, and Detachment: Their Role in Healing. Beginnings 3(8): 1–6, 1984
60. Larson DB, Greenwold-Milano MA: Are Religion and Spirituality Clinically Relevant in Health Care? Mind/Body Med 1(3): 147–157, 1995
61. Lawlis GF: Storytelling as Therapy: Implications for Medicine. Altern Therap in Health & Med 1(2): 40–45, 1995
62. Leskowitz E: Spiritual Healing, Modern Medicine and Energy. Advan Journ of Mind-Body Health 9(4): 50–53, 1993
63. Levin JS: Esoteric vs Exoteric Explanations for Findings Linking Spirituality and Health. Advan Journ of Mind-Body Health 9(4): 54–56, 1993
64. Levin JS: How Prayer Heals: A Theoretic Model. Altern Therapies in Health & Medic 2(1): 66–73, 1996
65. Lindgren KN, Coursey RD: Spiritual Support. Psychosocial Rehabilitation Journal 18(3): 93–111, 1995
66. Lippin RA: Alternative Medicine in the Workplace. Alternative Therapies in Health & Medicine 2(1): 47–51, 1996
67. Locke S, Colligal D: The Healer Within. Toronto, Fitzhenry and Whiteside Limited, 1986
68. Lu HC: Chinese System of Food Cures. New York, Sterling, 1986
69. Lukoff D, Lu FG, Turner R: Cultural Considerations in the Assessment and Treatment of Religious and Spiritual Problems. Psychiatr Clin North Am 18(3): 467–505, 1995
70. Mackey RD: Discover the Healing Power of Therapeutic Touch. AJN Nurse Practitioner Extra 95(4): 26–32, 1995

71. MacNutt F: The Power to Heal. Notre Dame, IN, Ave-Maria Press, 1992
72. Macrae J: Therapeutic Touch A Practical Guide. New York, Alfred A Knopf, 1988
73. Macrae J: Nightingale's Spiritual Philosophy and Its Significance for Modern Nursing. Image: The Journal of Nursing Scholarship 27(1): 8–10, 1995
74. May R: The Discovery of Being. New York, WW Norton, 1983
75. McClenon J: The Experiential Foundations of Shamanic Healing. J Med Philos 18(2): 107–127, 1993
76. Meadows K: Earth Medicine A Shamanic Way to Self Discovery. Longmead, Shattesbury, Dorset, England, Element Books, 1990
77. Montbrian MJ: Alternative Therapies as Control Behaviors Used by Cancer Patients. J Adv Nurs 22(4): 646–654, 1995
78. Moor N: Arizona Center for Health & Medicine: A Model of Integrated Healthcare. Altern Thera in Health & Medi 1(2): 17–18, 1995
79. Motz J: Healing Hopes Alternative Medicine in the Nation's Capitol. Advan Jour of Mind-Body Health 10(1): 68–74, 1994
80. Newham P: The Singing Cure An Introduction to Voice Movement Therapy. Boston, Shambhala, 1994
81. Nightingale F: Notes on Nursing: What It Is, and What It Is Not. Philadelphia, JB Lippincott, 1992
82. Park JH: Our Ministry of Cleansing Believing Prayer. Sharing Journal of Christian Healing 63(8): 6–24, 1995
83. Peters LG: Karga Pufa: A Transpersonal Ritual of Healing in Tamang Shamanism. Altern Therap in Health & Medic 1(5): 53–61, 1995
84. Quinn JF, Strelkauskas AF: Psychoimmunologic Effects of Therapeutic Touch on Practitioners and Recently Bereaved Recipients: A Pilot Study. Advanced Nursing Science 15(4): 13–26, 1993
85. Rew L: Awareness in Healing. Albany, Delmar, 1996
86. Roberts AH: The Powerful Placebo Revisited: Magnitude of Nonspecific Effects. Mind/Body Medicine 1(1): 35–43, 1995
87. Rosenthal NE: Light Therapy: Theory and Practice. Primary Psychiatry 31–33, 1994
88. Rossi F, Mangrella M, Loffreda A, Lampa E: Wizards and Scientists: The Pharmacologic Experience in the Middle Ages. Am J Nephrol 14: 4–6, 384–390, 1994
89. Rossman M: Working with Resistance. Atlantis Imagery Newsletter 1–2, 4, 8, 1995
90. Rowe KS: Synthetic Food Colourings and "Hyperactivity": A Double-Blind Crossover Study. Aust Paediatr J 24(2): 143–147, 1988
91. Rubik B: Can Western Science Provide a Foundation for Acupuncture? Alter Therap in Health and Medicine 1(4): 41–47, 1995
92. Samuels M: Art as a Healing Force. Altern Therap in Health & Medic 1(4): 38–40, 1995
93. Sancier KM: Medical Applications of Qigong. Altern Therap in Health & Medic 2(1): 40–46, 1996
94. Sanford A: The Healing Light. New York, Ballantine Books, 1972
95. Shames KH: Creative Imagery in Nursing. Albany, Delmar, 1996
96. Shealy CN: Miracles Do Happen. Rockport, MA, Element Books, 1995
97. Simonton OC, Hensor R: The Healing Journey. New York, Bantam Books, 1992
98. Somé MP: Ritual, Power, Healing and Community, Portland OR, Swan/Raven, 1993
99. Stein D: All Women Are Healers A Comprehensive Guide to Natural Healing. Freedom, CA, The Crossing Press, 1990
100. Stephens R: Imagery: A Strategic Intervention to Empower Clients. Clinical Nurse Specialist 7(4): 170–174, 1993
101. Sullivan WP: It Helps Me to Be a Whole Person: The Role of Spirituality Among the Mentally Challenged. Psychosoc Rehab Journ 16: 125–134, 1993
102. Tierney MJ, Minarik PA, Tierney LM Jr: Ethics in Japanese Health Care: A Perspective for Clinical Nurse Specialists. Clinic Nurse Spec 8: 235–240, 1994
103. Turner G: Indians of North America. New York, Sterling, 1992
104. Tyler VE: The Honest Herbal, 3rd ed. Binghamton, New York, Haworth Press, 1993
105. Villaire M: OAM Report. Altern Thera in Health & Medic 1(2): 12–13, 1995
106. Wallen J: Providing Culturally Appropriate Mental Health Services for Minorities. Journal of Mental Health Administration 19(3): 288–295, 1992
107. Watson J: Nursing's Caring-Health Paradigm As Exemplar for Alternative Medicine? Altern Therap in Health & Medic 1(3): 64–69, 1995
108. Weiss G: Attention Deficit Hyperactivity Disorders. In Lewis M (ed): Child and Adolescent Psychiatry: A Comprehensive Textbook. Baltimore, Williams and Wilkins, 1991
109. Wirth DP: Implementing Healing in Modern Medical Practice. Advan Jour of Mine-Body Heal 9(4): 69–81, 1993
110. Wirth DP, Barrett MJ: Complementary Healing Therapies. Int J Psychosom 41: 1–4, 61–67, 1994
111. Wirth DP, Cram JR: Multi-Site Electromyographic Analysis of Non-Contact Therapeutic Touch. Int J Psychosom 40: 1–4, 47–55, 1993
112. Wirth DP, Cram JR: The Psychophysiology of Nontraditional Prayer. Int J Psychosom 41: 1–4, 68–75, 1994
113. Wooten P: Humor An Antidote for Stress. Holis Nurs Pract 10(2): 49–56, 1996
114. Wright PA: The Interconnectivity of Mind, Brain, and Behavior in Altered States of Consciousness; Focus on Shamanism. Altern Therap in Health & Medic 1(3): 50–56, 1995

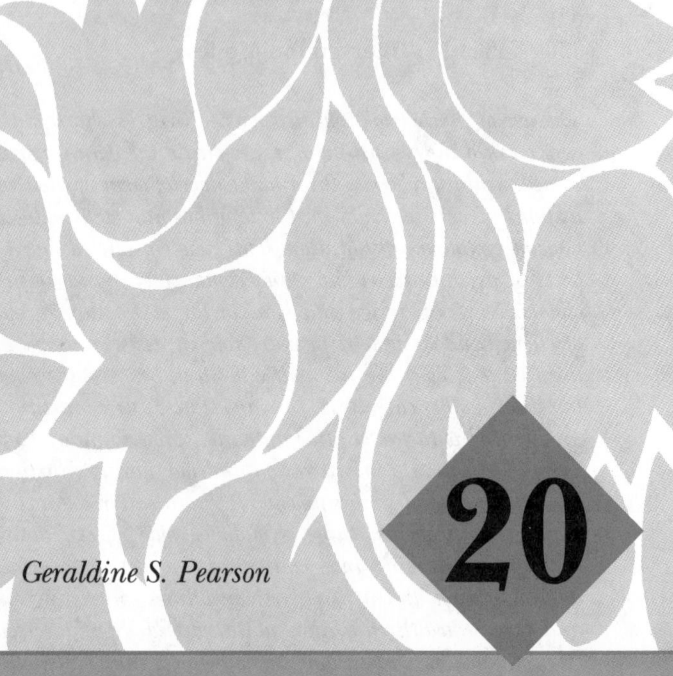

Psychopharmacology

Geraldine S. Pearson

20

Everything which succeeds is not the production of a scheme, or rules and of regulations made beforehand, but of a mind observing and adapting itself to wants and needs.

Florence Nightingale

The use of psychotropic medications to treat psychiatric disorders marked the beginning of a new era in the management of mental health problems. Prior to the development of these medications, clients were destined to long hospital stays with little hope of symptom amelioration. This new era altered many aspects of psychiatric nursing and community management of clients. Nurses manage and monitor the medication regimens of clients and assume a primary role in assisting them with these issues. They are frequently the link between the client's family and other caregivers. In many states, nurse practitioners are licensed with prescriptive authority, prescribing and managing medication administration and monitoring functions.

This chapter describes psychotropic medication according to major classifications, target symptoms, side effects, dosages, and specific nursing interventions. Principles of medication administration and nursing responsibilities concerning client and family health education are discussed. Specific circumstances, such as medication use with pregnant clients, clients with Alzheimer's disease or attention deficit disorder, and youthful or elderly clients, are also examined.

Learning Objectives

On completion of this chapter, you should be able to accomplish the following:

1. *Discuss the historical development of psychopharmacology and the role of the nurse in medication management.*
2. *Identify the nursing responsibilities in administration of psychotropic medication.*
3. *Identify principles of medication management with psychiatric clients.*
4. *Formulate a nursing care plan for a client whose treatment involves psychotropic medication.*
5. *Identify the actions, therapeutic dosages, uses, side effects, potential toxicity, administration, contraindications, and nursing implications of different types of psychotropic medications, including antipsychotic agents, antidepressants, anxiolytics, and medications used to treat manic conditions.*
6. *Identify nursing research issues relating to medication management by nurses.*

◆ Historical Perspective on the Development of Psychopharmacology

The first successful use of synthetic compounds occurred during the late 19th century and involved the use of bromides, chloral hydrate, and morphine. Modern psychopharmacology had its beginnings during World War II with the advent of barbiturates and amphetamines.[11]

During the 1950s, lithium was found to treat successfully manic agitation, and chlorpromazine was discovered as an effective tranquilizer.[11] In 1954, chlorpromazine was successfully used to treat schizophrenia in the United States. By 1970, 85% of all institutionalized psychiatric clients were receiving either chlorpromazine or other drugs from the phenothiazine family.[14] Because they were useful in managing individuals with schizophrenia, they became known as antipsychotic agents.

Monoamine oxidase inhibitors (MAOIs) were first used to treat individuals with tuberculosis but were successful in managing mood disorders. More importantly, the understanding that medication could influence brain chemistry marked the beginning of a realization that biological brain states influence mental status and mood. During the early 1960s, benzodiazepines were developed to treat anxiety disorders. Concurrent development of tricyclic antidepressant medication marked another milestone in the treatment of brain-based psychiatric disorders.[13]

The past several decades have marked a proliferation of new psychotropic medications used to treat psychiatric disorders. The advent of selective serotonin reuptake inhibitors (SSRIs), with their reduced side effects in treating affective disorders, and the development of neuroleptic medications with fewer side effects and greater effectiveness in treating psychosis have marked a new era in medication management. Nurses have a professional responsibility to remain current in their knowledge of new medications, clinical indications, and side effects. Clients taking psychotropic medications must be closely monitored for adverse side effects. Table 20-1 presents an adverse side effects index that should be used with all clients.

Peplau[30] notes that "the contemporary trend in psychiatry is to lean heavily toward nature for explanations and treatment of phenomena (symptoms) associated with mental illness."[30] She also notes that nurses tend to put more emphasis on psychotropic drugs as treatment for clients and focus less on psychosocial aspects of care.[31] The current status of psychiatric treatment makes it essential that nurses understand the importance of brain-based psychiatric illness but remain focused on the aspects of client care that tend to be ignored in a traditional medical model: health education, case management, family issues, client management, and advocacy.

◆ Antipsychotic Agents

Antipsychotic medications, also known as *neuroleptics,* are used to treat severe psychiatric disorders, such as psychotic disorders or schizophrenia (Case Study 20-1).

Table 20-1

Adverse Side Effects Index

The following side effects index can be used as a guide to assess a client's response to medication.

Client name:
Date of examination: Completed by:
Medication(s) and doses currently:
Pulse: Respiration: BP: Wt:

	No Problem				Severe Problem
GENERAL					
Decreased sleep:	0	1	2	3	4
Decreased appetite and weight loss:	0	1	2	3	4
Weakness, fatigue:	0	1	2	3	4
NEUROLOGIC					
Blurred vision:	0	1	2	3	4
Confusion:	0	1	2	3	4
Hallucinations:	0	1	2	3	4
Tics:	0	1	2	3	4
Dizziness:	0	1	2	3	4
Sedation:	0	1	2	3	4
Tremor:	0	1	2	3	4
CARDIOVASCULAR					
Palpitations:	0	1	2	3	4
Hypertension	0	1	2	3	4
Hypotension	0	1	2	3	4
GASTROINTESTINAL					
Nausea, vomiting	0	1	2	3	4
Constipation:	0	1	2	3	4
Diarrhea:	0	1	2	3	4
Dry mouth:	0	1	2	3	4
SKIN					
Rashes:	0	1	2	3	4

Used with permission of Towbin KE (personal communication).

(Pearson, G.S. Psychopharmacology. In Johnson, BS (ed): Child, Adolescent, and Family Psychiatric Nursing, pp. 410–423. Philadelphia, JB Lippincott 1995)

Psychiatric target symptoms include disorganized speech and behavior, flat or inappropriate affect, delusions, hallucinations, and catatonic behavior. They can also include acute and chronic thought disorders and confusion common to psychotic disorders, extreme aggressive behaviors, and dementia in the elderly. While predominantly used with clients exhibiting schizophrenia, these medications are also used as antiemetics, for treatment of intractable hiccoughs, and with individuals exhibiting Tourette's syndrome (vocal and motor tics).

Antipsychotic medications are subdivided into traditional and atypical agents (Table 20-2). Traditional agents block dopamine receptors in the brain and alter dopamine release and turnover; peripheral effects also include alpha-adrenergic blockade and anticholinergic properties.[43] Atypical antipsychotic drugs differ from traditional antipsychotic agents in their ability to be dopamine receptor blockers and significant serotonin receptor blockers. This simultaneous blocking may account for the increased efficacy of these drugs in improving the negative symptoms of schizophrenia with fewer extrapyramidal side effects.[9]

The mechanism of action for antipsychotic medication is complex and involves multiple neurotransmitters. Traditional and atypical antipsychotic agents have powerful side effects, including varying degrees of sedation, extrapyramidal reactions, and anticholinergic effects. Specific medications are chosen for the fewest side effects at the lowest dose with maximum alleviation of psychotic symptoms.

20-1 Case Study

Case Example: Mr. J.

Mr. J., a 23-year-old African American man, resided with his mother and several younger siblings in a public housing project in a large urban area. Diagnosed with paranoid schizophrenia in early adolescence, he had a long history of psychiatric hospitalizations, medication trials, and intermittent aggressive behavior.

His best symptom control was experienced with haloperidol 6 mg bid. This medication had been prescribed during his last hospitalization, and he continued to take it while in the community. Mr. J. had recently begun a job in the laundry of a local hospital and was working with community mental health outreach staff to establish his own apartment.

Unfortunately, Mr. J. began to develop extrapyramidal side effects evidenced by choreoathetotic movements in his tongue and stiffness in his extremities. He stopped taking haloperidol on his own without consultation with the nurse acting as his case manager. Within 2 weeks, he was brought by the police to the general hospital emergency room after threatening workers in a local coffee shop. He exhibited symptoms of paranoid ideation and admitted to auditory command hallucinations instructing him to kill his mother. He was transferred to the state psychiatric hospital for stabilization.

While there, Mr. J. agreed to a medication trial of risperidone. His mother agreed to assist him in monitoring the medication, and arrangements were made for continued follow-up in the community mental health center. Mr. J. showed a good response to risperidone and was discharged to his home.

Within 1 month, Mr. J. had reappeared at the emergency room exhibiting psychotic symptoms. He admitted to the nurse that he had "stopped that new drug because I couldn't 'make it' with my girlfriend."

After assessing his willingness to resume taking haloperidol with concomitant benzotropine, Mr. J. resumed his medication and began meeting or speaking with the nurse on a biweekly basis to assess side effects. He remained free of serious side effects and continued on his medication regime. He returned to his job in the laundry and began living independently.

Questions for Discussion

1. What collaborative relationship with Mr. J.'s supervisor in the laundry might have assisted him in avoiding psychiatric hospitalization?
2. What steps would the nurse take to develop a relationship with Mr. J. that would allow him to discuss his worries about medication rather than abruptly discontinue taking them.
3. Should clients be told about potential side effects, such as sexual dysfunction, before they agree to take a medication?
4. What role would the client's mother take in his care, and how would the nurse assess her relationship with her son?

ADVERSE SIDE EFFECTS OF TRADITIONAL AGENTS

Clients taking antipsychotic medication must be closely followed for adverse side effects. Unlike other psychotropic medications, such as antidepressants, there is a low risk of overdose from large doses of the medication. The incidence of lethality in neuroleptic medication is low.[18]

The greatest hazard involves the development of adverse side effects, such as extrapyramidal reactions and tardive dyskinesia. The risk of extrapyramidal symptoms is highest for clients with long-term use of older neuroleptic medications, such as haloperidol or perphenazine. Atypical antipsychotic medications, such as risperidone and clozapine, have a diminished incidence of severe movement disorders characterizing more established neuroleptics. Clozapine, in particular, can precipitate life-threatening agranulocytosis. They have a lower incidence of extrapyramidal symptoms (EPS) than older neuroleptics and show promise in improved management of psychotic symptoms.

Monitoring the development of movement disorders is a complex process that should involve the client and family. Prior to the initiation of any neuroleptic medication, the client must understand the risks and hazards of taking this medication. If the client is unable to participate in the process because of acute psychiatric symptoms, their family must be involved. Early diagnosis of beginning symptoms may result in prompt withdrawal of the neuroleptic or a change in medication. A thorough understanding of the symptoms and their cause will alleviate client and family anxiety if a movement disorder emerges.

Table 20-2

Motor Side Effects of Antipsychotic Medications

Symptoms	As Evidenced by	Treatment
EXTRAPYRAMIDAL SIDE EFFECTS		
Acute dystonic reactions	Tonic contractions of muscles in the mouth and torso that can last from minutes to hours; more often associated with high-potency neuroleptics (eg, haloperidol)	Intramuscular administration of diphenhydramine 25 mg
Parkinsonian reactions	Manifested by rigid, masklike facial expressions; shuffling gait; drooling; finger and hand tremors; or muscular rigidity (cogwheel phenomenon)	Intramuscular or intravenous administration of diphenhydramine or benzotropine
Akathisias	Restlessness or an inability to sit still, excitement, or agitation Usually develops in first 5 weeks of treatment; may appear as motoric hyperactivity Should be carefully noted by nurse	Changing to a different neuroleptic or decreasing the dose
TARDIVE DYSKINESIA		
	Results from prolonged use of neuroleptics Early signs: tongue movement or increased blinking Later signs: tongue protrusion and unusual mouth movements, such as sucking, smacking lips, or chewing jaw movements (rabbit syndrome).	Prevention (ie, regular reevaluation of drug dose and assessment for beginning side effects), along with maintenance on lowest effect dose of medication

Pearson, G.S. Psychopharmacology. In Johnson, BS (ed): Child, Adolescent, and Family Psychiatric Nursing, pp. 410–423. Philadelphia, JB Lippincott 1995.

Movement Disorders

Movement disorders occur most often with low-dose, high-potency phenothiazine medications, such as fluphenazine. Predominant movement disorders are summarized in Table 20-2 and include acute dystonic reactions, parkinsonism, akathisias, and the most serious, tardive dyskinesia. The most serious and potentially fatal side effect is *neuroleptic malignant syndrome*, characterized by severe muscular rigidity, altered consciousness, stupor, catatonia, hyperpyrexia, and labile pulse and blood pressure.[19] Treatment involves immediate discontinuation of the medication and hospitalization to stabilize acute symptoms.

Acute dystonic reactions generally occur within 5 days of initial administration of neuroleptic medication or after dose increases. Untreated, dystonic reactions can last minutes to hours and include muscular hypertonicity; tonic contractions of the neck, mouth, and tongue; and oculogyric crisis (eyes rolling upward and unable to move downward).[19] Concomitant treatment with anticholinergic and antiparkinsonian drugs, such as diphenhydramine and benztropine, usually results in rapid resolution of the acute dystonic reaction. Both medications may be given orally or intramuscularly as a response to the acute reaction. They may also be administered daily on a prophylactic basis along with the prescribed neuroleptic to prevent acute dystonic reactions.

Parkinsonism (also known as *pseudoparkinsonism*) presents with tremor, cogwheel rigidity, drooling, and a decrease in facial expressions. Maximum risk for developing symptoms occurs between 5 and 30 days after initiating neuroleptic medications. Parkinsonian symptoms generally respond to benztropine or trihexyphenidyl and resolve within days.[19]

Akinesia represents the most serious form of parkinsonism. Defined as a state of diminished spontaneity, with few gestures, apathy, and difficulty initiating activities, akinesia is difficult to differentiate from schizophrenia. Clients appear depressed, even if psychotic symptoms have begun to resolve, and social adjustment is compromised.

Akathisia, also called motor restlessness, usually occurs within 5 to 60 days after initiation of neuroleptic medication and is characterized by symptoms of uncomfortable restlessness, feelings of tenseness in the lower extremities with an irresistible urge to move them, inability to sit still, and foot tapping.[19]

Akathisia is characterized by the client's subjective feeling of restlessness and increased observed motoric activity. Clients are less likely to adhere to medication regimens when experiencing these uncomfortable side effects. Treatment of akathisia involves antiparkinsonian drugs, such as trihexyphenidyl; propanolol; benzodiazepines; clonidine; or changing medication.[19]

Neuroleptic Malignant Syndrome

Neuroleptic malignant syndrome is life-threatening and can occur after a single dose of neuroleptic medication but is more common within the first 2 weeks of administration or with an increase in dose.[19] Severe muscular rigidity, altered consciousness, catatonia, stupor, hyperpyrexia, and labile pulse and blood pressure are the most common symptoms. This syndrome can continue for up to 2 weeks after medication is discontinued, and treatment involves immediately stopping the neuroleptic followed by supportive treatment with dopaminergic agonists, such as bromocriptine and amantadine.[36]

Tardive Dyskinesia

Tardive dyskinesia (TD) represents the most serious side effect of long-term use of neuroleptics, because it is often irreversible and the symptoms tend to be severely disabling. The risk of developing irreversible TD increases with cumulative dose and duration of treatment. Fine wormlike movements of the tongue may the first signs of TD, and discontinuing the medication when this occurs may prevent development of the full-blown syndrome.[32]

While decreasing or discontinuing neuroleptic medication is the best treatment for TD, it can also precipitate the development of withdrawal dyskinesia. The symptoms of this are the same as the symptoms of TD, but they tend to resolve within a few weeks. Clients need help understanding that it may take time for the symptoms to resolve even if the medication has been discontinued.

Symptoms of TD usually include involuntary choreoathetotic movements affecting the face, tongue, perioral, buccal, and masticatory muscles. The neck, torso, and extremities may also be involved.

ADVERSE SIDE EFFECTS OF ATYPICAL AGENTS

Prior to the advent of clozapine, the only option for treating TD was discontinuation of antipsychotic medication and attempts at behavioral management of psychotic symptoms. Clozapine produces little or no TD and may significantly decrease or eliminate existing TD while the client takes the medication.[8,26] The symptoms of TD tend to return once clozapine is discontinued.

Use of clozapine requires weekly monitoring of white blood cell counts to assess for agranulocytosis. Clozapine suppresses the development of white blood cells in 1% to 2% of all clients who receive it. If white blood cell levels decrease significantly from baseline blood levels, immediate discontinuation of the medication is recommended. Older adults and women appear to be at higher risk for developing this side effect.[3] Clozapine should never be used with any other agent that suppresses white blood cell production, such as carbamazepine.

Unlike clozapine, risperidone does not cause agranulocytosis. While the incidence of extrapyramidal symptoms is less when compared with traditional antipsychotic medication, clients can experience these side effects. Neuroleptic malignant syndrome can also occur in clients receiving risperidone. Other negative side effects include orthostatic hypotension, dizziness, tachycardia, weight gain, sleep disturbance, constipation, and rhinitis. The increased risk of potentially life-threatening blood disorders makes this medication most appropriate for severely disturbed schizophrenic clients who have not responded favorably to other antipsychotic medications or who are at risk for worsening TD.[19]

◆ Antidepressant Agents

Antidepressants have been used primarily to treat affective or mood disorders, including bipolar disorder, major depressions, and dysthymias. They have also been used to treat obsessive-compulsive and anxiety disorders. Major depression represents a physiological illness that can be characterized by dysphoric mood, change in appetite and energy level, and anhedonia, or lack of interest in routine activities, difficulty concentrating, feelings of hopelessness, and suicidality.

Mood disorders can be divided into unipolar depressive disorders and bipolar disorders.[1] Both types of depression exist across the age span in children and adults. The Diagnostic and Statistical Manual of Mental Disorders, fourth edition, does not differentiate between adults and children with regard to the symptom manifestation of mood disorders. Both are responsive to antidepressant medications.

Antidepressant medications are generally divided into three categories: cyclic antidepressants, including tricyclic, heterocyclic, and atypical agents; MAOIs; and SSRIs.[11] The advent of new antidepressant medications has made precise classification difficult. The SSRIs represent the most recently developed agents used to treat depression.

While antidepressant medication is considered appropriate treatment for major depression, it should be used with caution in clients with a cardiac history or a history of seizure disorder.[28] A thorough physical assessment prior to beginning medication is essential to assess for cardiovascular irregularities. A baseline electrocardiogram is usually recommended prior to the initiation of antidepressant therapy.

All categories of antidepressant medication should be dispensed with caution in clients displaying a risk of suicide or self-injury. Outpatient providers frequently give only a few days to 1 week's worth of medication, requiring the client to return for evaluation before more medication is dispensed. Ingesting large amounts of antidepressant medication is potentially life-threatening.

TRICYCLIC ANTIDEPRESSANTS

Tricyclic medications are the oldest antidepressants. Their side effects include blood dyscrasias, cardiotoxicity, and a high risk of mortality with overdose. Clients with a suicide risk must be carefully monitored with regard to the amount of tricyclic medication they possess. Dispensing a few days of medication at a time in a clinic or outpatient setting and careful monitoring of need for hospitalization must accompany use of this type of medication to treat depression. Other side effects of tricyclics can include drowsiness, dizziness, tachycardia, skin rashes, dry mouth, constipation, and urinary retention. Impotence and changes in libido are also side effects clients might experience.[43] While tricyclics continue to be prescribed, their popularity is being eclipsed by new types of antidepressants with fewer side effects.

MONAMINE OXIDASE INHIBITORS

Monamine oxidase is an enzyme that inactivates more than 15 different monamines formed in the body that function as neurotransmitters, neuromodulators, and hormones.[27] The MAOIs were developed in the 1960s and were found to have antidepressant qualities.

These medications are as effective as other agents in treating depression but have severe side effects resulting from complex interactions with foods and other medications. This restricts their usefulness and contributes to diminished use in treating depression.

Clients taking MAOIs and their families require intensive health teaching about the foods and drugs that contain tyramine and produce a synergistic effect. Foods that interact in harmful ways include aged cheese, alcoholic beverages, yogurts, chocolates, pickled herring, and bananas. The concurrent use of MAOIs with amphetamines, methyldopa, epinephrine, or vasoconstrictors may precipitate a hypertensive crisis.[43] For this reason, careful monitoring of blood pressure is essential. Managing the nursing care of a client taking MAOIs requires thorough knowledge of lifestyle, family supports, and willingness to adhere to the strict guidelines of the medication.

SELECTIVE SEROTONIN REUPTAKE INHIBITORS

The SSRIs are a promising newer class of antidepressant and include fluoxetine, fluvoxamine, sertraline, and paroxetine. The SSRIs are chemically unrelated to and have fewer side effects than other antidepressants. The most common negative side effects include headache, nausea, vomiting, diarrhea, nervousness, sleep disturbance, and sexual dysfunction.[41] They are useful in treating psychiatric disorders other than depression, including eating disorders, obsessive-compulsive disorders, and Tourette's syndrome.

The powerful serotonergic effects of SSRIs are potentiated when tryptophan or lithium is concurrently prescribed. Serotonin syndrome may be characterized by nausea, headache, diarrhea, ataxia, seizures, or agitation.[41]

The American College of Neuropsychopharmacology endorsed the use of SSRIs to treat major depression, emergent suicidal ideation, and concomitant suicidality. It specifically noted that there is no evidence that the newer serotonin reuptake inhibitors trigger emergent suicidal ideation greater than the rates associated with other antidepressant medications. The importance of monitoring mental status with all antidepressant medications was cited.[24]

◆ Anxiolytics

Anxiolytic, or antianxiety, medications are used to treat generalized anxiety disorders and may provide relief for acute anxiety states. Symptoms of anxiety can include heart palpitations, sweating, trembling or shaking, shortness of breath, chest pain or discomfort, nausea, dizziness, feelings of unreality, fear of losing control or dying, chills, and numbness. These medications include buspirone, a novel anxiolytic, and benzodiazepines, such as diazepam and lorazepam.

Buspirone's exact mechanism of action is unknown; it lacks anticonvulsant, sedative, or muscle relaxant properties and binds serotonin receptors. Side effects include dizziness, headache, nervousness, insomnia, lightheadedness, nausea, dry mouth, vomiting, abdominal or gastric distress, and diarrhea. It should be given with caution in clients who use alcohol or other central nervous system depressants.[20]

In contrast, benzodiazepines share pharmacological effects of anxiolysis, sedation, centrally mediated muscle relaxation, and elevation of seizure threshold.[34] Side effects are the same as those of buspirone but also can include mild paradoxical excitatory reactions during the beginning of treatment. Drug dependence is also possible with occurrence of a withdrawal syndrome when the medication is discontinued. This most often occurs with higher doses of medication used for more than 4 months.[20]

These medications are generally considered safe and effective, and their adverse side effects are extensions of their central actions. They may be excessively sedating and are potentiated with narcotics and alcohol. Benzodiazepines have the potential for psychological and physical dependence and should not be used with other central nervous system depressants. They should be used cautiously with the elderly and with debilitated clients, depressed or suicidal clients, or clients with a history of substance abuse.[43]

Anxiolytic medications are not a cure for the psychological problems that underlie a client's psychiatric symptoms. Zarate and Agras[46] found that combining cognitive restructuring techniques with psychotropic medication offered the anxious, socially phobic client the best opportunity for effective treatment. Identifying the source of the anxiety or conflict may assist in dealing with the symptoms. Many clients view medication as a cure when it is used, especially with more psychologically based anxiety disorders, as an adjunct to psychotherapy or counseling.[46]

◆ Mood Stabilizers

Anticonvulsants and lithium are being increasingly used as mood stabilizers. Medications used for this include carbamazepine and valproic acid. Carbamazepine has been used for seizures, impulse-control disorders, and bipolar disorders.[13] Adverse side effects include dizziness, drowsiness, unsteadiness, nausea, and vomiting. More seriously, carbamazepine can cause fatal hepatitis with massive hepatic cellular necrosis and total loss of intact liver tissue.[18] Baseline and regular hepatic function tests are essential when monitoring the side effects of this medication. Valproic acid has similar side effects and may cause hepatic failure. Serum levels should be monitored carefully; acute toxicity is characterized by anorexia, nausea, vomiting, sedation, ataxia, and tremor.[13]

For several decades, lithium carbonate has been the drug of choice for clients with bipolar disorders, mania, and other types of mood disorder.[7,17] It is rapidly absorbed after oral administration, and peak blood levels emerge within 2 to 4 hours after initial dose.[38] It generally takes 2 to 3 weeks of gradually increasing doses to result in a therapeutic level of lithium.

Lithium has a notably low therapeutic index with only a slight difference between therapeutic and toxic levels. Toxicity is manifested by nausea, vomiting, diarrhea, tremor, headache, sedation, confusion, hypotension, and cardiac arrhythmia. Severe lithium toxicity is usually manifested at levels of 2.5 mEq/L; serum levels above 3.0 mEq/L require hemodialysis, and levels greater than 3.5 mEq/L are life-threatening.[38]

Before initial administration of lithium carbonate, a thorough physical examination with electrolyte studies, complete blood count, and thyroid function tests is recommended. Identification of preexisting physical problems provides a baseline for the nurse monitoring side effects of lithium carbonate. Client and family education are essential because excessive heat, diaphoresis, use of diuretics, and decreased salt intake can preclude the client to toxic blood levels. This occurs when the body's sodium levels are lowered and absorption is disrupted. Clients are encouraged to avoid the sun and potential overheating and to keep well hydrated with water. Weight gain and thyroid dysfunction are also side effects of lithium carbonate.

Weekly blood work is recommended while dose is being regulated, and monthly blood work is essential for monitoring lithium levels once a stable dose is established.[43] Blood levels are generally drawn 12 hours after the last dose of the medication is ingested.

Application of the Nursing Process to Medication Management

The nursing process is readily applied to principles of medication management. Each level is essential when providing quality nursing care to the client receiving psychotropic medications.

ASSESSMENT

Assessment involves careful reviewing of the client's history, experience with psychotropic medication, side effects, and efficacy. Acute and chronic psychiatric symptomotology must be differentiated. While assessment principles are similar with both types of psychiatric problems, the client with chronic problems (such as schizophrenia) or intermittently acute episodes (such as major depression) is more likely to have past experience with psychotropic medication. Chronic problems are also more likely to require long-term case management.

Clients with more acute disorders usually take medication for a prescribed time, and the crisis may be more traceable to a specific life event. These clients are also more likely to experience brief psychiatric hospitalization for their problems versus clients with chronic difficulties who may have longer and more frequent need for inpatient care.

Along with client life history, the presence or absence of established community and family supports must be assessed. Close collaboration between caregiver and family is needed. The locus of control should be shifted from institutions to communities and from providers to families. Family members can assist the client in deciding which medication might best serve their needs and be easiest to manage. Independent versus family living will influence the level of family involvement.

Assessment of target symptoms illuminates the symptoms that the medication will aim to improve or alleviate. By carefully assessing the client's perception of the problem and by evaluating the family's view of problematic symptoms, the prescriber can ascertain the best medication and dosage to address client dysfunction.

Assessment of the client's need for adjunct care is also important and involves willingness to participate in recommended treatment, such as individual, group, or family. Many chronically disturbed individuals are reluctant to be involved in prosocial activities, such as psychotherapy. They may be willing to participate in medication groups where the focus is specific and limited. Many communities provide drop-in centers for chronically involved clients to receive support, medication follow-up, and vocational counseling.

Stone and others[40] found that psychiatric care providers frequently included medicated individuals in their psychotherapy groups. This most often occurred with clients experiencing mood disorders, such as unipolar or bipolar depressions and dysthymia.

PLANNING

Ensuring client safety is the most important aspect of planning medication administration (Table 20–3). To do this, the nurse must know the following:

1. The prescribed dose and maximum dose that may be safely given to the client
2. Method of administration
3. Expected drug action
4. Side effects
5. Adverse effects (short and long term)
6. Nursing implications[4]

Planning for care also involves ascertaining the length of the medication trial, the client's need for follow-up, and monitoring of side effects. Part of this process is determining the best mode of medication administration. While many clients prefer oral tablets or capsules, for others taking neuroleptics for a long period, decanoate injectables (such as fluphenazine or haloperidol) are more convenient and eliminate the need to remember to take medication. Antipsychotic agents are the only medications available in decanoate form. Clients receiving decanoate medications should be more closely monitored for side effects during the first few administrations of the drug. Generally, decanoate medication is given every 4 to 6 weeks.[43]

Some clients may prefer liquid forms of their medication. Disadvantages of this include difficulties obtaining an accurate dose, risk of overdose, and need for juice or other liquid to mix with the medication. Many elderly clients receiving haloperidol or chlorpromazine in convalescent home settings are given their liquid medication in juice for ease of administration. Most of these clients do not independently pour their medication, so this function is performed by a nurse.

Side effects are best monitored through a combination of assessment techniques. Visual observation of the client will illuminate the overt presence of TD or other side effects of neuroleptics. The use of the Abnormal Involuntary Movement Scale (AIMS) is a more definite and precise way of evaluating abnormal movements.[33] The client's perceptions of response to medication are invaluable and should be carefully noted. An improvement in psychiatric symptoms (a positive response) might be accompanied by adverse side effects (negative). Careful processing with the client may need to occur to ensure that he or she continues with the medication. A careful review of the consequences of discontinuing medication is also essential.

INTERVENTION

Whenever possible, with client consent, family or significant others should be involved in implementation of a medication regimen. They can assist by monitoring symptoms, side effects, and efficacy of medication. They should also be included in the health teaching occurring for each drug an individual receives. Reinhard notes that "as the professional relinquished claim to exclusive authority, control is redistributed and families play an active role in decisions that affect them, such as changes in medication or living arrangements."[35] She further notes that providing family education promotes family coping rather than family pathology and will ultimately improve the family members' ability to provide care, if this is what the client needs.

Principles of client education include making the information available in a form that matches the reading and comprehension level of the client, making bilingual information available if needed, and providing follow-up to initial teaching sessions. Too often clients receive medicine without understanding the purpose, risks, or benefits. Nurses must make client and family education an integral part of their psychiatric practice, particularly with psychotropic medication.

Other aspects of intervention involve assessing

(text continues on page 347)

Table 20-3

Medication Guide to Psychotropic Medications

Please note: The following agents represent some of the psychotropic medications available for client use. They are given with adult doses; side effects and drug interactions are summarized. More detailed information on each medication can be found in the reference noted at the conclusion of the chart.

Generic	Trade	Dose	Route	Predominant Side Effects or Adverse Reactions	Drug Interactions
ANXIOLYTIC AGENTS					
alprazolam	Xanax	0.25–0.5 tid; should be individualized	PO	Initial transient, mild drowsiness; sedation, depression, lethargy, anger, hostility, confusion, constipation, diarrhea, dry mouth, nausea; drug dependence with drug withdrawal most common with abrupt withdrawal after 4 mo usage	Increased central nervous system (CNS) depression when taken with alcohol
buspirone	BuSpar	Initial 15 mg/d; not to exceed 60 mg/d after gradual increase in dose	PO	Dizziness, headache, nervousness, insomnia, lightheadedness, nausea, dry mouth, vomiting, diarrhea, gastric distress	Use with caution in clients taking alcohol or other CNS depressants; decreased effect if taken with fluoxetine
chlordiazepoxide	Libritabs/ Librium	Orally: up to 20–25 mg/tid Parenteral: up to 50–100 mg IM or IV initially for severe anxiety followed by 25–50 mg/tid	PO IM IV	Transient, mild drowsiness, sedation, depression, lethargy, apathy, fatigue, lightheadedness, disorientation, restlessness, confusion, constipation, diarrhea, bradycardia, tachycardia, incontinence, changes in libido, urinary retention, drug dependence with withdrawal syndrome; mild paradoxical excitatory reactions during first 2 wk of treatment, particularly with psychiatric clients	Increased CNS depression with alcohol; increased effects when given with cimetidine, disulfiram, and oral contraceptives; decreased effect if given with theophylline, aminophylline, dyphylline, or oxitriphylline
clorazepate	Tranxene	Orally: 30 mg/d in divided doses with upper range of 60 mg/d	PO	Initial transient, mild drowsiness, sedation, depression, lethargy, apathy, fatigue, lightheadedness, disorientation, anger, hostility, headache; constipation, diarrhea, dry mouth; mild paradoxical excitatory reactions during first 2 wk of administration	Increased CNS depression when taken with alcohol; increased effect with cimetidine, disulfiram, omeprazole, oral contraceptives; decreased effect with theophylline
diazepam	Valium	Oral: 2–10 mg bid/ qid Oral sustained release: 15–30 mg/d Parenteral: 2–20 mg IV or IM; injection may be repeated 1 h after first dose	PO IM IV	Initial transient, mild drowsiness, sedation, depression, lethargy, apathy, fatigue, lightheadedness, disorientation, restlessness, confusion, constipation, diarrhea, bradycardia, tachycardia, incontinence, urinary retention, changes in libido; drug dependence with withdrawal syndrome; mild paradoxical excitatory reactions during first 2 wk of treatment	Increased CNS depression with alcohol, omeprazole; increased pharmacological effects when given with cimetidine, disulfiram, oral contraceptives; decreased effects if taken with theophylline, ranitidine

hydroxyzine	Anxanil Atarax Vistaril	Oral: 50–100 mg qid IM: 50–100 mg stat and q4–6h prn	PO IM	Drowsiness, dry mouth	Increased CNS depression effects with alcohol, barbiturates, and opiates
lorazepam	Ativan	Oral: 2–6 mg/d in divided doses IM: 0.05 mg/kg up to 4 mg usually as preoperatively IV: initial dose of 2 mg or 0.044 mg/kg, whichever is smaller; total of 4 mg	PO IM IV	Initial transient, mild drowsiness, sedation, depression, lethargy, apathy, fatigue, lightheadedness, disorientation, anger, hostility, restlessness, confusion, crying, headache; constipation, diarrhea, dry mouth, nausea; drug dependence with withdrawal syndrome when drug is discontinued, more common with abrupt discontinuation of higher dosage used for longer than 4 mos	Increased CNS depression when taken with alcohol; decreased effectiveness if taken concurrently with theophylline
oxazepam	Serax	Oral: 10–15 mg up to 30 mg tid	PO	Initial transient, mild drowsiness, sedation, depression, lethargy, apathy, fatigue, lightheadedness, disorientation; constipation, diarrhea, dry mouth; incontinence, urinary retention; nasal congestion, hiccups, fever, diaphoresis	Increased CNS depression when taken with alcohol; decreased sedation when taken by heavy smokers or those taking theophyllines
ANTICONVULSANTS					
phenobarbital	Solfoton	Oral: 60–100 mg/d Parenteral for acute convulsions: 200–320 mg IM or IV repeated in 6 h if needed	PO IM IV	Somnolence, agitation, confusion, hyperkinesia, ataxia, vertigo, CNS depression, nightmares, lethargy, residual sedation, paradoxical excitement, nervousness, psychiatric disturbance, hallucinations, insomnia, anxiety, dizziness, thinking abnormality; nausea, vomiting, constipation, diarrhea, epigastric pain; bradycardia, hypotension, syncope; hyppoventilation, apnea, respiratory depression; pain at site of injection; withdrawal syndrome may be life-threatening	Increased serum levels when taken concurrently with valproic acid; increased CNS depression with alcohol; decreased effects of theophyllines, oral anticoagulants, beta-blockers, doxycycline, oral contraceptives, and estrogen when taken with phenobarbital
clonazepam	Klonopin	Oral: 1.5 mg divided into three doses; increase by 0.5–1 mg po q3d; maximum recommended dose of 20 mg/d	PO	Initial transient, mild drowsiness, sedation, depression, lethargy, apathy, fatigue, lightheadedness, disorientation; anger, hostility, restlessness, confusion, crying, headache, mild paradoxical excitatory reaction during first 2 wk of administration; constipation, diarrhea, dry mouth	Increased CNS depression when taken with alcohol; increased effect when given with cimetidine, disulfram, omeprazole, oral contraceptives; decreased effect with theophylline

continued

Table 20-3 (Continued)

Generic	Trade	Dose	Route	Predominant Side Effects or Adverse Reactions	Drug Interactions
phenytoin	Dilantin	Oral: usually begin with 100 mg/tid with dosage individualized after assessing serum levels; maintenance dose usually 300–400 mg/d Parenteral: 10–15 mg/kg by slow IV initially with maintenance at 100 mg IV q6–8h	PO IV	Nystagmus, ataxia, dysarthria, slurred speech, mental confusion, dizziness, drowsiness, insomnia, transient nervousness, motor twitchings, fatigue, irritability, depression, numbness, tremor, headache; nausea, gingival hyperplasia *The following side effects could be life-threatening:* liver damage, hematopoietic complications, gullous exfoliative or purpuric dermatitis, lupus erythematosus, and Stevens-Johnson syndrome	Phenytoin has numerous complex interactions with various drugs. Concurrent use of other medications should be carefully assessed before prescribing phenytoin
carbamazepine	Tegretol	Oral for epilepsy: 200 mg/bid increased gradually by up to 200 mg/d in divided doses q6–8h until maximum response; not to exceed 1,200 mg/d	PO	Dizziness, drowsiness, unsteadiness; nausea, vomiting *The following side effects could be life-threatening:* fatal hepatitis, fatal massive hepatic cellular necrosis with total loss of intact liver tissue, fatal cardiovascular complications, potentially fatal hematological disorders	Carbamazepine has numerous complex interactions with various drugs. Concurrent use of other medications should be carefully assessed before prescribing carbamazepine
primidone	Mysoline	Oral: graduated doses from 100–125 mg PO at bedtime to maximum dose of 250 mg tid or qid	PO	Ataxia, vertigo, fatigue, hyperirritability; nausea, anorexia	Toxicity when given with phenytoins; increased CNS effects, impaired hand–eye coordination, and death if taken with alcohol; multiple other medications interact with primidone and should be assessed carefully
ANTIDEPRESSANTS					
amitriptyline	Elavil	Oral: Initially, 100 mg/d in divided doses, increasing to 200–300 mg/d IM: 20–30 mg qid Replace with PO ASAP	PO IM	Sedation and anticholinergic effects, confusion, disturbed concentration; dry mouth, constipation; orthostatic hypotension	Amitriptyline has numerous complex interactions with various drugs. Concurrent use of other medications should be carefully assessed before prescribing amitriptyline

bupropion	Wellbutrin	Oral: begin with 100 mg bid; increase to 300 mg/d given as 100 mg/tid. Not to exceed 150 mg in any single dose	PO	Agitation, insomnia, headaches/migraine, tremor; dry mouth, constipation; dizziness, tachycardia; weight loss	Increased risk of adverse effects if taken with levodopa; increased toxicity if taken currently with MAO inhibitors; increased risk of seizures if taken with drugs that lower seizure threshold
clomipramine (tricyclic)	Anafranil	Oral: 25 mg/qid; gradually increase to 100 mg with a maximum dose of 250 mg/d; once a day at bedtime to minimize sedation	PO	Sedation, anticholinergic effects, confusion, disturbed concentration; dry mouth, constipation, orthostatic hypotension, menstrual irregularity, impotence, nasal congestion, laryngitis	Clomipramine has numerous complex interactions with various drugs. Concurrent use of other medications should be carefully assessed before prescribing clomipramine
desipramine (tricyclic)	Norpramin	Oral: 100–200 mg/d in single or divided dose; gradually increased to 300 mg/d if indicated	PO	Sedation and anticholinergic effects, confusion, disturbed concentration, dry mouth, constipation, nausea; orthostatic hypotension	Desipramine has numerous complex interactions with various drugs. Concurrent use of other medications should be carefully assessed before prescribing desipramine
doxepin (tricyclic)	Sinequan	Oral: Initial 25 mg/tid; optimum dose, 75–150 mg/d or total daily dose of 150 mg given at bedtime	PO	Sedation and anticholinergic effects; confusion, disturbed concentration, dry mouth, constipation, nausea, orthostatic hypotension	Doxepin has numerous complex interactions with various drugs. Concurrent use of other medications should be carefully assessed before prescribing doxepine
fluoxetine (selective serotonin reuptake inhibitor)	Prozac	Oral: Initial 20 mg/d up to 80 mg/d	PO	Headache, nervousness, insomnia, drowsiness, anxiety, tremor, dizziness, lightheadedness, nausea, vomiting, diarrhea, dry mouth, anorexia, dyspepsia, constipation, taste changes, upper respiratory infections, pharyngitis, painful menstruation, sexual dysfunction, frequency, sweating, rash, pruritus, weight loss, asthenia, fever	Increased therapeutic and toxic effects if taken with tricyclic antidepressants; decreased therapeutic effects if taken with cyproheptadine
imipramine (tricyclic)	Tofranil	Oral: Initial 100–150 mg/d in divided doses with gradual increase to 200 mg/d; may be increased to 250–300 mg/d Parenteral: IM at same doses as PO	PO IM	Sedation and anticholinergic effects, confusion, disturbed concentration, seizures; dry mouth, constipation, nausea; orthostatic hypotension	Imipramine has numerous complex interactions with various drugs. Concurrent use of other medications should be carefully assessed before prescribing imipramine

continued

Table 20-3 (Continued)

Generic	Trade	Dose	Route	Predominant Side Effects or Adverse Reactions	Drug Interactions
maprotiline (tricyclic)	Ludiomil	Oral: Initial 75 mg/d in outpatients up to 225 mg/d or 100–150 mg/d in hospitalized clients up to 300 mg/d	PO	Sedation and anticholinergic effects, confusion, disturbed concentration; dry mouth, constipation, nausea; orthostatic hypotension	Maprotiline has numerous complex interactions with various drugs. Concurrent use of other medications should be carefully assessed before prescribing maprotiline
nortriptyline (tricyclic)	Aventyl, Pamelor	Oral: 25 mg tid/qid up to 150 mg/d	PO	Sedation and anticholinergic effects, confusion, disturbed concentration; dry mouth, constipation, nausea; orthostatic hypotension	Nortriptyline has numerous complex interactions with various drugs. Concurrent use of other medications should be carefully assessed before prescribing nortriptyline
paroxetine (selective serotonin reuptake inhibitor)	Paxil	Oral: 20 mg/d up to 50 mg/d	PO	Somnolence, dizziness, insomnia, tremor, nervousness, headache, nausea, dry mouth, constipation, diarrhea, ejaculatory disorders, male genital disorders, sweatng, headache, asthenia	Increased levels and toxicity when taken with cimetidine monoamine oxidase (MAO) inhibitors will decrease effect of phenytoin, digoxin; decreased effect if taken with phenobarbital, phenytoin
phenelzine (monoamine oxidase inhibitor)	Nardil	Oral: Initial 15 mg/tid with increase to 60 mg/d; after maximum benefit, dose reduced slowly	PO	Dizziness, vertigo, headache, overactivity, hyperreflexia, tremors, muscle twitching, mania, hypomania, jitteriness, confusion, memory impairment, insomnia, weakness, fatigue, drowsiness, restlessness, overstimulation, increased anxiety, agitation, blurred vision, sweating; constipation, diarrhea, nausea, abdominal pain, edema, dry mouth, anorexia, weight changes *The following could be life-threatening:* Hypertensive crises after ingesting contraindicated food or drink containing tyramine	Phenelzine has numerous complex interactions with various drugs and foods. Concurrent use of other medications should be carefully assessed before prescribing phenelzine
sertraline (selective serotonin reuptake inhibitor)	Zoloft	Oral: Once a day beginning with 50 mg up to 200 mg/d	PO	Headache, nervousness, drowsiness, anxiety, tremor, dizziness, insomnia, vision changes, fatigue; nausea, diarrhea, dry mouth; rhinitis; painful menstruation; sweating	Serious, potentially fatal side effects if taken with MAO inhibitors

trazodone (atypical agent)	Desyrel	Oral: 150 mg/d with increase of 50 mg/d q 3–4 d	PO	Anger, hostility, agitation, nightmares/ vivid dreams, hallucinations, delusions, hypomania, confusion, disorientation, decreased concentration, impaired memory, impaired speech, dizziness, incoordination, drowsiness, fatigue; abdominal or gastric disorder, decreased or increased appetite, bad taste in mouth, dry mouth, hypersalivation, nausea, vomiting, diarrhea, flatulence, constipation; hypertension, shortness of breath, syncope, tachycardia, palpitations; decreased libido; allergic skin conditions, edema	Enhanced depressive effects if taken with alcohol; may decrease effectiveness of anticoagulant medications; may increase effects and toxicity of hydantoins
MOOD STABILIZING AGENTS					
lithium carbonate	Eskalith, Lithane, Lithonate, Lithotabs	Oral: Dosage must be individualized according to serum levels and clinical response; 300 mg/tid to produce a serum level of .6 to 1.2 mEq/L. Serum levels drawn q 2 mos before a dose or 8–12 hours from last dose	PO	Lethargy, slurred speech, muscle weakness, fine hand tremor; nausea, vomiting, diarrhea, thirst; polyuria	Increased risk of toxicity when given with thiazide diuretics; increased plasma levels with indomethacin and other NSAIDs; increased CNS toxicity when given with carbamazepine; potential encephalopathic syndrome when taken with haloperidol; increased risk of hypothyrodism when given with iodide salts
ANTIPARKINSONIAN AGENTS					
benztropine	Cogentin	Oral: initially 0.1–1 mg hs with daily total of 0.5–6 mg in two to four divided doses; may be given IM or IV in same doses as oral	PO IM IV	Dry mouth, constipation, nausea; urinary retention, urinary hesitancy; blurred vision; disorientation, confusion	May cause paralytic ileus when given with other anticholinergic drugs; additive adverse CNS effects with other drugs that have CNS anticholinergic properties; possible masking of persistent extrapyramidal symptoms (EPS), tardive dyskinesia (TD); may decrease effectiveness of antipsychotic medications
diphenhydramine	Benadryl	Oral: 25–50 mg q4–6h Parenteral: 10–50 IV or deep IM or up to 100 mg if required; maximum daily dose, 400 mg	PO IV IM	Drowsiness, sedation, dizziness, disturbed coordination; epigastric distress; thickening of bronchial secretions *The following could be life-threatening:* anaphylactic shock	Possible increased and prolonged anticholinergic effects if taken with MAO inhibitors

continued

Table 20-3 (Continued)

Generic	Trade	Dose	Route	Predominant Side Effects or Adverse Reactions	Drug Interactions
ANTIPSYCHOTICS					
risperidone (atypical agent)	Risperdal	Oral: 1 mg/bid with gradual increase to target dose of 3 mg/bid; when switching from other antipsychotics, minimize the overlap period and d/c other drugs before beginning risperidone	PO	Insomnia, anxiety, agitation, headache; nausea, vomiting, constipation *The following could be life-threatening:* TD, neuroleptic malignant syndrome	Increased therapeutic and toxic effects if taken with clozapine; decreased therapeutic effect if taken with carbamazepine; decreased effectiveness of levodopa if taken concurrently
haloperidol	Haldol	Oral: Initial 0.5–2.0 mg bid/tid up to 3–5 mg bid/tid IM: 2–5 mg q30–60 min or q4–8h IV: 2–25 mg q30 min or more at a rate of 5 mg/min	PO IV IM	Drowsiness, pseudoparkinsonism; dystonias, akathisia *The following could be life-threatening:* TD, neuroleptic malignant syndrome	Additive anticholinergic effects and possibly decreased antipsychotic efficacy with anticholinergic drugs; increased risk of toxic side effect if taken with lithium; decreased effectiveness if taken with carbamazepine
pimozide	Orap	Oral: 1–2 mg/d in divided doses, NTE 10 mg/d	PO	Lightheadedness, dizziness, sedation, headache, visual disturbances	May potentiate the CNS depressant effects of opiates, analgesics, anxiolytics, and alcohol
loxapine	Loxitane	Oral: Initial dose of 10 mg/bid up to 50 mg/d; usual dose, 60–100 mg/d IM: 12.5–50 mg q4–6h for acute agitation then change to PO	PO IM	Drowsiness, pseudoparkinsonism, dystonias, akathisia *The following could be life-threatening:* refractory arrhythmias, neuroleptic malignant syndrome	Additive CNS depressant effects with alcohol; barbiturates, narcotics, and anesthetics; decreased efficacy of levodopa; lithium will decrease plasma level; food and drinks containing caffeine will counteract antipsychotic effect
thiothixene	Navane	Oral: Initially 2 mg/tid or 5 mg/bid to usual optimum dose of 20–30 mg/d IM: 4 mg bid/qid with most clients controlled on 16–20 mg/d up to maximum dose, 30 mg/d	PO IM	Drowsiness, pseudoparkinsonism, dystonias, akathisia; photophobia, blurred vision; dry mouth, salivation, nasal congestion, nausea; urine discolored pink to red-brown *The following could be life-threatening:* refractory arrhythmias	Thiothixine has numerous complex interactions with various drugs. Concurrent use of other medications should be carefully assessed before prescribing thiothixene

chlorpromazine	Thorazine	Oral: Initial dose of 10 mg tid/qid or 25 mg bid/tid with increase of daily dosage by 20–50 mg semiweekly until optimum dose IM: Initial 25 mg with repeat in 1 h up to 400 mg q4–6h	PO IM	Drowsiness, insomnia, vertigo, extrapyramidal syndromes; dry mouth, salivation, nausea, vomiting, anorexia, constipation; hypotension, orthostatic hypotension; urinary retention; photophobia, blurred vision; urticaria; photosensitivity *The following could be life-threatening:* eosinophilia, leukopenia, leukocytosis	Additive anticholinergic effects and possibly decreased antipsychotic efficacy if taken concurrently with anticholinergic drugs; additive benefits of both drugs if concurrently with beta blockers; increased risk of tachycardia, hypotension if given concurrently with epinephrine, norepinephrine; increased risk of seizure if taken with metrizamide
fluphenazine	Prolixin	Oral: 0.5–10 mg/d in divided doses IM: Starting dose of 1.25 mg (range 2.5–10 mg) divided and given q6–8h Decanoate: 12.5–25 mg IM or SC q4 wk	PO IM SC	Drowsiness, dystonias, pseudoparkinsonism, akathisia *The following could be life-threatening:* autonomic disturbances, refractory arrhythmias, sudden death related to asphyxia or cardiac arrest	Additive CNS depression if taken with alcohol; increased likelihood of seizures with metrizamide (contrast agent used in myelography)
perphenazine	Trilafon	Oral: 4–8 mg PO tid; avoid doses greater than 64 mg/d IM: Initial dose 5–10 mg q6h NTE 15 mg/d ambulatory or 30 mg/d hospitalized clients	PO IM	Drowsiness, pseudoparkinsonism, dystonias, akathisia; photophobia, blurred vision, urine discolored pink to red-brown *The following could be life-threatening:* neuroleptic malignant syndrome, refractory arrhythmias, sudden death related to asphyxia	Additive CNS depression with alcohol; numerous complex interactions with other drugs; concurrent use of other medications should be carefully assessed
thioridazine	Mellaril	Oral: 50–100 mg PO tid with gradual increase to maximum of 800 mg/d; total daily dose, 200–800 mg divided into two to four doses	PO	Drowsiness, pseudoparkinsonism, dystonias, akathisia; photophobia, blurred vision, dry mouth, salivation, nasal congestion, nausea, urine discolored pink to red-brown *The following could be life-threatening:* neuroleptic malignant syndrome, refractory arrhythmias	Additive CNS depression with alcohol; numerous complex interactions with other drugs; concurrent use of other medications should be carefully assessed

continued

Table 20-3 (Continued)

Generic	Trade	Dose	Route	Predominant Side Effects or Adverse Reactions	Drug Interactions
trifluoperazine	Stelazine	Oral: 2–5 mg bid up to 15–20 mg/d IM: 1–2 mg by deep IM injection q4–6h prn up to maximum dose of 10 mg/d	PO IM	Drowsiness, pseudoparkinsonism, dystonias, akathisia; photophobia, blurred vision, dry mouth, salivation, nasal congestion, nausea, urine discolored pink to red-brown *The following could be life-threatening:* refractory arrhythmias	Additive CNS depression with alcohol; numerous complex interactions with other drugs; concurrent use of other medications should be carefully assessed
clozapine (atypical agent)	Clozaril	PO: 25 mg PO qid or bid; gradual increase with daily dosage increments of 25–50 mg/d to a dose of 300–450 mg/d; not to exceed 900 mg/d	PO	Drowsiness, sedation, seizures, dizziness, sycope, headache; nausea, vomiting, constipation; tachycardia, hypotension, fever	Increased therapeutic and toxic effects if taken with cimetidine; decreased therapeutic effect if taken with phenytoin, mephenytoin, ethotoin
STIMULANT AGENTS					
methylphenidate	Ritalin	Oral: Administer in divided doses bid/tid, 30–45 min before meals; dosage from 10–60 mg/d	PO	Nervousness, insomnia; anorexia, nausea, abdominal pain; increased or decreased pulse and blood pressure; tachycardia	Should not be given with MAO inhibitors, coumarin anticoagulants, and some anticonvulsants; increased effects if given with food or drink containing caffeine
pemoline	Cylert	Oral: Initial dose of 37.5 mg/d with gradual increase of 18.75 mg to mean effective dose of 56.25–75 mg/d not to exceed 112.5 mg/d	PO	Insomnia, anorexia with weight loss; stomachache	Caution is urged in taking pemoline with other medication; effects may be increased if taken with food or drink having caffeine

(Adapted from Karch AM: 1996 Lippincott's Nursing Drug Guide. *Philadelphia, JB Lippincott, 1996.)*

where and how the client will receive medication, need for follow-up appointments, and prescription renewal. Understanding the client's financial resources or insurance coverage for medications will help in implementation. Education about keeping medications out of the range of young children in the home should be provided if applicable.

EVALUATION

Evaluation of medication regimen involves reviewing the efficacy of the drug in improving functioning and the client's subjective perception of the medication. Regular monitoring of perceived response, feelings about the medication, and potential difficulties can ensure adherence, appropriate type, dose, and highest efficacy with least amount of psychotropic medication.

Clients may spontaneously discontinue medication without consulting with caregivers. Avoidance of criticism, rejection, or ultimatums is the best treatment strategy. However, the treatment team, including the nurse, will need to decide, after careful assessment of all factors, if care can continue if the individual chooses not to take psychiatric medication.

Through various functions, nurses assume an invaluable role in assisting clients and families to deal with psychotropic medication. The coordinator of an outpatient medication group for individuals with schizophrenia monitors symptoms, general functioning, and health needs of group members. A nurse practicing within a community outreach agency is likely to see clients in their home environments with family members. Nurses in inpatient settings provide the health teaching needed by the client and family in preparation for discharge to the community. Nurses are able to view multiple aspects of a client's life, monitoring response to medication, with continual needs assessment aimed at maximized functioning.

◆ Adherence to Medication Regimens

One of the most difficult aspects of psychiatric treatment with psychotropic medications involves adherence (or *compliance*) with recommended drug therapies. *Adherence* is defined as the willingness to receive recommended drug treatment as it is prescribed by a caregiver. Adherence involves the client's right to know and understand all aspects of the medication, potential side effects, benefits, and dangers. Some health care providers believe that complete knowledge of the medication may influence a client's nonadherence to the regimen. While this may be true, it is the client's right to refuse all treatments unless judged legally incompetent to make treatment decisions. Nurses have a responsibility to understand the specifics of legal competence and adherence to psychiatric care specific to their geographic area of practice. Legalities differ from state to state.

There are many reasons clients do not adhere to medication regimens. Most often, clients discontinue medication because of adverse side effects. Individuals with chronic psychiatric disturbances frequently feel they have little control in their lives and environment; refusing to take medication becomes a way to exert control. For many, taking psychotropic medication means they are "crazy" or "psychotic," even if they experience symptom relief and improved functioning as a result of the medication.

For some, the need for psychotropic medication means they can no longer deny their symptoms or problems. They may fear addiction to the medication, especially if they have a drug or alcohol abuse history and have received treatment for this.

Families may want their psychiatrically ill member to be "cured" or "fixed" by medication. When the symptoms abate and the client is no longer a management problem, they may agree to stopping the medication because the "cure" has occurred. However, with many chronic disorders, the need for medication may be long term. It is essential for clients and their families to understand this aspect of managing their disorder.[4] Unfortunately, many clients experience the social stigma of having a long-term psychiatric condition. They must be assisted in realizing that their condition is no different from other chronic physical conditions that require medication.

Clients may be influenced by their experiences with medications, including memories from childhood when they witnessed family members receive more primitive forms of psychiatric treatment. Some clients had difficult experiences as children and adolescents in the mental health system when long stays in state psychiatric hospitals meant custodial care and high doses of medication often used as a chemical restraint. Caregiver sensitivity to each client and his or her specific issues can positively influence adherence.[6]

The establishment of community and state hospitals in the late 1880s provided shelter and treatment to chronically disturbed individuals.[43] The last 2 decades have seen the deinstitutionalization movement dramatically alter the controlled living situations where clients received structured care. Clients who live in the community or on the streets are less likely to adhere to prescribed medication regimens. In one study, clients admitted to an acute care state hospital system who refused medication were found to have a higher number of previous admissions than nonrefusers. They were more often admitted involuntarily, and their refusal to adhere to a medication regimen generally led to a poorer clinical outcome, measured by length of hospitalization and incidence and duration of restraint episodes.[23]

Nurses can assist clients in complying with medication regimens in several ways. Keeping in close contact with the client in the community can provide an opportunity for early intervention if the client is experiencing adverse symptoms. Change in dose, time of administration, and medication may alleviate the difficulty and help the client continue with medication or at least discontinue taking the medication with the care providers' knowledge. Developing a therapeutic alliance, understanding community supports, and educating family members about indications and side effects are essential.

Nurses must clarify their own values about the benefit of psychotropic medication to treat psychiatric disorders. This clarification will influence the nursing care they provide to clients who may be refusing medication. Should clients be supported in their decision to refuse medication, even if refusal lowers their quality of life or increases the risk of psychiatric hospitalization or incarceration? Nurses must understand the multiple factors influencing their attitudes, including legal rights, institutional values of their working environment, and their personal value system about client care.(Case Study 20-2).

◆ Role of the Family in Medication Management

Family members play an essential role in medication management. Many adult clients depend on their parents and siblings for housing support, monetary assistance, and emotional guidance. The movement toward

20-2 Case Study

Mrs. C.

Mrs. C. is a 29-year-old woman with a history of chronic anxiety dating back to adolescence. Successfully treated, at intervals, with benzodiazepines, Mrs. C. has not taken medication for her anxiety in several years. Her use of relaxation techniques, biofeedback, and naturopathic medicine has successfully assisted her in dealing with her bouts of anxiety.

In the last year, Mrs. C. has attempted to conceive. Unsuccessful with this, her anxiety has increased markedly, and she is seeking medication. The nurse practitioner in the mental health clinic where she has sought care urges her to consider her options: postponing pregnancy and taking medication to alleviate the anxiety or attempting to manage the anxiety without medication and continuing trying to become pregnant.

After taking a thorough history from Mrs. C. and ascertaining that Mr. C. is supportive of his wife but concerned about her anxiety, the nurse realizes that her current disorder is based partly in her fears of parenting, her difficulties with her own mother, and her ambivalence about having a child. She recommends that Mrs. C. either join a weekly women's group meeting in the clinic or begin some brief individual psychotherapy for issues clarification. Mrs. C. chooses to join the group therapy and not take medication.

Questions for Discussion

1. What type of history would it be important to gather from Mrs. C.? What information about past medication might assist in understanding her current functioning?
2. What collaborative relationship might you want to establish with the naturopathic care provider who has taught Mrs. C. alternative means of dealing with her anxiety?
3. How would the nurse provide follow-up care for Mrs. C.? Outline the specific steps to accomplish this.

deinstitutionalization has necessitated more dependence on families and community-based models of care.[35] Further, the families of persistently mentally ill people are caring for the most disabled and underserved populations in society. Informal and formal networks of care available to the often aging parents of chronically disturbed adults are often inadequate. Medication management is usually a part of the care network and requires that the nurse approach case management with the client and family from a collaborative perspective that includes the family in a partnership of caring.[25]

Families may positively influence adherence to medication regimens, be the first line of assessment for adverse side effects, and supervise administration of the medication and refill of prescriptions. Any conflicts between client's confidentiality and the family's need for information must be resolved.[44] Family education about mental illness and the medications used to treat it should be focused on family coping rather than family pathology. "Family education programs constitute a structured, time-limited strategy to foster family-professional collaboration that supplement on-going collaboration with families."[35]

Although many adult clients may prefer that family members not be involved in medication management, Talbott notes that seven out of 10 people with severe mental illness had family members who could be involved in their care.[39] Including them in decision making regarding medication management, especially when they are actively assisting a psychiatrically ill family member, can only enhance the benefits of psychotropic medication and the client's positive response to this treatment.

◆ Medication Management With Special Populations

PREGNANT CLIENTS

Pregnant clients with psychiatric problems present special problems when they require psychotropic medication to stabilize symptoms. While there is mixed evidence on the teratogenic effects of psychotropic medications, most drugs, such as lithium, benzodiazepines, anticonvulsants, and neuroleptics, predispose the fetus to an increased risk of congenital malformation when their mothers used these medications during the first trimester of pregnancy.[2]

Unfortunately, the first trimester is the time when a women is most unaware of pregnancy. Nurses must conduct a thorough assessment of their clients of childbearing age who may be pregnant or planning to conceive. This is especially difficult if a client is in an acute psychotic state and unable to give an adequate or reliable sexual history.

In the third trimester, the major concern involves the transfer of medications across the placenta. The fetus is then unable to metabolize the medication or its byproducts safely. After delivery, the placenta is no longer available to assist with secretion, and drug toxicity may result.[43] Auerbach and others[5] looked at infants whose psychiatrically ill mothers had received antipsychotic and anxiolytic medications during the pregnancy. All of the infants (n = 12) exhibited poor neonatal motor functioning, including tremulousness, hypertonicity, and poor motor maturity. The authors speculate that this was related to a withdrawal syndrome.[5]

When it is imperative that the mother receive psychotropic medication, the lowest possible dose should be used, and careful monitoring of the fetus should be part of the nursing care plan. Hypervigilance to potential pregnancy will also assist in planning medication management.

Breast-feeding also poses dilemmas to mothers receiving psychotropic medication. All major classes of psychotropic medication will pass into maternal breast milk, transferring undetermined amounts of medication to the infant. Mothers are nearly always advised not to breast-feed if receiving psychotropic medication.[10]

CLIENTS WITH ATTENTION-DEFICIT DISORDER

Adult clients with diagnosed childhood-onset attention-deficit disorder may benefit from a trial of methylphenidate or other stimulants used to treat the same disorder in children. While there are few controlled studies of stimulant use in adults, Spencer and others noted, in a placebo-controlled, crossover study with 23 adult clients, that robust doses of methylphenidate were effective in treating attention-deficit disorder.[39]

Use of stimulants requires careful diagnosis of the disorder, use of the lowest possible effective dose, and careful monitoring of response. Stimulants, when used for illicit purposes, are considered valuable for resale. Like all controlled substances, they are prescribed in smaller amounts than other psychotropic medications.

PSYCHOTROPIC MEDICATION AND THE ELDERLY

The pharmacological actions of psychotropic medications change dramatically for people older than 60 years. This may be due to differences in drug absorption secondary to diminished gastrointestinal motility, low plasma proteins, decreased kidney function, or congestive heart failure. Other explanations might include normally occurring changes in body composition, lean body mass, muscle mass, or increase in fatty tissue.[43]

Regardless of the reasons, nurses need to be aware that elderly clients may respond differently than their younger counterparts to psychotropic medications. Because many older clients are taking several medication simultaneously for various physical ailments, there is an increased need for hypervigilance concerning side effects from polypharmacy. Coordination of medical and psychiatric providers is essential.

CLIENTS WITH ALZHEIMER'S DISEASE

Clients with dementia of the Alzheimer's type present as a special population of adults who may require treatment in inpatient or community psychiatric settings. Alzheimer's disease is a disorder of progressive brain deterioration resulting in cognitive decline and increasing impairment. It rarely occurs before age 65; until recently, research to develop effective therapeutic agents was largely unsuccessful.[22]

One palliative agent approved in 1993 by the U.S. Food and Drug Administration is tacrine (Cognex). This medication reversibly inhibits brain acetylcholinesterase, preventing the breakdown of acetylcholine from presynaptic neurons. In clients with Alzheimer's, tacrine increases the cholinergic transmission in undestroyed neurons.[14]

Tacrine may reverse cognitive changes back to functioning 6 months prior to initiation of the drug.[44] Although the drug has limited effectiveness with some clients, the benefits are short term, and further cognitive loss is probable.

For caregivers, the cost of the drug, the client's need for weekly blood work, and the uncertain hope generated by tacrine are considerations before initiation. Risk of liver toxicity, gastrointestinal upset, dizziness, headache, and agitation are potential side effects. Giving tacrine early in the disease process seems most helpful.[21]

CHILDREN AND ADOLESCENTS

Psychotropic medication has been used with children for several decades. While the standard of care for most practitioners makes this acceptable, there is much controversy and questioning about the need for these medications with a youthful population. Issues regarding efficacy, side effects, and long-term impact on development have been identified. Nurses must clarify their personal attitudes about the use of psychotropic medication with children and adolescents.[29]

The same principles of medication administration and management with adult clients are applicable to psychiatrically disturbed children and adolescents. Additionally, the nurse must be aware of the legal, physical, and emotional dependence children under the age of consent have on their parents or guardians. Informed consent principles and health education must be provided to youthful clients and their family members. Health teaching must be developmentally based and geared to the level of the client's understanding.

Medication management becomes more complicated with the involvement of school personnel, pediatric care providers, and afterschool or day care providers. Supervision of medication administration, assessment of efficacy through parent and school reports, and careful monitoring of family response to the youthful client's difficulties are present in a greater degree than with adult clients.

Psychotropic medications are useful when treating psychiatric disorders of children and adolescents.[19] While many are not approved by the Food and Drug Administration for use in children younger than a certain age, the American Medical Association has stated, "The prescription of a drug for an unlabeled (off-label) indication is entirely proper if the proposed use is based on rational scientific theory, expert medication opinion, or controlled clinical studies."[2]

A body of knowledge has accumulated showing that children and adolescents can benefit from particular drugs not approved for the age or symptom indicator.[19] These medications include tricyclic antidepressants, SSRIs, lithium, and clozapine. It is most important to understand that medication management in youthful populations is more complicated than that with adults and requires a developmental perspective for maximum clinical effectiveness.

◆ Implications for Research

Peplau considers the issue of biology versus environment an unresolved issue in nursing.[31] Because psychotropic medications are used to treat the biological and behavioral manifestations of psychiatric illness, it might follow that giving the drugs might become the treatment. However, Peplau pointedly notes the following:

> Clients are persons. They are more than biologic organisms. From birth to death persons live in an environment. They interact with other persons who, one way or another, influence them. . . . Persons have needs and psychosocial challenges, and they are shaped in meeting them. . . . Mental health personnel too often think they know clients' problems and rush to do something about them. The fact is that only clients know their existential state and look to psychiatric personnel to work with them in gradually becoming fully aware of and in resolving their difficulties.[30]

Understanding the psychosocial needs of clients who potentially benefit from psychotropic medications implies an awareness of their basic needs for food and shelter, their need for family and kinship, and the personal meanings of their psychiatric disorder. It means nurses must be willing to consider the prejudices and biases that are often leveled on individuals with chronic psychiatric problems, understand the role of gender and race in provision of psychiatric care, and consider whether or not psychotropic medication is in the client's best interests.[16]

Nurses are frequently an adjunct, albeit essential, part of research efforts initiated by physicians or pharmaceutical companies with specific roles in monitoring adherence to medication regimens and noting specific side effects. They should also be integrating their nursing research in which outcomes of health teaching or case management are studied and evaluated. Questions might include: ''Is this medication more effective in symptom management if a particular type of nursing care is delivered?'' ''What aspects of community management contribute to adherence in medication regimens?'' Puskar and others[34] are managing acutely psychotic individuals on a clinical research unit without the use of psychotropic medication. They evaluated how effective nursing interventions were in assisting a client in managing psychotic symptoms. Their work points to the need for nurses to consider pharmacological and nonpharmacological aspects of treating psychiatric clients.[34]

◆ Chapter Summary

It is a nursing responsibility to manage clients' use of psychotropic medication carefully and safely by thoroughly understanding side effects, doses, and the interpersonal meaning of psychotropic medication to the client and family. Integration of psychotropic medication into multiple aspects of nursing practice involving case management, health teaching, and family consultation requires creativity and sensitivity. Chapter highlights include the following:

1. The historical development of psychopharmacology has paralleled the increasingly important role of the nurse in medication management.
2. The administration of psychotropic medication involves specific nursing responsibilities.
3. Principles of medication management are applicable to psychiatric clients.
4. Particular psychotropic medications are characterized by side effects and administration guidelines. Medications should be used to treat psychiatric target symptoms for a specified time period.
5. Special client populations who may require psychotropic medication include the elderly, children and adolescents, and pregnant clients.
6. Families provide essential support to clients receiving psychotropic medication.
7. Nurses are able to blend an understanding of psychosocial needs with specific symptoms to provide optimal nursing care.
8. Nurses must engage in a research process that evaluates multiple effects of medication on a client's life and functioning.

Critical Thinking Questions

1. *Discuss the aspects of a biopsychosocial evaluation that must be considered before a client begins psychotropic medication.*
2. *Discuss the legal, ethical, and social issues involved when a patient with a chronic psychiatric illness refuses to adhere to a medication regime.*
3. *Elaborate the ways in which a nurse's personal attitudes about psychiatric medication might influence the care provided to clients.*

Review Questions

1. Which of the following groups of medications might be used to treat a client with a thought disorder?
   A. Risperidone, methylphenidate, pemoline
   B. Haloperidol, chlorpromazine, thiothixene
   C. None of the above
2. Which of the following foods are contraindicated in clients taking MAOIs?
   A. Bananas
   B. Alcoholic beverages
   C. Aged cheese
   D. All of the above
3. Psychotropic medication was first used in the early 1900s to treat manic depressive illness.
   A. True
   B. False
4. SSRIs are a class of antidepressants closely related to all other groups of antidepressants.
   A. True
   B. False
5. Which of the following statements is true?
   A. Antidepressants are rarely cardiotoxic if a client overdoses.
   B. The elderly client usually receives the same dose of psychotropic medication as younger individuals.
   C. Neuroleptic malignant syndrome can be life threatening.

D. A lithium level of 2.5 mEq/L is considered therapeutic.
E. None of the above

◆ References

1. Abramowitz I, Coursey R: Impact of an Educational Support Group on Family Participants who Take Care of Their Schizophrenic Relatives. J Consult Clin Psychol 57: 232–236, 1989
2. Altshuler LL, Szuba MP: Course of Psychiatric Disorders in Pregnancy: Dilemmas in Pharmacologic Management. Neurol Clin 12: 613–635, 1994
3. Alvir JMJ, Lieberman JA, Safferman AZ, Schwimmer JL, Schaaf JA: Clozapine-Induced Agranulocytosis: Incidence and Risk Factors in the United States. N Engl J Med 329: 162–167, 1993
4. Antai-Otong DJ: Psychopharmacology. In Johnson BS (ed): Psychiatric-Mental Health Nursing: Adaptation and Growth, 2d ed, pp 273–299. Philadelphia, JB Lippincott, 1992
5. Auerbach JG, Hans SL, Marcus J, Maeir S: (1992). Maternal Psychotropic Medication and Neonatal Behavior. Neurotoxicology and Teratology 14: 399–406, 1992
6. Baldessarini RJ: Enhancing Treatment With Psychotropic Medicines. Bulletin of the Menninger Clinic 58: 224–241, 1994
7. Baron M, Gershon E, Rudy V, Jonas W, Buchsbaum M: Lithium Carbonate Response in Depression. Arch Gen Psychiatry 32: 1107–1111, 1975
8. Birmaher B, Baker R, Kapur S, Quintant H, Ganguli R: Clozapine for the Treatment of Adolescents With Schizophrenia. J Am Acad Child Adolesc Psychiatry 31: 160–164, 1992
9. Borison RL, Pathiraja AP, Diamond BI, Beibach RC: Risperidone: Clinical Safety and Efficacy in Schizophrenia. Psychopharmacol Bull 28: 213–218, 1992
10. Buist A, Norm TR, Dennerstein L: Breastfeeding and Use of Psychotropic Medication: A Review. J Affective Dis 19: 197–206, 1990
11. Cade JJ: Lithium Salts in the Treatment of Psychotic Excitement. Med J Aust 3: 349–352, 1949
12. Ciraulo DA, Creelman WL, Shader RI, O'Sullivan RL: Antidepressants. In Ciraulo DA, Shader RI, Greenblatt DJ, Creelman W (eds): Drug Interactions in Psychiatry, 2d ed, pp 29–128. Baltimore, Williams & Wilkins, 1995
13. Ciraulo DA, Slattery M: Anticonvulsants. In Ciraulo DA, Shader RI, Greenblatt DJ, Creelman W (eds): Drug Interactions in Psychiatry, 2d ed, pp 249–310. Baltimore, Williams & Wilkins, 1995
14. Davison G, Neale JM: Abnormal Psychology: An Experimental Clinical Approach. New York, John Wiley and Sons, 1978
15. Gelenberg AJ: Tacrine in Alzheimer's Disease. Biological Therapies in Psychiatry Newsletter 17: 25–26, 1994
16. Gittelman M: Ensuring Public Health Care for the Mentally Ill by the Year 2000. International Journal of Mental Health 22: 36–45, 1993
17. Goodwin FK, Murphy DL, Dunner D, Bunney WE: Lithium Response of Unipolar Versus Bipolar Depression. Am J Psychiatry 129: 44–47, 1972
18. Goff DC, Baldessarini RJ: Antipsychotics. In Ciraulo DA, Shader RI, Greenblatt DJ, Creelman W (eds): Drug Interactions in Psychiatry, 2d ed, pp 129–174. Baltimore, Williams & Wilkins, 1995
19. Green WH: Child and Adolescent Clinical Psychopharmacology, 2d ed. Baltimore, Williams & Wilkins, 1995
20. Karch AM: 1996 Lippincott's Nursing Drug Guide. Philadelphia, JB Lippincott, 1996
21. Keltner NL: Tacrine: A Pharmacological Approach to Alzheimer's Disease. J Psychosoc Nurs 32: 37–39, 1994
22. Larrat EP: Update on the Treatment of Alzheimer's Disease. American Pharmacy 9: 59–66, 1992
23. Littrell RA, Mainous AG, Karem F, Coyle WR, Reynolds CM: Clinical Sequelae of Overt Noncompliance With Psychotropic Agents. Psychopharmacol Bull 30: 239–244, 1994
24. Mann JJ, Goodwin FR, O'Brien CP, Robinson DS: Suicidal Behavior and Psychotropic Medication: Accepted as a Consensus Statement by the ACNP Council. March 2, 1992. Neuropsychopharmacology 8: 177–183, 1993
25. Marsh D: Families and Mental Illness: New Directions in Professional Practice. New York, Praeger, 1992
26. Mozes T, Toren P, Chernauzar N, Mester R, Voran-Hegesh R, Bluemensohn R, Weizman A: Clozapine Treatment in very Early Onset Schizophrenia. J Am Acad Child Adolesc Psychiatry 33: 65–70, 1994
27. Murphy DL, Sunderland T, Cohen RM: Monoamine Oxidase-Inhibiting Antidepressants: A Clinical Update. Psychiatr Clin North Am 7: 549–562, 1984
28. Nakielny J: Seizures and Antidepressants. Br J Psychiatry 165: 272, 1994
29. Pearson GS: Psychopharmacology. In Johnson BS (ed): Child, Adolescent and Family Psychiatric Nursing, pp 410–423. Philadelphia, JB Lippincott, 1995
30. Peplau HE: Some Unresolved Issues in the Era of Biopsychosocial Nursing. Journal of the American Psychiatric Nurses Association 1: 92–96, 1995
31. Peplau HE: (1995a). Another look at schizophrenia from a nursing standpoint. In C. A. Anderson (ed.), Psychiatric Nursing 1974 to 1994: A report on the state of the art, (pp. 1-8). St. Louis, MO: Mosby-Year Book, 1995
32. Physicians' Desk Reference, 49th ed. Oradell, NJ, Medical Economics, 1995
33. National Institute of Mental Health: Abnormal Involuntary Movement Scale (AIMS). Special Feature: Rating Scales and Assessment. Psychopharmacol Bull 21 (4): 1077, 1985
34. Puskar KR, McAdam D, Burkhart-Morgan CE, Isadore RB: Psychiatric Nursing Management of Medication-Free Psychotic Patients. Archives of Psychiatric Nursing 4: 78–86, 1990
35. Reinhard SC: Perspectives on the Family's Caregiving Experience in Mental Illness. Image: Journal of Nursing Scholarship 26: 70–74, 1994
36. Sakkas P, Davis JM, Han J, Wang Z: Pharmacotherapy of Neuroleptic Malignant Syndrome. Psychiatric Annals 21: 157–164, 1991
37. Sands BF, Creelman WL, Ciraulo DA, Greenblatt DJ, Shader

RI: Benzodiazepines. In Ciraulo DA, Shader RI, Greenblatt DJ, Creelman W (eds): Drug Interactions in Psychiatry, 2d ed, pp 214–248. Baltimore, Williams & Wilkins, 1995
38. Sarid-Segal O, Creelman WL, Ciraulo DA, Shader RI: Lithium. In Ciraulo DA, Shader RI, Greenblatt DJ, Creelman W (eds): Drug Interactions in Psychiatry, 2d ed, pp 175–213. Baltimore, Williams & Wilkins, 1995
39. Spencer T, Wilens T, Biederman J, Faaraone SV, Ablon JS, Lapey K: A Double Blind, Crossover Comparison of Methylphenidate and Placebo in Adults With Childhood-Onset Attention-Deficit Hyperactivity Disorder. Arch Gen Psychiatry 52: 434–443, 1995
40. Stone WN, Rodenhauser P, Harkert RJ: Combining Group Psychotherapy and Pharmacotherapy: A Survey. Int J Group Psychother 41: 449–464, 1991
41. Sussman N: The Potential Benefits of Serotonin Receptor-Specific Agents. J Clin Psychiatry 55: 45–51, 1994
42. Talbott JA: The Chronic Mental client: What Have We Learned? American Journal of Social Psychiatry 2: 37–42, 1983
43. Townsend MC: Drug Guide for Psychiatric Nursing, 2d ed. Philadelphia, FA Davis, 1995
44. Woo JK, Lantz MS: Alzheimer's Disease: How to Give and Monitor Tacrine Therapy. Geriatrics 50: 50–53, 1995
45. Winker A: Tacrine for Alzheimer's Disease: Which Patient, What Dose? JAMA 271: 1023–1024, 1994
46. Zarate R, Agras WS: (1994). Psychosocial Treatment of Phobia and Panic Disorders. Special Issue: Psychosocial Treatments: Psychotherapy and Experience: Science, Subjectivity, and Society. Psychiatry of Interpersonal and Biological Processes 57: 133–141, 1994
47. Zipple AM, Langle S, Spaniol L, Fisher H: Client Confidentiality and the Family's Need to Know. Community Ment Health J 26: 533–545, 1990

Developmental Issues in Psychiatric-Mental Health Nursing

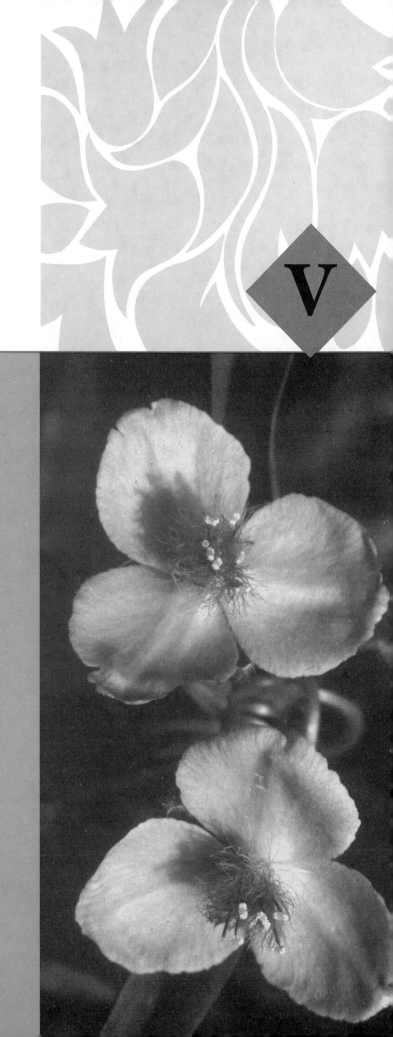

Development of the Person

Sylvia Anderson Whiting

21

To venture causes anxiety, but not to venture is to lose oneself.

Sören Aabye Kierkegaard

Complex factors and forces contribute to the development of personality, whereby traits are produced and exist as enduring behavioral patterns. These patterns convey emotions, gestures, and conduct. The person's unique personal dispositions and preferences are demonstrated through behavior that leads to successful or unsuccessful management of life and its circumstances.

Most adults can identify significant life events believed to have affected the present, but debate continues as to what conditions are most influential to the emergent personality. The nature-nurture controversy has continued and will most likely continue as long as there is human behavior to study.

The concept of facade *refers to the portrayed attitudes that differ distinctly from genuine attitudes and tendencies residing below the surface.*[16] *The more integrated and comfortable one is with the external world, the smaller the difference between the true self and the false self (facade). The facade is described as a "graft" of parents that with time has become "endorsed and assimilated" until it seems to belong to the self.*[16] *An example of facade development is seen when perfectionist parent models require their child to obey even when obedience makes absolutely no sense to the child. The child's initial tendency is to do what feels good (ie, do just the opposite of what the parents want and demand). However, the child is forced to comply through various parental mechanisms and ultimately accepts the parents' view of rightness, though it may not necessarily reflect what is the best decision in the situation.*

Temperament *is an innate quality.*[16] *One only has to observe any set of newborns in a nursery to note the differences in temperament. Mothers are often heard to say that one of their children is so different from their other children. The observed differences are the result of temperament, which may be described as sanguine (optimistic or hopeful), choleric (irritable), or melancholic (pessimistic, sad).*

Character *refers to the qualities acquired in response to a person's early environment.*[16] *From a psychoanalytic perspective, character has been understood as a manifestation of the operation of particular defense mechanisms. For example, people who are perfectionists use the defense mechanisms of intellectualization, rationalization, and affective isolation, whereas those who are more reactive—even hysterical—use repression to a great extent.*

From a neurobiological perspective, particular neural pathways and centers may influence development of personality. Specific regions in the brain are memory storage centers. These centers are significant in shaping what is known of personality by storing up experience memories and using them to formulate future responses. According to Singer and Salovey, memory contains "the seeds of long-term goals, strivings, or motives that may play a role in influencing our interests and choices."[15] *The cognitive system is thus viewed as a constant flow of internal and external interchange of conscious material.*

The personality is "the first line of psychological defense," a kind of stimulus barrier or boundary that protects the ego.[9] *If the barrier is too thin, the psyche is bombarded with stimuli excesses; if it is too thick, the psyche is prevented from receiving the stimuli it needs to respond effectively. Many of the mental disorders in the Diagnostic and Statistical Manual (DSM) represent "transient or chronic symptoms surfacing after the failure of personality to contain various stressors."*[16]

Because the newborn is an absolutely dependent individual, it is not long before the various forces of nature and nurture (environment) have begun the process of molding a distinct personality. In the past it was believed that by the time the child had reached school age, the personality was fixed. However, most authorities now ascribe to the belief that personality is a constantly unfolding process and that development of the person continues throughout the lifespan.

Nevertheless, there are personality types, and under certain stress-related circumstances, some individuals hold up very well and some succumb to the threat by the development of various conditions resulting in DSM diagnoses. Those who hold up very well are considered to be adaptive, *whereas those who succumb to the ravages of their stressors are considered to be* maladaptive. *Another important issue in relation to that of adaptation is* resilience. *There is great interest in determining the factors that enable one individual to withstand extreme difficulties, while another individual succumbs to much less difficult situations or conditions.*

The student at times may hear references to normal or abnormal development, but these terms are relative and depend on many factors. One must consider such factors as averages, statistical or social norms, individual response patterns, cultural influences, and the presence or absence of overt psychopathology.

This chapter reviews theories about human development from intrapsychic, interpersonal, social learning, neurobiological, cognitive, and behavioral perspectives.

Learning Objectives

On completion of this chapter, you should be able to accomplish the following:

1. *Differentiate between temperament and character.*
2. *Discuss the concept of facade, and give an example of how facade develops.*
3. *Describe some temperamental differences in people, and describe how they may influence future behavioral responses.*
4. *Describe how personality and defense mechanisms are related.*
5. *Relate the terms of adaptation, maladaptation, and resilience.*
6. *Discuss the influence of neurotransmitters in personality type development using Cloninger's model.*
7. *Discuss the phases of psychosexual development according to Freud's intrapsychic theory.*
8. *Describe the development of self-concept according to Sullivan's interpersonal theory.*
9. *Explain the developmental tasks of the eight stages of development described in Erikson's social learning theory.*

10. *Describe the thinking of children during each of the four periods of cognitive development according to Piaget's theory.*
11. *Discuss the effects of reinforcement on learning according to behavioristic theory.*
12. *Apply developmental criteria to the assessment of clients evidencing physical and emotional health problems.*
13. *Apply the nursing process to clients who have experienced difficulty in accomplishing developmental tasks.*

◆ Theories of Development

INTRAPSYCHIC THEORY

Sigmund Freud, deemed the father of psychiatry, was a Viennese physician who used hypnosis in the treatment of psychiatric clients and thus became interested in the processes of the unconscious. The art and science of psychoanalysis developed from his description of the unconscious, which is thought to contain the repressed memories of all experiences from the first 6 years of life. An extension of this concept states that although memories may be repressed, they continue to influence or drive all behavior.

Libidinal or instinctual drives influence behavior and are related to a person's attempt to gain pleasure or satisfaction through the mouth, anus, or genitalia. The three periods during which the infant and young child focus on these orifices are known correspondingly as the oral, anal, and phallic (or oedipal) phases of development.

The psychoanalytic theorist relates psychological (often called psychosexual) problems to the child's experiences during these three phases of development. Individuals with severe disturbances of the mind are believed to have experienced maladaptive maternal–child relationships during the early infantile period, the oral phase. Those with less severe mental disturbances are thought to have encountered difficulties during the later periods of early childhood; that is, during the anal phase (from about 18 months to 3 years) or during the phallic phase (from about 3 to 6 years).

Oral Phase

The development of the infant's ego strength depends on the mother's (or mothering person's) sense of personal security in the self and satisfaction in the mothering role. During the oral phase, the infant experiences whatever the mother feels; that is, the infant introjects the person of closest attachment and takes on the anxiety or serenity of that person.[12] When the anxiety of the mothering person is pervasive, the infant is particularly vulnerable and begins life with a deficit in adaptive abilities.

Anal Phase

The mothering person may encounter no difficulty during the period of infancy but may cope ineffectively with the mobile toddler. The anal phase challenges the mother's coping ability because she must allow the young child to move away—in effect, to seek freedom or a greater sense of self. Toilet training the toddler and other issues that arise during the anal phase often arouse psychological problems, particularly related to the rules of custom and culture.

While toddlers strive for mastery over certain aspects of life, they may not be ready to comply with the social expectations of their parents or other significant adults. The striving in two directions, compliance and noncompliance, is termed *ambivalence.* Toddlers may comply through proper elimination, thereby introjecting the values of parents, or they may not comply through retention or inappropriate discharge of feces, which then brings retribution and further anxiety. The "holding on" and "letting go" responses lead to various behaviors that psychoanalytic clinicians term *anal characteristics.*

Phallic Phase

As the child moves into the phallic (or oedipal) phase of development, the foundation for this stage has usually been well established. When anxiety has been present throughout the parent–child relationship, it is likely to continue to manifest itself in the ongoing relationship.

In addition, a problem of a different nature may evidence during the phallic phase, when the child begins to develop an awareness of gender. The child recognizes his or her own gender and manifests an interest in the sexuality of others. He or she may also engage in sexual exploratory play, which may cause parents considerable anxiety.

The term *oedipal* refers to the Greek myth about Oedipus Rex, who was separated from his mother in childhood, was reunited with her in adulthood, and not knowing that she was his mother, fell in love with her. Freud postulated that from 3 to 6 years, the child is unconsciously driven toward the parent of the opposite sex and in effect, desires to possess that parent for himself or herself. For the male child, the issue is less complex than it is for a female child, because the mother is the primary love object; for the girl, however, it means competing with mother, the young girl's primary love object. The child often resolves the oedipal complex by becoming like or identifying with the same-sex parent.

Latent and Genital Phases

Freud called the next two stages of development the *latent* and *genital* phases. His use of the term *latent* refers to his belief that sexuality in the child from 6 to 10 or 12 years does not disappear but becomes hidden. At this age, the child engages in the larger world and is absorbed by its challenges to such an extent that his or her libidinal drive seems to assume less importance and attention.

During the adolescent period, the oedipal strivings reawaken and stir a need for the adolescent child to rework and settle his or her libidinal drive toward the parent of the opposite sex. One way in which this is accomplished is by rechanneling his or her energies toward peers of the opposite sex.

An individual's responses during the infantile period or the early childhood period, if allowed to be carried into adulthood, may cause maladaptation and serious adjustment problems. A person who considers himself or herself to be in constant jeopardy is unable to turn energy away from the self to more productive activity, often resulting in problems of a sexual nature. In this way, a person may become self-absorbed and defensive in the protection of the self or ego. Defensive maneuvers arising from these early phases of development include repression, introjection, projection, denial, isolation, ambivalence, regression, and sublimation.

INTERPERSONAL THEORY

Harry Stack Sullivan, one of psychiatry's most influential thinkers, departed from Freudian concepts and used the term *integrating tendencies* to describe behavior by which one moves toward others.[17] These behaviors include smiling, eye contact, verbal communication, offering an object, and so on. This interpersonal relating of one individual to another takes place, according to Sullivan, to convert us "into human beings instead of merely members of the species by assimilating and becoming part of a vast amount of culture."[17]

Security and Self-Concept

Integrating tendencies are related to the pursuit or maintenance of security or the avoidance of insecurity so that the individual does not experience anxiety. The self comes into being through the young child's experiences. When the child experiences satisfactory fulfillment of needs, he or she senses a "good mother" who relaxes the tension of recurrent needs; this good mother becomes introjected as the "good me." When the child receives inadequate mothering and needs are not satisfactorily met, he or she senses the "bad or evil mother" associated with the experience of anxiety, which he or she then introjects as the "bad me."[18] If the maternal–child relationship is basically nonexistent, the child faces a more serious situation, from which there develops no sense of self or "not me." According to Sullivan's interpersonal theory, self-concept and anxiety are closely related to an individual's early life experiences and continue their influence throughout the lifespan.

SOCIAL LEARNING THEORY

Psychologist Erik Erikson has contributed a theory of development that has gained prominence during the last 3 decades. Erikson's theory is formulated according to three principles of organization—the somatic process, the ego process, and the societal process.

In the infantile period, the individual is influenced by somatic processes through exposure to pain, such as colic, earaches, and hunger pains, and by ego processes through exposure to anxiety, such as that introjected from the mothering figure. Through societal processes, such as the experience of a family crisis, the infant may be exposed to panic, which affects him or her through the method and quality of care administered by his or her caregiver.

Erikson describes the psychoanalyst as a kind of historian and the history of childhood as the basis for understanding human anxiety. According to this theory, anxiety is the outcome of the ongoing interaction of somatic, ego, and societal processes.

Developmental Tasks

The eight stages of developmental tasks or ego qualities devised by Erikson are as follows (Table 21-1):

1. Trust versus mistrust—infancy
2. Autonomy versus shame and doubt—toddlerhood
3. Initiative versus guilt—preschool years
4. Industry versus inferiority—school age
5. Identity versus role confusion—adolescence
6. Intimacy versus isolation—young adulthood
7. Generativity versus stagnation—middle adulthood
8. Integrity versus despair—older adulthood

Through satisfactory completion of the developmental task of each stage, the individual becomes ready to move on to each succeeding stage feeling strong and able to meet the requirements for that stage. An individual who experiences failure in any stage is likely to have greater difficulty achieving success in future stages of development. Each stage is also significant in its own right and results in satisfaction and need fulfillment to the individual who meets the challenges of that stage.

A further distinction of Erikson's social learning theory is his concept linking the developmental stages of individuals to certain social institutions or values. Success in living is described by Erikson in this way:

"Healthy children will not fear life if their elders have integrity enough not to fear death."[7]

NEUROBIOLOGICAL THEORIES

Several theorists have proposed multidimensional models of personality development. Cloninger (1986) focuses on the characteristics of novelty seeking, harm avoidance, and reward dependence in relation to the presence of certain neurotransmitters in an individual. (Table 21-2)[4] He correlates the following neurotransmitter conditions to personality types: low dopaminergic activity was associated with novelty-seeking, high serotonergic activity with harm avoidance, and low noradrenergic activity with reward dependence. Cloninger then used these neurotransmitter conditions as the bases for the eight personality types discussed in Table 21-1.

OTHER DIMENSIONAL MODELS

Torgerson has presented a three-dimensional model that incorporates the concepts of introversion and extroversion, neuroticism, and obsession and has suggested a fourth concept, reality weakness.[21] Torgerson, however, does not tie these types to neural pathways as Cloninger does. Another theorist, Eysenck, has developed a scale similar to Torgerson's and included extroversion and introversion, which he derives from the concepts of sanguineousness, melancholia, and phlegmatism; neuroticism from the concepts of emotionality and changeableness; and psychoticism as related to eccentricity and reality orientedness.[8]

Another dimensional model is presented by the theorist Millon who identifies eight dimensional patterns as follows: passive dependent (submissive), active dependent (gregarious), passive independent (narcissistic), active independent (aggressive), passive ambivalent (conforming), active ambivalent (negativistic), passive detached (asocial), and active detached (avoidant).[9] Stone further emphasizes that the opposites of any of the characteristics are not necessarily pathological.[16] For instance, independence is the opposite of dependence, but independence is not generally considered pathological (see Table 21-3). However, a nursing research study determined conditions in which independence is dysfunctional.[22] Stone refers to the "hermit or go-it-alone trailblazer" as examples of extreme independent types.[16]

COGNITIVE THEORY

Jean Piaget's theory of cognitive development states that motor activity involving concrete objects results in the development of mental functioning. For example, as an infant discovers that his or her hand is holding a rattle, he or she begins to recognize that a sound occurs every time she moves the hand with the rattle in it. Therefore, reflex activity drops out as repetition produces a result that the infant observes; activity begins to take on purpose. Eventually, the infant identifies the shaking rattle as a producer of sound. Later, the infant will realize that he or she is able to create the sound.

Piaget's four periods of cognitive development are as follows:

1. Sensorimotor (0–2 years), during which development proceeds from reflex activity to representation and sensorimotor learning
2. Preoperational (2–7 years), during which development proceeds from sensorimotor representation to prelogical thought
3. Concrete operational (7–11 years), during which development proceeds from prelogical thought to logical, concrete thought
4. Formal operational (11–15 years), during which development proceeds from logical, concrete thought to logical solutions to all kinds or categories of problems

Tenets of Piaget's Theory

Piaget's theory of cognitive development has four basic tenets:

1. Every child passes through each stage and substage of cognitive development in the same sequence, although not according to a given timetable.
2. Every child develops strategies for interacting with the environment and knowing its properties.
3. There is a gradual progression from one period of cognitive development to another, with the acquisition of each new operation building on already existing ones.
4. The process of development is one in which increasing differentiation and complexity are matched by increasing integration and coordination of schemata.[6]

Early Learning

According to Piaget, maximal learning occurs through the process of contemplative recognition, which precedes intentionality. From 4 to 8 months, the infant evidences interest in the results of his or her own behaviors on the environment and invents procedures to make interesting sights last. These reactions of the infant are forerunners of *contemplative recognition,* the function of recognizing and remembering that what has disappeared will reappear. In other words, the infant sees mother appear, disappear, and reappear frequently enough to anticipate a recurrence of the experience. This ability to recognize when an object has reappeared extends to many other objects. From approximately 6

Table 21-1

Erikson's Stages of Development with Adaptive or Maladaptive Characteristics Within Each Stage

INFANT			
Trust	**Versus**	**Mistrust**	**Societal Institution**
Ease in feeding Depth of sleep Relaxation of bowels The first social achievement allows mother out of sight without undue anxiety or rage		Withdrawal into schizoid and depressive states	Religious affiliation
TODDLER			
Autonomy	**Versus**	**Shame and Doubt**	**Societal Institution**
Self-control without loss of self-esteem Good will and pride Rightful dignity Lawful independence Sense of justice		Low self-esteem Secretiveness Feelings of persecution	Economic ethos
PRESCHOOLER			
Initiative	**Versus**	**Guilt**	**Societal Institution**
Loving Relaxed Bright in judgment Energetic Task-oriented		Hysterical denial Paralysis, inhibition, or impotence Overcompensatory showing off Psychosomatic disease Self-righteousness Moralistic surveillance	Law and order
SCHOOL-AGE			
Industry	**Versus**	**Inferiority**	**Societal Institution**
Productivity Task completion Steady attention Perseverance Manipulation of tools		Sense of inadequacy Mediocrity Self-restriction Constructed horizons Conformity	Technological ethos
ADOLESCENT			
Identity	**Versus**	**Role Confusion**	**Societal Institution**
Idealistic Integration of identifications with libidinal vicissitudes Integration of aptitudes with opportunity Confidence		Delinquency Psychotic episodes Doubt and sexual identity Overidentification with heroes, cliques, and crowds	Ideology and aristocracy
YOUNG ADULT			
Intimacy	**Versus**	**Isolation**	**Societal Institution**
Commitment Sacrifice Compromise True genitality Work productivity Satisfactory sex relations		Self-absorption Distancing behaviors Character problems	Ethical sense

continued

to 11 months, infants demonstrate this cognitive process when they repeatedly throw an object and wait expectantly for someone to pick it up. The game of peek-a-boo also reinforces this process.

Representational intelligence refers to the manipulation of mental representations of things and actions, the anticipation of events and consequences of actions, and the ability to evoke an image of an absent object rather than simply recognizing it when it appears. The development of representational intelligence leads to the preoperational stage, wherein objects are classified and categorized. Rudimentary cognitive function precedes language development.[6]

Piaget emphasizes the maturation of the nervous sys-

Table 21-1 (Continued)

MIDDLE-AGED ADULT **Generativity** Establishing and guiding the next generation Productivity Creativity	**Versus**	**Stagnation** Regression to an obsessive need for pseudointimacy Personal impoverishment Early invalidism Self-love Lack of faith	**Societal Institution** Ethos of generative succession
OLDER ADULT **Integrity** Assurance of order and meaning Experience conveying world order and spiritual sense New and different love of one's parents Defends the dignity of own lifestyle against threat Emotional integration Fellowship with others Acceptance of leadership	**Versus**	**Despair** Fear of death Sense of time as too short Disgust	**Societal Institution** Charity

(From Erikson EH: Childhood and Society. New York, WW Norton, 1968.)

tem in his theory of cognitive development. The abilities developed within each stage evolve according to the individual's unique timetable of maturation.

BEHAVIORISTIC THEORY

According to behavioristic theory, development is influenced by the stimulus–response interaction; behavior is shaped through the consistency of responding. Researchers have conducted studies to determine the effects of reinforcement of newborns' sucking behaviors, older infants' smiling behaviors, and other developmental skills, such as toilet training, sharing, helping, and cooperating.[11]

Reinforcement of Learning

The neonate is able to learn much more than is usually recognized by parents and professionals. Neonatal learning occurs through reinforcement that coincides with need satisfaction.[19] Perceptual discrimination and

Table 21-2

Cloninger's Three-Dimensional Personality Model

Dimensions			
Novelty Seeking	*Harm Avoidance*	*Reward Dependence*	*Personality Type*
1. High	Low	Low	Antisocial
2. High	Low	High	Histrionic
3. High	High	High	Passive-aggressive
4. High	High	Low	Explosive-schizoid
5. Low	Low	High	Cyclothymic
6. Low	High	High	Passive-dependent; avoidant
7. Low	High	Low	Obsessive-compulsive
8. Low	Low	Low	Imperturbable schizoid

(Adapted from Cloninger CR: A Unified Biosocial Theory of Personality and its Role in the Development of Anxiety States. Psychiatr Dev 3: 167–226, 1986.)

Table 21-3

Characteristics of Healthy Interdependence Versus Dysfunctional Independence

Healthy Interdependence	Dysfunctional Independence
Generally secure and self-assured; values self and others	Self-protective, fearful of appearing weak, expresses insecurity through defensiveness
Considers relationships meaningful and important	Prefers to be alone or in limited relationships; acts aloof and distant
Is flexible, open-minded, communicative, receptive, responsive, considerate, creative, mature, dependable	Is opinionated, rigid, wilful, oppositional, controlling, manipulative, domineering, dictatorial, sullen, pouty
Appropriately recognizes and acknowledges need for help; participates with individuals or groups to seek and give assistance, guidance, and support when needed or desired	Has problems accepting or asking for help from others, expressing needs for support; may take pride in not requesting help
Is responsive to needs of self and others; flexible enough to change roles and assist others when necessary	Demands compliance of others in family, work, or group situations; intimidates as a means of getting needs met or having own way; actions may be problematic for others
Tolerates differences of opinion and behaviour, able to relate to a variety of people	Is critical of others; has difficulty with differentness; adopts negative attitude toward many people and issues
Is emotionally caring and expressive; shows creativity and playfulness in relationships based on joy and humor	Has difficulty expressing and accepting love; views dependence and intimacy as weakness and fears or rejects them; overly cautious in interpersonal encounters
Interacts emotionally and intellectually; self-disclosing and empathically tuned to others	Communicates on superficial or overintellectual level instead of on an emotional level
Recognizes limitations and acknowledges own strengths and weaknesses	Has difficulty seeing self objectively and accepting criticism or feedback
Considers needs and plans of others and self; accepts responsibility for own actions without blaming others	Is self-absorbed and self-serving; shows little consideration to rights, needs, interests of others; does not admit mistakes
Enjoys working with others, able to ask for assistance or delegate as appropriate	Has difficulty working or collaborating with others, overextends self
Welcomes negotiation, has good negotiating skills	Reluctant to negotiate, may lack skills
Values equality, ethics, personal control, patience, and trust and growth in relationships	Uses poor judgment, persists in self-defeating activity; is unable to trust others; does not care for self physically or emotionally

active learning are possible for the newborn. Therefore, when a mothering person consistently appears along with a need-fulfilling stimulus (eg, the breast or bottle), the neonate relates the two and prefers that person over all others.

Differentiation between two faces and voices has been demonstrated during the first 2 weeks after birth. Furthermore, this recognition seems to be related to the neonate's development of social communication skills by means of bodily movements and within a short period of time, by means of the smile. These forms of social communication occur through mutual interaction of mother and neonate, which is reciprocally rewarding and reinforcing.

CURRENT DEVELOPMENTAL THEORY

Newer models of personality development discount theories that emphasize completion of development early in life. Today's theories assert that the human organism is complex and cannot be classified and categorized.

Flexibility and plasticity, two attributes of the human brain, allow for a developmentally significant variety of adaptive sequences.[20] Therefore, although early life experiences and influences are significant, they are not the sole producers of healthy or negative outcomes.

Consonance Versus Dissonance

An interactionist model of development focuses on the concept of *goodness of fit* and the related ideas of consonance and dissonance. This model demonstrates that development in a progressive direction occurs when *consonance* (or goodness of fit) exists and that *dissonance* (or poorness of fit) involves discrepancies between the individual and the environment. Such discrepancies result in distorted development and maladaptive functioning.[14] The goodness-of-fit concept implies that environmental demands and expectations are in accord with the individual's capacity to respond. This results in consonance or a sense of comfort, which makes progressive, optimal development possible.

Consider the following application of this concept: Mary is a shy, introverted individual who has just completed college with a bachelor's degree in biology. She restricts relationships to one or two people. She has two job opportunities from which to choose, one as a research assistant in a laboratory and the other as a public relations coordinator. They pay equitable and similar salaries. Using the goodness-of-fit concept, it is likely that Mary would be more comfortable and more adaptive as a research assistant than as a public relations coordinator and that her development would continue more smoothly.[19,20]

Numerous examples make a case for the goodness-of-fit model of development. Consider the situation of adoptive parents who appear as a set of ideal parents but who experience total failure in the outcome of one or more of the children they adopt. Consider parents who demonstrate completely irresponsible behavior but have children who become productive and healthy. Perhaps in other circumstances, the outcomes for all the children might have been different.

Nurses must maintain an open mind when dealing with parents who may be blamed because the children have turned out poorly or the opposite scenario of poor parents and healthy children. In some cases, problems may arise because the parent(s) "loved too much" and became overly invested and involved. In other cases, the neglectful parent may have provided, by their neglect, an opportunity for children to find and use their own resources. Many parents would like to do a good job of parenting, but for one reason or another, they lack the skills necessary to do so. Many of them imitate their own ineffective parental models, while others avoid the models they have had and make even worse decisions relative to childrearing.

Because children from an early age are able to produce certain desired responses in their parents, the parents may be totally confused by the roles that they play. Parents often have the idea that children should be more mature than their chronological age requires, and they often miss the fun of their children's experience. Consider the example in Box 21-1. In this example, Danny's view of the world and what is expected of him are becoming established. The pattern of belief about himself and his relationships, once set, becomes the schema of what can be expected in the future and predicts the view that the child begins to have of himself and the world (Box 21-2).

Each developmental stage requires adaptation particular to the demands of the child's chronological age and particular interests. For example, one 14-year-old may appear more as an adult than a child, whereas another 14-year-old may appear as a much younger child. Parents often refer to other parents for models, and this may cause confusion because there are so many conflicting examples of the correct way to parent. For instance, one 13-year-old may be allowed to drive and park the car in the yard, while another parent would not even consider allowing their child behind the wheel of the car. Problems are compounded by single-parent responsibilities that are faced by a growing number of families; a single parent might not be able to do what a couple might do under similar circumstances, or may do just the opposite. The provision of comfort, direction, and assistance to children is determined by parental resources and will influence outcomes in the children. Some youngsters may become angry, and others may become passive. In either case, the development of independence is likely to be hampered during the stage of adolescence when it is such a necessary precursor to future development. Interference with development of independence is likely to inhibit establishment of interdependence during adulthood (see Table 21-4). Many outcomes may be influenced by the childhood and adolescent periods.

◆ Developmental Issues in Nursing

Nurses must frequently assess developmental processes and progression in the course of implementing the nursing process. They frequently refer to one or a combination of theories to determine probable causes of behavior and interventions that will facilitate effective behavior change. Psychiatric-mental health nurses are

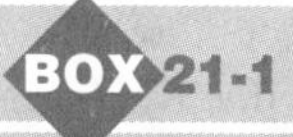

Matching Expectations to Abilities

Dan and Jane T are 27 and 25 years old, respectively. They are the parents of three children, 5-year-old Danny, 3-year-old Melanie, and 20-month-old Janet. Dan works as a printer and hopes to own his own business someday. He is working very hard to prove that he knows his job in case his employer who is nearing age 65 decides he wants to sell the business. Jane is a registered nurse who works 3 days a week "to make ends meet." She generally hires a baby sitter to care for their children but has had to change sitters frequently because she has not been pleased with them. One morning she arrived home after duty on the night shift and learned that the sitter was not able to come that day. Because Jane was tired, she told Danny, "I am going to go to sleep for 2 hours. I will put Janet in the playpen, and I want you to watch her and Melanie. Call Mommy if anything happens or if Melanie won't mind you." While Jane was asleep, Melanie attempted to crawl into the playpen and fell onto Janet. Janet screamed and awakened Jane. Janet continued screaming for an hour, so Jane decided she must take her to the emergency room to see if there were internal injuries. Emergency room personnel reprimanded Jane and told her that they must report the incident to child protective services. The chidren were removed from Jane's care and placed temporarily in the care of foster parents.

ANALYSIS

In this instance, Jane expected a child to carry out a responsibility that he is far too young to do. Danny is too young even to complain about the responsibility in a mature way. Danny is in need of caretaking himself. However, Jane was reared in a large family where all the children were expected to take care of each other. She apparently does not recognize that she is placing her children in a precarious position relative to physiological or safety needs. Danny is expected to carry out a function beyond his ability, but he will feel the weight of his mother's displeasure if something goes wrong. The children are in danger because Danny is too young to be a decision maker about most things. Ultimately, one of the children was hurt. They wakened their mother who had to take the baby to the emergency room, but in a less serious outcome, she may have become angry with the children because of sleepiness or unrealistic expectations. Maternal anger may further distance the children and their mother and place a weight of responsibility for thoughts and feelings with which the children should not have to deal at this time. Melanie is a toddler and likely to get into something dangerous. At this age, children are very active; it would be impossible for Danny to do a good job in this situation, and he will feel like a failure if things go badly. At this stage of development, Danny's "work" should be play activities or carrying out small chores under the direction of his mother. A 20-month-old toddler should not be out of the sight of an adult for more than a few minutes.

Unrealistic parental expectations, such as this one in Danny's life, can result in the following predictable pattern of events:

1. Parent places an unrealistic, age-inappropriate demand on a child.
2. Child feels responsible but also frightened, inadequate, and possibly angry.
3. Circumstances erupt, leading to frustration in Danny and inability to function adequately.

Even when parents place unrealistic expectations on their children, outcomes can vary depending on the parent's response, as shown in the following comparison:

Unhealthy Outcome	Healthy Outcome
Mother responds out of her lack of rest with tension, frustration, exasperation, or anger. ↓ Child responds with fear and tension because Mother is unhappy and expresses her displeasure. ↓ Danny feels like a failure, "bad," dissatisfied, and tense.	Mother recognizes that she has placed an unrealistic demand on her child and feels guilty. ↓ Mother responds with respectful concern, and Danny feels relief. ↓ Danny feels safe and satisfied. He feels important and loved by his mother.

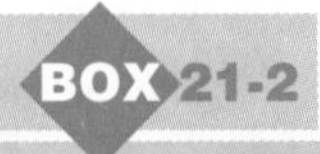

Therapeutic Dialogue: Impaired Parental Decision Making

Dan and Jane T, now faced with the involvement of Child Protective Services, have decided to seek the advice of an attorney. They want their children returned immediately and do not believe the authorities had any right to remove the children from their care. They fear that Danny, Melanie, and Janet have been separated from each other and that they probably are extremely upset. They appeal to their caseworker, Ms. Thompson, and ask her for information about the children who have now been gone for 2 days. Jane is distraught and has refused to eat or sleep since the children were taken. They call the Crisis Intervention Center for help and are told to come for an appointment that afternoon. The nurse assigned to them, Ms. Rogers, completes an assessment and notes that the parents are extremely guarded in their answers to her. The following interaction takes place between the parents and Ms. Rogers, R.N., C.S.

Jane: "I am a nurse; I know what I am doing with my own children."

Ms. Rogers: "Tell me what you usually do to manage your children's care."

Jane: "I had a sitter for them until last week, but the sitters don't know as much as Danny does. He knows what the rules are, and besides you don't know what a smart little guy he is."

Dan: "I would rather have Danny taking care of things than some of those bimbo-headed sitters we've had lately. You ought to see the mess Janet gets up to every time they are there."

Ms. Rogers: "What do you plan to do if you get the children back home?"

Jane: "I don't know; I guess I'll have to quit working."

Dan: "Jane, have you forgotten we have a house and a boat payment to make. Do you want to lose those things?"

Ms. Rogers: "Do you have any family who can help you out?"

Jane: "Well, Dan's parents are here, but I'd rather ask a stranger than to ask them for anything."

Dan: "Jane, if you wanted to, you could get along better with them."

Jane: "Well, I've tried everything I know how, and I can't make it work. Besides they don't like taking care of children."

Ms. Rogers: "What about your parents, Jane?"

Jane: "I don't speak to them any more than I have to."

Ms. Rogers: "Oh, it appears that there are problems in your relationships with your parents and in-laws. What about you, Dan; how do you get along with them?"

Dan: "Oh, I get along alright with all of them; it's just easier not to go around any of them since Jane and they always end up having some disagreement, and I get caught in the middle. I don't like having to make everyone feel better. It's bad enough trying to keep the kids in line."

Ms. Rogers: "The kids in line?"

Dan: "Yes. I try to keep them from upsetting their mother. It's not fun to live in a house when your wife is mad at you."

Ms. Rogers: "Jane, how do you feel about what Dan says?"

Jane: "I don't feel anything anymore. All I have time to do is cook and clean and baby sit and go to work. You don't know what it's like living in our situation. I'm just plain tired of it."

Ms. Rogers: "I'm going to do all that I can to help you. Meanwhile, I want you to go home and think about some things you can do to change your situation, and I'd like us to meet here again in 2 days. During that time, perhaps you can consider this a vacation and get some much needed rest. I will call Ms. Thompson and check on the children and will call you tomorrow just to check on you."

Jane: "OK. I won't promise that I'll get any rest, but I'll wait for your call."

Dan: "Well, maybe I can take my wife out to dinner somewhere, and we can discuss this whole thing. I do think we will need your help, though."

ASSESSMENT

1. Jane is a professional nurse, but she seems to have some deficits in her knowledge about child development.
2. Dan seems to share his wife's knowledge deficit about childhood needs.

continued

BOX 21-2 (Continued)

3. Jane views matters in an all-or-nothing manner, (ie, quitting work rather than finding a compromise.)
4. Dan's emphasis on having a boat may not be reasonable for the family at this point in their lives.
5. Jane is in conflict with both sets of parents and demonstrates no desire to resolve the conflict.
6. Dan expresses discomfort about Jane becoming upset by the children and about her relationship with their parents.
7. Jane is overwhelmed by the responsibilities of family and work responsibilities.
8. Jane complains of sleep deprivation.
9. Jane and Dan have a major dilemma relative to the loss of their children from their care.
10. Jane and Dan are not communicating effectively at this time.
11. Jane is distraught and deficient in problem-solving skills during this crisis.
12. The couple are in need of crisis intervention.

NURSING DIAGNOSIS

1. Impaired functioning in child care activities related to feelings of being overwhelmed
2. Crisis situation related to the loss of children to Child Protective Services
3. Lack of adequate support system related to communication difficulties with extended family systems
4. Impaired marital relationship related to system stress, financial overload, and loss of extended family support

CLIENT OUTCOMES

1. Jane and Dan will describe ways to reduce the stressors in their lives by (date).
2. Jane and Dan will report some immediate solutions to some of their problems so that they are better able to problem solve and make appropriate decisions by (date).
3. Jane and Dan will discuss with Ms. Rogers the issues that are causing estrangement between them and their parents and seek a resolution by (date).

4A. Jane and Dan will describe ways they can reduce their stress as related to financial distress and their lack of involvement with their extended family or other support systems by (date).

4B. Jane and Dan will report specific activities designed to improve marital relations by (date).

GOALS

1. Jane and Dan will demonstrate ability to problem solve in a mature manner so that their children will be safe, and the entire family wil experience feelings of satisfaction by (date).
2. Jane and Dan will prepare a budget that helps to eliminate the major stressors in their lives by (date).
3. Jane and Dan will have worked out a resolution of the problems between them and their extended family system by (date).
4. Jane and Dan will report greater marital satisfaction by (date).

INTERVENTIONS

1. In 2 days, meet with Jane and Dan to discuss how they can eliminate the current stressors that threaten their security at this time.
   Rationale: A short time was set to give the couple time to think about options and to experience hope and encouragement knowing that someone is available, willing, and able to provide assistance. During this period, the couple need directive therapy until their usual problem-solving skills are restored.
2. Assist Jane and Dan to list the specific stressors at the first meeting.
   Rationale: It will help the couple to engage in concrete problem-solving activities with the nurse's assistance until they can see the big picture.
3. Assist Jane and Dan to identify which conditions can be met to eliminate the current stressors in their lives.
   Rationale: If the couple can state some changes they are willing to make in the presence of a third person, it will help to hold them accountable.
4. Help Jane and Dan examine the relationship issues that contribute to the dysfunction between Jane and both sets of parents and between Jane and Dan in second and third meetings.
   Rationale: Jane has allowed relations between both sets of parents to deteriorate and may not know how to resolve the issues and still save face. With assistance, she can engage in the

continued

BOX 21-2 (Continued)

process in a less threatening way and gain the courage to confront issues after realizing that they are worth the effort. Restoration of the relationships will enhance the support system so badly needed by the family at this time. During a crisis, family members will often respond, and old hostilities are often more easily resolved.

5. Seek information about how the couple used their time together.
   Rationale: This is a helpful assessment technique for determining the couple's willingness and interest in going beyond the crisis that now faces them.
6. Help the couple determine what are appropriate developmental tasks for their children in the third and fourth meetings.
   Rationale: This technique assists the nurse to assess the couple's knowledge level and determine where to begin their instruction (ie, a referral to parenting classes versus the need for educational discussion within the therapy sessions).
7. Assist the couple to identify specific, appropriate child care options in fourth or fifth meetings.
   Rationale: This technique allows for assessment of couple's problem-solving skills and their ability to make appropriate decisions in preparation for the return of their children.
8. Serve as client advocate between Child Protective Service personnel and Jane and Dan throughout the process as long as Jane and Dan maintain a commitment to crisis intervention.
   Rationale: Clients often become discouraged and defeated during their involvement with Child Protective Services, sometimes with good reason, and they need assistance of a professional in negotiating the system.
9. Assist Jane and Dan to make appropriate plans for the eventual return of their children (ie, attendance at parenting classes, a written plan for child care in the future) from the fifth meeting until the crisis is resolved or the couple is involved in therapy.
   Rationale: Anticipatory guidance is a helpful technique for preparing a family's restoration to improved functioning.

EVALUATION

1, 2, and 3. Jane and Dan will give verbal evidence of having a clear perspective about their situation and will state a specific plan for resolving their dilemma.

4. Jane and Dan will demonstrate willingness to discuss family interpersonal issues and describe how the damaged relationships are preventing full use of a support system.
5. Couple will report at least one activity that helped them to feel relieved and connected to each other.
6. Couple will articulate their opinions and understanding about child rearing and identify ways in which they might improve child management.
7. Couple will present a plan by which to provide appropriate care for their children after the fifth meeting.
8. Couple will recognize that cooperation and participation with the nurse will assist them in achieving positive outcomes.
9. Couple will have begun participation in parenting classes or to have demonstrated their commitment to future resolution of their problems and restoration of their children.

necessarily interested in developmental issues, because physical and emotional health are in large part determined by adaptive or maladaptive responses along the developmental continuum.

One useful framework considers the presence of dependency, independence, or interdependency in progressive stages on a continuum (Table 21-4). This framework establishes that healthy, adaptive states are marked by progressive movement away from total dependency at birth to the ultimate adult condition of interdependency.[5] Some believe that in a fixated condition, one may get held up or hung up developmentally and fail to move past dependence or independence (see Box 21-2). Failure to move past these earlier developmental levels indicates dysfunction; dependent or independent behaviors may cause difficulty for the individual and significant others. Ongoing research is investigating the distinctions of dependence, independence, and interdependence.

The great struggle for independence occurs during the adolescent period and is responsible for creating marked disequilibrium. Ego crystallization, the crucial issue during adolescence, occurs through the process of developing a self-concept and achieving independence. This process is often reflected in the rebellion so typical of adolescence. When this process is incompletely experienced, it may need to be worked out in adulthood when other processes should be the focus and may hinder the development of those processes. A middle-aged adult behaving in a fashion typical of a

Table 21-4

Progression from Dependence to Interdependence

Infancy (0–1 y)	Childhood (1–12 y)	Adolescence *Early*	Adolescence *Middle*	Adolescence *Late*	Adulthood
Dependency	Decreasing dependency	Conflict in dependency	Struggle toward independence	Independence	Interdependency

much younger person may be attempting to complete the unfinished tasks of adolescence.

Dependency is closely related to anxiety and an emotionally restricted self. Manifestation of extreme dependency in adulthood generally is accompanied by a high level of anxiety as the person looks to others for caretaking. This is observed most typically in people with borderline personality disorder. Interdependency, on the other hand, characterizes people who are relatively free of anxiety and able to view themselves as capable individuals interacting with other capable individuals.

The overall goals of human development include social competence and mastery. Many believe that the first year of life is the most important; some would even propose that the first day of life may well be the most significant one.

The study and understanding of development are complex and multifaceted, even before the added influence of cultural differences. The development of a child in America and another in Samoa will demonstrate obvious differences in the manner in which tasks are mastered, the time when they occur, and the use of skills. Nevertheless, consistent sequential development occurs in numerous areas of functioning across cultures; the children within a given culture will evidence linear progression toward mastery of certain tasks expected within the cultural group.

To understand development, the nurse must consider genetic transmission, cultural transmission, temperament, motivation, physical endowment, stimulus provision, and interaction with others. The fact that these forces contribute to development lends credence to the notion that developmental outcomes are not the responsibility of one person. In the past, mothers were viewed as totally responsible for the child's healthy development. Fathers, siblings, extended family, and even the child were seen as mere bystanders in the scenario. Furthermore, the child's development was considered essentially complete in the first 6 years, and from 6 years on, the personality was only modified. Little attention focused on adult development, particularly on the middle- and late-age periods (see Nursing Care Plan 21-1).

Current developmental theories give rise to the hope that there is continuity in the process of development and that self-actualization may occur even in the late-age period. Many examples of people who achieved their greatest potential only after becoming older are available. Some adults appear to progress, regress, and progress according to life circumstances or crises. Late-age development was a less prominent issue in the past, when life expectancy did not exceed the middle-age period for most, but survival beyond 100 years is no longer uncommon. Generally, development in the elderly is not as much a matter of achieving a higher level of functioning as it is a qualitative transformation concerned with maintaining adaptive behavior governed by weakened physiological structure and increased egocentricity.[18] Adaptation requires considerable compensation for the individual whose sensory apparatus, from the fourth decade on, begins to limit function. As the seventh decade begins, the person's sensory and perceptual processes become slower, requiring more time to solve problems accurately. Research findings suggest that the major change in intellectual functioning from midlife to early old age is related to reaction time. An understanding of this concept is important if nurses are to avoid infantalizing the older individual who may respond to the label if he or she is regarded as incapable.[11] A common fallacy is that because elderly people do not function as well physically as the young person, they are also less capable intellectually. Nurses are in a position to reinforce the elderly individual as a person who has wisdom, responsibility, and prestige.[11]

◆ Chapter Summary

This chapter has presented an overview of six different developmental theories: intrapsychic, interpersonal, social learning, neurobiological, cognitive, and

Nursing Care Plan 21-1

Unresolved Developmental Issues and Conflicts

Normally, the developmental tasks and issues a person faces throughout life do not cause untoward turmoil or trauma. Although the transitional phases between the stages of development usually increase tension and stress to some degree, the person normally moves from one stage to another without major incident, achieving higher levels of growth.

Some people, however, do not make smooth transitions through these stages of development and thus are more vulnerable to future psychiatric disorders than those who make healthy adaptive transitions. Some researchers have asserted that certain variables—including biological predisposition, psychosocial and psychological stressors, and transitional issues—increase a person's susceptibility to affective disorders.[2] Others attribute some psychiatric disorders to early, unresolved issues. People at risk usually have difficulty dealing with social developmental issues and are at risk for crises and psychological turmoil with each transitional stage of development. This turmoil commonly is manifested by an affective disorder.

The following case history presents an example of a person who has experienced such developmental turmoil.

Stella S: Intimacy Versus Isolation

Stella S is a 25-year-old single woman who comes to the mental health center seeking help. She reveals that she has just moved to town and that she cannot get adjusted. She says that she is homesick and misses the people at home but cannot afford to leave her job and move back. She is especially distressed at having had to leave her therapist, whom she describes as "the mother I always wanted—I've looked for someone like her all my life." She confesses to having made numerous telephone calls (sometimes two or three times a day) to the therapist, who has told her that she must work at developing relationships where she is and to stop calling so frequently. She finds many reasons why she has not formed relationships with others close to her own age. She frequently responds with, "I can't because . . ." After several sessions, she has been diagnosed as having a borderline personality disorder. Stella seems to enjoy coming to therapy; she usually comes early and stays as long as possible.

Nursing Diagnosis

Ineffective Individual Coping related to dependence on others, particularly authority figures

Outcome

Client will begin to use coping measures as tools to increase self-reliance.

Intervention	Rationale
Help client identify areas in her life in which she relies on others rather than self.	Recognition of concrete instances in which over-reliance on other people occurred will aid in identification of scope of problem.
Assist client to identify own strengths and positive aspects of own functioning.	Identification of strengths will reinforce self-esteem and increase individual's sense of ability to handle problem situations.
Discuss methods of coping with problems, including relaxation techniques, stress management, and problem-solving.	Increased coping is a skill that can be learned. The use of the nurse–client relationship can help promote these skills.

Evaluation

Client's repertoire of adaptive coping skills increases.

continued

Nursing Care Plan 21-1 *(Continued)*

Nursing Diagnosis

Social Isolation related to lack of relationship skills secondary to fears of becoming close to people

Outcome

Client will develop a relationship with at least one peer in her age group.

Intervention	Rationale
Encourage client to describe concerns about forming relationships.	Discussion of fears and concerns will objectify the emotional responses client experiences when involved with others.
Assist client to identify at least three positive things about self that would enhance a friendship	This will assist client to accentuate strengths that can be brought to a relationship and diminish sense of worthlessness.
Encourage client to identify activities that would be enjoyable with another person.	This places responsibility on client to identify potential enjoyment with a peer.
Role play social situations with client.	Practicing situations prior to actual involvement will enhance confidence and provide client with skills necessary in social situations.

Evaluation

Client uses her social skills to develop friendship with at least one peer.

behavioristic. The integration of these theories has evolved into a body of knowledge permitting further study of developmental issues. Very little research has been done by nurses in the area of personality and its development. Some of the major points of the chapter are as follows:

1. Human development is a complex and multifactorial process involving a variety of forces that create unique personalities.
2. Development is a continuous process, unfolding throughout the lifespan, rather than being limited to a few early years in relationships with a limited number of people.
3. Responsibility for development is much larger in scope than just the mothering relationship; it is based on complex and interactive influences on the individual over time.
4. The last stage of life continues to have qualitative developmental experiences.
5. Neurobiological influences play a major role in personality development.
6. Healthy, adaptive adult functioning occurs at the interdependent level following the adolescent period when independence is established.

Critical Thinking Questions

1. *Discuss as many aspects of the nature-nurture controversy that you can, and state a personal position as to which, if either, you believe to be most significant.*
2. *Explain how an individual might develop a "pseudoself," and state the ways in which this could be problematic to the individual and to those who interact regularly with that individual.*
3. *Describe how Cloninger's neurobiological theory relates to behavior and the ultimate outcomes in the personality.*
4. *Discuss whether you believe an infant is acted on or is an actor in the relationship with the mother during the first 2 months of life.*
5. *Describe how defense mechanisms serve the ego, and relate your thinking to boundary protection.*
6. *Discuss what you think about the concept of "normal" or "abnormal" personality.*
7. *What are the influences that lead to the development of DSM diagnoses?*
8. *How are temperament and character related?*

Review Questions

1. Cloninger's neurobiological theory might be best linked to
   A. Freud's psychoanalytic theory.
   B. Erikson's social learning theory.
   C. Sullivan's interpersonal theory.
   D. Piaget's cognitive theory.
2. Erikson's stage of development that best suggests future problems in sexuality is
   A. trust versus mistrust.
   B. autonomy versus shame and doubt.
   C. initiative versus guilt.
   D. industry versus inferiority.
   E. identity versus role confusion.
3. Piaget's "contemplative recognition" is preceded by
   A. maximal learning.
   B. intentionality.
   C. formal operations.
   D. concrete operations.
4. "Representational intelligence" is a reference to
   A. sensorimotor functions.
   B. ability to figure out mazes.
   C. reinforcement of newborns' sucking behavior.
   D. manipulation of mental representations of things and actions.
5. Behaviorism implies the development of personality by
   A. shaping.
   B. reduction of anxiety that clouds the perceptual field.
   C. preference of one person over another.
   D. generalizing abstract mental representations.
6. Consonance refers to
   A. discrepancy.
   B. influence.
   C. good fit.
   D. generalization.
   E. challenge that is satisfactorily met.
7. Although infants and children are able to influence their environments, they must be cared for carefully for a considerable time in contrast to other species in the animal kingdom. In the case of Jane, Dan, and their children presented in this chapter, which is the best reason for removing the children from responsibility of the parents?
   A. The parents have to work and need a break.
   B. The parents are not very intelligent.
   C. The children are obviously undisciplined.
   D. The parents are abusive.
   E. The parents are neglectful.

◆ References

1. Akiskal HA, McKinney WT Jr.: Overview of Recent Research in depression: Integration of Conceptual Models into a Comprehensive Clinical Framework. Arch Gen Psychiatry 32 (March): 285–305, 1975
2. Bowlby J: Attachment and Loss, vol 2: Separation, Anxiety and Anger. London, Hogarth and Institute of Psychoanalysis, 1972
3. Brown GW, Prudo R: Psychiatric Disorder in Rural and Urban Population: Aetiology of Depression. Psychol Med 11 (August): 581–599, 1981
4. Cloninger CR: A Unified Biosocial Theory of Personality and its Role in the Development of Anxiety States. Psychiatr Dev 3: 167–226, 1986
5. Covey SR: The 7 Habits of Highly Effective People: Powerful Lessons in Personal Change. New York, Simon & Schuster, 1989
6. Drucker J: Development from One to Two Years: Ego Development. In Noshpitz JD (ed): Basic Handbook of Child Psychiatry, vol 1, pp 157–164. New York, Basic Books, 1979
7. Erikson EH: Childhood and Society, 2d ed. New York, WW Norton, 1963
8. Eysenck HJ: biological Basis of Personality. Springfield, IL, Charles C. Thomas, 1967
9. Millon T: The Disorders of Personality. In Pervin L (ed): Handbook of Personality Theory and Research, pp 339–370. New York, Guilford, 1990
10. O'Leary KD, Wilson GT: Behavior Therapy: Application and Outcome: Englewood Cliffs, NJ, Prentice-Hall, 1975
11. Plawecki H, Plawecki J: Act Your Age. Geriatr Nurs J 1 (September/October): 179–181, 1980
12. Roiphe H: A Theoretical Overview of Preoedipal Development During the First Four Years of Life. In Noshpitz JD (ed): Basic Handbook of Child Psychiatry, pp 118–127. New York, Basic Books, 1979.
13. Rosen H: Pathway to Piaget. Cherry Hill, NJ, Postgraduate International, 1977
14. Schaie KW: Psychological Changes From Midlife to Early Old Age: Implications for the Maintenance of Mental Health. Am J Orthopsychiatry 51 (April): 199–218, 1981
15. Singer JA, Salovey P: The Remembered Self. New York, Free Press, 1993
16. Stone MH: Abnormalities of Personality: Within and Beyond the Realm of Treatment. New York, WW Norton, 1993
17. Sullivan HS: Clinical Studies in Psychiatry. New York, WW Noton, 1956
18. Sullivan HS: The Fusion of Psychiatry and Social Science. New York, WW Norton, 1964
19. Thomas A: Current Trends in Developmental Theory. Am J Orthopsychiatry 51 (October): 580–609, 1981
20. Thomas A, Chess S: The Dynamics of Psychological Development. New York, Brunner/Mazel, 1980
21. Torgerson S: Temperamental Differences in Infants and 6-Yr. Old Children: A Follow-Up Study of Twins. In Strelau J, Farley FH, Gale A (eds): The Biological Basis of Personality and Behavior. Washington, DC, Hemisphere, 1985
22. Whiting S: A Delphi Study to Determine Defining Characteristics of Interdependence and Dysfunctional Independence as Potential Nursing Diagnoses. Issues in Mental Health Nursing, 15: 37–47, 1994

Children

Barbara Schoen Johnson

22

Modern living conditions have made it much more difficult for parents to create a setting in which both their own legitimate needs and the needs of their children can be satisfied with relative ease. That is why love is not enough and must be supplemented by deliberate efforts on the part of the parent. Fortunately most parents love their children and conscientiously strive to be good parents. But more and more of them become weary of the struggle to arrange life sensibly for their children, while modern pressures create more and more insensible experiences which are added to the life of the child.

Bruno Bettelheim,
Love Is Not Enough: The Treatment of Emotionally Disturbed Children, *1950*

Treating children whose behavior is troublesome is not a new phenomenon. In 1871 in the schools of New Haven, Connecticut, children with behavioral problems were labeled "contumacious aggressors" and segregated into their own special class. More than a century later, we are making progress in identifying and treating child mental disorders and in working with their families.

Nurses can have a significant impact on the mental health of children and their families. The nursing process is the problem-solving technique that helps nurses assess and diagnose mental health problems and plan, implement, and evaluate nursing interventions.

*This chapter examines the needs, problems, and challenges facing children with mental disorders and their families. It discusses the interventions and advocacy role of nurses and other mental health caregivers on behalf of children and families.**

Learning Objectives

On completion of this chapter, you should be able to accomplish the following:

1. *Discuss the incidence, prevalence, and causative or risk factors of mental disorders in children.*
2. *Describe the behavioral manifestations and dynamics of the mental disorders of childhood.*
3. *Assess the emotional, social, educational, and cultural needs and functioning of emotionally disturbed children within the context of their families.*
4. *Apply the nursing process to the care of mentally ill children and their families.*
5. *Identify measures to ameliorate the effects of multiple stressors and long-term exposure to stress on children's functioning.*
6. *Discuss the child advocacy role of psychiatric-mental health nurses.*

◆ Mental Illness in Children

INCIDENCE AND PREVALENCE

The problem of mental illness in children is a monumental one. Because various researchers use different criteria to measure childhood mental health or disorder, precise statistics regarding the amount and degree of mental illness in children are unavailable. Differences in the way disorder is defined, use of instruments, sampling, source of information, and ages examined also interfere with determining accurate incidence and prevalence of childhood mental illness. However, estimates of childhood disorder are possible.

The U.S. Congress Office of Technology Assessment in 1986 estimated that 12% to 15% of all children in the United States younger than 18 years (ie, about 7.5–9.5 million children and adolescents) need some level of psychiatric and mental health service, but only about 7% of these children receive the help they need.[65] In 1990, the U.S. Department of Health and Human Services reported that 17% to 22% of children (or 11–14 million children) suffer some type of diagnosable mental disorder.[66]

EFFECTS OF CHILDHOOD MENTAL ILLNESS

The effects of childhood mental illness are staggering. Many untreated children develop into seriously mentally ill adults.[65] Almost half of children with conduct disorder become antisocial adults. Untreated depression in children and young adolescents often results in chronic depression in later adolescence; chronic depression, especially in girls, often continues into adulthood.[66]

Other effects of these disorders are less obvious—guilt, shame, unfulfilled hopes of families, and unmet needs of siblings. Families and society bear the financial burdens of direct care costs and the costs of special education, physical health care, juvenile justice, and child welfare systems. More than 12 million children in the United States have limited or no access to health care because they lack health insurance.[10]

ETIOLOGY

The etiology of mental and emotional disorders is multifactorial; that is, no single causal agent is responsible for mental disorder in children. A risk factor or factors may cause a child to be vulnerable to disorder so that a particular situation may activate psychopathology.

Examining the rates of childhood psychiatric disorder according to the frequency of risk factors reveals that negative outcomes increase progressively. For example, if one risk factor is present in a family, studies show not much difference in incidence of disorder than if no risk factors are present. However, if two risk factors are present, there is a fourfold increase in the likelihood of a psychiatric disorder in children. The presence of four risk factors increases the likelihood of disorder 10-fold.[18] This evidence certainly reinforces the belief that multiple stressors and long-term exposure to stress have deleterious effects on children.

**Also see displays in Chapter 23, Adolescence, for additional DSM-IV criteria relevant to disorders of childhood.*

Risk Factors

The Office of Technology Assessment has identified seven specific groups of children at high risk for mental and emotional disorder:

1. Children of poverty
2. Children of mentally ill and substance-abusing parents
3. Children who are abused
4. Children of minority ethnic status
5. Children of teenage parents
6. Children in families with parental conflict or divorce
7. Children with chronic illness or disability[65]

Two other health threats with serious mental health consequences for children are acquired immunodeficiency syndrome and homelessness.[28]

Children of Poverty. Children are the poorest group of American citizens, and their numbers are growing. Of the nation's population younger than 6 years, 26% live below the federally established poverty level ($11,000 for a family of three and $14,000 for a family of four), according to a report from the National Center for Children in Poverty.[37] This figure means that the United States is now the only industrialized nation in the world whose children are the poorest segment of the population.[5] More than half of these children (57%) live in families in which one or both parents work but still cannot earn enough to lift them out of poverty.[37] Poverty cuts across ethnic groups, regions of the country, and family constellations.

Poverty should be seen as an indicator "that all is not well for the next generation and that strategic [public policy] steps should be taken" (p 175).[35] This would include providing access to health care, appropriate child care, employment training for the adult caretakers, and family support services for children.

Poverty compromises family functioning and increases the health risks of children.[5] Poverty denies children adequate housing, medical care, nutrition, and school and play environments. Parents in poverty live under chronic stress and have an increased likelihood of other risk factors for childhood mental and emotional disorders.[24]

Children of Mentally Ill and Substance-Abusing Parents. Children of mentally ill parents are at risk because their parents suffer a biological or biochemical brain disease; they also undergo multiple separations from their parents and are poorly stimulated in infancy. The severity and chronicity of the parent's illness, rather than the parent's diagnosis of schizophrenia, bipolar illness, or other disorder, are critical in predicting the child's level of functioning.[22]

In the United States in 1991, 375,000 newborns were exposed to drugs prenatally; 80% of these babies were exposed to cocaine. Recent research about the long-term effects of maternal crack cocaine addiction on children's development includes emotional neglect and abuse, including unavailability to and physical neglect of the children. The children of crack-addicted mothers show signs of behavioral and emotional problems, particularly aggression and withdrawal.[25] Effects of parental alcoholism on children include decreased intellectual ability, behavior disorders, substance abuse, criminality, depression, and suicide.

Children Who Are Abused. More than 2 million children are abused in the United States each year.[21] Physically, emotionally, and sexually abused children are at risk for many emotional and behavioral disorders throughout their lives, especially post-traumatic stress disorder and depressive disorders.[2] Other effects include shame, powerlessness, guilt, anxiety, low self-esteem, chemical dependency, sexual acting out, somatic complaints, poor school performance, sleep disorders, runaway and criminal behavior, and suicide attempts.[14]

Abuse in any form is in direct contrast to the ideal of nurturing, healthy environments for optimal child development. Abuse gives the child the messages that the world is not a safe place and that adults are not to be trusted (see Chapter 41, Violence Within the Family).

The exact incidence of sexual abuse of children is unknown but is estimated to be 60,000 to 100,000 cases per year and rising.[47] Sexual abuse may occur within or outside the family from people such as teachers or child care employees. Sexually abused children are particularly at risk for short- and long-term disorders, including post-traumatic stress and dissociative disorders.[61] Sexually abusive youths are usually victims of sexual abuse themselves; in a recent study, sexually abusive youth reported histories of physical and sexual abuse, neglect, and loss of a parental figure.[55]

Children of Minority Ethnic Status. Children of minority ethnic status experience adverse effects related to their ethnicity due to the double impact of poverty and racism in America. Nearly half of all African American children and more than 40% of Hispanic American children live in poverty. Fifty-four percent of young African-American children and 44% of young nonwhite Hispanic children live in poverty.[37] Children in the Native American and Native Alaskan populations have a high rate of mental and emotional disorder, especially substance abuse and adolescent suicide. Ethnicity and social class influence a child's developmental progress, attitudes about parenting, and parent–child interaction patterns. Minority children and their parents are a rapidly growing segment of the population whose mental health needs cannot be ignored.

Children of Teenage Parents. Every year more than 1 million teenagers become pregnant.[30] Estimates of projected teenage pregnancy and parenting rates are staggering and disheartening. Teenage parents are more likely to have premature or low–birth-weight infants and children with health problems. Moreover, teenage parents are less likely to have the physical, mental, and emotional maturity to deal constructively with the stressors that children add to family life.[31]

Children in Families With Parental Conflict or Divorce. Approximately 59% of children in the United States live at some point in their lives in a single-parent home. More than 15 million children and 54% of young poor children are living in a single-parent home.[42] A major factor in the rising number of poor women and children is divorce. The loss of a parent by death, divorce, or desertion is a significant one; the effect on the child may be overlooked or denied by the remaining, and often grief-stricken, parent.[43]

A recent study compared the psychosocial coping resources of elementary school children living with their sole-custody divorced parent to those of peers living with nondivorced parents. Children of divorce reported lower levels of self-esteem, self-efficacy, and social support and a restricted range of coping measures.[36]

Children With Chronic Illness and Disability. Most children with chronic conditions do not develop psychopathology; however, the chronic illness or disability is a life stressor that increases the risk of mental of disorder.[16] A child with epilepsy is five times more likely to have psychological problems than is a child without a chronic illness; a child with cerebral palsy, a speech impairment, or other handicapping conditions also has a higher risk of emotional problems.[7] Although it was previously believed that children with mental retardation were "untroubled" emotionally, it is now recognized that they are more likely to have emotional problems than are children with average intelligence.[67]

Sociocultural Factors

Identifying sociocultural factors in the development of childhood mental disorders has been elusive because the case finders may operate from middle-class biases. The reverse may be true: A behavior seen as a sign of a serious emotional problem in a middle-income child may be discounted in a child from a low socioeconomic group.

Sociocultural factors in the etiology of psychiatric disorders are probably less important in children than in adults, because most children function within a familial matrix that operates as a remarkably effective buffer to social change. Although children may be relatively undisturbed within the family environment when young, they increasingly come into contact with the larger society as they grow and develop. Stable, nurturing influences in the child's family life can safeguard him or her significantly; chronic and pervasive adverse influences produce adverse outcomes in children.[34]

Neurobiological Factors

Neuroimaging techniques have advanced the understanding of brain anatomy and function in children. Some of the neurobiological findings include the following:

1. In autism, regional structural abnormalities, such as localized parietal and frontal volume loss; possible neuronal migration abnormalities from the period of early central nervous system development, suggesting a pathophysiological insult in the first 6 months of gestation; possible hypermetabolism and abnormal cell metabolism in the prefrontal cortex; and possible increased cortical and ventricular cerebrospinal fluid (CSF)
2. In schizophrenia, decreased metabolism in the frontal cortex, probable reduced frontal cortex volumes, possible reduced amygdala and hippocampus volumes, possible reduced asymmetries of the temporal lobe and cortical surface, increased cortical CSF, increased size of the temporal horn of left lateral ventricle, larger basal ganglia, and decreased metabolism in basal ganglia
3. In attention-deficit hyperactivity disorder (ADHD), reduced cross-sectional area of copus callosum subregions, possible absence of normal caudate nucleus asymmetry, and possible sulcal widening[48]

Genetic influences may be evident in the development of disorders of childhood. Some people may have a genetic predisposition to handle stress poorly.

Stress

Although it is generally thought that multiple stressors impact negatively on the individual, it is possible that stress may inoculate some children against emotional disorders by causing them and their parents to develop effective coping responses.

One long-term study of children's development under stressful conditions found that children with greater assets—such as higher intelligence quotient (IQ), higher socioeconomic status, and positive family attributes of stability and cohesion—appeared to be more competent; under stress, they were more socially engaged with their peers and in their classrooms. Children with fewer assets, however, appeared to be more disruptive, especially when under stress. Higher IQ and higher socioeconomic status—and for girls, more positive family attributes—appeared to be protective factors against disruptive or aggressive responses to stress. Children in families with lower socioeconomic status and fewer positive qualities of stability, cohesion, and organization were more likely to be exposed to stressful life experiences and less likely to be intellectually able or competent to deal with these experiences. The effects of these stressful events and multiple risk factors appear to be cumulative.[18]

Parents and Families

Parents and families have a powerful effect on a child's growth and development. All parents bring their own concerns and anxieties to the task of child rearing. The parents' feelings of fear, guilt, depression, anxiety, love, and concern shape the child's developing sense of self and the world.

An important task of families is maintaining two essential family boundaries—the generational boundary and the division between the two sexes. The generational boundary divides the family into the parents, who nurture, lead, and direct, and the children, who are nurtured, follow, and learn. Division of the sexes results in gender awareness, identification, and security.

Disturbances in family functioning are multidimensional; a problem of one family member exists not in a vacuum, but as a function of family dynamics. There are five areas of family task deficiencies:

1. Individual disorder of a parent, such as a schizophrenic mother or alcoholic father
2. Deviant parental coalitions, such as chronic parental discord or triangling of relationships
3. Faulty nurturance, such as failure to promote the child's growth toward independence or child abuse
4. Faulty enculturation, such as parental behavior that is dramatically atypical of the surrounding culture and leads to the children's nonacceptance by others
5. Problems in independence, which are likely to surface in disturbance after the child has reached adulthood, married, and become a parent, thereby continuing the cycle of emotional disorder from one generation to the next

One of the unique features of parenting is that child development may be thought of not only as a result of parental actions, but also as an extension of the parent's self. What parents, including emotionally disturbed parents, believe about the world and their place in it may be extended to their children. For example, a parent who is depressed is likely to perceive himself or herself as helpless, and perhaps hopeless, and to perceive others in the environment, including his or her children, as victims of chance happenings. The effects of this cognitive pattern of helplessness on the child of a depressed mother would reinforce a depressive outlook on life.

◆ The Childhood Disorders

Some mental and emotional disorders are specific to childhood, such as conduct disorders and infantile autism. Others may be variations of adult disturbances. For example, many of the symptoms of depressive and bipolar disorders in young populations are similar to those of adults (see Chapter 29, Depressive and Bipolar Disorders); however, behaviors that are age dependent are presented in this chapter.

The eating disorders of anorexia nervosa and bulimia, which often surface in late childhood or adolescence, are discussed in Chapter 34, Eating Disorders. Chapter 33, Substance Abuse and Dependency, discusses the problems of psychoactive substance use disorders. The emotional and behavioral problems related to abuse of children are monumental; Chapters 32, Dissociative Disorders, and 41, Violence Within the Family, provide further information.

Criteria from the Diagnostic and Statistical Manual of Mental Disorders, fourth edition (DSM-IV), for several of the following disorders are found throughout this chapter.

ATTENTION-DEFICIT AND DISRUPTIVE BEHAVIOR DISORDERS

The grouping of attention-deficit and disruptive behavior disorders includes ADHD, oppositional-defiant disorder, and conduct disorder.

Attention-Deficit Hyperactivity Disorder

For more than 20 years, hyperactivity has been perhaps the most frequently diagnosed child psychiatric disorder. Formerly called *hyperkinetic reaction of childhood, minimal brain damage,* and *minimal brain dysfunction,* the disorder was eventually termed *attention-deficit hyperactivity disorder* (ADHD). This disorder is a persistent pattern of inattention or hyperactivity-impulsivity that is more frequent and severe than other children (or any-age individuals) of comparable developmental level.[2]

The diagnosis of ADHD requires that the child show signs of inattention or hyperactivity-impulsivity (Box 22-1). Symptoms of *inattention* include the following:

1. Failing to attend closely to detail or making careless mistakes
2. Difficulty attending to tasks or play
3. Not seeming to listen when addressed
4. Failing to follow through on instructions or to finish schoolwork and duties
5. Having difficulty organizing tasks and activities
6. Avoiding, disliking, or delaying tasks that require sustained mental effort, such as schoolwork

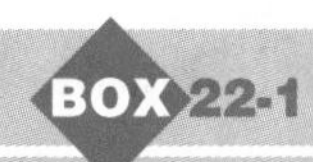

DSM-IV Diagnostic Criteria for Attention-Deficit/ Hyperactivity Disorder

A. Either (1) or (2):

(1) six (or more) of the following symptoms of **inattention** have persisted for at least 6 months to a degree that is maladaptive and inconsistent with developmental level:

Inattention

(a) often fails to give close attention to details or makes careless mistakes in schoolwork, work, or other activities
(b) often has difficulty sustaining attention in tasks or play activities
(c) Often does not seem to listen when spoken to directly
(d) often does not follow through on instructions and fails to finish schoolwork, chores, or duties in the workplace (not due to oppositional behavior or failure to understand instructions)
(e) often has difficulty organizing tasks and activities
(f) often avoids, dislikes, or is reluctant to engage in tasks that require sustained mental effort (such as schoolwork or homework)
(g) often loses things necessary for tasks or activities (eg, toys, school assignments, pencils, books, or tools)
(h) is often easily distracted by extraneous stimuli
(i) is often forgetful in daily activities

(2) six (or more) of the following symptoms of **hyperactivity-impulsivity** have persisted for at least 6 months to a degree that is maladaptive and inconsistent with developmental level:

Hyperactivity

(a) often fidgets with hands or feet or squirms in seat
(b) often leaves seat in classroom or in other situations in which remaining seated is expected
(c) often runs about or climbs excessively in situations in which it is inappropriate (in adolescents or adults, may be limited to subjective feelings or restlessness)
(d) often has difficulty playing or engaging in leisure activities quietly
(e) is often "on the go" or often acts as if "driven by a motor"
(f) often talks excessively

Impulsivity

(g) often blurts out answers before questions have been completed
(h) often has difficulty awaiting turn
(i) often interrupts or intrudes on others (eg, butts into conversations or games)

B. Some hyperactive-impulsive or inattentive symptoms that caused impairment were present before age 7 years.

C. Some impairment from the symptoms is present in two or more settings (eg, at school and at home).

D. There must be clear evidence of clinically significant impairment in social, academic, or occupational functioning.

7. Losing things necessary for tasks, such as books and papers
8. Being easily distracted by extraneous stimuli and forgetful in daily activities

Symptoms of *hyperactivity* include the following:

1. Fidgeting withhands or feet or squirming in seat
2. Often leaving seat in class or other situations in which remaining seated is expected
3. Running around or climbing excessively and inappropriately
4. Having difficulty playing or participating in leisure activities quietly
5. Being "on the go" often or acting as if "driven by a motor"
6. Often talking excessively

Symptoms of *impulsivity* include the following:

1. Often blurting out answers before hearing entire question
2. Often having difficulty awaiting turn
3. Often interrupting or intruding on others[2]

In addition, the child's behavior must cause significant impairment in two or more settings (ie, school and home) that affect social and academic functioning.[2]

Children with attention-deficit disorders are usually referred for treatment of the following problems:

1. Difficulty in learning, leading to school failure
2. Difficulty relating to peers
3. Difficulty complying with adult requests and commands

Children with ADHD are considered more difficult, aggressive, and disruptive than nonhyperactive children. They engage more frequently in risk-taking behavior, often resulting in accidents and injuries. They are more likely to be academic underachievers, although they do not score significantly lower on intelligence tests. However, their inability to sustain attention, control impulsivity, and control activity level leads to behavioral difficulties for the child and his or her family. The problem behaviors of impulsivity, distractibility, and excessive activity are inappropriate to certain structured environments, such as school.

Children of parents with childhood-onset ADHD are at high risk for the disorder. A study showed that 84% of adults with ADHD had at least one child with ADHD, and 52% had two or more children with the disorder.[6]

Treatment. Treatment includes providing structure and predictability within the home and school environment through routines. The child also is taught to slow down and think before speaking or acting, perhaps by using the image of a slow turtle who does his work slowly but carefully.

Other valuable approaches include compassionate understanding; role playing; relaxation; reinforcement of positive behaviors; consistency of expectations and in scheduling the day; a nonstimulating work environment; simple and clear instructions; logical consequences; positive self-expression; notes and lists to assist the child's memory; help in organizing schoolwork, room, and life; and provision of outlets for excess energy. Reframing of behavior is helpful; being a child "with lots of energy" is far preferable to being a hyperactive or impulsive child. Psychostimulant medication, such as methylphenidate (Ritalin), often improves the symptoms of inattention and impulsivity (Box 22-2).

Oppositional-Defiant Disorder

Oppositional-defiant disorder is a recurrent pattern of negativistic, defiant, disobedient, and hostile behavior toward authority figures. The child loses his or her temper, argues with adults, actively defies adults or refuses to comply with their requests, deliberately does things to annoy others, blames others for his or her own mistakes or misbehavior, and is touchy, easily annoyed by others, angry, resentful, spiteful, or vindictive.[2] The child resists directions from adults and is persistently stubborn and unwilling to compromise with adults or peers. He or she may test limits by ignoring orders, arguing, and refusing to accept blame for wrongdoings. Hostility is directed at adults and peers, often by verbal aggression. Usually the child does not engage in physical aggression, which is seen in conduct disorder.[2]

These behaviors occur more frequently than is typically observed in children of the same age. They cause significant impairment in the child's functioning at home and school and with peers. The disorder is more prevalent in boys than in prepubertal girls, but this is more equal after puberty.[2]

Treatment. Treatment requires providing consistent rules with logical consequences, helping the child identify anger and find acceptable ways to express it, and using a variety of behavioral interventions, including social skills training and role playing. Rational-emotive therapy may teach the child ways to manage anger[53] (Case Study 22-1).

Conduct Disorder

A repetitive and persistent pattern of behavior in which the child violates the basic rights of others or major age-appropriate social norms or rules is termed a *conduct disorder*.[2] The child with a conduct disorder displays antisocial behavior in the form of physical violence against another person, theft outside the home, fire setting, assault, or callous or manipulative behavior.

Children with conduct disorders may engage in the following behaviors:

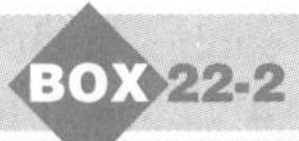

Example of: Medication Education for Families—Methylphenidate (Ritalin)

Use: Stimulant medications such as methylphenidate have been shown to be a safe and effective method of treatment of children with attention-deficit hyperactivity disorder (ADHD).

Purpose: Methylphenidate can reduce the symptoms of ADHD, which oftens results in improved relationships with family, teachers, and friends and improved performance on tasks such as school work.

Medication alone is not as powerful in reducing the symptoms of ADHD as the combination of behavior modification plus medication. Behavior modification includes structuring the child's daily activities, helping the child organize school work assignments and room, decreasing stimulation during tasks, using written notes and lists as reminders of responsibilities, and providing consistent assistance and expectations.

Drug holidays (periods when the child does not take the medication) should be taken at least yearly, usually in the summer, and some children stop taking the medication during weekends.

The usual dose of methylphenidate is 5 mg twice a day before breakfast and lunch, but if the child experiences decreased appetite, the medication may be taken with meals. Often the dose is raised until maximum benefits are seen. Some children require a third dose if they are having great difficulty with homework in the evening. The daily dose range is 5 to 60 mg/d.

Methylphenidate does not relieve ADHD symptoms in every child who takes the medication. It has a number of side effects, including nervousness, irritability, rapid heart beat, headache, insomnia, poor appetite with possible weight loss, unstable mood, and decreased physical growth. Height and weight should be monitored during treatment. Some of the side effects improve as the child continues to take the medication, or reduction of the dosage may help. Methylphenidate should never be taken by a child with a tic disorder. The child should be examined by the primary care provider yearly, including a physical examination, complete blood count, and liver function tests.

REFERENCES

Campbell M, Cueva JE: Psychopharmacology in Child and Adolescent Psychiatry: A Review of the Past Seven Years. Part I. J Am Acad Child Adolesc Psychiatry 34(9): 1124–1132, 1995

Pearson GS: Psychopharmacology. In Johnson BS (ed): Child, Adolescent and Family Psychiatric Nursing, pp 410–423. Philadelphia, J.B. Lippincott, 1995

Scahill L, Lynch KA: The Use of Methylphenidate in Children With Attention-Deficit Hyperactivity Disorder. Journal of Child and Adolescent Psychiatric Nursing 7(4): 44–47, 1994

1. Aggressive conduct causes or threatens physical harm to other people or animals. This behavior includes bullying, threatening, or intimidating others; initiating physical fights frequently; using a weapon that can cause physical harm to others, such as a bat, brick, knife, or gun; exhibiting physical cruelty to animals; forcing someone into sexual activity; exhibiting physical cruelty to people or animals; and stealing during a mugging, armed robbery, and so forth.
2. Nonaggressive conduct causes property loss or damage. This behavior includes deliberately setting fires to cause serious damage and destroying the property of others.
3. Deceitfulness or theft includes breaking into some-

Case Study

Designing Treatment for a Girl With Oppositional Behavior

Samantha is a 12-year-old girl who is admitted to a residential treatment center after her mother declared she could "no longer handle that girl!"

Samantha and her younger sister, now 9 years old, were born to a single mother who has had a history of recurrent depression. Throughout Samantha's life, her mother has had a number of "boyfriends" who have moved in and out of her home. Several times, at 6, 9, and 11 years, Samantha has been sexually abused by these men living in their home. At 9 and 11 years, Samantha told her mother about the abuse, but her mother did not believe her daughter. In the last 2 years, Samantha has become increasingly negative and rebellious, refusing to follow her mother's rules.

Most recently, Samantha has become irritable, stubborn, and verbally hostile. She argues with her mother and teachers, teases her sister, has angry outbursts, and refuses to comply with her mother's and teacher's requests.

Samantha arrived at the residential treatment center wearing heavy makeup, dyed black hair, a nose ring, a skin-tight top, and blue jeans. Throughout the interview, she spoke rudely to her mother and the admitting nurse.

Questions for Discussion

1. Based on Samantha's history, which childhood disorder most fits with her presenting behavior?
2. Identify nursing diagnoses that describe Samantha's symptoms and situation.
3. Create an initial nursing care plan for Samantha and her family.
4. Explain in lay terms the nature of Samantha's behavioral problems as though you were speaking to her mother.

one's home, building, or car and frequently lying to get favors or items of value without confronting a victim, such as forgery or shoplifting.

4. Serious violations of rules include staying out at night despite parents' prohibiting this behavior and before age 13, running away from home and being frequently truant.[2]

The behavior pattern causes significant impairment in the child's social and academic functioning.

One of the ways a child may act out feelings of rejection, isolation, and hostility is through cruelty to animals. This usually occurs concomitant with certain other symptoms, such as aggressiveness to younger siblings and other small children, fire setting, inappropriate interest in sex, enuresis, learning problems, hoarding, bulimia, and imperviousness to pain.[62] This behavior is seen most often in young and preadolescent boys (8–10 years). Although cruelty to animals and the associated symptoms may indicate a personality disturbance, they occur most commonly in children from chaotic homes with aggressive, violent parental models.[62]

Fire setting is a dangerous symptom that must be controlled rapidly. Children who set fires also typically display other forms of acting out, including running away, stealing, lying, truancy, and sexual acting out.

Treatment. Treatment is aimed at maintaining safety and helping the child develop internal limits, problem solving, and self-responsibility. It includes cognitive techniques of self-talk to decrease impulsivity; consistency in rules, expectations, and consequences; deescalation of aggressive episodes; parent training to avoid nagging, yelling, arguing, and angry interactions; and neuroleptic medication to decrease aggressive behavior (Nursing Care Plan 22–1).[11]

PERVASIVE DEVELOPMENTAL DISORDERS

The pervasive developmental disorders are characterized by severe and global impairment in communication and interpersonal skills or the presence of stereotypical behavior and activities.[2]

Autistic Disorder

Austistic disorder, sometimes called *early infantile autism, childhood autism,* or *Kanner's autism,* because it was first described by Leo Kanner in 1943, is a rare pervasive developmental disorder. The onset of autistic disorder occurs in infancy or childhood. Rates of autism are four to five times higher in boys. Mental retardation in the moderate range is often associated with the disorder.[2]

Autistic disorder is characterized by impaired social interaction and communication and a restricted repertoire of activity and interests.[2] The distinguishing characteristics are a lack of responsiveness to others, withdrawal from social contact, gross impairment in communication, and bizarre responses to the environment, such as a peculiar interest in or attachment to animate or inanimate objects and insistence on routines. The onset of these behaviors is evident before 3 years.

Nursing Care Plan 22-1

A Child With a Conduct Disorder

Twelve-year-old Michael was recently arrested for shoplifting $300 worth of merchandise from a local mall. This is his third arrest; at age 11 he was arrested for mugging an elderly woman to steal her purse, and earlier this year he pressured his peers to vandalize the school with him. His parents report that he has "no real friends," he "does whatever he wants," and that they fear his violent outbursts. Once he hit his father and has threatened to do it again.

Nursing Diagnosis

High Risk for Violence directed toward others.

Outcome

The child will not injure others.

Intervention	Rationale
Allow the child to role play a situation that "makes him mad" and see how anger is handled; teach acceptable ways to deal with angry feelings, such as using a punching bag, pounding a pillow, shooting baskets.	Consistency in expectations and consequences for behavior reinforces that unacceptable behavior, such as violence, is not tolerated.
Reinforce the child's use of verbal communication to express his feelings, instead of physical aggression.	Verbal expression of feelings is preferable to physical aggression.
Establish and consistently enforce rules about not hurting self, others, or property.	Safety for child and others is a priority.
Restrain the child physically when necessary.	
Interrupt a physical outburst before an aggressive act occurs; if the child does commit an aggressive act, have him or her "undo" the behavior as much as possible; for example, if he throws a chair, allow him a period of time to calm down, then have him pick up the chair and place it in its proper position.	De-escalation before aggressive, violent behavior occurs is preferable to restraining or secluding a child.
Provide a structured environment.	Structure places environmental limits on child's behavior.

Evaluation

Child does not display aggressive or violent behavior toward others.

Nursing Diagnosis

Ineffective Individual Coping related to poor frustration tolerance

Outcome

The child will delay gratification of needs and verbalize that he has thought about the consequences of an action before engaging in it at least 3 times a day.

continued

Nursing Care Plan 22-1 *(Continued)*

Intervention	Rationale
Help the child identify situations in which he had an angry or violent outburst.	Children with conduct disorder exhibit angry outbursts, in part, related to their poor tolerance of frustration.
Teach the child to think before acting; for example, by allowing a pause, which reinforces cause and effect	The child learns skills to cope with frustration by becoming aware of situations in which he is likely to become frustrated and learning to delay gratification

Evaluation

Child demonstrates increased tolerance of frustration and fewer episodes of violent behavior.

Nursing Diagnosis

Impaired Social Interaction related to manipulative relationships with peers

Outcome

The child will interact appropriately with peers.

Intervention	Rationale
Include child in a "social skills" class that teaches about productive interpersonal relationships through demonstration and role playing.	Demonstrations of healthy interpersonal skills and relationships role model expected social behavior for the child.
Point out to him when his interactions with peers involve behaviors that are manipulative or have other negative effects and discuss alternative ways to interact.	Helping the child identify his impaired social behaviors and alternative behaviors promotes social skill development.

Evaluation

Child interacts with peers without "using" or manipulating them.

Children with autistic disorder exhibit gross and sustained impairment in social interaction through markedly impaired awareness of others, lack of social or emotional reciprocity, lack of interest in seeking comfort or affection, and failure to develop peer relationships.

Autistic children also exhibit impaired communication, such as delayed or absent spoken language, abnormal nonverbal communication (stiffening when held), and abnormal pitch, rate, or rhythm of speech; stereotypical and repetitive use of language or idiosyncratic language; and absent or impaired imaginative play.

As infants, autistic children fail to respond to the sight or sounds of others. They give no evidence of a social smile or of pleasure in being with the mother or mothering figure. They do not physically reach out; they have no reaction to strangers. Because they are not demanding and do not fuss when separated from parents, these children are sometimes mistakenly called "very good babies." Social games, such as peek-a-boo, do not interest autistic children.

The autistic child fails to use speech for the purpose of communication. The child may not talk or may talk in a mechanical, parrotlike manner. Stereotypical or nonsensical phrases may be repeated, or what is said to the child may be echoed. If a certain word results in getting what the child wants, the word may be used over and over by the child—not according to its meaning. The child is unable to generalize word usage. These children may be so unresponsive that deafness is suspected. The child's response to sounds is likely to be inconsistent. If the autistic child has speech, it is likely to be echolalic and a private language. For example, a child may use the third-person pronoun to refer to himself, indicating poor differentiation of self from others, and may reverse other pronouns.

Restricted patterns of behavior and activities, such as an insistence on sameness, preoccupation with small objects, stereotyped body movements (hand flicking, spinning), and very restricted range of interests, are seen in children with autism.[2] The child may engage in rocking, twirling, other self-stimulatory or self-injurious behavior, such as head-banging.

The autistic child is usually fascinated with objects, especially those that spin, twirl, or reflect light and shadow. An important differentiation is that the normal child values a toy largely because it came from a parent; an autistic child finds joy in the toy's ability to be spun, manipulated, rolled, rocked, or put together (Box 22-3).

Autism is a long-term disorder. It seems to be due to biological factors because its occurrence is sometimes associated with maternal rubella, phenylketonuria (PKU), fragile X syndrome, encephalitis, and meningitis.[2] It is unclear whether the development of autistic children follows an erratic course, a steady rate, or a stable rate within a specific area of development with time.[60] About 75% of autistic children function at a retarded level.[2] Even when children are not retarded, their idiosyncratic speech and behavior may give the appearance that they are. Cognitive skill development

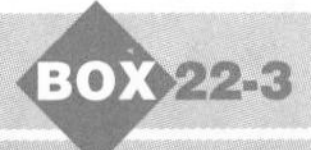
BOX 22-3

DSM-IV Diagnostic Criteria for Autistic Disorder

A. A total of six (or more) items from (1), (2), and (3), with at least two from (1) and one each from (2) and (3):
   - (1) qualitative impairment in social interaction, as manifested by at least two of the following:
     - (a) marked impairment in the use of multiple nonverbal behaviors, such as eye-to-eye gaze, facial expression, body postures, and gestures to regulate social interaction
     - (b) failure to develop peer relationships appropriate to developmental level
     - (c) a lack of spontaneous seeking to share enjoyment, interests, or achievements with other people
     - (d) lack of social or emotional reciprocity
   - (2) qualitative impairments in communication as manifested by at least one of the following:
     - (a) delay in, or total lack of, the development of spoken language (not accompanied by an attempt to compensate through alternative modes of communication, such as gesture or mime)
     - (b) in individuals with adequate speech, marked impairment in the ability to initiate or sustain a conversation with others
     - (c) stereotyped and repetitive use of language or idiosyncratic language
     - (d) lack of varied, spontaneous make-believe play or social imitative play appropriate to developmental level
   - (3) restricted repetitive and stereotyped patterns of behavior, interests, and activities, as manifested by at least one of the following:
     - (a) encompassing preoccupation with one or more stereotyped and restricted patterns of interest that is abnormal in intensity or focus
     - (b) apparently inflexible adherence to specific, nonfunctional routines or rituals
     - (c) stereotyped and repetitive motor mannerisms (eg, hand or finger flapping or twisting, or complex whole-body movements)
     - (d) persistent preoccupation with parts of objects

B. Delays or abnormal functioning in at least one of the following areas with onset prior to age 3 years: (1) social interaction, (2) language as used in social communication, or (3) symbolic or imaginative play.

C. The disturbance is not better accounted for by Rett's Disorder or Childhood Disintegrative Disorder.

may be impaired. The ultimate prognosis of individuals with autistic disorder is related to language skills and overall cognitive development.[2]

Treatment. Treatment of autistic and disintegrative behavior described in the following section consists of special education, extended day services, parent training, respite services for caregivers, a structured and stable environment, medication to manage behavioral problems, and play therapy through which the child can learn cognitive, social, and emotional skills.[45] Haloperidol (Haldol) and thioridazine (Mellaril) manage hyperactivity and stereotypical behavior[1] (Nursing Care Plan 22-2).

Childhood Disintegrative Disorder

Childhood disintegrative disorder is characterized by regression in many areas of functioning after at least 2 years of normal development and before the age of 10 years. The child may lose skill in language use, social skills, bladder or bowel control, play, or motor skills. This rare disorder is usually associated with severe mental retardation.[2]

This disorder is also characterized by behaviors similar to autistic disorder, such as impaired social interaction (lack of peer relationships, impaired nonverbal behaviors, lack of social and emotional reciprocity); impaired communication (delay or lack of spoken language, stereotypical and repetitive language, lack of make-believe play); and behavior, interests, and activities that are stereotyped and restricted.[2] Sometimes this loss of previously developed skills is preceded by increased activity, anxiety, irritability, and loss of speech (Box 22-4). It is a long-term and usually incapacitating disorder.

TIC DISORDERS

A *tic* is a sudden, repetitive movement, gesture, or utterance. Tics are of brief duration and frequently occur in bouts.[39] Although they are experienced as irresistible, they can be suppressed for varying amounts of time. They may be increased during periods of stress and lessened during absorbing activity.[2]

Simple motor tics include blinking the eyes, jerking the neck, facial grimacing, or coughing. *Complex motor tics* may be facial gestures, jumping, smelling an object, and stamping the feet. *Simple vocal tics* include clearing the throat, snorting, barking, and sniffing. *Complex vocal tics* may be repeating words or phrases out of context, coprolalia (using socially unacceptable words, often obscene), echolalia (repeating the sound or word last heard), or palilalia (repeating one's own words).[39]

Tic disorders include Tourette's disorder and chronic motor or vocal tic disorder.

Tourette's Disorder

Tourette's disorder is the most severe tic disorder. It is characterized by multiple motor tics and one or more vocal tics. The tics occur many times throughout the day for 1 year or more. The disorder impairs the child's functioning with peers and family and in school.[2]

Obsessions and compulsions, hyperactivity, disinhibited speech or behavior, and impulsivity may be associated with this syndrome. In addition, the child may suffer depression, school failure, and behavior problems (Box 22-5).[39]

Chronic Motor or Vocal Tic Disorder

Chronic motor or vocal tic disorder is characterized by the presence of motor or vocal tics but not both types. Motor tics of the upper extremities are the most common, and vocal tics are less common. Symptoms often develop between the ages of 6 and 10 years and have a waxing and waning course (Box 22-6).[39]

Treatment. Treatment of tic disorders involves education and supportive intervention with the child and family, school intervention, individual counseling or psychotherapy, family therapy and parent guidance, and pharmacotherapy with agents such as haloperidol, pimozide, clonidine, desipramine, fluoxetine, clomipramine, and sertraline.[39]

ANXIETY DISORDERS

Anxiety may be defined as a fear that is not justified by reality or as an extreme reaction to a real threat. The younger the child, the more difficult is the separation of inner and outer reality. Some symptoms of anxiety disorders are similar for adults and children; the differences are identified (see Chapter 25, Anxiety Disorders).

Obsessive-Compulsive Disorder

Obsessive-compulsive disorder (OCD) is characterized by the presence of recurrent intrusive thoughts (obsessions) and repetitive behaviors that the person realizes are senseless but necessary to perform (compulsions). Obsessions and compulsions consume hours of the day and are a source of distress to the child.[58]

Family and genetic studies have shown that the disorder occurs more frequently than expected in family members of people with OCD and Tourette's disorder, which indicates an inherited vulnerability to the disorder.[58]

Treatment. Treatment includes behavioral intervention within a highly structured environment. Particularly useful in treatment are *exposure* (deliberately confronting the client with stimuli that trigger obsessional

(text continues on page 390)

Nursing Care Plan 22-2

A Child With Autism

Seven-year-old Stanley spends his days in solitary activities, He ''jiggles'' pieces of paper, twirls the wheels on toy cars, rocks back and forth, and smiles. He shows no interest in playing with peers and appears to not notice when they are nearby. He rejects human touch and becomes very upset if his routine is disrupted in even the smallest way.

His language is usually echolalic, without understandable meaning, and delivered in a high-pitched voice. The quality of his school work is sporadic, but even at its best, it is far behind the level expected of a 7-year-old.

Nursing Diagnosis

Altered Sensory-perception related to diminished awareness of surroundings and interactions

Outcome

Child will remain safe.

Intervention	Rationale
Assess the child's judgment.	
Provide supervision to ensure safety; 1:1 supervision may be required.	Providing safety is an essential nursing responsibility while caring for a child with deficient self-protective behaviors.
Provide a predictable environment.	Child is more comfortable in a predictable environment.

Evaluation

Child is not injured.

Nursing Diagnosis

Ineffective Individual Coping related to ritualistic behavior, as evidenced by rocking, tearing paper, flipping a straw, twirling, placing shoes in a certain order, rubbing the rim of a glass before taking a drink

Outcome

The child will engage in ritualistic behavior for shorter periods each week.

Intervention	Rationale
Allow certain amounts of time to perform these rituals, then move the child into the expected activity.	Prohibiting the child from performing these rituals would increase his anxiety.
Do not reward rituals by smiling or laughing at the behavior.	Accepting, in a matter-of-fact manner, the child's need to engage in ritualistic behavior communicates respect for him and his level of functioning.

Evaluation

Child engages in ritualistic behavior for shorter periods of time.

continued

Nursing Care Plan 22-2 *(Continued)*

Nursing Diagnosis

Impaired Verbal Communication related to inadequate verbal skills, as evidenced by disjointed, inappropriate speech

Outcome

The child will imitate staff and parents who role model clear verbal communication.

Intervention	Rationale
Give specific instructions for behavior—at the table, in the classroom, and so on—and reward these behaviors. Reward attempts to communicate needs verbally and shape appropriate language.	Role modeling and rewarding the use of language promote the development of language skills.

Evaluation

Child increases his use of language to communicate with others.

Nursing Diagnosis

Social Isolation related to fear of others, as evidenced by lack of eye contact, staring at wall

Outcome

The child will interact with peers and adults.

Intervention	Rationale
Help the child discuss and identify feelings. Teach appropriate means of expressing feelings through words, physical activities. Include child in nonthreatening activities with peers.	Expanding the child's contact with peers in a safe environment and teaching about feelings diminishes his social isolation.

Evaluation

Child engages in social interactions with peers and adults in a less fearful manner.

Nursing Diagnosis

Impaired Social Interaction with other children related to isolation and withdrawal

Outcome

The child will interact with peers or a peer under supervision at least 1 hour per day.

Intervention	Rationale
Keep the child present in routine activities.	Keeping the child's attention and participation in activities and conversations prevents isolation.
Maintain eye contact with the child during conversations.	Eye contact promotes attending behavior.
Ask the child to look at the adult or other child while talking, and reinforce the child for this behavior.	Behavioral measures, such as reinforcing appropriate, desired behavior promotes its continuation.

Evaluation

Child demonstrates interpersonal skills while playing with peers.

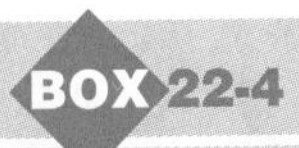

DSM-IV Diagnostic Criteria for Childhood Disintegrative Disorder

A. Apparently normal development for at least the first 2 years after birth as manifested by the presence of age-appropriate verbal and nonverbal communication, social relationships, play, and adaptive behavior.
B. Clinically significant loss of previously acquired skills (before age 10 years) in at least two of the following areas:
  (1) expressive or receptive language
  (2) social skills or adaptive behavior
  (3) bowel or bladder control
  (4) play
  (5) motor skills
C. Abnormalities of functioning in at least two of the following areas:
  (1) qualitative impairment in social interaction (eg, impairment in nonverbal behaviors, failure to develop peer relationships, lack of social or emotional reciprocity)
  (2) qualitative impairments in communication (eg, delay or lack of spoken language, inability to initiate or sustain a conversation, stereotyped and repetitive use of language, lack of varied make-believe play)
  (3) restricted, repetitive, and stereotyped patterns of behavior, interests, and activities, including motor stereotypies and mannerisms
D. The disturbance is not better accounted for by another specific Pervasive Developmental Disorder or by Schizophrenia.

thoughts and provoke the urge to perform rituals) and *response prevention* (either instructing the client to delay performing the ritual or blocking the performance of the ritual). The combination of exposure and response prevention allows the child to experience the rise and fall of anxiety.[58] Pharmacotherapy with clomipramine (Anafranil) and fluoxetine (Prozac) has been effective in treating the symptoms of OCD.[56]

Specific Phobia

Phobias are common anxiety disorders in children. A *phobia* is a morbid, irrational, and persistent fear. Childhood phobias are so common that mild, passing fears are considered part of normal development. The anxiety of a specific phobia in children may be expressed as crying, tantrums, or clinging.[2]

Frequently, the child may fear transportation (such as travel by car or plane) and animals. There may be exaggerated fears of burglars or kidnappers or concerns about dying. Many children fear dogs and become uncomfortable around them. The child with a phobia, however, is preoccupied with the prospects of meeting a dog, in a constant anticipatory anxiety state, and may not want to go to school or even out of the house to ensure that a dog is not encountered. A phobia can be incapacitating.

Treatment. Treatment approaches include preparing children for traumatic experiences and providing behavioral training, such as relaxation, desensitization, modeling, and psychotherapy.

Social Phobia

A child with *social phobia* exhibits excessive shrinking from social contact with unfamiliar people to the point of interfering with interpersonal functioning with peers. At the same time, the child desires increased contact with familiar peers or family members.

The child with this disorder appears socially withdrawn, embarrassed, self-conscious, and shy when in the company of strangers and very anxious if asked to interact, even minimally, with strangers. The avoidance

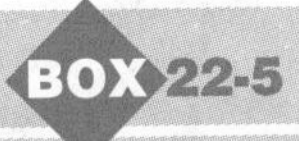

DSM-IV Diagnostic Criteria for Tourette's Disorder

A. Both multiple motor and one or more vocal tics have been present at some time during the illness, although not necessarily concurrently. (A *tic* is a sudden, rapid, recurrent, nonrhythmic, stereotyped motor movement or vocalization.)
B. The tics occur many times a day (usually in bouts) nearly every day or intermittently throughout a period of more than 1 year, and during this period there was never a tic-free period of more than 3 consecutive months.
C. The disturbance causes marked distress or significant impairment in social, occupational, or other important areas of functioning.
D. The onset is before age 18 years.
E. The disturbance is not due to the direct physiological effects of a substance (eg, stimulants) or a general medical condition (eg, Huntington's disease or postviral encephalitis).

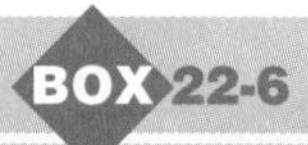

DSM-IV Diagnostic Criteria for Chronic Motor or Vocal Tic Disorder

A. Single or multiple motor or vocal tics (ie, sudden, rapid, recurrent, nonrhythmic, stereotyped motor movements or vocalizations), but not both, have been present at some time during the illness.
B. The tics occur many times a day nearly every day or intermittently throughout a period of more than 1 year, and during this period there is never a tic-free period of more than 3 consecutive months.
C. The disturbance causes marked distress or significant impairment in social, occupational, or other important areas of functioning.
D. The onset is before age 18 years.
E. The disturbance is not due to the direct physiological effects of a substance (eg, stimulants) or a general medical condition (eg, Huntington's disease or postviral encephalitis).
F. Criteria have never been met for Tourette's Disorder.

and anxious anticipation cause marked distress in new or forced social situations and impairment in the child's functioning at school and in play groups.[2]

Treatment. Supporting the child as he or she learns to extend himself to others, role playing and practicing social skills, reading books about children who have overcome their shyness, encouraging the child to take calculated risks, and reinforcing behavioral progress are means to treat social phobia in children.

Generalized Anxiety Disorder

Generalized anxiety disorder is marked by excessive or unrealistic anxiety or worry. The child with this disorder is extremely self-conscious and worries about both future and past events and his or her own competence and behavior. Concomitant physical symptoms of anxiety, headaches, gastrointestinal distress, nausea, shortness of breath, and dizziness also may be present. The child is particularly tense and unable to relax.[2] The child may be concerned about the quality of performance in schoolwork, sports, or hobbies and about issues such as money matters, punctuality, health, or appearance.

Treatment. Treatment of children with generalized anxiety disorder includes reassuring the child that he or she is safe and will receive care, helping the child to relax standards for his or her own performance to realistic levels, and providing parent training and relaxation training.

Separation Anxiety Disorder

A child with *separation anxiety disorder* exhibits excessive anxiety to the point of panic concerning separation from the person or people to whom the child is attached. When separated from significant others, the child may be preoccupied with morbid fears of accidents or illness or may be extremely homesick, almost to the panic level. The child feels distress when traveling independently away from the house and may refuse to visit or sleep at friends' houses, go on errands, or attend camp or school.[2]

Physical complaints, such as headaches, stomach aches, nausea, and vomiting, are common. The child may cling to, or *shadow,* the attachment figure. The child worries that attachment figures will be harmed, suffers nightmares about separation, and is reluctant or refuses to go to sleep without being near an attachment figure or to sleep away from home or parents.[2] An older term, *school phobia,* was actually a form of separation anxiety or perhaps a result of parents' difficulty in accepting the child's increasing independence.

Adolescents with separation anxiety disorder are likely to refuse to attend school and to voice somatic complaints. The prevalence of this disorder, however, drops as children approach adolescence (Box 22-7).[2]

Treatment. Treatment includes targeting populations at risk because of experiencing threatening events, providing educational training for parents and teachers, treating maternal depression, and using cognitive-behavioral strategies, such as self-talk, to handle anxiety.

Sleep Disturbances

Sleep disturbances are often tied to separation anxiety, because the very young child views sleep as separation. A transitory, common experience of sleep disturbance may be seen, for example, in 2- to 3-year-olds who fear loss of control over their bodies while asleep, resulting in bed wetting. The child may be afraid of sleep itself,

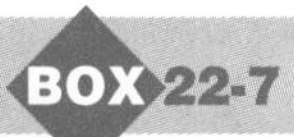

DSM-IV Diagnostic Criteria for Separation Anxiety Disorder

A. Developmentally inappropriate and excessive anxiety concerning separation from home or from those to whom the individual is attached, as evidenced by three (or more) of the following:
   (1) recurrent excessive distress when separation from home or major attachment figures occurs or is anticipated
   (2) persistent and excessive worry about losing, or about possible harm befalling, major attachment figures
   (3) persistent and excessive worry that an untoward event will lead to separation from a major attachment figure (eg, getting lost or being kidnapped)
   (4) persistent reluctance or refusal to go to school or elsewhere because of fear of separation
   (5) persistently and excessively fearful or reluctant to be alone or without major attachment figures at home or without significant adults in other settings
   (6) persistent reluctance or refusal to go to sleep without being near a major attachment figure or to sleep away from home
   (7) repeated nighmares involving the theme of separation
   (8) repeated complaints of physical symptoms (such as headaches, stomachaches, nausea, or vomiting) when separation from major attachment figures occurs or is anticipated

B. The duration of the disturbance is at least 4 weeks.

C. The onset is before age 18 years.

D. The disturbance causes clinically significant distress or impairment in social, academic (occupational), or other important areas of functioning.

E. The disturbance does not occur exclusively during the course of a Pervasive Developmental Disorder, Schizophrenia, or other Psychotic Disorder and, in adolescents and adults, is not better accounted for by Panic Disorder With Agoraphobia.

for fear that a horrible event, even death, may occur during sleep.

Nightmares peak between 4 and 6 years and may be the cause of the child's inability to remain asleep. A child awakens from nightmares feeling helpless and afraid and in need of comforting. At the extreme, night terrors leave the child feeling panicked and experiencing difficulty reorienting to reality, being comforted, and regaining self-control.

Treatment. Treatment involves calming activities before bedtime, attention to the child's fears and concerns, and parental reassurance.

MOOD DISORDERS

Depressive Disorders

Until recently, it was thought that children rarely, if ever, become depressed. We know now, however, that depression exists across age spans with some developmental differences and that children do experience depression.

Childhood depression often presents as headaches, chest pains, abdominal pain, and other somatic complaints. The child's behavior may mask the depression and may take the form of acting-out behavior or somatic complaints. The depressed child may express depressive themes in play, fantasy, dreams, and verbalizations. Depression may be seen more frequently in children and adolescents with chronic illnesses, gastrointestinal disorders, and chronic orthopedic problems.[26]

The various symptoms of depression are specific to the child's age or developmental level. For example, separation anxiety may be a sign of depression in a prepubertal child; a depressed adolescent boy may exhibit negativistic and antisocial behavior, sulkiness, social withdrawal, and school difficulties.

Some of the behaviors typically associated with depression in adults (see Chapter 29, Depressive and Bipolar Disorders) may or may not be seen in depressed children. The depressed mood of adults during a major depressive episode may not be seen in children and adolescents; rather, children may exhibit irritable moods.[2]

Feelings of depression are more prevalent in adolescence than in earlier childhood. Although psychosocial variables, such as family dysfunction, low self-esteem, and stressful life events, are associated with depressive disorders, in early adolescence, family environment may be a more important predictor of depressive symptoms than life events.[15,19]

Although clinical observations and evaluation measures, such as the Depression Self-Rating Scale and the Children's Depression Inventory, are invaluable tools for discerning the presence of depression in children, optimal assessment of the depressed child involves using multiple measures and informants.

Dysthymia in children is characterized by a depressed or irritable mood that lasts at least 1 year and can coexist with other disorders, such as ADHD or conduct disorder. Nurses may see children with dysthymia in school and clinics because their symptoms are not as debilitating as major depression.[44]

Bipolar disorder is rarely seen in prepubertal children. Those younger than 9 years present with irritability and affective lability, whereas the symptoms of adolescents resemble those of adults.[44]

Suicide

Suicide attempts in children younger than 12 years are relatively rare. However, rates of attempted and completed suicides in adolescents, beginning at 13 or 14 years, have risen dramatically in recent decades.[44] Children may fantasize suicide by stabbing themselves, jumping from heights, hanging themselves, and drowning themselves.

Suicidal behaviors are linked with depressive, substance use, and conduct disorders.[44] Other risk factors for suicidal behavior in children are preoccupation with death and suicidal tendencies or behaviors of the child's parents.

The family variables related to suicidal risk in childhood include parental separation or divorce, abuse (particularly abuse to the mother), ineffective communication patterns, crowding, family history of suicidal behaviors, and acute stressful events.

Treatment. Treatment of all mood disorders in children rests on the guiding principles of providing safety and a therapeutic environment; building self-esteem; using cognitive therapy, other psychotherapies, and medications to treat the symptoms; and participating in psychotherapy, family therapy, group therapy, and special education.

PSYCHOSIS IN CHILDREN

The child with psychosis may live in a world that is unavailable to anyone but himself or herself. The child may be preoccupied with sensory stimuli (visual, auditory, or kinesthetic) that have little thought content. For example, a toy car is fun for the psychotic child not because the child can pretend he or she is driving it, but because its wheels spin. Rather than engaging in make-believe, psychotic children exploit toys for their physical properties.

The child is often unable to differentiate between inner and outer reality; is often aggressive and unable to tolerate frustration; uses language associatively; displays stereotypic, compulsive behaviors; and perceives the world as persecutory.[59]

Childhood-Onset Schizophrenia

The DSM-IV requires that the same diagnostic criteria be met for schizophrenia in children as in adults, although the course of the illness may be more long-term and the symptoms more severe in children. Those with *childhood-onset schizophrenia* exhibit characteristic symptoms and deficits in adaptive functioning lasting at least 6 months.[45] The disorder is diagnosed before 12 years but rarely before 5 years.

Schizophrenia in children is characterized by delusions, hallucinations, and disorganized speech; catatonia; inappropriate or flat affect; avolition; alogia; and anhedonia.[2,45]

Treatment. Childhood-onset schizophrenia requires antipsychotic medication; a structured, therapeutic milieu; provision of safety; therapies and special education; parent, client, and family education and support.

ADJUSTMENT DISORDER

An adjustment disorder is characterized by clinically significant emotional or behavioral symptoms in response to an identifiable psychosocial stressor or stressors. The symptoms develop within 3 months after the onset of the stressor(s).[2] The course of adjustment disorders may be acute or chronic and may occur with depression, anxiety, or conduct disturbances.

In children, the maladaptive reaction is seen in an impairment in school functioning, usual social activities, or relationships with others or in symptoms that exceed a normal and expected reaction to the stressor. An example of this type of reaction occurs when a child becomes ill, is hospitalized, or is faced with surgery. While in the hospital, the child may exhibit regressed, fearful, and acting-out behavior. After discharge from the hospital and returning home, the child may continue to show increased anxiety, hostility, fearfulness, clinging to mother, and disruptions in meal, sleep, and toilet routines. Evidence of such behavior may gradually diminish 3 to 6 months after hospitalization.

Treatment. Understanding, continued support as the child works out feelings related to the stressors and encouragement to move past the event to adaptive coping are important in the treatment of children with adjustment disorder.

Application of the Nursing Process to Children With Mental Disorders

A child's referral for psychiatric-mental health treatment may have been initiated by the school, parents, health care providers, or court. A family crisis, acute or chronic physical illness, or other stressors may precipitate seeking therapeutic intervention for a troubled child. This section examines the steps of the nursing process applied to the care of children with mental illness and their families.

ASSESSMENT

Family Functioning

In child psychiatric-mental health nursing, the treatment team assesses the disturbed child and family and then collaboratively analyzes the information that has been gathered. Assessment sets the tone for the rest of the interaction and intervention with the child and family. It provides an opportunity to deal with the parents' fears and misinformation, support their desire to be good parents, and teach them to participate actively in their child's care. The nurse should answer the child's and family's questions honestly and with empathy.[32]

Assessment of the family, particularly members of the extended family who may help define the family's beliefs and values about childrearing, is best approached before the assessment of the child. This initial focus on the family, rather than on the child, gives a clear message to all involved that no one in the family is exempt from the problem and participating in problem solving.

The nurse or other mental health caregiver asks open-ended questions, such as, "How are things for the family?" This form of questioning allows the family to feel free to respond with whatever information they want to share. Usually, the parents respond first to opening questions and attempt to identify the problem.

Next, the nurse focuses on the child, who is typically the identified client in the family. Asking the child, "How are things going?" often brings a response of "I don't know," "Fine," or "My parents (or teachers) are mad at me."

Sources of Information. Although parents and teachers are probably better informants about the child's observable behavior, such as hyperactivity, academic problems, antisocial behavior, or difficulties with peers, the child is the best source of information about subjective symptoms. For example, the child should be assessed directly regarding suicidal ideation, disordered moods, feelings of guilt or low self-esteem, and hallucinations.

Throughout the assessment process, the nurse seeks information from the child, parents, siblings, extended family, teachers, and health care professionals. The nurse also notes the congruence or incongruence among the perceptions of each source of information.

Communication Patterns. During the initial assessment interview, the nurse observes the behavior of parents and children and determines what their body language is communicating, how the family members arrange themselves in the room, who speaks for whom, and who the primary spokesperson for the family is. In well-integrated, healthy family systems, each family member is free to speak—there is room for everyone's opinions and ideas.

Other ways of determining the openness of the family system are exploring extrafamilial interactions and influences, tolerance of differences of opinion among family members, clarity of the boundaries, and ability to deal with current issues (see Chapter 17, Families and Family Therapy).

Identifying the Problem. As the child and family define the problem, the nurse assesses its severity, duration, and effect on family functioning and for whom the problem is most distressing. For example, conduct disorders are likely to be very upsetting to parents, siblings, teachers, and other adults, whereas specific or social phobia may be most disturbing for the child.

The nurse also assesses how functional or dysfunctional the problem is. A child may be very manipulative with adults, and although the problem is distressing and adults do not feel comfortable with the child, growth and development continue satisfactorily.

Some mental health problems are dysfunctional for the child and family. For instance, when a child has anorexia nervosa, it is not uncommon for everyone in the family to try to placate the anorectic child. If a child exhibits aggressive behavior, as in a conduct disorder, the mother may interact with the child as the strict disciplinarian, while the father tries to create some positive interaction; this conflict may lead to marital problems.

Family Relationships. The nurse assesses the family members' genuineness of concern for each other. The family members are asked to describe their relationships and roles, including the child's role in the family. In addition, the family is often requested to perform a certain task, such as planning a family vacation. This experiential task demonstrates the actual relationships, roles, degree of autonomy or enmeshment, and empathy of family members.

Is the child functioning as a family scapegoat? In other words, is the child being blamed and held responsible for everything that goes wrong in the family? Who has power in the family? Who makes decisions? Does every family member have the chance to speak?

Perceptions of the Child. The parents' level of knowledge about the normal processes of child development and behavior influences how realistic their role expectations for the child are. For example, is the 6-year-old boy expected to be "the little man" of the family?

The nurse asks the parents about the level at which they think their child should be functioning now. They are asked to define what is different about this child and to assess the child's disposition or temperament, talents, and strengths. These will be incorporated into a plan to maximize the family's resources and strengths.

Sociocultural Influences. Socioeconomic and cultural information from the family provides another perspective about the family's childrearing practices and aftercare planning for the child. This information includes the parents' and other family members' education, occupations, incomes, and cultural beliefs and practices.

Sharing With Parents. During the assessment process, the nurse asks the family whose idea it was to seek help for the child and what intervention measures they have already tried. The nurse acknowledges the seriousness of the problem and compliments the family on their concern and love for the child.

To elicit information about the parents' values, expectations, culture, and attitudes and biases about parenting, the nurse can ask the question, "What do you wish your child were like now?" The parents are asked to describe what they hope the treatment team can do for them and their child. Their hopes for their child's future reveal what they believe about standards of behavior, relationships, and careers.

The parents need time to ask their own questions. They may fear they did something wrong that resulted in the child becoming hostile, aggressive, or withdrawn. The nurse should briefly explore with them the possibility of multiple factors in the development of a child's mental or emotional disorder.

The Child

History Taking. Taking a history of factors pertinent to the child's emotional problem includes the following information:

1. A history of psychiatric disorders, alcoholism and drug dependence, or organic illnesses in members of the nuclear and extended families
2. A thorough assessment of the growth and development of the child, including prenatal and perinatal factors
3. The time of onset of the problem and any significant events that occurred at or around this time
4. The child's health and social history

The parents, teachers, and child are asked to describe the child's strengths and weaknesses and his or her functioning at home, at school, and with peers. The child's social skills, interests and hobbies, and unusual or troublesome habits are noted.

Physical and Mental Assessment. A thorough physical examination should be conducted. The child's age, size, nutritional status, speech, hearing, and the presence of "soft" (subtle) neurological signs are assessed. A structured mental status assessment includes examining the following in the child:

1. Appearance: dress, gestures, posture, tics
2. Mood and affect: predominant feelings, mood fluctuations, ease or constriction in displaying feelings, appropriateness
3. Manner of relating to the examiner: perceptions of the reasons for the interview, rapport with or distance from the examiner, use of play, activity, verbalization, or relationships
4. Modes of thinking and intellectual skills: development of thinking, conceptualizations of causality, body image, memory, problem solving
5. Capacity for play and fantasy: amount and kind of involvement in play, use of play materials, themes of play, spontaneity of play, use of examiner in the play
6. Sensorimotor development: fine and gross motor activities, symmetry of movement, eye–hand coordination, and right and left discrimination[12]

The Mental Status Exam for a Child provides more information about mental assessment of children (Box 22-8).

Assessment Through Play. Because children's ability to express themselves verbally is limited, assessment is conducted primarily through the medium of play. A variety of play materials, including dolls, hand puppets, art materials (paint, clay, paper), movement toys (cars,

(text continues on page 400)

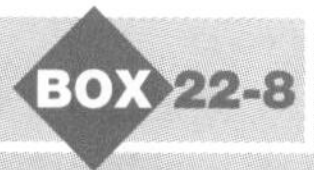

The Mental Status Exam for a Child

Nancy A. Moeller Sanchez, M.S., R.N., C.S.

When the nurse is conducting an assessment of a child, it is sometimes a great challenge to elicit data through the direct question-and-answer format used with adolescents or adults. It is vital that the nurse establish a sense of rapport and put the child at ease. One way to approach this is by allowing the child to explore the office and its contents—toys, games, and art supplies. While the child is examining the office, the nurse is able to make pertinent behavioral observations and ask some nonthreatening questions: "What's your name? How old are you? What grade are you in?"

As the child becomes more comfortable with the nurse, it is important to find out if the child is aware of why he or she is being brought in to talk to the nurse. Many children are unaware of the purpose of their visit to the nurse; parents may have made up an untrue reason for the visit to entice the child. Parents also may have told children they'd see a "doctor" or "nurse," and this may have frightened or worried them, especially if experiences with nurses or doctors have been negative or frightening.

At this point, the nurse should explain that to know the child better, it will be necessary for the nurse to ask some "silly" questions and to have the child use his or her imagination for a few minutes. Once the child indicates a willingness to respond more directly, the following questions may be helpful in evaluating the mental stuatus of the child:

ORIENTATION

What day/month/season is it today?
What would you like to be when you grow up?

SEXUAL PREFERENCE

If you had a chance to decide, would you rather be a boy or girl? Why?

RELATIONSHIPS

How do you get along with your family and friends?
Describe what you like to do with your friend(s).

FANTASY LIFE

Who would you like to take on a trip to the moon?
If you had three wishes, what would they be?
What animal would you like to be? Why?
What is your favorite daydream?
When you dream at night, what do you dream?
Do you ever have nightmares? [If yes] Tell me about them.
What are you most afraid of?
Do you ever see or hear things no one else can see or hear? [If yes] Please describe them.
Do you ever have strange thoughts or ideas?

AFFECT/MOOD

I'm going to name a feeling, and then you tell me when you feel that way.

I feel *sad* when
I feel *mad* when
I feel *happy* when
I feel *scared* when

What do you *do* when you feel

Sad?
Mad?
Happy?
Scared?

ASSESSMENT OF DRAWINGS

Now I want you to draw a few pictures. [Have blank $8\frac{1}{2}'' \times 11''$ paper and a No. 2 pencil available.] You don't have to be an artist, just do the best you can. [Ask the child questions about each picture as it is completed: "Who/what is in the picture?" "What is happening in the picture?"]

1. Draw a picture of a house.
2. Draw a picture of a tree.
3. Draw a picture of a person.
4. Draw a picture of you.
5. Draw a picture of a family doing something.

After the art assessment, ask the more difficult questions that follow.

RISK BEHAVIOR

Suicidal:

Do you ever feel like hurting yourself?
Have you ever tried to hurt yourself?

Homicidal:

Do you ever feel like hurting others? Who?
Have you ever tried to hurt them?

continued

BOX 22-8 (Continued)

Use of Chemicals:

Have you ever tried using any drugs? What? How often?

Have you ever tried drinking alcohol? How much? How often?

Abuse:

Has anyone ever touched you or made you touch them in the areas covered by your bathing suit (or private zones) [or point to genital, breast area on nurse]?

Did this make you feel funny or "not right"?

At the completion, the nurse should thank the child for cooperating and allow time for questions. If risk behavior is revealed, the nurse must explain that this information will help to be sure the child is going to be protected and safe.

Attached are samples of drawings done by chidren:

SAMPLE A

Drawn by a 6-year-old girl who has an average IQ, but whose drawings show signs of some emotional/developmental problems.

Notice absence of body parts

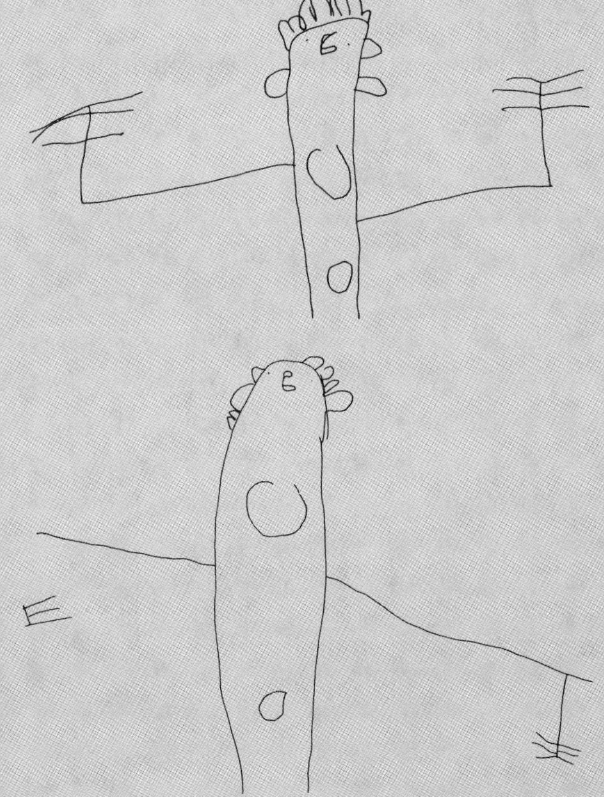

Notice disjointed drawing of house

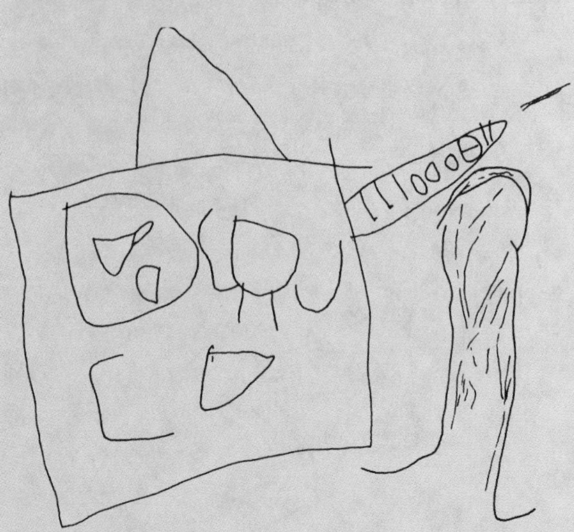

SAMPLE B

Drawn by a 7-year-old boy who has a low average intelligence, was very disturbed emotionally, and may have signs of organic impairment.

Notice the house's lack of shape or detail

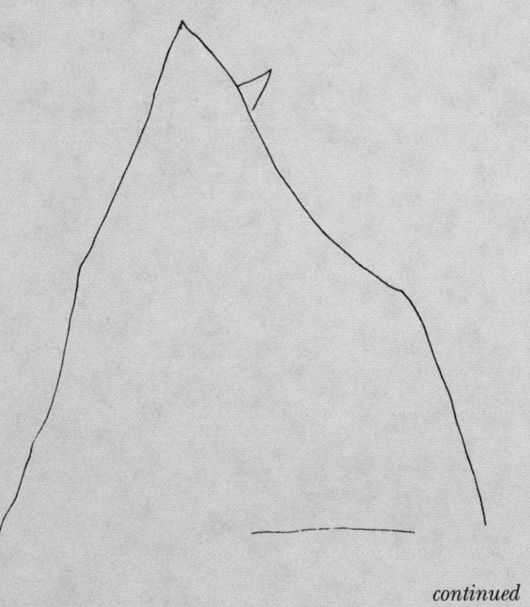

continued

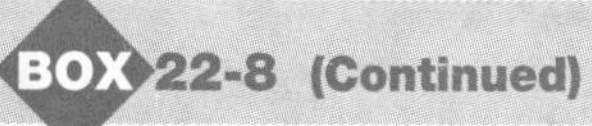

BOX 22-8 (Continued)

The drawings of people (boy and family) are disjointed, missing body parts

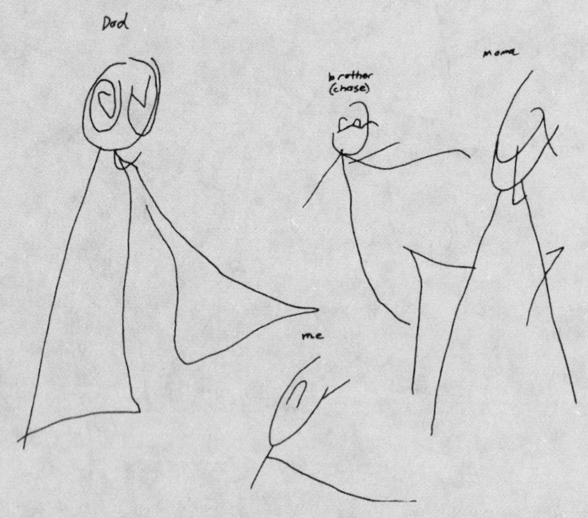

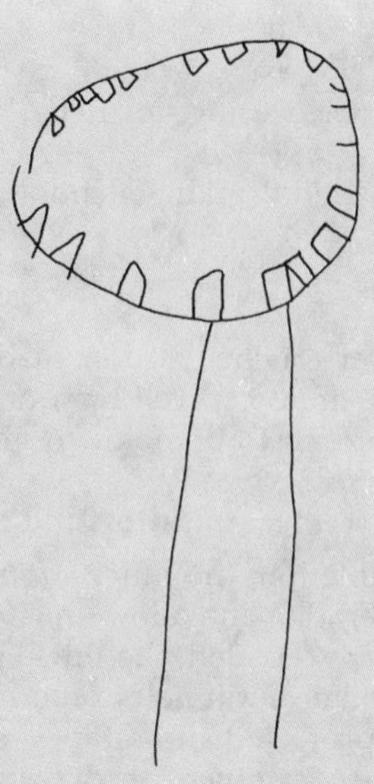

The kinetic family drawing shows the father whipping the child, saying, "Be quiet" to the child

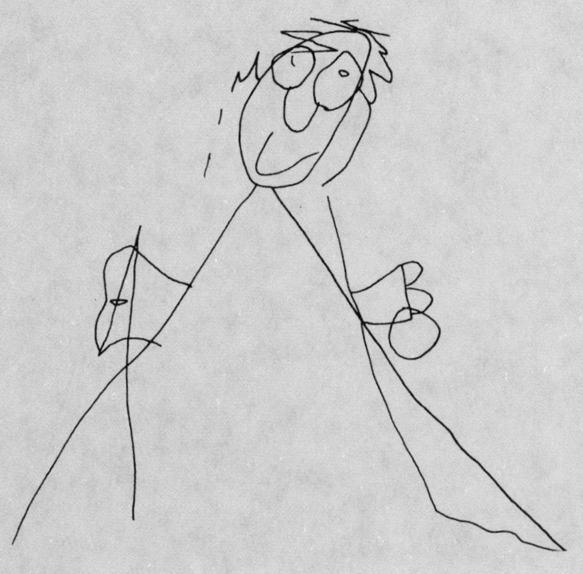

SAMPLE C: NORMAL SAMPLE

Drawn by a 7-year-old girl who has an average IQ and very few problems

Notice house and tree are fairly symmetrical

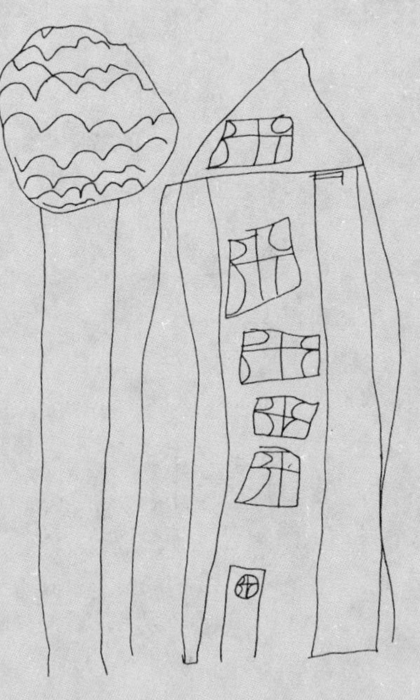

continued

BOX 22-8 (Continued)

The family seems happy as they are "camping out"

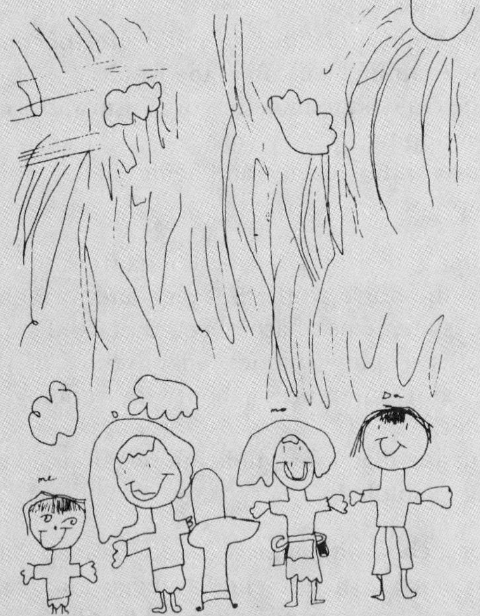

The man has all body parts

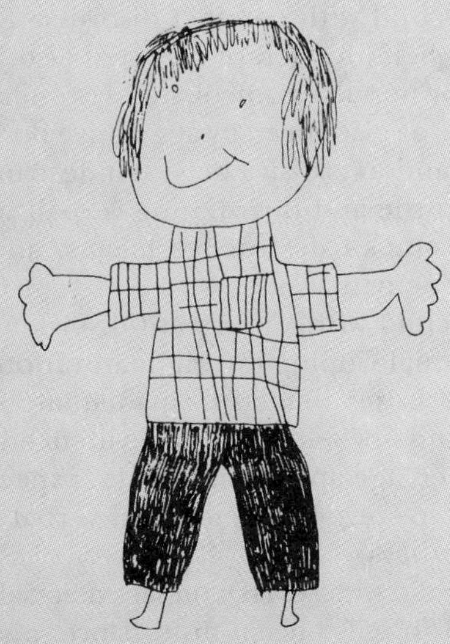

In addition, the mental status assessment should include the nurse's impressions of the following:

Appearance/dress
Motor activity
Nutritional status
Mannerisms
Tics

ATTITUDE AND GENERAL BEHAVIOR
(mark what is appropriate)

Anxiety ________ Fearful ________
Suspicious ________ Compliant ________
Alert ________ Cooperative ________
Relates well ________ Relates poorly ________

MENTAL ACTIVITY

Spontaneous ________ Blocked ________
Relevant ________ Tangential ________
Memory ________
Evidence of thought disorder ________

EMOTIONAL REACTIONS

Mood ________ Affect ________

IMPULSE CONTROL

At present:
Good ________ Fair ________ Poor ________
History:
Good ________ Fair ________ Poor ________

ORIENTATION

Time ________ Person ________ Place ________

Client's story about why he came to the mental health agency:

Nurse's summary of assessment process:

Tentative diagnosis:

Recommended further assessment needs:

(The author extends appreciation to Mr. Anthony Ravagnani, who prepared the children's art for publication.)

trucks, planes), and age-appropriate games (punching bag, toy telephone, rubber-tipped darts, and doll house and furniture) are provided for the child to tell his or her story.[12]

Assessment of Suicidal Intent. A child's suicide risk should be assessed to decrease the possibility of immediate self-harm and defuse the crisis situation. The nurse openly discusses with the child his or her self-harmful behaviors, thoughts, and tendencies.[49]

To assess suicide risk, the nurse must determine the presence of a suicide plan; the plan's lethality; the availability of lethal methods, such as a gun; and a history of substance abuse. An added risk factor is the child's exposure to suicidal people because of the potential for imitative suicidal actions.[49]

One approach to evaluating suicide risk focuses on the assessment of *imminent danger* rather than on the intensity of depression or hopelessness. The interviewer evaluates the youth's current suicidal plan or ideation. The presence of more than five of the following suicide-related factors places the child into a high-risk group: male sex, a suicide attempt with a method other than ingestion, more than one previous attempt, a history of antisocial behavior, a close friend who committed suicide or a family member who attempted suicide, frequent drug and alcohol use, depression, and incompatibility with the social environment.

The second phase of the interview is based on the youth's ability to behave in nonsuicidal ways, specifically the following:

1. The youth is able to promise in writing that he or she will not engage in suicidal behavior for a specific period of time, such as 2 weeks.
2. The youth is able to compliment himself or herself and others.
3. The youth is able to differentiate and assess his or her own feelings by placing them in a hierarchy of intense emotional states.
4. The youth is able to formulate specific plans to ward off suicidal situations.

A child or adolescent who is unable to perform these tasks is considered to be in imminent danger of suicide. Coping skills needed to fight off suicidal tendencies are not available.[54]

Use of Instruments. Using standardized instruments to evaluate children promotes an accurate nursing assessment. To be useful in the assessment of children with mental disorders, tools must provide standardized methods of administration, scoring, and interpretation.[40]

NURSING DIAGNOSIS

Developing nursing diagnoses for a child with a mental disorder is particularly difficult for several reasons:

1. A child is often inconsistent and unpredictable in behavior.
2. The child's relationship and degree of comfort with the examiner will affect the results.
3. The child is an immature organism and is constantly developing.
4. The child is affected and being shaped by his or her parents.

After gathering assessment data from the child and family, the nurse synthesizes data and formulates diagnostic statements that reflect the child's problems, strengths, coping abilities, adaptiveness of the symptoms, and inferences about the etiology of the disorder.[32]

Nursing diagnoses guide interventions, as in the following examples:

1. For a child with anxiety disorder: Sleep Pattern Disturbance related to child's anxiety and fears, as evidenced by interrupted sleep, difficulty falling asleep except when in presence of parent, listlessness, and lethargy during daytime activities
2. For a child with autistic disorder: Impaired Verbal Communication related to lack of reciprocal interaction with others and pathophysiological changes occurring in response to maternal rubella, meningitis, encephalitis, PKU, as evidenced by lack of speech, echolalia, or abnormal form or content of speech
3. For a child with conduct disorder: Risk for Violence: Self-directed or directed at others related to poor impulse control and dysfunctional family system, as evidenced by aggressive body language, overt and aggressive acts, self-destructive behavior, hostile and threatening verbalizations, rage, possession of destructive means, and increased motor activity
4. For a child with adjustment disorder: Ineffective Individual Coping during maturational and situational crises related to inadequate support systems and low self-esteem as evidenced by inability to meet age-appropriate role expectations, inability to solve problems, and verbal hostility toward others
5. For a child with ADHD: Impaired Social Interaction related to self-concept disturbance, poor attention and concentration, increased distractibility, excessive gross motor activity, as evidenced by observed discomfort in social situations, observed inability to communicate a sense of belonging or shared inter-

est, and dysfunctional interaction with peers and family

6. For any child with mental disorder: Altered Growth and Development related to existence of mental disorder, as evidenced by a variety of maladaptive behaviors[63]

Relational Problems

Whereas previous editions of the DSM focused exclusively on the diagnosis and treatment of mental disorders of individuals, in reality, many problems occur within the context of the family and other relational units. The DSM-IV has included these issues when they are a focus of clinical attention to provide a comprehensive approach to mental illness.

The DSM-IV relational problems appropriate for child clients include the following:

1. Parent–child relational problem
2. Sibling relational problem[2]

The DSM-IV problems related to abuse and neglect include the following:

1. Physical abuse of child
2. Sexual abuse of child
3. Neglect of child[2]

PLANNING

Planning with parents and the child is a collaborative effort. It begins with the assessment and analysis of the information about the child's developmental level and the needs and problems of child and family. It also involves sharing this information with the family.

Planning takes into account the nature of the mental disorder and the resources available.

Determining Client Goals and Outcomes

Goals of child and family mental health treatment may include the following:

1. The child and family will experience fewer symptoms of disorder and distress.
2. The child's development will proceed along normal lines.
3. The child will display increasing degrees of autonomy, initiative, and self-reliance.
4. The child's behavioral gains will be reinforced.
5. Therapeutic changes will occur in the child's home or school environment.

Client outcomes are more specific, measurable, and time limited than goals. The following are examples of client outcomes:

1. The child will name two feelings experienced during separation from parents while at school by a specific date.
2. The child will complete assigned chores at home each day and be rewarded by parents using a behavioral program.
3. The child will exercise outside (ride bike, shoot baskets) each day for 30 minutes after school.

Priority Setting

Planning also considers the priorities of psychiatric care. For example, a 13-year-old admitted to an inpatient treatment facility following a suicide attempt requires a treatment plan that first attends to physical safety. Caring for the child with a decreased level of consciousness, assessing blood levels of the drug ingested in an overdose attempt, and instituting antidotal therapy take precedence over psychosocial assessment of the child and family.

INTERVENTION

The type of psychiatric treatment depends on the needs and problems of the child and family. In the past, mentally disturbed children were treated with various methods of physiotherapy. As recently as the 1950s, shock treatments for psychotic children were attained through electricity, pentylenetetrazol, or insulin. Today's treatment methods are evolving. Tailoring interventions to address the individualized needs of children and families is part of the psychiatric nurse's role.

Prevention

The primary focus of intervention for mental disorders of childhood is prevention. *Primary prevention* refers to any activity undertaken before a child is identified as a client. Of the 7.5 to 9.5 million children needing psychiatric services, only 7% (usually the most disordered) receive the help they need.[65] Services to children and adolescents with mental disorders generally are inappropriate, inadequate, or unavailable.

Many children respond to difficult life experiences, such as parental abuse or the loss of a parent through divorce, death, abandonment, or illness, with symptoms of mental illness.[50] We know, however, that early identification of and intervention with children at risk can prevent more serious mental disturbance later in life. An example of this type of intervention is a group for children who have suffered the loss of a parent. Experiences with these groups demonstrate that children deal with this stressful event long after the loss itself.[38]

Unfortunately, preventive intervention has not been a priority of the American mental health care system. Until recently, it was thought that parenting required no special knowledge or skills; adolescents now often study parenting in school. Saving money by not providing preventive intervention is akin to being "penny wise but pound foolish."

Effective primary prevention programs must take into account the total sociocultural environment in which the child lives.[52] Brief exposures to interventions will not produce long-term effects in children who continue to live in a disturbed or chaotic environment.

The goals of preventive measures are as follows:

1. Reduce the incidence of new cases of the disorder.
2. Reduce the incidence of disabilities in the population.
3. Raise the immunity of individuals or groups to stress.
4. Decrease stress in the environment.
5. Improve the quality of life in a targeted population.
6. Improve the general health of children.[52]

Children and families at risk for mental disorder should be targeted for preventive efforts. The stress points in the life cycle that may require intervention to prevent disorder are pregnancy; birth (particularly prematurity); the maturational crises of adolescence, marriage, retirement, and dying; and situational crises, such as serious illness, divorce, and rape.

Wrap-Around Services

In today's mental health care market of brief treatment, it is essential to provide wrap-around services to children and families through a seamless delivery system. This means that the system provides what the child and family need, when and where they need it. To diminish interruption in child development and family life, this delivery model offers the following services: crisis stabilization in the home and hospital, day treatment, family support, case management, assessment, referral, therapeutic foster care, substance abuse treatment, school-based counseling, foster group home care, and prevention and early intervention.

Individual Therapy

Relationship Therapy. Therapy with a child with mental disorder focuses on the child's needs and problems. A therapist's effectiveness depends on the therapist–client relationship, and the therapist must respect the child's unique nature.[41] Approaching the child client may be difficult for nurses and other mental health care professionals due to what Anna Freud called "the fluidity of the child's personality."[17] The child is growing and developing; his or her needs are not constant.

The role of the therapist may be that of a participant-observer. The therapist hopes to become an important adult in the child's world, someone with whom the child can identify while moving along the growth process. Although Sullivan never treated children, his interpersonal theory has had far-reaching effects on child theory and therapy. His view of maturational processes centers on communication, skills of communication, and the factors that contribute to anxiety, thereby interfering with development.

Brief Psychotherapy. Elective, brief psychotherapy with children is a form of individual psychotherapy based on ego psychology. It is not a fragment of long-term therapy nor an attempt to condense long-term therapy into a short period of time.

The therapist and child identify a central issue that can be addressed in the available time. The goal of brief therapy focuses on the central issue or problem, which is openly discussed with the child and family.[64]

Play Therapy. Nondirective play therapy offers the child an opportunity to experience growth under the most favorable conditions. Because play is the child's natural medium for self-expression, therapy can offer the child a way to play out accumulated feelings of fear, tension, confusion, frustration, and aggression.

When the child plays out feelings, they are allowed to surface, and the child faces them and learns to control, accept, or abandon them. Through this process, children gradually realize that they are individuals in their own right and are capable of thinking and making decisions for themselves (Box 22-9).

Family Therapy

Family therapy is based on the premise that the behavior of an individual within the family cannot be understood or changed without understanding and effecting change within the entire family system. Because behavior does not occur in isolation, intervention is not directed only at the identified client, who is often a child.

The family therapist observes the family system in action, noting patterns of interaction among family members and determining what is maintaining the child's symptoms. The therapist intervenes to change the existing family behavior patterns to those that support new behavior, personal competence, and growth.

Successfully treating a child necessitates modifying the reinforcement patterns that are part of the child's environment. Therapeutic changes are unlikely to generalize without interventions that extend to the child's home environment. This involves training parents to become therapeutic agents of change. This training may occur in parent groups that focus on home-related problems and problem solving.

Milieu Therapy

Milieu therapy is the creation of a therapeutic living environment for the child that includes the setting, structure, and relationships with others. This environ-

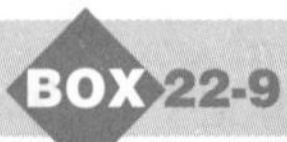

Play Therapy

Play is the child's work. Through play children learn to express their feelings and discover solutions to their problems. Through the intervention of play therapy, children can learn self-understanding, self-acceptance, self-mastery, and self-control. In addition, they can learn to identify, name, and deal with their feelings and to relate those feelings to behavior.

Play therapy is a special form of therapy which has been found to be most helpful to children. It teaches the child to open up and trust an adult within an atmosphere of unconditional positive regard. Although it usually takes place individually, some group therapies can use principles and techniques of play therapy with children.

Through play activities the therapist learns about how the child approaches new objects and experiences and expresses creativity, and identifies the themes—anger, conflict, sadness, and so on that emerge in the child's play. Models of play therapy, except for nondirective play therapy, use therapist behavior and/or selected play materials to guide the child's expression of feelings and behavior.

Play therapy goals and interventions are individualized according to the child's needs, conflicts, and problem behaviors. Stages of play therapy include: 1) the initial stage consisting of further assessment of the child; building of the therapeutic relationship, and encouragement of the child's free self-expression; 2) the middle stage which focuses on resolving conflict and problems and creating healthy personality change; and 3) the termination stage during which feelings of separation and rejection are worked through.

A play therapist is not a miracle worker. No therapist can force another person to change; however, through the medium of play the therapist's knowledge of children, experience, and skill can provide understanding and intervention that help the child change old ineffective patterns, develop new adaptive coping skills, and grow.

REFERENCES

Agler, L: Play Therapy: What's It All About? In Johnson BS, (Ed.) Psychiatric-Mental Health Nursing: Adaptation and Growth, 3rd ed., pp. 334–336. Philadelphia, J.B. Lippincott, 1993

Critchley, DL: Play Therapy. In Johnson BS, (Ed.) *Child, Adolescent, and Family Psychiatric Nursing,* pp. 335–350. Philadelphia, J.B. Lippincott, 1995

ment can be established in a treatment facility or in the child's own home.

In an effective therapeutic environment, every interaction becomes an opportunity for therapeutic intervention, and open, clear communication is modeled in all interactions.[33] These experiences include opportunities for learning, group socialization, reality testing, sublimation, and positive identification with adults.

Through the day-to-day living experiences of waking up, attending school, eating meals, participating in play and other activities, watching television, preparing bedtime snacks, and so forth, the child learns new and more effective ways to relate with others, deal with feelings, and manage daily activities. Music, dance, art, and other expressive activities may be incorporated into the milieu. The standard repertoire of milieu therapy with children includes negotiating, avoiding power struggles, talking a child down, and providing slow-down periods, relaxation techniques, self-soothing skills, coping and stress-reducing strategies, and safe, gentle holding.

Nurses and other caregivers who work in a therapeutic milieu become family surrogates for the child—supportive, respectful, cohesive adults who engage in open, healthy adult-to-adult and adult-to-child communication. The milieu staff, composed of child psychiatric-mental health professionals and paraprofessionals, constantly role model for the children.

The milieu environment provides safety, security,

structure, clear and reasonable limits, behavioral consequences, age-appropriate activities and expectations, pleasant surroundings, and the 24-hour availability of mature, caring, knowledgeable, ethical adults.

Seclusion and Restraint. Secluding a child to provide external control of disruptive behavior is a controversial intervention. On one hand, seclusion and restraint provide immediate containment of behavior, which safeguards the disruptive or assaultive client and other clients and staff who may be in danger. On the other hand, these measures limit client freedom. The literature demonstrates no link between seclusion and restraint and positive behavior change. There is no strong evidence that people learn more adaptive behavior as a result of being secluded or restrained.[68]

Time out, therapeutic holding, intensive care areas within treatment facilities, avoidance of power struggles, and ignoring negative behavior have all been suggested as alternatives to seclusion and restraint.[68] Early intervention and de-escalation of children is always preferable to the more intrusive methods of seclusion and restraint.

A recent study demonstrated that children who were more frequently secluded had organic involvement or developmental disabilities related to a high degree of impulsivity.[13] When placing a child in a seclusion room is not an alternative for inpatient staff, they are forced to use other methods to resolve crises, prevent escalation, and manage behavior.[29] If seclusion and restraint are aspects of the milieu, they should be used in a consistent manner and according to a well thought-out rationale.[20]

Behavior Therapy

Behavior therapy is based on the premise that emotional disorders represent learned behavior. Therefore, principles of learning are applied to the modification of these disorders. The desired client outcome is adaptive behavior change.[9]

Behavioral approaches to therapy for children with a mental disorder include the use of techniques such as token economies, time out (from positive reinforcement), and rewards for certain behaviors. This mode of treatment also uses less rigorously structured behavioral techniques. Teaching parents and teachers how to use these techniques necessitates that they be observant of child behavior, select the appropriate technique for the behavior, and apply it consistently.

An example of the use of behavior therapy is teaching the autistic child verbal imitation through differential reinforcement to shape verbal responses in the child. Another example of behavior therapy is parent training to help the parent manage a child's disruptive behavior.

Educational Approaches

A mentally disordered child's sense of failure is heightened by staying out of school, because attendance and accomplishment at school make up a significant aspect of the child's developmental strivings for completion. The school's dilemma may become how to manage the behavior of a child with mental illness while teaching the child the academics he or she needs.

The goals of special education for the emotionally disturbed child are as follows:

1. Decrease the child's deviant behavior.
2. Accelerate the child's rate of learning to enable him or her to remediate and progress.
3. Reintegrate the child into regular classes as soon as possible.

An important classroom technique when working with children with emotional disorders is to provide a high degree of structure. This lowers the child's anxiety by providing the security of defined limits and by making clear the expectations for the child's behavior. Another approach is to maximize the development of group cohesiveness and the use of peer pressure.

Children with mental disorder have experienced very little success in school. In the face of repeated failure, it is extremely difficult for the child to think positively about academic learning. The teacher's task is to provide a climate that helps the child become motivated. This is accomplished through awareness of the child's individual needs, teaching skills, and use of interesting materials and by not defining the child as a failure. Effective coordination between educational systems and the other systems of health care delivery is crucial.

Pharmacotherapy

Pharmacotherapy is one facet of a comprehensive therapeutic program. Giving a child medication does not alone solve emotional problems, but medication combined with family or parental counseling and education, individual therapy, and special educational plans increases the opportunity to improve the child's overall functioning.

Extra caution in administering these agents to children is required. Pharmacotherapy in children is different from that in adults. The child with mental disorder may resent medication and think that the drugs and their side effects are a punishment for bad behavior or a way to force compliance with adult authority.

Using medication alone to treat a child with mental disorder is ineffective because it does not help the child learn, understand, and practice social skills, academic information, or peer relationship skills. It does not replace developmental milestones that are not attained by the mentally disordered child, although some medications may help the child achieve developmental milestones by improving attention or decreasing psychomotor agitation.[46] Categories of psychoactive agents commonly used to treat children with mental disorders follow.

Antipsychotic Agents. This class of drugs includes the phenothiazines and related compounds. Their use in treating psychotic behavior began in the early 1950s.

- Examples of phenothiazines: chlorpromazine (Thorazine), prochlorperazine (Compazine), and trifluoperazine (Stelazine).
- Example of piperazines: fluphenazine (Prolixin).
- Example of piperidines: thioridazine (Mellaril).
- Example of butyrophenone: haloperidol (Haldol).

These agents have been used to sedate acutely agitated and psychotic children; decrease motor activity of hyperaggressive children; decrease impulsiveness, excitability, anxiety, and hyperdistractibility in children; and create a generally calming effect.

Although these medications are significant pharmacotherapeutic agents for psychotic and severely disturbed children, prolonged use can lead to serious complications, including tardive dyskinesia and withdrawal dyskinesia; therefore, they must be monitored carefully.

Anxiolytic or Antianxiety Agents. These drugs are prescribed for anxiety, phobic states, insomnia, irritability, and hyperactivity in children.

- Examples of diphenylmethane compounds: diphenhydramine (Benadryl), hydroxyzine (Vistaril); useful in treating children with behavior disorders and high anxiety levels

  Examples of benzodiazepine compounds: chlordiazepoxide (Librium), diazepam (Valium), lorazepam (Ativan)

The sedative action may be useful in mild to moderate anxiety states or hyperactivity.

Stimulants. These drugs are used to manage hyperactive behavior in conjunction with environmental management and parental education. They are used to treat hyperactivity, hyperaggressivity, and hyperdistractibility of children with ADHD. Examples include methylphenidate (Ritalin) and pemoline (Cylert).

Stimulants increase alertness, concentration, and motor activity; decrease fatigue and sleepiness; and suppress appetite.

Methylphenidate, a short-acting stimulant with a 1- to 4-hour duration, is considered safer than other stimulants, although side effects may include insomnia, loss of appetite, irritability, mood instability, nervousness, and tachycardia. It has presynaptic and postsynaptic effects on norepinephrine and dopamine, although its precise mechanism of action is unknown.[57]

Antidepressants. Examples of antidepressants include imipramine (Tofranil), amitriptyline (Elavil), nortriptyline (Aventyl), trazodone (Desyrel), doxepin (Sinequan), and fluoxetine (Prozac).

These drugs are used to treat depression, with or without anxiety, in children by elevating mood and improving sleep and appetite patterns. They are also used to treat enuresis in children. Sometimes imipramine is more effective in the treatment of children with attention deficit disorder than the central nervous system stimulants, particularly in children with high levels of anxiety or depression.

Antimanic Agents. Lithium is a metal ion effective in treating bipolar disorder. Trade names include Lithobid, Lithonate, Lithane, or Eskalith. Because there is narrow range of therapeutic level of lithium, regular serum lithium levels should be determined in all clients taking the medication. Side effects of lithium treatment occur frequently in children younger than 6 years, especially during the initial phase of treatment. Lithium is used with great caution in children.[23]

Anticonvulsants. Examples of anticonvulsants include diphenylhydantoin (Dilantin), valproic acid (Depakene), and carbamazepine (Tegretol).

These drugs are used to treat childhood behavior disorders with or without associated seizures. The anticonvulsants are also used to treat bipolar illness, particularly the rapid cycling form.

Combined Pharmacotherapy

Although mental health clinicians hope that children will respond favorably to single agents, increasingly medications are being used in combination to treat mental disorders in children and adolescents. This is indicated because disorders may occur comorbidly and because of the synergistic, or more powerful, effects of multiple agents.[69]

The following are examples of these combined agents that have been useful:

1. Stimulants, antidepressants, and clonidine (Catapres)
2. Methylphenidate and clonidine to control aggressive symptoms of ADHD with oppositional defiant or conduct disorder
3. Two antidepressants from different classes or the addition of antianxiety medications for children with chronic depression that does not respond to usual agents
4. Fluoxetine, benzodiazepines, and mood stabilizers[69]

Medication Education

Medication education must be provided for the child client and his or her family, teachers, and caregivers. Information about the medication must include its name, purpose, amount, dosing, desired effects, and side or toxic effects. The steps to take in the case of an untoward reaction must be made clear to all those involved in the child's care and to the child himself. (Box 22-2 offers an example of a medication education plan for Ritalin.)

EVALUATION

The effectiveness of child psychiatric treatment is determined by the treatment, therapist, child and family, specific problem for which treatment was sought, and treatment circumstances.

Evaluating effectiveness of intervention requires deciding how to define success and how to measure therapeutic change. Does success mean reducing the symptoms (maturation alone can alter those), reducing the child's anxiety, or improving academic performance? Does psychopathology mean normal development gone awry so that success in treatment means a return to an appropriate developmental course?

Research that evaluates the outcomes of child therapy must rely on objective observations and information provided by significant others, such as parents and teachers. The child's progress within therapy, however, does not ensure similar progress outside of therapy. Nontreatment factors, such as the child's school, may play an important role in his or her behavioral change and must be considered when evaluating the outcome of intervention.

Evaluating psychiatric care of emotionally disturbed children and their families includes examining the behaviors of children and families following the implementation of therapeutic measures and determining with the client and family whether treatment goals have been reached.

Various therapeutic modalities are available to children and families, and often a combination of approaches provides the optimal effect for children. Periodic reassessment of treatment techniques and their effectiveness is needed. The nurse and other members of the mental health team must be able to change approaches to maximize the benefits for the child and family.

NEED FOR RESEARCH

Research into childhood mental illness was identified as a national mental health priority in the late 1980s. Without this research and knowledge, preventive measures, adequate recognition, and prompt and effective treatment of childhood disorders are not possible. Early in 1995, however, the Institute of Medicine reviewed the progress being made in research into childhood and adolescent mental disorders and found that the dissemination of research findings was severely lacking.[27]

Nursing research also needs to strengthen its attention to the development and treatment of childhood disorders and evaluation of its outcomes. The Association of Child and Adolescent Psychiatric Nurses promotes research into child and adolescent mental health and illness and quality clinical services for children and adolescents.

◆ Advocacy for Emotionally Disturbed Children and Their Families

The child is not a miniature adult, but a developing person within a family system. The child's needs are not those of an adult, but those of an individual in an emotional and often confusing world.

Children have legal rights and physical and emotional needs. Under British law, children did not have recognized rights separate from their parents. In recent decades, the courts have significantly expanded the rights of children and have affirmed that children have many of the constitutional rights of adults. The rights of physically and mentally disabled children are especially important. These include the following:

1. Equal educational opportunity provided by public schools
2. Freedom from involuntary sterilization
3. Equal access to quality medical care
4. Independent legal counsel in any proceeding that could lead to the child's institutionalization
5. Care and treatment in the least restrictive setting

Advocacy for children's rights may be formal, such as appearing in a court case on a child's behalf. Often, however, the advocacy is informal, in the form of promoting the respect of children's rights. Strategies that inform parents, professionals, and institutions of children's rights; attempts to overcome budget restrictions; recognition of individuals' rights; and cooperation with other advocates for children and families (eg, case workers, attorneys) are examples of informal advocacy for children.

Child psychiatric-mental health nurses are in a unique position to advocate for the welfare of children and families; whether a nurse assumes this responsibility is an individual ethical choice.

◆ Chapter Summary

This chapter has focused on the incidence, prevalence, causative factors, dynamics, behavioral manifestations, and treatment of children with mental disorders and their families. Chapter highlights include the following:

1. The primary intervention in childhood mental disorders should be prevention.
2. Mental and emotional disorders in children constitute a serious mental health problem in the United States; estimates suggest that 12% to 15% of children are in need of psychiatric-mental health services.
3. Many theories of childhood mental and emotional disorder postulate an interactive effect of genetic, biological, physical, intrapsychic, familial, sociocultural, and environmental factors.
4. Assessment of emotional disorders of childhood requires an examination of the child and family environment in which the child lives.
5. Treatment planning is a collaborative activity involving the child, family, and mental health team.
6. Nursing intervention for children with mental disorders requires maturity, thoughtfulness, advocacy, and an ethical orientation to psychiatric-mental health care.
7. Research must continue into the multiple factors that contribute to the development of mental disorders in children and the interventions that bring about positive change and emotional growth.

Review Questions

1. Which of the following is *not* a group at high risk for mental disorder?
   - **A.** Children with first-degree relatives with mental illness or chemical dependence
   - **B.** Children whose parents are in therapy
   - **C.** Children who have been sexually abused
   - **D.** Children whose parents are teenagers
2. A child who exhibits physical violence against other people, sets fires, and commits theft is diagnosed as having
   - **A.** oppositional defiant disorder.
   - **B.** attention-deficit hyperactivity disorder.
   - **C.** criminal delinquent behavior.
   - **D.** conduct disorder.
3. A long-term disorder marked by idiosyncratic language and behavior and mental retardation that is evident soon after birth is termed
   - **A.** autism.
   - **B.** childhood disintegrative disorder.
   - **C.** pervasive retardation.
   - **D.** Tourette's disorder.
4. Which of the following statements is true about separation anxiety disorder?
   - **A.** The child experiences panic when left alone.
   - **B.** Somatic complaints occur rarely.
   - **C.** Psychoanalytical approaches offer the best hope of treatment for these children.
   - **D.** The child worries about the safety of attachment figures.
5. Name five areas of mental health assessment of children.
6. In today's health care market, psychiatric services for children must be
   - **A.** long-term and intensive.
   - **B.** provided in a seamless delivery system.
   - **C.** oriented toward inpatient care.
   - **D.** through pharmacotherapeutic agents.
7. Identify indications for behavioral therapy techniques with children.
8. Which of the following statements is false?
   - **A.** Prolonged use of antipsychotic medications can lead to tardive and withdrawal dyskinesias.
   - **B.** Antidepressants elevate mood and improve sleep and appetite patterns in children.
   - **C.** Stimulants such as methylphenidate are used to treat ADHD.
   - **D.** Lithium is a safe medication for children with depression.

◆ References

1. Aman MG, Van Bourgondien ME, Wolford PL, Sarphare G: Psychotropic and Anticonvulsant Drugs in Subjects With Autism: Prevalence and Patterns of Use. J Am Acad Child Adolesc Psychiatry 34 (12): 1672–1681, 1995
2. American Psychiatric Association: Diagnostic and Statistical Manual of Mental Disorders, 4th ed. Washington, DC, American Psychiatric Association, 1994
3. Asarnow J, Thompson M: Childhood-Onset Schizophrenia: A Follow-Up Study. Schizophrenia Bulletin 20 (4): 559–617, 1994
4. Baggett JM: Attention Disorders. In Johnson BS (ed): Child, Adolescent and Family Psychiatric Nursing, pp 207–220. Philadelphia, JB Lippincott, 1995
5. Bassuk E: In Support of Children and Youth: Encouraging Research Dissemination. Am J Orthopsychiatry 65 (2): 172–173, 1995
6. Biederman J, Faraone SV, Mick E, Spencer T, Wilens T, Kiely K, Guite J, Ablon JS, Reed E, Warburton R: High Risk for Attention Deficit Hyperactivity Disorder Among Children of Parents With Childhood Onset of the Disorder: A Pilot Study. Am J Psychiatry 152 (3): 431–435, 1995
7. Bishop SM: Educating for Parenthood in the 1990s: Preventive Intervention for High-Risk Youth. J Child Adolesc Psychiatr Ment Health Nurs 3 (1): 1–2, 1990
8. Brooks RB: Children at Risk: Fostering Resilience and Hope. Am J Orthopsychiatry 64 (4): 545–553, 1994
9. Brunett NM, Cutbirth S: Behavior Management. In Johnson BS (ed): Child, Adolescent and Family Psychiatric Nursing, pp 392–409. Philadelphia, JB Lippincott, 1995
10. Children's Defense Fund: Children 1990: Report Care,

Briefing Book, and Action Primer. Washington, DC, Children's Defense Fund, 1990

11. Conley JF: Conduct Disorders. In Johnson BS (ed): Child, Adolescent and Family Psychiatric Nursing, pp 221–231. Philadelphia, JB Lippincott, 1995
12. Critchley DL: Mental Status Examinations With Children and Adolescents. Nurs Clin North Am 14 (September): 429–441, 1979
13. Earle KA, Forquer SL: Use of Seclusion With Children and Adolescents in Public Psychiatric Hospitals. Am J Orthopsychiatry 65 (2): 238–244, 1995
14. Finkelhor D, Browne A: Initial and Long-Term Effects: A conceptual Framework. In Finkelhor D (ed): A Sourcebook on Child Sexual Abuse, pp 180–198. Newbury Park, CA, Sage Publications, 1986
15. Fleming JE, Offord DR: Epidemiology of Childhood Depressive Disorders: A Critical Review. J Am Acad Child Adolesc Psychiatry 29 (4): 571–580, 1990
16. Francis S: Disability and Chronic Illness. In Johnson BS (ed): Child, Adolescent and Family Psychiatric Nursing, pp 146–173. Philadelphia, JB Lippincott, 1995
17. Freud A: Normality and Pathology in Childhood: Assessments of Development. New York, International Universities Press, 1965
18. Garmezy N: Stress, Competence, and Development: Continuities in the Study of Schizophrenic Adults, Children Vulnerable to Psychopathology, and the Search for Stress-Resistant Children. Am J Orthopsychiatry 57 (April): 159–174, 1987
19. Garrison CZ, Jackson KL, Marsteller F, McKeown R, Addy C: A Longitudinal Study of Depressive Symptomatology in Young Adolescents. J Am Acad Child Adolesc Psychiatry 29 (4): 581–585, 1990
20. Garrison WT: Aggressive Behavior, Seclusion and Physical Restraint in an Inpatient Child Population. J Am Acad Child Psychiatry 23 (July): 448–452, 1984
21. Gill CD: Protecting Our children: Where Have We Gone and Where Should We Go From Here? J Psychosoc Nurs 33 (3): 31–35, 1995
22. Gross DA: Children of the Mentally Ill. In Johnson BS (ed): Child, Adolescent and Family Psychiatric Nursing, pp 101–113. Philadelphia, JB Lippincott, 1995
23. Hagino OR, Weller EB, Weller RA, Washing D, Fristad MA, Konntras SB: Untoward Effects of Lithium Treatment in Children Aged Four through Six Years. J Am Acad Child Adolesc Psychiatry 34 (12): 1584–1590, 1995
24. Halpern R: Poverty and Early Childhood Parenting: Toward a Framework for Intervention. Am J Orthopsychiatry 60 (1): 6–8, 1990
25. Hawley TL, Halle TG, Drasin RE, Thomas NG: Children of Addicted Mothers: Effects of the "Crack Epidemic" on the Caregiving Environment and the Development of Preschoolers. Am J Orthopsychiatry 65 (3): 364–379, 1995
26. Hughes MC: Recurrent Abdominal Pain and Childhood Depression: Clinical Observations of 23 Children and Their Families. Am J Orthopsychiatry 54 (January): 146–155, 1984
27. Institute of Medicine: Report Card on the National Plan for Research on Child and Adolescent Mental Disorders: The Midway Point. Washington, DC, 1995
28. Institute of Medicine: Research on Children and Adolescents with Mental, Behavioral, and Developmental Disorders. Research Rep. No. IOM-89-07. Washington, DC, National Academy Press, 1989
29. Irwin M: Are Seclusion Rooms Needed on Child Psychiatric Units? Am J Orthopsychiatry 57 (January): 125–126, 1987
30. Johnson BH: A Call to Action in Behalf of Children and Families. Child Health Care 20 (3): 185–188, 1991
31. Johnson BS: Mental Health of Children, Adolescents, and Families. In Johnson BS (ed): Child, Adolescent and Family Psychiatric Nursing, pp 1–14. Philadelphia, JB Lippincott, 1995
32. Johnson BS, Baggett JM: Applying the Nursing Process to Children, Adolescents, and Families. In Johnson BS (ed): Child, Adolescent and Family Psychiatric Nursing, pp 15–31. Philadelphia, JB Lippincott, 1995
33. Johnson CM: Therapeutic Environments. In Johnson BS (ed): Child, Adolescent and Family Psychiatric Nursing, pp 424–438. Philadelphia, JB Lippincott, 1995
34. Killeen MR: Problems in Parenting. In Johnson BS (ed): Child, Adolescent and Family Psychiatric Nursing, pp 32–44. Philadelphia, JB Lippincott, 1995
35. Knitzer J, Aber L: Young Children in Poverty: Facing the Facts. Am J Orthopsychiatry 65 (2): 174–176, 1995
36. Kurtz L: Psychosocial Coping Resources in Elementary School-Age Children of Divorce. Am J Orthopsychiatry 64 (4): 554–563, 1994
37. Li J, Bennett N: Young Children in Poverty: A Statistical Update. New York, National Center for Children in Poverty, Columbia University School of Public Health, 1994
38. Lohnes KL, Kalter N: Preventive Intervention Groups for Parentally Bereaved Children. Am J Orthopsychiatry 64 (4): 594–603, 1995
39. McSwiggan-Hardin MT: Tic disorders. In Johnson BS (ed): Child, Adolescent and Family Psychiatric Nursing, pp 285–300. Philadelphia, JB Lippincott, 1995
40. Meyer EC, Edwards GH, Rossi JS: Evaluation and Selection of Standardized Psychological Instruments for Research and Clinical Practice. Journal of Child and Adolescent Psychiatric Nursing 8 (3): 24–31, 1995
41. Moustakas CE: Psychotherapy With Children: The Living Relationship. New York, Ballantine Books, 1959
42. National Center for Children in Poverty: Five Million Children: A Statistical Profile of Our Poorest Young Citizens. New York, National Center for Children in Poverty, 1990
43. Opie ND: Issues Facing Child Psychiatric Nursing in the 1990s: Response and Recommendations. Journal of Child and Adolescent Psychiatric Mental Health Nursing 3 (2): 68–71, 1990
44. Pearson GS: Mood Disorders. In Johnson BS (ed): Child, Adolescent and Family Psychiatric Nursing, pp 253–269. Philadelphia, JB Lippincott, 1995
45. Pearson GS: Pervasive Developmental Disorders. In Johnson BS (ed): Child, Adolescent and Family Psychiatric Nursing, pp 270–284. Philadelphia, JB Lippincott, 1995
46. Pearson GS: Psychopharmacology. In Johnson BS (ed):

Child, Adolescent and Family Psychiatric Nursing, pp 410–423. Philadelphia, JB Lippincott, 1995

47. Peters SD, Wyatt GE, Finkelhor D: Prevalence. In Finkelhor D (ed): A Sourcebook on Child Sexual Abuse, pp 15–19. Newbury Park, CA, Sage Publications, 1986
48. Peterson BS: Neuroimaging in Child and Adolescent Neuropsychiatric Disorders. J Am Acad Child Adolesc Psychiatry 34 (12): 1560–1576, 1995
49. Pfeffer CR: Assessment of Suicidal Children and Adolescents. Psychiatr Clin North Am 12 (4): 861–872, 1989
50. Pothier PC: The Issue of Prevention in Psychiatric Nursing. Archives of Psychiatric Nursing 1 (June): 143–144, 1987
51. Proctor JT: Hysteria in Childhood. Am J Orthopsychiatry 28 (April): 394–406, 1958
52. Rae-Grant N: Prevention. In Stenhauer PD, Rae-Grant Q (eds): Psychological Problems of the Child in the Family, 2d ed, pp 591–610. New York, Basic Books, 1983
53. Raynor CM: Managing Angry Feelings: Teaching Angry Children to Cope. Perspectives in Psychiatric Care 28 (2): 11–14, 1992
54. Rotheram MJ: Evaluation of Imminent Danger for Suicide Among Youth. Am J Orthopsychiatry 57 (January): 102–110, 1987
55. Ryan G, Miyoshi TJ, Metzner JL, Krugman RD, Fryer GE: Trends in a National Sample of Sexually Abusive Youths. J Am Acad Child Adolesc Psychiatry 35 (1): 17–25, 1996
56. Scahill L, Lynch KA: Clomipramine and Obsessive-Compulsive Disorder. Journal of Child and Adolescent Psychiatric Nursing 8 (2): 42–45, 1995
57. Scahill L, Lynch KA: The Use of Methylphenidate in Children with Attention-Deficit Hyperactivity Disorder. Journal of Child and Adolescent Psychiatric Nursing 7 (4): 44–47, 1994
58. Scahill L, Walker RD, Lechner SN, Tynan KE: Inpatient Treatment of Obsessive Compulsive Disorder in Childhood: A Case Study. Journal of Child and Adolescent Psychiatric Nursing 6 (3): 5–14, 1993
59. Sloate PL, Voyat G: Cognitive and Affective Features in Childhood Psychosis. Am J Psychotherapy 37 (July): 376–386, 1983
60. Snow ME, Hertzig ME, Shapiro T: Rate of Development in Young Autistic Children. J Am Acad Child Adolesc Psychiatry 26 (6): 834–835, 1987
61. Swegle J, Personett R: Victimization of Children and Adolescents. In Johnson BS (ed): Child, Adolescent and Family Psychiatric Nursing, pp 129–145. Philadelphia, JB Lippincott, 1995
62. Tapia F: Children Who Are Cruel to Animals. Child Psychiatry Human Dev 2 (Winter): 70–77, 1971
63. Townsend MC: Nursing Diagnoses in Psychiatric Nursing: A Pocket Guide for Care Plan Construction, 2d ed. Philadelphia, FA Davis, 1991
64. Turecki S: Elective Brief Psychotherapy with Children. Am J Psychother 36 (October): 479–488, 1982
65. U.S. Congress, Office of Technology Assessment: Children's Mental Health: Problems and Services—A Background Paper (Report No. OTA-BP-H-33). Washington, DC, U.S. Government Printing Office, 1986
66. U.S. Department of Health and Human Services: National Plan for Research on Child and Adolescent Mental Disorders. Rockville, MD, National Institute of Mental Health, 1990
67. Varley CK, Furukawa MJ: Psychopathology in Young Children with Developmental Disabilities. Child Health Care 19 (2): 86–92, 1990
68. Walsh E, Randell BP: Seclusion and Restraint: What We Need to Know. Journal of Child and Adolescent Psychiatric Nursing 8 (1): 28–40, 1995
69. Wilens TE, Spencer T, Biederman J, Wozniak J, Connor D: Combined Pharmacotherapy: An Emerging Trend in Pediatric Psychopharmacology. J Am Acad Child Adolesc Psychiatry 34 (1): 110–112, 1995

23

Adolescents

Celeste M. Johnson

"Who are you?" said the caterpillar. Alice replied rather shyly, "I–I hardly know, sir, just at present—at least I know who I was when I got up this morning, but I must have changed several times since then."

Lewis Carroll,
Alice's Adventures in Wonderland

This chapter addresses an increasingly important and complex mental health problem—mental and emotional disturbance in adolescents. Normal adolescent development, theories of adolescent disturbance, and the incidence and significance of the problem are presented. The dynamics of several important disorders occurring during adolescence are discussed.

*The steps of the nursing process are applied to adolescent disorders. Emphasis is on assessing the adolescent based on knowledge of developmental variables, planning with the adolescent and his or her family (including discharge planning), intervention through various treatment modalities, and evaluating the outcomes of interventions. Mental health professionals are encouraged to examine their feelings and attitudes about working with people in this group.**

Learning Objectives

On completion of this chapter, you should be able to accomplish the following:

1. *Describe the primary and secondary changes of normal adolescent development.*
2. *Discuss various theories of adolescent development.*
3. *Describe the incidence of various adolescent disorders.*
4. *Discuss the variables of family communication, parenting style, personality, social pressures, and stressors that may contribute to the disorder.*
5. *Identify the dynamics of adolescent disorders.*
6. *Apply the nursing process to mentally and emotionally disturbed adolescent clients.*
7. *Discuss how a nurse's feelings affect interaction with an adolescent client and family.*

◆ Adolescent Development

Adolescence is a transitional developmental period between childhood and adulthood that is characterized by more biological, psychological, and social role changes than any other stage of life except infancy. Adolescents vary considerably with respect to the onset, duration, and intensity of the changes they experience. Nurses need to take into account developmental theory when assessing and planning care for adolescents.

One framework for understanding adolescent development includes primary and secondary changes.[32] The biological, cognitive, and social role changes of adolescence are viewed as "primary changes" because they are universal across culture and occur prior to the secondary changes of adolescence. The "secondary changes" refer to identity, achievement, sexuality, intimacy, autonomy, and attachment. Primary changes have an impact on the secondary changes through the contexts in which adolescents develop, namely, family, peer, school, and work settings.

PRIMARY CHANGES OF ADOLESCENCE

The primary changes of adolescence include biological or pubertal changes, psychological or cognitive changes, and social redefinition.

Biological or Pubertal Changes

Substantial physical growth and change occur during adolescence. Boys experience changes in body proportions, facial characteristics, voice, body hair, strength, and coordination; girls experience changes in body proportions, body hair, breast growth, and menarchal status. Peak pubertal development occurs 2 years earlier in girls than in boys. Awareness of these physical changes may be pleasing or horrifying to the adolescent. A lack of information about puberty and sexuality contributes to emotional upset. The response of family and peers to the adolescent's advancing development impacts on how such events are experienced.[32]

The onset of different pubertal changes within the individual also varies. This variation among individuals in the time of onset, duration, and termination of the pubertal cycle has social consequences. For example, a 14-year-old boy who has experienced puberty early may be preferred for athletic activities and social events over a same-age peer who has not yet begun pubertal changes. However, there is no relationship between physical development and cognitive development. A boy who is more physically mature than the majority of his peers is not necessarily able to think more abstractly or complexly than others his age. Nurses and parents should not assume that physical changes indicate development in cognitive or psychological areas.[32]

Psychological or Cognitive Changes

Though not as easily seen, cognitive changes in adolescence are as dramatic as the physical changes. Adolescence is the period of formal operational thinking in which adult-level reasoning takes place.[50,51] Adolescents who achieve such thinking abilities are able to think more complexly, abstractly, and hypothetically and are able to think realistically about the future. These cognitive changes have important implications for parent–adolescent relationships. Adolescents are increasingly able to discuss and argue about issues with their parents, see the flaws in their parents' arguments, imagine what it would be like to have different parents, and think

**Also see displays in Chapter 22, Children, for additional DSM-IV criteria relevant to disorders of adolescence.*

about their parents' marital relationship separate from their own relationships with their parents.[32]

A parent of an adolescent may need to be educated about typical adolescent behavior. Parents may use their own adolescence as "the norm," thus biasing their attributions about their child's behavior. Parents have the additional task of integrating their own expectations with the norms of their child's peer group. Particularly for parents who are dealing with adolescence for the first time, the nurse can help them bring their expectations in line with what is known about normative behaviors during the adolescent period.

Social Redefinition

The social status of children changes during adolescence and varies greatly in different cultures. In nonindustrial societies, rites of passage take place soon after the onset of puberty. In western industrialized societies, the transition is less clear, but changes in social status do take place. Changes occur across four domains: *interpersonal* (eg, changes in familial status), *political* (eg, late adolescents are eligible to vote), *economic* (eg, adolescents are allowed to work), and *legal* (eg, late adolescents can be tried in adult court systems).[32]

Adolescents vary in their ability to adapt to changing societal expectations for acceptable behavior. There is little consensus about what constitutes "normal" behavior for adolescents in western culture. The media frequently present conflicting messages concerning sexuality and substance abuse. Given a lack of role clarity, the adolescent's failure to sort through conflicting expectations may contribute to psychopathology.[32]

Contextual Changes of Adolescence

Contextual changes during adolescence occur across the following settings: family, peer, school, and work.

Changes in Family Relationships. Adolescence is a time of transformation in family relationships. Scholars who have written about adolescence from a psychoanalytic perspective have viewed this developmental period as a time of storm and stress when extreme levels of conflict with parents result in reorientation toward peers. Recent research has not supported these early storm and stress notions. Only 20% of adolescents have such relationships with their parents.[32] Despite the lack of a traumatic relationship during early adolescence, a period of increased emotional distance and conflict in the parent–adolescent relationship peaks during pubertal change. Increases in conflicts between parents and adolescents usually are about mundane issues rather than basic values. Most adolescents negotiate this period without severing ties with parents or developing serious disorders.[32]

The nurse should be aware that transformations in attachments to parents are expected during adolescence and that normal familial problems may arise because of difficulties managing this transition. The nurse must evaluate whether an adolescent's difficulties are actually continuations of problems that began in early or middle childhood or are difficulties in managing the transition to adolescence.

One of the major tasks for parents during this developmental period is to be responsive to the adolescent's needs for increasing responsibility and decision-making power in the family while maintaining a high level of cohesiveness in the family environment. Parents who lack flexibility and adaptability during this developmental period tend to have teenagers with less successful outcomes.[24] Interventions planned for the family can facilitate parental adaptability and developmental sensitivity.

Changes in Peer Relationships. One of the strongest predictors of adult difficulties is poor peer relationships during childhood and adolescence.[32] Child–child relationships have positive effects on all spheres of development.[32] Sullivan[56] provides a stage theory for the development of peer relationships. Similar to Piaget, Sullivan stresses the importance of interpersonal relationships and the differences between child–child and parent–child relationships. Sullivan describes the notion of "chumship" in adolescence and maintains that this typically same-sex friendship is a critical developmental accomplishment. With this relationship, the adolescent learns about intimacy, and this friendship is the basis for later close relationships. Nurses may facilitate the development of such "chumship" relationships in young adolescents who have few friends either by increasing the adolescent's involvment in extracurricular activities or by including the adolescent in group therapy.[32]

Families and peers each provide unique contributions to development and adjustment. Healthy family relationships provide a secure base for an adolescent's exploration into the world of peers. Adolescents usually adhere to their parents' values even during increases in peer involvement. In fact, parent and peer values are typically similar, especially concerning important issues. Differences between parent and peer values are more likely when adolescents have distant relationships with their parents and when they associate with peers who endorse antisocial behaviors.[32] Nurses need to assess the status and quality of their clients' peer relationships and the manner in which the family and peer environments intertwine. Nurses may involve peers or older siblings in treatment to provide opportunities for the adolescent to practice social skills.

Effects of the School Context. School is an important environment for the development of the adolescent's personality, values, and social relationships.[58] Movement between schools can be stressful, with multiple school transitions producing negative effects. Children, particularly girls, who switched from an elementary school into a junior high school (as opposed to staying in a kindergarten through eighth grade school) showed decreased self-esteem, which was partially attributable to movement from a protected environment like elementary school to the impersonal environment of junior high school.[58]

Other aspects of the school's impact on adolescent development are physical setting, limitations in resources, philosophies of education, teacher expectations, and curriculum characteristics. Interactions between teacher and student also are related to a variety of adolescent outcomes.[32] The high rate of dropouts in some school districts indicates that the school environment and student needs have not been well matched. On a positive note, larger schools provide larger numbers and more variety of peers with whom the adolescent can interact. Nurses should assess the nature and quality of their adolescent clients' school environments; practitioners can enhance or minimize aspects of the school environment, depending on their impact.

Effects of Working. More than 80% of all high school students in this country work before they graduate.[32] Although adolescents who work tend to develop an increased sense of self-reliance, they also tend to develop cynical attitudes about work, spend less time with their families and peers, and are less involved in school. They are more likely to abuse drugs and commit delinquent acts. Working may preempt time for self-exploration and identity development. These problems may be because of the monotonous and stressful nature of jobs open to adolescents. Nurses need to encourage balance between work and other aspects of an adolescent's life.

SECONDARY CHANGES OF ADOLESCENCE

The secondary changes of adolescence are identity, achievement, sexuality, intimacy, autonomy, and attachment.[32]

Identity

A major psychological task of adolescence is the development of an identity.[18] Adolescents develop identity through role explorations and commitments. One's identity is multidimensional and includes self-perceptions and commitments across a number of domains, including occupational, academic, religious, interpersonal, sexual, and political. Research in the area of identity development has defined at least four types of identity status with respect to the dimensions of commitment and exploration[32]:

- Identity moratorium: exploration with no commitment
- Identity foreclosure: commitment with no exploration
- Identity diffusion: no commitment and no systematic exploration
- Identity achievement: commitment after extensive exploration

An adolescent's status can change with time, reflecting increased maturation or conversely, regression to some less adaptive identity status. Most importantly, an adolescent's identity status also varies depending on the domain under consideration (eg, academic versus interpersonal).

The nurse must recognize that the process of identity formation is different for boys and girls. Identity development in boys involves struggles with autonomy and themes of separation, whereas identity development in girls is more likely to be intertwined with the development and maintenance of intimate relationships.[32]

Achievement

Decisions made during adolescence can have serious consequences for the future. For the first time, the student has a choice of classes in high school. Some adolescents decide to drop out of school; others graduate from high school and seek full-time employment; and some decide to continue their education in college or graduate school. These decisions present the adolescent with new opportunities but also limit the range of future options. Choices that affect the future usually are accompanied by anxiety. The nurse can use the issues to help parents serve as guides or models for the adolescent, rather than as authority figures. Given the complexity of achievement decisions, adolescents who have developed advanced cognitive abilities (ie, the ability to use future-oriented thinking, abstract reasoning, and hypothetical thinking) are at an advantage when they begin to make decisions related to their education and career.

Sexuality

Most children have mixed reactions to becoming a sexually mature adolescent. Parents also have conflicting reactions to such increasing maturity. Very little is known about normal adolescent sexuality, primarily due to the difficulty in conducting studies on this topic. Factors that are associated with the onset and maintenance of sexual behavior include pubertal changes, ethnic and religious differences, personality characteristics, and social factors.[32]

The increasing rates of sexually transmitted diseases among adolescents and the fact that many young adults with acquired immunodeficiency syndrome probably became infected as adolescents suggest that adolescent sexuality deserves attention from mental health practitioners working with adolescents. Family life education is beginning to make a positive difference in teenagers' sexual behavior. Education programs have led teenagers to postpone sexual activity or to use contraceptives.[10] Given the often conflicting nature of adolescent, peer, and parental responses to sexuality, nurses may be educators about sexual matters. Practitioners must be clear, direct, and thorough in their evaluation of adolescent sexual behaviors. This requires nurses to be aware of their own conflicts associated with sexual issues.

Intimacy

During adolescence, friendships have the potential to become intimate. An intimate relationship is characterized by trust, mutual self-disclosure, a sense of loyalty, and helpfulness. Intimate sharing with friends increases during adolescence.[32]

All relationships become more emotionally charged during the adolescent period, and adolescents are more likely to engage in friendships with opposite-sex peers than they were as children. Girls' same-sex relationships are more intimate than boys' same-sex relationships. Having intimate friendships is adaptive; adolescents with such friendships are more likely to have high self-esteem.[32]

Autonomy

There is more than one type of adolescent autonomy.[55] *Emotional autonomy* is the capacity to relinquish childlike dependencies on parents.[23] Adolescents deidealize their parents, see them as people rather than simply as parenting figures, and are less dependent on them for immediate emotional support.

When adolescents are *behaviorally autonomous*, they have the capacity to make their own decisions, to be less influenced by others, and to be more self-governing and self-reliant. Being behaviorally autonomous does not mean that adolescents never rely on the help of others. Instead, they become increasingly able to recognize situations in which they have the ability to make their own decisions versus situations in which they will need to consult with a peer or parent for advice. Susceptibility to peer pressure increases to a peak in early adolescence due, in part, to an increase in peer pressure prior to early adolescence and an accompanying decrease in susceptibility to parental pressure. The nurse should be particularly attentive to the following autonomy-related issues as they arise during treatment:

1. To what degree is the adolescent responsible in managing the level of autonomy he or she has been granted?
2. Do parent and child have realistic expectations for the level of autonomy to be granted in the future?
3. Is there a discrepancy between the amount of autonomy the parent is willing to grant and the amount of autonomy the adolescent is able to manage?
4. What is the parental response to the adolescent's attempts to be autonomous (ie, do they have the ability to foster healthy levels of autonomy in their children?)
5. How flexible are parents in changing their parenting related to autonomy issues?[32]

Attachment

One task of adolescence is to gain increasing levels of behavioral autonomy without sacrificing the attachment with primary caregivers. Parental disapproval about issues of importance to the adolescent is more difficult than peer disapproval. During adolescence, the attachment relationship between parent and adolescent is transformed from one of unilateral authority to one of mutuality and cooperation.[55]

◆ Adolescent Disturbance

INCIDENCE AND SIGNIFICANCE

In adolescents, true psychopathology is relatively rare. The percentage of adolescents showing symptoms is between 10% and 20%.[32] Difficulties arise in distinguishing normal adolescent behaviors from serious disturbance. Overdiagnosis and underdiagnosis can result from a lack or erroneous knowledge of developmental norms. If the seriously disturbed teenager does not receive appropriate treatment, the chances are remote that he or she will grow out of the problem.[32]

Approximately half of all adolescent disorders are continuations of those seen in childhood; however, the nature of the disorders may vary in adolescents. For example, the impulsivity and inattentiveness components of attention-deficit hyperactivity disorder (ADHD) are much more likely to be evident during adolescence than is the hyperactivity component. Moreover, the manner in which impulsivity and inattentiveness are exhibited changes as children move into adolescence.[32]

Rates of depression, bipolar affective disorders, attempted suicide, completed suicide, and schizophrenia increase during adolescence. Antisocial activities increase in frequency but not in the number of individuals committing the acts. Agoraphobia and social phobias become more common during adolescence.[32]

The incidence of acting-out behaviors in adolescents continues to rise. The juvenile violent crime arrest rate increased by 50% from 1985 to 1991.[3] Violent crimes include homicide, forcible rape, robbery, or aggravated assault. Approximately the same proportion of youth are committing violent acts with about the same frequency as 10 years ago, but the lethality of that violence has increased: Victims are being killed rather than injured. Researchers attribute much of the increased lethality to the growing use of handguns.

The teenage violent death rate reflects deaths from homicide, suicide, and accidents among 15- to 19-year-olds. In 1991, this rate rose to 71.1 per 100,000, a 13% increase over the 1985 rate of 62.8. Thirty-three states and the District of Columbia followed the national trend toward a worsening teenage violent death rate. This trend is even more disturbing in light of the steady decline in auto-related fatalities. The overall growth in this indicator is due almost entirely to a doubling in the incidence of teenage homicide victims since 1985. Firearms are involved in more than half of all adolescent homicides and suicides.[57]

Violence by juveniles is most often inflicted on other juveniles. The Justice Department estimates that nearly 1 million 12- to 19-year-olds are raped, robbed, or assaulted each year, most often by their peers.[57] This rate is twice that of the general population.[59] Adolescents from 12 to 19 years have the highest victimization rates for crimes of violence and theft. As evidence of this disturbing rise in violence, some teenagers are now planning their own funerals, suggesting their clothing, attendees, and music.

The issue of whether or not to use drugs is virtually universal in American society and is a developmental problem faced by adolescents and their families. Two separate surveys released in 1994 document an increase in teenage drug and alcohol use between 1992 and 1993.[10] The percentage of 12th-grade students who said they had used an illicit drug within the previous 30 days rose from 14.4% in 1992 to 18.3% in 1993, with marijuana use increasing most sharply. Among eighth-grade students, marijuana use increased by 60% between 1992 and 1993. The percentage of teenagers 12 to 17 years old using illegal drugs rose from 6.1% in 1992 to 6.6% in 1993. Alcohol use jumped 15% among 12- to 17-year-olds between 1992 and 1993. More than one in four eighth-grade students and more than one in two high school seniors reported currently drinking alcohol in 1993. That year, more than one in eight eighth-grade students and more than one in four seniors said they had engaged in "binge" drinking, defined as consuming five drinks or more in a row, within the previous 2 weeks.[10]

One challenge that girls face in early adolescence is an increased risk of sexual abuse. Overall rates of sexual abuse increase substantially for girls between 10 and 14 years old.[48] Girls 14 to 15 years old have the highest risk of being raped of any age group. In turn, rape and sexual abuse are associated with a greatly increased risk for depression, particularly in female victims, shortly after and long after the abuse. Boys are also victims of rape and other forms of sexual abuse, but young girls and adolescent girls are at least two to three times more likely than boys to be the victims of abuse.[58] Childhood sexual or physical abuse is highly traumatic and has profound significance for the psychological development and behavior of its victims. Such abuse is not necessarily a precursor of psychiatric disorders, but it may be a risk factor.[25]

Comorbidity, or co-occurrence, of psychiatric disorders in adolescents is of special relevance to the nurse because it affects the majority of adolescent clients.[39] All psychiatric disorders in adolescents appear to show some degree of comorbidity, although the degree to which any two disorders are comorbid varies. For example, adolescents with substance use disorders are more likely to have a comorbid disruptive behavior disorder than they are to have an anxiety disorder.[39]

Comorbidity has implications for diagnosis, theories of etiology, and clinical issues. Comorbidity in adolescents is associated with increased mental health service use, impaired role functioning, likelihood of suicidal behavior, academic problems, and increased conflict with parents.[39]

When conducting an initial assessment, the nurse should probe for disorders other than those suggested by the referral. The high degree of comorbidity expected in clinical practice with adolescents also emphasizes the importance of interventions that address a multiplicity of problems. The high rate of comorbidity in adolescents may partially explain why it is difficult for clinicians to achieve outcome results as good as those reported in clinical trials because samples often exclude clients with comorbid disorders. The high rate of comorbidity in referred clients also emphasizes the importance of addressing the unanswered question of which disorder should by the primary target for the intervention.[39]

ETIOLOGICAL THEORIES

Several theorists have identified factors related to the cause of adolescent disturbance. These formulations are important in assisting nurses to understand how disturbance develops and how it might be prevented, diagnosed, and treated. Although the theories provide different views about the causes of the disorders, they are not mutually exclusive. Adolescent disturbance is multifactorial and involves biological and psychological theories.[8]

The factors associated with depression illustrate the complexity of etiological theories of adolescent disturbance. Etiological models of depression are based on different theoretical frameworks, each suggesting potentially helpful treatment strategies. Biological models emphasize familial and biochemical factors that influence preventive and medical treatment. Psychosocial theories suggest different types of interventions, such as psychoanalytical, behavioral, or cognitive techniques. Biopsychosocial models influence assessment and treatment by fusing physiological and psychosocial considerations.

Biological models indicate that adolescent depression may result from the underactivity of nerve cells whose neurotransmitters are the biogenic amines, such as serotonin or norepinephrine.[53] Findings from twin, adoption, and family studies support the influence of genetics among the causes of depression. There is an increased incidence of depression in adoptees whose biological parents had an affective disorder.[8]

Psychoanalytic and cognitive-behavioral theories of depression hold that relying on the acceptance and approval of others for self-esteem puts a person at risk for depression because the approval of others is not always reliable.[48]

◆ Dynamics of Adolescent Disorders

ADJUSTMENT DISORDERS

Reactive or situational in nature, adjustment disorders are evidenced by significant emotional or behavioral symptoms in response to identifiable psychosocial stressors.[1] Stress temporarily overwhelms the capacity of the individual to solve problems. The stressor may be a single event (eg, termination of a relationship) or multiple events (eg, move to a new city and parental divorce). Stressors may be recurrent (eg, associated with holidays) or continuous (eg, living in a high-crime neighborhood). Stressors may affect the adolescent, the adolescent's entire family, or a larger group or community (eg, as in a natural disaster). Some stressors accompany specific developmental events (eg, going to college). Symptoms of adjustment disorders express a conflict about dependence and independence issues.

The prevalence of adjustment disorders in outpatient mental health centers ranges from 5% to 20%.[1] Adjustment disorders occur in any age group, and males and females are equally affected. Adolescents from disadvantaged life circumstances experience a high rate of stressors and are at increased risk for the disorder.[1]

The subjective distress or impairment in functioning associated with adjustment disorder is frequently manifested as decreased school performance or attendance and temporary changes in social relationships. Adjustment disorders are associated with an increased risk of attempted and completed suicide. Adjustment problems often complicate the course of illness in an adolescent with a physical disorder and may be demonstrated by decreased compliance with recommended medical regimens.

The nature, meaning, and experience of the stressors and the evaluation of the response to the stressors vary across cultures. Nurses should consider the context of cultural setting when evaluating whether the adolescent's response to the stressor is maladaptive and if the associated distress seems excessive. Cognitive and behavioral interventions may help the adolescent cope with actual stressors or change perceptions about stressors. Medications may be indicated to treat comorbid medical conditions or reduce anxiety.

DISRUPTIVE BEHAVIOR DISORDERS

Attention-Deficit Hyperactivity Disorder. The occurrence of ADHD is as common in adolescents as it is in children. It is characterized by symptoms such as distractibility, impulsivity, inattention, and disruptive behaviors. Without hyperactivity to call attention to them, adolescents with ADHD are often ignored, underdiagnosed, and undertreated. As many as 9% of children and adolescents have ADHD. Long-term outcomes indicate that most symptoms remain throughout life.[19]

The results of ADHD are impaired school performance, limited participation in extracurricular activities, increased risk of delinquency, and harmed social relationships and family interactions. Without effective treatment, ADHD often results in increased risk of trauma, substance abuse, and conduct, anxiety, and affective disorders during adolescence.[19,65] Difficulties in evaluation of adolescents with ADHD are the misdiagnosis of other recognizable disorders as ADHD and the failure to recognize comorbid disorders.[62] The phenomenological overlap between bipolar disorder and ADHD often makes it difficult to distinguish between these two syndromes because the core symptoms of both conditions include impaired attention, racing thoughts, distractibility, motor hyperactivity, and impulsive behavior.[62,63]

No standardized formal tests establish the diagnosis of ADHD in adolescents.[63] Rating scales can identify an adolescent who is hyperactive, distractible, or impulsive, but these may not discriminate between ADHD and other possible causes of the behavior.[63] Clinical history and observational data from teachers and family are effective in identifying ADHD. Useful tools include the Child Behavior Checklist (CBCL) for 12- to 16-year-olds, the CBCL Youth Self-Report for 11- to 18-year-olds, the CBCL for parents and teachers, the Connors scales, and the Child Attention Problems Scale.[63] No specific physical or neurological findings consistently establish the diagnosis, but a positive response to methylphenidate (Ritalin) is suggestive.[63]

Treatment for adolescents with ADHD includes medication, individual and family psychotherapy, education, and support for parents, families, and school personnel.[63] The combination of these interventions varies with the needs of the adolescent and family.

Stimulant medications reduce hyperactivity, distractibility, inattentiveness, and oppositionality and may improve motor, impulse, and self-control; mood; sociability; personal relationships; and academic success.[63] Distractible adolescents on medication may be able to organize their ideas better when speaking or writing, increase concentration and stay on task, benefit more from psychotherapy because they can reflect before responding, and use cognitive strategies for learning. Common side effects include diminished appetite, stomachache, headache, and marked hyperactivity and insomnia when the medication wears off.[63] A second dose of medication in the afternoon or early evening resolves the rebound hyperactivity. Children followed into adulthood show stimulant drug therapy to be effective and safe without apparent long-term side effects.[63]

Tricyclic antidepressants are effective alternatives to stimulants and are particularly useful if the adolescent with ADHD is also depressed.[63] The most common side effect of tricyclic antidepressants is drowsiness, which can be reduced by administering medication at bedtime and by starting with a low dose and gradually increasing the dosage. These antidepressants have a longer duration of action than the stimulants, can be monitored by plasma drug levels, and have less risk of abuse or dependence.[63]

Although some adolescents do well without pharmacotherapy, the best results are derived from a combination of medication and counseling. Absence of medication for ADHD, despite other treatment modalities, correlates closely with a poor outcome in adolescence and early adulthood.[63]

Psychoeducational counseling, behavioral management techniques, cognitive therapy, school interventions, family therapy, biofeedback, and social skills training have each been used alone and in combination with variable success.[63]

The first step in treatment is educating the adolescent with ADHD and the parents. Each must understand the disorder and recognize that the limitations imposed by the disorder are as debilitating as any other chronic physical condition. Counseling helps the family and adolescent cope more effectively with the consequences of ADHD and the need for special interventions, including medications.

Because an adolescent with ADHD has trouble controlling impulses, focusing attention, and following rules, parents and teachers need guidance in ways to manage these behaviors. Behavior management and cognitive therapy have been used successfully at home and at school.[63]

Individual counseling or psychotherapy can make ADHD less damaging to self-esteem and reduce morbidity in half. At a time when adolescents are shaping their identity, counseling helps them define their strengths, assume responsibility for their medication, and accept the limitations ADHD imposes on them.[63]

Family therapy aims to form strategies to handle disruptive behaviors and develop positive ways of addressing sibling concerns and conflicts. It promotes family communication and cohesion, changes members' perceptions and expectations, and improves styles of interacting and roles within the family.[63]

Biofeedback training has been successful with adolescents with ADHD. After being taught biofeedback techniques using computer games, adolescents with ADHD improved their concentration, scanning, and tracking skills.[63]

Adolescents with ADHD tend to be rejected or neglected by their peers. Social skills training helps these adolescents increase social competence and improve social relations. Training techniques include direct coaching, role playing, observing videotapes of successful peer interactions, and practicing methods for resolving conflicts.[63]

Adolescents with ADHD have difficulty remembering sequential information because their distractibility interferes with concentration. Laptop computers and electronic notebooks can help them keep track of assignments and appointments. Extra time on tests, small group classes, curriculum modifications, tutoring in study skills, and multiple choice tests benefit some adolescents. Teachers should participate in the treatment planning for adolescents with ADHD to achieve optimal outcomes, or they may unknowingly sabotage treatment.[63]

Oppositional-Defiant Disorder

Oppositional-defiant disorder (ODD) is one of the most common disorders presented by adolescents for treatment. Resistant, hostile, and belligerent, the adolescent with ODD does not grow out of the symptoms without treatment and usually does not come to treatment willingly [1] (Box 23-1).

Prevalence rates of ODD range from 2% to 16%.[1] The disorder is more common in boys who, in preschool years, had problematic temperaments or high motor activity. The disorder is more prevalent in boys than girls before puberty but equally prevalent in both genders after puberty. Symptoms in boys and girls are similar except that boys have more confrontational behavior and more persistent symptoms.

Adolescents with ODD manifest negativistic and defiant behaviors through stubbornness, resistance to directions, and unwillingness to negotiate with adults or peers. They persistently test limits, usually by ignoring

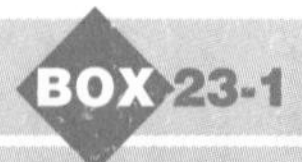

DSM-IV Diagnostic Criteria for Oppositional Defiant Disorder

A. A pattern of negativistic, hostile, and defiant behavior lasting at least 6 months, dursing which four (or more) of the following are present:
   (1) often loses temper
   (2) often argues with adults
   (3) Often actively defies or refuses to comply with adults' requests or rules
   (4) often deliberately annoys people
   (5) often blames others for his or her mistakes or misbehavior
   (6) is often touchy or easily annoyed by others
   (7) is often angry and resentful
   (8) is often spiteful or vindictive

B. The disturbance in behavior causes clinically significant impairment in social, academic, or occupational functioning.

C. The behaviors do not occur exclusively during the course of a Psychotic or Mood Disorder.

D. Criteria are not met for Conduct Disorder, and, if the individual is age 18 years or older, criteria are not met for Antisocial Personality Disorder.

directions, arguing, or failing to accept responsibility for behavior. Hostility is directed at adults or peers by deliberately annoying others or by verbal aggression. Symptoms of this disorder are usually present at home, especially in interactions with adults or peers whom the adolescent knows well but may not be seen at school or in the community. Adolescents with ODD do not see themselves as oppositional or defiant but justify their behavior as a response to unreasonable demands or circumstances.[1]

Low self-esteem; mood lability; low frustration tolerance; swearing; precocious use of alcohol, tobacco, or illicit drugs; and interpersonal conflicts are associated with ODD in school-age children. Adolescents and their parents often get caught in a vicious cycle of bringing out the worst in each other. This disorder is prevalent in families in which child care is disrupted by a succession of different caregivers or in families with harsh, inconsistent, or neglectful parenting practices. Learning and communication disorders and ADHD are associated with ODD.[1] Youth with ODD are at risk for developing conduct disorder.[41]

Oppositional behavior in adolescents is common and may be a sign of the process of normal individuation rather than a symptom of ODD. When interviewing the adolescent, the nurse should assess the following:

1. Do these behaviors occur more frequently and have more serious consequences than typically seen in other adolescents?
2. Have the behaviors caused significant impairment in social, academic, or occupational functioning?

Behavior modification techniques are effective in changing behaviors, such as room care, personal hygiene, completion of chores, verbal and physical abusiveness, and safety violations (eg, curfew violations and reporting whereabouts).[54] When parents and adolescents are involved together, behavior modification programs can be more effective than traditional talk therapy.

Conduct Disorder

Conduct disorder is one of the most frequently diagnosed conditions in outpatient and inpatient mental health facilities for adolescents.[1] Prevalence rates range from 6% to 16% in boys younger than 18 years; for girls, rates range from 2% to 9%. The onset of conduct disorder is usually in late childhood or early adolescence, rarely occurring after 16 years (Box 23-2).

Early age of onset of conduct disorder symptoms is predictive of the persistence of the symptoms and is one of the best predictors of chronic offending.[41] As the number of conduct problems increases, the disorder becomes more severe and the prognosis for recovery worse.[33] Adolescents with a conduct disorder often are unmanageable at home and disruptive in the community.

Adolescents with conduct disorder may have little empathy and concern for the feelings and well-being of others. In ambiguous situations, aggressive adolescents with this disorder frequently misinterpret the intentions of others as more hostile and threatening than is the case and respond with aggression that they then feel is reasonable and justified. They may be callous and lack appropriate feelings of guilt and remorse. These individuals learn that expressing guilt may reduce or prevent punishment, making it difficult to evaluate whether displayed remorse is genuine. Adolescents with conduct disorder often blame others, including their companions, for their misdeeds. Behind a projected image of toughness is low self-esteem.

Low frustration tolerance, irritability, temper outbursts, and recklessness are frequently associated with conduct disorder. Accident rates are higher in adolescents with conduct disorder than in those without it due to risk-taking behaviors, such as drinking, smoking, using illegal substances, and experimenting with sexual behavior and other reckless acts. Use of illegal drugs

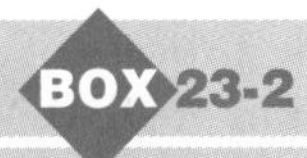

DSM-IV Diagnostic Criteria for Conduct Disorder

A. A repetitive and persistent pattern of behavior in which the basic rights of others or major age-appropriate societal norms or rules are violated, as manifested by the presence of three (or more) of the following criteria in the past 12 months, with at least one criterion present in the past 6 months:

Aggression to people and animals
- (1) often bullies, threatens, or intimidates others
- (2) often initiates physical fights
- (3) has used a weapon that can cause serious physical harm to others (eg, a bat, brick, broken bottle, knife, gun)
- (4) has been physically cruel to people
- (5) has been physically cruel to animals
- (6) has stolen while confronting a victim (eg, mugging, purse snatching, extortion, armed robbery)
- (7) has forced someone into sexual activity

Destruction of property
- (8) has deliberately engaged in fire setting with the intention of causing serious damage
- (9) has deliberately destroyed others' property (other than by fire setting)

Deceitfulness or theft
- (10) has broken into someone else's house, building, or car
- (11) often lies to obtain goods or favors or to avoid obligations (ie, "cons" others)
- (12) has stolen items of nontrivial value without confronting a victim (eg, shoplifting, but without breaking and entering; forgery)

Serious violations of rules
- (13) often stays out at night despite parental prohibitions, beginning before age 13 years
- (14) has run away from home overnight at least twice while living in parental or parental surrogate home (or once without returning for a lengthy period)
- (15) is often truant from school, beginning before age 13 years

B. The disturbance in behavior causes clinically significant impairment in social, academic, or occupational functioning.

C. If the individual is age 18 years or older, criteria are not met for Antisocial Personality Disorder.

increases the risk that conduct disorder will persist. Conduct disorder behaviors often lead to school suspension or expulsion, work adjustment problems, legal difficulties, sexually transmitted diseases, unplanned pregnancy, and physical injury from accidents or fights.[1]

Conduct disorder may be associated with ADHD, learning disorders, anxiety disorders, mood disorders, and substance-related disorders.

Conduct disorder remains a poorly understood disorder for which no clear etiological factors or agents have been identified; however, risk factors have been extensively studied. These risk factors include parental rejection and neglect; difficult infant temperament; inconsistent child-rearing practices with harsh discipline; physical or sexual abuse; lack of supervision; early institutional living; frequent changes in caregivers; large family size; association with a delinquent peer group; the presence of ADHD, ODD, or learning disability; and familial psychopathology, including parental substance abuse.[1,41] Physical aggression is significantly related to the early onset of conduct disorder.[41]

Outcome studies are needed for the treatment of conduct disorders. Despite innovations brought about in recent years by behavioral and social learning models, the psychosocial treatment of delinquent behavior has not been consistently successful in the long run.[64] There remains a need for programs to allow longitudinal growth of social skills and social awareness, with psychiatric, educational, and neuropsychological interventions as needed.[43]

Psychopharmacological intervention for adolescent conduct disorder has not been widely researched. Some clinicians treat associated psychopathology with medication. Lithium and haloperidol decrease symptoms of aggression and impulsivity in conduct disordered boys.[11] Antidepressant therapy decreases symptoms in children diagnosed with a comorbid depression.[11] Pharmacological treatment of conduct disorders needs further study.

SUBSTANCE ABUSE

Among adolescents, the prevalence of alcohol and drug use disorders is 32%.[28] In adolescent populations at high risk for social impairment, such as those with psychiatric problems, the prevalence is even higher. Adolescents with a substance abuse disorder often have comorbid psychopathology. Substance abuse is highly associated with mood disorders, anxiety disorders, and disruptive behavior disorders.[28] Conduct problems are strongly related to concurrent substance use in adolescence; a greater number of symptoms of conduct disorder in children predicts a greater rate of substance abuse disorder in adolescence.[28,29]

Demographical, social, behavioral, and individual risk factors have been found to lead to adolescent substance abuse.[6] While the presence of these factors does not guarantee that adolescents will drink or use drugs, it does make them more susceptible.

Age and gender can predict the course of substance abuse. Boys have a higher rate of alcohol or illicit drug use than girls.[6] The greatest risk for developing a substance use disorder occurs between 15 and 19 years.[28]

Social risk factors involve the influence of the family, peers, and the environment.[6] Adolescents in families that frequently use alcohol and other drugs are more likely to become involved.[5,37] Adolescents from dysfunctional or disturbed families are more likely to become substance abusers[6] as are those whose peer group is involved with alcohol and other drugs.[6]

Environmental factors that affect adolescents' attitudes toward drinking and drug use include a lack of appropriate law enforcement and mixed messages from society.[6] In communities where law enforcement is lax, teenagers may be encouraged to have weekend "beer bashes."[40] Finally, mixed messages about drinking and drug abuse received by adolescents from their environment also contribute to the problem. Adolescents are adept at spotting hypocrisy and have difficulty understanding and abiding by a policy of "Just say 'no' to drugs" in a society where the use of alcohol and other drugs is not only accepted, but often is glorified.

Behavioral risk factors can also lead to adolescent substance abuse. The use of certain substances, such as alcohol and marijuana, can lead to the use of "harder" drugs.[6] Substance abuse is also associated with a tendency to engage in other problem behaviors, such as rebelliousness and precocious sexual and delinquent activities.[6] Abuse of alcohol, marijuana, or cocaine, used alone or in combination, significantly contributes to the prevalence of adolescent suicide, homicide, accidental death and disability, fighting, robbery, rape, and assault.[59]

A final category of risk factors is individual characteristics. Low academic aspirations and poor achievement influence alcohol and other drug use.[2,37] Adolescents who do poorly in school may feel like they are failures, and this feeling may be reinforced by teachers' or parents' responses. Conversely, adolescents who are heavily involved with alcohol and other drugs place little value on academic performance, because the urge to drink and use drugs takes precedence.[6]

Psychological variables, such as self-esteem, motivation, developmental factors, and depression, can also be factors.[6] Teenagers who use chemical substances have a difficult time with the developmental tasks of adolescence, which include forming an identity and separating from the nuclear family. Adolescents may abuse substances to escape from the negative feelings they have about themselves as a result of these psychological and developmental difficulties.

Finally, students who are employed during the school year are more susceptible to substance use and abuse than those who do not work.[6] Adolescents who work have more money to spend on alcohol and illicit drugs and they must simultaneously deal with the pressures of work and school.[6]

Denial of substance abuse or the belief that it is the cause of other problems in the adolescent's life is common in early treatment. Assisting adolescents to associate substance abuse with resulting problems in their lives and challenging faulty logic promote insight into defensive behavior. Group process is especially helpful in confronting defenses, such as denial and rationalization.[66] Attending self-help groups, such as Alcoholics Anonymous or Narcotics Anonymous, helps maintain treatment gains. Regular aftercare, self-help group attendance, and treatment completion are associated with successful outcomes.[66]

DEPRESSION AND SUICIDE

Depression among adolescents is a serious problem that not only afflicts the individual, but often threatens cohesion and even the survival of the family. The prevalence rate for major depression in adolescents ranges from 0.4% to 6.4%.[52] Before adolescence, boys tend to have more depressive symptoms than girls. However, by 13 or 14 years, girls are twice as likely than boys to have these symptoms.[48,49] Gender differences in personality or behavioral style that are present before early adolescence are risk factors that may make adolescent girls more prone to depression when faced with the increased challenges of early adolescence.[48]

A common thread in the literature on depression in adolescence is a distinction between depressed mood and depressive disorders.[46] Depressed mood occurs within the context of expected reactions to life events, whereas depressive disorder occurs when the affective symptoms are out of proportion to the environmental stressors and cause functional impairment.[46] Moderate levels of depression can have a significant negative impact on adolescents. Moderate levels of depression may persist for months in some adolescents and are associated with significant impairment in school and peer functioning.[48] Adolescents with moderate levels of depressive symptoms are also at high risk for major depressive disorders.[48] Thus, even though moderate levels of depressive symptoms may not meet criteria for a psychiatric disorder, they are of concern.

The fourth edition of the Diagnostic and Statistical Manual of Mental Disorders (DSM-IV) lists the criteria of two common depressive disorders of adolescence: dysthymic disorder and major depressive disorder [1] (see Chapter 29, Depressive and Bipolar Disorders). Both are characterized by depressed mood, decreased or increased appetite, sleep disturbance, fatigue or loss of energy, diminished interest or pleasure in usual activities, poor concentration, indecisiveness, low self esteem, feelings of hopelessness, and social withdrawal. Suicidal ideation or behavior may also be present. In major depressive disorder, these symptoms are more acute, dramatic, and functionally impairing than in dysthymic disorder.

Identifying depressive disorder in adolescents is often difficult because of the frequency of mood swings common to that age. Symptoms of depression in adolescence are acting-out behaviors, such as substance abuse, truancy and school dropout, running away from home, antisocial behavior, and self-injury. Suicide is acting out in the extreme. Acting out is seen for several reasons—the adolescent's intolerance for intense feelings, learned behavior, or a lack of verbal skills. Adolescents who are ambivalent about dependency needs may feel that requesting help is a regression to childhood.

Suicide is the second leading cause of death among 15- to 19-year-olds.[15] Of the estimated 400,000 teenagers in the United States who attempt suicide every year, 5,000 to 10,000 succeed. For individuals attending college, the risk may be significantly greater than for those who are not.[31] Fifty percent of college students surveyed reported seriously considering suicide or having attempted suicide sometime in the past.[31]

Verbal and behavioral clues before suicide attempts vary widely. Any markedly different behavior in a teenager is a possible warning sign of a suicide attempt and should be investigated. The teenager who is unable to express feelings clearly requires a caring, knowledgeable professional who will take seriously the suicidal ideation or attempt. The threat of suicide should always be taken seriously. Factors associated with increased risk of suicide include high intelligence; male gender; self-esteem deficits; depression; impulsive, angry, and aggressive behavior; feelings of hopelessness; history of death or loss; and recent school or social problems.[49]

Mental health professionals have become increasingly interested in accurate means of assessing depressed adolescents. The nursing interview should focus on recent changes in school performance, peer and family support systems, and substance abuse. If significant problems are identified, further evaluation of the vegetative symptoms (eg, sleep disturbance, appetite changes, and persistent fatigue) is indicated. Adolescents can best report inner symptoms of depression that may escape the detection of others.[8]

Several empirically validated instruments exist for identifying depression.[8] The Beck Depression Inventory is the most widely used tool. This tool is heavily weighted on cognitive items, whereas the Hamilton Rating Scale focuses on biological features. The Schedule for Affective Disorders and Schizophrenia for School-Age Children and Adolescents successfully identifies previously undetected bipolar adolescents.[8]

Treatment of depressed adolescents includes pharmacotherapy, cognitive-behavioral therapy, and family therapy.[8,16] Family, school, and social environments are all affected. The primary aim of treatment is to shorten and decrease the negative consequences of episodes of depression.

The adolescent should be carefully evaluated before starting antidepressant medication. The mood disorder must be persistent and cause disability. Up to 30% of adolescents improve with evaluation alone or with minor psychosocial intervention.[16]

Depressed adolescents often are treated with tricyclic antidepressants, such as imipramine, desipramine, amitriptyline, and nortriptyline. The choice of antidepressant medication is based largely on side-effect profiles.

Adolescents respond to antidepressants that inhibit serotonin reuptake more than to those inhibiting noradrenergic uptake.[16] Selective serotonin reuptake inhibitors, such as fluoxetine, paroxetine, and sertraline, are newer antidepressants that are well tolerated by adolescents and have fewer side effects.[16] Findings of one controlled study in depressed adolescents indicate that fluoxetine is safe and effective in adolescents with major depressive disorder.[17]

Cognitive-behavioral therapy decreases cognitive errors and improves age-appropriate developmental skills. Nurses can help depressed adolescents use the following techniques:

1. Writing about activities or rating their moods in a notebook
2. Scheduling activities and planning the day to foster a sense of control
3. Using self-talk or coping self-statements to respond appropriately to certain situations

Through individual and group therapies, nurses can assist adolescent clients to focus on their strengths and interests instead of negative self-perceptions. Nurses can encourage involvement in activities that are successful for clients, which positively reinforces their success.

Working with the family of depressed adolescents is important. Parents can be helped to recognize the manifestations of their adolescent's low self-esteem and helplessness and their role in improving these feelings. Adolescent clients and their parents are encouraged to identify events that lead to these feelings. Nonthreatening support of the parents reduces their feelings of guilt and enhances their cooperation and assistance with their child's treatment[8] (Nursing Care Plan 23–1).

EATING DISORDERS

The eating problems of adolescents range from mild to severely debilitating. Although large numbers of teenagers have disordered eating, they may not meet the DSM-IV criteria for either anorexia nervosa or bulimia nervosa.[1] However, they may suffer as much psychological distress as those who meet the criteria.[21] This chapter examines the two major eating disorders of adolescence: *anorexia nervosa,* a starvation syndrome, and *bulimia,* a binge-purge syndrome (see Chapter 34, Eating Disorders).

Although many anorectic clients in the United States are white, well-educated, and come from middle- and upper-income families, authors in the last decade have noted that anorexia and bulimia are detectable in all social classes.[21] The onset of illness is often associated with a stressful life event, such as leaving home for college.[1] Hospital admissions for eating disorders have increased up to 300% from 1970 to 1990.[4] Of individuals admitted to university hospitals, the long-term mortality is more than 10%.[1] Death most commonly results from starvation, suicide, or electrolyte imbalance.

Incidence rates for anorexia nervosa have increased steadily among those 10 to 19 years old.[21] The reported prevalence rate for anorexia nervosa of 0.48% among girls 15 to 19 years old in the United States makes it the third most common chronic condition among adolescent girls after obesity and asthma.[21] The prevalence of bulimia nervosa among adolescent girls is approximately 1% to 3%; the rate of occurrence in boys is one-tenth that of girls.[1] Prevalence rates for bulimia nervosa are higher in college-age women than in high school students.[21]

Weight loss, one of the diagnostic criteria for anorexia nervosa in an older adolescent with a stable premorbid weight and height, is not necessarily present in younger adolescents with the disorder. Because growth is a dynamic process, severe nutritional deficits can occur in the absence of weight loss in early adolescence.[21] Appropriately, the DSM-IV diagnostic criteria for *anorexia nervosa* include the failure to achieve expected weight gain during a period of growth.

A fear of not being in control is the central issue in anorexia nervosa. What makes anorexia nervosa especially interesting and difficult to treat is the lack of clarity as to how much of the manifestation, medically and psychiatrically, is a reflection of the effects of hunger and starvation.[21] Three main areas of disturbed psychological functioning in anorectics are body image; misinterpretation of internal and external stimuli, especially hunger; and overwhelming feelings of ineffectiveness.

Cognitive development of anorectics is characterized by egocentricity and magical thinking. Developing new ways of acting and thinking, which are a normal part of adolescence, can be frightening to the anorectic. The person with anorexia acts out the conviction that by being skinny and in need of protection, she ensures eternal love and care from her parents.[21] Amenorrhea further fosters the illusion of prolonging childhood.

The adolescent who becomes anorectic is usually described as previously being loving, devoted, and well behaved. Compliance probably concealed the fact that she was deprived of living a life of her own. Throughout childhood, her parents failed to acknowledge or confirm the developmental progress she initiated, so her parents perceive growth and development as their accomplishment, not hers. Other characteristics of the anorectic are excessive involvement in preparing, cooking, and talking about food; excessive exercise; and food refusal. Often the young person has been socially isolated during the year preceding the onset of the disorder.[9]

An individual's family may foster excessive concern

Nursing Care Plan 23-1

A Depressed and Suicidal Adolescent

Fifteen year old Sarah was transferred from a general pediatric to an adolescent psychiatric unit after medical stabilization for a suicide attempt by means of Tylenol ingestion. Sarah reported feeling depressed and hopeless after unsuccessfully trying to convince her parents that she did not want to return to her private boarding school several hours away from home. She stated, "My parents don't understand. I just don't want to go back to that school. I've been depressed since school started five weeks ago." She said that she was tremendously homesick and had a difficult time adjusting to the rigorous curriculum at the school. She had a conflict with her new roommate and felt isolated and alone at school.

As the semester progressed she became more depressed, isolated, socially withdrawn, and anhedonic. On her visits home, she was irritable and resisted returning to the private school. On the weekend prior to her overdose, she refused to get in the car when asked to return to school and argued with her parents for most of the trip. Back at school, she began to feel very hopeless and without alternatives. Throughout the evening, she took 50 to 60 Tylenol and Advil pills. After taking the pills, she became nauseated, then went to sleep. When she began vomiting in the morning, she still refused to disclose the overdose, but after remaining sick for another hour, she told the school nurse what she had done.

Sarah was admitted to a pediatric unit where she was treated for the physical effects of the overdose. During that time she was seen by a psychiatrist and psychiatric clinical nurse specialist. Transfer to the adolescent psychiatric unit was recommended because she remained dysphoric and information was elicited that she had never reported a prior suicide attempt. Because her parents insisted that she return to the private school, she felt that no one was really listening to her. She chose to be treated in the psychiatric program because she felt nothing had changed despite her overdose. Although she said that she really had no intention of killing herself, she had wished that something would prevent her from having to attend the private school.

Sarah, the oldest of four siblings, has always been an excellent student without academic difficulties. However, she had not been challenged as much as she had at the private school. Having completed ninth grade at the public school in her hometown of 4000 people, her parents enrolled her in a boarding school because they disapproved of her friends and activities. Her mother is a homemaker who had previously been a teacher; her father is a veterinarian. Sarah is very close to her younger sister and youngest brother but says she gets along best with her mom who seems to be very similar to her emotionally. Sarah has a conflicted relationship with her father but states that they are close as well.

In the admission interview, Sarah was cooperative but difficult to engage. Her speech was soft, but fluent and coherent. She exhibited psychomotor retardation. Her mood was depressed and dysphoric; her affect was very restricted. Her thought processes were logical, goal-directed, and coherent. Her thinking was abstract and her intellect above average. There was no evidence of psychosis. Thought content was remarkable because she continued to deny suicidal ideation, despite the two suicide attempts.

Nursing Diagnosis

Risk for Self-Directed Violence related to feelings of depression and powerlessness

Outcome

Sarah will not harm herself.

Intervention	Rationale
Determine level of suicide precautions for Sarah and institute them on admission; continually assess suicidal potential.	Clients at high risk for suicidal behavior need constant supervision and removal of potentially harmful objects, while those at lower risk may require less intensive supervision. Suicidal potential may change with time.
Explain suicide precautions and their purpose to Sarah.	Explanations convey that Sarah is a participant in her care.

continued

Nursing Care Plan 23-1 *(Continued)*

Intervention	Rationale
Observe Sarah closely, especially when antidepressant medication effects an improvement in mood or dramatic behavior change occurs.	Risk of suicide increase as the client's energy level increases with medication. Sudden behavior change may indicate that the client has decided to kill herself.
Encourage Sarah to express feelings and reinforce that all feelings are acceptable.	Expression of feelings may relieve feelings of despair, hopelessness, sadness, anger, and so on.

Evaluation

Sarah does not engage in self-injurious behaviors.

Nursing Diagnosis

Ineffective Individual Coping related to conflicts with parents, withdrawal, anxiety about new school, and identification of limited alternatives other than overdose

Outcome

Sarah will identify and use effective ways to deal with stress and emotional problems.

Intervention	Rationale
Teach Sarah about causative factors, behaviors, and effects of depression.	Education about depression increases the client's knowledge and insight into her behavior and feelings.
Encourage Sarah to express feelings and fears verbally and through journal writing. Use role playing to practice expressing her feelings, especially to her parents.	Ventilating feelings helps the client identify, accept, and work through those feelings even though they are uncomfortable to her. Role playing allows the client to try out new behaviors in a supportive environment.
Help Sarah write a list of supportive people she knows outside of the hospital and how to contact them.	Having an identified support system strengthens the client's available resources.
Plan with Sarah how she will recognize and deal with feelings and situations that precipitated suicidal behavior and feelings in the past, including whom to contact, where to go, and what to do to alleviate suicidal feelings.	Concrete plans help to avert a crisis or suicidal behavior. Risk of suicide is decreased when client is not socially isolated.

Evaluation

Sarah demonstrates an array of positive coping strategies and seeks out supportive others.

with bodily needs. Members of the families often are overinvolved in each other's lives, with a resultant loss of individuation.[45] Transactional patterns in these families are characterized by enmeshment, overprotectiveness, rigidity, and lack of conflict resolution.

When seriously underweight, adolescents with anorexia manifest depressive symptoms, such as depressed mood, social withdrawal, irritability, and insomnia. These symptoms meet criteria for major depressive disorder but are the psychological sequelae of semistarvation.[1] The best antidepressant agent in anorexia nervosa often is the treatment of the eating disorder itself.[30,60]

Bulimia is an episodic, uncontrolled, rapid ingestion of large quantities of food in a short time (binge eating), resulting in feelings of physical and emotional discomfort. These episodes are typically ended by exhaustion, social interruption, self-induced vomiting, or misuse of laxatives and diuretics. The person with anorexia typically denies hunger, while the bulimic person gives in to impulses and then controls body size through purging.[60] Definite precipitating factors are unknown, but onset often occurs during the senior year in high school, which is a transitional period. Severe weight loss does not occur in bulimia as it does in anorexia nervosa, and amenorrhea seldom occurs.[1,60]

Most of the bulimic's life revolves around disturbed eating habits. Major physical problems associated with bulimia stem from self-induced vomiting, laxative abuse, and diuretic use. These include hypokalemia, alkalosis, hypochloremia, hyponatremia, dental enamel erosion, parotid and salivary gland enlargement, lazy bowel syndrome, and malabsorption.[21,60]

Compared with anorectics, bulimic clients are more anxious, depressed, interpersonally sensitive, and somatically inclined. Mood and anxiety disorders occur more frequently in adolescents with bulimia.[1] Bulimics may improve in response to antidepressants. Also, because families of bulimic people often are significantly disturbed and disturbing to live with, family therapy may be an important treatment modality.

Early hospitalization for younger adolescents who do not yet have a chronic form of the disease may prevent the multiple hospitalizations characteristic of an older adolescent with chronic anorexia. Hospitalization is indicated when weight loss has been so prolonged or so rapid that life-threatening complications must be averted or when weight loss continues despite outpatient treatment.[21] The sooner the weight loss is stopped, the greater the chances of a more complete recovery.

Clients with bulimia nervosa require hospitalization when they have not responded to outpatient treatment or if there is dehydration, electrolyte disturbance, cardiac dysrhythmia, or gastrointestinal bleeding. Hospitalization also breaks the binge-purge cycle.

The goals of treatment are to help the client achieve physical and emotional health. For both types of eating disorders, the best inpatient care is provided within a group milieu in which clients are expected to finish the meals provided for them with or without a nutritive supplement. Nasogastric feedings may be needed when the client is unable to tolerate enough food orally to gain adequate weight. Increasing energy levels are usually provided during the course of the hospitalization at a rate the client can physically and psychologically tolerate.[21,60] Nutritional rehabilitation must be performed slowly to avoid cardiac failure and the refeeding syndrome.[21] Weight gain at the rate of 0.25 to 0.5 lb/day has been shown to be safe in adolescents with anorexia nervosa. Basic information about health, energy metabolism, medical complications, and nutrition should be provided as part of treatment. This information should be developmentally appropriate and should be repeated during the course of treatment. Long-term active guidance prepares recovering adolescents to nourish themselves adequately for the rest of their lives.[21] Specific adolescent issues, including autonomy, conflict resolution, assertiveness, educational achievement, social skills, family interaction, substance use, and sexual behaviors, should be addressed as part of treatment.

Psychopharmacological agents may have limited use and may cause complications of the disease during the refeeding stage in anorexia nervosa. Antidepressants are indicated when there is clinical evidence of depression.[21]

Involving parents in the treatment alliance is essential, because young adolescents are not emotionally or situationally autonomous. Later in the course of treatment, family therapy centers on issues like separation and individuation, family expression of feelings, and conflict resolution.[21]

Adolescents with anorexia nervosa generally have a better prognosis than adults. Poorer outcomes are related to later onset and longer duration of illness. Lower minimum weight, failed previous treatment, disturbed premorbid personality, social difficulties, difficult family relationships, increased somatic or obsessional concerns, and premorbid history of obesity, bulimia, vomiting, or laxative abuse are other predictors of poor outcomes.[21]

SCHIZOPHRENIA

Although schizophrenia rarely occurs in children younger than 12 years, its incidence increases steadily during adolescence to achieve adult rates of approximately 0.1% new cases per year.[42] Early-onset schizophrenia (onset before 18 years) occurs twice as often in men as women. As age increases, this ratio tends to even out.

Premorbid personality abnormalities, such as withdrawal, oddness, and isolation, are seen in 54% to 90% of adolescents with early-onset schizophrenia. Multiple developmental delays, including lags in cognitive, motor, sensory, and social functioning, are also seen. Early-onset schizophrenia has the same range of outcomes as reported in adults, although most adolescents have some degree of chronic impairment. Poor outcomes relate to the increased frequency of poor premorbid functioning and developmental delays. The risk of suicide or accidental death directly due to behaviors caused by psychotic thinking is at least 5%.[42]

Because of the prognosis and social stigma associated with schizophrenia, clinicians may be hesitant to make this diagnosis, even when there is sufficient evidence to do so. This potentially denies the adolescent and family access to appropriate treatment, knowledge about the disorder, and specialized support services. The diagnostic criteria for schizophrenia are outlined in the DSM-IV.[1] (See Chapter 30, Schizophrenia, for DSM-IV criteria.) Even when the diagnostic criteria are met, the initial diagnosis may be inaccurate because of the overlap in symptoms between schizophrenia, affective disorders with psychotic features, and personality and dissociative disorders.[42] Adolescents and their families should be educated about these diagnostic issues, and the client must be reassessed periodically to ensure accuracy. Structured interviews, symptom scales, and diagnostic decision trees can help the clinician make a reliable diagnosis.

Approximately one-half of adolescents with bipolar disorder are originally misdiagnosed as having schizophrenia.[42] Organic etiological agents that may cause psychosis include delirium, seizure disorders, central nervous system lesions (eg, head trauma, brain tumors), neurodegenerative disorders, metabolic disorders, toxic encephalopathies (eg, alcohol and other abusable substances), and infectious diseases. In adolescents, the first psychotic break often occurs with comorbid substance abuse, which is a triggering factor rather than a primary etiological agent.[42]

To manage schizophrenia successfully, it is important to understand its usual course as one of cycles of acute psychosis, followed by longer periods of recuperation, and then remission or residual phases. Treatment of schizophrenia is specifically aimed at the symptoms and addresses the psychological, social, educational, and cultural needs of the adolescent and family resulting from the disorder.[42] Therapeutic resources include inpatient or day treatment psychiatric programs with developmentally appropriate psychiatric, neurological, and medical services; community programs with comprehensive case management services, including medication, psychotherapy, education, family support, and vocational and rehabilitative assistance; and in some cases, long-term residential programs. Adolescents with schizophrenia usually need a specialized classroom with low levels of stimulation, an individualized curriculum addressing their cognitive impairments, and teachers trained to deal with emotionally disturbed youth.[42]

The only specific treatment of documented efficacy in schizophrenia is antipsychotic (neuroleptic) medication. In acutely psychotic adolescents, haloperidol and loxapine are effective compared with placebo.[42] Clozapine is an atypical antipsychotic agent effective in treating adolescent schizophrenics who have not responded to traditional neuroleptic therapy.[38,42] Clozapine does not produce extrapyramidal symptoms or tardive dyskinesia. However, it has potential adverse reactions that include weight gain, agranulocytosis, and seizures. Clozapine has been prescribed safely in conjunction with extensive blood-monitoring program.[38,42]

Treatment plans that integrate medication management and family and supportive psychotherapies are effective at reducing morbidity and decreasing relapse rates in schizophrenic adolescents.[42] The goal of therapy is not only to help the adolescent return to premorbid level of functioning, but also to proceed with age-appropriate developmental tasks. Comprehensive plans address the individual's needs and include comorbid psychiatric conditions (eg, substance abuse), control of stressors, and other factors complicating recovery.

Family intervention programs, in conjunction with social skills training and medication therapy, have significantly decreased schizophrenia relapse rates.[42] Unlike more traditional family therapies, these interventions primarily provide family members with an understanding of the illness, its potential causes and treatments, and intervention strategies for dealing with the symptoms of schizophrenia. Social skills training helps the adolescent develop strategies for dealing with conflict; identify the correct meaning, content, and context of verbal messages; and enhance socialization and vocational skills.[42]

OBSESSIVE-COMPULSIVE DISORDER

Obsessive-compulsive disorder (OCD) usually begins in adolescence or early adulthood. One-third to one-half of adults with OCD report the onset of symptoms during childhood or adolescence.[44] There is much disagreement about the incidence of OCD in adolescents. Misdiagnosis may result in the client being seen as psychotic, severely depressed, or oppositional.

This disorder is characterized by recurrent obsessions or compulsions that are time consuming, cause distress, or impair functioning.[1] *Obsessions* are persistent ideas, thoughts, impulses, or images that are intrusive, inappropriate, and cause anxiety or distress. Common obsessions are repeated thoughts about contamination, repeated doubts, a need to have things in a particular order, aggressive impulses, and sexual imagery. *Compulsions* are repetitive behaviors or mental acts that serve to reduce anxiety or distress. The adolescent feels driven to perform the compulsion to reduce the distress that accompanies an obsession. Common compulsions include washing and cleaning, counting, checking, requesting or demanding assurances, repeating actions, and ordering. Gradual declines in schoolwork occur secondary to impaired ability to concentrate. Like adults, adolescents are more likely to engage in rituals at home than in front of peers, teachers, or strangers.

At some point during the course of the disorder, the adolescent recognizes that the obsessions or compulsions are excessive or unreasonable. However, the individual's insight varies across times and situations. For example, the adolescent may recognize a compulsion as unreasonable when discussing it in a "safe situation" (eg, in the therapist's office) but yield to the compulsion when feeling anxious. The person may avoid situations that involve the content of the obsessions. For example, the adolescent with obsessions about dirt may avoid public restrooms or shaking hands with strangers.

Treatment for OCD includes pharmacotherapy and behavior therapy.[44] Serotonin reuptake inhibitors, including fluoxetine, clomipramine, sertraline, and paroxetine, are the most useful pharmacological treatments for adolescents with OCD.[14] Improvement is seen in 37% of adolescent clients treated with clomipramine, but relapse commonly follows medication discontinuation.[13] Behavioral therapy in the form of exposure and response prevention has been effective in preventing relapse when medications are discontinued.[44]

Application of the Nursing Process to Mentally and Emotionally Disturbed Adolescents

ASSESSMENT

The assessment of the adolescent brought for treatment sets the tone for the rest of the interaction and intervention with the teenager and family. It provides an opportunity to deal with the parents' fears and misinformation, support their desire to be "good parents," and encourage them to participate actively in their adolescent's care. The nurse answers the adolescent's and family's questions and offers them information and options with empathy and honesty. This assessment period is a time of sharing between the nurse and the adolescent and family, rather than a one-sided interaction.

The nurse gathers data from which nursing diagnoses will be formulated by means of therapeutic use of self, information from the adolescent and family, and specific techniques or tools. Means of collecting assessment data about the adolescent client include interviews with the adolescent and parents; behavior rating scales completed by parents, teachers, or significant adults; physical examination, including neurological assessment; and laboratory and psychological tests. Data obtained from multiple assessment methods are more reliable than those from a single source.[12,36]

By having the initial contact between mental health professionals and the entire family, the "identified" adolescent client is given the message that the whole family is involved in the problem, easing some of the pressure on the adolescent. The family intake interview is valuable for learning about family feelings and dynamics. Adolescents can hear what parents are saying and can offer their points of view and versions of the situations presented by parents. The nurse needs to address the adolescent first and ask who they believe requested the assessment, the reasons they believe the person had for the request, and if they agree with that opinion. The nurse asks what goals or expectations the adolescent and family have for treatment and helps the adolescent and family set realistic goals.

Data are gathered from multiple sources; this prevents preconceived notions about a problem from leading to a premature focus on a particular area to the exclusion of other relevant information. Sources may include members of the nuclear and extended family, teachers, other health care professionals, and the adolescent. Consistency of information among the sources is assessed. In many settings, the multidisciplinary team collaboratively assesses, diagnoses, and plans treatment with the adolescent and family.[12,36]

Throughout the assessment interview, data are gathered about the nature of the adolescent's problem: its onset, severity, duration, and impact; perceptions of the problem; and any significant concomitant events. Information is collected about the adolescent's developmental stage, temperament, developmental stressors, sociocultural influences, relationships with family and peers, patterns of behavior, strengths and weakness, experiences of traumatic events, and academic performance. Assessment of the adolescent also includes the teenager's sense of identity, independence, self-image, impulsiveness, drug and alcohol use, and sexuality. The nurse must convey respect for adolescents' confidentiality and privacy. They might not want to talk about some areas with the family present.

Assessing suicidal risk for adolescents is important to prevent self-harm and defuse the crisis situation. A focused mental status examination helps to evaluate judgment, impulsiveness, signs of psychosis, organicity, intoxication, and suicidal tendencies.[36] Open discussion with the adolescent about self-harmful behaviors, thoughts, and tendencies; the availability of lethal methods of suicide; and history of substance abuse help to plan for safety.

The validity of a nursing diagnosis, resultant plans, and interventions depend on the accuracy of assessment information. The accuracy of assessment data can be verified by observing the adolescent in more than one setting, reviewing previous health and school records, using standardized tests or assessment tools, and discussing observations and impressions with the adolescent, family, teachers, and other health professionals.

NURSING DIAGNOSIS

The purpose of assessment is to determine nursing diagnoses that specify treatment interventions. To formulate a nursing diagnosis, the nurse synthesizes data and reaches conclusions about the adolescent's problems, strengths, coping abilities, adaptiveness of the symptoms, and inferences about the etiology of the disorder. Knowledge of developmental norms is a basis for making sound diagnostic judgments, assessing the need for treatment, and selecting the appropriate treatment. When working with adolescent clients and their families, the nurse may formulate many different nursing diagnoses to guide care.

There is controversy about the appropriateness of using nursing diagnoses versus stating the problem in language that is jargon free, meaningful to all treatment disciplines, and understandable to the adolescent client and family. Planning by various disciplines as a team unites effort for effective treatment. Parallel systems of assessment and intervention by individual disciplines separates the team and may cause conflicts and inefficiency.

PLANNING

The skillful matching of appropriate interventions with an adolescent's problems and developmental level is as important as an accurate assessment.

Planning takes into account the following questions:

1. What alternative services are appropriate to meet the client's assessed needs?
2. What outcome can be expected from each alternative?
3. Which alternative is most cost-effective?
4. Are some alternatives less restrictive than others?
5. Do the alternatives allow the adolescent to continue education, be in contact with peers, and work on psychosocial growth tasks?
6. How long is treatment expected to be necessary?

Client and family involvement in the planning process helps to prevent noncompliance or sabotage and strengthens family support.

Goals

General goals for adolescent clients include the following:

1. Fewer and less intense symptoms of the mental disorder
2. Improvement in mood
3. Greater autonomy and self-esteem
4. Improved problem-solving ability

Client Outcomes

Outcome statements help nurses to evaluate whether goals are being met. Also called behavioral outcomes, they should be specific, measurable, attainable, realistic, time limited, and client focused. The following are examples of client outcomes:

1. The adolescent will make two positive self-statements by (date).
2. The adolescent will gain 0.25 lb/day.
3. The adolescent will complete a journal daily and discuss with individual therapist.
4. The family will plan and carry out one "fun" activity every 2 weeks in which all members participate.

Discharge Planning

Discharge planning for the hospitalized adolescent begins at the time of admission to a treatment facility. It involves decisions about placement if the adolescent is not to return home, self-management of symptoms, readjustment to the school and community, carryover of the benefits of inpatient treatment to home life, and follow-up with aftercare services. Discharge planning is a collaborative process involving the adolescent, family, and treatment team.

INTERVENTION

Modalities available to the nurse who intervenes with adolescent clients include family, group, and individual therapies and behavioral strategies. Other milieu interventions may include communication and interpretation of daily events, limit setting, and analysis of the outcome of personal interactions.

Psychotherapy with adolescents focuses on building a relationship, helping the client experience mutual trust, and reality testing to correct inaccurate perceptions of the self, environment, and consequences of action. These goals may be achieved in family, group, or individual psychotherapy.

Family Therapy

Family involvement is an essential aspect of treatment for the adolescent client. Early aspects of family therapy provide parents with input, support, and an opportunity to express their feelings. Family therapy aims at forming strategies to handle disruptive behaviors and develop positive ways of helping and addressing members' concerns and conflicts. It promotes family cohesiveness and offers members opportunities to express perceptions and expectations and to replace styles of interacting with more successful ones. Family therapy facilitates healthy functioning to cope with developmental crises and stress and decreases the adolescent's symptoms.

Group Therapy

Groups are naturally occurring phenomena for adolescents. Therefore, group interventions may be more like the norm and less threatening than individual therapy. Peer interactions provide opportunities for psychological development, such as the formation of close relationships with other people, development of social skills that promote positive interactions, and understanding of self and others. Additional benefits include feedback about behaviors that are annoying or pleasing to others, knowledge of cognitions that are self-defeating or self-enhancing, toleration of others, and opportunities to practice new behaviors, such as giving and receiving critical feedback and advice. Group therapy provides members with support, identification with others in similar circumstances, and the confidence to discuss problematic issues.[26]

Group themes may focus on special problems experienced by adolescents, such as sexual abuse, substance abuse, identity issues related to adoption, bereavement, chronic illness, or the teenager's attitude about relevant current events. The purpose of these homogeneous groups is to attack directly a problem of concern to all clients in the group. Homogeneous groups can penetrate defenses quickly by helping members experience feelings of being understood and accepted. The individual's sense of discrimination, isolation, and defensiveness is lessened.[26]

Individual Therapy

Individual therapy may be useful if other modalities are not available, if the adolescent needs an intense relationship with a significant other to develop trust, or if the adolescent refuses to communicate in the presence of family members or group members. The particular focus of individual psychotherapy depends on the identified needs of the client.

It is a therapeutic challenge to gain adolescents' trust and to motivate them to change. Therapists must demonstrate that symptomatic behavior is self-defeating. The therapist determines whether the goal of individual therapy is supportive, educational, or directed toward the integration of newly learned adaptive patterns.

Broad outcomes of therapeutic relationships include improved self-understanding, symptom reduction, development of a consistent sense of self, ability to use foresight and have fun, recognition of the desire to be with others, ability to be alone, and enhancement of the ability to make wholesome choices.[61] The nurse may pursue these outcomes by discussing topics identified in the assessment and by encouraging the client to address areas of concern not previously verbalized. The choice of topic during therapy sessions is less important than the atmosphere in which the discussion occurs.

Nursing interventions help the clients connect behaviors and feelings, such as self-criticism and low self-esteem. Therapeutic communication helps the adolescent differentiate between thoughts, feelings, and behaviors. The client is encouraged to express genuine feelings, and the nurse-therapist unconditionally accepts the client and his or her feelings.

Behavioral and Cognitive Strategies

Because many adolescent clients with mental disorders are not at the intellectual stage of formal operations (ie, using logic and making abstractions) and because of the high energy and propensity for acting out characteristic of this age, it is often useful to emphasize behavior and observable events, rather than inferred mental states and constructs.

Behavior modification analyzes an adolescent's acceptable and unacceptable behaviors and designs programs to maximize the former while minimizing the latter. Techniques of behavior modification that may be used with adolescents include systematic desensitization, positive reinforcement, extinction, role-modeling, and role-playing. Adolescents may lose interest in rewards and penalties quickly. Therefore, these should be evaluated and varied regularly. Furthermore, involving adolescents in devising behavioral contracts helps increase compliance with the treatment plan.

Behavioral therapy is a philosophy of motivation by rewards. Tokens, or *reinforcers*, are given for certain behaviors, and behaviors are tied to privileges the adolescent may earn. Expectations for positive behavior are clearly spelled out, as are consequences for maladaptive behaviors. Movement through a treatment program with increasing levels of responsibility and freedom is monitored, planned, and reevaluated in relation to the individual's behaviors. Behavior modification programs are matter of fact: Rewards and consequences for noncompliance are based on well-defined behaviors and not on emotional reactions. Manipulative behavior between client and staff is decreased because expectations and outcomes are known to everyone and agreed to in advance.

Cognitive therapy may be more suitable for older adolescents because they may view any system of behavior management or modification as an issue of control and a threat to their independence, autonomy, and self-esteem. Interventions help the adolescent assess the circumstances, plan ahead more accurately, develop effective techniques to solve problems, and recognize negative self-perceptions that detour thought into dysfunctional pathways.[19]

Therapeutic Milieu

Because hospitalizing adolescents takes them out of their usual developmental mainstream, the decision to admit an adolescent is not taken lightly. When a decision is made to hospitalize an adolescent, an inpatient unit staff must pay particular attention to the effect of the milieu on a given client. The milieu is the total context in which treatment occurs. The physical setting, the atmosphere generated by interpersonal exchanges, and the opportunities available to experience challenge and growth are important therapeutic tools. Whether the therapeutic environment is an acute inpatient unit, a day or partial hospital, or a residential treatment center, several program components characterize all therapeutic milieus. These include distributed power, physical setting, structure, treatment modalities, and therapeutic interactions between clients and staff, disciplines, and treatment team members.[35]

Distributed Power. In therapeutic milieus, adolescent clients are active, responsive participants who share in the decision-making process. This process conveys to clients that they must help themselves, rather than wait for answers from staff. Clients identify their own problems, set their own goals, and decide on a plan to reach those goals with the assistance and support of peers and staff.[35]

Physical Setting. Because the physical setting is an integral part of the psychosocial climate, it should be given as much consideration as other elements of the treatment program. The value assigned to clients is reflected in the physical space planned and prepared for them. An adolescent in crisis cannot be supported in an environment that subliminally, and perhaps overtly, says, "You are really not that important."

Inpatient adolescent units should create a homelike environment. Activity rooms should include game tables and materials appropriate for the age and developmental level of the adolescents who live there. Large common areas can be subdivided into smaller conversation pits simply by furniture arrangement. Casual, easily movable furniture encourages informal, flexible behavior and activities by staff and clients. Several activities involving small groups of adolescents and staff can occur simultaneously. This design not only fosters interaction, but also requires fewer staff members to monitor clients safely. A staff member having a one-to-one talk with a client also can be aware of what is occurring around him or her in the environment and is easily available if the situation requires intervention.[35]

Structured Treatment Program. Because adolescents who require inpatient or partial psychiatric hospitalization often need additional protection, structure, or boundaries, the total environment is consciously structured to provide this. Three basic components contribute to the overall structure of a therapeutic milieu: philosophy; rules, limit setting, and consequences; and treatment level system.

The philosophy provides the framework against which all client behavior and treatment plans are evaluated. Because the family is an integral part of the child's life, adolescent programs are often based on a family systems model with a developmental perspective. When the adolescent is treated in the context of the family, his or her behavior may be viewed as a symptom of a malfunctioning family system. The adolescent also is evaluated for accomplishment of developmental tasks, so one aspect of treatment may be to help the adolescent complete uncompleted tasks.[35]

Just as in a family, an inpatient or partial hospital program has basic rules to follow and *consequences* for noncompliance. Written program guidelines help the adolescent learn what is expected and help staff members develop consistency. Consistency in application of rules and consequences is important for adolescents because different consequences for the same behavior can be confusing. These guidelines provide an objective reference point when clients or staff have questions about the rules.

A peer or "buddy" system may help adolescents adapt to the milieu culture and learn the rules and routines. The buddy system serves a dual purpose: The adolescent new to treatment feels more comfortable with a peer who shares similar problems and is "in the same boat," and the buddy feels needed and important with the responsibility of orienting a new client, resulting in increased competency and self-esteem. The positive changes the buddies have made are strengthened as they reexperience where they have been, realize how far they have come, and describe where they are now in the treatment and growth process.

The milieu's overall structure must be responsive to each client's individual needs. *Limit setting* is critical because it reinforces the predictability of the environment; that is, for certain actions, there will be a consequence, and clear feedback is given regarding the results of the behavior. Milieu staff are charged with the daily responsibility of maintaining the therapeutic structure of the treatment milieu by setting appropriate limits. As external limits are set, the adolescent is assisted in developing a functional set of internal controls. In addition, milieu staff are responsible for educating the adolescent and parents about appropriate limit setting so that positive behavioral changes achieved in treatment can be generalized to the home.

The therapeutic milieu stresses positive reinforcement rather than punishment. Adolescents are rewarded for following rules and routines and attaining daily goals. In programs using a behavioral system, the number of points earned determines the adolescent's level and privileges for the next day. Higher points indicate a higher level and more privileges.

Treatment Modalities. The therapeutic environment promotes active involvement in treatment. Each adolescent is expected to participate in the daily activities, with clear, appropriate consequences if the adolescent chooses not to participate. Examples of activities include community meeting; goals group; school; individual, group, and family therapy; and therapeutic recreation.

Therapeutic Interaction. Confrontation is a central feature of the therapeutic milieu. Sharing experiences and feelings involves forcing the adolescent to confront and recognize the use of habitual responses that cause unmanageable problems to occur and perhaps cause deep hurt. Analyzing interactions helps the adolescent see that usual ways of coping are ineffective in getting needs met and that to continue in the same way means more failure and loneliness. Reframing is used to help adolescents see situations that formerly seemed hopeless from perspectives that may be more positive. Milieu therapy provides the supportive ambiance for the adolescent to apply new behavioral responses.

The therapeutic environment works most effectively when the staff is cohesive, and all disciplines work collaboratively. Conflicts between disciplines, shifts, or individuals are noticed easily by clients who may try to split the staff or pit one group against another. To maintain staff cohesiveness, milieu staff must be alert to the warning signals and be able to identify and resolve problems among themselves quickly and thoroughly. Open communication is the best antidote for splitting.

Conflicts are inevitable within the work group but can be resolved by open and direct communication. Staff must be willing to take the same risks that they expect clients to take—work on relationships, negotiate, communicate openly and honestly, accept responsibility for their own choices, and be vulnerable and feel "feelings."

Pharmacological Treatment

Psychopharmacology in adolescents is changing from a nonspecific modifier of behavior to medications that affect areas of the brain and neurotransmitters. The medical treatment is specific to diagnostic categories. Medications may have a shorter mean half-life in adolescents than in adults, so in some cases, a higher dosage may be required for adolescents.

Changes in body composition at puberty, especially the distribution of body fat, are important determinants of the metabolism, disposition, and storage of many drugs. Women usually have twice as much fat per unit of body weight as men. Therefore, if a drug is distributed largely in body water, the dose for boys may be higher than for girls after puberty. If the drug is fat soluble, mature girls might require a higher dose than younger girls or mature boys. The more fat present in the body, the greater the amount of the drug distributed, particularly if the drug is highly lipid soluble, such as imipramine.[20]

Failure to detect drug effect may reflect lack of efficacy; however, it may also be due to medication noncompliance. Medication compliance may become a struggle of adolescent autonomy and independence.[16,20] Noncompliance also may be related to the following:

1. Forgetfulness
2. Unwillingness to be a "guinea pig"
3. Unwillingness to take pills during school hours because it makes the adolescent feel "different" from peers
4. Inability to swallow pills
5. Undesirable side effects
6. Inadequate education regarding medications
7. Attention seeking from parents
8. Lack of motivation
9. Interference with other activities[20]

Although informed consent is required from parents, compliance may be encouraged by providing information and obtaining assent from the teenager. Adolescents who are uncomfortable about taking medications often will agree to a time-limited trial of medications. Once medication is initiated, systematic rating of symptoms by the adolescent and clinician can demonstrate the benefits.[16]

EVALUATION

Evaluation of the adolescent's progress toward attaining specific behavioral outcomes as a result of nursing interventions is not a difficult step in the nursing process if the outcomes are clearly stated at the start of treatment. Adolescent progress often involves movement of "one step forward and two steps back;" therefore, stating outcomes in small increments, rather than major changes, aids in evaluating the adolescent's progress.

◆ The Nurse's Feelings

Nurses considering working with adolescents should carefully examine memories of their own adolescence. It might even be helpful to evaluate to what extent each of the adolescent growth tasks were completed by the nurse. The nurse's own self-awareness, by whatever means attained, is the best way to avoid being caught off guard emotionally or intellectually when interacting with adolescents. Nurses who can be honest with themselves are most likely to be honest with clients.

Impulsiveness, emotional lability, and issues of self-control and sexual identity may cause nurses to have emotional reactions. Adolescent conflicts within the nurse may be reawakened. If nurses are not secure in their own sexual identity, they may project that insecurity by overreacting to situations or by not providing limits when an adolescent is testing parameters. The nurse also may become frightened of the adolescent with tenuous self-control. It is hard to be on the receiving end of a barrage of hostile remarks, and the nurse may feel like retaliating against the belligerent adolescent. By being aware of these potential reactions, the nurse may be able to avoid inadvertently encouraging the adolescent to act out.

Because of the necessity to set limits, the nurse may have exaggerated feelings of authority and a tendency to engage in power struggles with the adolescent. An example of this is evident in an adolescent's description of events leading to seclusion.

> I woke up in a bad mood because last night I was mad at one of the staff. I felt like nothing was going right with me this morning. For everything I did, I'd get a consequence. Since I didn't get my clothes last night from the washer, my clothes were locked up for 24 hours. I didn't mind the 24 hour lock-up but then she [the nurse] changed it. She gave me my clothes back but she gave me another consequence. I had to sit by myself at lunch and not talk to anyone. I got real angry and I said, "Well, that sucks" and she just said, "That's another hour [of not talking to peers] you've got too." And I said the same thing, "Well, that sucks because I feel like everything I do I'm getting a consequence for. I think that's stupid." And she said, "You've got another hour." And I said the same thing again. And she said, "Okay, that's seclusion."[34]

The epithet, "Well, that sucks," after receiving a consequence from the nurse could have been converted into a learning experience by the nurse questioning the meaning of the comment. The nurse, in turn, would have known more about the client.

Positive expectations must be emphasized when working with adolescents. The adolescent can choose whether or not to try new ways of acting if the nurse clarifies which behaviors are likely to lead to satisfying relationships and increased self-esteem. Adolescents want to be accepted, loved, and understood. Their message may be, "Do not lead, I may not follow; do not push, I may give up; walk beside me and help me discover my way."

◆ Chapter Summary

This chapter has introduced some of the parameters of normal adolescent development. Several theories providing frameworks for understanding adolescence are presented. The chapter's major points include the following:

1. The adolescent undergoes marked physical change with individual differences within each sex almost as great as the differences between the sexes.
2. Adolescence is the period of formal operational thinking when adult-level reasoning takes place.
3. The social status of adolescents changes across four domains: interpersonal, political, economic, and legal.
4. The secondary changes of adolescence include identity, achievement, sexuality, intimacy, autonomy, and attachment.
5. The incidence of adolescent emotional disorders is difficult to identify because of varying diagnostic biases.
6. Etiological theories of adolescent disturbance examine the variables of family communication, parenting style, personality, social pressures, and stressors.
7. In the assessment phase of the nursing process, the nurse gathers data about the nature of the adolescent's problem: its onset, severity, duration, and impact; perceptions of the problem; and any significant concomitant events.
8. In the nursing diagnosis phase, the nurse synthesizes data and reaches conclusions about the adolescent's problems, strengths, coping abilities, adaptiveness of the symptoms, and inferences about the etiology of the disorder.
9. In the planning stage, the nurse collaborates with the adolescent and family to determine client outcomes and goals based on assessed needs.
10. Various intervention strategies for working with disturbed adolescents may include family, group, individual, and milieu therapies; behavioral and cognitive strategies; and psychopharmacology.
11. Stating outcomes in small, measurable increments, rather than as major changes, aids in evaluating the adolescent's progress toward goals.
12. Working with adolescents requires a firm awareness of self and a willingness to confront issues such as identification, separation, sexuality, and self-control.

Review Questions

1. Describe the primary and secondary changes of normal adolescent development. Describe a social consequence that can result due to the variation in development among individuals.
2. Discuss Piaget's and Sullivan's contributions to adolescent development.
3. Describe the incidence of adolescent disturbance and one reason why clinicians may overdiagnose or underdiagnose adolescent disturbance.
4. Give three examples of how the variables of family communication, parenting style, personality, social pressures, or stressors may contribute to adolescent disorder.
5. Which of the following are risk factors for adolescent substance abuse. (Circle as many as apply.)
   A. Demographics: age and gender
   B. Social: parental substance abuse or family dys-

function, peer group who is involved in drugs or alcohol

C. Environmental: mixed messages from society about drugs and alcohol

D. Individual: low academic aspirations, low self-esteem

6. John is distractible, impulsive, and inattentive in school. He has difficulty staying on task in class and completing assignments. He often blurts out answers without waiting to be called on by the teacher. What do you suspect is his DSM-IV diagnosis? What tools can aid your assessment? What interventions would you suggest for John?
7. What must the nurse do to avoid being caught off guard emotionally or intellectually when interacting with adolescents?

◆ References

1. American Psychiatric Association: DSM-IV: Diagnostic and Statistical Manual of Mental Disorders, 4th ed. Washington, DC, American Psychiatric Association, 1994
2. Andrews J, Smolkowski K, Hops H, Tildesley E, Ary D, Harris J: Adolescent Substance Use and Academic Achievement and Motivation. Paper presented at the Annual Convention of the American Psychological Association, San Francisco, CA, 1991
3. Annie E: Kids Count Data Book: State Profiles of Child Well-Being. Baltimore, MD, Casey Foundation, 1994
4. Ash JB, Piazza E: Changing Symptomatology in Eating Disorders. International Journal of Eating Disorders 18 (1): 27–38, 1995
5. Barrett H: Drug Use in Rural Kansas Fifth and Sixth Graders. Kansas, Fort Hays State University (ERIC Document Reproduction Service No. ED 339 955), 1990
6. Beman DS: Risk Factors Leading to Adolescent Substance Abuse. Adolescence 30 (117): 201–208, 1995
7. Berndt TJ, Savin-Williams RC: Peer Relations and Friendships. In Tolan PH, Cohler BJ (eds): Handbook of Clinical Research and Practice With Adolescents, pp 203–220. New York, John Wiley, 1993
8. Brage DG: Adolescent Depression: A Review of the Literature. Archives of Psychiatric Nursing 9 (1): 45–55, 1995
9. Bruch H: The Golden Cage: The Enigma of Anorexia Nervosa. Cambridge, MA, Harvard University Press, 1978
10. Children's Defense Fund: The State of America's Children Yearbook. Washington, DC, Children's Defense Fund, 1995
11. Conley JF: Conduct Disorders. In Johnson BS (ed): Child, Adolescent, and Family Psychiatric Nursing, pp 221–229. Philadelphia, JB Lippincott, 1995
12. Clunn PL: Assessment of the Adolescent. In Hogarth CR (ed): Adolescent Psychiatric Nursing, pp 133–175. St. Louis, CV Mosby, 1991
13. DeVeagh-Geiss J, Moroz G, Biederman J: Clomipramine Hydrochloride in Childhood and Adolescent Obsessive-Compulsive Disorder: A Multicenter Trial. J Am Acad Child Adolesc Psychiatry 31: 45–49, 1992
14. Drost LM, Ross LS: Anxiety Disorders. In Johnson BS (ed): Child, Adolescent, and Family Psychiatry Nursing, pp 193–206. Philadelphia, JB Lippincott, 1995
15. Eggert LL, Thompson EA, Herting JR: A Measure of Adolescent Potential for Suicide (MAPS): Development and Preliminary Findings. Suicide and Life-Threatening Behavior 24 (4): 359–381, 1994
16. Emslie GJ, Kennard BD, Kowatch RA: Affective Disorders in Children: Diagnosis and Management. J Child Neurol 10 (1): S42–S49, 1994
17. Emslie GJ, Rush AJ, Weinberg WA, Kowatch RA, Hughes CW, Carmody T, Rintelmann J: A Double-Blind, Randomized Placebo-Controlled Trial of Fluoxetine in Depressed Children and Adolescents. Arch Gen Psychiatry. Paper presented at American Academy of Child and Adolescent Psychiatry Annual Meeting, New Orleans, LA, October, 1995
18. Erikson E: Identity: Youth and Crisis. New York, Norton, 1968
19. Faigel HC, Sznajderman S, Tishby O, Turel M, Pinus U: Attention Deficit Disorder During Adolescence: A Review. Journal of Adolescent Health 16 (3): 174–184, 1995
20. Finkelstein JW: The Effect of Developmental Changes in Adolescence on Drug Disposition. Journal of Adolescent Health 15: 612–618, 1994
21. Fisher M, Golden NH, Katzman DK, Kreipe RE, Rees J, Schebendach J, Sigman G, Ammerman S, Hoberman HM: Eating Disorder in Adolescents: A Background Paper. Journal of Adolescent Health 16 (6): 420–437, 1995
22. Freud A: Adolescence. Psychoanalytic Study of the Child 13: 231–258, 1958
23. Fuhrman T, Holmbeck GN: A Contextual Analysis of Emotional Autonomy and Adjustment in Adolescence. Child Dev 66: 793–811, 1995
24. Fuligni AJ, Eccles JS: Perceived Parent-Child Relationships and Early Adolescents' Orientation Toward Peers. Developmental Psychology 29: 622–632, 1993
25. Fullerton DT, Wonderlich SA, Gosnell BA: Clinical Characteristics of Eating Disorder Patients Who Report Sexual or Physical Abuse. International Journal of Eating Disorders 17 (3): 243–249, 1995
26. Gilbert C: Group Therapy. In Johnson BS (ed): Child, Adolescent, and Family Psychiatric Nursing, pp 369–380. Philadelphia, JB Lippincott, 1995
27. Green WH, Padron-Gayol M, Hardesty AS, Bassiri M: Schizophrenia With Childhood Onset: A Phenomenological Study of 38 Cases. J Am Acad Child Adolesc Psychiatry 31: 968–976, 1992
28. Grilo CM, Becker DF, Walker ML, Levy KN, Edell WS, McGlashan TH: (1995). Psychiatric comorbidity in adolescent inpatients with substance use disorders. Journal of the American Academy of Child & Adolescent Psychiatry, 34(8), 1085-1091, 1995
29. Henry B, Feehan M, McGee R, Stanton W, Moffitt TE, Silva P: The Importance of Conduct Problems and Depressive Symptoms in Predicting Adolescent Substance Use. J Abnorm Child Psychol 21 (5): 469–480, 1993

30. Herpertz-Dahlmann BM, Wewetzer C, Remschmidt H: The Predictive Value of Depression in Anorexia Nervosa: Results of a Seven-Year Follow-up Study. Acta Psychiatr Scand 91 (2): 114–119, 1995
31. Hirsch J, Ellis JB: Family Support and Other Social Factors Precipitating Suicidal Ideation. Int J Soc Psychiatry 41 (1): 26–30, 1995
32. Holmbeck GN, Updegrove AL: Clinical-Developmental Interface: Implications of Developmental Research for Adolescent Psychotherapy. Psychotherapy 32 (1): 16–33, 1995
33. Kazdin AE: Prevention of Conduct Disorder. Paper presented at the National Conference on Prevention Research, Bethesda, MD, National Institute of Mental Health, 1990
34. Johnson C: Adolescent Patients' Perceptions of the Seclusion Experience: A Phenomenological Study. Unpublished master's thesis, Arlington, The University of Texas at Arlington, 1991
35. Johnson C: Therapeutic Environments. In Johnson BS (ed): Child, Adolescent, and Family Psychiatric Nursing, pp 424–438. Philadelphia, JB Lippincott, 1995
36. Johnson BS, Baggett JM: Applying the Nursing Process to Children, Adolescents, and Families. In Johnson BS (ed): Child, Adolescent, and Family Psychiatric Nursing, pp 15–31. Philadelphia, JB Lippincott, 1995
37. Johnson CA, Pentz MA, Weber MD, Dwyer JH, Baer N, MacKinnon DP, Hansen WB, Flay BR: Relative Effectiveness of Comprehensive Community Programming for Drug Abuse Prevention With High-Risk and Low-Risk Adolescents. J Consult Clin Psychol 58 (4): 447–456, 1990
38. Kowatch RA, Suppes T, Gilfillan SK, Fuentes RM, Grannemann BD, Emslie GJ: Clozapine Treatment of Children and Adolescents With Bipolar Disorder and Schizophrenia: A Clinical Case Series. Journal of Child and Adolescent Psychopharmacology 5 (4): 241–253, 1995
39. Lewinsohn PM, Rohde P, Seeley JR: Adolescent Psychopathology: III. The Clinical Consequences of Comorbidity. J Am Acad Child Adolesc Psychiatry 34 (4): 510–519, 1995
40. Linden MF: Attitudes Toward Alcohol Use and Abuse in a Rural School. Paper presented at the annual meeting of the Southwest Educational Research Association, Houston, TX (ERIC Document Reproduction Service No. ED 341 001), 1992
41. Loeber R, Green SM, Keenan K, Lahey BB: Which Boys Will Fare Worse? Early Predictors of the Onset of Conduct Disorder in a Six-Year Longitudinal Study. J Am Acad Child Adolesc Psychiatry 34 (4): 499–509, 1995
42. McClellan JM, Werry JS: Practice Parameters for the Assessment and Treatment of Children and Adolescents With Schizophrenia. J Am Acad Child Adolesc Psychiatry 33 (5): 616–635, 1994
43. McManus M: Conduct Disorder. In Hsu LKG, Hersen M (eds): Recent Developments In Adolescent Psychiatry, pp 269–288. New York, John Wiley & Sons, 1989
44. March JS, Mulle K, Herbel B: Behavioral Psychotherapy for Children and Adolescents With Obsessive-Compulsive Disorder: An Open Trial of a New Protocol-Driven Treatment Package. J Am Acad Child Adolesc Psychiatry 33 (3): 333–341, 1994
45. Minuchin S, Rosman B, Baker L: Psychosomatic Families. Cambridge, MA, Harvard University Press, 1978
46. Mufson L, Moreau D, Weissman M, Klerman G: Interpersonal Psychotherapy for Depressed Adolescents. New York, Guildford Press, 1993
47. National Institute of Mental Health: Suicide Fact Sheet. Washington, DC, U.S. Government Printing Office, 1992
48. Nolen-Hoeksema S, Girgus JS: The Emergence of Gender Differences in Depression During Adolescence. Psychol Bull 115 (3): 424–443, 1994
49. Overholser JC, Adams DM, Lehnert KL, Brinkman DC: Self-esteem Deficits and Suicidal Tendencies Among Adolescents. J Am Acad Child Adolesc Psychiatry 34 (7): 919–928, 1995
50. Piaget J: Piaget's Theory. In Mussen PH (ed): Manual of Child Psychology, 3d ed, pp 703–732. New York, John Wiley, 1970
51. Piaget J: Intellectual Evolution From Adolescence to Adulthood. Human Development 15: 1–12, 1972
52. Powell JW, Denton R, Mattsson A: Adolescent Depression: Effects of Mutuality in the Mother-Adolescent Dyad and Locus of Control. Am J Orthopsychiatry 65 (2): 263–273, 1995
53. Rawlins R: Hope-Hopelessness. In Rawlins R, Williams S, Beck C (eds): Mental Health-Psychiatric Nursing: A Holistic Life-Cycle Approach, 3d ed, pp 257–284. Chicago, CV Mosby, 1993
54. Stein DB, Smith ED: The "REST" Program: A New Treatment System of the Oppositional Defiant Adolescent. Adolescence 25 (100): 891–903, 1990
55. Steinberg L: Interdependence in the Family: Autonomy, Conflict, and Harmony in the Parent-Adolescent Relationship. In Feldman SS, Elliott GL (eds): At the Threshold: The Developing Adolescent, pp 255–276. Cambridge, MA, Harvard University Press, 1990
56. Sullivan HS: The Interpersonal Theory of Psychiatry. New York, Norton, 1953
57. Texas Commission on Children and Youth. Safeguarding Our Future: Children and Families First. Austin, TX, Texas Commission on Children and Youth, 1994
58. Trickett PK, Putnam FW: Impact of Child Sexual Abuse on Females: Toward a Developmental Psychobiological Integration. Psychological Science 4: 81–87, 1993
59. Valois RF, McKeown RE, Garrison CZ, Vincent ML: Correlates of Aggressive and Violent Behaviors Among Public High School Adolescents. Journal of Adolescent Health 16 (1): 26–34, 1995
60. Waller D: Eating disorders. In Parmelee DX (ed): Child and Adolescent Psychiatry for the Clinician. St. Louis, CV Mosby, 1996
61. Weeks SM: Individual Therapy. In Johnson BS (ed): Child, Adolescent, and Family Psychiatric Nursing, pp 351–357. Philadelphia, JB Lippincott, 1995
62. Weinberg WA, Emslie GJ: Attention Deficit Hyperactivity Disorder: The Differential Diagnosis. J Child Neurol 6 (Suppl): S21–S34, 1991

63. West SA, McElroy SL, Strakowski SM, Keck PE, McConville BJ: Attention Deficit Hyperactivity Disorder in Adolescent Mania. Am J Psychiatry 152 (2): 271–273, 1995
64. White JL: The Troubled Adolescent. New York, Pergamon Press, 1989
65. Wilens TE, Biederman J, Spencer TJ, Frances RJ: Comorbidity of Attention-Deficit Hyperactivity and Psychoactive Substance Use Disorders. Hosp Community Psychiatry 45 (5): 421–433, 435, 1994
66. Woodard VA: Chemical Dependency. In Johnson BS (ed): Child, Adolescent, and Family Psychiatric Nursing, pp 315–328. Philadelphia, JB Lippincott, 1995

Mental Health of the Aging

Patriciann Furnari Brady

24

From "An Old Lady Has The Last Word" What do you see, nurse, what do you see?
What do you think when you're looking at me?
A crabby old woman, not very wise,
Uncertain of habit, with faraway eyes,
Who dribbles her food and makes no reply
When you say in a loud voice, "I do wish you'd try."
Who seems not to notice the things that you do,
And forever is losing a stocking and shoe.
Who, resisting or not, must do as you will.
Is that what you're thinking: is that what you see?
Then open your eyes, nurse, you're not looking at me.
. . .inside this old carcass a young girl still dwells,
And now and again my battered heart swells.
I remember the joys, I remember the pain,
And I'm loving and living life all over again.
I think of the years, all too few, gone too fast,
And accept the stark fact that nothing can last.
So open your eyes, nurse. Open and see.
Not a crabby old woman: look closer—See Me.

Author Unknown

The elderly constitute a significant portion of our society. The number of individuals over the age of 65 has tripled from 4% in 1900 to 12.6% in 1990 and the actual number has increased 10-fold to 31.2 million.[11, 24, 29] *The number of individuals in their 70s and 80s has been steadily increasing and it has been projected that they will continue to grow.*[11]

Recognizing the needs of elderly adults and understanding the physiological, psychological, and social changes they experience are essential skills for all nurses. This chapter focuses on helping nurses to identify their own attitudes about the elderly and to incorporate their knowledge about the physical, psychological, and social changes of aging in applying the nursing process to the care of elderly clients.

Learning Objectives

On completion of this chapter, you should be able to accomplish the following:

1. *Identify those persons in our society who are labeled elderly.*
2. *Discuss nurses' attitudes toward the elderly.*
3. *Describe adaptation to the normal physiological, psychological, and social changes during the aging process.*
4. *Identify means for promotion of health and positive adaptation to aging.*
5. *Discuss common geropsychiatric problems and their mental health care.*

◆ The Elderly and Nursing

IDENTIFYING THE POPULATION

Individuals who reach the age of 65 have been identified by our society as the elderly. Gerontologists have defined chronological categories of the "young old" (65-74), the "middle old" (75-84) and the "old old" (age 84 and older).[25] At present, there are about 30.3 million individuals at 65 years or older, including 2.9 million aged 85 years or older. Individuals are unique and so are their aging processes. As a greater proportion of the population lives longer, relatively rare challenges of the past are now becoming more common.[12] The care of the elderly person is possibly the most complex area of nursing.[7]

Old age is a period of continued development. Developmental tasks of aging include conservation of strength and resources, when necessary, and adaptation to those changes and losses that occur as part of the normal aging process. The ability to adapt and thrive is contingent on physical health, personality, early life experiences, and societal support, such as adequate finances, shelter, medical care, social roles, and recreation.[5]

The picture of an old person sitting in a wheelchair in a nursing home does not describe the elderly adult of today. Only about 5% of the older population reside in nursing homes at any given time. Elderly individuals, aged 65-74, constitute only 1% of the nursing home population.[24] Therefore, the environments vary in which nurses come in contact with elderly clients, and frequently include the community.[4]

THE NURSE'S ATTITUDES

In June 1966, geriatric nursing was first recognized as a vital speciality by the American Nurses' Association (ANA), and in 1970 the ANA established the Standards of Geriatric Nursing Practice. In 1976 the Geriatric Nursing Division changed its title to Gerontological Nursing Division.

Nursing care of the elderly has not commanded the prestige of many other areas of clinical nursing practice. In the past, being a geriatric nurse implied that the nurse was inferior in capabilities or could not handle the demands of the acute-care setting. It is now recognized that nurses working with the elderly provide both skilled nursing care for individuals during illness and guidance in maximizing their capabilities throughout the aging process.

Care of the elderly has become a highly sophisticated area of practice. There has been a profound growth in the number of nurses who have focused their practice on the care of the elderly. Several hundred nurses every year achieve American Nurses Association certification in gerontological nursing.[11] The specialty has advanced rapidly and will continue to grow as the challenges of and demand for specialized nursing of the elderly become more apparent.

Care of the elderly should include the use of scientific principles and rationales for care. The following principles guide nursing care of the elderly:

1. Aging is a common and natural process.
2. Various factors influence the normal aging process.
3. Knowledge of the aging process and knowledge of nursing science are combined in providing care for the elderly.
4. The nursing process is used in providing care for the elderly.
5. The focus of gerontological nursing is to provide planned, organized and therapeutic nursing actions.[10]

BARRIERS TO MENTAL HEALTH CARE

Elderly adults who experience mental health problems have been largely neglected by our society.[10] The incidence of mental illness is higher in the elderly than in the young.[11] Epidemiological studies since the 1950s have documented a 15-25% prevalence of serious mental disorders in those over the age of 65. It is estimated that approximately one fourth of the elderly in the community and more than one half of the elderly in nursing homes have symptoms of mental illness.

Two factors make identifying and treating mental disorders in the elderly especially challenging. On the one hand, failure to distinguish disease-related psychiatric symptoms from manifestations of normal aging may blur the understanding of mental functioning in the healthy elderly.[24] Mental health problems of the elderly cannot be addressed when the behavior exhibited is viewed as normal aging. It is often difficult, for example, to determine if an individual is experiencing dementia or depression. The distinction is important, however, since, unlike dementia, depression in the elderly can be successfully treated.[35] On the other hand, dementia and depression may be misdiagnosed as physical problems[5,8,27,35] because mental and physical illness in older people often occur simultaneously, and each tends to mimic or exacerbate the symptoms of the other.[29]

Often medical conditions are the focus of care of an elderly individual rather than considering mental health issues. If an elderly individual suddenly begins to refuse to leave the home, panic disorder with agoraphobia should be considered. A complete assessment might reveal panic symptoms and reduced activity associated with agoraphobia related to medical conditions that occur frequently in this age group.[22]

The elderly are often reluctant to seek assistance, particularly to seek treatment for mental or emotional disorders.[10] The need for self-determination and independence often impedes their willingness to seek care. They may endure problems as a sign of independence and those with cognitive disturbances may not be motivated or aware of the need for care.[10]

Approximately 60% of all nursing home residents suffer from a chronic mental condition.[10] Nursing home staff are frequently not prepared to deal with the challenging needs of the mentally ill elderly. A combined consultation and training program has been used to meet these clients' needs which, although it cannot completely replace direct professional intervention, may help nursing home staff effectively manage behavioral problems.[30]

◆ The Aging Process

All individuals, including the elderly, develop at varying rates. Some elderly persons are highly independent, whereas some are dependent on others for aspects of care. Manifestations of illness are less predictable in the elderly, causes are more variable, and consequences are farther reaching.[25] The propensity for multiple health problems further complicates nursing care.

Holistic mental health care of elderly clients must use the nursing process and focus on three areas:

1. Physiological changes of aging
2. Geropsychiatric problems
3. Changes of aging requiring adaptation

PHYSIOLOGICAL CHANGES OF AGING

The aging process begins at birth and is an expected outcome of living. Infants become toddlers, pubescent children blossom into young women and men, and adolescents develop into responsible adults.[11] Elderly adults move to a stage of evaluation of life and adaptation to the changes that occur in a body that has served itself for many years. The rapidity of aging depends on a person's heredity, amount and regularity of exercise, past illnesses, presence of chronic illnesses, and the stresses experienced throughout life.[16] The result is not only individual variations but also differences in the pattern of aging of various body systems within the same individual.[11]

Changes attributed to aging include the following:

1. Decreased rate of cell dimension in specialized cells that regenerate (e.g., epithelial)
2. Deterioration of more specialized nondividing cells, particularly neurons and skeletal muscle cells, leading to decreased functional capacity
3. Changes in connective tissue, leading to increased rigidity and loss of elasticity, producing changes in organ systems
4. General loss of reserve functional capacity in all organ systems.[16]

Functional impairment, or a decreased ability to meet one's needs, is a common outcome of many disorders of the elderly.[19] Common physical conditions of community-based elderly include arthritis, hypertension, hearing and visual impairment, heart disease, cataracts, orthopedic impairments, sinusitis, and diabetes.[29] These illnesses may precipitate a hospital admission, which further threatens the aging person's functional ability. As many as 75% of functionally independent elderly people are no longer independent on discharge from an acute-care hospital.[20] Difficulties with mobility, cognition, continence, and nutrition require a problem-oriented approach and must include functional assessment as well as traditional clinical medical care.[24] Nursing interventions at the time of hospitalization that reduce the incidence of functional impairment of the elderly include the following:

1. Adequate nursing and support staff to rehabilitate the geriatric patient

2. Acute-care nursing practices that support the principles of geriatric rehabilitation
3. Comprehensive assessment of premorbid and current functional abilities
4. Specialized programs that promote continence and mobilization.[24]

The nurse can help the elderly client determine which physiological changes of aging are normal and which signal illness. The nurse working with elderly clients focuses on assisting them to understand the normal aging process, to maintain the body through diet, rest, sleep and exercise, and to cope with physiological changes through adaptation (see Nursing Care Plan 24-1).

The nurse's understanding of the normal aging process facilitates the elderly client's adaptive skills. Three major age-related changes include: 1) altered thought processes; 2) altered sensory perception; 3) sleep pattern disturbances. Planning and implementing nursing care to enhance the client's ability to cope effectively with these changes is the nurse's goal. Most physiological changes of aging bring with them psychological components that cannot be negated, including threat to self-image, self-esteem, personal identity, and role performance. The nurse addresses these aspects of the elderly client's psychological well-being in providing holistic care (see Nursing Care Plan 24-2).

GEROPSYCHIATRIC PROBLEMS

An elderly person's sense of self and security may be threatened when it becomes necessary to adapt to various personal changes. Changes in physical status, loss of significant other, hospitalization, or movement to a long-term care facility have a profound effect on the elderly person's sense of independence. Uncharacteristic behaviors may emerge or existing personality traits may be exaggerated in acute-care settings, or when the client is in a crisis state or receiving treatment and medications.[10]

The elderly have an advantage over those in other age groups because they have experienced many life situations which have helped them develop a variety of coping skills. Nevertheless, the elderly may experience a variety of mental health problems, including depression, anxiety, paranoia, alcohol abuse, and hypochondriasis. Today, greater numbers of people are reaching old age, and they may bring with them a variety of lifelong mental health problems.[11]

Depression

Depression represents the most common psychiatric disorder in the elderly.[8] It is difficult to differentiate the behaviors exhibited by elderly clients as either dementia or depression. Although major depression presents differently in different individuals, symptoms generally involve loss of interest in pleasurable activities. However, depressive symptoms may not always manifest as sadness, but rather as irritability, anxiety, and anger.[8]

Late life depression impairs memory function to a greater degree than that seen in the normal aging process. A thorough history and mental status examination are crucial and must include questioning about affective symptoms and testing for cognitive impairment.[27] Depressed older adults require cognitive support at both encoding and retrieval to demonstrate memory facilitation.[1] The Mini-Mental Status Exam may be effective in determining the type of mental impairment present in an elderly client and in differentiating depression (see Chapter 8). Cognitive processing, immediate recall, and recent recall can be assessed by the Mini-Mental Status Exam; however, past and remote recall cannot be assessed.[2] Depressed elderly store more information when it is presented slowly and respond with retrieval clues.[1]

Depression in the elderly may be caused by a variety of physical and psychological factors. As part of a comprehensive assessment of the elderly, the nurse needs to consider the following influences on the development of depression:

1. Chemical imbalance in the brain (information obtained through a family history of depression)
2. Unresolved or dysfunctional grieving in response to a loss
3. Existence of specific diseases:
   a. Hypothyroidism
   b. Alzheimer' disease
   c. Sensory deprivation
4. Drug toxicity (history of taking more than three medications)[8]

Suicide

As the elderly attempt to cope with the changes of aging, normal adaptation skills may be effective. Failure of adaptation skills, however, may lead to depression which, in turn, may lead to suicide.[25] The rate and nature of physical decline, under the influence of depression, can reflect the will to live or die in the elderly.[25]

Elderly persons make fewer suicide attempts, communicate intention of suicide less frequently, use more lethal methods of suicide, and are more successful in their suicide attempts than younger individuals.[25] Effectiveness of coping abilities and strength of will to live appear to be crucial factors in determining who among the elderly will attempt suicide.[25] In an era when suicide among the elderly is increasing, caregivers need to understand ways in which to address intent and to follow through on statements that are serious in nature.[35]

Nursing Care Plan 24-1

The Aging Client Who Somatizes His Feelings

Mr. F, a 76-year-old retired lawyer, lives in a retirement community. He has a history of hypertension, monitors his blood pressure, and takes antihypertensive medication. Mr. A, his best friend, has just been diagnosed with pancreatic cancer. Increasingly, since the illness of his friend, Mr. F has complained of epigastric distress, has self-medicated with over-the-counter antiacids, and has refused to go out to dinner, a former source of enjoyment. Although his wife and children have been preparing his favorite food to encourage eating, he is beginning to lose weight. Mr. F was seen by his family physician and when a complete gastrointestinal (GI) evaluation indicated no physical cause, he was referred to a geriatric nurse specialist who developed with him a plan of care to decrease his indigestion and to decrease his focus on physical symptoms.

Nursing Diagnosis

Ineffective Individual Coping related to his fears about his gastrointestinal functioning

Outcome

Client will experience no further epigastric distress

Intervention	Rationale
Complete a physical assessment of client's gastrointestinal system.	Physical assessment assures an holistic approach to nursing care
Assist client and his family to plan a nutritious diet and eliminate acid- and gas-producing foods.	A nutritious diet without irritating foods decreases GI distress and irritability.
Help client identify activities he enjoys	Participation in enjoyable activities decreases his preoccupation with bodily functions.
Spend time in conversation unrelated to physical complaints.	Interaction not centered on symptoms demonstrates that one can receive attention without focusing on to physical complaints.
Assist family members to understand that his physical complaints are related to mental state.	Education of family helps them reinforce positive behavior and not be manipulated by the client's symptoms.

Evaluation

Client participates in conversation and activities that are not focused on physical complaints.

Suicide is actually a means of reacting to one or more of the changes brought about by the aging process. In making assessments, the nurse should consider the client's attitude about death. Persons who have a healthy attitude about death, that is, perceive life and death as a challenge and not a threat, are thought to be less vulnerable to depression.[9]

The finality of suicide should make the nurse aware of the importance of accurate assessment. When interviewing an elderly client, the nurse should clarify suicide intent by specifically questioning the client to determine the existence and lethality of a suicide plan. Nursing interventions include staying with the client to lend support and strength and prevent institution of a plan.[35] Individualized plans of care will assist in the prevention and early detection and treatment of depression in the elderly.[9] Specific nursing interventions addressing depression may be reviewed in Chapter 29, Depressive and Bipolar Disorders.

Anxiety Disorders

Many of the physical, psychological, and social changes of aging cause symptoms of anxiety. Anxiety reactions, not uncommon in older persons, may be manifested in

Nursing Care Plan 24-2

Dealing With Normal Problems of Aging

Mr. and Mrs. J live in a high-rise apartment for the elderly. Mr. J has been discharged from the rehabilitation center following treatment after surgery to repair a fractured hip. The community health nurse is making a home visit to assess the home environment and to address the learning needs of Mr. and Mrs. J regarding health maintenance. During the visit, the nurse assesses that the apartment is clean and nicely furnished, although somewhat cluttered. In discussion with Mr. and Mrs. J, they express concerns regarding prevention of any other falls and complain about difficulty sleeping.

The nurse prepares a nursing care plan to address the normal problems of aging, oriented toward maintaining health.

Nursing Diagnosis

Risk for Injury related to decreased balance and sensory changes secondary to aging process

Outcome

Client(s) will remain safe in the home environment.

Intervention	Rationale
Teach client(s) measures to minimize risk of falling and to compensate for age-related changes.	Educating the elderly about the expected changes in aging and compensation for these will help maintain health and independence.
1. Change position slowly.	1. Postural hypotension is common in the elderly, especially in those who take medication affecting cardiovascular system.
2. Walk slowly with feet in wide stance.	2. Balance can be enhanced by using a slow gait with a wide base of support.
3. Remove scatter or throw rugs from walking areas.	3. Loss of muscle tone and proprioception sense occurs in elderly; falls can occur by tripping on loose rugs.
Teach measures to adapt to sensory changes, such as decreased vision.	
1. Maintain adequate lighting and place objects within reach and visual field	1. Visual accommodation and peripheral vision alter or decrease with aging.
2. Wear prescription glasses or contact lenses.	2. Visual acuity and corneal sensitivity decrease with aging.
3. Use a magnifying glass for very small print, especially medication labels.	3. Adaptation to decreased visual acuity can be enhanced by simple measures such as use of magnifying glass.

Evaluation:

Client maintains safety in home environment.

Nursing Diagnosis

Ineffective Individual Coping related to frustration secondary to increased length of time to complete tasks

Outcome

Client will allow increased time to perform activities.

continued

Nursing Care Plan 24-2 (Continued)

Intervention	Rationale
Teach client to plan added time to perform activities of daily living	Response and reaction time decrease with age which increases frustration
Teach client(s) that although response times are increased, intelligence and ability are not decreased as part of normal aging.	Maintaining and reinforcing self-esteem and encouraging independence are important for healthy adaptation to aging.

Evaluation

Client completes tasks without verbalizing frustration.

Nursing Diagnosis

Sleep Pattern Disturbance related to difficulty falling asleep and awakening often during the night

Outcome

Client(s) will verbalize measures to promote sleep.

Intervention	Rationale
Teach client(s) to decrease use of caffeine.	Caffeine has psychostimulant effects and prevents restful sleep.
Encourage client(s) to provide a relaxing environment prior to bedtime.	A warm bath or warm milk promote relaxation leading to drowsiness.
Teach client to get out of bed and read, watch TV, or engage in other quiet activity if sleep does not come.	Remaining in bed awake increases tension and worry about one's sleep problems.
Encourage client(s) to keep a sleep chart and to record the times that they awaken.	Accurate data help the client identify specific sleep problems on which to base further interventions.
Encourage client(s) to go to bed and awaken at the same time each day.	A specific routine will support body's normal rhythms.

Evaluation

Client reports 6 hours of uninterrupted, restful sleep.

various ways, including somatic complaints, rigidity in thinking and behavior, insomnia, fatigue, hostility, restlessness, chain smoking, pacing, fantasizing, confusion, and increased dependency.[11] A number of medical conditions, such as hyperthyroidism, cardiac arrhythmias, pulmonary edema, or embolism, may be mistakenly diagnosed as anxiety.[24]

An accurate assessment will help the nurse determine the source of the client's anxiety. Assessment information should include:

1. Recent changes or new stressors
2. Use of stimulants (ie, caffeine, alcohol, nicotine, over-the-counter medications including cold medications)[11,34]

Nursing interventions for clients experiencing anxiety disorders are discussed in Chapter 25.

Paranoia

Paranoia refers to unfounded fear and suspiciousness which may be generalized or specific to certain persons and situations.[10] Paranoia may occur in the elderly related to the following factors:

1. Sensory losses, common in later life, cause the environment to be misperceived.
2. Illness, disability, living alone, and a having a limited budget promote insecurity
3. Overt and subtle forces within society may underscore a message of the undesirability of the old.
4. The elderly are frequently victims of crime and unscrupulous practices.[11]

The initial consideration in working with paranoid older individuals is to explore interventions that could reduce insecurity and misperceptions.[11] Corrective lenses, hearing aids, supplemental income, improved housing, and a stable environment help prevent the client's socially isolative behavior.[11]

Interventions to diminish paranoid and suspicious behavior include: establishing a therapeutic relationship; protecting the client from harm; determining the reality of the fears and suspicions; including the client in developing a daily schedule; establishing consistent expectations; reinforcing effective coping skills; providing opportunities for participating in decision making; providing information prior to instituting action; and avoiding competitive activities and situations.[10,11] The nurse, other healthcare providers and family must not take the client's behavior personally, but rather recognize it as a symptom of a disorder.

Alcohol Abuse

Alcohol abuse in the elderly is increasing in incidence. It is expected to become more prevalent with the aging of currently middle-aged persons whose alcohol use has been greater than that of former generations.[24] Only 1.4% of the elderly have been diagnosed as alcoholic, compared with 3.9% of those persons under the age of 60.[10] Nevertheless, alcohol use in the elderly represents a significant health problem. Given the relatively complete absorption of alcohol, the smaller volume of distribution, and increased organ dysfunction, older adults who drink alcohol regularly are subject to more toxic effects.[24]

Most often, late-life alcoholics report psychosocial stressors as the cause of their alcohol abuse.[10] Elderly persons who abuse alcohol may have a history of previous abuse; individuals tend to use the same patterns of behavior to cope as they did in their earlier life. Persons who become alcoholic in old age, like those of any age, are usually those who find it difficult to cope with various problems and resort to alcohol as a means of escape.[34] The combination of various medications and alcohol can cause great difficulty for elderly persons. Alcohol-medication interactions are often overlooked or unrecognized. Elderly persons often use alcohol to help them sleep; however, alcohol-induced sleep lacks restorative benefits and thus interferes with coping behavior. Although alcohol may induce drowsiness as an initial effect, it is known to suppress REM sleep and increase nighttime awakening.[25]

Alcohol abuse also challenges various systems and impairs the ability to adapt to the aging process. Alcoholism strains available resources, interferes with sexual functioning, increases the risk of serious injury, and affects nutritional status by reducing appetite.[25] Nurses must be aware of the cycle of alcohol and depression; alcohol causes depression and depression leads to alcohol abuse.[25]

Hypochondriasis

Hypochondriacal symptoms are often associated with depression in the elderly. Hypochondriasis is a somatoform psychiatric disorder characterized by physical symptoms related to morbid anxiety that cannot be attributed to any physical disorder.[24] Elderly clients may complain of symptoms but lack apparent distress.[24]

Elderly individuals are experiencing a stage in their life when friends and loved ones are often diagnosed with illness. Adapting to the loss of relationships, the elderly may begin to focus on their own personal well-being. Since our society does not value the elderly and tends to view the elderly as ill rather than well, illness-related behavior in the elderly is reinforced. Although hypochondriasis is often associated with depression, for some it may be an attention-getting mechanism.[11]

Pseudodementia Versus Dementia

Dementia is a deterioration of intellectual function and other cognitive skills leading to a decline in the ability to perform activities of daily living.[24] Alzheimer's disease and other structural changes within the brain may cause behavioral changes in the elderly. Dementia is a common disorder, affecting approximately 15% of persons 65 years of age and as many as 50% of persons 85 years of age.

Nurses and other healthcare providers must determine which behaviors or mental functions are caused by organic changes in the brain and which are related to the normal process of aging. Personality, attitude, morale, and self-esteem are usually stable throughout the life span; changes in these characteristics tend to be associated with health problems or reaction to life events.[11]

Care of individuals with pseudodementias involves treating the actual condition that is being manifested as a dementia so that the clients can return to their pre-illness behavior. An accurate diagnosis is essential; dementia is a condition that implies a guarded prognosis, so mislabeling a client can have tragic consequences. Because dementia can often lead health care providers to treat clients in a stereotypically demeaning manner, many facilities have care units that focus on the quality of life.[10]

MENTAL HEALTH NURSING INTERVENTIONS

Maintaining independence and control are critical issues in the care of the elderly, whose mental health problems commonly relate to their perception of personal integrity, space, and control. Living a life characterized by personal integrity and self-esteem is important to all of us. The elderly are confronted daily with issues of loss and change.

The nurse's goals, in caring for the elderly client experiencing mental health problems, should be to reinforce the client's own coping skills. The nurse should seek to strengthen the client's capacity to manage problems and stress, in part by eliminating or minimizing the limitations imposed by age-related problems and stress, and to assist elderly clients to be actively involved in their care to the best of their ability.[11] See Table 24-1 for a sample clinical pathway.

Nurses, other healthcare providers, and family members must foster independence in the elderly. Regardless of their mental health problems, the elderly need social support and respectful care. They may participate in mental health day care programs that provide mental health treatment and reintegration into a supportive setting. Well-meaning staff and families may deny older adults their dignity by infantilizing or patronizing them.[32] Nurses are in a position to identify and discourage such behavior. Nurses can offer positive alternatives and, through their interactions, model behaviors and attitudes that demonstrate respect for and promote dignity among older adults.[32]

Medications may be useful in the treatment of mental disorders but are weighed against the incidence and severity of side effects. See Chapter 20 for information about psychotropic medication. The elderly should be given the lowest possible doses to effect the desired action. Indications for and reactions to these medications should be closely monitored and accurately documented.[6,11]

As health care delivery systems change, nurse practitioners are poised to assume the monitoring of medication needs of the elderly.[23] Guidelines of psychotropic drug therapy follow:

1. Complete alleviation of symptoms may be unrealistic if the necessary dosage leads to harmful side effects.
2. One drug at a time should be added to a therapeutic regimen.
3. The initial dose of most psychotropic drugs should be reduced by 30%-50% for an elderly individual. The dosage can then be titrated slowly to achieve maximal benefit with minimal side effects.
4. Periodic attempts should be made to further reduce the dosage or discontinue the medication entirely.[35]

◆ Social Adaptation to Aging

The developmental period of aging challenges the resources of elderly individuals. The changes that come with aging demand multiple adjustments requiring stamina, adaptability, and flexibility.[11] For most people, late life is a period of transition which includes retirement, bereavement, and relocation.[24]

One common challenge of late life is the task of maintaining hope in the face of loss.[18] Strategies that foster hope include the following:

1. Connecting with self, others, and the world as a source of encouragement
2. Engaging in purposeful activities that focus on the needs of others versus self
3. Savoring uplifting memories provided through looking back at positive experiences
4. Consciously using cognitive strategies to transform perceptions into a positive frame
5. Cherishing inanimate objects that possess a meaning beyond the concrete
6. Measuring time by relationships to provide a new focus
7. Cultivating lightheartedness, aliveness, and playfulness of the inner spirit
8. Engaging in spiritual beliefs and practices that are affirmed[18]

Social support is an important variable in assisting elderly individuals to adapt to the changes of aging. Nurses assess a client's social support needs and resources and intervene to promote the quality and availability of needed social support.[32] Various social support organizations such as Senior Citizens Centers bring together a group of contemporaries experiencing similar transitions. Senior citizens' programs strengthen and enhance the support system of their members and thus are important referral resources for nurses engaged in working with older adults.[32]

RETIREMENT

One of the first adjustments facing the elderly is retirement. About 33% of retirees have difficulty adjusting to certain aspects of retirement, such as reduced income and altered social roles and prestige within the community[24] Many individuals base their sense of identity on the position they hold in the work force. Friendships and social relationships often include those who share a common work experience. Occupational identity is largely responsible for a person's social position and for the social role attached to that position.[11]

Retirement may include the reestablishment and renegotiation of roles between spouses. Each spouse, whether working outside the home or not, has had a daily routine that provided a sense of identity and accomplishment. Retirement requires significant adjustments for both partners. Preparing for retirement is a preventive intervention that helps individuals plan for

Table 24-1 Clinical Pathway: Geriatric—Geropsychiatric Inpatient

Patient Name: ______________ **Case Manager:** ______________

Admit date: ______ Expected LOS: ______________ UR days certified: ______

Task	Day 1	Day 2	Day 3
Assessment and Evaluations	Nsg. Asses., Nutr. screen, H&P, Soc. HX, Dr. Initial TX Plan/ Admit Note; Precautions Eval., V/S.	Precaution Eval., ADL Assess., Diet. Consult, Baseline skin integriy AIMS, falls assessment	Psych Eval done, Social HX on chart Precaution Evaluation
Procedures	Lab ordered-Admit profile UA, UDS, EKG, Other:	Lab results checked Abnormals called to Dr.	Follow-up for abnormal lab results
Consults	GT ordered Y/N FT ordered Y/N	GT started Passar Screening done	Passar faxed to assessment center
Treatment Planning	N1: ______ Axis III ______	Potential Sleep Dist. Potential Self-Care Defecit	Pot./Actual Impaired Comm., MTP done
Interventions	Assess S/H/Aggr.	Monitor sleep patterns Assist with ADL PRN	Encourage pts. attempts to communicate
Medications	Meds ordered, Informed Consent	Consider orthostatic V/S daily	Drug interaction checked by Pharm. Dr. signs Informed consent
Level	Level ordered	Least restrictive milieu	Reevaluate level
Teaching	Pts. Rights, Advanced directive, orient to Unit.	Orient to program Provide written schedule	Medication teaching
Nutrition/Diet	Diet Ordered:	I&O consider suppl.	I&O
Care Continuum	Initial D/C plans	Outcome Survey	Placement Search
Patient Outcomes	Control S/H/Aggr.	6–8 hours sleep	Pt. func. more independ.

Abbreviation Key: ADL = Activities of Daily Living; AIMS = Assessment of Involuntary Movement Scale; D/C = Discharge; EPS = Extraphysical Symptoms; FT = Family Therapy; GT = Group Therapy; LOS = Length of Stay; I/O = Intake and Output; MR = Medical Record; MTP = Master Treatment Plan; NI = Nurse Identified Problem; Passar = part of psychiatric assessment for a geriatric patient; PHP = Partial Hospitalization Program; RX = Medication; S/H/Aggr. = Suicide, Homicide, Aggression; TX = Treatment; UA = Urinalysis; UDS = Urine Drug Screen; UR = Utilization Review; V/S = Vital Signs

transitions and maximizes the potential for health and well-being in old age.[11] (see Box 24-1)

BEREAVEMENT

Losses experienced during the aging process vary from the loss of significant others to the loss of social status. Older women outnumber older men and the mortality rate for women has declined rapidly over the past 40 years.[24] The mortality rate is related to the adjustment of men and women to the loss of a spouse or significant other.

Men's and women's responses to the loss of significant relationships differ. In the two year period following the death of a spouse, men tend to have a higher mortality rate then women.[24] In the first 3 months following the death of a spouse, the mortality rate increases 48% in men over the age of 65 and 22% in women over the age of 65.[24]

Widowhood, the death of friends, and the recognition of declining functions make older persons more aware of the reality of their own death.[11] Before helping the elderly deal with death and bereavement, nurses must acknowledge their own feelings about death. Contemplating one's mortality and working through the grief process assists individuals to find meaning in the life that still remains for them. Nursing care and health promotion for the elderly is most effective when it focuses on maximizing the desire for independence and self-reliance and minimizing dependency and learned helplessness.[21] Nurses need to assess cultural values, personal characteristics, health beliefs, health practices, and social support systems to achieve optimal functioning and quality of life in this age group.[21,26,27]

Discussing the past is therapeutic and necessary for the elderly to feel their life has had meaning. Through the life review, unresolved guilt, unachieved aspirations,

Physician: ______________________ **Medical Record #** ______________________

______________ Discharge Date: ______________ Actual LOS: ______________

Day 4	Day 5	Day 6	Day 7
	Assess for level of care	Assess for goals achieved	Assess for readiness for discharge.
	Medication levels if applicable		
Follow-up on Passar	Discharge planner interview family		
Pot./Actual Impaired Memorization	MTP update/revised Treatment Team mtg.		
Encourage reminiscence focus on accomplishments	Assess client support network	Written info re: MTP and Meds sent to Caregiver	Transportation arrangements
Meds evaluated/readjusted Assess EPS, other side effects and document		Discharge instructions for medication to pt. and family	Reinforce discharge med instructions
Reevaluate level	Reevaluate level	Consider PHP	
Devise methods to assist pt. with memory deficit	Meds reinforced		D/C inst. documented in nurses note
I&O	I&O and weight	I&O	Diet D/C instructions
D/C plan update/revised	Aftercare Plan written		Outcome Survey
Enhance self-esteem	Broaden support base	Continuity of care	Comm. w/support sys.

perceived failures, and other aspects of unfinished business can be better understood and resolved.[11]

RELOCATION

Giving up one's home and moving into a nursing home or a long-term care facility is one of the transitions often experienced in later life. The probability of nursing home placement within a person's lifetime is closely related to age; for those aged 65-74 the probability is 17%, but for those over the age of 85 it is 43%.[24]

Moving to a nursing home is often seen as relinquishing independence and assuming a dependent role. Older adults faced with loss of loved ones, multiple health problems, and decreasing ability to care for themselves need to have the support of hope. Sources of hope include religious symbols, relationships with others, and activities.[27] A well designed environment can influence feelings of hopefulness; elderly clients should be encouraged to choose or plan their new environments as much as possible.[27]

Many older individuals cannot deal with the loss of independence after moving to a nursing home and become depressed. Individuals who see themselves as hardy, that is, committed, in control, and challenged are less likely to experience depression upon institutionalization in a nursing home.[9] Therefore, care planning in the nursing home must involve clients in the planning process. An older person placed in a long-term care facility, faced with an unscheduled life event which may be permanent, needs all possible resources to cope with stress and avoid depression.[9]

Many nursing homes do not have mental health nurses available to help nursing staff deal with client adjustment to the nursing home environment. Psychiatric-mental health nurses can positively influence the

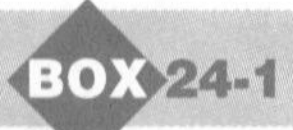

Preretirement Plans

1. Establish and practice good health habits, such as following a proper diet and regular exercise program and avoiding alcohol, drug, and tobacco use.
2. Develop interests unrelated to work, such as leisure activities, hobbies, and participation in civic, church, or senior groups.
3. Develop roles outside of the employment area. Use experiences to assist others. Develop the role of a community or volunteer helper.
4. Recognize the realities versus the fantasies of retirement. Establish goals and routines to provide stability for the future.
5. Establish financial security. Develop a budget that is realistic yet provides for leisure activities.
6. Begin to establish renegotiated roles for married individuals, and plan for sharing household activities and responsibilities. Provide for separate and joint activities.

day-to-day care of elderly clients and assist them with their transition to the nursing home by acting as teachers, resource persons, facilitators, and role models.[30]

By participating in decisions related to relocation, the elderly client will retain a sense of control in an event that otherwise may seem out of control.[19] Methods of assisting individuals to maintain control include planning for social, spiritual, and physical care needs. Providing spiritual care for aging clients requires an understanding of where they are on their spiritual journey through life, and assists them to adapt to losses and find spiritual meaning in late-in-life struggles.[3] (see Chapter 11, Spiritual Aspects of Care)

Adult children of the elderly are often faced with assisting in decisions about nursing home placement. This is a difficult time for the adult children as they experience feelings of guilt and fears about abandoning their parents. The set of circumstances surrounding placement of a parent in a nursing home is complex and unique to each family.[33] The role of the nurse should extend to the adult children as they grieve the loss of ability to care for a parent. Preplacement education and weekly support groups for adult children can lessen the stress of placing a parent in a nursing home.[33] Using these strategies, the movement to the nursing home can be a positive experience for both the elderly and their family members.

◆ Chapter Summary

This chapter focuses on the holistic mental health care of elderly clients, specifically the physiological changes of aging, geropsychiatric problems, and social changes requiring adaptation. Chapter highlights include the following:

1. Aging is a process of continuous physiological and developmental changes.
2. Nurses are urged to identify their attitudes about the elderly and how these influence care.
3. Through an understanding of the normal aging process, the nurse can help elderly clients comprehend and adaptively cope with the inherent physiological and psychological changes of aging.
4. The elderly experience a variety of mental health problems and needs which can be addressed through proper assessment and interventions.
5. Elderly clients need nursing assistance to adapt to the social changes associated with aging

Critical Thinking Questions

1. *Discuss possible causes leading to the tendency in our society to neglect mental health problems in the elderly.*
2. *What factors can interfere with accurate mental status assessment of geriatric patients?*
3. *What stigmas surrounding the geriatric client influence the client's ability to access appropriate mental health care?*

Review Questions

Barbara, a 73 year old widow, moved into an assisted living apartment following the death of her husband three months ago. The home health nurse has been visiting Barbara to monitor her hypertension and diabetes. Over the last two weeks, Barbara has forgotten to take her anti-hypertensive medication and has been skipping meals. She complains of waking up early in the morning and has stated that she does not know how much longer she can live this way.

1. Which of the following is a significant contributing factor of the behavior observed in Barbara by the home health nurse?
   A. The elderly frequently are noncompliant in taking medication as directed by physicians.
   B. Optimal living arrangements for the elderly require admission to a long-term care facility.

C. Unresolved or dysfunctional grieving in response to a loss is a major contributing factor in depression among the elderly.
D. Family members must be involved in assuring medication compliance in the elderly.

2. From the information provided in the situation, which would be a priority nursing diagnosis for Barbara:
   A. Social isolation
   B. Dysfunctional grieving
   C. Sensory-perceptual alteration
   D. Altered thought process
3. Which of the following would be a priority nursing intervention for the home health nurse to implement when working with Barbara?
   A. Spend time in conversation unrelated to illness.
   B. Assist family members to understand the dynamics of the elderly.
   C. Accept Barbara's negative behavior
   D. Assist Barbara to discuss the death of her husband.
4. A common outcome of many physical disorders of the elderly is:
   A. Altered thought processes
   B. Functional impairment
   C. Sensory-perceptual alteration
   D. Social isolation
5. A primary principle which serves as a guide for providing care for elderly experiencing mental health problems is:
   A. Strengthen the elderly's capacity to manage problems and stress.
   B. Provide opportunities for socialization
   C. Encourage the participation in an adaptation group
   D. Foster the development of the opportunity for spiritual growth.

◆ References

1. Backman L, Forsell Y: Episodic Memory Functioning in a Community-Based Sample of Old Adults With Major Depression: Utilization of Cognitive Support. J Ab Psych 103 (2): 361–370, 1994
2. Baker FM: Screening Tests for Cognitive Impairment. Hospital and Community Psychiatry 40(4): 339–340, 1989
3. Berggren-Thomas P, Griggs M: Spirituality in Aging: Spiritual Needs or Spiritual Journey? J Gerontol Nurs: 23(3) 5–10, 1995
4. Buckwalter KC: Geropsychiatry: On Care of the Older Adult: Are You Really My Nurse, or Are You a Snake Sheriff? J Psych Nurs 31 (6): 33–34, 1993
5. Butler RN: Successful Aging and the Role of Life-Review. J Am Ger Soc 22 (12): 529–535, 1974
6. Cantu TG, Korek JS: Prescription of Neuroleptics for Geriatric Nursing Home Patients. Hospital and Community Psychiatry 40 (6): 645–647, 1989
7. Carroll M, Brue LJ: A Nurses' Guide to Caring for Elders. New York, Springer, 1989
8. Cosgray RE, Hanna V: Physiological Causes of Depression in the Elderly. Perspectives in Psychiatric Care 29 (1): 26–28, 1993
9. Cataldo JK: Hardiness and Death Attitudes: Predictors of Depression in the Institutionalized Elderly. Archives of Psychiatric Nursing 8(9): 326–332, 1994
10. Ebersole, P. Caring for the Psychogeriatric Client. New York: Springer, 1989.
11. Eliopoulos, C. Gerontological Nursing. Philadelphia: J.B. Lippincott. 1993
12. Fine J.K., Rouse-Bane, S. Using Validation Techniques to Improve Communication with Cognitively Impaired Older Adults. Journal of Gerontological Nursing 20(6) 39-45, 1995.
13. Fingeld, D.L. Becoming & Being Courageous. Issues in Mental Health Nursing 16 (1) 1-11, 1995.
14. Flaskerud, J.H., Kviz,F.J. Rural Attitudes Toward and Knowledge of Mental Illness and Treatment Resources. Hospital and Community Psychiatry 34(3) 229-233, 1983.
15. Gaskins, S., Forte,L. The Meaning of Hope: Implications for Nursing Practice and Research. Journal of Gerontological Nursing. 219(3) 17-24, 1995.
16. Graves, M. Physiological Changes and Major Diseases in the Older Adult. In Hogstel, MO (ed) Nursing Care of the Older Adult: In the Hospital, Nursing Home and Community. New York: John Wiley and Co. 1981.
17. Hamilton L, Lyons PS: A Nursing-Driven Program to Preserve and Restore Functional Ability in Hospitalized Elderly Patients. Journal of Nursing Administration 25(4): 30–37, 1995
18. Herth K: Hope in Older Adults in Community and Institutional Settings. Issues in Mental Health Nursing 14 (2): 139–156, 1993
19. Johnson RA, Hlava, C: Translocation of Elders: Maintaining the Spirit. Geriatric Nursing 15(4): 209–212, 1994
20. Lamont CT, Sampson S, Mathias R, et al: The Outcome of Hospitalization for Acute Illness in the Elderly. J Am Ger Soc 31 (5): 282–288, 1983
21. Laferriere RH, Bissell-Hamel BP: Successful Aging of Oldest Old Women in the Northeast Kingdom of Vermont. Image: Journal of Nursing Scholarship 26(4): 319–323, 1994
22. Luchins DJ, Rose RP: Late-Life Onset of Panic Disorders with Agoraphobia in Three Patients. Am J Psych 146 (7): 920–921, 1989
23. Mahoney DF: Appropriateness of Geriatric Prescribing Decisions Made By Nurse Practitioners and Physicians. Image: Journal of Nursing Scholarship 26(1): 41–46, 1994
24. The Merck Manual of Geriatrics 2nd ed. Abrams, W et al (eds), New Jersey, Merck Co. Inc, 1995
25. Miller CA: Nursing Care of the Older Adult: Theory and Practice. Glenview, Scott Foresman, 1990
26. Nelson PB: Social Support, Self-Esteem, and Depression in the Institutionalized Elderly. Issues of Mental Health Nursing 10: 55–68, 1989
27. Oxman TE: Delayed Recall: Demented, Depressed or Treated? Lancet 344: 213–214, 1994

28. Porter EJ: Older Widows' Experience of Living Alone at Home. Image: Journal of Nursing Scholarship 26(1): 19–24, 1994
29. Richards BS: Geropsychiatric Nursing: Present Issues and Challenges. Nursing Clinics of North America 29(1): 49–56, 1994
30. Smith M, Mitchell S, Buckwalter KC, Garand L: Geropsychiatric Nursing Consultation: A Valuable Resource in Rural Long-Term Care. Arch Psych Nurs 8(4): 272–279, 1994
31. Sullivan Marx EM: Delirium and Physical Restraint in the Hospitalized Elderly. Image: Journal of Nursing Scholarship 276(4): 295–300, 1994
32. Sutherland D, Murphy E: Social Support Among Elderly in Two Community Programs. J Gerontol Nurs 21(2): 31–38, 1995
33. Tipton-Smith S, Tanner GA: Coping With Placement of a Parent in a Nursing Home Through Preplacement Education. Geriatric Nursing 15(6): 322–326, 1994
34. Weiner MF, Simmons JH: Differentiating Depression From Dementia in the Elderly: How to Proceed When Cognitive Dysfunction is the Complaint. Consultant 589–595, 1994
35. Whal A: Assessing Suicidal Intent. J Gerontol Nurs 13 (8): 36–37, 1987
36. Yurick AG, Spier BE, Robb SS, Ebert NJ: The Aged Person and The Nursing Process. Norwalk, CT, Appleton and Lange, 1989

Application of the Nursing Process to Disordered Behaviors

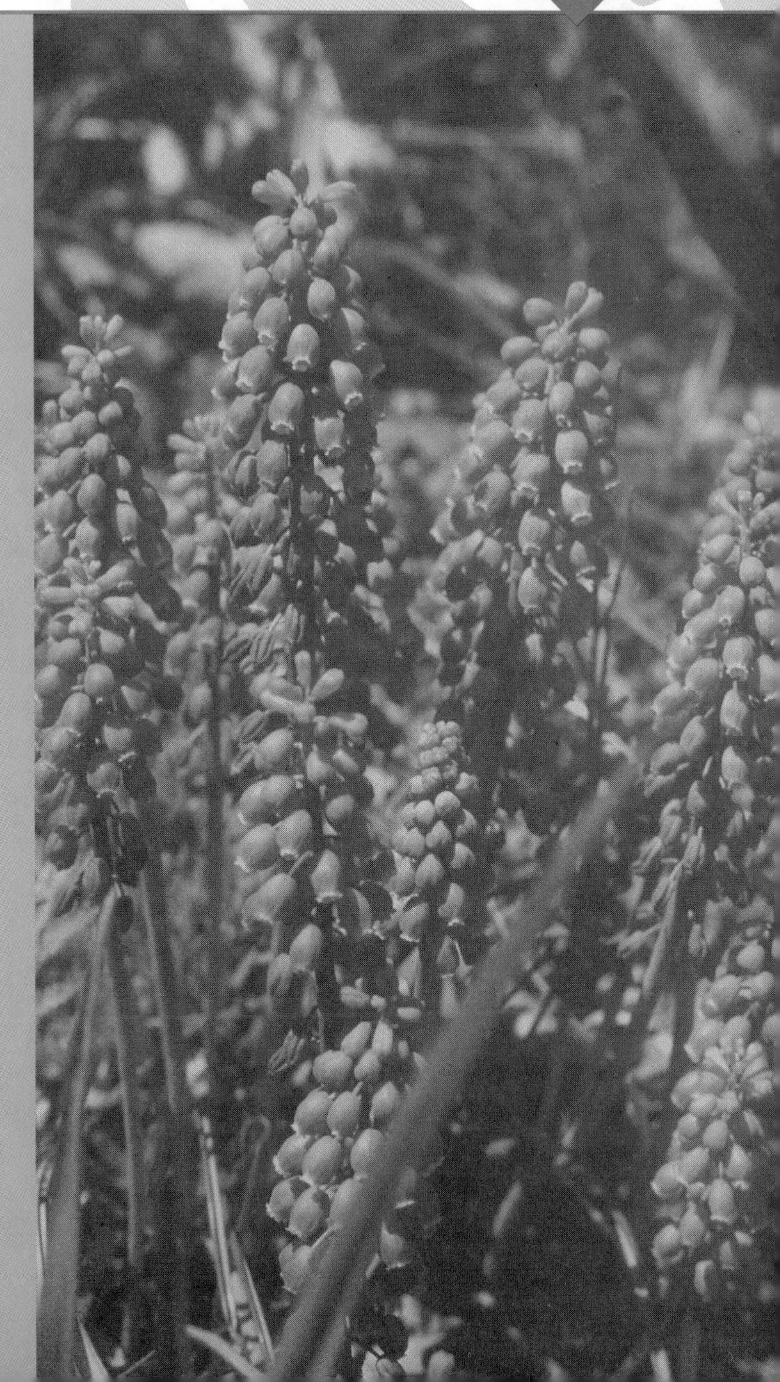

Anxiety Disorders

Judith A. Greene

25

Grief has limits, whereas apprehension has none. For we grieve only for what we know has happened, but we fear all that may possible happen.

Pliny the Younger,
Letters

The phenomenon of anxiety is not new. People in every historical era and in every culture have experienced it. To feel anxious occasionally for brief periods is a natural part of human life. However, when anxiety persists, cannot be dismissed, and begins to interfere with daily existence, then an anxiety disorder is present.

A clinical feature of almost every psychiatric syndrome, anxiety is the primary symptom of the anxiety disorders. Although anxiety disorders generally are considered to be less serious than the personality disorders and major psychoses, they can be as disabling as these other disorders.

Learning Objectives

On completion of this chapter, you should be able to accomplish the following:

1. *Define the term anxiety.*
2. *Discuss the concept of anxiety and its physiological, perceptual, cognitive, and behavioral effects.*
3. *Define the term anxiety disorders.*
4. *Identify how anxiety manifests in selected anxiety disorders.*
5. *Discuss the major signs and symptoms of anxiety disorders.*
6. *Apply the nursing process—assessment, nursing diagnosis, planning, intervention, and evaluation—to clients with selected anxiety disorders.*

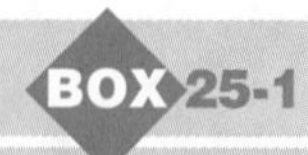

25-1

Behavior Patterns Used to Cope With Anxiety

People commonly attempt to cope with anxiety by using the following major behavioral patterns:

1. Withdrawal: behavioral or psychological retreat from anxiety-provoking experiences
2. Acting out: discharge of anxiety through aggressive behavior
3. Psychosomatization: visceral or physiological expression of anxiety
4. Avoidance: management of anxiety-laden experiences through evasive behaviors
5. Problem solving: using anxiety in the service of learning adaptive behavior

With the exception of problem solving, these behavior patterns are considered maladaptive because they replace feelings of anxiety with feelings of pleasure and comfort at the expense of accurate reality perception and growth toward maturity. Thus, the primary goal of treatment in anxiety disorders and other psychiatric syndromes is to help clients use anxiety to increase their commitment to reality and growth toward maturity.

◆ Anxiety Defined

According to Hildegard Peplau, *anxiety* is the initial response to a psychic threat.[16,17] Because anxiety is a form of energy, it is not accessible to direct observation. It must be ascertained mainly through a client's self-report. An anxious client may describe the subjective experience of anxiety as involving varying feelings of vague discomfort, uncertainty, self-doubt, diffuse apprehension, dread, restlessness or jumpiness, jitteriness, helplessness, powerlessness, and irrationality.[16]

On a more objective basis, the effects of anxiety may be inferred from verbal and nonverbal behaviors and physiological responses. Behaviors and responses indicating anxiety occur along a continuum ranging from mild, moderate, and severe degrees of anxiety to panic.[16,17] Box 25-1 lists behaviors used to cope with anxiety.

PHYSIOLOGICAL EFFECTS OF ANXIETY

Anxiety causes certain physiological responses. Initially, epinephrine and norepinephrine are released from the adrenal medulla, and cortisone is secreted by the adrenal cortex. These hormones increase heart rate, elevate blood pressure, and increase rate and depth of respirations. Other physiological effects accompanying anxiety include excessive perspiration, increased muscle tension, changes in the menstrual cycle, sexual dysfunction, decrease in the blood's clotting time, and release of glycogen by the liver. The extent of these physiological effects depends largely on the degree and duration of anxiety. Generally, mild and moderate anxiety enhance these physiological responses, whereas severe anxiety and panic tax the capacity for them.[16]

PERCEPTUAL EFFECTS OF ANXIETY

Anxiety also affects the ways a person perceives and processes sensory input. *Mild anxiety* actually heightens sensory awareness—sight, hearing, taste, smell, and touch. *Moderate anxiety,* on the other hand, dulls perception, although the individual can attend to greater sensory input if directed to do so.[16] In *severe anxiety,* perception becomes increasingly distorted, sensory input is reduced, and processing of sensory stimuli occurs in a scattered, disorganized manner. In *panic* level anxiety, perception becomes grossly distorted.[16] At this point, the person is incapable of differentiating between real and unreal stimuli.

EFFECTS OF ANXIETY ON COGNITION

Cognition—the ability to concentrate, learn, and solve problems—is greatly influenced by anxiety. Mild and moderate anxiety levels are more conducive to concentration, learning, and problem solving. A person of average intelligence who is mildly to moderately anxious discerns relationships between and among concepts with relative ease and can concentrate and problem solve without undue difficulty.

In contrast, severe anxiety hinders cognitive function. The severely anxious person has difficulty concentrating and may fail to discern even obvious relationships between and among concepts. The panic-stricken person suffers even greater cognitive impairment; concentration, learning, and problem solving are virtually impossible during panic episodes.[16]

EFFECTS OF ANXIETY ON VERBAL AND NONVERBAL BEHAVIOR

In mild anxiety, speech content and form reflect heightened sensory awareness and cognitive function. Thoughts are logically verbalized; speech rate and volume are appropriate to content and communication context. The mildly anxious person typically appears alert, confident, and relatively secure.

Verbal behavior of the moderately anxious person is commonly marked by frequent changes of topic, repetitive questioning, joking, and wordiness. *Blocking*, or loss of train of thought, may also occur. Speech rate often accelerates, and speech volume often increases. The moderately anxious person may change body position frequently, use excessive hand gestures, and assume aggressive body postures toward others. Furthermore, because moderately anxious people do not perceive and process sensory input as efficiently as mildly anxious people, they tend to hesitate and procrastinate in meeting routine social and vocational expectations. Such behaviors often present an overall picture of restlessness and discontent that may provoke in others feelings of irritation toward the person.

The severely anxious person displays verbal behavior that indicates highly distorted perceptual and cognitive function. The person may verbalize emotional pain through such assertion as, "I can't stand this" or "I can't think" or by vociferously demanding help and relief. Nonverbal behavior typically involves fine and gross motor tremors, facial grimaces, and other forms of purposeless activity, such as pacing and hand wringing.[16] Severely anxious people present an overall picture of extreme emotional discomfort and behavioral disorganization.

Panic level anxiety results in even greater emotional pain and behavioral disorganization. Verbal and nonverbal behaviors suggest a psychotic-like state in which the panic-stricken person is virtually helpless and cannot negotiate simple life demands. The person may scream and run wildly or may cling tenaciously to something or someone accurately or inaccurately perceived as a source of safety and security. Protective and calming measures must be initiated promptly, because a prolonged panic state is incompatible with life.[16,17]

◆ Anxiety Disorders

The term *anxiety disorder* refers to a psychiatric condition characterized by the emotion of intense terror.[12,19,23] This emotional state is accompanied by thoughts of impending catastrophe and prevails over substantial time periods. People with anxiety disorders rigidly cling to maladaptive perceptual behavioral styles as they futilely attempt to reduce or eliminate their painful state.[3] Failure to achieve the desired relief usually increases the severity of symptoms.

Anxiety disorders include panic, phobic, generalized anxiety, obsessive-compulsive, and stress disorders. Physiological, perceptual, cognitive, and behavioral effects follow a distinct pattern in each of these disorders. Despite these differences, however, these disorders share some common features:

1. The person is distressed by a single symptom or group of symptoms.
2. The person perceives the symptom or symptoms as intensely uncomfortable.
3. Reality testing, the ability to perceive reality accurately, is grossly intact.
4. The disorder endures or recurs without treatment.
5. The disorder cannot be attributed to an organic factor or cause.[12]

A person with an anxiety disorder may receive primary and secondary gains from these symptoms. The *primary gain* is defense against and reduction of the emotional pain associated with anxiety. *Secondary gains* acquired because of symptoms may include relief from responsibility and receiving extra attention or monetary rewards. Receiving primary and secondary gains tends to reinforce symptoms and maladaptive behavioral styles associated with anxiety disorders.[22]

ETIOLOGY

Various possible predisposing factors are connected with the development of anxiety disorders, including hereditary predisposition; persistent neurochemical abnormalities in the brain; physical diseases producing continual fears of death, as in the case of mitral valve prolapse; developmental traumas producing special vulnerabilities; inadequate social or interpersonal experiences necessary for acquiring mature coping mechanisms; counterproductive cognitive patterns in the form of unrealistic goals, values, or belief sets; and exposure to extreme psychological stressors.[3,8,15]

Additional factors that may contribute to the onset of anxiety disorders include chronic physical illness; exposure to stimulants, such as marijuana, cocaine, or amphetamines; use of caffeine and alcohol even in moderation; continuous exposure to a harsh environment; repeated exposure to physical or psychological danger; chronic, insidious exposure to subtle criticism, threats, and disapproval; and specific external stressors impinging on specific emotional vulnerabilities, as in the case of an autonomous person being forced to conform to the strict norms of a rigid, regimented group.[3,10] Any of the preceding factors alone or in combination with others could be the cause of an anxiety disorder.

INCIDENCE AND PREVALENCE

Statistics concerning the incidence and prevalence of anxiety disorders vary considerably.[3] According to Horowitz, 10% to 15% of the general population has experienced what might be classified as an anxiety disorder at some time.[8] Pasnau, on the other hand, estimates the incidence at only 2% to 4% of the population.[15] Other researchers have speculated that 5% of the population currently suffers from an acute or chronic anxiety disorder.[12] A more recent nationwide survey revealed that 12.6% of the U.S. population is affected by an anxiety disorder within a 12-month period.[11]

Based on available information, anxiety disorders affect twice as many women as men. Also, anxiety disorders tend to run in families. No reliable information indicates that the incidence of anxiety disorders has increased significantly.[12]

Application of the Nursing Process to Anxiety Disorders

ASSESSMENT

Phobic Disorder

A *phobia* is a persistent, irrational fear attached to an object or situation that objectively does not pose a significant danger.[3,8] The person experiences a compelling desire to avoid the dreaded object or situation, even though he or she usually recognizes that the fear is unreasonable or excessive in proportion to the actual threat.[15] Unlike panic attacks, phobias are always anticipated and never occur unexpectedly. When phobias occur along with panic attacks, the condition is diagnosed as a panic disorder.[10]

Agoraphobia. *Agoraphobia* is a marked fear of being alone or in a public place from which escape would be difficult or help would be unavailable in the event of suddenly becoming disabled.[1] As such, it is the most severe and pervasive form of phobic disorder.[8] It can begin abruptly after severe stress or can arise for no apparent reason. It can also develop slowly in associa-

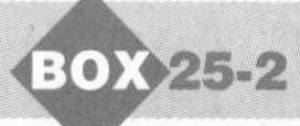

DSM-IV Diagnostic Criteria for Agoraphobia

A. Anxiety about being in places or situations from which escape might be difficult (or embarrassing) or in which help may not be available in the event of having an unexpected or situationally predisposed Panic Attack or panic-like symptoms. Agoraphobic fears typically involve characteristic clusters of situations that include being outside the home alone; being in a crowd or standing in a line; being on a bridge; and traveling in a bus, train, or automobile.
B. The situations are avoided (eg, travel is restricted) or else are endured with marked distress or with anxiety about having a Panic Attack or panic-like symptoms, or require the presence of a companion.
C. The anxiety or phobic avoidance is not better accounted for by another mental disorder, such as Social Phobia (eg, avoidance limited to social situations because of fear of embarrassment), Specific Phobia (eg, avoidance limited to a single situation like elevators), Obsessive-Compulsive Disorder (eg, avoidance of dirt in someone with an obsession about contamination), Posttraumatic Stress Disorder (eg, avoidance of stimuli associated with a severe stressor), or Separation Anxiety Disorder (eg, avoidance of leaving home or relatives).

DSM-IV Diagnostic Criteria for Social Phobia

A. A marked and persistent fear of one or more social or performance situations in which the person is exposed to unfamiliar people or to possible scrutiny by others. The individual fears that he or she will act in a way (or show anxiety symptoms) that will be humiliating or embarrassing. **Note.** In children, there must be evidence of the capacity for age-appropriate social relationships with familiar people and the anxiety must occur in peer settings, not just in interactions with adults.
B. Exposure to the feared social situation almost invariably provokes anxiety, which may take the form of a situationally bound or situationally predisposed Panic Attack. **Note.** In children, the anxiety may be expressed by crying, tantrums, freezing, or shrinking from social situations with unfamiliar people.
C. The person recognizes that the fear is excessive or unreasonable. **Note.** In children, this feature may be absent.
D. The feared social or performance situations are avoided or else are endured with intense anxiety or distress.
E. The avoidance, anxious anticipation, or distress in the feared social or performance situation(s) interferes significantly with the person's normal routine, occupational (academic) functioning, or social activities or relationships, or there is marked distress about having the phobia.
F. In individuals under age 18 years, the duration is at least 6 months.
G. The fear or avoidance is not due to the direct physiological effects of a substance (eg, a drug of abuse, a medication) or a general medical condition and is not better accounted for by another mental disorder (eg, Panic Disorder With or Without Agoraphobia, Separation Anxiety Disorder, Body Dysmorphic Disorder, a Pervasive Developmental Disorder, or Schizoid Personality Disorder).
H. If a general medical condition or another mental disorder is present, the fear in Criterion A is unrelated to it, eg, the fear is not of Stuttering, trembling in Parkinson's disease, or exhibiting abnormal eating behavior in Anorexia Nervosa or Bulimia Nervosa.

tion with chronic severe anxiety. The agoraphobic person usually is excessively dependent on others and may become symptomatic for the first time when faced with the loss of a significant relationship.[5]

Agoraphobia typically is most intense in enclosed spaces, such as stores, restaurants, theaters, airplanes, subways, or other situations involving crowds. The agoraphobic person perceives such situations as dreadfully frightening. Cognitively, the person is preoccupied with avoiding the situation or when in the situation, with finding an escape route or exit.[1] Besides severe anxiety, the agoraphobic person also feels embarrassment and humiliation about being unable to bear a situation that usually is well tolerated or enjoyed by others.[14] Eventually, the limitations imposed by agoraphobia may lead to depression.[15]

Agoraphobia also affects interpersonal behavior. Often the agoraphobic person is conspicuously dependent on a spouse or close family member. This dependency is closely bound with the person's sense of security, especially if he or she must leave home to face the dreaded situation. Eventually, the agoraphobic person may even become housebound and insist on the constant companionship of this significant other.[8] In such a case, normal life activities are greatly constricted for the agoraphobic person and his or her companion.

The level of adaptation achieved by an agoraphobic person usually is seriously impaired unless treatment is received. Prolonged remissions are rare, and spontaneous cures almost never occur. Complications such as substance dependence and major depression are common[8] (Box 25-2, p. 456).

Social Phobia. A *social phobia* represents a persistent irrational fear of and compelling desire to avoid situations in which the person may be exposed to the scru-

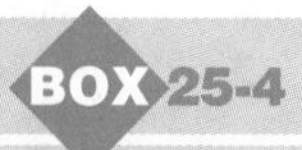

BOX 25-4

DSM-IV Diagnostic Criteria for Specific Phobia

A. Marked and persistent fear that is excessive or unreasonable, cued by the presence or anticipation of a specific object or situation (eg, flying, height, animals, receiving an injection, seeing blood).
B. Exposure to the phobic stimulus almost invariably provokes an immediate anxiety response, which may take the form of a situationally bound or situationally predisposed Panic Attack. **Note:** In children, the anxiety may be expressed by crying, tantrums, freezing, or clinging.
C. The person recognizes that the fear is excessive or unreasonable. **Note:** In children, this feature may be absent.
D. The phobic situation(s) is avoided or else is endured with intense anxiety or distress.
E. The avoidance, anxious anticipation, or distress in the feared situation(s) interferes significantly with the person's normal routine, occupational (or academic) functioning, or social activities or relationships, or there is marked distress about having the phobia.
F. In individuals under age 18 years, the duration is at least 6 months.
G. The anxiety, Panic Attacks, or phobic avoidance associated with the specific object or situation are not better accounted for by another mental disorder, such as Obsessive-Compulsive Disorder (eg, fear of dirt in someone with an obsession about contamination), Posttraumatic Stress Disorder (eg, avoidance of stimuli associated with a severe stressor), Separation Anxiety Disorder (eg, avoidance of school), Social Phobia (eg, avoidance of social situations because of fear of embarrassment), Panic Disorder With Agoraphobia, or Agoraphobia Without History of Panic Disorder.

tiny of others.[1] Additionally, the person harbors the fear of behaving in a manner that may prove humiliating or embarrassing. The person will experience marked anticipatory anxiety if confronted with such a situation and will attempt to avoid it.[15]

Usually symptoms of social phobias occur in personal rather than impersonal situations.[5] In such a situation, the person may perceive others as threatening sources of criticism and the self as small and insignificant in comparison. Thought patterns may become disturbed or blocked, as evidenced by garbled speech or the inability to speak or write. Besides feeling severe anxiety, other symptoms may include shaking, trembling, blushing, vomiting, and vertigo. As these symptoms worsen, the person tends to avoid friendships and other close associations. Consequently, social phobia causes isolation. Examples of social phobias include fear of speaking in public, writing in the presence of others, or using public restrooms.[15]

Adaptation achieved by people with social phobias is severely restricted. This condition is a chronic illness and interferes with normal life routines and occupational and academic pursuits. Although spontaneous remission may occur, treatment with psychotherapy and psychochemotherapy is almost always indicated[8] (Box 25-3, p. 457).

Specific Phobia. A *specific phobia* (also called *simple phobia*) is a persistent, irrational fear of and compelling desire to avoid a circumstance or thing other than those specific to agoraphobia or social phobia.[1,8] Common specific phobias include acrophobia (fear of heights), claustrophobia (fear of closed spaces), blood phobia (fear of the sight of blood or injury), and fear of birds, cats or furry animals, house dust, microbes, snakes, or insects.[8,15]

Exposure to the dreaded circumstance or thing causes anxiety that may reach the panic level. Before probable exposure, a person with specific phobia may behave in a manner similar to people in crisis situations. For example, the person may seek a great deal of information before committing to action, become hypervigilant, or experience disbelief and psychic numbing.[8]

The nature of a person's specific phobia greatly determines the level of adaptation achieved.[1] Impairment may be minimal or almost nonexistent if the dreaded object or circumstance is rare in the environment and can be easily avoided (eg, snakes in a large city). On the other hand, a fear of riding elevators can be disabling in a large city. Usually, an adult who has had a specific phobia since childhood or who has acquired one requires treatment to reach an optimal adaptation level (Box 25-4).

Panic Attack and Panic Disorder

Panic disorder involves recurrent panic attacks that occur unexpectedly.[1,10,15] Although panic attacks are unpredictable in onset, they may occur in a specific situation, such as driving. Attacks do not necessarily occur every time the person confronts the situation, however. Moreover, anxiety attacks may occur in other circumstances as well. This feature is helpful in distinguishing panic attacks from phobias.

Panic attacks typically are characterized by a sudden onset of tense apprehension or terror and are often associated with feelings of doom.[8] The clinical picture closely approximates the alarm reaction described in Selye's general adaptation syndrome, involving psychological and physiological overresponse to stressors. For example, the person experiencing a panic attack incorrectly perceives his or her circumstances as life-threatening; therefore, he or she experiences such physiological reactions as dyspnea, chest pain, palpitations, choking or smothering sensations, dizziness, vertigo, paresthesias, hot and cold flashes, sweating, and fainting. The person may also report feelings of depersonalization, derealization, and fears of dying, going crazy, or behaving in an uncontrolled manner.[15] Attacks typically last for several minutes and reach a peak within 10 minutes.[8,10]

During panic attacks, the person may make extreme efforts to escape from what is perceived to be causing the panic. Consequently, social and work relations may be disrupted by the apparently strange behavior.[8] Between panic attacks, the person often remains moderately to severely anxious in anticipation of the next panic attack.[10,15] Thus, the level of adaptation may be seriously thwarted unless treatment is sought (Box 25-5).

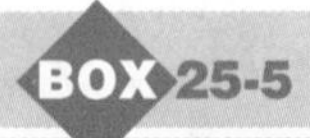

DSM-IV Diagnostic Criteria for Panic Attack

A discrete period of intense fear or discomfort, in which four (or more) of the following symptoms developed abruptly and reached a peak within 10 minutes:

1. palpitations, pounding heart, or accelerated heart rate
2. sweating
3. trembling or shaking
4. sensations of shortness of breath or smothering
5. feeling of choking
6. chest pain or discomfort
7. nausea or abdominal distress
8. feeling dizzy, unsteady, lightheaded, or faint
9. derealization (feelings of unreality) or depersonalization (being detached from oneself)
10. fear of losing control or going crazy
11. fear of dying
12. paresthesias (numbness or tingling sensations)
13. chills or hot flushes

Generalized Anxiety Disorder

Generalized anxiety disorder is usually characterized by chronic anxiety that is uncomfortable to the point of interfering with daily life.[1] Seldom do people suffering from this disorder experience eruptions of acute anxiety.[12] Rather, they persistently exhibit signs of severe anxiety, such as motor tension, autonomic hyperactivity, and apprehensive expectation.[15] Some people may also exhibit chronic hypervigilance for potential threats. Displays of impatience and irritability and complaints of feeling on edge are common.[8]

Due to this tense hyperarousal, the person may be unable to concentrate, suffer chronic fatigue, and experience sleep pattern disturbances. Additionally, he or she may exhibit tenseness and distractibility in social situations. For these reasons, this disorder eventually may lead to depression.[8] Because of these symptoms, a person with generalized anxiety disorder usually seeks treatment to improve his or her adaptation level (Box 25-6).

Obsessive-Compulsive Disorder

In *obsessive-compulsive disorder,* the person experiences recurrent obsessions or compulsions.[15] The term *obsession* as used in this diagnosis refers to recurrent, intrusive, persistent ideas, thoughts, images, or impulses. The person with this disorder does not voluntarily produce obsessions but feels invaded by the obsessive thoughts and often finds them repugnant or meaningless. Despite efforts to ignore or dismiss them, the person remains preoccupied with unbidden ideations.[8,15]

Compulsions, on the other hand, are ritualistic behaviors that the person feels compelled to perform either in accord with a specific set of rules or in a routinized manner. The ritual is designed to prevent or reduce anxiety associated with some future event the person wants to prevent or produce.[15] At the same time, the person invests the compulsive act with symbolic significance by unrealistically believing that the act magi-

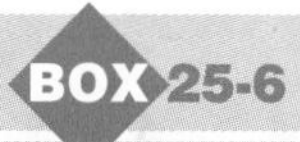

DSM-IV Diagnostic Criteria for Generalized Anxiety Disorder

A. Excessive anxiety and worry, (apprehensive expectation), occurring more days than not for at least 6 months, about a number of events or activities (such as work or school performance).
B. The person finds it difficult to control the worry.
C. The anxiety and worry are associated with three (or more) of the following six symptoms (with at least some symptoms present for more days than not for the past 6 months). **Note.** Only one item is required in children.
   1. restlessness or feeling keyed up or on edge
   2. being easily fatigued
   3. difficulty concentrating or mind going blank
   4. irritability
   5. muscle tension
   6. sleep disturbance (difficulty falling or staying asleep, or restless unsatisfying sleep)
D. The anxiety, worry, or physical symptoms cause clinically significant distress or impairment in social, occupational, or other important areas of functioning.
E. The disturbance is not due to the direct physiological effects of a substance (eg, a drug of abuse, a medication) or a general medical condition (eg, hyperthyroidism) and does not occur exclusively during a Mood Disorder, a Psychotic Disorder, or a Pervasive Developmental Disorder.

cally solves problems or atones for past misdeeds.[8] If the affected person or others intervene to stop the compulsive act, anxiety results[8,13,15] (Box 25-7).

At one time, there was speculation that this anxiety disorder was closely related to obsessive-compulsive personality disorder. More recent evidence, however, suggests there is no real relationship between the two. To illustrate, the person with obsessive-compulsive personality disorder does not experience symptoms of this disorder as uncomfortable, distressful, or bothersome. Moreover, people with obsessive-compulsive personality disorder do not have actual obsessions or compulsions. People with the anxiety disorder of obsessive-compulsive disorder, however, experience their symptoms as alien to themselves and threateningly intrusive.[10]

Symptoms of obsessive-compulsive disorder may be mild to severe. Whatever the degree of severity, symptoms that interfere with occupational pursuits and quality of life usually lead the affected person to seek help. If treatment is not sought or is unsuccessful, the person may become so uncomfortable that he or she becomes depressed and often suicidal.[5] Because of these factors, the adaptation level achieved by obsessive-compulsive people varies (Nursing Care Plan 25-1, p. 462).

Posttraumatic Stress Disorder

Posttraumatic stress disorder is defined as the development of characteristic symptoms after exposure to a severe or extraordinary stressor.[1,10] Unlike other psychiatric conditions, which are causally linked to an individual's psychosocial and biological makeup, posttraumatic stress disorder occurs only in response to a traumatic life experience.[13]

Traumatic events capable of causing posttraumatic stress disorder include natural disasters, accidental human-made disasters, and intentional human-made disasters (Box 25-8, p. 463).[9] With all these stressors, there must be actual or threatened death or serious injury or maiming to the self or others. Additionally, these stressors must be capable of producing intense fear, helplessness, or horror in people exposed to them.

Characteristic symptoms of posttraumatic stress disorder include the following (see Box 25-9, p. 464):

1. Psychic numbing and denial
2. Reexperiencing the traumatic event through intrusive recollections, dreams, or suddenly feeling and acting as if the event is recurring[15]
3. Perceptual distortions, including illusions, intrusive

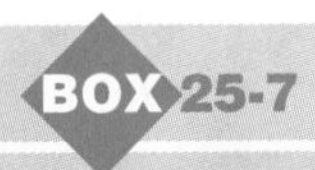

DSM-IV Diagnostic Criteria for Obsessive-Compulsive Disorder

A. Either obsessions or compulsions:
Obsessions as defined by (1), (2), (3), and (4):
1. recurrent and persistent thoughts, impulses, or images that are experienced, at some time during the disturbance, as intrusive and inappropriate and that cause marked anxiety or distress
2. the thoughts, impulses, or images are not simply excessive worries about real-life problems
3. the person attempts to ignore or suppress such thoughts, impulses, or images, or to neutralize them with some other thought or action
4. the person recognizes that the obsessed thoughts, impulses, or images are a product of his or her own mind (not imposed from without as in thought insertion)

Compulsions as defined by (1) and (2):
1. repetitive behaviors (eg, hand washing, ordering, checking) or mental acts (eg, praying, counting, repeating words silently) that the person feels driven to perform in response to an obsession, or according to rules that must be applied rigidly
2. the behaviors or mental acts are aimed at preventing or reducing distress or preventing some dreaded event or situation; however, these behaviors or mental acts either are not connected in a realistic way with what they are designed to neutralize or prevent or are clearly excessive

B. At some point during the course of the disorder, the person has recognized that the obsessions or compulsions are excessive or unreasonable. **Note:** This does not apply to children.

C. The obsessions or compulsions cause marked distress, are time consuming (take more than 1 hour a day), or significantly interfere with the person's normal routine, occupational (or academic) functioning, or usual social activities or relationships.

D. If another Axis I disorder is present, the content of the obsessions or compulsions is not restricted to it (eg, preoccupation with food in the presence of an Eating Disorder; hair pulling in the presence of Trichotillomania; concern with appearance in the presence of Body Dysmorphic Disorder; preoccupation with drugs in the presence of a Substance Use Disorder; preoccupation with having a serious illness in the presence of Hypochondriasis; preoccupation with sexual urges or fantasies in the presence of a Paraphilia; or guilty ruminations in the presence of Major Depressive Disorder).

E. The disturbance is not due to the direct physiological effects of a substance (eg, a drug of abuse, a medication) or a general medical condition.

images, pseudohallucinations, and actual hallucinations[9,10]

4. Feelings of being pressured, confused, or disorganized when thinking about the event
5. Memory impairment, especially with regard to aspects of the trauma
6. Overgeneralization of other sensory inputs so that they seem related in some way to the event
7. Hypervigilance and exaggerated startle reactions
8. Somatic symptoms, such as fatigue, headache, and muscular pain
9. Alterations in activity pattern, including compulsively repeating actions associated with the event, frantic overactivity, withdrawal, and indecision about how to respond to the consequences of the event

Nursing Care Plan 25-1

The Client With Obsessive-Compulsive Disorder

Situation: A client is diagnosed with obsessive-compulsive disorder. The client engages in ritualistic handwashing every 15 minutes while awake. At night, the client insists on sleeping in latex gloves to prevent contamination of her hands. This compulsive behavior interferes with the client's other activities of daily living.

Nursing Diagnosis

Ineffective Individual Coping related to preoccupation with repetitive, ritualistic behavior, which interferes with activities of daily living.

Outcome

Client will decrease performance of ritual to 1 to 2 times per hour after 3 days of treatment and complete activities of daily living.

Intervention	Rationale
Assess client for attending to stimuli that distract from performance of the ritual.	Distraction can be useful to gradually extinguish ritualistic behavior.
Assess the client's anxiety level when exposed to the distracting stimulus; if the anxiety level does not increase, present the distracting stimulus at gradually shorter time intervals until the ritualistic behavior is extinguished. Negotiate with the client a schedule for performing the ritual that allows time for performing self-care activities.	Negotation surrounding the ritual interjects the idea that behavioral paterns can be more flexible and that change does not have to be overwhelmingly threatening.
Do not overtly stop the client's performance of the ritual.	Stopping the ritual without offering an alternate behavior can produce a state of 4+ anxiety and possible depression.

Evaluation

Client's performance of ritual decreases and completion of self-care activities increases.

10. Alterations in social role due to loss of a reality-based relatedness with the ongoing world
11. Paranormal experiences, such as déjà vu, precognition, telepathic dreams, transpersonal experiences, and other altered states of consciousness[1,9]

A latency period of hours, weeks, months, or even years may separate exposure to the traumatic stressor and the onset of symptoms. When symptoms appear within less than 4 weeks of exposure to the trauma, a variation of posttraumatic stress disorder, called *acute stress disorder,* can be diagnosed (Box 25-10, p. 465). This form of posttraumatic stress disorder usually lasts less than 3 months. When symptoms appear within 6 months of the trauma, the chronic form of posttraumatic stress disorder exists. If symptoms begin more than 6 months after the traumatic event, the condition is called a delayed posttraumatic stress disorder.[1] Of the three subtypes of posttraumatic stress disorder, delayed posttraumatic stress disorder is thought to have the worst prognosis.[10]

In any of the three subtypes of posttraumatic stress disorder, the person's adaptation level can be positively or adversely affected. With effective treatment, people with this disorder may recover and gain increased psychological resilience and coping capacity. In other cases, however, the disorder may increase vulnerability to development of other anxiety disorders, substance abuse and dependence, and depression.[9] Prompt, effective treatment seems crucial to helping the person attain an optimal adaptation level (see Nursing Care Plan 25-2, p. 466 and Case Study 25-1, p. 467).

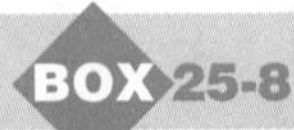

Traumatic Events Capable of Producing Posttraumatic Stress Disorder

Natural Disasters

Earthquakes
Floods
Hurricanes
Tornadoes
Volcanic eruptions

Accidental Human-Made Disasters

Nuclear plant accidents
Auto crashes
Industrial accidents
Airplane crashes
Train derailments

Intentional Human-Made Disasters

Military combat
Rape
Muggings
Armed robbery
Assault
Stalking
Hazing
Abuse of all kinds—verbal, physical, sexual, emotional

NURSING DIAGNOSIS

Formulating nursing diagnoses for clients manifesting symptoms of anxiety disorders is a challenging nursing responsibility. Some of the many nursing diagnoses that may apply to a client with an anxiety disorder include the following:

1. Sensory/Perceptual Alterations related to severe anxiety
2. Altered Thought Processes related to severe anxiety
3. Altered Thought Processes related to decisional conflict
4. Ineffective Breathing Pattern related to hyperventilation associated with severe anxiety
5. Impaired Memory related to preoccupation with repetitive, ritualistic activity
6. Diversional Activity Deficit related to preoccupation with repetitive, ritualistic activity
7. Self Care Deficit related to preoccupation with repetitive, ritualistic activity
8. Altered Thought Processes related to repetitive, intrusive thoughts
9. Fear of being alone related to feelings of impending harm
10. Anticipatory Anxiety of severe proportion related to preparing for excursion outside home
11. Ineffective Individual Coping related to chronic moderate anxiety
12. Ineffective Individual Coping related to extreme fear of being observed by others
13. Impaired Verbal Communication related to severe anxiety
14. Impaired Social Interaction related to psychic numbing
15. Altered Thought Processes related to reexperiencing a traumatic event

PLANNING

Despite the differences among the anxiety disorders, the major goals for nursing care apply to all of them. Concerned primarily with the client learning about anxiety and how to cope with it, the goals are as follows:

1. Accept the experience of anxiety as natural and inevitable
2. Increase self-awareness with regard to fluctuations in anxiety level
3. Reduce shame about exhibiting signs of anxiety
4. Learn and apply self-help techniques designed to reduce anxiety
5. Learn how to remain calm in anxiety-producing situations
6. Increase problem-solving and coping skills

Clients who meet these goals develop not only an increased tolerance of anxiety, but also an increased awareness of their strengths and limitations.

INTERVENTION

To help the client accomplish the preceding goals, the nurse needs to establish a supportive therapeutic relationship. This relationship is characterized by trust, empathy, respect, and calmness on the part of the nurse. Displaying these attributes to the client consistently will lay the groundwork for successful therapy.

Clarifying the Issues

To defuse the client's emotionally charged state, the nurse needs to remain calm because anxiety is transmitted easily through interpersonal contact.[20] Because the perceptual and cognitive processes of a client may be disturbed due to high anxiety levels, nurses should position themselves centrally in the client's visual field

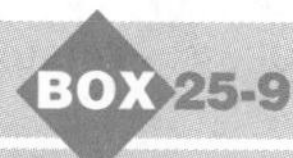

DSM-IV Diagnostic Criteria for Posttraumatic Stress Disorder

A. The person has been exposed to a traumatic event in which both of the following were present:
   1. the person experienced, witnessed, or was confronted with an event or events that involved actual or threatened death or serious injury, or a threat to the physical integrity of self or others
   2. the person's response involved intense fear, helplessness, or horror. **Note:** In children, this may be expressed instead by disorganized or agitated behavior

B. The traumatic event is persistently reexperienced in one (or more) of the following ways:
   1. recurrent and intrusive distressing recollections of the event, including images, thoughts, or perceptions. **Note:** In young children, repetitive play may occur in which themes or aspects of the trauma are expressed.
   2. recurrent distressing dreams of the event. **Note:** In children, there may be frightening dreams without recognizable content.
   3. acting or feeling as if the traumatic event were recurring (includes a sense of reliving the experience, illusions, hallucinations, and dissociative flashback episodes, including those that occur on awakening or when intoxicated). **Note:** In young children, trauma-specific reenactment may occur.
   4. intense psychological distress at exposure to internal or external cues that symbolize or resemble an aspect of the traumatic event
   5. physiological reactivity on exposure to internal or external cues that symbolize or resemble an aspect of the traumatic event

C. Persistent avoidance of stimuli associated with the trauma and numbing of general responsiveness, (not present before the trauma), as indicated by three (or more) of the following:
   1. efforts to avoid thoughts, feelings, or conversations associated with the trauma
   2. efforts to avoid activities, places, or people that arouse recollections of the trauma
   3. inability to recall an important aspect of the trauma
   4. markedly diminished interest or participation in significant activities
   5. feeling of detachment or estrangement from others
   6. restricted range of affect (eg, unable to have loving feelings)
   7. sense of a foreshortened future (eg, does not expect to have a career, marriage, children, or a normal life span)

D. Persistent symptoms of increased arousal, (not present before the trauma), as indicated by two (or more) of the following:
   1. difficulty falling or staying asleep
   2. irritability or outbursts of anger
   3. difficulty concentrating
   4. hypervigilance
   5. exaggerated startle response

E. Duration of the disturbance (symptoms in Criteria B, C, and D) is more than 1 month.

F. The disturbance causes clinically significant distress or impairment of social, occupational, or other important areas of functioning.

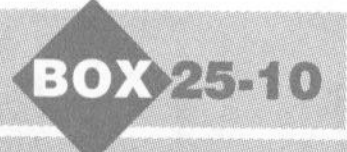

DSM-IV Diagnostic Criteria for Acute Stress Disorder

A. The person has been exposed to a traumatic event in which both of the following were present:
   1. the person experienced, witnessed, or was confronted with an event or events that involved actual or threatened death or serious injury, or a threat to the physical integrity of self or others
   2. the person's response involved intense fear, helplessness, or horror

B. Either while experiencing or after experiencing the distressing event, the individual has three (or more) of the following dissociative symptoms:
   1. a subjective sense of numbing, detachment, or absence of emotional responsiveness
   2. a reduction in awareness of his or her surroundings (eg, "being in a daze")
   3. derealization
   4. depersonalization
   5. dissociative amnesia (ie, inability to recall an important aspect of the trauma)

C. The traumatic event is persistently reexperienced in at least one of the following ways: recurrent images, thoughts, dreams, illusions, flashback episodes, or a sense of reliving the experience; or distress on exposure to reminders of the traumatic event.

D. Marked avoidance of stimuli that arouse recollections of the trauma (eg, thoughts, feelings, conversations, activities, places, people).

E. Marked symptoms of anxiety or increased arousal (eg, difficulty sleeping, irritability, poor concentration, hypervigilance, exaggerated startle response, motor restlessness).

F. The disturbance causes clinically significant distress or impairment in social, occupational, or other important areas of functioning or impairs the individual's ability to pursue some necessary task, such as obtaining necessary assistance or mobilizing personal resources by telling family members about the traumatic experience.

G. The disturbance lasts for a minimum of 2 days and a maximum of 4 weeks and occurs within 4 weeks of the traumatic event.

and speak clearly using a low voice volume and tone. Doing so will help the client perceive accurately what the nurse is saying. For the same reason, the nurse needs to ask short, simple questions to aid the client's articulation of the specific issues associated with the symptoms of anxiety. Once the issues surrounding the anxious state are revealed and clarified, the nurse can begin intervening to help the client understand the connections between identified issues and the experience of anxiety.

For example, a client came to the emergency room exhibiting near panic level anxiety and complaining of being terrified of driving. Shortly after her admission to the mental health unit, she revealed that her adult son had moved back home about 2 months ago with his wife and infant, creating upheaval in her household. She confided that she would like to "run away from home." Because the client had become terrified of driving, she had few choices except to stay in her home or seek refuge in the hospital. After assisting the client to clarify the issues associated with the onset of her anxious state, the nurse was able to help her learn how to cope and problem solve more effectively.

Accepting the Inevitability of Anxiety

The nurse needs to explain the concept of anxiety to the client in simple terms and emphasize that all people feel anxious from time to time. Doing so can reduce the client's anxiety about being anxious by "normalizing" this experience to some degree.[3] Also, this intervention may help assuage the shame that the client may feel about losing control of his or her emotions.

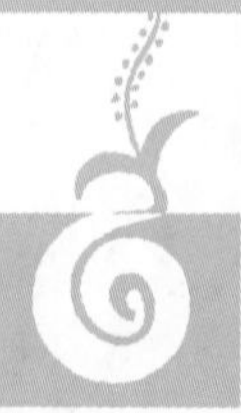

Nursing Care Plan 25-2

The Client With Posttraumatic Stress Disorder

Situation: The client reports being assaulted by his coworker and supervisor 12 hours before reporting to the emergency room. The client reports that this assault was preceded by verbal abuse in the form of threats, hazing, and ridicule for many weeks. The client is severely anxious and expresses the fear of going crazy due to experiencing intrusive thoughts.

Nursing Diagnosis

Posttrauma response related to severe anxiety secondary to reexperiencing traumatic event by way of unbidden images, terror, and pseudohallucinations

Outcome

Client will verbalize decreased anxiety and decreased experiences of intrusive images.

Intervention	Rationale
Reassure the client that these experiences are common occurrences after a traumatic event and are not serious portents of psychosis (ie, "going crazy").	This intervention reduces anxiety by presenting factual information while meeting the client's emotional needs for understanding and validation.
Stay with the client until these experiences subside; offer reassurance and empathy as needed.	Presencing, reassurance, and empathy support the client through these experiences.

Evaluation

Client reports decreased anxiety and less frequent experiences of intrusive images.

Increasing Self-Awareness

In the preceding example, the client may have viewed the change in her household situation as merely coincidental with the development of panic episodes associated with driving. To assist the client to recognize the highly probable connection between the two events, the nurse should engage the client in self-awareness activities, such as the following:

1. Ask clients to maintain a diary in which they record when they feel anxious, what they are doing at the time, what they are thinking, and who is with them. This may help clients begin to recognize what triggers their anxiety.
2. Ask clients to maintain a graph, with anxiety levels on one axis and the time measured in 30-minute intervals on the other axis (Fig. 25-1) for a 24-hour period. This activity in combination with keeping a diary may assist clients to develop awareness of when and under what circumstances their anxiety is mild, moderate, severe, or of panic proportions. Discussing and analyzing the findings with clients is crucial in this process.[2]
3. Ask clients to participate in a family conference in which family members or significant others enter the conference group one at a time. As each person enters the room, ask the client to rate his or her anxiety level and to record the findings on a small piece of paper. The results can be discussed in the family conference and in subsequent individual interactions with the client. The client and family need careful preparation for this exercise. The purpose must be explained as helping the client and family to identify how they affect each other. Additionally, the client and family need to know that this exercise is to help all involved become more responsible for their own feelings and behavior and not to blame each other.

Learning Self-Help Skills

Once the client has identified the factors associated with uncomfortable symptoms of anxiety, the nurse needs to help the client identify ways of reducing anxiety to a tolerable level. In the situation previously mentioned, the client connected the onset of her symptoms with the upheaval created by her adult son and his family moving into her home. Additionally,

Case Study

Caring for the Client With Posttraumatic Stress Disorder

Ms. S was brought to the hospital emergency room by a friend. Ms. S was in a stunned, dazed state; had difficulty attending to questions or statements addressed to her; and was disoriented to time and place. She was, however, oriented to her own identity and that of her friend. Ms. S also seemed unable to appreciate the significance of her having been brought to the emergency room for examination and possible treatment. Her general appearance was within normal limits; she appeared well nourished, neat, clean, and appropriately dressed.

Her friend reported that Ms. S answered her door reluctantly when she made an impromptu visit earlier and that when she was finally allowed to enter, Ms. S's home was in disarray. The friend further reported that she realized Ms. S's home had been forcibly entered. She called the police for assistance. Blood-stained clothes were discovered in Ms. S's bathroom by the police, and the friend expressed the fear that Ms. S had been raped.

When a male physician approached Ms. S in the examination room, she displayed an exaggerated startle response and muscular stiffening. Additionally, Ms. S recoiled and began to mumble nonsensical statements as she struggled to distance herself from the male physician.

A nurse clinical specialist with expertise in rape crisis counseling was then called to help Ms. S. The nurse was able to defuse Ms. S's extreme state of anxiety by acknowledging that she must have been terribly hurt by someone and that it was normal to be upset about being hurt. As Ms. S began to attend to the nurse, she was able to admit finally that a man had hurt her. Gently, the nurse asked her if she had been raped. Although Ms. S cried out loudly and at first was incoherent, she eventually acknowledged that she had been raped. After crying and vividly recounting details of the incident and her attempt to make herself forget by taking several baths, Ms. S was able to undergo the necessary examination and procedures needed by rape victims.

Ms. S was discharged from the emergency room and referred to the local mental health center for intensive rape crisis counseling. For 6 months, Ms. S received individual and group therapy. The primary focus of the treatment was aimed at helping her view herself as an effective survivor rather than a helpless victim.

Within 6 months, Ms. S was completely recovered. She was able to serve as an effective witness in the identification and prosecution of the perpetrator of the crime committed against her.

she was able to articulate her anger about her son's refusal to contribute money to pay for household expenses and his inattention to his wife and child. The client's anger was frightening and unacceptable to her, because it meant that she had failed in her role as the "good mother." Rather than express her anger directly to her son, she repressed and suppressed her feelings. When these defense mechanisms failed to shore in her emotions, they appeared in the form of severe to panic level anxiety. Because the client unconsciously wanted to escape from her anxiety-producing situation yet simultaneously realized that she could not do so because of fear of appearing irresponsible, she began to experience anxiety attacks, especially when she attempted to drive.

To assist the client to express her feelings openly and honestly without losing control, the nurse encouraged the client to learn assertiveness skills. The client attended an assertiveness training class daily for 5 days, and in role-play exercise with other clients, she practiced expressing her feelings (positive and negative) to her son and practiced making behavior change requests to her son. At the end of the 5 days, the client was able to use assertiveness skills effectively with her son and other family members in a family therapy session led by the nurse.

Although the client had gained a great deal of knowledge and insight into her condition and had become more assertive with her family and associates, she still expressed doubt about her ability to drive without becoming overly anxious. To help prepare the client for resuming this activity, the nurse taught her how to use positive coping statements to allay her self-doubt and anxiety about driving. The nurse asked the client to compose reassuring statements that she could say aloud or silently to herself whenever she felt anxiety or self-doubt about driving. The client was then asked to repeat these statements continuously until she experienced relief.

The nurse then asked the client to sit, close her eyes, and imagine herself in her car; she then imagined herself driving, feeling alert and calm, and being successful and

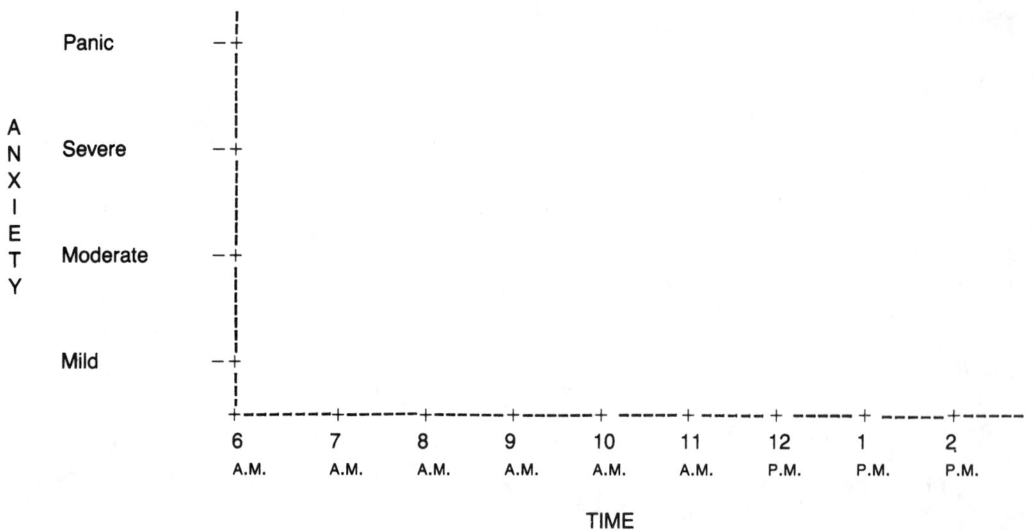

Figure 25-1. Graph of anxiety levels.

in control. The client was asked to repeat this exercise, known as *covert rehearsal,* at least three times each day.

Relaxation therapy was also used to assist the client in learning how to control her anxiety. The client learned to use progressive muscular relaxation and deep breathing exercises to decrease anxiety. Using this form of therapy through audiotape instruction each morning and evening helped the client to control her anxiety.

The nurse also suggested that the client read self-help books and pamphlets written by individuals who had successfully overcome anxiety disorders similar to hers, a form of treatment known as *bibliotherapy.*[6,7] Additionally, the client attended a self-help group, Emotions Anonymous, daily. Through these experiences, the client developed an understanding of herself and her anxiety disorder and eventually accepted her tendency to feel anxious occasionally.

Increasing Problem-Solving and Coping Skills

Besides learning self-help skills, clients with an anxiety disorder can also benefit from individual and group psychotherapy designed to help identify emotions and automatic behaviors used to relieve uncomfortable feelings. When clients are able to identify their emotions and behaviors, they can engage in problem solving with regard to the following:

1. The extent to which their appraisal of stressors as dangerous is correct

Table 25-1

Common Antianxiety Medications

Generic Name	Brand Name	Usual Adult Dosage Range for Anxiety Disorder (mg/d)
Diazepam	Valium	4–40
Clorazepate	Tranxene	7.5–60
Lorazepam	Ativan	1.5–6
Alprazolam	Xanax	0.5–6
Buspirone	BuSpar	10–40

(Reference: Preston J, O'Neal J, Talaga M: Handbook of Clinical Psychopharmacology for Therapists. Oakland, CA, New Harbinger Publications, 1994)

2. Whether their emotional responses exceed the degree of anxiety expected in view of the actual danger posed by stressors
3. The effectiveness and appropriateness of the relief behavior
4. Alternative ways of perceiving and appraising stressors
5. Alternative coping mechanisms for allaying and discharging anxious feelings

Having completed this, clients can test alternative coping mechanisms in therapy to enhance their ability to generalize them to life situations.

Administering Antianxiety Agents

Ideally, antianxiety agents are prescribed for a client during the initial phase of treatment. Because many people with anxiety disorders are at risk for substance abuse or dependence, antianxiety agents that have addictive properties are administered sparingly and on a short-term basis. Antidepressant medications with little or no addictive properties have been useful in treating anxiety disorders and can be prescribed on a longer term basis without fear of the client becoming addicted. Whether antianxiety or other drugs are prescribed for anxiety disorders, these drugs do not cure anxiety disorders. Rather, these agents calm clients sufficiently to enable them to engage in and benefit from therapies that may be beneficial, if not curative in some cases (Tables 25-1 and 25-2).[18]

More recently, *biofeedback* has been used to teach clients to self-regulate their reactions to stressful events or processes. This technique involves the client learning to remain relaxed to prevent the hyperarousal physiological state produced by anxiety.[21] Additionally, psychiatric-mental health nurse clinical specialists with training in administering biofeedback can use this technique in combination with family systems psychotherapy to effect dramatic relief for individuals with anxiety disorders.

EVALUATION

Evaluating whether nursing care for a client with an anxiety disorder is effective is based on the client's report of his or her feeling state and observed changes in behavior. Behavior changes indicating improvement—such as decreased muscular tension and tremors, increased appetite, normal physiological indices, and increased attention span and concentration—may be the first signs of improvement. The reduction of cardinal symptoms associated with anxiety disorders and their replacement with adaptive behaviors also signifies improvement, as does the development of increased self-awareness and ability to cope with anxiety-producing situations, as evidenced by self-disclosures and behavioral patterns. More importantly, the client's acceptance of anxiety as an inevitable part of human existence and commitment to live life effectively in spite of this represent major advances toward recovery of adaptive mental health.

◆ Chapter Summary

This chapter has provided an overview of anxiety as a natural part of human existence. It has discussed the more severe levels of anxiety that persist, cannot be dismissed, and interfere with the person's life—the anxiety disorders. Specifically, this chapter has made the following points:

1. Anxiety is a clinical feature of almost every psychiatric syndrome.
2. Anxiety occurs as the initial response to psychic stressors and is ascertained through the client's self-report, such as feelings of dread, apprehension, restlessness, and jitteriness, and through physiological signs, such as increased heart rate and blood pressure, excessive perspiration, sexual dysfunction, and increased rate and depth of respiration.

Table 25-2

Antidepressant Medications Useful in Treating Obsessive-Compulsive Disorder and Other Anxiety Disorders

Generic Name	Brand Name	Usual Adult Dosage Range for Anxiety Disorder (mg/d)
Clomipramine	Anafranil	200–300
Fluoxetine	Prozac	20–80
Sertraline	Zoloft	50–200
Paroxetine	Paxil	20–50

(Reference: Preston J, O'Neal J, Talaga M: Handbook of Clinical Psychopharmacology for Therapists. Oakland, CA, New Harbinger Publications, 1994)

3. Levels of anxiety range from mild to moderate, severe, and panic.
4. An anxiety disorder is a psychiatric condition characterized by intense terror and thoughts of impending catastrophe persisting for some time.
5. Phobic disorders commonly seen in clinical practice include agoraphobia, social phobia, and specific phobia.
6. A panic disorder is an anxiety disorder characterized by recurrent anxiety attacks of panic proportions that occur unpredictably.
7. Generalized anxiety disorder is characterized by chronic anxiety that is so uncomfortable that it interfere with daily life.
8. A person with obsessive-compulsive disorder experiences recurrent obsessions (persistent thoughts, images, or impulses) and compulsions (ritualistic behaviors performed in a routinized manner).
9. Posttraumatic stress disorder is the development of certain characteristic symptoms after exposure to a severe, extraordinary, traumatic life experience.
10. Planning and implementing nursing care for a client with an anxiety disorder center on helping the client accept anxiety as natural and inevitable, increase self-awareness of variations in anxiety levels, reduce shame about exhibiting signs of anxiety, learn and apply self-help techniques to reduce anxiety, and improve problem-solving and coping skills.

Review Questions

1. Which of the following statistics accurately reflects the percentage of U.S. citizens affected by acute or chronic anxiety disorders within a given 12-month period?
   - **A.** 25.5%
   - **B.** 5.5%
   - **C.** 18.6%
   - **D.** 12.6%
2. Which of the following phrases most accurately defines the term phobia?
   - **A.** A persistent, irrational fear of an objectively nonthreatening object or situation
   - **B.** Repetitive, persistent, intrusive ideas, thoughts, images, or impulses
   - **C.** A specified set of rules governing the performance of ritual-like behaviors
   - **D.** A tendency to exhibit an exaggerated startle response even in nonthreatening situations
3. An individual experiences chronic anxiety that is uncomfortable and intense, along with tension and somatic manifestations. This person eventually seeks treatment. Which of the following diagnoses is most likely applied to this individual?
   - **A.** Panic attack
   - **B.** Panic disorder
   - **C.** Generalized anxiety

◆ References

1. American Psychiatric Association: Diagnostic and Statistical Manual of Mental Disorders, 4th ed. Washington, DC, American Psychiatric Association, 1994
2. Andreason N: Posttraumatic Stress Disorder. In Kaplan H, Saddock B (eds): Comprehensive Textbook of Psychiatry, 7th ed. Baltimore, Williams & Wilkins, 1994
3. Beck A, Emery G, Greensburg R: Anxiety Disorders and Phobias. New York, Basic Books, 1986
4. Gordon M: Manual of Nursing Diagnosis. New York, McGraw-Hill, 1985
5. Gray M: Neurosis. New York, Von Nostrand Reinhold, 1978
6. Green M: Living Fear Free. New York, Warner Books, 1985
7. Handley R, Neff P: Anxiety and Panic Attacks. New York, Fawcett Crest, 1985
8. Horowitz M: In Goldman H (ed): Review of General Psychiatry, pp 362–375. Los Altos, CA, Lange Medical, 1984
9. Horowitz M: A Review of Posttraumatic and Adjustment Disorders. Hosp Community Psychiatry (March): 241–249, 1986
10. Maxmen J, Ward N: Essential Psychopathology and Its Treatment, 2d ed, Revised for DSM-IV. New York, WW Norton, 1995
11. Narrow W, Regier D, Rae D, Marderscheid R, Locke B: Use of Services by Persons with Mental and Addictive Disorders. Archives of General Psychiatry 50 (2): 95–107, 1993
12. Nemiah J: Neurotic Disorders. In Kaplan H, Saddock B (eds): Comprehensive Textbook of Psychiatry, 7th ed. Baltimore, Williams & Wilkins, 1994
13. Nemiah J: Obsessive-Compulsive Disorders. In Kaplan H, Saddock B (eds): Comprehensive Textbook of Psychiatry, 7th ed. Baltimore, Williams & Wilkins, 1994
14. Nemiah J: Phobic Disorders. In Kaplan H, Saddock B (eds): Comprehensive Textbook of Psychiatry, 7th ed. Baltimore, Williams & Wilkins, 1994
15. Pasnau R: Diagnosis and Treatment of Anxiety Disorders. Washington, DC, American Psychiatric Press, 1984
16. Peplau H: A Working Definition of Anxiety. In Burd S, Marshall M (eds): Some Clinical Approaches to Psychiatric Nursing. New York, Macmillan, 1963
17. Peplau H: Interpersonal Relations in Nursing. New York, GP Putnam's Sons, 1952
18. Roy-Byrne P, Katon W: An update on Treatment of the Anxiety Disorders. Hosp Community Psychiatry (August): 835–843, 1987
19. Reusch J: Disturbed Communication. New York, WW Norton, 1972
20. Reusch J: Therapeutic Communication. New York, WW Norton, 1973
21. Rosenbaum L: Biofeedback Frontiers. New York, AMS Press, 1989
22. Smith S, Karasik D, Meyer B: Review of Psychiatric and Psychosocial Nursing. Los Altos, CA, National Nursing Review, 1984
23. Stern V, Stern E: Keeping Faith With the Terrorized Patient: A Dialogue. The Psychotherapy Patient 1 (4): 3–10, 1985

Somatoform Disorders

Suzanne Doscher

26

We are not ourselves
When nature, being oppress'd,
Commands the mind
To suffer with the body

Shakespeare,
King Lear, *Act II, Scene 4*

Early beliefs that humans are composed of a dichotomous mind and body have given way to a view of the human being as a system composed of interrelated parts. This chapter focuses on the interrelated parts, or systems—psychological, biological, and familial—that affect a person's unintentional *choice to communicate physical symptoms that suggest a general medical disorder but have no discernible biological basis. The individual experiences distress in social, interpersonal, occupational, or other areas of functioning, but physical pathology does not reveal evidence of bodily impairment.*

The overview of somatoform disorders relates the incidence, possible causes, and examples of responses that are somatoform in nature. Later sections address application of the nursing process to clients experiencing medically unexplained physical symptoms that are related to psychological distress.

Learning Objectives

On completion of this chapter, you should be able to accomplish the following:

1. *Define the term somatoform disorder.*
2. *Describe characteristic features of specific somatoform disorders.*
3. *Differentiate between somatoform disorders and physical disorders with an organic basis in which psychological factors affect the physiological condition.*
4. *Describe possible psychological, neurobiological, and familial etiologies of somatoform disorders.*
5. *Identify possible emotional themes exhibited by clients with somatoform disorders.*
6. *Apply primary prevention nursing strategies to the care of clients and families at risk for somatoform disorders.*
7. *Apply the steps of the nursing process—assessment, nursing diagnosis, planning, intervention, and evaluation—to clients who exhibit somatoform disorders.*
8. *Identify measures to deal with your own feelings and attitudes when caring for clients with somatoform disorders.*

◆ Mind–Body Interrelationship

For years, terms such as *psychosomatic* or *psychophysiological* were used to describe individuals who manifested clinically significant physical signs and symptoms that appeared to be associated with psychological distress. It was presumed that certain physical diseases, such as bronchial asthma, essential hypertension, peptic ulcer, ulcerative colitis, and rheumatoid arthritis, had primarily a psychologically based etiology; other diseases were primarily biological in origin and had no psychological overlay. This view strongly suggested a mind–body dualism in humans.

These early beliefs have rapidly given way to a view of humans as a composite of interrelated systems in which disruption in any one system affects the whole system. This view transcends the boundaries of discrete disease entities and focuses on the interrelationship between psychosocial and physiological factors present in every person. Additionally, the interrelationship of all aspects of the person suggests a connection of the whole of life experiences—those in current life linked with those of the past. Experiences in the present and the past interrelate with emotional responses and bodily processes that a person communicates at any time.

◆ Somatoform Disorders: Types and Characteristics

While the symptoms of somatoform disorders are physical, they are classified as a group of mental disorders in the fourth edition of the Diagnostic and Statistical Manual of Mental Disorders (DSM-IV) because demonstrable organic pathology found in laboratory tests or physical examination is absent. The roots of the somatic symptoms are linked to psychological rather than biological findings.[1] These disorders, which are real to the person, appear to articulate the relationship between the discomfort of emotional stress and physical symptoms. More than 20% and as many as 75% of all clients in nonpsychiatric primary care settings present psychological problems through somatic symptoms without any organic disease.[10]

The DSM-IV identifies numerous disorders as somatoform. Unfortunately, negative labels, such as "attention seeker" and "doctor shopper," have been attached to people with somatoform disorders. Such labeling is tragic, because the affected person does not intentionally cause the physical symptoms and has no conscious or voluntary control over them. The absence of voluntary control is in contrast to the symptoms of a person who is diagnosed with factitious disorder or malingering. *Malingering*, for example, involves conscious deception and communication of false symptoms.

SOMATIZATION DISORDER

Somatization disorder historically has been called hysteria or Briquet's syndrome. It begins before age 30, has persistent recurring patterns of somatic complaints, and is a polysymptomatic disorder involving various body systems. Diagnostic features of somatization are listed in Box 26-1.

Individuals living with somatization disorder usually present exaggerated, inconsistent, yet complicated medical histories. Seeking treatment from numerous health care providers is common. The interrelationship

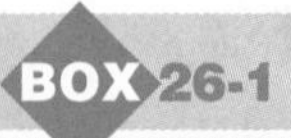

DSM-IV Diagnostic Criteria for Somatization Disorder

A. A history of many physical complaints beginning before age 30 years that occur over a period of several years and result in treatment being sought or significant impairment in social, occupational, or other important areas of functioning

B. Each of the following criteria must have been met, with individual symptoms occurring at any time during the course of the disturbance:
   (1) *Four pain symptoms:* a history of pain related to at least four different sites or functions (eg, head, abdomen, back, joints, extremities, chest, rectum, during menstruation, during sexual intercourse, or during urination)
   (2) *Two gastrointestinal symptoms:* a history of at least two gastrointestinal symptoms other than pain (eg, nausea, bloating, vomiting other than during pregnancy, diarrhea, or intolerance of several different foods)
   (3) *One sexual symptom:* a history of at least one sexual or reproductive symptom other than pain (eg, sexual indifference, erectile or ejaculatory dysfunction, irregular menses, excessive menstrual bleeding, vomiting throughout pregnancy)
   (4) *One pseudoneurological symptom:* a history of at least one symptom or deficit suggesting a neurological condition not limited to pain (conversion symptoms, such as impaired coordination or balance; paralysis or localized weakness, difficulty swallowing or lump in throat; aphonia; urinary retention; hallucinations; loss of touch or pain sensation; double vision; blindness, deafness; seizures; dissociative symptoms, such as amnesia; or loss of consciousness other than fainting)

C. Either (1) or (2):
   (1) After appropriate investigation, each of the symptoms in criterion B cannot be fully explained by a known general medical condition or the direct effects of a substance (eg, a drug of abuse, a medication).
   (2) When there is a related general medical condition, the physical complaints or resulting social or occupational impairment is in excess of what would be expected from the history, physical examination, or laboratory findings.

D. The symptoms are not intentionally produced or feigned (as in Factitious Disorder or Malingering)

between the medically unexplained and unintentionally expressed physical symptoms and the psychological well-being of individuals with somatization disorder is dramatic; this is underscored by the fact that approximately two-thirds of these individuals have suffered from recurrent major depression.[8,9,20–22]

In addition to the positive correlation between somatization disorders and the affective disorder of depression, many individuals who have symptoms that meet the diagnostic criteria of somatization disorder also suffer with anxiety disorders, such as panic disorder or generalized anxiety disorder.[17]

UNDIFFERENTIATED SOMATOFORM DISORDER

The persistent, unexplained physical symptoms that characterize *undifferentiated somatoform disorder* last for at least 6 months. They do not fully meet the criteria for somatization disorder or any other somatoform disorder. Common complaints include fatigue, loss of appetite, and gastrointestinal or urinary symptoms.

Individuals suffering with this disorder do not feign the symptoms and do experience negative ramifications in interpersonal, occupational, or other aspects of functioning. The presented history, physical examination, or laboratory tests do not explain or verify the physical symptoms or disruption in life experiences.[1]

CONVERSION DISORDER

The predominant feature of *conversion disorders* is a loss in voluntary motor or sensory functioning that appears to represent physiological dysfunction but instead relates psychological conflict or need. The onset of the nonfeigned symptoms follows an event or experience perceived as a major stressor. The symptoms are a way of assisting the individual to defend against the intrapsychic anxiety generated by the event or experience. Conversion symptoms are defined as "pseudoneurological" because they cannot be explained by medical tests or laboratory findings. Examples of such symptoms include paralysis or localized weakness, impairment in balance, aphonia, urinary retention, and difficulty swallowing.[1] See Box 26-2 for diagnostic criteria.

Conversion of intrapsychic conflict to physical symptoms is an unconscious mechanism. The psychological conflict is symbolically expressed through physical processes. People diagnosed with conversion disorder manifest little anxiety about the physical symptoms or the attendant disruption to their lives, a characteristic termed *la belle indifference.* This lack of concern is in contrast to the preoccupation with the "serious disease" manifested by individuals who suffer with hypochondriasis.[1] While the symptoms of conversion disorder may be severe and may significantly affect life functioning, they tend to involve less long-term morbidity and disability than do human responses associated with somatization disorder.[11]

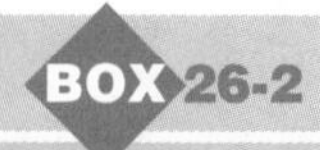

DSM-IV Diagnostic Criteria for Conversion Disorder

A. One or more symptoms or deficits affecting voluntary motor or sensory function that suggest a neurological or other general medical condition.
B. Psychological factors are judged to be associated with the symptom or deficit because the initiation or exacerbation of the symptom or deficit is preceded by conflicts or other stressors.
C. The symptom or deficit is not intentionally produced or feigned (as in Factitious Disorder or Malingering).
D. The symptom or deficit cannot, after appropriate investigation, be fully explained by a general medical condition, or by the direct effects of a substance, or as a culturally sanctioned behavior or experience.
E. The symptom or deficit causes clinically significant distress or impairment in social, occupational, or other important areas of functioning or warrants medical evaluation.
F. The symptom or deficit is not limited to pain or sexual dysfunction, does not occur exclusively during the course of Somatization Disorder, and is not better accounted for by another mental disorder.

Primary and Secondary Gain

Symptoms associated with conversion disorder provide the individual with *primary gain* in that psychological conflict or anxiety is blocked from conscious awareness. Also, the expression of physical symptoms offers *secondary gain,* such as releasing the person from fulfilling expected responsibilities and receiving increased attention from others. In many cases, the symptoms provide the person with a way to communicate intense dependency longings and to meet such needs.

PAIN DISORDER

The characteristic symptom in *pain disorders* is the nonintentional presence of physical pain. Individuals suffering with pain disorders experience the pain as a major focus in their lives and are likely to frequent health care services and to take medication for the symptoms. Pain disorder is not linked with a definable medical condition but appears to be linked with emotional disorders, such as mood and anxiety disorders.[1] See Box 26-3 for diagnostic criteria.

HYPOCHONDRIASIS

The DSM-IV describes the individual experiencing *hypochondriasis* as having an unwarranted fear or belief that his or her body houses a serious disease in the absence of significant pathology.[1] Heightened attention to the body and preoccupation with bodily sensations lead to the misinterpretation and overreaction to physical signs and symptoms that are usually prolonged and chronic. Much of the person's psychic energy may be bound in unrealistic fears that diagnoses, such as cancer, cardiac disease, or sexually transmitted diseases, are being missed by health care professionals (Box 26-4).

People with hypochondriasis frequently seek medical care, often from numerous sources. Disruption in social relationships and work may occur because of the person's preoccupation with bodily distress and attendant expectations that others focus on his or her physical well-being. In contrast to the lack of anxiety dis-

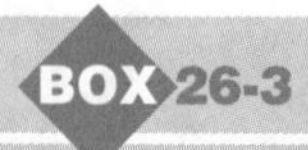

DSM-IV Diagnostic Criteria for Pain Disorder

A. Pain in one or more anatomical sites is the predominant focus of the clinical presentation and is of sufficient severity to warrant clinical attention.
B. The pain causes clinically significant distress or impairment in social, occupational, or other important areas of functioning.
C. Psychological factors are judged to have an important role in the onset, severity, exacerbation, or maintenance of the pain.
D. The symptom or deficit is not intentionally produced or feigned (as in Factitious Disorder or Malingering).
E. The pain is not better accounted for by a Mood, Anxiety, or Psychotic Disorder and does not meet criteria for Dyspareunia.

played by people with conversion disorders, those with hypochondriasis appear anxious about their symptoms and can acknowledge that their fear of a dreaded disease is unfounded. However, they are unaware of the underlying psychic issues or conflicts represented by the symptoms, as described in Box 26-4.

The outcomes of hypochondriasis are variable. More severe symptoms, longer duration of illness, and coexisting psychiatric illness (eg, anxiety disorder, especially panic disorder with agoraphobia, and depressive disorders) predict a more unremitting course and a worse long-term outcome.[14] The dual diagnoses of depression and hypochondriasis are frequently described in the literature[2,12,15,23]; however, some people suffer from hypochondriasis alone (Case Study 26-1).[2]

BODY DYSMORPHIC DISORDER

The primary feature of *body dysmorphic disorder* is preoccupation with an imagined defect in appearance when no abnormality or disturbance is present. Individuals suffering with this disorder tend to obsess about imagined defects, such as facial flaws, wrinkles, spots on the skin, facial asymmetry, or excessive facial hair. Other body parts, such as the genitals, breasts, buttocks, hands, or feet, may be the focus of distress and embarrassment for the individual. Thinking that others are noticing the imagined flaw may be an associated feature of the disorder (Box 26-5).

Because of being extremely self-conscious regarding the imagined defect, the individual may retreat from usual activities and resort to social isolation.[1] Research on body dysmorphic disorder is limited. Obsessive-compulsive disorder has been observed in a number of individuals with body dysmorphic disorder.[4]

SOMATOFORM DISORDER NOT OTHERWISE SPECIFIED

This category in the DSM-IV includes disorders that do not meet criteria for other specific somatoform disorders. Physical symptoms are present for less than 6 months and include conditions such as pseudocyesis (a false belief of being pregnant) and unexplained physical symptoms of fatigue or body weakness.[1]

◆ Psychological Factors Affecting Medical Conditions

This chapter emphasizes information pertinent to caring for individuals who present psychosocial distress through physical symptoms that have no organic basis. Whereas somatoform disorders occur in the absence of medically diagnosed pathology, the diagnostic classification *psychological factors affecting medical condition* refers

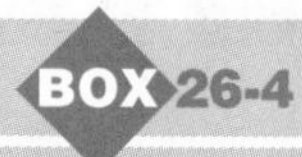

DSM-IV Diagnostic Criteria for Hypochondriasis

A. Preoccupation with fears of having, or the idea that one has, a serious disease based on the person's misinterpretation of bodily symptoms.
B. The preoccupation persists despite appropriate medical evaluation and reassurance.
C. The belief in Criterion A is not of delusional intensity (as in Delusional Disorder, Somatic Type) and is not restricted to a circumscribed concern about appearance (as in Body Dysmorphic Disorder).
D. The preoccupation causes clinically significant distress or impairment in social, occupational, or other important areas of functioning.
E. The duration of the disturbance is at least 6 months.
F. The preoccupation is not better accounted for by Generalized Anxiety Disorder, Obsessive-Compulsive Disorder, Panic Disorder, a Major Depressive Episode, Separation Anxiety, or another Somatoform Disorder.

26-1 Case Study

Planning Care for the Client Diagnosed With Hypochondriasis

Mr. J, 53 years old, has had repeated visits to several physicians in the last 2 years. His complaints focus primarily on his cardiovascular system and have included tightness in his chest, palpitations, chest pain on exertion, dizzy spells, and brief periods that he describes as "feeling like I've had a stroke." Extensive diagnostic testing has revealed no organic basis for Mr. J's complaints.

About 6 months ago, Mr. J took an early retirement from his job of 21 years. A major reorganization of his work system approximately 2 years early had cost several of his coworkers their jobs. During his last year at work, Mr. J often used sick leave time to "stay home to rest" because of his symptoms or to keep doctor's appointments. Mr. J truly believes that he has some major cardiovascular problem.

Mr. J's wife, a chemical engineer, received a job promotion about 1 year ago. This promotion requires her to travel out of town 2 to 3 days every other month. Mr. J has increasingly withdrawn from social engagements that he and his wife used to enjoy together. For example, according to his wife, when they are invited out to parties or supper, very often he will tell her "You go on. I'm too sick to go; I just know that I have some heart disease the doctors just can't find."

Questions for Discussion

1. Discuss your values, attitudes, and beliefs that might affect your care of Mr. J.
2. What possible feelings might you and other health care professionals have in response to Mr. J? How might these feelings impact your relationship with him?
3. What gains do the physical symptoms supply for Mr. J? What emotional needs do the physical symptoms communicate?
4. What etiologic factors possibly contribute to Mr. J's somatoform disorder?
5. Based on the data, formulate one nursing diagnosis and appropriate outcomes and nursing interventions.

to clinical associations between psychological factors and clinically diagnosed medical conditions.[1] Psychological factors, such as depression and anxiety, may adversely affect the course of physical disorders affecting any body system.

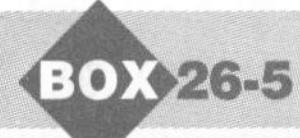

BOX 26-5 DSM-IV Diagnostic Criteria for Body Dysmorphic Disorder

A. Preoccupation with an imagined defect in appearance. If a slight physical anomaly is present, the person's concern is markedly excessive.
B. The preoccupation causes clinically significant distress or impairment in social, occupational, or other important areas of functioning.
C. The preoccupation is not better accounted for by another mental disorder (eg, dissatisfaction with body shape and size in Anorexia Nervosa).

Depression has been found to be the strongest psychological factor associated with the course and outcome of physical dysfunction. For example, the presence of depression adversely affects the course and prognosis of conditions such as multiple sclerosis, epilepsy, myocardial infarction, certain cancers, rheumatoid arthritis, psoriasis, irritable bowel syndrome, and peptic ulcer disease.[19]

◆ Etiology of Somatoform Disorders

Given similar life situations, why does one person communicate psychological distress through bodily symptoms that have no organic basis, and another person does not? Susceptibility to respond in such a way depends on many factors. Few authors would support a single explanation for the *unintentional* style of communicating psychological distress and needs through the body; rather, multifactorial causation with a complex interaction of psychological, neurobiological, and familial factors is at the root of somatoform disorders.

PSYCHOLOGICAL FACTORS

Careful history taking about the physical illness may reveal life changes that have been stressful. Studies indicate that various illnesses correlate positively with a high life-change profile.[5] Marriage, death of a loved one, retirement, trouble at work, buying a house, and financial changes are a few of the common and often inevitable events that occur in life. The psychological impact of one or more of these events varies.

After analyzing 5,000 case histories of clients' life situations at the onset of illness, Holmes and Rahe developed a Social Readjustment Rating Scale that focuses on life-change events at the onset of illness (Table 26-1).[6] The scale assigns a value of 11 to 100 life change units (LCUs) for each life event. The authors found that the higher a person's number of LCUs, the greater the likelihood that the person would develop a physical illness. Almost 80% of people with more than 300 LCUs in a year soon become physically ill.

Although Holmes and Rahe's major contribution to understanding the relationship between life experiences and physical distress focused on the quantity of life-change events, one must never lose site of the fact that a person's perception of events is crucial to his or her reactions or responses. Some people may succumb to their interpretation of certain life experiences as debilitating burdens, whereas others may interpret similar life experiences as opportunities for growth and change.

Aside from stress reactions being a possible underlying psychological dimension of somatoform disorders, in some instances physical suffering becomes a primary way for a person to obtain gratification and attention. Also, unresolved experiences of abuse, loneliness, or bereavement may be camouflaged by physical illness. Likewise, the individual may have extreme difficulty with direct expression of dependency longings and anger within interpersonal relationships, so the body becomes an avenue for such expression.[16]

Depression is commonly discovered at the root of somatoform disorders. Often loss or conflict precipitates the depression. The individual is unaware of the concomitant feelings and presents with physical symptoms, such as fatigue or pain.[16]

NEUROBIOLOGICAL FACTORS

According to biological theories, physiology plays a key role in the development of somatoform disorders. Cannon's studies in the 1920s led to the discovery of the adaptive function of adrenalin in assisting the body to strive for homeostasis when experiencing stress.[3] In the 1940s, Hans Selye focused on the role of the pituitary-adrenal mechanism in the body's reaction when defending against stress. Selye called this reaction the *general adaptation syndrome.*[18] Cannon and Selye believed that if the body experiences a prolonged adaptive struggle to combat stress, the person is likely to develop a "physical disease of adaptation."

Abnormal central nervous system regulation of incoming sensory information may be a key factor in some cases. This alteration may lead to inhibition of sensory input, causing a decreased awareness in the connection between mind and body or an exaggeration of focus on bodily symptoms. Another neurobiological theory addresses deficiency in communication between brain hemispheres that impedes awareness and expression of emotion.[7]

FAMILIAL FACTORS

Mechanisms for adapting to stress commonly are learned in the family arena. Children are greatly influenced by how their parental role models react and adapt to stressors, such as conflict, loss or change, or disappointment. Also, at times of stress, each child and each parent plays a distinct, separate role in the family system.

For some families, the primary mode of adaptation to emotional tension is through physical disorders. Generally, one child is the physical symptom bearer and communicates the emotional pain of the entire system. Years ago, when describing the "psychosomatic family," Minuchin asserted that the family has distinct characteristics that are absent from a nonpsychosomatic family.[13] These families are frequently overinvolved (enmeshed) with one another, deny the existence of conflict, have a poor ability to resolve differences, and have a narrow, rigid, and often ineffective repertoire of responses when faced with change.

Application of the Nursing Process to Somatoform Disorders

The nurse participates in all levels of preventive care. Through primary prevention, the nurse intervenes to assist a client to become more aware of potential stressors and to develop or maintain functional methods of adaptation. Secondary prevention focuses on interventions that demonstrate genuine caring and support; the nurse assists the client to improve physical health, adapt to stress, enhance self-knowledge, examine methods used to express needs and feelings, and consider alternatives for coping other than becoming physically ill. Through tertiary prevention, the nurse supports the cli-

Table 26-1

The Social Readjustment Rating Scale

Rank	Event	Value	Score
1	Death of spouse	100	_
2	Divorce	73	_
3	Marital separation from mate	65	_
4	Detention in jail or other institution	63	_
5	Death of a close family member	63	_
6	Major personal injury or illness	53	_
7	Marriage	50	_
8	Being fired at work	47	_
9	Marital reconciliation with mate	45	_
10	Retirement from work	45	_
11	Major change in the health or behavior of a family member	44	_
12	Pregnancy	40	_
13	Sexual difficulties	39	_
14	Gaining a new family member (eg, through birth, adoption, oldster moving in)	39	_
15	Major business readjustment (eg, merger, reorganization, bankruptcy)	39	_
16	Major change in financial state (eg, a lot worse off or a lot better off than usual)	38	_
17	Death of a close friend	37	_
18	Changing to a different line of work	36	_
19	Major change in the number of arguments with spouse (eg, either a lot more or a lot fewer than usual regarding childrearing, personal habits)	35	_
20	Taking out a mortgage or loan for a major purchase (eg, for a home, business)	31	_
21	Foreclosure on a mortgage or loan	30	_
22	Major change in responsibilities at work (eg, promotion, demotion, lateral transfer)	29	_
23	Son or daughter leaving home (eg, marriage, attending college)	29	_
24	In-law troubles	29	_
25	Outstanding personal achievement	28	_
26	Wife beginning or ceasing work outside the home	26	_
27	Beginning or ceasing formal schooling	26	_
28	Major change in living conditions (eg, building a new home, remodeling, deterioration of home or neighborhood)	25	_
29	Revision of personal habits (eg, dress, manners, association)	24	_
30	Troubles with boss	23	_
31	Major change in working hours or conditions	20	_
32	Change in residence	20	_
33	Changing to a new school	20	_
34	Major change in usual type or amount of recreation	19	_
35	Major change in church activities (eg, a lot more or a lot less than usual)	19	_
36	Major changes in social activities (eg, clubs, dancing, movies, visiting)	18	_

ent as new means of expressing needs and feelings and coping with stress are attempted.

PRIMARY PREVENTION

Promoting health and striving to reduce the incidence and prevalence of disease are at the forefront of nursing care in these last years of the 20th century. Accompanying this charge to nursing is the charge to every person in western society: to cope with a world of mounting stress and challenge. For nurses, the charge is dual: to take care of themselves and to assist others to discover ways of adapting that facilitate emotional and physical well-being.

Some people adapt to stress or express emotional needs by becoming physically ill. Bottling up feelings, being frightened or unsure of how to express needs, and receiving reinforcement for such responses may be at the root of many physical illnesses.

In primary prevention, nurses must direct intervention to the family as a target of care. All people begin the journey of growth and development in the family unit and learn patterns of behavior that are either functional or dysfunctional. Families at high risk for communicating psychological distress through physical symptoms are those in which one or both parents express needs and feelings in this way. Regardless of the setting, a thorough nursing assessment and analysis may reveal information suggesting that the client is at risk for using physical symptoms as a means of coping. Early preventive measures may be influential in choices made as growth and development progress.

Another vulnerable group for somatoform disorders are people who have experienced multiple life changes. Changes are inevitable in life, yet the nurse engaging in primary prevention can offer information that assists people to cope functionally with change and stress, rather than relinquishing control to the event or stressor.

Planning and Intervention

The following goals are directed at the primary prevention of somatoform disorders:

1. Family relationship patterns that do not foster the use of somatoform behaviors
2. Functional adaptation to life changes

The nurse practicing in any setting can share knowledge and skill by role modeling, teaching, and supporting parents and entire families to foster functional relationships with one another. The nurse uses interventions that facilitate the prevention of somatoform disorders and the promotion of functional family relationships by assisting families to do the following:

1. Create an atmosphere within the family that is caring, accepting, safe, and supportive.
2. Develop and nourish communication patterns that are open and honest and that permit direct expression of feelings and needs.
3. Accept, encourage, and respect differences in ideas and opinions.
4. Negotiate and cooperate at times of conflict.
5. Use a flexible approach to problem solving.
6. Achieve a balance between belonging needs and separation needs (autonomy).
7. Establish supportive resources beyond the family matrix.

Promoting functional adaptation to life changes may occur in various settings. Opportunities for nursing practice in primary prevention far surpass those in the traditional hospital setting. Speaking at Parent Teacher Organization meetings, participating in health fairs, teaching prenatal and postnatal classes, and working with people experiencing life transitions are some of the settings in which anticipatory guidance may be practiced. With the myriad of life changes, perceptions of the effect of similar events may vary from person to person. The nurse assists people to prepare for changes and consider options for coping when stress mounts. Active nursing involvement may help people cope with the stress in ways other than becoming physically ill.

SECONDARY PREVENTION

By the time the nurse meets the client in need of secondary prevention, the somatoform disturbance is already present. Through the nursing process—assessment, nursing diagnosis, planning, implementation, and evaluation—the nurse helps to shorten the duration of the existing disorder, thereby reducing the prevalence of the disorder.

Because most people in need of treatment for somatoform responses do not seek psychiatric care, the nurse usually meets them in outpatient and inpatient nonpsychiatric care settings.

Assessment

A holistic approach to assessment is especially critical when caring for individuals with somatoform disorders. Viewing the client as a system greater than the sum of its parts, or subsystems, assists the nurse to assess the whole person rather than focusing only on the most obvious—the physical body. The nurse's knowledge of possible multiple causes of the illness facilitates a comprehensive assessment that includes psychological, social, and family influences on the client. Analysis of assessment data focuses on a thorough examination of the possible interrelationships of all systems assessed. While assessing the client, the nurse simultaneously practices therapeutic use of self and conveys behaviors that exemplify understanding of therapeutic relationships.

Nursing assessment of the client exhibiting psychophysiological behavior addresses the following major areas:

1. Physical examination
2. Health history (physiological, psychological, and family life)
3. Emotional themes

Physical Examination. Even 20 years ago, nurses did not perform thorough examinations. In most nursing curricula today, the nursing student begins to develop and master physical assessment skills. These skills, linked with knowledge of the physical sciences, enable the nurse to monitor the client's physiological status and plan appropriate nursing interventions.

Health History. During history taking, the nurse elicits information relative to the client's current and past health status. Because the client's awareness of the relationship between bodily dysfunction and psychosocial or familial factors is absent, specific focus on this area is pertinent. Attention to issues such as the client's perception of self, perception of changes in lifestyle associated with health status, emotional responses to health, and relationships with others is significant.

Psychosociocultural assessment includes the following significant areas:

1. What are the client's attitudes toward physical illness? What does the client know about the illness? How does the client feel about being ill?
2. What does the client perceive as his or her strengths and limitations?
3. How does the client usually adapt to stress or tension?
4. Have any of the client's significant others used similar behaviors when adapting to stress?
5. What events preceded or precipitated this physical illness?
6. What relationship does the client perceive between his or her physical illness and emotions or behavior?
7. What tasks has the illness kept the client from performing?
8. In what ways has the physical disorder changed the client's or family's lifestyle?
9. What roles have changed in the client's family because of the physical illness?
10. How does the client generally meet emotional needs?
11. What interpersonal resources are available to the client?

Based on the client's physical status and the nurse's perception of the client's comfort and trust level, the nurse may decide that pursuit of psychosocial assessment is inappropriate during the initial contact. As the client's physical status improves and trust and rapport are built between the nurse and client, the nurse encourages the client to think about and disclose pertinent psychosociocultural history.

Emotional Themes. Within the context of a caring, nonthreatening nurse–client relationship, information is obtained about the client's ways of behaving within interpersonal relationships, including expressing needs and feelings, and intrapersonal experiences that focus on emotional life. Because depression and anxiety may be at the root of the physical symptoms, the nurse must be particularly sensitive to assessment strategies that focus on these areas. Additionally, because people with somatoform disorders often have difficulty with direct expression of needs and feelings, assessment needs to focus on areas such as dependent personality traits and hostility.

Underlying depression may be outside the client's awareness. Hence, the nurse assesses the possible presence of this mood disorder by focusing on possible symptoms experienced by the client. For example, encouraging and caring queries about possible feelings of loneliness, helplessness, hopelessness, and self-doubt may assist the client in associating these feelings with communication through the body. Have others commented to the client about perceiving him or her as being depressed? Has the client experienced difficulty in concentrating, thinking clearly, completing tasks, or enjoying usual activities, including sex and sleep?[16]

In terms of anxiety, is the client aware of excessive worry, dread, fear, apprehension, or rigid or obsessional thinking? Are physical signs and symptoms, such as restlessness, diaphoresis, palpitations, shortness of breath, or muscle tension, present?[16] If any of these are "owned" by the client, encourage the description of specific experiences.

Because the person may be ill equipped to meet dependency needs appropriately, focus on how the client receives gratification, nurturance, and attention. Sensitive questions and comments that assist the client to reflect on and disclose data about perceptions of self-sufficiency or perhaps possible codependency problems can be useful. Similarly, the nurse uses approaches that may lead to uncovering narcissism or a tendency to be demanding within interpersonal relationships.

Repression or denial of anger may be comingled with depression and the inability to meet dependency needs appropriately. Assessment of anger is pertinent. The individual, for example, may "swallow-down" anger out of fear of rejection or abandonment. Guilt and an overriding sense of powerlessness may be present, masked by the veneer of physical illness.

Nursing Diagnosis

When formulating nursing diagnoses for a client with a somatoform disorder, the nurse faces the challenge of addressing the client's holistic nature. As the client suffering with a somatoform disorder strives to adapt to stress and anxiety, various diagnoses that reflect physical and emotional responses may emerge from the analysis of assessment data. For example, based on an assessment of a client with somatoform disorder, the following diagnoses may become the focus of nursing care:

1. Anxiety
2. Ineffective Individual Coping
3. Ineffective Denial
4. Self Esteem Disturbance
5. Spiritual Distress
6. Diarrhea or Constipation
7. Pain

Regardless of the type of somatoform disturbance, a nursing diagnosis of particular relevancy in most cases is Ineffective Individual Coping. This diagnosis addresses the fact that the client is experiencing a human response of impairment or disruption in adaptation to stress.

Planning and Intervention

When planning care, the nurse must prioritize nursing diagnoses and intervene accordingly. In some instances, the client may be acutely physically ill, which mandates that the nurse direct attention primarily to physical care. The therapeutic use of self allows the nurse to minister to the client's physical needs while simultaneously responding to verbal and nonverbal cues that may indicate underlying emotions, such as hopelessness or anxiety. The nurse is likely to find that the most important aspect of intervention is using the self in a manner that communicates openness, empathy, caring, and acceptance. These behaviors are likely to facilitate the client's decision to adapt in more functional and satisfying ways. The focus needs to be on care, not cure.

Because somatoform behavior is communicated by means of various bodily systems, assessment and analysis may reveal that specific outcomes and interventions need to be directed toward the care of affected bodily organs—cardiovascular, gastrointestinal, or any other. In addition, outcomes of care must address the client's emotional life (Nursing Care Plan 26–1).

When intervening to help the client achieve outcomes other than those associated with specific physical needs, the nurse recognizes that the client is frequently unaware of the relationship between physical and emotional aspects of being. Frequently, the mental mechanisms of denial, repression, and suppression are operating, and the client has no awareness of feelings and their effect on behavior and choices. These defenses often are strong and important for the client. Therefore, the nurse uses care and caution when helping the client gain insight and change.

A good principle of therapeutic practice is never to remove a client's defense unless a replacement that is more functionally sustaining can be offered. Sometimes, zealous health care providers think they know the answers to the client's problems and eagerly "lay the cards on the table." This type of zeal can be destructive and may reinforce the client's dysfunctional modes of adaptation. Instead, attitudes and behaviors that convey a genuine willingness to help the client discover options for solving problems are far more constructive and useful. This requires patience and a belief in the client's capability to unfold self-understanding, meaning, and healing.

Because the emotional themes of unmet dependency needs or unexpressed anger frequently underlie the client's somatoform disorder, specific nursing approaches are recommended. Nursing interventions for unmet dependency needs include the following:

1. Be aware of your own feelings and how you allow these to affect your behavior. Because the client's need is often communicated by means of a facade of independence and demanding or manipulative behavior, you may react with anger and resistance. Develop an awareness and understanding of this dynamic. Work within a health care team context to deal with your own feelings.
2. Accept the client's feelings. Clients quickly pick up on nonacceptance, which tends to reinforce their maladaptive position.
3. Begin by meeting clients' dependency needs, then gradually help them meet more of their own needs. Developmentally, the client may be in a position like a young child who needs consistent caring and nurturing. You are in a position to offer the needed care while recognizing the client as a responsible individual. Set limits in a context that conveys belief and positive affirmation of the client's abilities.
4. Anticipate the client's dependency needs. Clients often strongly deny their dependency needs or feel that it is not acceptable to ask directly to have those needs met. Expecting that they will quickly give this up is apt to lead to feelings of anger, distance, and resistance in nurses and feelings of anger and anxiety in clients. Therefore, recognition and anticipation of needs early in the relationship are useful in meeting the client's needs and building a solid foundation of trust within the relationship. This trust becomes an especially valuable vehicle for helping the client develop greater insight, self-acceptance, and functional independence and for you to communicate care and confront the client.
5. As the trusting relationship progresses, support and encourage any cues of functional independence. Assist clients if needed, but do not usurp their responsibility and ability to think and do for themselves. Of great importance is your support, caring, and willingness to follow through with your commitment and acceptance.
6. Throughout the process, use yourself in modeling and facilitating open communication. Assist the client in thinking and talking about thoughts and feelings. With greater awareness of dependent behavior and movement toward independence, the client is likely to experience feelings of anger, shame, guilt, or anxiety. Encourage the client to identify and work through these feelings.

Nursing interventions for unexpressed anger include the following:

Nursing Care Plan 26-1

A Client With Somatoform Disorder

Ms. S is a twenty-seven year old graduate student on her summer break. She presents with complaints of severe abdominal pain and cramping, at times so severe that she cannot stand up. She also has sleep disturbance, headaches, and anhedonia. After medical investigation, and change of diet, there does not seem to be any physical cause for her symptoms. She is afraid that she may have cancer, and expresses fears of "being handicapped, and not knowing why—I want to get back to work!" Ms. S admits to "being depressed lately," and attributes this to not knowing anything definite about the source of her abdominal pain.

Upon inquiry, she reveals that her father had died two months ago from stomach cancer. She had been estranged from her father, and had not visited him in several years, though he lived an hour away. Ms. S had been unaware that her father was ill, and learning of his death was a surprise.

Nursing Diagnosis

Anxiety related to presence of physical symptoms without organic basis

Outcome

Client will report decrease in physical symptoms and increase in sense of well-being.

Intervention	Rationale
Listen nonjudgmentally to client complaints about physical symptoms.	Physical symptoms are real to client despite having no identifiable physiological basis.
Establish trusting nurse–client relationship.	Trust forms the basis for therapeutic interventions.
Avoid reinforcing secondary gains client may receive from physical symptoms.	Secondary gains serve to maintain somatoform symptoms and decrease level of client functioning.
Assist client to verbalize and identify sources of current life stress.	Defense mechanisms of denial and displacement are used in somatoform disorders to avoid dealing with uncomfortable issues.
Teach client problem solving methods that may be used to deal with stress related issues.	Use of problem solving methods reduces anxiety and need for physical symptoms as method of coping.

Evaluation

Client reports feelings of well-being and decreased physical symptoms.

Nursing Diagnosis

Ineffective Individual Coping related to unresolved issues surrounding death of father

Outcome

Client will take steps to resolve issues regarding relationship with father.

Intervention	Rationale
Encourage client to verbalize feelings regarding relationship with father.	Verbalization of feelings allows them to be examined and explored.
Accept nonjudgmentally client's choice to avoid visiting father.	Acceptance of client helps her accept her own behavior and diminishes guilt.

continued

Nursing Care Plan 26-1 *(Continued)*

Intervention	Rationale
Encourage client to write letter to her father expressing thoughts and feelings she would have wished to say.	Use of letter writing as therapeutic tool can aid client in coming to terms with unresolved issues.
Encourage client to establish contact with family members who are supportive.	Re-establishing family contact will decrease sense of isolation.
Encourage client to visit father's gravesite.	Visiting the gravesite facilitates the grieving process and provides an opportunity for client to resolve her feelings about her father's death.

Evaluation

Client states that she is actively resolving her feelings about her father.

1. Be aware of your own feelings and how you allow these to affect your behavior. Considering that the client's expression of hostility is usually passive or diverted outwardly to an inappropriate source, you may react with frustration, avoidance, or anger. Allowing these feelings to influence your behavior negatively is likely to prevent clients from exploring their real feelings and the source of these feelings.
2. Accept clients and their feelings. Acceptance is likely to help clients to develop a higher level of insight and eventually adapt in a more functional manner. Clients fear rejection and abandonment if they deal directly with feelings; therefore, nonacceptance may reinforce their fears. Repressing or denying anger is a client's primary way of adapting. These mechanisms are usually strong and serve as significant protection. Patience and acceptance are important approaches as a relationship builds and develops.
3. Assist clients to recognize their anger, identify the source of anger in current situations, and explore alternative ways of dealing with anger. This may be a slow process because clients have learned maladaptive behavior over a long time. Through a trusting nurse–client relationship, the client may begin an open, direct examination of feelings that affords a welcome release from the anxiety and tension experienced when feelings are bottled up.
4. Clients may direct anger toward you by means of criticism, profanity, or other derogatory ways. Set limits on the behavior while accepting the clients and their feelings.

In addition to individual care for the client, the family must be a focus of nursing care. Keeping in mind that clients did not exist or develop in a vacuum when they developed somatoform responses as a mode of adaptation helps nurses broaden their perspective toward the family. There is therapeutic value in the nurse developing a relationship with the family and intervening as needed. The nurse also assists the family to examine how the whole family system affects the client's physical status and how the client's physical status affects the family.

Aside from the nursing approaches for the specific dimensions of unmet dependency needs and unexpressed anger, several other general interventions may be applicable:

1. Education should be provided regarding relaxation training and stress reduction techniques, such as deep breathing, progressive muscle relaxation, and imagery.
2. Supportive counseling should come from a health care provider who believes that the focus of the relationship is on trusting care and not cure. Such a model of counseling de-emphasizes the focus on bodily symptoms and grants the person the chance to receive acceptance, respect, reassurance, and supportive guidance that may be a newfound experience in life.
3. Medication management, including education, may be warranted if an underlying depression or anxiety disorder is diagnosed and treated with medication as one strategy. Additionally, if medications are prescribed for the physical symptoms, the nurse must be particularly attuned to monitoring for dependency on medications.
4. In a primary care setting, scheduling of frequent, brief, regular appointments is strongly advised. This arrangement helps grant the client a sense of secu-

rity and decreases the intensity and creation of symptoms.[16] Dependability and a sincere interest in listening and caring are crucial aspects during contacts with the client.

Evaluation

Evaluation is an ongoing process occurring in each phase of the nursing process. Because clients living with somatoform disorders communicate their needs through various body systems, evaluation of the effect of care on the client's physical status is contingent on the bodily system involved and the progression or regression of the physical malady. Regarding the effect of nursing care on the client's emotional well-being, the nurse–client relationship is a valuable tool for measuring the effectiveness of care. For example, does the client show evidence of being more self-reliant, of being able to set internal limits on seeking attention and reassurance?

During evaluation, the nurse focuses on goals and outcomes. For example, has the client been able to identify thoughts and feelings relative to physical illness? When evaluating whether this goal has been met, the nurse examines interactions with the client and cites progress, regression, or status quo. Evaluation allows the nurse to continue or adjust the plan of care and is crucial to quality nursing care.

TERTIARY PREVENTION

The major focus of tertiary prevention may be to support the client who is considering whether or not to make changes that could reduce the likelihood of physical response to stress. It is not uncommon for clients who experience somatoform disorders to resist change in lifestyle, attitudes, and behavior. Along with change comes loss of a customary, familiar way of adapting—physical illness—and the sense of security it provides. The idea of change is frightening, but the nurse can offer support while assessing the client's readiness to consider change; the client chooses whether or not to move through the problem-solving process.

Planning and Intervention

The major goal for tertiary prevention of somatoform behavior is to develop functional adaptation to life stressors without physical behavior. When planning interventions, the nurse must remember that patterns of adaptation are not changed readily. Behavior changes slowly, and nurses must monitor their expectations of themselves and of the client. Expecting too much of themselves or the client hinders nurses from helping the client consider more functional methods of adaptation. An important goal for nurses may be to eradicate any expectations that they might hold. This would free nurses to be themselves and to assist clients in being realistic as they examine themselves. Working within a team approach is critical also.

Nursing interventions for tertiary prevention focus predominately on the change process:

1. Assist clients in examining and clarifying values and goals.
2. Assist clients in examining realistically how they cope with stress, express feelings, and have needs met. Help the client consider what, if any, congruence there might be between these aspects and their values and goals.
3. Be honest in sharing your perceptions regarding the negative consequences of the client's current coping pattern.
4. Assist clients with considering alternative modes of coping. Facilitate identifying pros and cons of all alternatives, and help clients consider ramifications for themselves and significant others.
5. Offer support, care, and belief in the client as he or she decides to change.
6. Positively reinforce functional change, and do not abandon clients if they regress to old modes of adaptation.

Evaluation

When evaluating the care offered during the tertiary phase of prevention, the nurse focuses on the modes of adaptation the client incorporates. The nurse may consider the following questions:

1. What evidence suggests that the client views stress as a growth-producing experience rather than a destructive one?
2. What change in lifestyle, attitude, and behavior does the client exhibit?
3. Has the client given up physical illness as a mode of adapting?
4. How is the client adapting now?
5. Is the client open with expressing and dealing with feelings in interpersonal relationships?
6. Is problem solving easier for the client?
7. What changes are evident in the family's style of relating?

Answers to these and similar questions may indicate whether the client has decided to adopt a more functional coping pattern and is striving to exercise self-control instead of allowing events and situations to control life choices.

◆ Chapter Summary

This chapter has focused primarily on a view of somatoform disorders as a mode of communicating emotional unrest. Suggestions for nursing care during primary, secondary, and tertiary prevention have been offered. The following ideas have been highlighted:

1. The human being is a composite of interrelated systems; therefore, the mind and the body cannot be divorced.
2. There is no single cause for somatoform responses; etiological theories include psychological, neurobiological, and familial factors.
3. Physical illness may be a means of communicating feeling states and needs, such as anxiety, anger, and dependency.
4. The nurse has a responsibility to participate in primary, secondary, and tertiary care aimed at preventing somatoform disturbance.
5. During the primary prevention of somatoform response, the nurse aims to promote functional family relationships and functional adaptation to life changes.
6. Many clients in need of secondary prevention for somatoform disorder also need supportive psychiatric care.
7. Assessment, intervention, and evaluation for the somatisized disturbed client focus on physical and psychosocial life and on the expressions of emotional needs and feelings.
8. The emotional themes of unmet dependency needs or unexpressed anger frequently underlie somatoform disorders.
9. During the tertiary prevention of somatoform behavior, the client's engagement in the process of change is the focus of nursing practice.

Review Questions

1. How do somatization disorder, conversion disorder, and body dysmorphic disorder differ?
2. Describe three possible responses to a client who tearfully states that "everyone tells me that the pain I complain about is not real."
3. How would you equip yourself to deal with a client who seems to have a somatoform disorder but discusses the physical pain and experiences with the health care system in an angry way, using shouting, paranoid statements, and aggression?
4. What are the theories about the possible neurological basis of somatoform disorders?
5. What is the possible role of family therapy in treating a client suffering from hypochondriasis?

◆ References

1. American Psychiatric Association: Diagnostic and Statistical Manual of Mental disorders, 4th ed, pp 445–469. Washington, DC, American Psychiatric Association, 1994
2. Barsky AJ, Wyshak G, Klerman GL: Hypochondriasis: An Evaluation of the DSM-III Criteria in Medical Outpatients. Archives of General Psychiatry 43: 493–500, 1986
3. Cannon WB: Bodily Changes in Pain, Hunger, Fear and Rage. New York, Appleton, 1920
4. Hollander E, Neville D, Frenkel M, Josephson S, Liebowitz MR: Body Dysmorphic Disorder. Diagnostic Issues and Related Disorders. Psychosomatics 33 (2): 156–165, 1992
5. Holmes TH: Life Situations, Emotions, and Diseases. Psychosomatics 19 (December): 747–754, 1978
6. Holmes TH, Rahe RH: The Social Readjustment Rating Scale. Journal of Psychosomatic Research 11: 213–218, 1967
7. Kaplan C, Liplin M Jr, Gordon GH: Somatization in Primary Care: Patients With Unexplained and Vexing Medical Complaints. J Gen Intern Med 3: 177–190, 1988
8. Katon W, Buchwald D, Simon G, et al: Psychiatric Illness in Patients With Chronic Fatigue and Rheumatoid Arthritis. J Gen Intern Med 6: 277–285, 1991
9. Katon W, Egen K, Miller D: Chronic Pain: Lifetime Psychiatric Diagnoses and Family History. Am J Psychiatry 142: 1156–1160, 1985
10. Katon W, Ries RK, Kleinman A: The Prevalence of Somatization in Primary Care. Comprehensive Psychiatry 25: 208–215, 1984
11. Kent D, Tomasson K, Coryell, W: Course and Outcome of Conversion and Somatization Disorders. Psychosomatics 36 (2): 138–144, 1995
12. Mabe PA, Hobson DP, Jones LR, Jarvis RG: Hypochondriacal Traits in Medical Inpatients. Gen Hosp Psychiatry 10: 236–244, 1988
13. Minuchin S, Roseman B, Baker L: Psychosomatic Families: Anorexia Nervosa in Context. Cambridge, MA, Harvard University Press, 1978
14. Noyes R, Roger K, Fisher M, Phillips B, Suelzer M, Woodman C: One-year Follow-up of Medical Outpatients with Hypochondriasis. Psychosomatics 35 (6): 533–545, 1994
15. Robbins JM, Kirmayer LJ: Cognitive and Social Factors in Somatization: Research and Clinical Perspectives. Washington, DC, American Psychiatry, 1991
16. Roberts SJ: Somatization in Primary Care. Nurse Practitioner 19 (5): 47–56, 1994
17. Russo J, Katon W, Sullivan M, Clark M, Buchwald D: Severity of Somatization and its Relationship to Psychiatric Disorders and Personality. Psychosomatics 35 (6): 546–555, 1994
18. Selye H: The Stress of Life. New York, McGraw-Hill, 1956
19. Stoudemire A: Psychological Factors Affecting Physical Condition and DSM-IV. Psychosomatics 34 (1): 8–11, 1993
20. Sullivan M, Katon W, Dobie R, et al: Disabling Tinnitus: Association With Affective Disorder. Gen Hosp Psychiatry 10: 285–291, 1988
21. Walker E, Harrop-Griffith J, Holm L, et al: Chronic Pelvic Pain: The Relationship to Psychiatric Diagnoses and Childhood Sexual Abuse. Am J Psychiatry 145: 75–80, 1988
22. Walker E, Roy-Byrne P, Katon W: Irritable Bowel Syndrome and Psychiatric Illness. Am J Psychiatry 147: 565–572, 1990
23. Zonderman AB, Hegt MW, Costa PT: Does the Illness Behavior Questionnaire Measure Abnormal Illness Behavior? Health Psychology 4: 425–436, 1985

Cognitive Disorders

Cheryl Detwiler

27

It is no easy matter to accept that one is growing old, and no one succeeds in doing it without first overcoming his spontaneous refusal. It is difficult, too, to accept the growing old of someone else, of one's nearest and dearest. That of a mother whose kindness, welcome, and understanding used to seem inexhaustible, and with whom one begins to hesitate to share one's intimate confidences, because they no longer arouse in her the warm, lively echo they used to. The aging of a father whose judgment and advice always used to seem so sound, but whom one can no longer consult because he must not be worried, or because his faculties are failing. The aging of a friend to whom one no longer talks as one used to, because it would be necessary to shout out loud things that used to be said quite quietly. It is hard to accept the decay of conversation into banality, empty optimism, and insignificance.

Paul Tournier,
Learn To Grow Old, *1972*

This chapter discusses mental disorders in which primary afflictions lie within the cognitive performance of the brain. The effects of the various disorders are considered in terms of their incidence and occurrence in the general population. Etiological factors and clinical manifestations of the cognitive disorders are discussed. Nursing interventions, as derived from the application of the nursing process, are provided, with the goal of achieving optimal care for clients affected by these disorders and their families.

Learning Objectives

On completion of this chapter, you should be able to accomplish the following:

1. *Define the term cognitive mental disorder.*
2. *Discuss the incidence and significance of the cognitive disorders.*
3. *Compare the possible etiologies of the cognitive disorders.*
4. *Identify the behaviors associated with various cognitive disorders.*
5. *Apply the steps of the nursing process to clients with cognitive disorders.*

◆ Defining Cognitive Disorders

Cognitive mental disorders are a group of disorders characterized by the disruption of or deficit in cognitive functioning. The specific Diagnostic and Statistical Manual of Mental Disorders, fourth edition (DSM-IV), categories within this disorder include 1) delirium, dementia, amnestic, and other cognitive disorders; 2) mental disorders due to a general medical condition; and 3) substance-related disorders. Previously these disorders were clustered by the DSM-III-R into the category of organic mental disorders. This group of disorders is no longer recognized as the only mental disorders with the origin attributable to the biologically malfunctioning or diseased brain. Rather, the disorders' distinguishing landmarks are pathologically driven changes in *cognition* that can be recognized clinically as notable deficits or impairments.[2] An example of this is a memory deficit where none was present before. Specific disease entities associated with each of the previous categories are discussed later in the chapter.

The etiology of the cognitive disorders is primarily biological. The disturbed behavior seen in these disorders is secondary to the brain's resulting transient or permanent dysfunctional or diseased state. The key to these diagnoses lies in the tangible proof of an organic problem affecting the brain tissue, obtained from the clinical history, physical examination, laboratory findings, or classic description of the syndrome. This organic factor may be a primary disease of the brain, a systemic influence originating in another body system, or an exogenous substance that is currently affecting the brain tissue or has left some residual, chronic deficit.

In some situations, a client with a cognitive disorder realizes that something is wrong and becomes extremely frustrated and emotionally distraught. This emotional reaction may escalate to the point that the person demonstrates actual psychotic behavior. In this scenario, the ensuing disturbed behavior is a result of two etiologies. This is not an uncommon finding, but it is a complex problem that necessitates the laborious procedure of collecting and sifting data to support the diagnosis of a disease state in the brain that has no definitive therapy and to guide medical treatment of potentially correctable maladies.[34]

Collecting data for a definitive diagnosis of a cognitive disorder is difficult, but the implications for treatment make it imperative. The brain in these disorders is not a healthy intact organ, and to not attempt to discover the basis of the problem is to misdirect the subsequent treatments and therapies and possibly incur permanent damage.

INCIDENCE AND SIGNIFICANCE

The incidence of organic mental disorders continues to increase in the mushrooming geriatric population, in the chronic disease survivor population, and in the population of acute care facilities. More than 1 million people, or 5% of the American population older than 65 years, are affected significantly enough by dementia to deter independent living. This means that 60% of the residents of nursing homes manifest some sort of cognitive mental disorder. In addition, another 10% of the American population older than 65 years is so affected by intellectual impairment that only semiindependent living is possible.[14]

Medical intervention that has prolonged the lives of clients requiring critical care and disease chronicity with all of its system disturbances sets the stage for iatrogenic cerebral damage and dysfunction. Systemic metabolic disturbances originating in the cardiovascular, respiratory, renal, or other body systems may affect brain homeostasis. Drug therapies, antineoplastic therapies, post-trauma resuscitation, and other sophisticated therapeutic modalities can and do result in a rising psychiatric morbidity.[16] Whether the mental impairment is couched in the temporary effects of a delirium or the permanent effects of a dementia, there is a change in the cognitive functioning.

ETIOLOGICAL FACTORS

Cognitive disorders usually result from the following:

1. A primary brain disease
2. The brain's response to the influences of systemic disturbances

3. The brain tissue's unique reaction to an exogenous substance
4. The residual effects or withdrawal of an exogenous substance[2]

The etiological factor(s) responsible for any one disorder may determine whether the cognitive deficits can be reversed. For example, the two most commonly seen neuropsychiatric disorders of delirium and dementia generally have different prognoses. *Delirium* is often caused by the disruption of brain homeostasis. When the cause of that disruption is eliminated or subsides, the cognitive deficits will usually resolve. *Dementia*, on the other hand, is caused by primary brain pathology, which is usually less amenable to treatment resolution, and recovery.[3] Thus, in some situations, there is an optimistic prognosis with reversal or slowing of cognitive defects. In other cases, there is minimal chance for improvement regardless of what changes are made in the physiological environment, and the prognosis for the reversal of cognitive deficits is poor.

The plausible list of etiological factors of cognitive disorders is exhaustive. When more than one element is present, the problem of identification is compounded. For example, by itself, an exogenous substance, such as a medication may be innocuous, but in combination with another medication or a food, it may become toxic. Another possible phenomenon is that the aftermath of exogenous substance exposure sometimes can be more devastating than the initial effect. Withdrawal of an exogenous substance may produce unique physiological responses in neuronal structures of the brain. Accordingly, when the acute response to the substance subsides, the remaining chronic deficits may still be harmful. Finally, in some situations, the presenting symptomatology is that of an acute problem, such as delirium, wherein underlying symptomatology may coincide, such as that present in vascular dementia. Thorough, persistent, investigative screenings must be the hallmark of the clinical path to determine the diagnosis and possible etiological culprit of any of the conditions in the cognitive disorders.

◆ Delirium

Delirium connotes a group of cognitive disorders that has as its hallmark a rapid onset of cognitive dysfunction and disruption in consciousness. In the clinical area, delirium has often been called intensive care unit psychosis, acute brain syndrome, acute confusion, or acute psychosis.[17]

The elderly are especially susceptible to this group of disorders because of an aging neurological system. In addition, delirium is often concomitant with, or a harbinger of, physical illness in the geriatric client. Estimates are that up to 80% of the hospitalized elderly will experience this disorder, though they may not be recognized by the attending clinicians.[8]

ETIOLOGICAL FACTORS

In general, the causes of delirium include conditions affecting metabolic balance, such as postoperative conditions or metabolic disorders; withdrawal of substances, such as alcohol; and the toxicity of drugs or other exogenous substances. Metabolic disturbances in the brain result in a decrease in cerebral metabolism and disrupted neurotransmissions.[17] These metabolic disruptions can occur with metabolic illness that causes electrolyte imbalances and hypoprofusion of the brain, or hypoxia. The withdrawal of substances of abuse, such as alcohol or cocaine, can interrupt cerebral homeostasis, resulting in delirium. Probably the most prevailing cause of the metabolic disturbances in the brain is the toxic effects of exogenous substances. Not surprisingly, medications are the primary exogenous offenders, especially in the elderly.[17,31] Box 27-1 delineates some of the specific causes of delirium, and Box 27-2 lists categories of delirium.

CLINICAL FEATURES

The three salient features of delirium are disordered cognition, attention deficit, and reduced level of consciousness. The main disorders of cognition include the aspects of thinking, perception, and memory. The *thinking* aspect of the individual's cognition is disorganized. The individual appears to be in a confused state with minimal or absent problem-solving abilities. This results in an apparent inability to comprehend the situation. Speech is frequently pressured, rambling, bizarre, and even incoherent. Individuals with delirium are unable to distinguish reality from imagery and dreams. They do not readily assimilate new information with prior knowledge. Persecutory delusions are not uncommon.[17,31]

The *perceptual* aspect of the individual's cognition is disturbed. Hallucinations and illusions are frequent manifestations of this disturbance. If present, the hallucinations, which can be auditory, tactile, or visual, are often graphic and can induce a state of great trepidation. The client may assume a fight or flight stance to elude their unfounded perceptions and can be very combative with whomever or whatever they see as thwarting their efforts to escape.[17,31]

The *memory* aspect of the individual's cognition is impaired. Short-term memory is especially affected. The person experiences antegrade and retrograde amnesia, and these sequelae do not resolve quickly.

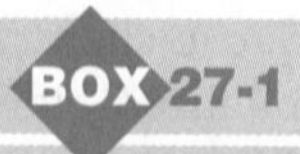

Specific Causes of Delirium

PRIMARY BRAIN DISEASE

Tumors
Head injury: concussion, contusion, hemorrhage, vascular obstruction

SYSTEMIC DISEASES SECONDARILY DISRUPTING BRAIN HOMEOSTASIS

Acid–base imbalance
Cancer
Dehydration
Endocrine disorders: diabetes (hypoglycemia), Hypothyroid or hyperthyroid
Epilepsy
Fever due to any cause
Hypothermia or hyperthermia
Hypokalemia
Hypoprofusion of the brain: myocardial infarction, dysrhythmia, congestive heart failure, vascular hypotension
Hypoproteinemia
Hypotension with cerebral ischemia
Hypoxia producing chronic obstructive pulmonary disease, anemia, gastrointestinal bleeding
Infections: bacteremia, septicemia, urinary tract infection, upper respiratory infection
Malnutrition
Organ failure: hepatic, renal, pulmonary
Postoperative state
Sodium depletion
Stroke
Trauma: burns, hip fracture
Uremia
Vitamin deficiencies

WITHDRAWAL OF EXOGENOUS SUBSTANCES OF ABUSE

Alcohol
Barbiturates
Sedative-hypnotics
Tranquilizers

BRAIN TOXIC EXOGENOUS SUBSTANCES

Antidysrhythmic drugs: lidocaine, amiodarone propranolol, digitalis
Anticholinergic drugs
Antidepressants: amitriptyline, doxepin
Antipsychotics: chlorpromazine, thioridazine
Antidiarrheal: diphenoxylate
Antihistamines
Antihypertensives: methyldopa
Antiparkinsonian agents
Antimicrobials
Cimetadine
Corticosteroids
Digitalis glycosides
Diuretics
Narcotic analgesics: meperidine, pentazocine
Nonsteroidal anti-inflammatory agents: indomethacin
Neuroleptic
Over-the-counter cold/cough medications
Psychiatric medications: diazepam, flurazepam, tricyclic antidepressants, benzodiazepines
Xanthines: caffeine, theophylline

(Compiled from Lipowski,[17] Tueth and Cheong,[31] and Ludwig.[18])

Another salient feature of delirium is *attention deficit*. Individuals have difficulty directing their attention and can neither focus nor shift their attention readily. In addition, they are frequently distracted by the stimuli in their environment. This occurrence of diminished ability to control attention focus and attention span fluctuates during the day but is predictably more pronounced at night. With the disturbances in cognition and attention, the individual is frequently disoriented to time, if not place and person. In more severe cases of delirium, the unfamiliar are mistaken for familiar, and not uncommonly, hospital personnel are seen as the more familiar brother, sister, husband, wife, or child.[17,22,31]

Concomitant with the salient features of delirium, there is also a reduced level of consciousness, a disturbance of sleep-wake cycle, and an abnormality of psychomotor behavior. The change in the level of consciousness may present itself in a fluctuating continuum of alert yet easily distracted to barely able to rouse. The individual often reverses the sleep-wake cycle, being drowsy and napping throughout the day only to be extremely agitated and sporadically "cat napping" at night.

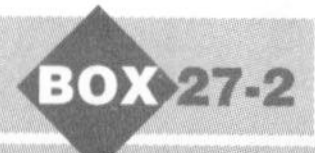

DSM-IV Categories of Delirium

Delirium Due to . . . [Indicate the General Medical Condition]
Substance Intoxication Delirium
Substance Withdrawal Delirium
Delirium due to Multiple Etiologies
Delirium Not Otherwise Specified

The psychomotor activity of the individual ranges from hypoalert, hypoactive (which is typical of a metabolic state) to hyperalert, hyperactive (which is typical of a drug withdrawal state) or any combination thereof. The client in the hypoalert, hypoactive scenario is stuporous with slow response to any requests and minimal activity; this person is often mistakenly seen as depressed. The client in the hyperalert, hyperactive scenario is very animated to the point of agitation and exhibits loud and pressured speech (Case Study 27-1).[17,31]

◆ Dementia

Dementia denotes a group of specific cognitive disorders in which many progressive, cognitive deficiencies occur, the most conspicuous of which is memory loss. In addition to memory loss, usually there are deficits in thought process functioning, agnosia, aphasia, or apraxia.[23] The impairment is not just an annoying inconvenience one might associate with aging, but rather is rigorous enough to significantly impact the social or occupational arena of the individual's life (Table 27-1).[2]

The *memory impairment* that occurs in dementia encompasses the individual's ability to learn new material (short-term memory) and to recall previously learned material (long-term memory).[2] Initially, environmental prompts and social amenities may hide the failing recollections, but the final outcome is blatant eradication. The sad scenario of this progressive loss of both types of memory depicts an individual who initially forgets the names of people he or she just met, ultimately forgetting the name and identity of the person to whom he or she has been married for 50 years or more. The person may even become a stranger in his or her own mind, forgetting his or her own personhood (Case Study 27-2).

The individual may also incur the insult of *agnosia,* not being able to recognize or identify familiar objects (such as the parts of a telephone); *aphasia,* not being able to use the forgotten words, requiring a painstaking game of charades until others guess the forgotten word (such as referring to Thanksgiving Day as the time of the turkey or pumpkin); or *apraxia,* not being able to carry out motor tasks, such as brushing the teeth and combing the hair despite intact motor function.[2,23]

Finally the individual may exhibit deficits in thought process functioning so that abstract thinking is hindered. Problems in this area may manifest themselves in circumstances in which the individual has to adjust to new situations. In dementia, the thought processes are so impaired that the individual cannot abstractly take old behaviors and adjust them to the new situations.[2]

CATEGORIES OF DEMENTIA

Dementia is the result of many entities. Box 27-3 reveals the categories of dementia according to the DSM-IV. Several of the disease entities are discussed separately.

Alzheimer's Disease

Alzheimer's disease is the most prevalent of the dementias. It is estimated that 4 million Americans are victims of dementia, Alzheimer's type (DAT),[32] which occurs

Case Study

Delirium

Meredith had been thrown from a horse and experienced a broken leg and a concussion. The evening following surgery to pin her femur, Meredith asked the nurse, whom she called by her sister's name, to close the barn door and latch it before the squeaking mice could climb up her leg. She was very insistent, and when she was oriented by the nurse to her present situation, Meredith became more agitated. She pleaded for anyone to chase the mice off her leg. She began to whimper and suddenly began to beat the bed and the cast on her leg shouting "Get off. Don't bite me. Go hide in the hay!" After this, she rambled incoherently for some time before finally "drifting off to sleep."

Questions for Discussion

1. What type of hallucinations is Meredith experiencing?
2. What is the probable physical basis for her delirium?
3. Are the features of her disordered cognition related to the circumstances of her recent injury and in what way?

Table 27-1

Comparison of Delirium and Dementia

Indicator	Delirium	Dementia
Onset	Rapid development	Gradual and insidious
Duration	Brief duration—1 mo or less depending on resolving cause	Long with progressive deterioration
Course	Diurnal alterations, more nocturnal exacerbations	Stable progression of symptomatology
Thinking and short-term memory	Disorganized and impaired	Short- and long-term impairments—eventual complete loss
Orientation	Markedly decreased, especially to environmental cues	Progressively decreases
Language	Rambling, pressured, irrelevant	Difficulty recalling the correct word; later may lose language
Perceptual disturbance	Environment unclear progressing to illusions, hallucinations, and delusions	Often absent but can progress to paranoia, delusions, hallucinations, and illusions
Level of consciousness	Cloudiness that fluctuates; inattentiveness to hyperalert with distractibility	Not affected
Sleep	Day-night reversal, insomnia, vivid dreams and nightmares	Piecemeal
Psychomotor actions	Sluggish to hyperactive; change of range unpredictable	Not affected
Emotional status	Anxious with changes in sleep; fearful if experiencing hallucinations; weeping; yelling	Depression/anxiety when insight into condition present; late in pathology, anger with outbursts, restless with pacing

(Compiled from Lipowski Z: Delirium in the Elderly Patient. N. Eng J Med 320 (9): 578–582, 1989; American Psychiatric Association: Diagnostic and Statistical Manual of Mental Disorders, 4th ed. (DSM-IV) Washington, DC: APA, 1994).

more frequently in women. Demographic studies reveal unequivocal risk factors of age and familial aggregation. The incidence and prevalence of Alzheimer's disease directly correlates with increased age; Alzheimer's is present in approximately 6%, or one in 26 people 65 years and older, rising to 45%, or one in two people 85 years and older.[32] Studies have also shown a positive relationship between Alzheimer's disease and the familial aggregates of Down syndrome, Parkinson's disease, older age of mother, incidence of head trauma, and incidence of depression or hypothyroidism.[25,32]

The etiology of Alzheimer's disease is unknown, although noteworthy findings have generated several theories. Physiological studies indicating degenerative changes in the cholinergic neurons and biochemical changes involving the biosynthetic enzyme for acetylcholine give credence to an etiology of a neurotransmitter deficiency (Box 27-4).

Other metabolic aberrances have also been noted. Higher than normal amounts of aluminum deposits have been detected in the brains of Alzheimer's clients; some researchers believe that these deposits may be a cause or a result of the disease. Other studies have shown abnormally high antibody titers, raising the possibility of an immunological defect. A higher incidence of Alzheimer's has been associated with adult Down syndrome clients and with close relatives of Alzheimer's clients, leading to the theory of a probable defect in chromosome 21 or another chromosome. Other genetic links have also been proposed. Finally, some groups believe that DAT may be composed of a group of disorders that had been seen as one disease entity.[1,36]

The microscopic findings of senile plaques and neurofibrillary tangles present in the brains of people with Alzheimer's closely resemble the pathological changes documented in people whose brains exhibit "normal" aging. This resemblance is so close that differentiation between the disease state of the brain in Alzheimer's and the state of the brain in normal aging is not always substantiated in the histological findings at autopsy. Sometimes the disease can be authenticated only by the person's documented aberrant behaviors.

Vascular Dementia

The second most common form of dementia is vascular dementia. Though the incidence of this form of dementia is thought to be considerably less than DAT, some allege that it may be the most common demen-

Case Study

Memory Deficit

Mandy W lives 650 miles from her 82-year-old father. Mr. W is a very independent widower of 12 years who lives alone in a small farming community where he has lived all of his life. Mandy calls her father on a weekly basis and goes to see him every Thanksgiving. During her last visit, everything seemed fine, though she noticed that her father's house was becoming more cluttered and he had yet to use the new videocassette recorder she had given him for his birthday; she teased him when she found out that "Mr. Electronics" himself hadn't yet figured out how to program his new toy. She was initially hurt when she did not receive a card or the traditional birthday phone call from her father, but then she became concerned when her father's only sister called to complain that he had forgotten her birthday too.

Mandy flew to see her father when one of his neighbors called to tell her that her father had a small fire in the house after he had gone to bed without turning off the stove's gas burner. When she arrived at his home she found unpaid bills lying throughout the house and received phone calls from the family dentist and eye doctor asking her to reschedule her father's unkept appointments. Mandy took her father for an appointment to get a thorough checkup in spite of his insistence that he was fine.

Questions for Discussion

1. What procedure would the physician more than likely follow during the checkup of Mandy's father?
2. If the memory deficit present in Mandy's father proved to be a dementia, what would be the prognosis?
3. What type of arrangements might Mandy make for her father to ensure his safety and well-being?

tia in those older than 85 years. In vascular dementia, cognitive deficits arise from multiple infarcts in the cortex and the white matter seen as the aftermath of hemorrhage or ischemia inherent in a cerebrovascular disorder. Risk factors for this dementia parallel those for stroke and include hypertension, smoking, hyperlipidemia, atrial fibrillation, and diabetes. The physical evidence of brain pathology is often verified by computed tomography and magnetic resonance imaging. Historically, the stepwise deterioration and focal neurological signs present in the client complete the picture for the diagnosis.[4] The exact symptomatology seen with this dementia often depends on which sectors of the brain are affected and to what extent. There will, however, be problems with impaired memory (learning new and recalling old information) and the manifestation of aphasia, apraxia, agnosia, or executive functioning.

Parkinson's Disease

Parkinson's disease is a neurodegenerative illness that progresses slowly without the interference of a known cure. It affects 1 million Americans and though its predominate clinical picture is that of immobility, the cognitive decline of dementia runs concurrently with more than 40% of its victims. The heart of the pathology of the disease resides in the decreasing number of cells in the substantia nigra with a resultant depletion of the neurotransmitter dopamine. The client displays involuntary muscle movements at rest accompanied by overall slowness and rigidity. Most often seen in clients who display postural instability and gait disturbance, the intellectual deficits are varied, though their progression is predictably insidious and progressive. This disease does not ravage the language of its victim as do many other dementias, but memory retrieval and executive functioning are not spared. The dementia seen

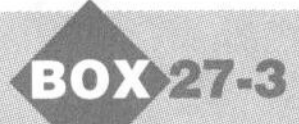

DSM-IV Categories For Dementia

Dementia of the Alzheimer's Type, With Early Onset
- Uncomplicated
- With Delirium
- With Delusions
- With Depressed Mood

Dementia of the Alzheimer's Type, With Late Onset
- Uncomplicated
- With Delirium
- With Delusions
- With Depressed Mood

Vascular Dementia
- Uncomplicated
- With Delirium
- With Delusions
- With Depressed Mood

Dementia Due to HIV Disease
Dementia Due to Head Trauma
Dementia Due to Parkinson's Disease
Dementia Due to Huntington's Disease
Dementia Due to Pick's Disease
Dementia Due to Creutzfeldt-Jakob Disease
Dementia Due to ... [Indicate the General Medical Condition not listed above]
---.-- Substance-Induced Persisting Dementia**
---.-- Dementia Due to Multiple Etiologies (code each of the specific etiologies)
Dementia Not Otherwise Specified

in Parkinson's disease is unique and different from that seen in Alzheimer's, though sadly, some who have Parkinson's disease probably have Alzheimer's disease also.[26]

Huntington's Chorea

Huntington's chorea is a familial disease passed on by an autosomal dominant trait. Children of affected parents have a 50% chance of inheriting the trait-carrying gene. Men and women are affected equally, though white Americans have a preponderance of incidence with 4.1 to 7.5 cases per 100,000 as opposed to 1.5 for African Americans. In people with the trait, the disease inevitably manifests between 35 and 45 years. The course of the disease from onset to death is approximately 15 years.[15] A genetic marker for Huntington's chorea makes presymptomatic and prenatal testing possible; however, the test is not always available. Moreover, when the test is available, it produces a high anxiety quotient for the at-risk person. People identified as carrying the autosomal dominant trait often face a dilemma as to what course of action to take for their future and for that of their children.[12] The clinical history is the most reliable diagnostic finding, although autopsy typically reveals frontal cerebral atrophy. Research laboratory findings suggest that this disease may be the result of biochemical changes within the brain cells.[34]

The victim of this disease experiences choreic movements that are intensified during stress as simple as having to wait for a need to be met. The jerking movements usually zenith in about 10 years after onset and then stabilize or decrease. The dementia seen with this disease lacks aphasia, agnosia, and apraxia but does manifest in the form of memory deficits, slowed thinking, problems with sustained attention span, and deficiency in judgment. An emotional component is apparent by the time the client reaches his or her 20s or 30s. As the frontal lobe begins to deteriorate, the client becomes labile, impulsive, easily frustrated, irritable, hostile, and aggressive. The illness becomes more relentless with time, with the victim often exhibiting affective or intermittent explosive disorders.[15]

Pick's Disease

Pick's disease is another degenerative cognitive disorder that resembles Alzheimer's disease in clinical picture, although it occurs less frequently. Pick's disease occurs equally in men and women in their early to mid-50s. The actual cause is unknown, but genetic tendencies are suspected. General microscopic findings include atrophy of the frontal and temporal brain portions. Why this atrophy occurs is not clearly understood, but it is believed to be associated with the aberrant behaviors seen in Pick's disease.[29]

Creutzfeldt-Jakob Disease

Creutzfeldt-Jakob disease is a rare disease that causes a cognitive disorder by targeting the central nervous system. With an incidence of about 1 new case per 1 million people per year, this rapidly progressive and ultimately fatal disease has been thought to be caused by a virus. Though the exact etiology is somewhat in dispute, the disease is termed "spongiform" because of the spongy appearance of cerebral and cerebellar cortex. Creutzfeldt-Jakob disease is seen most frequently in the middle-aged to elderly and is often misdiagnosed as Alzheimer's disease.

The symptomatology of Creutzfeldt-Jakob disease passes through three distinct stages. Initially, a dementia is present in which the mental changes are most pronounced with a rapidly progressing dementia. Later, a jerking is then followed by a generalized myoclonus. In many clients, ataxia, dysarthria, and other cerebellar signs

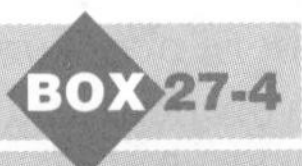

TACRINE THERAPY

One of the findings in Alzheimer's disease (AD) is diminished activity in the cholinergic system. Some researchers believe that anything that will activate or augment whatever activity remains in the cholinergic system will benefit cognitive function. Tacrine is a centrally acting, noncompetitive inhibitor of acetylcholinesterase, which helps to elevate the level of acetylcholine (ACh) in the system by decreasing the binding sites of acetylcholinesterase. This lengthens the potential for cholinergic activity. Tacrine is effective as long as there are at least some cells producing ACh; consequently, Tacrine is most efficacious in mild to moderate cases of AD. Even then, the effects of this drug on cognition are temperate with only small improvements and possible slowing of deterioration of cognition.

Tacrine is rapidly absorbed and metabolized by the liver; therefore, the liver is most vulnerable to the drug's toxicity. Clients' liver function, especially alanine aminotransferase (ALT) must be monitored every week for the first 18 weeks. If it is necessary to increase the dosage, ALT must be monitored for 6 weeks. Once the dose is stable, monitoring is done monthly.

The most common side effects involve the gastrointestinal system with nausea and vomiting being the most prevalent complaints and elevated ALT being the most common sign. Clients should be monitored for the development of peptic ulcer disease because the drug can increase gastric secretions. Cimetadine should not be given concomitantly to dissuade the development of ulcers, but antacids may be given, especially if there is a history of ulcer disease or the taking of nonsteroidal anti-inflammatory drugs.

Tacrine is contraindicated in any client sensitive to tacrine or acridine derivatives, with a history of liver disease or elevated ALT levels, or with a total bilirubin greater than 3.0 mg/dL. Clients with a history of strokes, subdural hematomas, or hydrocephalus are not candidates for this drug therapy.

Tacrine should not be given along with other drugs that have anticholinergic effects. Clients taking theophylline must be monitored carefully because theophylline levels can be elevated as a result of taking these two drugs concurrently.

Though the effects of Tacrine are palliative and not curative, it is the only pharmacological hope offered to the AD victim. Therefore, Tacrine will probably be seriously considered in most of the appropriate cases of dementia in spite of its troublesome side effects.[7,35]

are present. Extrapyramidal signs, disruption in many of the senses, and seizures are other manifestations found during the middle phase of this disease. The final phase is usually marked by coma with the client succumbing to infections and respiratory problems.[5]

◆ Amnestic Disorders

Amnestic disorders include conditions in which short-term memory loss is a hallmark. The deterioration of the memory is so great that it deters the individual from functioning at previous levels of social and occupational performance. The client typically may not have any recollections of events as recent as 2 minutes prior and is seriously deterred from learning new information. These individuals may have some difficulty recalling what they formerly knew to be a fact, be it events or knowledge. Remote memory recall acuity, however, varies with individuals. As with most amnesias, the brain damage that causes the condition leaves the individual disoriented to some degree as to time and place.[2,23] The classifications of this disorder are listed in Box 27-5.

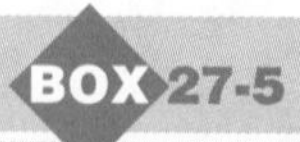

BOX 27-5

DSM-IV Categories of Amnestic Disorders

Amnestic Disorder Due to:
(Specify if: Transient or Chronic)
General Medical Condition
Substance-Induced, persisting
Amnestic Disorder Not Otherwise Specified

WERNICKE-KORSAKOFF SYNDROME

This amnestic disorder, one of the substance-induced persisting amnestic disorders, has been know for years as Korsakoff's syndrome. The most prominent feature of the Wernicke-Korsakoff syndrome is that the client's compulsion for ingestion of alcohol supersedes the need for nutritional intake.[20] This syndrome is usually found in the 40- to 70-year-old alcoholic with a steady and progressive alcohol intake. In time, this person develops a vitamin B_1 (thiamine) deficiency that directly interferes with the production of the brain's main nutrient, glucose.[19]

◆ Behaviors Associated With Cognitive Disorders

The behavioral manifestations associated with cognitive mental disorders are many and varied. No essential features are predictably present in every client. Frequently, the most significant behavioral problems are due to emotional reactions occurring when the client becomes aware of the cognitive deficits resulting from his or her condition.[2]

Behavior refers to a person's responses to continual changes in the internal and external environment. The physiological soundness of the brain is a necessary ingredient for the successful adaptation of human behavior to these changes. When the organic integrity of the brain is interrupted or interfered with, maladaptive behavior often will follow.[49] Some of the dementias have commonalities of behavior as listed in Table 27-2.

SENSORIUM AND ATTENTION DEFICITS

Deficits in the sensorium stem from the client's inability to use the information collected by the five senses to discern the environment. If this discernment does not take place, the client experiences confusion that affects attentiveness to the environment and ultimately level of consciousness. As the level of consciousness decreases, the client is unable to concentrate on any specific event. The attention span decreases, and the client becomes easily distracted.

DISORIENTATION

Disorientation occurs when a client is hampered from successfully receiving and centrally integrating the data obtained from the internal and external environments. When the sensory inputs fall below the minimum need requirements and when the brain is affected structurally in such a way that it can no longer perceive and interpret the stimuli adequately, decreased orientation results. Disoriented clients do not know where they are, how they came to be there, why they are there, or how they fit into the environmental milieu.

PERCEPTUAL AND MEMORY DISTURBANCES

Many of the conditions in the cognitive disorders cause clients to experience the perceptual abnormalities of illusions and hallucinations (see Chapter 30, Schizophrenia).

Memory disturbances are the most common deficits in the conditions of the cognitive disorders. Recent memory impairment is the most prevalent finding; however, remote memory also may be impaired. The inability to register, retain, and retrieve accumulated information is a key clinical manifestation of cognitive disorders and may affect the client's intellectual capability.[2]

The deficits in recent memory associated with delirium are recounted in the clinical features. Many of the behaviors seen as a result of the memory impairment tend to worsen during the hours after sunset, a phenomenon termed the *sundown effect.* Often the personnel in the evening and night will have to deal with clients who mistake them for a significant other, are combative, and hallucinate, after receiving a report from the day shift that the client was quiet or dozed through the day.

DEGENERATIVE IMPAIRMENTS

Many of the cognitive disorders with a chronic dimension tend to have behavioral manifestations that are predictively associated with their degenerative nature, especially when the disease has a known irreversible pathology. Many degenerative conditions are difficult to diagnose. Their impairments are global, and the intellectual deterioration is often concealed by the client's well-preserved social skills and mastery of confabulation.[23]

Table 27-2

Comparative Assessment for Cognitive Disorders

Cognitive	Level of Consciousness	Memory	Appearance	Emotional
ALZHEIMER'S DISEASE				
Global intellectual impairment Insidious onset characterized initially by "mistakes in judgment," progressing to inability to comprehend, agraphia, aphasia, and finally to unresponsiveness.	Clouding late in disease	Short-term memory loss initially Progressing to both short and long-term loss	Progressive loss of grooming habits due to forgotten social behaviors and decreasing coordination required to dress	Initally depression and anxiety about recognized regression Progressing to loss or severe dampening of emotions Subtle loss of interest in work Inability to recognize family members
PICK'S DISEASE				
Intellect intact Lack of insight into disease process	Not affected		Slovenly	Dramatic personality changes Socially inappropriate behavior Flip beyond reasonable propriety
HUNTINGTON'S CHOREA				
Insight into the psychological deteriorative changes		Increasingly a problem as pathology progresses but without aphasia, agnosia, or apraxia	Choreiform movements Sloppy	Mood swings from apathy to agressive behavior Inappropriate behavior Despair about changes taking place Suicidal Decreased interest in job
WERNICKE-KORSAKOFF SYNDROME				
Cannot learn new information due to inability to retain facts	Alert	Suspended in time Recall limits to 2–3 min Extensive memory loss	Unsteady gait due to peripheral neuropathies	Communication impaired related to memory gaps Confabulation
VASCULAR DEMENTIA				
	Not affected	Cannot learn new material or recall previously learned; proceeds in a stepwise progression as ministrokes occur Does not handle new situations well	Deterioration of hygenic standards	Depression or pseudodepression

◆ Application of the Nursing Process to Clients With Cognitive Disorders

The nurse can facilitate recovery or improve the quality of life for a client with a cognitive disorder. The first step in determining treatment and nursing approaches for this client is a clinical screening for any treatable physical causes of the problem. This involves extensive history taking, physical examination, and laboratory workup. Laboratory and diagnostic evaluation often includes the tests listed in Table 27-3.

If the results of screening tests prove noncontributory, the physician, nurse, and other health care providers may look to other, more subjective factors. Is

Table 27-3

Screening Tests

Test	Clinical Importance
1. WBC with differential	1. Infection
2. Sedimentation rate	2. Infection or vasculitis
3. Urine examination and toxicology test	
a. Sugar and acetone	a. Diabetes
b. Leukocytes	b. Infection
c. Barbiturates and other toxic substances	c. Toxicity
d. Albumin	d. Renal failure
e. Porphyria screen	e. Renal failure
4. Serum tests	
a. Blood urea nitrogen	a. Renal failure
b. Creatinine	b. Renal failure
c. Sugar	c. Diabetes, hypoglycemia
d. T_3, T_4	d. Thyroid disease
e. Electrolytes	e. Evaluation for imbalance including Na^+, K^+, Ca^{2+}, Cl^-, PO_4 =, parathyroid-induced changes in calcium, phosphorus
f. Mg^+, Br^+	f. If available, bromides are still present in some common drugs and overuse may inadvertently lead to toxicity
g. Serum folate level	g. Nutritional problems, thiamine deficiency
h. SGOT, SGPT	h. Liver failure
i. VDRL	i. Syphilis
j. Drug levels—specific search for evidence of drugs—ETOH, etc.	j. Barbiturate, other drug overdose
5. Routine radiographs	
a. Chest	a. Infection, heart failure
b. Skull	b. Evidence of increased intracranial pressure, fractures, etc.
6. EEG	6. Ictal phenomenon
7. CT scan	7. Brain tumor, subdural hematoma, infection, hemorrhage
8. Spinal tap	8. Infection, hemorrhage
9. Invasive neuroradiologic procedures	9. Suspicion of tumors, vascular lesions, hydrocephalus

(From Staub R, Black F: Organic Brain Syndromes, pp 109–110. Philadelphia, FA Davis, 1981)

there pain? Is the client recovering from surgery? Is there inordinate stress and anxiety from personal losses? Is the client a victim of sleep and sensory deprivation or overload? Although the behavior seen with psychological stress is attributed to the dysfunction of the brain, removal, or at least amelioration, of the psychological factors may lessen the load to be handled by the dysfunctional brain.

ASSESSMENT

Nursing assessment focuses on the client's behavior (Box 27-6). The client's family is one of the most reliable sources of information because the client may not know when the behavior began or have insight into its sequential progression. The nurse gathers and compiles behavioral reports, because the client's disruptive behavior may at first be overlooked by the family or be regarded as an idiosyncrasy of age.

The nurse attempts to break down the component parts of the client's behavior and assess the deficits or intactness of each component. Intellectual or cognitive deficits may be assessed by using the various measurements listed in Table 27-4. The classic assessment tool used to assess intellectual or cognitive deficits is the short, portable mental status questionnaire (SPMSQ) developed by Pfeiffer (Box 27-7).

The examiner administering these tests can observe

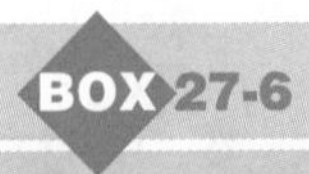

Assessment Guide

I. Subjective Data
   A. Behavioral changes (often asked of the family)
      1. Is there a change in behavior? If so,
         a. How does the present behavior differ from former behavior?
         b. When was this change in behavior first recognized?
   B. Emotional changes
      1. Are any of the following present?
         a. Depression
         b. Anxiety
         c. Paranoia
         d. Agitation
         e. Grandiosity
         f. Confabulation
      2. Does the client have insight into the fact that "things are not right"?
      3. Is the client complaining of many physical ailments for which there are no bases?
      4. Are certain previous personality traits becoming predominant or exaggerated?
   C. Social changes
      1. Is the client exhibiting embarrassingly loud and jocular behavior?
      2. Is there sexual acting-out beyond the bounds of propriety?
      3. Have the following developed?
         a. Short-temperedness
         b. Irritability
         c. Aggressiveness
      4. Is there an increasing inability to make social judgments?
   D. Intellectual behavior
      1. Has the ability to remember recent events decreased?
      2. Has the ability to problem solve decreased? (This might be especially apparent in the work or job area.)
      3. Do new environments or even old environments result in the client's disorientation?
      4. Is it difficult for the client to carry out complex motor skills? Do his or her efforts result in many errors?
      5. Are any of the following language problems present:
         a. Has the client's language changed?
         b. Does the client's language ramble and wander from the point of the conversation?
         c. Is the point of the conversation never clearly stated?
         d. Is there difficulty comprehending complex material?
         e. Does the client have trouble remembering names of people and objects?
         f. Does the client have difficulty writing?

II. Objective Observations
   A. Level of consciousness
      1. Is the client confused, sleepy, withdrawn, adynamic, apathetic?
   B. Appearance
      1. Is there decreased personal hygiene?
   C. Attention
      1. Does the client have decreased ability to repeat digits after the interviewer?
      2. Do other stimuli in the environment easily distract the client from the interviewer?
      3. Does the client focus on only one of the stimuli in the environment and is he unable to turn attention from the one stimulus?
   D. Language
      1. Outflow of words decreases.
      2. Patterns of repetitive, tangential, or concrete speech appear.
      3. Writing skills decrease more rapidly than the spoken word.
   E. Memory
      Tests client's ability to remember four unrelated words and recent events. (Confabulation and anger will often be used by the client to move the interviewer away from questions related to memory.)
   F. Constructional ability
      The client is instructed to copy a series of line drawings; the client is often unable to do this or the ability to do so will decline dramatically over a period of time.
   G. Cortical function
      1. The client's ability to perform arithmetic is faulty, reveals many errors
      2. Proverb interpretation—usually, the client will give only a concrete interpretation of the proverb.
      3. Similarities—The client will often deny similarities between two objects and give instead a concrete answer. For example, when asked, "What is the similarity between a tiger and a cat?" the client may reply, "One is small and one is large. There is no similarity."

Table 27-4

Testing for Cognitive Deficits

Focus of Test	Name of Test	What Is Measured	Analysis Potential
Intelligence, verbal performance	Wechsler Adult Intelligence Scale (WAIS)	Crystallized and fluid intelligence	Notes if client can pay attention and use memory
Memory	Wechsler Memory Scale-Revised California Verbal Learning Test		Alzheimer's Sensitive in early dementia If single finding, may indicate amnestic disorder
Language skills	Boston Diagnostic Aphasia Exam	Aphasia subtest—word finding ability—common in dementia	Alzheimer's Single finding may indicate focal deficit
Conceptualization	WAIS-R Similarities subtest	Abstract versus concrete thinking	
Visuospatial skills	Benton Visual Retention Test Block Design subtest of the WAIS-R		Alzheimer's
Attention	Digit Span subtest of the WAIS-R		Single finding may indicate delirium disorder, focal frontal lesion

(Compiled from Jutagir K, Peterson M: Psychological Aspects of Aging: When Does Memory Loss Signal Dementia? Geriatrics 49(3): 45–51, 1994)

the psychomotor skills used by the client during each test. The data substantiate problem areas when analyzed carefully, each finding in light of each other. The nurse observes and documents the client's *level of consciousness* and *sensorium.* The amount of stimulation required to elicit a response from the client is also assessed. This stimulation may range from simply calling the client's name in a normal tone of voice to shaking the client vigorously and shouting his or her name. *Attention span* may be simply appraised by asking the client to repeat six or seven digits forward, or to cross out all the a's in a paragraph the client is asked to read. Failure to perform tasks such as these indicates that the client is having difficulty concentrating.

Information concerning *perceptual* disorders may be gained by direct observation of the client's behavior and by asking about any strange or unusual feeling or sensory experiences that the client has mentioned. The family may also be able to contribute information about observing such behavior or hearing the client voluntarily express concerns about the bugs, roaches, and so forth that he or she sees.

Assessment includes evaluating the client's orientation to person, environment, time, and date. In doing so, the nurse must ask the questions in a way that does not embarrass the client who has enough intellectual function left to become insulted by the questions. The nurse should couch the questions in a conversational manner or be prepared to assuage the frustration or anger of the client. The client's family also should be questioned to ascertain if the client experiences the sundown effect.

Those living with or in daily contact with the client are able to provide much information concerning his or her ability to care for self and personal affairs. Social interaction between the family and the client should be observed and described; it will reveal many of the client's social assets and deficits.

The nurse spends time with the client to determine the quality of communication efforts. Many social skills remain long after intellectual deterioration occurs. When talking, people give many verbal cues to one another that indicate the proper response. For example, cues such as nodding and smiling indicate a positive atmosphere in which a reciprocal nod or smile is appropriate. However, this is an automatic, learned response, and the nurse needs to ask the client questions that solicit more than a yes or no answer.

The client's memory is also evaluated during the nursing assessment. Incidents evoking remote memory

BOX 27-7

Short, Portable Mental Status Questionnaire

Instructions: Ask question 1 through 10 in this list and record all answers. Ask question 4A only if patient does not have a telephone. Record total number of errors based on 10 questions.

+	−	
		1. What is the date today? ____________ Month Day Year
		2. What day of the week is it? ____________
		3. What is the name of this place? ____________
		4. What is your telephone number? ____________
		4A. What is your street address? ____________ (Ask only if patient does not have a telephone.)
		5. How old are you? ____________
		6. When were you born? ____________
		7. Who is the President of the U.S. now? ____________
		8. Who was President just before him? ____________
		9. What was your mother's maiden name? ____________
		10. Subtract 3 from 20 and keep subtracting 3 from each new number you get all the way down

For white subjects with at least some highschool education, but no more than high school education, the following criteria have been established:

0–2 errors	Intact intellectual functioning
3–4 errors	Mild intellectual impairment
5–7 errors	Moderate intellectual impairment
8–10 errors	Severe intellectual impairment

(Source: Pfeiffer E: A Short Portable Mental Status Questionnaire for the Assessment of Organic Brain Deficits in Elderly Patients. J Am Ger Soc 23:433–441)

are usually easy to elicit from the client. Recent memory may be assessed by evaluating the client's response to questions that ask for recall of the events of the previous day or week.

NURSING DIAGNOSIS

There are as many nursing diagnoses for the client with cognitive disorders as there are possibilities of symptoms. Although nursing diagnoses must reflect the uniqueness of each client, a plan of care might include some of the following:

1. Altered Thought Processes related to decreased ability to interpret external stimuli
2. Risk for Violence: Self-directed related to awareness of mental deterioration
3. Impaired Social Interaction related to inability to use effective communication
4. Dressing/Grooming Self Care Deficit related to deficit in motor skills that enable hygienic tasks to be accomplished
5. Powerlessness related to inability to halt the debilitating progress of the disorder or disease
6. Ineffective Family Coping: Disabling related to financial and spiritual bankruptcy by the relentlessness of the disease's or disorder's debilitating progress
7. Risk for Injury related to lack of retention of any memory for personal actions maintaining personal safety
8. Altered Role Performance related to inability to maintain mental acuity defined by role in work performance and family position

PLANNING

Developing the plan of care should involve members of the client's family, which may include the spouse and adult children. If the client's prognosis is continued degeneration, family participation becomes even more crucial as family members assume increasing responsibility for care.

The conflict and stress brought about by changes in family dynamics and the debilitating effects of the cognitive disorder compel those involved in planning care to include measures that will encourage family cohesiveness and stability. Discharge planning must be initiated early in the treatment process. It must be decided what responsibilities family members can assume and what relief people, such as neighbors, friends, and respite care providers, may be secured to prevent exhaustion of the future primary caregivers.

Goal Setting

The general goals of care and subsequent outcomes for the person with a cognitive disorder are threefold:

1. Goal 1: To eliminate the organic etiology, if possible
   Client outcome: The client will demonstrate no signs or symptoms originating from an active organic etiology and minimal residual symptoms from a formerly active organic etiology.
2. Goal 2: To prevent the acceleration of symptomatology
   Client outcome: The client will exhibit no or minimal increase in signs and symptoms.
3. Goal 3: To preserve the client's dignity
   Client outcome: The client will at all times command the respect of caretakers, family, and friends as a fellow human being.

These goals are facilitated by the following supportive goals and outcomes:

1. To maintain peak physical health, with the outcome that the client will demonstrate the highest level of health on the wellness continuum that he or she is capable of reaching
2. To promote a structured environment, with the outcome that the client will operate in an environment that is safe for decreasing mental and physical capabilities
3. To promote socialization, with the outcome that the client will continue to participate within the social context as faculties allow
4. To promote independent functioning, with the outcome that the client will actively care for self to the extent that mental and physical resources allow
5. To preserve the family unit, with the outcome that the family will continue to support the active participation of the client as a member and be supported in its efforts to maintain its normality by the cooperative efforts of the health team

INTERVENTION

General interventions for clients with cognitive disorders are presented. Nursing Care Plan 27-1 illustrates the nursing process for a client with Alzheimer's disease.

Maintaining Peak Physical Health

One of the most essential nursing actions for the client with a cognitive disorder is to facilitate optimal functioning by maintaining physical health. Because exogenous substances can initiate or exacerbate aberrant behavior, the nurse must be sensitive to the client's response to prescribed medications. Besides knowing the side effects and toxic reactions of the specific drugs the client is receiving, the nurse also must be alert to possible drug interactions.

The nurse also assesses the client daily for any symptoms of an ensuing physical disorder. Prompt recognition of symptoms and appropriate intervention may prevent acceleration of the client's existing mental dysfunction.

The nurse also attempts to minimize any sensory impairment. Poor vision necessitates well-fitting eye glasses that the client actually wears, not carelessly sets aside. Diminished hearing requires a hearing aid or giving louder, slower, uncomplicated instructions while standing directly in front of the client. The client may participate in activities but may require a slower pace or simpler instruction before the activity to allow sufficient time to compute the significance of the input from faulty sensory organs.

Structuring the Environment

The nurse may need to structure the client's immediate environment to increase or decease sensory input. When clients cannot tolerate the sensory level in their environment, they need to be moved to quieter areas or private rooms where environmental stimuli are at a level with which the client can cope and where they can rest or sleep. The nurse may place orientation clues in the environment; clocks, calendars, and seasonal pictures provide sensory input and can help maintain the client's orientation to time and place. The number of family members, friends, and hospital personnel entering the environment should be controlled to provide for stimulation with which the client can optimally cope. The people and objects within the environment should be as familiar to the client as possible. This means that the same hospital personnel need to care for the client on a consistent basis (Box 27-8).

The perceptual difficulties of hallucinations or illusions may be decreased simply by controlling the light in the environment. Light may easily eradicate the sundown effect. Any environmental hazards must be elim-

Nursing Care Plan 27-1

A Client With Alzheimer's Disease

Mr. B is an 83-year-old man with Alzheimer's disease who was admitted two months ago to a nursing home facility. He has had gradually increasing memory loss with loss of judgment over a 3 year period. His spouse describes that he has become increasingly childlike and easily angered.

Since admission to the nursing facility, he has not slept through the night. When he hears people talking in the hall, he becomes agitated. If left alone, he would wear pajamas all day and ignore hygienic needs. When staff try to assist him in daily care, his agitation escalates. When his schedule varies, he begins to pace the halls. At mealtimes he is overwhelmed by a variety of foods on his plate and subsequently his intake has decreased and his weight has dropped 20 lbs since admission.

Before retirement, Mr. B owned his own successful business. He had been actively enjoying his retirement until the symptoms of his dementia began to interfere with his daily activities. Presently his wife and children visit regularly but he does not consistently recognize them.

Nursing Diagnosis

Altered Nutrition: Less than body requirements related to inability to make decisions about which food to eat

Outcome

Client will demonstrate adequate nutritional status as evidenced by a weight gain of 1 pound/wk until normal weight is restored.

Intervention	Rationale
Place only one food and one utensil on the table at mealtime.	Limiting choices decreases frustration over food selection.
Don't comment or fuss over client's eating habits or responses during meals.	Stewing over his eating habits may increase his frustration and overload his executive functioning.
Weigh client every Monday before breakfast.	Weight changes are more likely noted on a weekly basis; weekly weighing de-emphasizes the problem.

Evaluation

Client gains 1 pound/week until a normal weight is reached and maintained.

Nursing Diagnosis

Ineffective Individual Coping related to over-response to stress

Outcome

Client will evidence fewer incidents of agitation.

Intervention	Rationale
Respond to the client calmly and gently.	Responding in a calm, gentle manner creates a safe environment and helps him mirror the behavior.
Determine the cause of the behavior and remove or modify the cause if possible. If precipitating factor is unavoidable, slow down the activity or reduce it into simple parts that are within client's capabilities.	If the object of agitation is removed, the job simplified, or the task is understood, the stress threshold of the client may be able to handle the remaining activities.

Evaluation

Client completes his tasks throughout the day with minimal agitation.

continued

Nursing Care Plan 27-1 (Continued)

Nursing Diagnosis

Sleep Pattern Disturbance related to confusion and misperception of environmental stimuli

Outcome

Client will re-establish regular sleep patterns as evidenced by sleeping an 8-hour period without awakening.

Intervention	Rationale
Place client in an uncluttered room.	Clutter lends itself to misinterpretation of the objects in the cluttered area.
Leave a night light on in his room.	Lighting the room enhances his ability to interpret his environment correctly.
Keep his important possessions where he can see them and let him keep these possessions on his person if necessary.	Letting him keep his possessions visible or on his person gives him a sense of security and reduces anxiety.
If medication is necessary to diminish sleep problems or agitation, administer a low dose.	Sleep deprivation can augment the metabolic disturbances within the brain to cause a delirium to be added onto the dementia.

Evaluation

Client sleeps 6–8 hours per night without awakening.

Nursing Diagnosis

Bathing/Grooming Self-care Deficit related inability to remember to bathe, dress daily

Outcome

Client will maintain a routine of self-care with minimal daily reminders and assistance.

Intervention	Rationale
Have one person help client with self-care and adhere to a regular schedule.	Consistency of routine carried out by one person lessens demands on executive functioning.
Minimize decisions the client must make (eg, appropriateness of clothing).	Minimal decision-making decreases frustration and dignity is maintained through appropriate dress.

Evaluation

Client participates in self-care with minimal assistance and lessened agitation.

inated. An agitated client may become panic stricken if medical safety devices are used to ensure safety. In this situation, the client might benefit from environmental structuring in which someone from the hospital or family remains with the client to prevent self-injury by such acts as climbing over the bed rails, pulling out tubes, or removing dressings.

Promoting Socialization

Promoting the client's socialization may be approached in various ways. The client who is exhibiting signs of fairly severe disorientation may benefit from reality orientation therapy. Through this technique, the nurse consistently bombards the client with four or five concrete reminders of who the client is, where

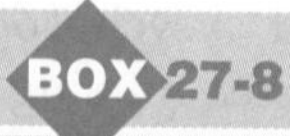

Therapeutic Dialogue: Reality Orientation—Presenting Concrete Information

Nurse: (Seated beside the client in her room, looking directly at her, with one of the nurse's hands touching the client's arm.) Good morning, Mrs. S. I see that you have just finished your bath.

Mrs. S.: (Nodding vigorously and smiling.) Yes, yes. (Pats the nurse's hand.)

Nurse: Mrs. S., it is 11:00 in the morning, so would you like to walk with me to the day room in this hospital to see the beautiful sunshine?

Mrs. S.: Yes, oh my yes.

Nurse: Mrs. S., because you are here in St. Luke's hospital, I will walk with you. It is such a pretty day outside. I want you to enjoy the sunshine before noontime when you will eat your lunch.

Mrs. S.: Yes dear. Oh my. (Remains sitting until the nurse stands and gently pulls upward on her arm and begins to walk with her to the door.)

Discussion

Often the client with a cognitive disorder retains impressive social skills even though she has lost cognitive capability to understand and orientation to person, time, and place.

In this dialogue, the nurse constantly reminds Mrs. S. who she is and where she is going. The nurse also reminds the client of the time through specific facts and references to the sunshine, lunch, and so on. All of which help orient Mrs. S. to time. Note that none of this interaction took place in a manner demeaning to the client. Particularly helpful during this conversation were the "signals" given to Mrs. S., by means of touch and body language that she should stand and walk. Without these signals, she would have understood less of the conversation.

he or she is, why he or she is here, and what is expected of him or her.[24] This reeducative program has come under scrutiny, because it does not consistently produce significant improvement in clients' mental status. Validation therapy may be an alternative approach in long-term facilities. Through validation therapy, psychiatric care attempts to identify the personal meaning of each situation for the client, then try to relate emotionally with the client in the context of that definition.[30]

The client can be included in group work to promote socialization. The group provides a safe, empathetic atmosphere in which clients may be motivated to use all faculties to their remaining potential.

Promoting Independent Functioning

The nurse promotes the client's independent functioning by maintaining peak physical health and by helping the client to accomplish the activities of daily living. Making the materials for daily care available and accessible, keeping the routine of care simple and consistent, and giving the client time to complete tasks that can be completed are supportive nursing actions.

Preserving the Family Unit

The nurse must not forget the importance of preserving the family unit. Discussing with the family ways in which relief may be provided by interested neighbors or by home health aides provides a respite for the family from the heavy responsibilities of full-time care for the client with a cognitive disorder. Day care for the client is one possibility that would allow family members to continue with their daily activities and responsibilities. Through day care, the spouse may be able to retain his or her job and income and have the energy to care for the client during evening and weekend hours. Some communities have overnight respite care to give the caregiver welcomed time alone. Family support groups and individual family counseling may help some families experiencing undue stress or having difficulty coping with the situation and its demands. One of the most effective nursing interventions is to educate the family members in the necessary skills and knowledge to give care to their loved one. Families are also empowered when the nurse can work with them to increase their problem-solving skills. Showing the family that they have some options and linking them up with community-based services are tremendous contributions of the nurse to the family that is trying hard to deal with their situation.[6] The family's stress and responses to a member with a cognitive mental disorder are discussed in Box 27-9.

EVALUATION

Because the client with a cognitive mental disorder is constantly changing, nursing actions must be regularly evaluated for their successful outcome and rel-

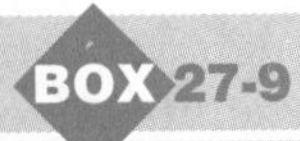

Alzheimer's Disease: Caring for Client and Family

The devastation of Alzheimer's disease is not limited to the client alone. Throughout the course of the disease, the client's family suffers greatly, both from the anguish of seeing the demise of their loved one and from the stress of caring for him or her. They often feel inept and have feelings of guilt. They worry about the relationship that they have with their loved one as the dynamics of that relationship change to caregiver and care receiver; they are anxious about long-term care issues and how to deal with the extended family and their own coping skills.[28]

The adversity encountered while caring for a person with Alzheimer's disease often produces major health problems in caregivers.[17] The nurse can help alleviate some of the family's difficulties by providing continuous education about the disease process and by assisting with problem solving of the situational difficulties and crises that arise.

Adult care centers in some communities may offer families the opportunity for a few hours of respite care. Relatives responsible for or actually administering care should be aware of helpful books, such as *The 36-Hour Day: A Guide to Caring for Persons with Alzheimer's Disease and Related Dementing Illnesses*[21] and *Understanding Alzheimer's Disease* (Aronson). They should also get in touch with the Alzheimer's Disease and Related Disorders Association (70 East Lake Street, Chicago, IL, 6061-5997; 1-800-621-0379). Alzheimer's disease support groups are found throughout the country in large and small communities. Family members can find the support group closest to them by calling the Alzheimer's Association Chapters, which are usually listed in the phone book; by calling the Alzheimer's Association toll-free telephone number (1-800-272-3900, fax: [312] 335-1110) for a Chapter referral; or by calling their Area Agency on Aging. Families may also receive the *Alzheimer's Association Newsletter* to keep abreast of developments in research, legislation, and techniques of care.

The nurse must remember that the family needs as much nursing care as does the victim of dementia, especially because the disease progresses in such an agonizingly slow manner. By providing emotional support and counseling and serving as a coordinator of available community resources, the nurse can significantly help relieve the stress on the family caregiver.

evance. The client's physical and psychosocial changes may make previously successful nursing efforts ineffectual. The nurse also realizes that when dealing with the degenerative aspects of cognitive disorders, success may be measured in terms of slowing down the process rather than stopping or curing the problem.

◆ The Nurse's Attitudes and Feelings

Working with clients who have cognitive disorders may be discouraging for the nurse. In certain situations, neither the institution nor the medical staff desire or are able to provide the supportive environment and milieu that the client needs. For example, the client with an acute episode of aberrant behavior may receive attention to physical needs only, and psychological needs are merely tolerated. The chronically deficient client may elicit pity from the staff, not the dynamic intervention that is reserved for the "curable" client. Such attitudes may pervade the environment in which the nurse works, making it difficult for the nurse's own feelings or philosophy to prevail.

Few clients have more intensive needs in physical and psychological realms than clients with cognitive disorders. These clients present a tremendous challenge for which nurses must draw on all of the resources available within them and available to them.

◆ Chapter Summary

This chapter discusses one of today's mushrooming problems, cognitive disorders. These disorders appear not only in the aging population, but in the general population as well and are becoming increasingly prominent in the health care scene. Some of the major emphases of this chapter are as follows:

1. The possible etiologies of cognitive disorders include primary brain disease, systemic disturbances, influences of exogenous substances, and withdrawal and residual effects of exogenous substances.
2. Aberrant behaviors associated with these disorders may include deficits in the sensorium, attention span, orientation, perception, and memory.
3. Symptoms of cognitive disorders may be approached in terms of acute onset and chronic progression.

4. Gathering and analyzing assessment data for a client with a cognitive disorder requires participation of family members or friends who have been in close contact with the client.
5. Goal setting for the client with an organic disorder focuses on eliminating the organic etiology, preventing acceleration of symptoms, and preserving dignity.
6. Specific nursing interventions strive to maintain the client's optimal physical health, structure the environment, promote socialization and independent functioning, and preserve the family unit.

Review Questions

1. What is the salient finding present in a client diagnosed with a cognitive mental disorder?
2. What are the main factors influencing the incidence and significance of most cognitive disorders?
3. What are the four general etiologies of cognitive disorders?
4. Which client would be most likely to exhibit a hyperalert as well as a hypoalert state?
   A. A client with Alzheimer's disease
   B. A client with Pick's disease
   C. A client with delirium tremors
   D. A client 18 hours post surgery

◆ References

1. Abraham I, Neundorfer M: Alzheimer's: A Decade of Progress, A Future of Nursing Challenges. Geriatr Nurs (May-June): 116–119, 1990
2. American Psychiatric Association: Diagnostic and Statistical Manual of Mental Disorders, 4th ed. Washington, DC, American Psychiatric Association, 1994
3. Breitner J, Welsh K: Diagnosis and Management of Memory Loss and Cognitive Disorders Among Elderly Persons. Psychiatric Services 46 (1): 29–35, 1995
4. Butler R, Ahronheim J, Fillit H, Rapoport S, Tatemichi T: Vascular Dementia: Stroke Prevention Takes on New Urgency. Geriatrics 49 (11): 32–42, 1993
5. Chipps E, Paulson G: Creutzfeldt-Jakob Disease: A Review. J Neurosci Nurs 26 (4): 219–223, 1994
6. Collins C, Given B, Given C: Interventions With Family Caregivers of Persons With Alzheimer's Disease. Nurs Clin North Am 29 (1): 195–207, 1994
7. Davis K, Powchik P: Tacrine. Lancet 345 (8950): 625–630, 1995
8. Foreman M: Complexities of Acute Confusion. Geriatr Nurs 11 (3):139–139, 1990
9. Gomez G, Gomez E: Delirium. Geriatr Nurs 8 (6): 330–332, 1987
10. Guze S: Acute Brain Syndrome. Hospital Medicine 13 (4): 63–69, 1977
11. Holt J: How to Help Confused Patients. Am J Nurs 32–36, 1993
12. Jackson L: A Predictive Test for Huntington's Disease: Recombinant DNA Technology and Implications for Nursing. J Neurosci Nurs 19 (5): 244–250, 1987
13. Jutagir R, Peterson M: Psychological Aspects of Aging: When Does Memory Loss Signal Dementia? Geriatrics 49 (3): 45–51, 1994
14. Katzman R: Early Detection of Senile Dementia. Hosp Pract 16 (June): 61–67, 1981
15. Kovach C, Stearns S: Understanding Huntington's Disease: An Overview of Symptomatology and Nursing Care. Geriatr Nurs 14 (5): 268–271, 1993
16. Lipowski Z: A New Look at Organic Brain Syndrome. Am J Psychiatry 137 (June): 674–677, 1980
17. Lipowski Z: Delirium in the Elderly Patient. N Engl J Med 320 (9): 578–582, 1989
18. Ludwig L: Acute Brain Failure in the Critically Ill Patient. Critical Care Nurse 9: 62, 1990
19. Lukasiewicz-Ferland P: When Your I.C.U. Patient Can't Sleep. Nursing 87 (November): 51–53, 1987
20. McKinney A: Appropriate Investigations of Stroke and Dementia. Geriatrics 36 (June): 41–48, 1981
21. Mace N, Rabins P: The 36-Hour Day: A Family Guide to Caring for Persons With Alzheimer's Disease and Related Dementing Illnesses (revised edition). Baltimore, Johns Hopkins University Press, 1991
22. Mantes J: A Nursing Protocol to Assess Causes of Delirium: Identifying Delirium in Nursing Home Residents. Journal of Gerontological Nursing 21 (2): 26–30, 1995
23. Morrison J: DSM IV Made Easy: The Clinicians Guide to Diagnosis. New York, The Guilford Press, 1995
24. Nursing Services, Tuscaloosa Veterans Administration Hospital: Guide for Reality Orientation. Tuscaloosa, AL, 1974
25. Rocca W: Frequency, Distribution, and Risk Factors for Alzheimer's Disease. Nurs Clin North Am 29 (1): 101–111, 1994
26. Scharre D, Mahler M: Parkinson's Disease: Making the Diagnosis, Selecting Drug Therapies. Geriatrics 49 (10): 14–23, 1994
27. Seltzer B, Sherwin I: Organic Brain Syndromes: An Empirical Study and Critical Review. Am J Psychiatry 135 (January): 13–20, 1978
28. Smith G, Smith M, Toseland R: Problems Identified by Family Caregivers in Counseling. Gerontologist 31 (1): 15–22, 1991
29. Staub R, Black F: Organic Brain Syndromes. Philadelphia, FA Davis, 1981
30. Stolley J: When Your Patient Has Alzheimer's Disease. Am J Nurs August: 34–40, 1994

31. Tueth M, Cheong J: Delirium: Diagnosis and Treatment in the Older Patient 48 (3): 75–80, 1993
32. Ugarriza D, Gray T: Alzheimer's Disease: Nursing Interventions for Clients and Caretakers. J Psychosoc Nurs 3 (10): 7–10, 1993
33. Weksler M: Alzheimer's Disease: How Research is Changing Primary Care Management. Geriatrics 49 (7): 47–51, 1994
34. Wells C: Chronic Brain Disease: An Overview. Am J Psychiatry 135 (January): 1–11, 1978
35. Wood J, Lantz, M: Alzheimer's Disease: How to Give and Monitor Tacrine Therapy. Geriatrics 50 (5): 50–53, 1995
36. Yi E, Abraham I, Holroyd S: Alzheimer's Disease and Nursing. Nurs Clin North Am 29 (1): 85–99, 1994

Personality Disorders

Judith A. Greene

28

Judge not, that ye be not judged. For what judgement ye judge, ye shall be judged: and with what measure ye mete, it shall be measured to you again. And why beholdest thou the mote that is in thy brother's eye, but considerest not the beam that is in thine own eye? Or how wilt thou say to thy brother, Let me pull out the mote out of thine eye; and behold, a beam is in thine own eye? Thou hypocrite, first cast out the beam out of thine eye; and then thou shalt see clearly to cast the mote out of thy brother's eye.

Matthew 7:1–5,
King James Bible

We live in what has become known as the age of narcissism.[7,8] *Narcissism, an exaggerated love for and overinvolvement with the self, stands in contrast to love for humanity. Given that many popular life philosophies advocate individual growth and survival at the expense of others, the term narcissism appropriately describes the current state of human society.*[7,8]

With this change in how people view themselves in relation to others, the incidence of psychiatric syndromes also has changed. Unlike the age of anxiety (1930s–1950s), when people succumbed to various neuroses (now called anxiety disorders), the age of narcissism is associated with an increased incidence of personality disorders.[7]

Although diagnostic criteria for personality disorders have undergone many changes, making it impossible to ascertain valid statistics regarding their actual incidence, experts agree that personality disorders constitute a significant psychiatric-mental health problem.[7,8,22,23]

Learning Objectives

On completion of this chapter, you should be able to accomplish the following:

1. *Define the terms personality and personality disorder.*
2. *Identify common characteristics of personality disorders.*
3. *Discuss perceptual, cognitive, affective, and behavioral disturbance; adaptation levels; and mental health-seeking behaviors of selected personality disorders.*
4. *Apply the nursing process to clients with personality disorders.*

◆ Personality and Personality Disorder Defined

Personality may be defined as the totality of a person's unique biopsychosocial and spiritual traits that consistently influence behavior. Personality is as indispensable to self-identity as is physical appearance. In fact, personality may be considered the psychological equivalent of physical appearance in that neither are amenable to more than minimal changes over time. An individual's personality may be adaptive or maladaptive. When a person's personality is maladaptive, the designation *personality disorder* is appropriately applied.

COMMON CHARACTERISTICS

Although several distinct types of personality disorder exist, the following characteristics are common to all of the disorders:

1. A deeply ingrained, inflexible, maladaptive response to anxiety
2. Maladaptation that is most apparent in an interpersonal or social context
3. The capacity to cause others to feel extreme irritation and annoyance
4. A self-centered, inflexible approach to work and interpersonal relationships[22]

Adjectives or descriptive phrases applicable to many people with personality disorders include the following: narcissistic, unempathetic, inordinate sense of entitlement, dependent, lack of self-insight while giving evidence of pseudo self-knowledge, unable to self-evaluate, cynical, pessimistic, depressed, subjective, lack of self-control, egocentric, selfish, lonely, immature, manipulative, aggressive, impulsive, hostile, and suspicious.[2,8,22] While these terms concretize to some extent the four characteristics associated with all personality disorders, they also indicate the severity of these disorders.

Personality disorders can occur in minimal, mild, moderate, or severe forms.[9,23] Whatever their classification, personality disorders pose a serious mental health problem in today's society. Box 28-1 provides the general Diagnostic and Statistical Manual of Mental Disorders, fourth edition (DSM-IV) diagnostic criteria for a personality disorder.

ETIOLOGY

Because diagnostic criteria for personality disorders have changed frequently, the precise etiology remains unverified. It is commonly believed that genetic, constitutional, maturational, and environmental factors play a part in their emergence.[23] The social fabric of today's world, with its emphasis on indulgences of all kinds, also is thought to play a major part in the development of some personality disorders.[7,8]

COURSE AND PROGNOSIS

Because little information is available about the prevalence of personality disorders, determining an accurate prognosis is difficult.[23] Based on reported clinical observations, the following outcomes are likely:

1. Personality disorders may become permanent and worsen with time.
2. Some people with personality disorders may mature and thereby develop more adaptive coping styles.
3. Others may drop out of treatment, thus preventing further follow-up of treatment outcome.
4. Many others with personality disorders may never seek mental health care and thus remain a totally unknown variable in the study of these disorders.[1,23]

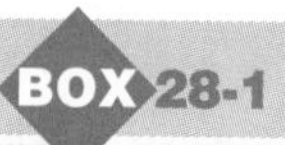

BOX 28-1 DSM-IV Diagnostic Criteria for a Personality Disorder

A. An enduring pattern of inner experience and behavior that deviates markedly from the expectations of the individual's culture. This pattern is manifested in two (or more) of the following areas:
   1. Cognition (ie, ways of perceiving and interpreting self, other people, and events)
   2. Affectivity (ie, the range, intensity, lability, and appropriateness of emotional response)
   3. Interpersonal functioning
   4. Impulse control

B. The enduring pattern is inflexible and pervasive across a broad range of personal and social situations.

C. The enduring pattern leads to clinically significant distress or impairment in social, occupational, or other important areas of functioning.

D. The pattern is stable and of long duration, and its onset can be traced back at least to adolescence or early adulthood.

E. The enduring pattern is not better accounted for as a manifestation or consequence of another mental disorder.

F. The enduring pattern is not due to the direct physiological effects of a substance (eg, a drug of abuse, a medication) or a general medical condition (eg, head trauma).

Application of the Nursing Process to Personality Disorders

ASSESSMENT

Perceptual, cognitive, affective, and behavioral disturbances accompany all of the personality disorders. The DSM-IV has grouped the personality disorders into three clusters according to descriptive similarities.[1] Cluster A, which includes paranoid, schizoid, and schizotypal personality disorders, represents individuals whose behavior is odd or eccentric. Cluster B includes antisocial, borderline, histrionic, and narcissistic personality disorders; individuals with these disorders often appear dramatic, emotional, or erratic. Cluster C, including avoidant, dependent, and obsessive-compulsive personality disorders, represents individuals with anxious or fearful behavior.[1]

Cluster A: Paranoid, Schizoid, and Schizotypal Personality Disorders

Paranoid Personality Disorder

The term *paranoid personality* applies to people who display pervasive and long-standing suspiciousness. This suspicious pattern affects perceptual, cognitive, affective, and behavioral functions in specific ways. Alterations in these functions reflect the great effort that these people must make to counter the anxiety they experience in everyday life. See Box 28-2 for DSM-IV criteria.

Perception. In people with paranoid personalities, perception is extremely acute, intense, and narrowly focused in search of "clues" or the "real" meaning behind others' behavior or life events in general. To a great extent, paranoid people perceive the world as being composed of clues to hidden or special messages; hence, they disregard or even disdain manifest reality. Moreover, they perceive unexpected or unpredictable events and behaviors as highly threatening.[19]

Paranoid people generally perceive others as dishonest, full of trickery, and out to undermine them.[1] Their extreme distrust of others stems largely from their distorted perception of self. They usually view themselves as self-sufficient, objective, rational, emotionally balanced, and very important.[11] This inflated view of self usually represents a defense against low self-esteem.

Cognition. The great perceptual distortion present in paranoid personality disorder significantly influences cognitive function. Cognitive disturbances may range from transient ideas of reference to overvalued ideas resembling delusions, in which they grossly misinterpret trivial events or achievements to fit their grandiose self-perceptions. These overvalued ideas may also be of a persecutory nature, in which they believe that others are being unduly critical or purposefully deceptive or

BOX 28-2

DSM-IV Diagnostic Criteria for Paranoid Personality Disorder

A. A pervasive distrust and suspiciousness of others such that their motives are interpreted as malevolent, beginning by early adulthood and present in a variety of contexts, as indicated by four (or more) of the following:
   1. Suspects, without sufficient basis, that others are exploiting, harming, or deceiving him or her
   2. Is preoccupied with unjustified doubts about the loyalty or trustworthiness of friends or associates
   3. Is reluctant to confide in others because of unwarranted fear that the information will be used maliciously against him or her
   4. Reads hidden demeaning or threatening meanings into benign remarks or events
   5. Persistently bears grudges (ie, is unforgiving of insults or slights)
   6. Perceives attacks on his or her character or reputation that are not apparent to others and is quick to react angrily or to counterattack
   7. Has recurrent suspicions, without cause, about fidelity of partner

B. Does not occur exclusively during the course of Schizophrenia, a Mood Disorder With Psychotic Features, or another Psychotic Disorder and is not due to the direct physiological effects of a general medical condition.

malicious toward them. Paranoid people are hypercritical of others and are prone to collect real or imagined injustices. Often they seek retribution for such injustices through the legal system. While these people criticize others freely, they regard criticism by others as signs of betrayal, jealousy, envy, or persecution.[1,11] Their cognitive function thus deals primarily with making the imagined real and the real invalid.

Affect. The paranoid person's affective domain reflects a lack of basic trust. Extreme suspiciousness, vigilant mistrust, guardedness, and hostility characterize this lack of basic trust. Other affective attributes include abrasive irritability, defensiveness, envy, jealousy, serious mindedness, and emotional coldness. Typically, paranoid people assume a callous, unsympathetic approach to others in an effort to purge themselves of any tendencies to experience humor or affectionate and tender feelings. Moreover, others' expressions of affection or tenderness likely will arouse fears of entrapment, deceit, and domination.[11] When confronted with humorous situations, they often react with anger, hostility, and extreme suspiciousness.

Paranoid people experience profound emotional constriction and are virtually unable to reach out or connect with other people in an emotional sense. Consequently, they experience little if any interpersonal or sensual pleasure. Furthermore, they must resort to fault finding and projecting their own shortcomings onto others to preserve their own sense of self-esteem.[19] Through projection and psychological and social withdrawal, they control their fears and anxieties. Their behavior patterns reflect these maladaptive approaches to anxiety control.

Behavior Patterns. Paranoid people appear hypervigilant, mobilized, and prepared for attack. Rarely do they seem relaxed or unguarded. For the most part, they remain coldly reserved and on the periphery of events, seldom mixing smoothly with people in social situations, instead remaining withdrawn, distant, and secretive. Because they lack the capacity for spontaneity and abandonment, their nonverbal behaviors appear very deliberate, tense, and at times, even rehearsed.[11,19]

Paranoid people often engage in verbal exchanges designed to test others' honesty. The nature and lengthiness of these interchanges may cause others to become quite exasperated and angry. Besides testing the trustworthiness of others, people with paranoid personalities also may display argumentative, contentious, intimidating, and cajoling verbal behaviors.[11] The content of their verbalization usually reflects themes of blame, deceit, control, persecution, and self-aggrandizement.[1]

Level of Adaptation. Most people with paranoid personalities experience lifelong effects of the disorder. In some, this disorder may precede the development of schizophrenia. In others, paranoid personality disorder may remit with maturity and reduction of life stressors.[22] Few people with paranoid personalities voluntarily seek mental health services. When they do appear for treatment, it usually is at the insistence of family members or associates.[11]

Individual rather than group psychotherapy is usually indicated.[22] Trust between client and therapist is the basis for other therapeutic techniques.[11] Genuineness, respect, courtesy, and a formal (instead of warm) approach facilitates the establishment of trust.[22] After trust is established, cognitive restructuring or psychoanalytic techniques may be beneficial.[10] Behavioristic techniques usually are contraindicated because of their intrusive nature.[22] Such therapeutic interventions stabilize, rather than change, the paranoid personality structure.[11]

Schizoid Personality Disorder

Socially detached, shy, and introverted people may be described as having *schizoid personality disorder.* This classification refers to people exhibiting perceptual, cognitive, affective, and behavioral patterns that fall within the more adaptive end of the schizophrenic spectrum.[22] This personality disorder differs from the schizotypal personality disorder in that the latter's symptomatology more closely resembles schizophrenia. In contrast to schizotypal and schizophrenic people, schizoid personalities do not demonstrate odd or eccentric perceptual, cognitive, and behavioral patterns.[22] See Box 28-3 for diagnostic criteria.

Perception. People with schizoid personalities exhibit a distorted pattern of perception, characterized by a reduced ability to attend, select, differentiate, and discriminate adequately between and among interpersonal and social sensory inputs. Consequently, they tend to blur or mix up these inputs, resulting in disorganized perceptual function. This perceptual dysfunction appears largely confined to interpersonal social contexts.[11] Because illusions and hallucinations do not occur as part of this dysfunction, these people remain able to recognize reality, despite their faulty interpersonal or social perception.

Cognition. The cognitive pattern of schizoid personality types is consistent with their perceptual style. With regard to interpersonal and social situations, schizoid people demonstrate vague, impoverished thought processes; that is, in the social realm, they possess little social intelligence.

These people are more apt to apply their cognitive abilities to mechanical problems, artistic pursuits, or metaphysical questions, and they sometimes excel in these areas.[16,17,22] Inanimate objects and ideas, instead of people, occupy the schizoid's intellectual pursuits.

Affect. Indifference characterizes the affect of the schizoid personality and manifests itself in various ways. These people seem indifferent to the thoughts and feelings of other people, appearing emotionally constricted, aloof, and inappropriately serious. Some clinicians believe that fear underlies this aloofness.[22] Even in the face of considerable provocation, these people rarely express anxiety, anger, or depression.[22] Although they seldom become emotionally involved with others, they invest emotionally in imaginary friends and in various cognitive activities.[22]

Behavior Patterns. Characteristic nonverbal and verbal behaviors reflect a socially detached life pattern that can be described as under-responsive. Prominent nonverbal behaviors include blank, affectless facial expression; inability to tolerate eye contact; lethargic, awkward body movements; social withdrawal and aloofness; and

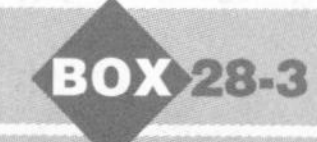

DSM-IV Diagnostic Criteria for Schizoid Personality Disorder

A. A pervasive pattern of detachment from social relationships and a restricted range of expression of emotions in interpersonal settings beginning by early adulthood and present in a variety of contexts, as indicated by four (or more) of the following:
   1. Neither desires nor enjoys close relationships, including with family
   2. Almost always chooses solitary activities
   3. Has little, if any, interest in having sexual experiences
   4. Takes pleasure in few, if any, activities
   5. Lacks close friends or confidants other than first-degree relatives
   6. Appears indifferent to the praise or criticism of others
   7. Shows emotional coldness, detachment, or flattened affectivity

B. Does not occur exclusively during the course of Schizophrenia, a Mood Disorder With Psychotic Features, another Psychotic Disorder, or a Pervasive Developmental Disorder and is not due to the direct physiological effects of a general medical condition.

unfashionable dress.[22] Often, schizoid people appear so drab and inconspicuous that they escape the attention of others altogether.

Verbally, these people are unproductive. Although speech is goal directed, verbal emissions are short and to the point. They avoid spontaneous conversation and usually remain silent.[22] Their slow, monotonous speech may contain an occasional odd metaphor or word selection.[11]

Level of Adaptation. People with schizoid personality types live out their lives in a socially detached way; they neither desire nor enjoy social interaction. They prefer to be alone and keep other people and life experience at arm's length.

Very few schizoid people ever seek mental health services. Their social isolation and indifference reduce their motivation for doing so. For those who do seek help, treatment is similar to that for paranoid personality disorder. Unlike paranoid people, schizoid people eventually may tolerate and even profit from group psychotherapy.[11,22]

Schizotypal Personality Disorder

A lifelong history of interpersonal deficiencies that severely limit the capacity for emotional closeness with others describes the *schizotypal personality disorder.*[10] People with this disorder are almost always friendless, anxious around strangers, and have a suspicious nature. These individuals appear odd and usually stand out in a bizarre way in a crowd.[1] Additionally, these individuals tend to gravitate toward cults and other extremist groups due to their eccentricities. See Box 28-4 for diagnostic criteria.[10]

Perception. Schizotypal personality disordered individuals perceive life, themselves, and others through a "bizarre" lens. Their distorted perceptual style often results in their claiming to have received special messages telepathically or through their "sixth sense."[1] In addition to these claims, the person with schizotypal personality disorder often repeats odd perceptual experiences, such as tuning in to the presence of a supernatural, celestial, or extraterrestrial entity.[1,10] Somatic illusions of strength or power associated with some unusual practice or consumption of a highly unconventional substance or diet may also be reported by the person with schizotypal personality.[10]

Cognition. The thought content and form of schizotypal personalities reflect their bizarre perceptual style. Their thought content centers around superstitions and weird, odd beliefs that are inconsistent with cultural norms.[1] Their thought form is odd, illogical, and loosely connected to reality.[1,10]

Affect. Emotionally, the schizotypal personality is often depressed, anxious, and suspicious.[1,10] Individuals with these personalities often experience strong feelings of alienation due to paranoid ideation or ideas of reference. Feelings of alienation in addition to their other eccentricities place schizotypal personalities at risk for recruitment to cults and other extremist groups of all kinds.[10] Overall, the affect of the schizotypal personality can be described as inappropriate or constricted.[1]

Behavior Patterns. The verbal and nonverbal behaviors of the schizotypal person reflect the perceptual and cognitive styles associated with this personality disorder. Nonverbally, the person with schizotypal personality disorder is withdrawn and eccentric and demonstrates a lack of social skills. The speech pattern of the schizotypal person is vague, circumstantial, tangential, and often metaphorical.[1] Additionally, the schizotypal personality often displays an impoverished vocabulary and unusual or inappropriate word usage. Their verbal content usually centers around fanatic, eccentric, or even racist beliefs.[10]

Level of Adaptation. Unlike the schizoid personality, people with schizotypal personalities are more likely to display eccentricities and bizarre behaviors.[1,10] Additionally, they appear to be at greater risk for developing transient psychotic states or full-blown schizophrenia. If schizophrenia develops, the schizotypal diagnosis is dropped. It is generally believed that schizophrenia should be suspected in people younger than 35 years with diagnosed schizotypal personality disorder.[10]

People with schizotypal personalties often seek mental health services for issues related to depression and alienation associated with paranoid ideations or ideas of reference. Supportive individual therapy of a nonexploratory nature is usually recommended for this personality disorder. Like people with paranoid personalities, those with schizotypal personalities experience group therapy as overly threatening and intrusive.[9]

Psychoeducational approaches, such as social skills training, may also be helpful in assisting the schizotypal personality to feel more comfortable with others. Additionally, some clinicians recommend low-dose antipsychotic medications, such as thiothixene (Navane) and perphenazine (Trilafon), to alleviate anxiety and cognitive symptoms displayed by schizotypal personalities.[10]

Cluster B: Antisocial, Borderline, Histrionic, and Narcissistic Personality Disorders

Antisocial Personality Disorder

The term *antisocial personality* refers to an aggressive behavioral pattern. This aggressive personality type is the acting out kind of person, "the adventurer," and the delinquent and criminal.[17] Although people with antisocial personalities use action as a primary form of expression, they also possess characteristic ways of per-

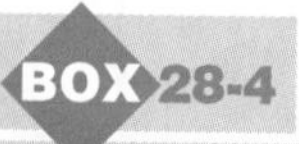

DSM-IV Diagnostic Criteria for Schizotypal Personality Disorder

A. A pervasive pattern of social and interpersonal deficits marked by acute discomfort with, and reduced capacity for, close relationships and by cognitive or perceptual distortions and eccentricities of behavior, beginning by early adulthood and present in a variety of contexts, as indicated by five (or more) of the following:
1. Ideas of reference (excluding delusions of reference)
2. Odd beliefs or magical thinking that influences behavior (eg, superstitiousness, belief in clairvoyance, telepathy, or "sixth sense"; in children and adolescents, bizarre fantasies or preoccupations)
3. Unusual perceptual experiences, including bodily illusions
4. Odd thinking and speech (eg, vague, circumstantial, metaphorical, overelaborate, or stereotyped)
5. Suspiciousness or paranoid ideation
6. Inappropriate or constricted affect
7. Behavior or appearance that is odd, eccentric, or peculiar
8. Lack of close friends or confidants other than first-degree relatives
9. Excessive social anxiety that does not diminish with familiarity; tends to be associated with paranoid fears rather than negative self-judgments

B. Does not occur exclusively during the course of Schizophrenia, a Mood Disorder With Psychotic Features, another Psychotic Disorder, or a Pervasive Developmental Disorder.

ceiving, thinking, and feeling. See Box 28-5 for diagnostic criteria.

Perception. Antisocial personalities perceive others and the world as hostile, harmful, and out to undermine them. Consequently, they expect to experience malice, humiliation, and betrayal at every turn.[11] Viewing the world and other people through such a hostile lens causes feelings of being continually threatened.

People with antisocial personalities view others as threats to their independence because they perceive themselves as superindependent people capable of negotiating life's demands alone.[11] More specifically, these people see themselves as assertive, self-sufficient, tough minded, competitive, powerful, and superior. Valuing these characteristics highly, they reject attributes associated with warmth, caring, or tenderheartedness in themselves and others.

Cognition. Their hostile perceptual style influences what antisocial personalities believe about themselves and others in drastic ways. To illustrate, the slogans "might makes right" and "beat the other guy to the punch" could serve as life mottoes for these people. More simply, antisocial people believe that human beings are basically evil; therefore, they are entitled to take a highly antagonistic stance toward other people and society in general. Holding these beliefs, they use their cognitive capacities for the most part, to design schemes, tactics, or strategies to outwit and punish their perceived adversaries. The terms rigid, devious, and cunning describe the cognitive style of these people.[10,11]

Affect. Affectively, antisocial people appear hostile, punitive, and vengeful.[1] Because these people project their own malevolent attributes onto others, they mistrust others—especially those who display warm, caring, or tender behaviors, who are seen as being insincere, deceitful, and out to undermine them.[11]

Antisocial people also experience anxiety, particularly when they cannot control or get rid of people or situations perceived as threatening.[11] To reduce anxiety and increase feelings of power and control, they act out in various ways.

Behavior Patterns. Behavioral manifestations of antisocial personality disorder reflect the characteristic perceptual, cognitive, and affective patterns. Nonverbally, antisocial people appear cold, callous, and insensitive to others' feelings and values. Although they periodically may display gracious, cheerful, and socially clever behaviors, they express neither warmth nor compassion toward others.[11]

Because these people become easily bored, restless, and frustrated when faced with the tedium of day-to-day routines and responsibilities, they often impulsively

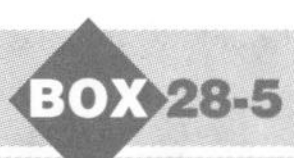

DSM-IV Diagnostic Criteria for Antisocial Personality Disorder

A. There is a pervasive pattern of disregard for and violation of the rights of others from age 15 years, as indicated by three (or more) of the following:
   1. Failure to conform to social norms with respect to lawful behaviors as indicated by repeatedly performing acts that are grounds for arrest
   2. Deceitfulness, as indicated by repeated lying, use of aliases, or conning others for personal profit or pleasure
   3. Impulsivity or failure to plan ahead
   4. Irritability and aggressiveness, (ie, repeated physical fights or assaults)
   5. Reckless disregard for safety of self or others
   6. Consistent irresponsibility, as indicated by repeated failure to sustain consistent work behavior or honor financial obligations
   7. Lack of remorse, as indicated by being indifferent to or rationalizing having hurt, mistreated, or stolen from another

B. The individual is at least 18 years old.

C. There is evidence of Conduct Disorder with onset before 15 years.

D. The occurrence of antisocial behavior is not exclusively during the course of Schizophrenia or a Manic Episode.

seek thrills and dangers to buffer these feelings. Examples of such acting-out behaviors include aggressive sexual behavior, vandalism, fighting, dangerous sports, outbursts of explosive anger, substance abuse, and exploitation of others.[22]

Verbal behaviors reflecting the antisocial personality style include derogating, humiliating, belligerent verbalizations directed to or about people perceived as threatening; vicious argumentation and insults; and other forms of violent, verbal abuse. Such verbal behaviors betray these people's tendency to become furious and vindictive when faced with threats to their power and control over others. That is, their first inclination is to attack the perceived threat by resorting to demeaning, violent, or controlling behavior.[11,14,23]

Although most antisocial people manifest abrasive, rude, or callous behavior, some are capable of sensitively detecting the subtleties of human interaction.[10] This ability, however, is not actually empathy because there is an absence of caring and concern. More specifically, while these people are keenly aware of the moods and feelings of others, they use this awareness to manipulate, exploit, and control others. In short, antisocial personalities use verbal and nonverbal behaviors to accrue power and independence and to cope with anxiety.

Level of Adaptation. At one time, the term antisocial personality primarily suggested criminal and delinquent behaviors.[14,20] More recently, clinicians have come to the realization that the prison population represents only a small proportion of these people. Actually, many of these people receive societal reinforcement and reward for their tough, competitive approach to life and find socially valued positions in business, politics, or the military. However, many find their place in society as harsh, abusive parents or spouses; manipulative and exploitative clergy; or vengeful administrators, bosses, or teachers.[11]

In any case, antisocial people seldom seek mental health services. Even if they do so, they are unlikely to make significant progress in the direction of adaptive mental health.

Borderline Personality Disorder

People with *borderline personality disorder* exhibit a cross-section of almost all the perceptual, cognitive, affective, and behavioral disturbances present in the other personality disorders. In many ways, borderline personality disorder corresponds to the infantile personality described by Ruesch.[16,17] These people typically cannot tolerate anxiety and use the major maladaptive coping behaviors—avoidance, withdrawal, acting out, and psychosomatization—to defend themselves against it. See Box 28-6 for diagnostic criteria.

Perception. An outstanding feature of the borderline personality type's perceptual pattern is the tendency to view other people in either-or categories, for example, as either all good or all bad or kind, rewarding, and supportive or hateful, distant, and punitive.[1,9,11,22] This tendency to pigeonhole people into all

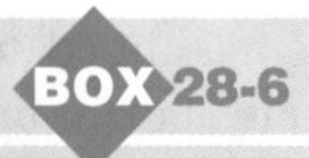

DSM-IV Diagnostic Criteria for Borderline Personality Disorder

A pervasive pattern of instability of interpersonal relationships, self-image, and affects and marked impulsivity beginning by early adulthood and present in a variety of contexts, as indicated by five (or more) of the following:

1. Frantic efforts to avoid real or imagined abandonment.
2. A pattern of unstable and intense interpersonal relationships characterized by alternating between extremes of idealization and devaluation
3. Identity disturbance: markedly and persistently unstable self-image or sense of self
4. Impulsivity in at least two areas that are potentially self-damaging (eg, spending, sex, substance abuse, reckless driving, binge eating)
5. Recurrent suicidal behavior, gestures, or threats or self-mutilating behavior
6. Affective instability due to a marked reactivity of mood (eg, intense episodic dysphoria, irritability, or anxiety usually lasting a few hours and only rarely more than a few days)
7. Chronic feelings of emptiness
8. Inappropriate, intense anger or difficulty controlling anger (eg, frequent displays of temper, constant anger, recurrent physical fights)
9. Transient, stress-related paranoid ideation or severe dissociative symptoms

good or all bad categories is called *splitting*.[22] As mentioned later, this phenomenon also occurs in the narcissistic personality disorder (idealization alternating with devaluation).[1]

These people's self-perceptions also are distorted. Often they lack a clear, internal picture or image of who they are as individuals. Consequently, borderline personalities often suffer identity disturbances with regard to self-image, sexual orientation, and social and occupational roles.[22]

Cognition. The perceptual distortion evident in borderline personality disorder significantly affects cognitive function. Because these people tend to perceive others in narrow, rigid ways, their cognitive function is altered. Holding diametrically opposed and rapidly shifting beliefs about the "goodness" or "badness" of others contributes to an almost constant state of cognitive confusion.[11] The lack of a clear self-perception results in a confused self-concept.

People with borderline personalities also manifest cognitive dysfunction in that they fail to learn from life experiences.[11] For this reason, they continue to repeat their mistakes. Their ability to problem solve—that is, to cope adaptively with anxiety—is seriously impaired.

Affect. Affective instability, marked by shifts from normal mood to anger or depression with the return to normal mood often within only a few hours, is a cardinal sign of borderline personality disorder.[11] Another striking feature is intensity of affect.[9] Anger, loneliness, depression, emptiness, impatience, self-pity, low self-esteem, and deficient self-confidence are some of the emotions that these people experience intensely and erratically.[2,3] They may experience fears of loss and abandonment and intense dependency longings and feelings of entitlement to special care or privileges.[1] Furthermore, when authority figures do not provide immediate relief for their uncomfortable feelings, these people may become enraged, hostile, and jealous.[9]

Subjectively, these people report feeling scattered, unintegrated, and incapable of following chosen pursuits and principles.[11] Instead, they depend on others to give their lives direction and meaning. Thus, the borderline personality type may be described as having an external locus of control. In this sense, the borderline personality type bears an exaggerated resemblance to Reisman's "other-directed person" and as such, stands as a tragic caricature of the average person in today's society.[15]

Behavior Patterns. The behavior of those with borderline personalities dramatically reflects the perceptual, cognitive, and affective disturbances associated with this disorder. Nonverbally, these people display their changeable and intense affect through such impulsive behaviors as extravagant spending, sexual promiscuity, hyperingestion of food and mood-altering substances, and sometimes, antisocial behaviors, such as lying and stealing.[1,11] During stressful periods, they commonly exhibit self-mutilating behaviors.[1-3] To a great extent, whimsical or rageful acting out characterizes the nonverbal behavior of borderline personalities.

Characteristic verbal behaviors are self-critical, demanding, whining, threatening, manipulative, argumentative, complaining, ingratiating, and blaming.[11] Periodically, these people even become verbally abusive to others.[3]

These verbal and nonverbal behaviors anger others. Often, others feel imposed on or manipulated by the person with borderline personality disorder and may want to retaliate with punishment. The characteristic verbal and nonverbal expression of intense emotions also tends to arouse feelings of fear in others. Sometimes families, friends, and associates actually may fear for their safety. However, borderline people seldom become physically assaultive.[3]

Level of Adaptation. The life histories of people with borderline personalities reveal a series of beginnings and endings. Numerous intense interpersonal relationships, checkered school and work records, and drastic lifestyle changes reflect the person's overall unstable pattern. Getting into and out of difficulty becomes a way of life for these people; consequently, they seldom realize their full potential. Some even may succumb periodically to brief psychotic episodes.[1] Their major strength lies in their ability to recruit sufficient interpersonal or social support to make another beginning.[11]

Many people with borderline personality disorder seek mental health care services. Commonly, they present with symptoms of depression, psychosis, or suicidal crisis. Short-term hospitalization may be needed in these instances. Treatment is aimed at reducing the presenting symptoms. Because borderline personality disorder is a deeply ingrained pattern, it resists treatment and requires intensive and prolonged psychotherapy to effect behavioral changes.[3,8,11]

Histrionic Personality Disorder

Perception. People with *histrionic personalities* tend to perceive others, the world, and especially themselves through a dramatic, imaginative lens. They focus on novel, exciting stimuli and become easily bored. Their perception is impressionistic, and they are quite suggestible. Histrionic personalities are virtually unable to focus on or deal with details and facts. See Box 28-7 for diagnostic criteria.[10]

Cognition. Cognition in the histrionic personality reflects an impressionistic, superficial mindset. Moreover, individuals with this disorder lack an interest in intellectual achievement or analytical pursuits.[10] Histrionic personalities are therefore more concerned with impressions than facts and have considerable difficulty with problem solving.

Affect. Underlying the histrionic personality type's impressionistic, superficial mindset is a basically shallow and rapidly shifting emotionality that spills out onto others in the immediate environment in an effort to become the center of attention. In fact, histrionic personalities become emotionally uncomfortable in situations in which they are unable to capture the attention of others. Because these individuals have deep feelings of helplessness and dependence, they require constant reassurance and affirmation.[10]

BOX 28-7

DSM-IV Diagnostic Criteria for Histrionic Personality Disorder

A pervasive pattern of excessive emotionality and attention seeking, beginning by early adulthood and present in a variety of contexts, as indicated by five (or more) of the following:

1. Is uncomfortable when he or she is not the center of attention
2. Interaction with others often characterized by inappropriate sexually seductive or provocative behavior
3. Displays rapidly shifting and shallow expression of emotions
4. Consistently uses physical appearance to draw attention to self
5. Has a style of speech that is excessively impressionistic and lacking in detail
6. Shows self-dramatization, theatricality, and exaggerated expression of emotion
7. Is suggestible (ie, easily influenced by others of circumstances)
8. Considers relationships to be more intimate than they actually are

Behavior Patterns. The histrionic personality type's verbal behavior reflects the disorder's characteristic perception, thoughts, and feelings. The person displays a speech style that is excessively impressionistic and lacking in detail. The content of verbalizations commonly centers on self-dramatizations and exaggerations designed to draw attention to the self.[1] Nonverbally, the histrionic personality displays theatrics and often behaves seductively in an effort to control others, gain attention, or enter into dependent relationships.[1] Often, these individuals present an overall behavioral pattern of vitality and charm that initially may be appealing. Later, the initial charm gives way to emotional excitability, irrational outbursts, and temper tantrums. Interpersonally, histrionic personalities often inaccurately assess relationships as being more intimate than they actually are and consequently, experience unhappiness and dissatisfaction when their expectations are not met.[10]

Level of Adaptation. Histrionic people usually report their subjective distress in global generalities. They rarely exhibit insight regarding the origins of their distress.[10] Moreover, these individuals seem relatively unaware of their behaviors and how they affect others in their immediate environment.

Although histrionic personalities often complain and overdramatize their difficulties, they do not seek adaptive solutions through problem solving and learning. Rather, these people often attempt to manipulate their family members and friends by making suicidal threats, gestures, and attempts. To histrionic people, the solution to life's problems lies in their ability to control others and enter into dependent relationships in which others are forced or manipulated to meet their needs. Additionally, these individuals use sexual and romantic fantasy and sexually provocative behavior to cope and gain needed satisfaction. Because their sexuality is often constricted and immature, they often experience dissatisfaction and unhappiness.[10]

Treatment of individuals with histrionic personality disorder presents a difficult challenge. Traditionally, psychoanalytic therapy has been used to treat individuals with this disorder. Additionally, supportive therapy emphasizing a problem-solving approach or cognitive techniques is used to assist histrionic personalities to cope more effectively with their distorted thinking and excessive emotional outpouring.[10] Because substance abuse often accompanies this disorder, addiction counseling may also be indicated.

Narcissistic Personality Disorder

Perception. Narcissistic personalities perceive themselves through the lens of grandiosity. Specifically, this grandiosity takes the form of an exaggerated sense of self-importance or uniqueness.[1] Other people often view the narcissistic personality as "conceited." Viewing themselves through this lens of grandiosity results in narcissistic personalities overestimating their accomplishments and talents and their failures.[10] In short, the narcissistic personality insists on viewing the self as godlike and incapable of common human frailties and mistakes. See Box 28-8 for diagnostic criteria.

Cognition. Cognitively, the narcissist is preoccupied with fantasies and dreams of brilliance, success, beauty, wealth, and other such ideals. Additionally, this personality disorder believes that he or she is special and unique and thus deserving of only the best in terms of associates and social status. Narcissists are also prejoccupied with their physical appearance and social standing.[10]

Affect. Emotionally, the narcissist craves attention and universal admiration and praise. Behind this requirement for excessive attention and admiration is a profound sense of low self-esteem that results in the narcissist's intolerance to criticism and rejection. Feeling states aroused by criticism include rage, anger, humiliation, negativism, and depression.[10] Selfishness, disdain, envy, and jealousy also occur in the narcissist when he or she is faced with criticism or frustration in achieving goals.[1]

Behavioral Disturbance. Because narcissists are self-centered and selfish, they produce interpersonal difficulties in all social contexts. These difficulties arise from the narcissist's tendency to act with a sense of entitlement in which unrealistic expectations for compliance with his or her wishes are placed on others. Because narcissistic personalities lack empathy, as evidenced by their unwillingness or inability to identify with the feelings and needs of others, they relate to people as if they were their personal servants. Additionally, narcissists engage alternately in idealization and devaluation of their associates. This tendency to idealize or worship others in one instance only to despise them moments later is called splitting.[10]

Level of Adaptation. Individuals with narcissistic personality disorder infrequently seek treatment because they consider themselves perfect. If they seek treatment, it is usually because they have become depressed or developed a physical condition that threatens their grandiosity. Treatment of narcissistic personalities focuses on respecting their need for an exaggerated sense of self-importance while gently assisting them to place this need into perspective. Long-term psychotherapy is recommended for these individuals, even though the probability of achieving significant change is considered minimal.[10]

Cluster C: Avoidant, Dependent, and Obsessive-Compulsive Personality Disorders

Avoidant Personality Disorder

The term *avoidant personality disorder* is relatively new in psychiatric literature. In fact, this category was new in DSM-III.[1] To date, this diagnosis is seldom applied in clinical practice and appears uncommon compared

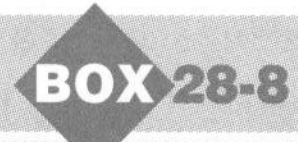

DSM-IV Diagnostic Criteria for Narcissistic Personality Disorder

A pervasive pattern of grandiosity (in fantasy or behavior), need for admiration, and lack of empathy, beginning by early adulthood and present in a variety of contexts, as indicated by five (or more) of the following:

1. Has a grandiose sense of self-importance (eg, exaggerates achievements and talents, expects to be recognized as superior without commensurate achievements)
2. Is preoccupied with fantasies of unlimited success, power, brilliance, beauty, or ideal love
3. Believes that he or she is "special" and unique and can only be understood by, or should associate with, other special or high-status people (or institutions)
4. Requires excessive admiration
5. Has a sense of entitlement (ie, unreasonable expectations of favorable treatment or automatic compliance with his or her expectations)
6. Is interpersonally exploitative (ie, takes advantage of others to achieve his or her own ends)
7. Lacks empathy; is unwilling to recognize or identify with the feelings and needs of others
8. Is often envious of others or believes that others envy him or her
9. Shows arrogant, haughty behaviors or attitudes

with other personality disorders. See Box 28-9 for diagnostic criteria.[10]

Perception. People with avoidant personalities tend to view the world and other people as rejecting. Similarly, they view themselves as worthy of the rejection of others.[10] Thus, the person with avoidant personality views life through the "lens of rejection."

Cognition. Viewing life through the lens of rejection, thought processes are concerned primarily with devising ways of avoiding disapproval and gaining ap-

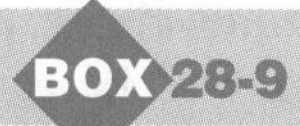

DSM-IV Diagnostic Criteria for Avoidant Personality Disorder

A pervasive pattern of social inhibition, feelings of inadequacy, and hypersensitivity to negative evaluation, beginning by early adulthood and present in a variety of contexts, as indicated by four (or more) of the following:

1. Avoids occupational activities that involve significant interpersonal contact because of fears of criticism, disapproval, or rejection
2. Is unwilling to get involved with people unless certain of being liked
3. Shows restraint in intimate relationships; fears being shamed or ridiculed
4. Is preoccupied with being criticized or rejected in social situations
5. Is inhibited in new interpersonal situations because of feelings of inadequacy
6. Views self as socially inept, personally unappealing, or inferior to others
7. Is unusually reluctant to take personal risks or to engage in any new activities because they may prove embarrassing

proval. Despite being convinced of their inferiority, avoidant personalities intensely desire to relate to other people.[1,10]

Affect. The individual with avoidant personality is painfully shy and hypersensitive to criticism and rejection. The person will become involved with others only when acceptance is virtually guaranteed. Once involved with another, the person with avoidant personality remains inhibited and restrained for fear of embarrassment, ridicule, or shame. The avoidant personality's low self-esteem coupled with an intense desire for affection and acceptance often produces anxiety, frustration, and anger in this individual.[1,10]

Behavior Patterns. Like the schizoid personality, the person with avoidant personality is a loner. The individual with avoidant personality, unlike the schizoid personality, however, wants to develop relationships with others.[10] Despite an intense desire for friends, the person with avoidant personality is retiring in social situations. Often, the avoidant personality is overly ingratiating in an attempt to escape criticism or negative social evaluation.[10]

Furthermore, the avoidant personality disordered person avoids occupational and recreational activities that involve a high degree of interpersonal contact to escape possible humiliation or disapproval. While most people with avoidant personality disorder may also be diagnosed with social phobia, the majority of people with social phobia do not qualify for the diagnosis of avoidant personality disorder.[10] That is, avoidant personality disorder pervades *all* social situations, while social phobia is confined to specific situations (eg, public speaking or eating in public).

Level of Adaptation. Individuals with avoidant personality disorders seldom seek mental health services. Many people with this disorder are able to marry and work. When they do seek assistance from mental health professionals, it is usually for anxiety, depression, or substance abuse associated with loss of their support systems.[10]

Dependent Personality Disorder

Perception. Individuals with *dependent personality disorder* view themselves as virtually helpless and incapable of self-care. Perceiving themselves in this manner and others as their source of support, dependent personalities require the advice and care of others to function in everyday life. See Box 28-10 for diagnostic criteria.[1,5]

Cognition. In keeping with these perceptions, the dependent personality has difficulty making routine decisions without an excessive amount of advice and reassurance from others. Believing that their own cognitive abilities and judgment are lacking, people with dependent personalities have difficulty initiating and completing projects.[1,5,10]

Affect. The individual with dependent personality has an excessive fear of abandonment and separation. Consequently, people with this disorder experience intense anxiety when thrust into independent or leadership positions. If forced to be alone, individuals with dependent personality disorder experience feelings of discomfort and helplessness. Typically, people with this disorder lack self-confidence and often have unrealistic preoccupation and worry about losing the people on whom they desperately depend.[10]

Behavior Patterns. Individuals with dependent personalities behave in a passive, submissive, clinging manner, thereby allowing others to assume responsibility for major areas of their lives. Because they fear abandonment, these individuals have great difficulty expressing disagreement with others. Those with dependent personalities will go to extreme measures to obtain nurturance and support from others, including volunteering for unpleasant tasks and in some instances, even tolerating substantial physical or emotional abuse. If these individuals lose someone on whom they depend, they will urgently seek out another to provide their required care and support.[1,10]

Level of Adaptation. Dependent personality disordered people seldom if ever seek mental health services for dependency; they do, however, often seek the assistance of mental health professionals when they lose those on whom they depend. Because these individuals dread autonomy, they become subordinate to and dependent on others. Seemingly, they prefer to be other-reliant rather than self-reliant.[5,10]

Individuals with this disorder are at increased risk for other psychiatric complications. Agoraphobia, generalized anxiety disorder, major depressive disorder, and substance abuse may occur concomitantly with dependent personality disorder.[10]

Treatment of individuals with dependent personality disorder may involve psychochemotherapy, psychodynamic psychotherapy, supportive group therapy, and assertiveness training. The selection of appropriate treatment modalities is based on the extent to which the individual is psychologically minded and capable of tolerating firm limits regarding contact with the therapist between scheduled appointments[10] (Nursing Care Plan 28-1).

Obsessive-Compulsive Personality Disorder

Perception. Perceptual disturbances associated with *obsessive-compulsive personality disorder* include inattention to new facts or different viewpoints, sharp focus on selected details, and inability to focus on casual or peripheral details.[1] In short, individuals with this disorder perceive the parts while missing the "big picture." See Box 28-11 for diagnostic criteria.

Cognition. This narrow perceptual focus leads to

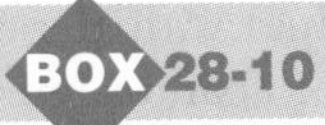

BOX 28-10

DSM-IV Diagnostic Criteria for Dependent Personality Disorder

A pervasive and excessive need to be taken care of that leads to submissive and clinging behavior and fears of separation, beginning by early adulthood and present in a variety of contexts, as indicated by five (or more) of the following

1. Has difficulty making everyday decisions without an excessive amount of advice and reassurance from others
2. Needs others to assume responsibility for most major areas of his or her life
3. Has difficulty expressing disagreement with others because of fear of loss of support or approval. **Note:** Do not include realistic fears of retribution.
4. Has difficulty initiating projects or doing things on his or her own; lacks self-confidence in judgment or abilities rather than motivation or energy
5. Goes to excessive lengths to obtain nurturance and support from others, to the point of volunteering to do things that are unpleasant
6. Feels uncomfortable or helpless when alone because of exaggerated fears of being unable to care for himself or herself
7. Urgently seeks another relationship as a source of care and support when a close relationship ends
8. Is unrealistically preoccupied with fears of being left to take care of himself or herself

various cognitive disturbances. Intellectual rigidity, or the inability to voluntarily shift attention and concentration to another topic, is prominent in the obsessive-compulsive personality.[19] The associated cognitive content usually centers around rules, standards, or codes of a moralistic or legalistic nature.[11] Consequently, the obsessive-compulsive personality is often described as dogmatic.

Affect. The obsessive-compulsive personality's narrow, yet tenaciously sharp perceptual focus also reflects an underlying affective disturbance. Anxiety and indecision lie at the heart of this disturbance. Specifically, the person with obsessive-compulsive personality experiences anxiety concerning the ability to control various desirable, but forbidden, emotions and impulses. Moralistic or legalistic injunctions defend the obsessive-compulsive personality against those feelings and impulses.[1,11] Thus, the person avoids experiencing anxiety by tenaciously clinging to a set of fixed beliefs or injunctions.

Emotional constriction, evidenced by a lack of humor, affection, lust, or frivolity, occurs as an outgrowth of this concentrated focus on rules and regulations and represents another feature of the affective disturbance. Also, others' whimsical or frivolous behavior often precipitates feelings of resentment and contempt in the person with an obsessive-compulsive personality.[19]

Behavioral Disturbance. Behavioral disturbances exhibited by people with obsessive-compulsive personalities include inflexible stubbornness; blind conformity and obedience; excessive prudence, neatness, and cleanliness; and undue preoccupation with work, efficiency, and productivity.[1,11] In interpersonal relationships, obsessive-compulsive personalities show little ability to give and take. Instead, these people insist on doing things the "right" way, that is, their way.[22] Issues of control and dominance take precedence over issues of human care and concern. These people often are perceived as cold, self-centered, and demanding. Because they often display verbal and nonverbal disapproval of people whose behavior departs from their standards, these perceptions have some grounding in reality.[19]

Additionally, people with obsessive-compulsive personalities engage in various behaviors aimed at convincing others to conform to their personal rules and regulations. This need to control others stems from an unconscious battle to control the self.[19] In other words, the person with obsessive-compulsive personality seeks to control the self through controlling others.

Level of Adaptation. Despite the perceptual, cognitive, affective, and behavioral disturbances, obsessive-compulsive personality disorder is adaptive and even rewarded in some occupational settings. Thus, affected people rarely are viewed as mentally ill.[11] At worst, they

Nursing Care Plan 28-1

The Client With Dependent Personality Disorder

Mrs. D, age 35 years, came to a psychiatric clinic for an evaluation. She was tearful and demanded help with "getting my husband back." She explained that her husband had left her, "running away with his secretary" and taking their life savings with him. As the interview progressed, Mrs. D became increasingly distressed, clinging dependently to the therapist and exclaiming, "I'll kill myself if you don't help me get my husband back."

Mrs. D was admitted to the crisis stabilization unit to insure her safety and avoid an unnecessary and expensive hospitalization. She disrupted the entire unit by clinging to personnel and demanding their constant assistance and direction. She repeatedly said, "Tell me what to do! I don't know what to do!"

The psychiatric nurse formulated a care plan to help stabilize this client.

Nursing Diagnosis

Ineffective individual coping related to extremely dependent behavior secondary to abandonment by husband

Outcome

Client will display no clinging or demanding behavior, engage in appropriate self-care, and voice no suicidal threats when demands for assistance are not met.

Intervention	Rationale
Assist client to identify others on whom she relies besides estranged spouse; limit the frequency of demands placed on staff.	Client is assisted to use problem-solving to identify other social/emotional supports and to manage her own emotions.
Direct client to pursue constructive, independent action and present reality about her ability to care for herself.	Pointing out reality about her self-care abilities promotes independence in self-care.
Present reality that no one can force her spouse to return to her. Do not bargain about her unrealistic demands.	This information reinforces that neither she nor others can force her spouse to meet her dependency needs.
Provide environmental security and protection to prevent suicide attempts.	Milieu of the crisis stabilization unit implements safety measures to protect client from self-harm.
Point out client strengths, positive aspects of independent thinking, feeling and acting, and any signs of client's beginning acceptance of her loss.	Reinforcing client strengths and progress encourages her to confront the reality of her situation.
Help client locate community resources to follow-up on an out patient basis.	After effective use of crisis stabilization services, client is ready to continue working on her independence and recovery.

Evaluation

Client displays independent decision-making and self-care behavior, without signs of self-harm, and is discharged within 15 hours.

are considered obstinate and boring; at best they are seen as ideal, efficient workers.

Moreover, people with obsessive-compulsive personalities are not drawn to seek therapy, which would necessitate change. Because change is threatening, these people usually seek therapy only if they experience unanticipated stress that overwhelms their coping mechanisms.[11] When people with obsessive-compulsive personalities do seek treatment, they commonly present with psychophysiological discomforts, anxiety, sexual problems, exhaustion, depression, or substance abuse.[11,12,23] Treatment, therefore, centers

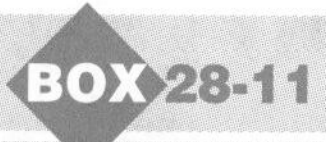

BOX 28-11

DSM-IV Diagnostic Criteria for Obsessive-Compulsive Personality Disorder

A pervasive pattern of preoccupation with orderliness, perfectionism, and mental and interpersonal control at the expense of flexibility, openness,and efficiency, beginning by early adulthood and present in a variety of contexts, as indicated by four (or more) of the following:

1. Is preoccupied with details, rules, lists, order, organization, or schedules to the extent that the major point of the activity is lost
2. Shows perfectionism that interferes with task completion (eg, is unable to complete a project because his or her own overly strict standards are not met)
3. Is excessively devoted to work and productivity to the exclusion of leisure activities and friendship (not accounted for by obvious economic necessity)
4. Is overconscientious, scrupulous, and inflexible about matters of morality, ethics, or values (not accounted for by cultural or religious identification)
5. Is unable to discard worn out or worthless objects even when they have no sentimental value
6. Is reluctant to delegate tasks or to work with others unless they submit to exactly his or her way of doing things
7. Adopts a miserly spending style toward both self and others; money is viewed as something to be hoarded for future catastrophes
8. Shows rigidity and stubbornness

around reducing or controlling the presenting symptoms rather than dealing with the obsessive-compulsive disorder itself.

Behavior Patterns Common to all Personality Disorders

Several behavior patterns are common to personality disorders with different diagnostic labels.[23] These include the following:

1. Splitting: The inability to evaluate and then synthesize and accept the imperfections of significant others both past and present. Instead, many individuals with personality disorders tend to divide individuals into all good or all bad categories.
2. Projection: The attribution of one's own feelings and experiences onto others. Additionally, personality disordered individuals resort to excessive fault finding, criticism, and confrontation to reduce their own feelings of inadequacy.
3. Passive-aggression: The tendency to turn anger against the self in a provocative manner with the underlying motive of forcing others to comply with their wishes and needs.[23] This tendency is behaviorally expressed through such acts as wrist cutting, nonlethal drug overdoses, and eating disorders. Eating disorders often seen in personality disordered individuals include obesity, anorexia nervosa, and bulimia nervosa.[4]
4. Acting out: The direct behavioral expression of a wish or conflict that allows the individual to avoid the conscious experience of the thoughts and emotions accompanying it
5. Narcissism: The tendency to perceive the self as all powerful and important and therefore entitled to criticize and belittle others. This individual often gives the impression of being vain and arrogant.
6. Dependency: The expression of incessant, unrealistic wishes, wants, and needs in a demanding manner, while at the same time, strenuously denying dependent behavior
7. No-win relationship style: The tendency to seek out relationships that offer a promise of something for nothing. Individuals manifesting this behavior thus feel entitled to take without giving and usually find themselves in relationships that are difficult to end.[23]

Because clients with personality disorders display these behavioral characteristics, they are often labeled as crocks, grumps, complainers, and manipulators. Nurses and other mental health personnel need to remember that personality disordered individuals suffer greatly and need careful assessments and well-planned and executed treatment plans.

NURSING DIAGNOSIS

Because clients with personality disorders demonstrate distinct disturbances associated with perceptual, cognitive, affective, and behavioral functioning, nursing diagnoses should target particular areas of dysfunction. Nursing diagnoses can be classified as follows:

1. Perceptual disturbances
   a. Ineffective Individual Coping due to use of splitting
   b. Body Image Disturbance related to eating disorders
   c. Body Image Disturbance related to gender confusion
2. Cognitive disturbances
   a. Decisional Conflict related to unclear life goals or ineffective problem-solving skills
   b. Impaired Thought Processes related to substance abuse
   c. Personal Identity Disturbance due to social withdrawal
3. Affective disturbances
   a. Ineffective Individual Coping related to labile affect
   b. Ineffective Individual Coping related to depression
   c. Ineffective Individual Coping related to suspiciousness
   d. Powerlessness related to extreme dependency needs
4. Behavioral disturbances
   a. Social Isolation related to suspiciousness of others
   b. Impaired Verbal Communication related to social withdrawal
   c. Noncompliance with medication regimen related to manipulative behavior

PLANNING AND IMPLEMENTATION

Planning and implementing of nursing care for personality disordered clients is one of the greatest challenges in psychiatric-mental health nursing. These clients inevitably trigger a negative counter-transference in therapists and other health care providers. The associated behavior patterns are not only annoying, but also difficult to change. Consequently, nurses and other mental health personnel often become irritated, frustrated, and rejecting while working with these clients.

Self-Awareness

To plan and implement effective care for personality disordered clients, the nurse needs to develop a high degree of self-awareness. Nurses and other mental health care providers often experience emotional reactions to these clients indicative of negative counter-transference phenomena, such as anger toward the client, defensiveness, wanting to control and dominate the client, excessive preoccupation with the client, and becoming frustrated, confused, and unable to concentrate during interactions with the client.[22] Learning to work through these phenomena requires that the nurse be able to tolerate and accept these feelings as natural reactions to personality disordered clients and at the same time to refrain from acting on these feelings. Discussing emotional reactions to these clients with a knowledgeable and trusted nurse colleague can increase the nurse's self-awareness and emotional control.

Trust Development

Because many personality disordered clients tend to mistrust others, the nurse needs to exercise special care to establish trust. A straightforward, matter-of-fact approach, as opposed to an overly warm approach, is indicated when working with these clients. Punctuality, honesty, respect, and genuineness also add significantly to trust formation.

In verbal interactions with personality disordered clients, the nurse should avoid interpreting the client's behavior, because mistrustful clients tend to view interpretations as intrusive and controlling. Instead, the nurse should use open-ended questions designed to assist these clients to focus on their behavior and its consequences. The nurse also must maintain congruence between verbal and nonverbal behaviors; incongruent behavior by the nurse often causes these clients to become more suspicious.[22] Some clients may attempt to use such discrepancies to manipulate the nurse and other health care providers.

Counter-projection

When working with a suspicious personality disordered client who uses projection extensively, the nurse needs to avoid interjecting doubt into the client's assertions. To dispute the client merely reinforces and increases the use of projection. Instead, the nurse needs to acknowledge that the client's assertions are within the realm of possibility, if not probability. The nurse can then use empathy techniques to encourage the client to talk about real feelings or motives, even though they are attributed to others rather than to the self (Box

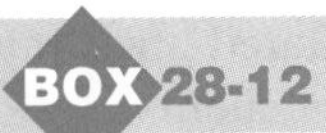

Therapeutic Dialogue: Using Counter-projection

Mr. Barton has been hospitalized for a slight head injury due to a fall at home. From the outset of hospitalization, he has asserted that someone tampered with his stepladder, causing his fall. He later informs his nurse that be believes his wife's lover had secretly entered their home and tampered with the ladder. All diagnostic tests with regard to his mild head injury are negative; there is no organic factor accounting for his paranoid thoughts. Moreover, his wife informs the nurse that she has no lover. She does report, however, that Mr. Barton has always been jealous of her and is very suspicious of others. He has had several disputes and grievances with former employees, whom he had accused of undermining his authority and position. She also states that he has threatened her with physical abuse.

The psychiatric liaison nurse is asked to assess Mr. Barton for possible transfer to the psychiatric-mental health services offered by the hospital. After several sessions with Mr. Barton, the nurse decides to use counter-projection in an effort to gain his trust and willingness to seek treatment.

Nurse: How do you feel when you say that your wife's lover is responsible for your falling from the ladder?

Client: (With a look of distrust.) What do you mean? He is crazy and will do anything to get me out of the picture so he can be with her.

Nurse: That's a scary, frightening thought. (Stated with empathy.) Why do you think he'd be so desperate to have your wife?

Client: He's jealous of me and wants to humiliate me. The best way to do that would be through my wife.

Nurse: You're a successful man and can take pride in your accomplishments, and you can find the inner resources to help stay on top of this situation with some assistance. You and I can agree that it's important that you not let this situation weaken your position.

Client: Yes. I'm a strong man, but sometimes I get worried about my marriage and my business. Sometimes I think my wife and employees might try to make a fool out of me—like if I lose control and hurt someone or destroy the business I've spent so long to build. I need help, but I know what is best.

Nurse: I can understand your concern about getting the help you need and want to handle your problems.

Client: Well, I don't want to hurt anyone or what I've accomplished, but I've got all these troublemakers at work to handle, plus my wife, I'm going to have to do something. (When the nurse empathizes with the client and suggests their collaboration, Mr. Barton reveals his fear of losing control.)

Nurse: May I tell you about some services offered here that might help you decide how you can best cope with your situation so you can stay on top of it? (The nurse uses a matter-of-fact and respectful approach to avoid triggering distrust or insulting a client who is obviously paranoid and narcissistic.)

Client: Yes.

By using the above approaches, the nurse is able to engage Mr. Barton in a therapeutic pact and gain his cooperation in exploring mental health treatment.

28-12). By using empathy rather than confrontation, trust is promoted, which eventually may lead to the client revealing emotions and feared impulses.[23]

Time Out

Breaking off interactions or postponing the next interaction is called taking time out and may be useful for clients who refuse to help themselves or use passive-aggressive tactics to gain attention or sympathy.[23] It can break the pattern of struggle whereby the client attempts to force the nurse to do all the work during therapy. Additionally, this technique can underscore the point that passive-aggressive techniques result in less, not more, attention.[23] An extra benefit of this technique is that it gives the nurse time to become more self-aware and emotionally controlled (Box 28-13).

Confrontation

Confrontation may be necessary to work effectively with some personality disordered clients who attempt to use manipulation.[22] Pointing out a client's problematic behavior may assist the client to become more self-aware. Keys to effective confrontation include the following:

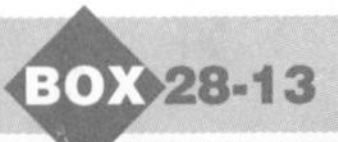

Therapeutic Dialogue: Using Time Out

A psychiatric nurse has been having daily one-to-one sessions with Ms. Samson. This client is diagnosed as having a narcissistic personality disorder and has a history of lashing out angrily in an attempt to devalue others. Ms. Samson has been late to meals, group therapy, and activities. She now has been late for her session with the nurse.

Nurse: (In a neutral tone of voice.) I notice that you seem to have some difficulty getting to therapy today.

Client: So, I think I'm doing you a favor just to be here. (Her face reddens, and she holds her head and torso in an arrogant almost haughty posture.)

Nurse: (Remains silent, because further comments would possibly be interpreted as defensiveness.)

Client: What's wrong with me marching to the beat of my own drummer?

Nurse: Being right or wrong has nothing to do with your punctuality. The unit rules that I, other staff, and clients agree to follow state that everyone will do their best to be on time for all therapies and activities.

Client: I suppose you think I'm just another client. Well, do I have news for you. I'm not, and you need to act accordingly. (Her voice volume increases, and she steps up closer to the nurse.)

Nurse: From your voice tone and facial expression, I can see that you and I aren't accomplishing anything worthwhile. I'm not going to pursue this with you any further. Perhaps, later when you and I are less emotional, we can try again. (She calls time out to avoid further verbal abuse from the client and to allow both of them to regain their composure.)

1. Pointing out the behavior as soon as possible after its occurrence
2. Being specific when describing the behavior
3. Using a nonaccusatory, nonjudgmental, matter-of-fact manner
4. Focusing on the client's actual behavior rather than on the client's explanation of it

Confrontation should occur in a setting in which the client feels safe and supported. The nurse must exercise sound and sensitive judgment when planning and implementing confrontations (Box 28-14). A trusting relationship between the nurse and client is a prerequisite.

Limit Setting

A client's manipulative, dependent, and acting-out behaviors may necessitate the use of limit setting. The nurse must remember that limit setting includes more than merely telling a client to stop a particular behavior. Specifically, limit setting involves the following:

1. Identifying the behavior that the client needs to control
2. Offering an appropriate, alternate behavior for the client to pursue
3. Anticipating that the client will test nurses to determine if they will back down
4. Remaining steadfast and consistent in the use of limit setting

Limit setting must be applied sensitively and judiciously to ensure effectiveness. Vacillation and backing down after setting limits with a client seriously jeopardize the development and maintenance of a trusting nurse–client relationship (Box 28-15).

Setting limits with clients can pose significant problems for nurses who lack maturity, self-confidence, and the ability to control their own anger and acting-out tendencies. Similarly, nurses who meet their own emotional needs by seeking approval and affection from clients are unable to set limits effectively. Effective limit setting requires clinical skill and personal maturity.

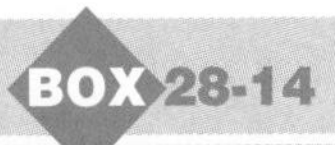

Therapeutic Dialogue: Using Confrontation

Mr. Samuels has been receiving partial hospitalization treatment for alcohol abuse. In addition, Mr. Samuels displays some behaviors associated with borderline personality disorder, such as erratic and intense moodiness, dependence, hyperingestion of alcohol, and splitting. Despite Mr. Samuels' tendency to split staff into two groups, "the good guys and the bad guys," he has come to trust his nurse therapist, Mr. Brown.

When Mr. Brown noticed that Mr. Samuels had missed attending the partial hospitalization treatment program for substance abuse the previous day, he decided to confront Mr. Samuels after conferring with the other treatment team members.

Nurse: I noticed that you were absent yesterday and did not notify us in advance of your absence.

Client: (In a whining tone.) I guess I didn't think all of you would notice.

Nurse: Why would you think that?

Client: I've got to start looking for another job.

Nurse: I was trying to speak with you about your absence yesterday, and you started talking about getting a job. (He refocuses client on the topic of his behavior—not showing up for treatment.)

Client: (Sounding somewhat defensive and irritable.) Really? I'm just worried about not having a job. Besides what difference does it make to you? After all, this place has already got its money for my treatment.

Nurse: I don't know whether it makes a difference or not. I do know that you have a serious illness, alcoholism, and that your physical health and occupational success have suffered in the past due to your alcohol abuse. (He points out the effects of the client's behavior.)

Client: Yeah, so I've drunk too much in the past; I'm not going to anymore, so don't accuse me of being drunk yesterday and laying out. (The client is loud and angry as he makes this statement.)

Nurse: (He remains silent. Further talking would merely repeat what he has already said. The nurse also needs the opportunity to deal with his own feelings about having been verbally attacked in an angry manner)

Client: Yeah, so I had a drink yesterday. So what?

Nurse: What are you going to do about it? (The nurse places the responsibility for the client's behavior onto the client.)

Client: I don't know. Maybe I need more help than I've been willing to admit.

The goal of this confrontation is to increase Mr. Samuels' awareness regarding the effects of his noncompliance with attendance to partial hospitalization for alcohol abuse.

Other Approaches

The nurse can enhance therapeutic effectiveness for personality disordered clients by following these guidelines:

1. Require the client to be responsible for his or her own behavior; blaming or punishing the client is seldom, if ever, effective.
2. Avoid assuming responsibility for the client's behavior; more specifically, do not attempt to rescue the client or encourage dependency.
3. Encourage the client's involvement in appropriate self-help groups, such as Alcoholics Anonymous, Narcotics Anonymous, Emotions Anonymous, or Overeaters Anonymous. Such involvement assists the client to offer appropriate help to others who may be more needy.

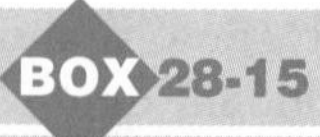

Therapeutic Dialogue: Using Limit Setting

Ms. Masters has been recently admitted to a day treatment program for eating disorders. She is 5 ft, 9 in tall, and weighed 190 lb on admission to the day treatment program. Having attended the day treatment program for 2 weeks, she now weighs 200 lb. Ms. Masters expresses disbelief that she could have gained 10 lb in 2 weeks. Her nurse therapist, however, has noticed that Ms. Masters often has been seen by other staff and clients retreating to a secluded area of the facility to eat high-calorie foods in private.

Client: (Eating a candy bar and chips in the lobby of the facility.)

Nurse: I've noticed that you often come here to eat food not allowed in the treatment area. I'm also aware that you have continued to gain weight. (The nurse points out the behavior that the client needs to control in a neutral, nonaccusatory manner.)

Client: I feel just awful. I used to eat to make myself feel better. Now, eating just makes me feel worse. What should I do? (appeals to nurse to assume responsibility for her behavior.)

Nurse: What do you want to do? (Responds in a way to assist client to retain responsibility for self.)

Client: Find something else to make me feel better that won't hurt me.

Nurse: In the past, can you recall anything else that has helped you feel less anxious and better about yourself?

Client: Talking with someone who cares and understands.

Nurse: Well, what about the next time you feel the urge to eat food not allowed on your diet, you talk to an understanding person here or if you are at home, call your Overeaters Anonymous sponsor?

Client: Yes, yes. I'll try that.

Two days later, the nurse again finds Ms. Masters in the lobby eating a cake. The nurse is not surprised, having expected the client to test the limit set.

Nurse: (Firmly yet good naturedly.) I thought you decided to seek comfort from talking to someone you trust rather than by eating. I expected you would really stick to that decision.

Client: This is the first time I've done this, and, you can see I've only had a bite. I guess I just really wanted to know that you really meant what you said.

Nurse: Yes. I meant what I said. I'm also confident that you can do what you said you wanted to do. (Remains consistent and steadfast.)

4. Present the idea that behavioral change is within the realm of possibility rather than demanding behavioral change.
5. Ask questions that assist the client to think through actual or intended behaviors. Gaining the ability to predict behavioral consequences in advance of behavior promotes more healthful adaptation.
6. Behave as naturally as possible to promote trust development.
7. Avoid requesting or recommending the use of psychotropic medications routinely, because these drugs cannot alter personality structure.[23]

EVALUATION

The nursing care administered to personality disordered clients cannot be evaluated solely on the basis of achieved client outcomes. Despite effective care, these clients may not improve to any great extent. Thus, other criteria must be used to measure the quality of nursing care. For instance, the extent to which nurses identify their own counter-transference reactions and successfully work through them is one important way of measuring effective clinical performance. The effectiveness with which nurses set realistic limits is another. Most important in the evaluation process is the extent to which nurses grow in terms of their own emotional maturity and objectivity in attempting to provide professional nursing care to difficult and often uncooperative clients.

◆ Chapter Summary

This chapter presents the concepts of personality and personality disorder. These concepts provide the necessary background for discussing the perceptual, cognitive, affective, and behavioral disturbances evident in the obsessive-compulsive, histrionic, narcissistic, antisocial, paranoid, schizoid, and borderline disordered personality disorders. Major points of the chapter include the following:

1. Maladaptive personality patterns or styles may be described as personality disorders.
2. The behavior of people with personality disorders is often narcissistic, dependent, depressed, egocentric, immature, hostile, and manipulative.
3. Paranoid personalities display pervasive suspiciousness and cognitive disturbances ranging from ideas of reference to highly valued ideas.
4. Schizoid personality disorder is marked by social withdrawal and extremely shy behavior, impoverished thought processes, indifference, and underresponsiveness.
5. The individual with schizotypal personality disorder speaks and behaves in an "odd" manner; this individual is often superstitious, believes in telepathy, and is at risk for gravitating toward extremist groups.
6. Antisocial personality disorder is characterized by hostility, antagonism, punitiveness, mistrust, callousness, and insensitivity.
7. The person with borderline personality disorder uses many maladaptive patterns to avoid anxiety: splitting, avoidance, withdrawal, acting out, and psychosomatization.
8. The person with histrionic personality disorder perceives the world and the self through the lens of drama and imagination, is attention seeking, is often sexually provocative and impressionistic, is prone to exaggerated expressions of emotion, and is unable or unwilling to deal with facts.
9. Narcissistic personality disordered individuals typically perceive the world through the lens of grandiosity and are preoccupied with fantasies of unlimited success, beauty, power, and other such ideals while lacking emotional depth or the capacity to empathize with others.
10. People with avoidant personality disorder have a pervasive fear of *all* social situations, especially fearing negative social evaluations.
11. Dependent personality disordered individuals behave in a passive, clinging manner and allow others to assume responsibility for major areas of their lives; these individuals will urgently seek to replace someone on whom they depended and then lost.
12. Obsessive-compulsive personality disorder is marked by narrow perceptual focus, intellectual rigidity, anxiety and indecision, lack of mirth, inflexible stubbornness, and attempts to control others.
13. Nursing care of personality disordered clients requires nurses to develop a high degree of self-awareness, personal maturity, and clinical skill.

Review Questions

1. Which of the following statements most accurately reflects the personality disordered individual's approach to seeking mental health care?
   A. Help-seeking for self
   B. Help-rejecting for self
   C. Help-rejecting for other
   D. Help-seeking for other and self
2. Which of the following statements best describes the individual with an obsessive-compulsive personality disorder?
   A. The individual experiences recurrent obsessions or compulsions.
   B. The individual experiences symptoms as threatening.
   C. The individual does not experience the symptoms as distressful.
   D. The individual experiences life fully from a broad perspective.
3. Which of the following does *not* describe borderline personality disorder?
   A. Either-or, black and white thinking
   B. Clear internal picture or image of who they are
   C. Narrow, rigid perception
   D. Affective instability and recurrent suicidal or self-mutilating behavior

◆ References

1. American Psychiatric Association: Diagnostic and Statistical Manual of Mental Disorders, 4th ed. Washington, DC, American Psychiatric Association, 1994
2. Chessick R: The Borderline Patient. In Arieti A (ed):

American Handbook of Psychiatry, vol 3, 2d ed, pp 808–819. New York, Basic Books, 1975.

3. Dubovsky S: Psychotherapeutics in Primary Care. New York, Grune & Stratton, 1981
4. Herzog D: Advances in Psychiatry: Focus on Eating Disorders. New York, Park Row, 1987
5. Johnson S: Character Styles. New York, WW Norton, 1994
6. Kernberg O: Internal World and External Reality. New York, Jason Aronson, 1980
7. Lasch C: The Culture of Narcissism. New York, WW Norton, 1978
8. Marin P: The New Narcissism. Harper's (October): 45–56, 1975
9. Masterson J: Psychotherapy of the Borderline Adult. New York, Brunner/Mazel, 1976
10. Maxmen J, Ward N: Essential Psychopathology and Its Treatment, 2d ed, Revised for DSM-IV. New York, WW Norton, 1995
11. Millon T: Disorder of Personality. New York, John Wiley & Sons, 1981
12. Parsons R, Wicks R (eds): Passive-Aggressiveness: Therapy and Practice. New York, Brunner/Mazel, 1983
13. Peck S: People of the Lie. New York, Simon & Schuster, 1983
14. Rappaport J: Antisocial Behavior. In Arieti S (ed): American Handbook of Psychiatry, vol 3, 2d ed, pp 253–269. New York, Basic Books, 1975
15. Reisman D: The Lonely Crowd. New Haven, Yale University Press, 1961
16. Ruesch J: Disturbed Communication. New York, WW Norton, 1957
17. Ruesch J: Therapeutic Communication. New York, WW Norton, 1973
18. Salzman L: Other Characteristic-Personality Syndromes: Schizoid, Inadequate, Passive-Aggressive, Paranoid, Dependent. In Arieti S (ed): American Handbook of Psychiatry, vol 3, 2d ed, pp 224–234. New York, Basic Books, 1975
19. Shapiro D: Neurotic Styles. New York, Basic Books, 1975
20. Stanton A: Personality Disorders. In Nicholi A Jr. (ed): The Harvard Guide to Modern Psychiatry, pp 283–295. Cambridge, MA, Belknap Press of Harvard University Press, 1978
21. Tupin J, Halbrich U, Pena J (eds): Transient Psychosis: Diagnosis, Management, and Evaluation. New York, Brunner/Mazel, 1984
22. Vaillant G, Perry J: Personality Disorders. In Kaplan H, Freeman A, Sadock B (eds): Comprehensive Textbook of Psychiatry III, vol 2, 3d ed, pp 1562–1590. Baltimore, William & Wilkins, 1980
23. Vaillant G, Perry J: Personality Disorders. In Kaplan H, Freeman A, Sadock B (eds): Comprehensive Textbook of Psychiatry, 4th ed, pp 958–986. Baltimore, Williams & Wilkins, 1985

Depressive and Bipolar Disorders

Nancy Kupper

29

Mysterious and in ways that are totally remote from normal experience, the gray drizzle of horror induced by depression take on the gravity of physical pain.

William Styron,
Darkness Visible, A Memoir of Madness

Perhaps more than any other response to stress, disturbances of mood or affect illustrate that human feeling and behaviors exist on a continuum with no clear demarcation between "normal" and "abnormal" or between health and illness. This chapter focuses on the feelings, thought, behaviors, and physical states that characterize people with depressive and bipolar disorders. The overview of depressed and manic behavior discusses the incidence, possible causes, and types or diagnostic categories used to facilitate the care and treatment of clients with depressive and bipolar disorders. A major emphasis is the application of the nursing process—assessment, nursing diagnosis, planning, implementation, and evaluation—to these clients and their families.

Learning Objectives

On completion of this chapter, you should be able to accomplish the following:

1. *Compare biological and psychosocial theories on the etiology of depressive and bipolar disorders.*
2. *Contrast the incidence and symptomatic behaviors of mania and depression.*
3. *List the types of depressive and bipolar disorders according to current diagnostic classification.*
4. *Discuss primary prevention of depressive and bipolar disorders.*
5. *Apply the nursing process to the care of clients with depressive and bipolar disorders.*
6. *Recognize and discuss the nurse's feelings and behaviors that may influence therapeutic use of self with depressive and bipolar clients.*

◆ Incidence and Significance

Depression may be a temporary normal human emotional response to a loss, disappointment, or failure. It may also be pathological, causing a persistent intense state of unhappiness. Depressive illnesses affect people for months or even years and involve the body, mood, and thoughts. The National Institutes of Health estimate that 15 million Americans will become seriously depressed in any given year.[14] Other studies estimate lifetime prevalence to be much higher, up to 26% for women and 12% for men.

At least 50% of suicides can be attributed to a major depressive disorder. One of every five teenagers has suffered from at least one major depression by the time they are 18 years old.[20] The suicide rate among the elderly (80–84 years) is more than double the rate for the general population.[3] In the United States, depressive disorders rank within the top 10 most costly diseases and account for 70% of psychiatric hospitalizations. In addition, mood disorders, such as depression, are associated with an increased rate of substance abuse (especially alcohol), medical hospitalizations, somatic illnesses, and outpatient medical use.

Depression and bipolar disorder (formerly called manic-depressive illness) are disturbances in mood. Manic episodes are characterized by the triad of unstable mood, pressured speech, and increased motor activity.

Depression can occur at any age and seems unrelated to the pressures produced by any civilization or period of history. Mood disorders have been described for more than 40 centuries, with ancient victims such as Nebuchadnessar, Saul, and Herod. Hippocrates (460–377 BC) subscribed to the idea that black bile (melancholia), a toxic product of digestion, caused depression. This belief probably constitutes the first "biological" causal theory of depression. The pain of depression has been felt by such notables as Dostoyevsky, Edgar Allen Poe, Nathaniel Hawthorne, Abraham Lincoln, and Winston Churchill. More recent victims include William Styron, Vincent Foster, Rod Steiger, Mike Wallace, Kitty Dukakis, Joan Rivers, Rona Barrett, and first ladies Betty Ford and Barbara Bush.

Children develop depressive symptoms similar to those found in adults. Infants may exhibit signs of *anaclitic* (which means "leaning on") depression when deprived of a warm, close experience with another person. As a response to this neglect, infants may fail to thrive, lack social responsiveness, and have an apathetic mood. Depression in children and adolescents may be difficult to recognize. Children and adolescents develop some symptoms similar to those found in adults, but other symptoms may be more subtle or developmentally related. The child or adolescent may have difficulties with schoolwork, lack enthusiasm and energy, be socially withdrawn, and have impulsive, angry outbursts with more disobedience than normal. Children may experience anxiety and hyperactivity, whereas adolescents may have more diffuse symptoms, such as drug abuse, violence, and sexual acting out. Approximately 400,000 children yearly suffer from depression, and teenage depression and suicide rates have risen dramatically within the past few years. Suicide is the third leading cause of death of 15- to 19-year-olds in the United States.

An adult who enters a depressive episode often describes the mood as sad, hopeless, black, and helpless. Low self-esteem and decreased physical and psychic energy lead to apathetic withdrawal from the environment. There is, however, another dimension to depression experienced by a significant number of adults who express anxiety, irritability, restlessness, and anguished feelings.

Depression is the most common psychiatric disorder in the elderly population. Depression in people 65 years or older is a complex phenomenon that has many social and psychological causes. The elderly sustain many losses: meaningful work, income and structured routine, friends and loved ones, and physical strength. In American society, the elderly may feel superfluous, isolated, and alone. Other precipitants to depression may be medical illnesses or the drugs used to treat them. The elderly client often reports less change in mood and attitude and more somatic complaints, such as constipation, headaches, and fatigue. Moreover, the elderly depressed client may appear confused, have memory loss, and be agitated. This is sometimes called *pseudodementia* and may be mistaken for a true dementia. Approximately 12% of the elderly diagnosed as suffering from dementia may have pseudodementia arising from untreated depression.[24]

◆ Etiological Theories

Many recent advances in genetic, biological, and psychological research may provide clues to the cause of depression and bipolar disorder. No definitive cause of these mood disorders has been discovered, but research has predominantly focused on neurobiology. A genetic marker has not yet been identified for major depression, but one has been found for specific bipolar disorders. There is reason to believe that genetic, psychological, and other environmental forces are operating to influence the development and course of mood disorders.

GENETIC INFLUENCES: DEPRESSIVE AND BIPOLAR ILLNESS IN FAMILIES

Depression and manic-depressive disorders occur in families. Evidence confirms the heritability of these disorders. Studies of twins have shown that if an identical twin develops a major depressive illness, the other twin has a 70% chance of developing the disorder.[12] The risk decreases to about 15% with siblings, parents, or children of the afflicted person. Studies also consistently show that the incidence of bipolar illness (7%–10%) and unipolar illness (8%–10%) in adults is much higher in first-degree relatives than in the general population.[12] Neurobiological researchers continue searching for a genetic marker that could be linked to these disorders. Recently discovered is a gene that lies along a short stretch of chromosome 18 that seems to create a predisposition to manic-depression.[22] Genetic studies may provide the knowledge to help identify those most susceptible, which will allow primary preventive efforts.

Biochemical Influences

A biological basis for the depressive and bipolar disorders was first proposed when clients who were being treated for hypertension with a biogenic amine-depleting agent, reserpine, became depressed. In contrast, iproniazid, a biogenic enhancing agent used to treat tuberculosis, was causing euphoria in some clients. The biogenic amines are neurotransmitter substances known as *norepinephrine* and *serotonin*; they have shown to be mood regulators. Subsequently, the monoamine oxidase inhibitors (MAOIs) were found to be effective antidepressant agents by interfering with the degeneration of the biogenic amines. The tricyclic antidepressants (TCAs) were then found to block the reuptake of the amines into the presynaptic neurons.[16]

These observations gave rise to the original biogenic amine hypothesis of depression and bipolar disorder. Researchers believe these neurotransmitters are excessively imbalanced at critical effector sites in the central nervous system. These neurotransmitters, located in the limbic-diencephalic system near the center of the brain, control behavior, feelings, and thoughts. Serotonin generally serves inhibitory functions in the brain, and disturbances in its functioning may underlie the irritability, anxiety, and sleep disturbances common to depression. Norepinephrine is involved in the maintenance of arousal, alertness, and euphoria. Disturbances in norepinephrine function are thought to underlie lack of energy and depressed mood.

Research continues to find causal agents for depression and bipolar disorder. Other neurotransmitter substances under investigation include acetylcholine, dopamine, amino acids, glutamic acid, τ-aminobutyric acid (GABA), and peptides, such as substance p, neuropeptide Y, and endorphins. Recently, investigation has focused on the effect of lithium at the level of gene expression; this may reveal insights into the molecular basis of bipolar and unipolar mood disorders.[24] The results of biochemical research could further prevention and enhance treatment of these disorders.

Biophysical Influences

Besides chemical disturbances, certain physiological changes are associated with depression. Muscle tension and heart and respiration rates may increase. Cells retain more salt than usual, which may cause an imbalance within the electrical system in the body. Alcohol and drug abuse are often related to depression. Certain medications ,such as hormones, sedatives, and some antibacterials, may cause secondary depression. Medical illnesses, such as multiple sclerosis, Epstein-Barr virus, hepatitis, and acquired immunodeficiency syndrome, have been associated with depression.

Hormone secretion is influenced by neurotransmitters in limbic centers, and conversely, alterations in neurotransmitter function affect hormone secretion. Many depressed clients exhibit a blunted thyroid-stimulating hormone level in response to being challenged with thyrotropin-releasing hormone infusion, but they have otherwise normal thyroid profiles. The hypothalamic-pituitary-adrenal axis that controls the release of cortisol does not appear to function correctly in depression. Many depressed clients demonstrate cortisol hypersecretion in the dexamethasone-suppression test.

The influence of circadian body rhythms, which occur approximately every 24 hours and are influenced by changes of the light-dark cycle, may be associated with mood disorders. Circadian rhythmicity impacts sleep, body temperature, cortisol, thyrotropin, and melatonin hormone secretion. Mood disorders follow cyclical and seasonal patterns in their exacerbation; the Diagnostic and Statistical Manual of Mental Disorders, fourth edition (DSM-IV), has added a subtype of bipolar disorder with a seasonal pattern[1] (Box 29-1).

PSYCHOSOCIAL AND ENVIRONMENTAL INFLUENCES

Interpersonal Theory

Interpersonal theory identifies the cause of depression as beginning in childhood when a person suffers the real or perceived loss of a valued object, such as the loss of parental love through death or divorce. After such a loss, if the adaptive grieving process does not occur, a person can develop a profound depression. Repression of ambivalent feelings of guilt and hate develops in an attempt to hide feelings of grief. The depressed person responds to these negative feelings with anger, hostility, and agression, which are turned inward. Disappointment and frustration ensue when attempts are made to establish intimate relationships.

BOX 29-1

DSM-IV Diagnostic Criteria for Seasonal Pattern Specifier

A. There has been a regular temporal relation1ship between the onset of Major Depressive Episodes in Bipolar I or Bipolar II Disorder or Major Depressive Disorder, Recurrent, and a particular time of the year (eg, regular appearance of the Major Depressive Episode in the fall or winter).

B. Full remissions (or a change from depression to mania or hypomania) also occur at a characteristic time of the year (eg, depression disappears in the spring).

C. In the last 2 years, two Major Depressive Episodes have occurred that demonstrate the temporal seasonal relationships defined in Criteria A and B, and no nonseasonal episodes have occurred during that same period.

Psychoanalytic Theory

Psychoanalytic theories of depression have focused on unexpressed and unconscious rage as a reaction to being helpless or dependent on others or to loss of a loved one. In such situations, the client cannot express anger either because it would antagonize the person on whom the client is dependent or because the client does not want to recognize that the relationship with the deceased was not entirely positive. According to psychoanalytic theory, this unexpressed anger is turned inward, producing feelings of depression. Mania is believed to be a defense against depression.

Behavioral Theory

Seligman proposed the theory of *learned helplessness* as an antecedent to depression. People susceptible to depression have encountered a lifetime of experiences that have taught them that they are ineffective and lack the ability to influence their sources of suffering and gratification. Behaviors that define learned helplessness, such as passivity, negative expectations, and feelings of helplessness, hopelessness, and powerlessness, are also symptoms of major depression.[27]

Cognitive Theory

Cognitive theory states that clients experience depression because of errors in thinking and unrealistic attitudes about themselves and the world. The cognitive view holds that cognitive (thinking) errors precede changes in mood. These cognitive errors involve undervaluing oneself, having a negative view of one's ability to achieve goals, and being pessimistic, resulting in low self-esteem and the inability to experience pleasure. Self-depreciation and unrealistic expectations cause recurrent dissatisfaction, which leads to depression.[31]

Aaron Beck developed cognitive therapy, a time-limited, structured approach based on the proposition that a person's moods and emotions are determined by thoughts and ideas. Believing that affect can be influenced by altering thoughts and ideas, Beck formulated a treatment model in which the therapist takes an active and directive position to help the client uncover distorted thinking and use reality-based judgments to formulate experience.[31] The cognitive approach to treating depression has implications for nursing intervention with moderately depressed clients and is discussed later in this chapter.

Neurobiological researchers continue to investigate the causes of depressive and bipolar disorders. Whether the physical and mood changes associated with these disorders are caused by biochemical factors is unknown. A biochemical imbalance may represent a genetic vulnerability set in motion by some psychosocial or environmental factors.

The nurse treating and caring for a client with a depressive or bipolar disorder must ask several questions:

1. What made the client vulnerable?
2. What triggered the disturbance?
3. Why did the client's defenses fail?
4. What kinds of intervention will help the client adapt and grow?

◆ Types of Mood Disorders

The mood disorders can be categorized in various ways. The category types vary in regard to the number of symptoms, their severity, and persistence. However, these theoretical categorizations should not interfere with offering effective help based on specific knowledge of the client, family, and community.

If depression is perceived as existing on a continuum from health to illness and as sometimes serving a useful function, the reaction of grief and the process of mourning would be placed at the healthy end of the continuum. Most people respond to losses in fairly predictable ways. Denial, usually short-lived, progresses to a developing awareness of the loss, followed by anger and sadness. Finally a resolution occurs, characterized by acceptance of the loss and perhaps idealization of the lost object or individul. Grief in response to a psychic wound, such as the death of a loved one, can be compared to the pain that accompanies a physical wound. The mourning process, which may take as long as 1 year or more, can be compared to the healing of a physical wound. This ability to resolve loss varies greatly among people and depends on previous interpersonal experiences, ego strength, and the support and resources available. Some depressions can be linked to unresolved grief.

DEPRESSIVE DISORDERS

The depressive disorders include major depressive disorder, dysthymia, and depressive disorder not otherwise specified (NOS).[1]

Major Depressive Disorder

According to DSM-IV criteria, a client diagnosed with *major depression* must have either a depressed mood or an inability to derive pleasure from previously enjoyable activities. Symptoms must be present most of the day nearly every day for at least 2 weeks, and they must cause significant distress or impairment in functioning. A client's bereavement that persists for longer than 2 months after the loss of a loved one may be diagnosed as major depression.[1] Depressive episodes are classified according to severity as mild, moderate, or severe and can occur singly or in a recurrent pattern. Episodes are also categorized as occurring with or without accompanying psychotic features, that is, hallucinations or delusions.

Typically, major depressive episodes last from several weeks to several months and are followed by periods of relatively normal mood and behavior. The average major depressive episode lasts about 4 months; however, it can last for 12 months or more without remitting. Studies suggest that people with depression will have at least one subsequent episode of depression in their lifetime[30] (Box 29-2).

Large-scale studies indicate that rates of depression are increasing rapidly across the life span in the United States and abroad. Many reasons have been suggested for the increase, including alcohol and drug use, decreased work opportunities, job layoffs, and societal stressors, such as threats of violence, single-parent homes, and increased divorce rates. The highest rates of major depression are in 18- to 44-year-olds and in those who are separated, divorced, or unhappy in their marriage.[6]

Mental health professionals who work with depressed clients may encounter descriptors of mood disorders used to enhance understanding of the client's situation and condition. Major depression is also called unipolar depression. Major depression occurring after childbirth is called postpartum depression. When it occurs around the sixth decade of life, it may be termed involutional melancholia. The depressed client who is agitated may have agitated depression; the client who is almost inert may be described as having retarded or vegetative depression. Depression that seems to occur without any relationship to external events is sometimes called endogenous depression. This is in contrast to a reactive or exogenous depression, the cause of which is evident from the client's history.

The many terms used to label depression are the result of the efforts of mental health caregivers to provide accurate descriptions of the depresssive process. Accurate classification and descriptions of depression aid in diagnosis, guide treatment, and facilitate professional communication and research efforts.

Dysthymic Disorder

The word dysthymia comes from the Greek prefix *dys,* meaning difficult or bad, and *thymos,* meaning mind. The DSM-IV considers dysthymia a milder form of depressive illness in which the symptoms are not as severe as depressive disorder but may be chronic. According to the DSM-IV, diagnostic criteria include depressed or irritable mood for most of the day, occurring more days than not for at least 2 years (1 year in children and adolescents). During this time, the client has had no more than 2 months in

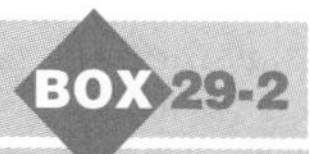

DSM-IV Diagnostic Criteria for Major Depressive Episode

A. Five (or more) of the following symptoms have been present during the same 2-week period and represent a change from previous functioning; at least one of the symptoms is either (1) depressed mood or (2) loss of interest or pleasure.
   (1) depressed mood most of the day, nearly every day, as indicated by either subjective report (eg, feels sad or empty) or observation made by others (eg, appears tearful). **Note:** In children and adolescents, can be irritable mood.
   (2) markedly diminished interest or pleasure in all, or almost all, activities most of the day, nearly every day
   (3) significant weight loss when not dieting or weight gain, or decrease or increase in appetite nearly every day. **Note:** In children, consider failure to make expected weight gains.
   (4) insomnia or hypersomnia nearly every day
   (5) psychomotor agitation or retardation nearly every day (observable by others, not merely subjective feelings of restlessness or being slowed down)
   (6) fatigue or loss of energy nearly every day
   (7) feelings of worthlessness or excessive or inappropriate guilt (which may be delusional) nearly every day (not merely self-reproach or guilt about being sick)
   (8) diminished ability to think or concentrate, or indecisiveness, nearly every day
   (9) recurrent thoughts of death (not just fear of dying), recurrent suicidal ideation without a specific plan, or a suicide attempt or a specific plan for committing suicide

B. The symptoms cause clinically significant distress or impairment in social, occupational, or other important areas of functioning.

C. The symptoms are not due to the direct physiological effects of a substance or a general medical condition.

D. The symptoms are not better accounted for by Bereavement, ie, after the loss of a loved one, the symptoms persist for longer than 2 months or are characterized by marked functional impairment, morbid preoccupation with worthlessness, suicidal ideation, psychotic symptoms, or psychomotor retardation.

which symptoms are not present and has not experienced a manic or depressive episode[1] (Box 29-3).

The chronic nature of this disorder is cause for concern because it is often accompanied by a lifelong struggle against depression that can assume various maladaptive forms. In an attempt to escape negative self-esteem, feelings of self-depreciation, emptiness, low energy and fatigue, pessimism about the future, and hopelessness with suicidal ideations, the client may engage in certain activities to generate excitement. Gambling, criminal behavior, promiscuity, and unplanned pregnancy may be examples of acting out. Intensification of work, spending money, sexual behavior, and religious and mystic involvement may be used in a struggle against depression. The depressed client may turn to substance abuse or food to dull or escape psychic pain. Dysthymia often predates the appearance of major depression by as much as 3 years.[1] Nurses practicing in acute-care settings and in the community play a crucial role in primary prevention by identifying these clients.

Depressive Disorder Not Otherwise Specified

Depressive disorder NOS includes disorders with depressive features that do not meet the criteria of other depressive disorders. Examples include premenstrual dysphoric disorder, a minor depressive disorder, and postpsychotic depressive disorder of schizophrenia.

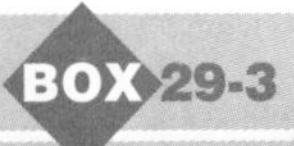

DSM-IV Diagnostic Criteria for Dysthymic Disorder

A. Depressed mood for most of the day, for more days than not, as indicated either by subjective account or observation by others, for at least 2 years. **Note:** In children and adolescents, mood can be irritable and duration must be at least 1 year.

B. Presence, while depressed, of two (or more) of the following:
   (1) poor appetite or overeating
   (2) insomnia or hypersomnia
   (3) low energy or fatigue
   (4) low self-esteem
   (5) poor concentration or difficulty making decisions
   (6) feelings of hopelessness

C. During the 2-year period (1 year for children or adolescents) of the disturbance, the person has never been without the symptoms in Criteria A and B for more than 2 months at a time.

D. No Major Depressive Episode has been present during the first 2 years of the disturbance (1 year for children and adolescents); or Major Depressive Disorder, In Partial Remission.

E. There has never been a Manic Episode, a Mixed Episode, or a Hypomanic Episode and criteria have never been met for Cyclothymic Disorder.

F. The symptoms are not due to the direct physiological effects of a substance or a general medical condition.

G. The symptoms cause clinically significant distress or impairment in social, occupational, or other important areas of functioning.

BIPOLAR DISORDERS

The bipolar disorders include bipolar I disorder, bipolar II disorder, cyclothymic disorder, and bipolar disorder NOS.[1]

Bipolar I Disorder

Bipolar I disorder has a clinical course characterized by one or more manic episodes, usually alternating with major depressive episodes. Manic episodes are periods of abnormally and persistently elevated, expansive, or irritable mood. These episodes usually begin suddenly and last from a few days to a few months. While in a manic phase, the person does not often realize he or she is behaving strangely and may resist treatment. It is common for the client to have abrupt mood changes, with rapid shifts from euphoria to anger or depression. The former name for this illness was manic-depressive disorder because of the diametrically opposite symptoms. The client may have a hypomanic episode or a relatively mild manic phase occurring with a severe depression.

Bipolar I disorder is further categorized according to whether it occurs with a single manic episode or whether the most recent episode was hypomanic, manic, depressed, or mixed (manic and major depression).[1] Bipolar I is a recurrent disorder; 90% of people with one manic episode have future episodes (Box 29-4).

Bipolar II Disorder

Bipolar II disorder is characterized by one or more major depressive episodes and at least one hypomanic episode but without a history of a true manic episode.[1] Most hypomanic episodes in bipolar II disorder occur immediately before or after a major depressive episode (Box 29-5).

First-degree biological relatives of individuals with bipolar disorders have elevated rates of bipolar I and bipolar II disorders and major depressive disorder compared with the general population.[1]

Research continues into the genetic causes of bipolar disorder. Recently, investigators have found that either dominant or recessive alleles are a major susceptibility locus for bipolar disorder on chromosome 21.[7] National Institute of Mental Health researchers have proposed a cellular model for bipolar illness. They propose that a reduction in the activity of the sodium, potassium, and ATpase pump increases membrane excitability and decreases neurotransmitter release. These cellular changes lead to mania and depression.[22] Fur-

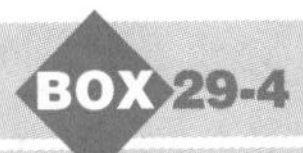

DSM-IV Diagnostic Criteria for Bipolar I Disorder Variants

BIPOLAR I DISORDER, SINGLE MANIC EPISODE

A. Presence of only one Manic Episode and no past Major Depressive Episodes

BIPOLAR I DISORDER, MOST RECENT EPISODE HYPOMANIC

A. Currently (or most recently) in a Hypomanic Episode.
B. There has previously been at least one Manic Episode or Mixed Episode.
C. The mood symptoms cause clinically significant distress or impairment in social, occupational, or other important areas of functioning.

BIPOLAR I DISORDER, MOST RECENT EPISODE MANIC

A. Currently (or most recently) in a Manic Episode.
B. There has previously been at least one Major Depressive Episode, Manic Episode or Mixed Episode.

BIPOLAR I DISORDER, MOST RECENT EPISODE MIXED

A. Currently (or most recently) in a Mixed Episode.
B. There has previously been at least one Major Depressive Episode, Manic Episode, or Mixed Episode.

BIPOLAR I DISORDER, MOST RECENT EPISODE DEPRESSED

A. Currently (or most recently) in a Major Depressive Episode.
B. There has previously been at least one Manic Episode or Mixed Episode.

Note: For all Bipolar I Disorders, the Manic Episode is not better accounted for by Schizoaffective Disorder and is not superimposed on Schizophrenia, Schizophreniform Disorder, Delusional Disorder, or Psychotic Disorder Not Otherwise Specified.

ther investigation of bipolar disorders is needed to allow better diagnosis and treatment for this population.

Cyclothymic Disorder

Clients experiencing repeated periods of nonpsychotic depression and hypomania for a least 2 years (1 year for children and adolescents) are described as having a cyclothymic disorder. Hypomania or mania may be considered a defense or reaction formation against the painful experience of depression. Manic behavior has also been associated with an increase or surplus of neurotransmitter amines in the brain. The opposing manifestations of depression and hypomania are seen in the following pairs of symptoms: feelings of inadequacy (during depressed periods) and inflated self-esteem (during manic periods); social withdrawal and uninhibited people seeking; sleeping too much and not sleeping enough; diminished productivity at work and increased productivity. Cyclothymic disorder is diagnosed only if a major depressive or manic episode has never been present (Box 29-6).

Bipolar Disorder Not Otherwise Specified

Bipolar disorder NOS includes disorders with bipolar features that do not meet the criteria for any specific bipolar disorder. Examples of this diagnostic category include a rapid alteration (over days) of depressive and manic behavior that does not meet the criteria for major depression or manic episodes or recurrent hypomanic episodes without depression.

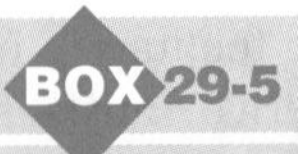

BOX 29-5

DSM-IV Diagnostic Criteria for Bipolar II Disorder

A. Presence (or history) of one or more Major Depressive Episodes
B. Presence (or history) of at least one Hypomanic Episode
C. There has never been a Manic Episode or a Mixed Episode
D. The symptoms cause clinically significant distress or impairment in social, occupational, or other important areas of functioning

Application of the Nursing Process to Clients With Depressive and Bipolar Disorders

Nursing care for clients with depressive and bipolar disorders focuses on primary prevention (ie, the maintenance of mental health) and on secondary and tertiary prevention through the provision of care and treatment to those already identified as mentally ill.

Rapid changes in society, with the concomitant stresses and losses of traditional support systems, such as family, church, and neighborhood, may contribute to the increased incidence of depression. Factors that increase the vulnerability to depressive disorders include the following:

1. Being a young, single mother of small children who is head of a household living in poverty[26]; being a young adult[2]; or being elderly[7]
2. Experiencing a prior loss or trauma, financial problems, social isolation, parental or marital discord
3. Being without employment outside of the home and lacking an intimate relationship
4. Having three or more children living at home or caring for an elder in the home
5. Seeking feelings of love, respect, recognition, and worth in life through another person or group

Primary prevention cannot be achieved solely through biological intervention. At this time, there are no specific physical tests predict vulnerability, or to diagnose or treat mood disorders. In the absence of these predictors, psychosocial and developmental factors must be considered to reduce the incidence and prevalence of mood disorders.

PLANNING PRIMARY PREVENTION

Two major goals in primary prevention of mood disorders follow:

1. The development of a positive self-concept, as demonstrated by self-confidence, self-respect, and striving for self-actualization
2. Healthy adaptation to loss

Nurses can help clients realize these goals in acute-care settings and in the community when caring for clients across the life span.

Children

A person's self-concept has its foundation in infancy and childhood and reflects parental perceptions and messages. Parents teach their children overtly and covertly about their ability to master the environment. It is important to assess if a child can initiate ideas and follow through with an activity, because these abilities are recognized and reinforced. The child may instead perceive that his or her efforts are inadequate, useless, and not wanted. Rejection can be devastating to the development of a positive self-concept. Children who experience rejection sometimes conclude that they can elicit love and approval from significant others only if

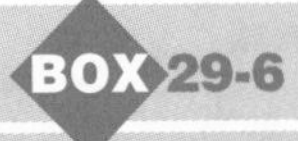

BOX 29-6

DSM-IV Diagnostic Criteria for Cyclothymic Disorder

A. For at least 2 years, the presence of numerous periods with hypomanic symptoms and numerous periods with depressive symptoms that do not meet criteria for a Major Depressive Episode. **Note:** In children and adolescents, the duration must be at least 1 year.
B. During the above 2-year period (1 year in children and adolescents), the person has not been without the symptoms in Criterion A for more than 2 months at a time.
C. No Major Depressive Episode, Manic Episode, or Mixed Episode has been present during the first 2 years of the disturbance.
D. The symptoms are not due to the direct physiological effects of a substance (eg, a drug of abuse, a medication) or a general medical condition (eg, hyperthyroidism).
E. The symptoms cause clinically significant distress or impairment in social, occupational, or other important areas of functioning.

they assume guilt or punishment themselves. Children who do not learn to love themselves may become adults who measure their own worth solely according the perceptions of others.

Adolescents

Adolescence is often a time of emotional turmoil, mood swings, and rebelliousness. Substance abuse may result in a missed diagnosis of depression. Researchers have identified basic elements of temperament, including an agitated activity level, lack of adaptability, intensity of reaction, and negative mood that may be signs of impending depression. This type of temperament leads to frequent conflicts with parents and an unhealthy parent–child relationship. The poor relationship results in the lack of a firm sense of identity and a poor self-concept, which increase the adolescent's vulnerability to suicidal behavior.

The Elderly

The elderly sustain many losses: meaningful work, death of loved ones, financial hardships, changes in lifestyle, loneliness, and loss of purpose. Retirement may contribute to depression because of lost social networks, isolation, and aloneness. Also, many age-related illnesses, and many medications taken by the elderly, such as drugs for hypertension or arthritis, can trigger depression.

PROMOTING ADAPTATION TO LOSS

Nurses function in many practice settings in which children, adult clients, and families are experiencing growth, development, change, and loss. Hospitalization can result in loss of status, loss of self-determination, loss of usual family relationships, and perhaps loss of wage-earning ability. In addition, the client may be adapting to a changing body image, a changing lifestyle, and even the loss of life. Some of these losses can be anticipated, and clients can be helped to adapt through anticipatory guidance and other supportive nursing actions that allow for verbalization, sharing of feelings, and problem solving. Events such as rape, or situations involving loss, such as death of a child or spouse, can become crises for the people involved. The nurse's ability to recognize a crisis and intervene or arrange for others to do so may facilitate adaptive behaviors and prevent depression. Chapter 39, Crisis Theory and Intervention, provides more information on helping clients deal with overwhelming stressors.

Nurses who participate in health education programs (Box 29-7), such as prenatal and postnatal education, sexuality and family planning, genetic counseling, age-specific parenting groups, and support groups for those in transition (eg, widows, divorcees, retirees) are providing knowledge and exploring feelings to help clients maintain control over and derive satisfaction from their own lives. Nurses who practice in community health agencies, doctors' offices, well-baby clinics, homes, and pediatric care settings have many opportunities to promote healthy parent–child and parent–adolescent relationships. The nurse can share knowledge of growth and development to help parents understand their children's behavior and, just as importantly, feel more positive about themselves.

PROMOTING SECONDARY AND TERTIARY PREVENTION

Secondary prevention of depressive and bipolar disorders aims to reduce the prevalence of mental disorder by providing intervention that decreases the number of stressors and shortens the duration of disequilibrium. Tertiary prevention refers to measures used to reduce the disabilities, such as social defects, that result from mental disorder. This type of prevention often includes rehabilitation and readaptation to the environment.

The nurse participates in secondary and tertiary prevention by applying the nursing process—assessment, nursing diagnosis, planning, implementation, and evaluation—in client care settings. Although people with affective disorders can be found virtually anywhere, the following discussion focuses on the client in a psychiatric care setting. However, the nursing process is never bound by a location or setting.

ASSESSMENT

Nursing assessment of depressive and manic behaviors involves systematic, thorough consideration of the client's affect, thought processes, intellectual processes, and physiological and psychomotor activity. The nurse identifies the client's actual or potential problems in these areas of functioning, formulates nursing diagnoses, and specifies client behavior outcomes that guide planning of interventions.

The following discussion includes observations that the nurse commonly makes when encountering clients with manic or depressive disorders. No two clients present the same history and behavior, and the nurse should avoid the tendency to perceive clients with a mind-set created by textbook descriptions.

Affective Changes

Affect in Depression. One area of assessment that provides essential data is the client's affect. Because depression and mania manifest primarily as disturbances in mood or affect, the client's emotional tone may be the most obvious deviation from healthy be-

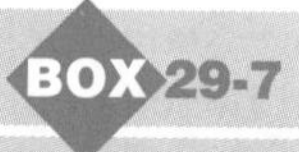

DSM-IV Diagnostic Criteria for Manic and Hypomanic Episodes

MANIC EPISODE

A. A distinct period of abnormally and persistently elevated, expansive, or irritable mood, lasting at least 1 week (or any duration if hospitalization is necessary).
B. During the period of mood disturbance, three (or more) of the following symptoms have persisted (four if the mood is only irritable) and have been present to a significant degree:
   (1) inflated self-esteem or grandiosity
   (2) decreased need for sleep (eg, feels rested after only 3 hours of sleep)
   (3) more talkative than usual or pressure to keep talking
   (4) flight of ideas of subjective experience that thoughts are racing
   (5) distractibility (ie, attention too easily drawn to unimportant or irrelevant external stimuli)
   (6) increase in goal-directed activity (either socially, at work or school, or sexually) or psychomotor agitation
   (7) excessive involvement in pleasurable activities that have a high potential for painful consequences (eg, engaging in unrestrained buying sprees, sexual indiscretions, or foolish business investments)
C. The symptoms do not meet criteria for a Mixed Episode.
D. The mood disturbance is sufficiently severe to cause marked impairment in occupational functioning or in usual social activities or relationships with others, or to necessitate hospitalization to prevent harm to self or others, or there are psychotic features.
E. The symptoms are not due to the direct physiological effects of a substance or a general medical condition

HYPOMANIC EPISODE

A. A distinct period of persistently elevated, expansive, or irritable mood, lasting at least 4 days, that is clearly different from the usual nondepressed mood
B. Same mood disturbances as in Manic Episode occur.
C. The episode is associated with an unequivocal change in functioning that is uncharacteristic of the person.
D. The episode is not severe enough to cause marked impairment in social or occupational functioning, or to necessitate hospitalization, and there are no psychotic features.
E. The symptoms are not due to the direct physiological effects of a substance or a general medical condition

havior. Depressed clients appear sad, dejected, apathetic, and uncomfortable in their painful suffering, but they usually do not exhibit bizarre behavior. They feel hopeless and helpless to do anything about the situation. They may verbalize feelings of guilt, anger, or hostility and the inability to feel pleasure (anhedonia) or experience joy.

These verbalized (and perhaps nonverbalized) feelings are consistent with the client's physical appearance. There is frequently a disregard for grooming, cleanliness, and personal appearance. Stooped posture and dejected facial expression are other nonverbal messages of depression. While observing and communicating with the depressed client, the nurse may perceive that depression actually can be a defense against sadness and grief. Depression seems to raise the threshold for psychic pain, thereby serving as a protective mechanism for the client.

Age-Related Signs of Depression

Depression in Children and Adolescents. Researchers believe that depression is an underdiagnosed condition in childhood because the expression of depression may be different than in adults and may be related to the developmental level of the child. Anger, aggressiveness, hyperactivity, delinquency, and school problems may indicate depression more than sad, tearful faces, withdrawal from activities, and verbal expression of poor self-esteem. An adolescent with low self-esteem may turn to drugs and alcohol to feel good. This often leads to risk-taking behavior and sexual promiscuity.

Depression in the Elderly. The elderly who are depressed often report fewer mood changes and more somatic complaints, such as constipation, headaches, and fatigue. They may appear confused, have memory loss, and be agitated, resulting in the misdiagnosis of dementia.

Affect in Mania

The manic client's mood is in direct contrast to that of the depressed client's. Manic clients are self-satisfied, confident, and aggressive, feel on top of the world, and feel in control of their destinies. These clients' flights into the external world may be a defense against sadness and grief. Anger, sarcasm, and irritability become evident when the nurse attempts to set limits on clients' behavior or when clients are frustrated by other people or objects in the environment.

The degree of the client's affective change is one of the most important judgments the nurse makes. Is the client mildly depressed, severely depressed, exhibiting retarded depression, or in depressive stupor? The mildly depressed client requires a less intensive approach than the severely depressed client, who sees no reason to continue living. The nurse must also observe for changes in the client's affective state, which indicate that the client is responding to other modes of therapy.

Thought Content and Processes

Thought Content and Processes in Depression. The thoughts of depressed or manic clients are congruent with their feelings; there is no dichotomy between thought and affect. Depressed clients ruminate about their unhappy situations, discussing them repeatedly and asking the same questions, to which no one can give a satisfactory answer. Thinking may be difficult and slow; content becomes limited to a few topics. Replies to the nurse's questions may be delayed and condensed, and clients do not reveal their private thoughts.

Delusions. In depression, there often is a heightened awareness of inner sensations and a reduced awareness of external events. This inability to mobilize attention to events in the outside world may lead to delusional thinking. These delusions or false beliefs are consistent with the client's affective state. Delusional content is frequently characterized by self-deprecation, guilt, and remorse. There may also be a suspicious and persecutory trend to the ideas; that is, clients may believe they are being persecuted by others. Delusions also may be hypochondriacal. Clients may believe they have a consuming illness that is destroying them from within.

Thinking in Absolute Terms. Depressed clients think they are failures and are totally pessimistic about the future. They believe that life will not improve, and they will not be convinced otherwise. Filled with self-reproach, they think in absolute terms and become averse (rather than simply indifferent) to opportunities for change.

Suicidal Ideation. Because depression is characterized by negative thoughts and accompanying feelings of self-hate and hostility, one of the most crucial areas for the nurse to assess is the degree of the client's suicidal ideation. What thoughts does the client have about taking his or her own life? How great is the risk of an attempt to do so? An accurate assumption for the nurse to make is that all depressed clients are potentially suicidal; the question is to what degree the client is suicidal.

Although a database for assessment of suicide risk has not been scientifically established, statistics point toward some generalizations. Of those who attempt suicide, 7% to 10% kill themselves, and 60% to 70% of those who talk about suicide to relatives or friends attempt it within 6 months.[8]

The severity of depression is directly related to the degree of suicidal risk. In addition, the nurse must assess other behaviors or symptoms. Anxiety, hopelessness, withdrawal, disorientation, and hostility indicate an increased risk of suicide. Clients who do not have social and personal resources, such as housing, transportation, money, employment, and available significant others, are also at higher risk for suicide. A history of alcohol and drug abuse is another factor in increased suicide potential. Clients who have a history of multiple, high-lethality suicide attempts are also at greater risk. Verbalization of a desire to die, having a specific plan, or hearing voices commanding the client to hurt himself or herself requires immediate intervention.

Depression, like suicide, is an attempt to communicate a state of deprivation. The client has lost all hope and feels overwhelmed and helpless. When these feeling become too painful to communicate, the depressed client feels that suicide is a logical answer. Suicide can be viewed as a last desperate cry for help or love when no other avenues of communication exist (see Chapter 42, Suicide).

Thought Processes and Content in Mania. Nursing assessment and diagnosis of the hypomanic or manic client's thought processes reveal different kinds of material. In all degrees of mania, there is little introspection.[1] Manic clients evade thinking and are occupied with phonetics rather than meaning in their thinking and speech. Their stream of thought is characterized by a rapid association of ideas, termed flight of ideas, with rhyming and word play. Although these thoughts seem illogical, the manic client's remarks are similar to free associations prompted by unconscious thoughts and feelings. When flight of ideas is severe, the client's speech may be disorganized and incoherent:

> How do I feel? I feel with my hands. How do you feel? No, seriously, everything is wonderful; couldn't be better. Going "from bed to worse" Benchley said. Really, honey, this is a marvelous place you've got here. Mar-vel-ous. Mar-vel-ous. Vel. I really must shampoo my hair.

In a euphoric or elated state, the manic client is full of ambitious schemes and exaggerations that belie reality. Delusions are usually expansive, fleeting, and wish fulfilling. Clients may erroneously believe that they have great wealth and power. They are too busy to submit ideas and impressions to critical examination. A client's desperate need to convince others of his or her grandiosity should alert the nurse to the strong feelings of inadequacy that the client is trying to overcome.

Intellectual Processes

Characteristic intellectual processes of mood disorder are disordered perception, consciousness, and orientation. In conjunction with the changes in affect and thinking previously described, these disordered processes often leave the client with decreased powers of judgment and decision making. In such instances, the nurse must determine whether it is necessary to assume decision making for the client and when this action is therapeutically warranted. Although autonomous behavior is a long-term goal for every client, at times during acutely severe depression and mania, the nurse must make decisions for clients because they are unable to do so for themselves.

Perception. The perception of depressed clients may be distorted because of their intense affective states. They perceive the world as strange and unnatural. For instance, a client with deep guilt feelings may interpret the sound of wind in the trees as reproaching voices. This misinterpretation of a real sensory experience is called an illusion. The severely depressed client may less frequently experience hallucinations, perceptions that occur when there is no impulse created by the stimulation of a receptor. Auditory hallucinations, the most frequent form of perceptual disturbance, usually represent projections of affective distress. For example, clients may hear voices blaming them or telling them that they are worthless.

Hallucinations may occur in manic excitement but are not common. As in depression, perceptual disorders in mania usually take the form of illusions.

Consciousness. Among disturbances of consciousness are those imposed by disordered attention. Attention is the conscious, selective reaction by which a person examines the external world for useful data. Feelings and attitudes influence attention, and depressed and manic clients may exhibit problems in the area of attention. The attention of depressed clients may be so tenaciously directed toward a limited mental content that nothing will divert their energy elsewhere.

Severely depressed clients may be so fearful of some impending disaster that they may actually become confused. Retarded or vegetative depression, in which stream of thought and psychomotor activity are inhibited, may result in stupor. In depressive stupor, there is almost complete immobility (catatonia), a clouded sensorium, and intense preoccupation.

The manic client, on the other hand, is easily distracted by people, noises, and activity in the environment. Because of this inattention or distractibility, the manic client may fail to discriminate among objects and people. The most severe form of mania, delirious mania, is characterized by purposeless and continuous activity.

Orientation. Disorientation as to who one is, where one is, and what time it is may occur in any mental disorder involving extensive impairment of memory, the extent or accuracy of perception, or attention. Because the intensely depressed or manic client may experience impairment orientation, the nurse should assess clients' understanding of their environment and how they locate themselves within it.

Assessment of intellectual processes also includes insight. Insight, or self-knowledge, depends on perceptual accuracy and consciousness and refers to the ability of clients to observe and understand themselves. Depressed clients are acutely aware of their suffering, know they are ill, and usually demonstrate some desire to end their suffering. Unfortunately, their ambivalence and mistrust of others may interfere with effective use of the resources available. Manic clients, on the other hand, deny their many conflicts and are not aware that they are coping with them in an unhealthy way.

Physiological and Psychomotor Activity

Depression and mania are physical and psychological states. Assessment of the client with a depressive or bipolar disorder would be incomplete without a thorough consideration of physiological status and psychomotor activity.

Physical Effects of Depression. In the depressed client, a deficit in psychic energy is accompanied by a decrease in physical energy. Physiologically, depression manifests itself in various ways. The client may have difficulty sleeping or may sleep excessively with unpleasant and frightening dreams. Anorexia with significant weight loss or increased appetite and significant weight gain can occur. Sexual desire is often decreased; the male client may be impotent. The client may feel continually fatigued and may complain of physical symptoms for which no organic basis can be found. Depressed clients who are delusional may refuse to eat or drink, because they believe they are undeserving of sustenance.

Unless agitated by anxiety, most depressed clients are lethargic and withdrawn and resist social contacts. The depressed client lacks interest in personal hygiene and normal grooming and hygiene routines. Hair and clothes may be unkempt, and the body may need bathing.

Physical Effects of Mania. The manic client presents some of the same problems for care but for different reasons. Nutritional deficits may exist because the client will not take the time to eat or cannot attend to this activity. Dehydration may occur for the same reasons. Because continuous activity may not result in a feeling of fatigue, exhaustion may result.

The manic client may dress bizarrely, use makeup inappropriately, and not attend to personal hygiene. Acute manic episodes may be accompanied by signing, shouting, writing, or destroying clothing and property. The client may intrude on the activities of others or may collect objects. Although this overactivity is purposeful, the client does not attain an objective or goal because tasks or projects are not completed.

Nursing assessment of the client with a depressive or bipolar disorder must be a continuous process. The client's mood may change quickly, and the potential for suicide is great. Physical illness may complicate client care. The disturbances in affect, thought, intellect, and psychomotor activity described should be general guidelines. When clients begin to receive treatment, especially with medication or electroconvulsive therapy (ECT), their behavior may change. Somatic treatment of depression, although helpful for the client, can make nursing assessment more complex.

NURSING DIAGNOSIS

The nurse analyzes the assessment data to form the bases for nursing diagnoses, which guide planning, implementing, and evaluating nursing intervention.

The following nursing diagnoses may apply to clients with depressive and bipolar disorders:

1. Ineffective Individual Coping
2. Hopelessness
3. Spiritual Distress
4. Social Isolation
5. Impaired Social Interaction
6. Self Esteem Disturbance
7. Altered Thought Processes
8. Powerlessness
9. Risk for Violence: Self-directed
10. Sensory/Perceptual Alterations
11. Self Care deficits
12. Risk for Injury
13. Sleep Pattern Disturbance
14. Altered Family Processes
15. Sexual Dysfunction
16. Constipation
17. Altered Nutrition: Less than body requirements
18. Altered Nutrition: More than body requirements

PLANNING

The nurse can plan for the clients with a mood disorder with a legitimate feeling of optimism. Mania and depression are time-limited conditions; in most instances, the nurse will see the client return to a healthier state of functioning. This does not mean that nursing and medical care are not needed. Both can shorten the intensity and length of these affective states and perhaps even save the client's life.

There is no single way to approach depressed or manic clients. The nurse must perceive the client as an individual. Collaboration, by sharing and comparing preceptions with other health team members, is essential. Identification of the client behavior outcomes should be a combined effort of those involved in client care, including the client and family when possible (Nursing Care Plans 29-1 and 29-2).

Outcomes for the Depressed Client

Frequently, assessment of the depressed client's behavior will identify client outcomes related to the following needs:

1. Physical safety and health
2. Expression of painful negative feelings
3. Love, acceptance, and a feeling of belonging rather than one of isolation
4. Feelings of being useful and needed
5. Opportunities to achieve worthwhile accomplishments
6. Opportunities for autonomy and self-actualization

These needs are a direct consequence of the essence of depression—a lonely, loveless, and hopeless state. They are appropriate for the nurse to address because they all depend on relationships with other human beings. These needs also transcend the experience of hospitalization.

(text continues on page 552)

Nursing Care Plan 29-1

The Depressed Client

Nursing Diagnosis

Risk for Violence: Self-directed related to feelings of worthlessness

Outcome

Client will agree to and sign a "no self-harm" contract.

Intervention	Rationale
Establish a trusting nurse–client relationship.	A relationship built on trust helps meet client's dependency needs, reduce anxiety, and monitor risk of suicide.
Implement suicide precautions according to treatment program's policy and procedure.	Prevention of self-harm activities ensures client safety.
Monitor safety of client's environment including: control of dangerous items, monitoring medication ingestion, constant observation.	Safety provisions are part of nursing's legal and ethical responsibility.
Administer medication for target symptoms and institute medication education with client and family.	Relief of symptoms and education promote compliance with medication regime.
Focus on client's emotional state and strengths rather than intent to harm self.	Focusing on client's feelings communicates caring.

Evaluation

Client complies with "no self-harm" contract and remains safe.

Nursing Diagnosis

Feeding/Bathing/Dressing, Self Care Deficit related to decreased interest in daily activities and low energy level

Outcome

Client will eat, bathe, and dress independently.

Intervention	Rationale
Expect client to eat regular meals and allow plenty of time for client to eat; feed client if necessary.	A depressed person may neglect to eat or perform other self-care activities.
Bathe client daily if necessary and supervise related activities, such as mouth and hair care.	Meeting client's hygiene need when he is unable to do so validates his worth and dignity.
Offer client limited clothing choices or select clothes for him.	Offering simple choices helps the client become more independent.
Reinforce any self-care efforts of client.	Behavior that is reinforced is more likely to continue.

Evaluation

Client performs self-care activities independently.

continued

Nursing Care Plan 29-1 (Continued)

Nursing Diagnosis

Sleep Pattern Disturbance related to early morning awakening and/or difficulty falling asleep

Outcome

Client will sleep at least 5 hours per night.

Intervention	Rationale
Establish regular hours for sleeping and wakefulness.	Establishment of sleep–wake routines encourages sufficient rest.
Encourage client to participate in physical exercise daily; prohibit daytime sleeping.	Exercise increases sense of well-being by stimulating endorphin release, and contributes to fatigue at bedtime.
Establish sleep chart record.	Data related to sleep and awake patterns aids in determining further interventions.
Promote relaxation at bedtime by offering soothing bath and warm milk to drink and decreasing environmental stimuli.	Relaxation measures promote sleep.

Evaluation

Client reports adequate amount of restful sleep.

Nursing Diagnosis

Self Esteem Disturbance related to feelings of dejection

Outcome

Client will identify two positive attributes about self and use positive self-talk.

Intervention	Rationale
Schedule regular items with client that ensure privacy, and communicate client's importance as an individual.	Client's worth is validated when nurse spends time and offers self.
Point out to client that self-deprecating comments block communication.	Cognitive approaches present reality by challenging negative beliefs about self.
Do not allow client to ruminate about failures; redirect to present problems or involve in another type of activity.	Focusing on the present promotes effective coping.
Help client recognize opportunities to congratulate self-achievement.	Self-worth is enhanced by recognizing own achievements and abilities.
Include client in group activities that provide for success.	Successful group participation reinforces client's achievement and continuation of participation.

Evaluation

Client reports positive sense of self-worth.

continued

Nursing Care Plan 29-1 *(Continued)*

Nursing Diagnosis

Powerlessness related to client's sense of inadequacy and nonassertive behavior

Outcome

Client will make decisions regarding care, treatment, and future plans.

Intervention	Rationale
Support client's attempts at decision making.	Positive reinforcement enhances decision-making.
Encourage and role model use of problem-solving process in decision making.	New behavior can be learned through modeling.
Allow sufficient time for client to think and act.	Client with depression may have sluggish or slowed thinking and behavioral responses.
Clearly communicate what is expected of client.	Clear expectations of behavior provide guidelines for self-motivation.
Help client formulate written plan of activity, first on day-to-day basis, then for longer periods.	Written activity plans foster feelings of control.

Evaluation

Client reports improved decision-making skills.

Nursing Diagnosis

Ineffective Individual Coping related to feelings of depression and lack of energy

Outcome

Client will verbalize feelings and identify and use effective coping skills.

Intervention	Rationale
Initiate interaction with client on a regular basis.	Individuals with depression lack the energy and drive to make interpersonal contact.
Encourage verbalization of feelings, as in "You look very annoyed this morning."	Verbalization of feelings allows client to examine relationships between feelings, event, and behaviors.
Encourage physical expression of feelings, such as striking pillows or a punching bag and hammering appropriate objects.	Feelings can be expressed nonverbally, as well as verbally.
Avoid impulse to cheer up clients or try to talk them out of the depression.	Nurses' good intentions to talk clients our of their depression has no effect on lifting it.
Explore with client what is helping to maintain the feeling of depression. (What are the secondary gains?)	Client may need help exploring the feelings of guilt, inadequacy, etc. that underlie depression.

Evaluation

Client expresses feelings and reports use of effective coping skills.

Nursing Care Plan 29-2

The Client With Bipolar Disorder, Manic Type

Nursing Diagnosis

Risk for Injury related to overactivity and impulsive behavior

Outcome

Client will remain free of injury.

Intervention	Rationale
Keep environmental stimuli to a minimum.	Decreased stimuli decrease potential for impulsive, acting-out behavior. Client may have to be removed from company of other clients if infringing on their rights.
Provide client sufficient room in which to move.	Increased energy levels can be channeled through activities such as walking or pacing.
Assist client to engage in activities, such as writing and drawing, to dissipate energy.	Writing and drawing channel energy and allow client to express feelings.
Set and maintain limits on acting-out behavior.	Clear limits on behavior are necessary to provide external controls when client lacks internal controls.

Evaluation

Client remains physically safe.

Nursing Diagnosis

Feeding/Bathing/Toileting Self-care Deficit related to excessive energy level and distractibility

Outcome

Client will perform self-care activities of eating, bathing, toileting independently.

Intervention	Rationale
Provide finger foods which client can carry around; don't expect client to sit for meals.	Client with manic behavior is "driven by motor" and distractible and needs to eat foods while moving constantly.
Provide 6–8 glasses of fluid per day.	Increased metabolic demands associated with client's constant movement may lead to dehydration.
Choose foods for the client that provide needed additional calories.	Client's excessive movement requires additional calories and foods high in nutritive value.
Maintain an intake and output record, if warranted.	Nursing must monitor adequacy of client's intake and output.
Remind client to bathe, brush teeth, use toilet, and assist as necessary.	Client may be too distractible and "busy" to groom and toilet self unless reminded or assisted.
Help client select clothing appropriate to climate and situation.	Client with manic behavior may wear suggestive or otherwise inappropriate clothing unless directed otherwise.

continued

Nursing Care Plan 29-2 *(Continued)*

Evaluation

Client performs self-care activities of eating, bathing, and toileting adequately.

Nursing Diagnosis

Impaired Social Interaction related to impatience with others and inability to tolerate frustration

Outcome

Client will identify problems in relating with others and behavior that interferes with socialization.

Intervention	Rationale
Assist client to interact with nurse and one other person in social situation.	Interaction with a group may be too stimulating for client. Limited social interaction is preferable.
Plan situations in which client experiences successful interaction with another; choose activities such as participating in a cooking or art project.	Client with manic behavior has difficulty cooperating; therefore, controlled situations in which client has a specific role in a project can promote improved social interaction.
Use persuasion rather than force.	Use of force leads to increased angry and defiant behavior.
Point out behaviors that lead to rejection by others, (such as demanding privileges, controlling others, manipulation) in a nonblaming manner.	Discussing problematic behaviors helps client explore their effect on others.
Reinforce use of effective social skills, such as consideration of others, being helpful, taking turns.	Behavior that is reinforced is more likely to continue.

Evaluation

Client and others report client's use of more productive social skills.

Nursing Diagnosis

Sensory-perceptual Alteration related to "racing thoughts" and sensory overload

Outcome

Client will report diminished sensory overload and incidence of racing thoughts.

Intervention	Rationale
Minimize environmental stimuli.	Decreased stimuli reduces client's distractibility.
Clarify reality for client.	Sensory overload and excessive activity may lead to reality confusion for client.
Inform client when conversation is not understandable; help client focus on one thing at a time.	Client with flight of ideas needs help in completing one activity or conversation at a time.

Evaluation

Client reports less disturbance from racing thoughts and sensory overload.

continued

Nursing Care Plan 29-2 (Continued)

Nursing Diagnosis

Altered Thought Processes related to grandiose beliefs about self

Outcome

Client will differentiate between reality and delusions.

Intervention	Rationale
Reinforce reality by not talking or arguing about client's delusions.	Delusional beliefs are reinforced by discussions or challenges.
Respect client by not laughing at behavior that is occurring during manic phase.	Respectful treatment maintains client dignity and protects from others' ridicule.
Protect client from self-harm and giving away possessions.	Safety interventions are essential nursing responsibilities.

Evaluation

Client distinguishes reality from delusions.

Outcomes for the Manic Client

Assessment of the manic client will result in a different list of needs during the manic state:

1. Physical safety and health
2. Opportunities to channel physical and psychic energy
3. Accurate perception of reality

The manic client has the same underlying needs for love and autonomy that the depressed client exhibits in a more obvious manner. During the manic episode, however, the client's strong denial necessitates that the nurse postpone most interpersonal actions that may help the client meet these needs.

Discharge Planning

Most clients with depressive and bipolar disorders have functioned in society as adult family members and will be able to do so again in the future. Planning, therefore, must extend beyond the time and place of hospitalization. The client's family must be incorporated into the plan of care to prevent the client from feeling abandoned and alone.

Other resources, such as church, work, and social groups, must be maintained if at all possible. What employment opportunities will be available to the client? What opportunites for socialization will present themselves to the client? To whom can the client turn when under stress? These and similar questions must be answered as the nurse and other members of the mental health team plan with clients and family for the return to home and community.

INTERVENTION FOR THE CLIENT WITH DEPRESSION

After identifying nursing diagnoses and behavior outcomes for the client with a depressive disorder, the nurse identifies nursing actions designed to achieve these outcomes. Behavior changes slowly, and the client may have periods of regression. Realistic expectations about behavior change must accompany the nurse's actions. Even minor changes in the client's behavior should be considered significant; nursing approaches should not be discarded prematurely (Case Study 29-1).

Physical Safety and Health

Decreasing Suicide Risk. The depressed client's needs for physical safety and health require that the nurse maintain a constant vigil for the possibility of suicide and other self-destructive behaviors. Once the nurse has determined that the client is suicidal, several actions are warranted. The client should be observed frequently or continuously on a one-to-one basis. The nurse must make sure that the environment is as free from potential danger as possible. Belts, razor blades, scissors, and other sharp objects should be removed. The nurse should be very aware of the medications that the client is taking and the possiblity of the client hoarding dosages for future lethal ingestion. Pill overdose is the most common form of successful suicide and suicidal gesture.[9] If these clients leave the unit or hospital for any reason, they and their belongings should be carefully

Case Study

Major Depression

Mrs. A was admitted to the unit by her older brother, who summarized her life for the nurse. Although Mrs. A was born at a time of parental financial difficulty, her life was uneventful until she was 7 years old, when her mother died and she assumed many household chores. While her father cared about her, he worked hard and spent little time with her. She assumed the responsibilities of cooking for her father and older brother and making household decisions. Mrs. A finished high school and business college, having limited social activities because of caring for her father and brother. However, she met a young man in the office where she worked, and they eventually married. Mrs. A told her brother she experienced happiness for the first time since early childhood. She was a good mother to her two children and enjoyed her home and family. When her oldest child, a son, married and left home, she felt a great sense of sadness and loss. However, she continued to care for her daughter and husband and at times enjoyed activities and her home.

Two years after the son married, Mrs. A's husband died. This was six months before her admittance to the hospital. At first, Mrs. A had shown very little grief and did not cry.

On admission, Mrs. A cried frequently and reported feelings of guilt and worthlessness. She had lost interest in her friends and social events. Her older brother brought her to the physician with complaints of constipation, anorexia, difficulty falling asleep and he was afraid she would harm herself. Mrs. A's history, general appearance, crying spells, and potential for self harm led the physician to believe hospitalization was warranted. She has no previous psychiatric hospitalizations.

After talking with Mrs. A in the quietness of her room the following data base was obtained, nursing diagnosis derived and care plan implemented (see Nursing Care Plan for the Depressed Client, 29-1).

I. Objective data
  A. General appearance, attitude, and activity
    1. Appearance: wearing a wrinkled house dress, hair uncombed, no make-up
    2. Attitude: appears sad, gloomy, answers questions very slowly
    3. Activity: looks at the floor, sits for long periods without looking up or moving, moves slowly when encouraged
  B. Communication patterns
    1. When encouraged to talk, dwells on how guilty and worthless she is
    2. Communication is understandable
  C. Contact with the environment
    1. Oriented to time, place and person
    2. Not distracted by sights or sounds in the room
  D. Sensorium and intelligence
    1. Memory is accurate for recent and remote events
    2. Somewhat detached and inattentive, and states she would like to rest
  E. Thought processes
    1. Coherent
  F. Thought content
    1. Continually dwells on her own self-worthlessness, and wonders why she should go on
    2. No delusions or hallucinations reported
  G. Social Assessment
    1. Mrs. A is in the upper-middle-class socioeconomic group and a high-school graduate, with business school training.
    2. Her parents are deceased: mother died when she was 7 years old. Her husband died 6 months ago. Living relatives: married son, older brother and a 16-year-old daughter who lives at home
    3. The children do not seem surprised by their mother's condition; however, they are concerned. Her older brother, who brought her in, states she has been sad off and on through the years, but never this bad.
    4. The family plans daily visits, wants to participate in family conferences or therapy, and are anxious for Mrs. A to be discharged.

continued

Case Study (Continued)

H. Physical Assessment
1. Reports constipation, bowel sounds present but hypoactive
2. Weight is 110 lbs, reports weight loss of 8 lb in one month and states she is nau seated at the sight of food
3. Sleeping only 3–4 hs./night, complains of difficulty getting to sleep and early morning awakenings.

II. Subjective data

A. Present Illness

Mrs. A states her reason for coming to the hospital is "My brother was worried about me not eating, sleeping and my lack of energy. I cry most of the time, and I would like some medicine to get rid of this con stipation."

B. Precipitating Event

Mrs. A tells of her husband's death six months ago, and states he was her hope in life, her love, and her security. She, however, does not relate this loss to her present crying, nausea, insomnia or constipation. She states she has had "sad spells off and on for as long as she can remember."

Questions for Discussion

1. Explore the role of unresolved grief/bereavement as a precipitator of depression.
2. What psychosocial considerations does the nurse need to be cognizant of regarding planning care with Mrs. A and her family?
3. How would the nurse facilitate the patient gaining insight into her problems?
4. What is Mrs. A's highest priority need on admission to the hospital?
5. What community resources would you provide the client and family on discharge?

searched on return. Psychiatric facilities should have a detailed written description of suicide precautions to be implemented when clients are identified as suicidal. The nurse should be familiar with these and assume responsibility for their initiation, enforcement, and modification.

There is a close relationship between suicide and crisis theory. The nurse may view the suicidal state as a therapeutic opportunity. The client may be ready to learn new coping skills that can be used after the crisis has subsided. If the nurse has not already established a relationship with the client, it is imperative that the nurse or some other health care team member do so at this time. If suicide is a cry for love, help, and attention, clients must feel that someone perceives these needs and cares for them. The nurse may determine that the risk of suicide is so great that the client should not be left alone, even in the bathroom. Important interventions are acknowledging the client's stressful situation and offering support and help in controlling these impulses. Gratifying dependency needs during this acutely stressful period may reduce the client's level of anxiety, which in turn decreases the risk of suicide.

In addition to meeting dependency needs, the nurse should use the therapeutic relationship to help depressed clients gain an understanding of the crisis, become aware of and accept their feelings (which may be hostile), and explore coping mechanisms other than self-destruction.

Nurses base their reactions to the suicidal client on the beliefs that clients who talk about suicide do commit suicide and that threats and attempts must be taken seriously. Nurses must not deny the client's feelings by shying away from discussing suicidal thoughts. Such discussions will not cause clients to commit suicide or make them more suicidal; rather, they will probably reduce some of the anxiety. Suicidal clients are ambivalent about dying, and the nurse should maximize arguments the client accepts or offers for living. The client who commits suicide is not necessarily psychotic or even mentally ill. In many instances, the risk of suicide is greatest when the client is emerging from the depths of depression and appears to be improving. The client then has the physical and mental energy to conceive a plan and carry it out. The client may actually feel and communicate relief on finding a final solution (ie, suicide) to problems (see Chapter 42, Suicide).

Ensuring Physical Health. Severely depressed clients may not have the energy to attend to bodily needs. The nurse should do the following as long as clients cannot do them for themselves:

1. Bathing the client
2. Assisting with the client's grooming, such as care of hair and nails
3. Selecting appropriate clothing
4. Ensuring the intake of nutritious food, which may mean sitting with clients as they eat

5. Clearing the environment of potential hazards, such as misplaced furniture, slippery rugs, and poorly lighted areas
6. Maintaining a record of sleeping patterns, bowel function, and menstrual function
7. Identifying the need for further nursing and medical actions

Promoting Physical Activity. The depressed clients should be encouraged to engage in physical activity to expel energy and produce feelings of physical well-being, control, and accomplishment (see Box 29-8). Because joy accompanies activity, clients should participate in active behaviors that were previously reinforcing, such as jogging, tennis, or housekeeping, even if they do not want to do them. Clients progress from solitary activity to noncompetitive activity with others to competitive activity with others.

Monitoring Side Effects of Medication. If the depressed client is receiving antidepressant medication, the nurse should be familiar with the side effects of these medications. These may include constipation, dry mouth, sedation, loss of visual accommodation, headache, dizziness, nausea and vomiting, increased perspiration, and weight gain or loss. These side effects can be minimized or avoided by gradually increasing the dosage to the optimal therapeutic level.[16] The nurse should discuss possible side effects with the client and encourage the client to report any that occur.

Expression of Feelings

Exploration of Anger and Sadness. Depressed clients fear open communication and intimacy; nevertheless, feelings that rage inside them need some form of expression. In every phase of its development, depression includes a component of anger, whether that anger is visible or invisible, conscious or unconscious. Regardless of whether clients appear angry, they need someone with whom they can share sadness and verbalize guilt. The nurse must not be intimidated or discouraged by these interactions. Sometimes nurses mistakenly assume that it is a nursing responsibility to make things better for a client. Even if clients profess extreme helplessness, the nurse must not approach them as though they were helpness beings.

The nurse may find it useful to explore with the client what is helping to maintain the depression. Once the client identifies depression-reinforcing behaviors used to elicit sympathy from others, such as crying, the client may decide to stop engaging in these behaviors and stop talking about the depression.

Therapeutic Communication. The nurse engages in active listening and demonstrates acceptance of whatever feelings and thoughts the client communicates (Box 29-9). If the nurse withdraws or more overtly rejects clients or the feelings they express, clients are reinforced in the belief that it is not safe to express themselves and that others do not care about them. Nurses should not try to talk clients out of their sadness by being imappropriately cheerful and optimistic or by offering false reassurance.

Cultural Influences. Overt expression of feelings is influenced by cultural heritage. People from Southern European and Latin American cultures tend to be very expressive: those from Northern European and Asian cultures are not. Some people believe that expressing feelings is a sign of weakness to be avoided at all costs. This

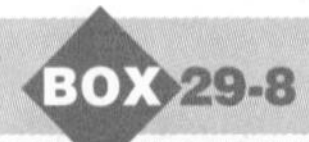

The Brain–Body Phenomenon

Physical exercise, such as walking, jogging, bicycling, swimming, and aerobic dance, may be powerful antidotes to depression and anxiety for the following reasons:

1. Exercise produces a sense of enhanced mental energy and concentration. Joggers express feelings of heightened mental acuity and hours of clear headedness after running.
2. Exercise relieves tension. Strenuous activity is all-absorbing, not allowing the participant to worry about anything else. Tension may not return until hours after exercise. Stress on one body system may help relax another.
3. Exercise is adult play, accompanied by joy and lightheartedness.
4. Exercise produces a sense of self-worth. Participants set progressive goals that are achievable and not in competition with others. It is hard to feel sorry for yourself and exercise at the same time.
5. Exercise produces a sense of control. It gives the participant freedom not experienced in other aspects of life. The cyclist or jogger does not depend on anyone else for exercise.
6. Exercise can symbolize active participation in life and serve as a socially acceptable way of asserting oneself.

Mental energy, lightheartedness, self-worth, autonomy, and assertiveness are the antitheses of depression. Movement, through physical exercise, may be a prescription of choice for mood disturbances.

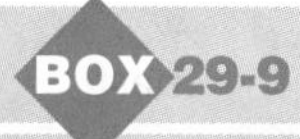

Therapeutic Dialogue: Encouraging Expression of Feelings

Nurse: Sarah, you mentioned you were in the hospital because you attempted suicide; tell me more about that. (sitting on a bed next to the client, maintaining eye contact, leaning toward the client)

Client: I took an overdose of Elavil. I ended up in Intensive Care for 4 days. I just couldn't take it anymore. I had to get out of the house. (looking at the nurse, speaking calmly and deliberately)

Nurse: Then you didn't intend to kill yourself? (asked in a questioning manner, trying to make eye contact with the client)

Client: No, it was the only way I could get away from my parents. (The client, Sarah, is a 32-year-old woman with muscular dystrophy who is confined to a wheelchair.) They don't support me; they didn't even come to see me when I was in Intensive Care. (maintaining intermittent eye contact with the nurse, wiping tears off cheek).

Nurse: You wanted them to care? (speaking softly)

Client: Yes. You know it's hard watching your body deteriorate a little bit at a time. Every day I lose something. I remember when I could dance like everybody else. (affect very sad, still maintaining intermittent eye contact) I'm depressed, but I've got a good reason to be depressed. There's no cure for me; I'm just getting worse.

Nurse: It's a heavy burden for you. (maintaining eye contact with the client).

Client: Yes. (nodding head) So I've got to use my mind. That's the only thing I have left.

Discussion

Sarah voluntarily mentioned her suicidal behavior to the nurse who did not hesitate to explore this further. Suicide is accompanied by an intense feeling state; there is a need to verbalize and share.

The nurse attempts to clarify Sarah's feelings and the meaning of her suicidal behavior. Sarah expresses ambivalent feelings toward her parents; she wants to leave them, but she wants them to care. The nurse has not yet begun to explore the origin of these feelings, nor the alternative ways to express them.

The nurse conveys a sincere interest in the meaning of, and the feelings associated with, the client's behavior. The nurse neither moralizes about the act of suicide nor challenges the client with the possibility that she really had no intent to take her own life.

As Sarah has explained, her depression can be associated with a very real, ongoing loss. She seems to be communicating that she needs more help to cope with the feelings of anger and frustration inherent in her situation. The nurse identifies this need, which will become an important focus in Sarah's plan of care.

belief is demonstrated in the subculture of sex. In many societies, it is acceptable for girls and women to express their feelings, but not for boys and men. As the nurse implements care, these cultural differences must be considered.

Positive Reinforcement. Another helpful approach in the treatment of depression is the concept of positive reinforcement. The nurse may advocate the use of an antidepression kit, which contains pleasuring items, memorabilia of happy times, or reminders of future activity. Clients create this kit and turn to it when they feel depressed.

Effects on the Caregiver. Depression is contagious, and depressed people tend to drive others away from them. Depressed clients are repetitively negativistic and sometimes clinging and manipulative. Nurses often feel frustrated and angry at themselves in return. Planning and sharing the client's care with other health team members give nurses a means of group support and an opportunity to express and explore their feelings. The client's family, who may have been likewise frustrated, may be encouraged by learning that depression is self-limiting and that they can look forward to a time when the client will return to a more normal level of functioning. Family members' involvement in the client's treatment may help determine the degree of adaptation and growth that the entire family is able to achieve as a result of the depressive episode.

Feelings of Acceptance and Belonging

The nurse can initiate a therapeutic relationship with the depressed client to facilitate feelings of acceptance and belonging. The nurse may schedule regular meeting times, thereby ensuring privacy and communicating that the client is important as an individual. These individual appointments should be arranged only if the nurse can realistically implement and follow through with them. The nurse's trustworthiness and consistency are paramount issues in providing care for the depressed client.

The nurse must also maintain a sensitivity to the environment and constantly question how other clients and staff influence the depressed client. Is the client being included in activities? Is he or she relating to others, and if so, on what level? The psychiatric-mental health nurse generally has more opportunity to make such observations and manipulate the environment to the client's benefit than does any other health team member.

Feelings of Being Useful and Needed and Feelings of Accomplishment

Illness and hospitalization, whether for mental or physical reasons, usually cause the client to experience a certain degree of helplessness and dependency. Consequently, it is often difficult to promote feeling of being useful and needed in the client. Nevertheless, the nurse should use whatever opportunities arise to develop and reinforce these feelings. As soon as clients are ready, they should participate in groups that share in decision making for the unit or facility in which care is being given. Clients also should be encouraged to assume some responsibility for planning and carrying out social activities and sharing in other unit tasks.

A severely depressed client is drawn into a state of lethargy and inactivity and may not be able to function as an effective member of a group; expecting such a client to do so may reinforce a negative self-view. The nurse must assess the client carefully before communicating expectations. The severely depressed client may benefit from an initial one-to-one relationship that gradually expands to include a larger sphere of people with whom the client feels comfortable.

Nursing actions intended to mobilize depressed clients into activity have been designed using Beck's cognitive framework.[31] His approach of acceptance, reactivation, and cognition is based on the assumption that the way we think about, evaluate, or predict events around us determines how we feel and behave. The aim is to relieve such symptoms as apathy, self-criticism, and thoughts of suicide. Behavioral techniques to counteract helpless thinking patterns are graded task assignments, activity schedules, and mastery-pleasure monitoring.

Graded task assignments consist of breaking up large tasks into small manageable steps that allow the client to focus on behaviors associated with grooming, eating, and socialization. Daily activity scheduling entails an hourly designation of activities for the client intended to counteract the inactivity associated with negative ruminations and sadness. With the mastery-pleasure technique, the client keeps a running account of and rates experiences that provide for mastery or pleasure. This provides evidence for clients that they have certain competencies and that not everything is without some degree of pleasure.

Once the client is able to engage in constructive activities, cognition is increasingly emphasized.[4] Lethargy-inducing patterns of thought, such as, "I have nothing important to share with anyone," are analyzed and tested by the client and nurse. Questioning assumptions and identifying distortions in thinking, such as, "I have to be perfect to be loved," may be enough to disprove self-defeating ideas and allow the client to identify alternative thoughts that focus on strengths.

Successful experiences in the hospital may help clients believe that they also can be effective outside the hospital. Discharge planning must include a consideration of what in the client's future life will permit feelings of being needed and useful. Are there family members to whom the client is important? Is there an occupation in need of his or her talent? To whom or what does the client make a difference?

Opportunities for Autonomy and Self-Actualization

Autonomy and self-actualization are frequently identified as characteristics of mentally healthy people.[9] Autonomy, a component of self-actualization, implies a relative independence of the physical and social environment. Autonomous people are not dependent for their main satisfactions on other people and their opinions and affections. Self-actualization is exhibited by people who must do what they are fit to do and must be true to their own nature. Autonomy and self-actualization are long-term goals toward which many people strive throughout life.

Learned helplessness and dependency, the opposites of autonomy and self-actualization, are frequent companions of depression. Severely depressed clients may not be able to take care of their own bodily needs, decide how to dress in the morning, or choose what to have for breakfast. They are even less able to make decisions about relationships, financial needs, or occupational matters. In some situations, the nurse must make such decisions for the client until the anxiety level decreases and decision-making ability increases. The nurse does what must be done to mobilize the client; this frequently requires a directive approach. For example, the client is not asked if he or she would like to have breakfast but is told that it is time for breakfast. In this instance, the nurse may appear to be taking away the client's autonomy; however, a client cannot be deprived of autonomy when it has already been surrendered to depression.

As clients progress, the nurse encourages them to

listen to themselves and to make more decisions. The nurse's own problem-solving skills provide both support and a corrective educational process for clients. What does the client perceive as his or her problems? What are the possible outcomes of such solutions? What puts the client in control of self and situation? The client who can recognize the potential for self-direction and development is taking a step toward health and away from a mode of thinking that plays a central role in depression.

Pharmacotherapy

Antidepressant Medication. Antidepressant and antimanic drugs may alleviate the client's syptoms but do not resolve the psychosocial issues that may have precipitated, or result from, these disorders. Drug therapy lessens the overwhelming agitation, anxiety, and sadness the client is suffering, making him or her more amenable to psychotherapy.

Antidepressant drugs are the primary classification of drugs prescribed for a client with a depressive episode. These drugs are *mood regulators,* which work by altering the brain's response to neurotransmitter substances (norepinephrine, serotonin, dopamine). The benefits of using these medications include improved sleep and energy, appetite regulation, improved ability to cope, and decreased irritability and anxiety.

There are three main classifications of antidepressants:

1. TCAs, which alter the brain's responses to the neurotransmitters norepinephrine ans serotonin
2. MAOIs, which block the action of an enzyme that breaks down the transmitters norepinephrine and dopamine
3. *Selective serotonin reuptake inhibitors* (SSRIs), which enhance the activity of serotonin by preventing its reabsorption at nerve endings

The TCAs, such as amitriptyline (Elavil) and imipramine (Tofranil), are still commonly prescribed, but their use is declining because of side effects and the availability of alternatives. The MAOIs, such as phenelzine (Nardil) and tranylcypromine (Parnate), may be useful for clients who cannot tolerate the side effects of TCAs or have an atypical depression.[16] The MAOIs can produce hypertension when taken at the same time as tyramine, a substance found in aged cheese, red wine, and certain other foods. The nurse must teach the client dietary precautions to avoid this serious interaction.

The SSRIs, such as fluoxetine (Prozac), sertraline (Zoloft), nefazodone (Serzone), trazodone (Desyrel); the tetracyclics bupropion (Wellbutrin) and maprotiline (Ludiomil); and the newer nonselective uptake inhibitor antidepressants fluvoxamine (Luvox) and venlafaxine (Effexor) are as effective as the TCAs. However, these drugs do not cause the weight gain, urinary retention, blurred vision, and heart dysrhythmias associated with the TCAs.

The SSRIs do have associated nausea, nervousness, insomnia, headache, and sexual dysfunction as potential side effects. The nurse should be knowledgeable about the therapeutic dose ranges, half-life, side effects, and drug interactions for any antidepressant a client is taking. An essential aspect of nursing care is client and family education regarding drug management. The goal should be to minimize any adverse side effects of the drug on the client's lifestyle.

Antidepressants must be taken for 3 to 4 weeks for a significant therapeutic response to be evident. Suicidally depressed clients can become motivated and begin to look better before their subjective depressive feeling and suicidal thoughts are relieved. It is estimated that more than 50% of depressed outpatients who begin treatment with antidepressant medication experience complete remission of their depressive symptons, and 65% to 85% show marked improvement.[15,16]

Client and Family Medication Education

An essential aspect of nursing care is client and family education regarding medication management. The goal should be to minimize adverse side effects of the drug on the client's lifestyle. For example, constipation can be alleviated by increasing the client's fluid and fiber intake. Fall prevention precautions are indicated for orthostatic hypotension or dizziness. Seizure precautions should be initiated for clients with preexisting seizure disorders. Elderly clients and those with cardiac disease require surveillance. The nurse must observe clients carefully to verify that they are taking their medication. A client with depressive or bipolar disorder may believe that drugs are not necessary or are even harmful.

INTERVENTION FOR THE CLIENT WITH MANIA

Nursing care of the manic client is focused primarily on maintaining physical health until the manic state subsides. A client in a manic state seeks to release tension through physical activity and may not be aware of other physical or psychological needs. The client's flight of ideas prevents significant interpersonal contact.

Physical Safety and Health

The manic client's increased mobility ranges from mild motor excitement to incessant activity. The client's talking, singing, dancing, and teasing are frequently accompanied by anorexia, weight loss, insomnia, and constipation. The nurse intervenes by keeping environmental stimuli to a minimum, for example, keeping the client away from areas where others are engaging in noisy physical activity. The client is extremely distractible and reacts to almost any stimulus in the environment.

Unrealistic client demands are also a potential problem and are best approached with partial fulfillment of the demand whenever possible. The nurse tries to avoid direct confrontations by letting clients know what they can do rather than what they cannot do. A client's request to go outside at night, for example, could be answered with the information that he or she will have the opportunity to go out in the morning, if this is true. This approach encourages the client to focus on positive aspects, rather than on the limitations placed on behavior.

At times it may be necessary to use clients' distractibility to ease them out of a troublesome situation. The euphoric mood of manic clients can change quickly to irritation or even rage when others do not respond to their enthusiasm or do not react in accordance with their expectations.

Promoting Physical Health. If excitability is not aggravated, the nurse may find it easier to attend to the client's physical needs. The client cannot be expected to sit down for complete meals but can be given foods and liquid to carry around and eat. These foods should be high-calorie and high-protein substances because of the increased energy expenditure. The nurse also should monitor the client's sleeping and elimination patterns, which may be neglected. Nursing or medical intervention may be necessary to promote proper rest and elimination. Clients also should be observed carefully for signs of illness; they may be in a debilitated state and may ignore or be unaware of developing symptoms of physical disease.

Channeling Physical and Psychic Energy

A creative nursing approach to the manic client is crucial in planning treatment. The nurse attempts to reduce the client's accelerated manner of thinking and speaking by presenting accurate feedback. For example, when a client moves rapidly from one topic to the next, the nurse states that what the client has said is not understood and asks for clarification. When interacting with this client, the nurse may find it necessary to refocus or redirect the conversation so that only one topic is discussed at a time. Although these approaches may meet with limited success, the nurse has an obligation to provide accurate information to clients about how they are being perceived by others. It is usually best to avoid long discussions with the manic client.

If manic clients have access to paper and pen or pencil, they often will write voluminously. Writing may in fact provide a therapeutic benefit to the client who can use this medium to express feelings. The nurse may involve the client in gross motor activities, such as sweeping, mopping, or other tasks, and some noncompetitive physical exercises to channel hyperactivity. Because the client's attention span is short, participation in games and sports that require sustained interest and adherence to rules usually is unsuccessful. Monitoring and directing the client's activity are essential to prevent exhaustion.

Reinforcement of Reality

Manic clients are expansive in thinking and may be delusional. They may believe they exert great power and control and possess great wealth. They may identify with the influential people in the environment; for example, the manic client may be found making rounds with the doctors or nurses. Nurses mirror reality for these clients by responding to them as the people they are. The client's beliefs are not challenged; nonetheless, delusional thinking is not encouraged.

Consistency in Approach

Because of the manic client's propensity to manipulate people in the environment, those responsible for care must communicate with one another and respond to the client in a consistent manner. The client can be argumentative and demanding; the nurse should not respond in kind. The nurse and other mental health caregivers set limits on the client's behavior consistently and with confidence, knowing that they have planned and chosen the most appropriate interventions according to the client's needs.

Drug Therapy

Lithium. Lithium is the drug of choice for mania, and when it is used preventively, it protects a client by reducing the recurrence of cycles of mania and depression. It effectively decreases the client's excessive elation, hyperactivity, and accelerated thinking and speaking.

Lithium, a relatively dangerous drug because of its narrow therapeutic dose range, is 80% effective in treating the manic episodes of bipolar disorder.[13] The narrow margin of safety between therapeutic and toxic levels requires frequent blood tests to monitor lithium levels. The initial stabilization phase may be followed by a maintenance phase during which the dose is reduced.

At the start of treatment, blood lithium levels are monitored every few days. Once drug levels stabilize, monitoring is at 1- to 3-month intervals. Lithium treatment takes 5 days to 2 weeks to become effective. Clients may be maintained on lithium for an indefinite period, depending on the recurrence, severity, and duration of each manic episode.

Because lithium is almost entirely eliminated from the body by the kidneys, laboratory tests of kidney function are done before and during therapy. Thyroid function tests are usually evaluated because lithium can cause goiter or hypothyroidism. An electrocardiogram and electrolyte panel may also be considered.

Initially a client may be given an antipsychotic to control aggressive behavior until the lithium reaches therapeutic levels. During this lag phase in the treatment, the nurse should keep in mind that high doses of antipsychotics will mask the nausea and vomiting of lithium toxicity.

The nurse should ascertain what the client and family understand about the need for the lithium and help them accept the likelihood of continuing therapy for an extended time. The client's family should also be alerted to the effects and side effects of the lithium and the importance of monitoring the reappearance of manic behavior.

Lithium may interact with a number of other drugs, resulting in decreases or increases in lithium levels; the client should not take any other medications without consulting the nurse or physician.

The nurse should instruct the family on early side effects, such as nausea, vomiting, diarrhea, thirst, and fine hand tremor. Simple measures, such as taking the drug on a full stomach or with a glass of milk, are effective for the gastrointestinal symptoms. The nurse should make sure the client's family is knowledgeable about the signs of impending lithium toxicity and the need to notify the physician (see Chapter 20, Psychopharmacology).

Individuals with a form of bipolar disorder that cycles rapidly from depression to mania represent 13% to 20% of the bipolar population. Although lithium remains the treatment of choice for classic bipolar disorder, failure rates as high as 72% to 82% have been reported for lithium among those who have the rapid cycling form of bipolar disorder.

Treatment alternatives for these clients include the use of the anticonvulsant divalproex sodium (Depakote).[5] Divalproex and valproic acid (Depakene) probably increase the brain levels of GABA. The client should have liver function tests and prothrombin times at baseline and at monthly intervals for the first 6 months.[15] Carbamazepine (Tegretol) seems to work by inhibiting nerve impulses, thus limiting the influx of sodium ions across the cell membrane in the motor cortex. Blood levels of both drugs are monitored frequently in the beginning of treatment and every 3 months or so afterwards.

Client and Family Medication Education. The client should be warned that use of carbamazepine with MAOIs may cause a hypertensive crisis. Also, carbamazepine interferes with the contraceptive ability of the birth control pill. Liver enzymes should be monitored for elevation and thyroid function for decreased values.

The nurse should instruct clients to consult with their care provider before taking any other drug because of the possibility of numerous drug interactions.

The nurse may refer the client and family to a local chapter of the National Depressive and Manic-Depressive Association[23] for continued support.

Other Therapies

Various other therapies for the client with a mood disorder include drugs, ECT, light therapy, and psychotherapy.

Electroconvulsive Therapy. First used in 1938, ECT involves the application of a small dose of electricity to one or both sides of the brain to induce a seizure. Exactly how ECT works remains unclear, but the seizure probably modifies the metabolism of the neurotransmitters believed to contribute to depression.[21] This is considered effective for clients with severe delusional or endogenous depression, acute mania, and schizophrenia of short duration with concurrent affective illness.

A relatively safe procedure, ECT sounds more ominous than it is. Nevertheless, the nurse should keep in mind that it may elicit strong feelings of fear and anxiety in clients and families. The client may envision electrocution or death or may anticipate permanent intellectual changes. The physician and nurse must carefully explain what the treatment is like and prepare the client and family for the aftereffects.

The client is prepared for ECT in a manner similar to preparation for surgery. The nurse ensures that the client takes no food or drink the morning of the treatment, voids just before the procedure, removes dentures, and wears a hospital gown or loose clothing. The client must give informed consent, and the appropriate form must be signed. A complete physical examination is required, including a spinal x-ray. Vital signs are monitored before and after treatment.

Electroconvulsive therapy is usually administered in a room designated for this purpose. The client is placed on a stretcher or firm bed, and a rubber mouthpiece is inserted in the mouth to maintain an airway. Usually the client is given a short-acting anesthetic, such as methohexital (Brevital), and a muscle relaxant, frequently succinylcholine (Anectine), just before the electric shock is administered. Electrodes are applied unilaterally or bilaterally to the client's temples, and the shock is administered. The client experiences a typical grand mal seizure with tonic and clonic phases. The nurse and others in attendance should not attempt to restrain the client's body but should guide the extremities to prevent injury during the seizure activity.

When the seizure ends, oxygen may be given as a safety measure because apnea may occur physiologically in any general convulsive seizure. Airways and equipment for oxygenation should be readily available in the treatment area.

Once the client is transferred to the recovery area, consciousness will be regained quickly. The client should be positioned on his or her side while awakening to prevent aspiration of oral secretions. The nurse monitors the client's vital signs during the recovery period. It is usual for the client to be confused. The client must be observed carefully to ensure his or her safety and must be reoriented to surroundings.

The client may or may not be hospitalized for ECT treatments. The treatments are usually given three times a week; the number of treatments a client receives depends on the results obtained. The nurse's observations of the client during this time are important in the decision making regarding the number of future treatments.

A frequent aftereffect of ECT is memory impairment, ranging from a mild tendency to forget details to severe confusion. This may persist for weeks or months after treatment. The nurse prepares the client and family for this confusion and assures them that it is expected and that full return of memory will eventually occur. Evidence that unilateral treatment (administering electric current to only one side of the brain) produces less confusion and memory loss than bilateral treatment (administering current to both sides) is being investigated.

Light Therapy. Some major depressive episodes may have a seasonal pattern; the person becomes depressed when the days shorten, probably related to light and melatonin production. Treatment is provided with artificial-light therapy (also called phototherapy) and generally lasts from one-half to 3 hours one or twice a day.[10] Nurses can promote health in clients by teaching about the relationship between light and moods and the benefits of daily sunshine. They can also advocate better lighting in workplaces.

Psychotherapy. Psychotherapy is beneficial in treating depression, usually accompanied by treatment with medication. Cognitive and interpersonal therapies are particularly effective means to assist clients with mood disorders. These therapies may take place in individual or group contexts.

Cognitive and Behavioral Therapy. The goal of cognitive therapy is to assist the client to identify and correct distorted, negative, and catastrophic thinking, thereby relieving depressive symptoms. There is evidence that using cognitive therapy can reduce subsequent relapse after the period of initial drug treatment has been completed.[28] The goal of behavioral therapies is to modify maladaptive behaviors through homework assignments, structured schedules, and various other techniques. Chapter 18, Behavioral Approaches, provides further information about cognitive therapy.

Interpersonal Therapy Interpersonal therapy involves assisting clients to clarify various interpersonal difficulties, such as social isolation and role disruptions. Including the spouse or significant other in therapy reduces depressive symptoms.[29]

The nurse may provide or assist with these therapies to improve symptoms. The client can be given nursing guidance on current problems, methods to enhance social supports, and reinforcement of coping strengths and resources. Chapter 15, Individual Psychotherapy, provides information about a variety of interpersonal approaches to clients.

EVALUATION

The nurse evaluates care of the client with a depressive or bipolar disorder by observing the client's behaviors and comparing them with previously formulated client behavior outcomes. The nurse also collects data relating to the client's behavior by talking with the family and other health team members who are involved in care. The nursing process is cyclical: Evaluation results in reassessment of the client, formulation of new or modified nursing diagnoses and client behavior outcomes, and specification of additional or modified nursing interventions aimed at bringing the client closer to optimal health.

As the client interacts with the nurse and others during this evaluation phase, the nurse can consider the following questions:

- Has the client's self-concept become more positive? Is there any indication of suicidal ideation?
- Has the client's outlook become more optimistic?
- Has dependency decreased?
- Is decision making easier?
- Does the client interact more frequently with others?
- Does the client sleep more and complain less of fatigue and other physical maladies?
- Is appetite improved?
- Is weight being gained?
- Is the client attending to personal hygiene and grooming?

Positive responses to questions such as these usually indicate that the client has begun to assume control of life and is motivated to participate in activities of daily living.

When evaluating care of the manic client, the nurse may ask the following questions:

- Are the client's psychomotor activity and speech becoming slower and more regulated?

- Is the client less distractible?
- Is there a more realistic self-perception of influence and abilities?
- Is the client more introspective?
- Are dress and use of makeup more appropriate?
- Is the client sleeping more and able to monitor personal physical needs?

A return to a healthier state depends on the efforts of all health care team members, including family members, friends, and the clients themselves. When clients return home, these resources must still be accessible as they encounter many stressors that will test their newly acquired confidence. Clients may have new living arrangements to which they must adapt, a new job in which they must succeed, and altered or new relationships to establish and maintain. Clients must continue to have someone with whom to share feelings and validate perceptions and problem-solving skills.

◆ Chapter Summary

This chapter has focused on the characteristics of two different but related behavioral patterns—depression and mania—and the nursing care indicated for each. Chapter highlights include the following:

1. Depressive and bipolar disorders, described early in recorded history, are a major mental health problem in the United States.
2. Depression and mania are extreme feeling states with cognitive and physical components that differ primarily in degree, rather than in kind, from those experienced by healthier people.
3. The cause or causes of depressive and bipolar disorders have not been established with certainty; etiological theories include biological and psychosocial influences.
4. Depressive and bipolar disorders can be chronic and acutely psychotic and can be masked by various maladaptive behaviors, such as alcoholism and promiscuity.
5. The nurse has a responsiblity to participate in the primary prevention of mood disorders and in secondary and tertiary prevention.
6. The nurse is a collaborator with other members of the health care team, including the client and family, and assumes an influential role in client care and treatment, which have psychosocial and biological components.
7. Nursing assessment and intervention for the depressed client focus on the client's physical health and safety, feelings about self and others and expression of these feelings, and distorted perceptions and false beliefs about the environment and self.
8. Suicide, frequently an outcome of depression, can be prevented but not in every case.
9. Nursing assessment and intervention for the manic client focus on the client's energy, environmental manipulation, and reinforcement of reality.
10. Somatic therapy, including drug therapy and ECT, is a vital component of the treatment plan for a client with a mood disturbance.
11. Nurses and other mental health professionals need opportunities to express, explore, and resolve the feelings, including anger and frustration, that may develop as a result of their work with depressed and manic clients.

Review Questions

1. When planning care for a client with a depressive disorder, priority should be given to
   - **A.** planning appropriate activities.
   - **B.** structuring a pleasant milieu.
   - **C.** preventing suicidal behavior.
   - **D.** assisting the client to express repressed anger.
2. When working with a withdrawn client, which of the following techniques would be useful?
   - **A.** Insist that client communicate and participate in activities.
   - **B.** Use alternative communication techniques, such as painting or music.
   - **C.** Fill the silence with environmental descriptions.
   - **D.** Tell the client to approach you when ready to talk.
3. A client in a manic state often has intrusive behavior; which of the following would be essential to include in the care plan?
   - **A.** Encouragement to express emotions
   - **B.** Calling attention to self-deprecating remarks
   - **C.** Protecting her from attack
   - **D.** Preventing her from talking about her problems
4. A depressed client tells the nurse, "I'm no good. I deserve to die." Which of these responses would be most emotionally supportive?
   - **A.** Assurance that everyone has value and reminders that the client held a job until admission
   - **B.** Telling the client that everyone dies sooner or later and one's worth has nothing to do with it
   - **C.** Acknowledging feelings and then engaging the client in helping the nurse with a simple task
   - **D.** Admitting that the client probably has things to be ashamed of and helping to identify them

5. An overactive client says, "My name is BJ, but you can call me Cool Dude. I'm a flyer with unrestricted license. My CIA status is 007—licensed to kill. $2,000, that's what this suit cost. I got this blind eye when my rodeo chute wouldn't open." This speech pattern is
   - **A.** flight of ideas.
   - **B.** perseveration.
   - **C.** clang association.
   - **D.** associative looseness.
6. Electroconvulsive shock therapy is likely to produce which of the following side effects?
   - **A.** Tardive dyskinesia
   - **B.** Memory loss
   - **C.** Oculogyric crisis
   - **D.** Waxy flexibility
7. A behavior that suggests the greatest improvement in a client experiencing manic behavior would be
   - **A.** sitting through a group meeting.
   - **B.** commenting about the environment.
   - **C.** initiating interactions with others.
   - **D.** expressing dissatisfaction directly to the nurse.

◆ References

1. American Psychiatric Association: Diagnostic and Statistical Manual of Mental Disorders, 4th ed. Washington, DC, American Psychiatric Association, 1994
2. Brage DG: Adolescent Depression: A Review of the Literature. Archives of Psychiatric Nursing 9 (1): 45–55, 1995
3. Buckwalter K: How to Unmask Depression. Geriatric Byeaubfm July/August: 179–181, 1990
4. Butler ST, Chalder M, Ron BW et al: Cognitive Behavior Therapy in Chronic Fatigue Syndrome. J Neurol Neurosurg Psychiatry 54: 153–158, 1991
5. Calabrese JR, Woyshville MJ: Medication Algorithm for Treatment of Bipolar Rapid Cycling? J Clin Psychiatry 56 (3): 11–18, 1995
6. Coryell W, Endicott J, Keller M: Major Depression in a Nonclinical Sample: Demographic and Clinical Risk Factors for First Onset. Archives of General Psychiatry 49: 117–125, 1992
7. Craddock N, Owen M: Is there an Inverse Relationship Between Down's Syndrome and Bipolar Affective Disorder? Journal of Intellectual Disability Research 36 (Pt 6): 613–620, 1994
8. Cronkite K: On the Edge of Darkness, p 117. New York, Dell Publishing, 1995
9. Depression Guidelines Panel: Depression in Primary Care: Detection, Diagnosis, and Treatment. Quick Reference Guide for Clinicians, Number 5. Rockville, MD, U.S. Department of Health and Human Services, Public Health Service, Agency for Health Care Policy and Research Publication No. 93-0552
10. Dunham KL: Seasonal Affective Disorder: Light Makes Right. Am J Nurs December: 45–46, 1992
11. El-Mallakh RS, Wyatt RJ: The Na, K-ATPase Hypotheses for Bipolar Illness. Biological Psychiatry 37 (4): 235–244, 1995
12. Gold et al: Manifestations of Depression. N Engl J Med Aug. 11, 319 (6): 1988
13. Grinspoon L: Depression and Mood Disorders. The Harvard Mental Health Letter 11 (7): 1–3, 1995
14. Hall RC, Wise MG: The Clinical and Financial Burden of Mood Disorders. Cost and Outcome. Psychosomatics March-April, 36 (2): 8–11, 1995
15. Handbook of Psychotropic drugs, pp 6–7, 30. Springhouse, PA, Springhouse Corporation, 1992
16. Janicak PG, Savis JM, Preskorn SH, Ayd FJ: Principles and Practice of Psychopharmacotherapy, 280-290. Baltimore, Williams and Wilkins, 1993
17. Kennedy GJ: The Geriatric Syndrome of Late-Life Depression. Psychiatr Services 46 (1): 43–48, 1995
18. Kim MT: Cultural Influences on Depression in Korean Americans. J Psychosoc Nurs Ment Health Serv 33 (2): 13–17, 1995
19. Kovacs M, Akiskal HS: Childhood Onset Dysthymic Disorder: Clinical Features and Prospective Naturalistic Outcome. Arch Gen Psychiatry 51: 365–374, 1994
20. Lewinsohn PM, Hops H, Roberts RE Jr., Andrews JA: Adolescent Psychopathology: I. Prevalence and Incidence of Depression in Other DSM III-R Disorders in High School Students. J Abnorm Psychol 102: 133–144, 1993
21. Mann JJ, Kapur S: Elucidation of Biochemical Basis of the Antidepressant Action of Electroconvulsive Therapy by Human Studies. Psychopharmacol Bull 30 (3): 445–453, 1994
22. NARSAD Research Newsletter (National Alliance for Research on Scizophrenia and Depression) Summer: 4, 1994
23. National Depressive and Manic-Depressive Association, Chicago, IL
24. Papolos D, Papolos J: Overcoming Depression, rev ed, p 225. New York, Harper Collins, 1992
25. Potter WZ, Rudorfer MD, Manji RW: Drug Therapy. N Engl J Med 325 (9): 633–642, 1991
26. Romito P: Work and Health in Mothers of Young Children. Int J Health Serv 24 (4): 607–628, 1994
27. Seligman MP, Friedman RJ, Katz MM (eds): Depression and Learned Helplessness In the Psychology of Depression: Contemporary Theory and Research, pp 83–125. New York, John Wiley & Sons, 1974
28. Tastily JD, Segal Z, Williams JM: How Does Cognitive Therapy Prevent Depressive Relapse and Why? Behav Res Ther 33 (1): 25–39, 1995
29. Waring EM: The Role of Marital Therapy in the Treatment of Depressed Married Women. Can J Psychiatry 39 (9): 568–571, 1994
30. Wittchen H, Knauper B, Kessler RC: Lifetime Risk of Depression. Br J Psychiatry December (26): 23–30, 1994
31. Wright JH, Thase ME: Cognitive and Biological Therapies: A Synthesis. Psychiatric Annals 22: 451–458, 1992

Schizophrenic Disorders

Barbara Schoen Johnson

30

While I was at Grace Hospital, it was my sense of hearing which was the most disturbed. But soon after I was placed in my room at home, all of my senses became perverted. I still heard the "false voices"—which were doubly false, for Truth no longer existed. The tricks played upon me by my senses of taste, touch, smell, and sight were the source of great mental anguish.

Clifford Beers,
A Mind that Found Itself: An Autobiography, *1923*

This chapter focuses on a cluster of disorders marked by disturbed reality orientation, thought processes, and social involvement that collectively is known as schizophrenia. *These serious and often persistent mental disorders cause an untold burden on human lives.*

The overview of schizophrenic disorders describes their incidence, etiological theories, and types or diagnostic categories. The chapter discusses application of the nursing process—assessment, nursing diagnosis, planning, intervention, and evaluation—to clients with schizophrenia and to their families and communities.

Learning Objectives

On completion of this chapter, you should be able to accomplish the following:

1. *Discuss biological and psychosocial theories of the etiology of schizophrenia.*
2. *Identify the types of schizophrenia.*
3. *Describe the characteristic behaviors of schizophrenic disorders, including thought, affective, and social or behavioral disturbances.*
4. *Apply the nursing process to clients with schizophrenic disorders.*
5. *Discuss the effects and value of pharmacotherapeutic agents on the lives of clients with schizophrenia.*
6. *Describe the impact of a schizophrenic member on the family, community, and society.*
7. *Intervene educationally and therapeutically with the family of a schizophrenic client.*
8. *Identify interventions for populations at risk for developing schizophrenic disorders.*
9. *Evaluate your own feelings and attitudes when caring for clients with schizophrenia and their families.*

◆ Schizophrenic Disorders

Schizophrenia is a common and unsolved mental health problem in the world today. It is estimated that 1% of the United States' population (ie, 2–3 million people) is, has been, or will be affected by the disorder. Its onset usually occurs early in life--adolescence or young adulthood—and may become a progressive and disabling condition, although the course of schizophrenia need not be progressive and chronic. Recovery is possible.[62] See Box 30-1 for Diagnostic and Statistical Manual of Mental Disorders, fourth edition (DSM-IV), criteria for schizophrenia.

Economic, family, and community factors influence the lives of severely disturbed clients and their loved ones. The stigma of schizophrenia makes it more tragic, because clients and families must bear the stigma as well as the disease. "Schizophrenics," says Dr. Fuller Torrey, "are the lepers of the 20th century."[63] Unparalleled as a stigmatizing disease, schizophrenia reaps the societal consequences of personal shame, family burden, and inadequate support of clinical care, research, and rehabilitation.

The remarkable thing about schizophrenia as a disease, says Torrey, is how little attention it has received, given its prevalence and severity. Its cost in the United States has been estimated at $10 to $20 billion annually, including the costs of hospitalization, social security benefits for the disabled, welfare payments, and lost wages. Demographically, it is the most expensive of all chronic diseases, because the person is well during rearing and education and then becomes ill and dependent on society just when he or she would have become a contributing wage earner.[63]

Although multiple etiological theories have been proposed and studied, the definitive causes of schizophrenia remain unknown. Current methods of prevention and treatment are often inadequate—a clear case of "too little, too late."

Some types of schizophrenia exist worldwide, in all populations, regardless of culture.[30] There are, however, different incidence rates of schizophrenia when compared cross-culturally. See Box 30-2, p. 568, for DSM-IV criteria for the six types of schizophrenia.

Most likely, schizophrenia is not a single disease, but a *heterogeneous disorder*, that is, a group of several distinct disorders or a collection of disorders with some common features. These common features include disturbances in thinking and preoccupation with the self and inner fantasies. The person with a schizophrenic disorder may live in a private world—a world inhabited by voices that condemn or accuse the person of vile acts and by visions of frightening animals, monsters, or scenes. The person may be totally withdrawn from the external environment and may be preoccupied with an internal fantasy life. The person may regress to such an extent that personal hygiene, activities of daily living, interpersonal contacts, and even the presence of physical illness or pain are not managed.

COURSE AND PROGNOSIS

After the initial year of symptoms, the client's schizophrenia may be classified as *episodic, continuous,* or *in partial or full remission.*[1] There is growing evidence of heterogeneity in the long-term outcome of schizophrenia. Unfortunately, historical expectations of progressive deterioration of the person with schizophrenia have guided clinical teaching, diagnosis, treatment planning, and policy decisions for decades and have robbed many clients and their families of hope for recovery.

Schizophrenic disorders have symptoms (such as thought disturbances) and outcomes that change over

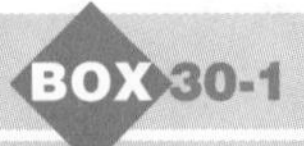

DSM-IV Diagnostic Criteria for Schizophrenia

A. Characteristic symptoms: Two (or more) of the following, each present for a significant portion of time during a 1-month period (or less if successfully treated):
   (1) delusions
   (2) hallucinations
   (3) disorganized speech (e.g., frequent derailment or incoherence)
   (4) grossly disorganized or catatonic behavior
   (5) negative symptoms, i.e., affective flattening, alogia, or avolition

B. Social/occupational dysfunction: For a significant portion of the time since the onset of the disturbance, one or more major areas of functioning such as work, interpersonal relations, or self-care are markedly below the level achieved prior to the onset (or when the onset is in childhood or adolescence, failure to achieve expected level of interpersonal, academic, or occupational achievement).

C. Duration: Continuous signs of the disturbance persists for at least 6 months. This 6-month period must include at least 1 month of symptoms (or less if successfully treated) that meet Criterion A (i.e., active-phase symptoms) and may include periods of prodromal or residual symptoms. During these prodromal or residual periods, the signs of the disturbance may be manifested by only negative symptoms or two or more symptoms listed in Criterion A present in an attenuated form (e.g., odd beliefs, unusual perceptual experiences).

D. Schizoaffective and Mood Disorder exclusion: Schizoaffective Disorder and Mood Disorder With Psychotic Features have been ruled out because either (1) no Major Depressive, Manic, or Mixed Episodes have occurred concurrently with the active-phase symptoms; or (2) if mood episodes have occurred during active-phase symptoms their total duration has been brief relative to the duration of the active and residual periods.

E. Substance/general medical condition exclusion: The disturbance is not due to the direct physiological effects of a substance (e.g., a drug of abuse, a medication) or a general medical condition.

F. Relationship to a Pervasive Development Disorder. If there is a history of Autistic Disorder or another Pervasive Developmental Disorder, the additional diagnosis of Schizophrenia is made only if prominent delusions or hallucinations are also present for at least a month (or less if successfully treated).

time. In the past, mental health professionals were pessimistic about the the prognosis for a person with schizophrenia; however, long-term studies have found that one-half to two-thirds of subjects with schizophrenia significantly improve or recover at at 20-, 30-, or 40-year follow-up periods.

Clients who are frequently readmitted to psychiatric hospitals are sometimes called "revolving door" clients. A recent study demonstrated that the two most important factors related to frequency of hospitalization were alcohol and drug problems and noncompliance with medication regimens.[25] There is a high comorbidity of cocaine abuse in clients with schizophrenia.

Hope is an essential ingredient in the recovery from schizophrenia, according to personal accounts of former clients (Box 30-3, p. 569). Psychiatric rehabilitation emphasizes the important role that nurses and other practitioners play in instilling hope in clients. A recent study identified stigma and the effect of symptoms as negatively affecting the development of hope.[31]

ETIOLOGICAL THEORIES

Schizophrenic disorders are due to uncertain causes, although numerous etiological theories exist. Box 30-4 (p. 571) traces early ideas about schizophrenia and its origins. Two main groups of theories include biologi-

(text continues on page 570)

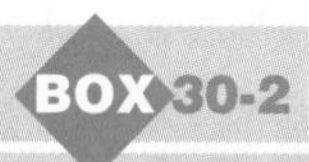

DSM-IV Diagnostic Criteria for Schizophrenia and Related Disorders

Diagnostic Criteria for Schizophrenia, Paranoid Type

A type of Schizophrenia in which the following criteria are met:

A. Preoccupation with one or more delusions or frequent auditory hallucinations.

B. None of the following is prominent: disorganized speech, disorganized or catatonic behavior, or flat or inappropriate affect.

Diagnostic Criteria for Schizophrenia, Disorganized Type

A type of Schizophrenia in which the following criteria are met:

A. All of the following are prominent:
   (1) disorganized speech
   (2) disorganized behavior
   (3) flat or inappropriate affect

B. The criteria are not met for Catatonic Type

Diagnostic Criteria for Schizophrenia, Catatonic Type

A type of Schizophrenia in which the clinical picture is dominated by at least two of the following:

(1) motoric immobility as evidenced by catalepsy (including waxy flexibility) or stupor

(2) excessive motor activity (that is apparently purposeless and not influenced by external stimuli)

(3) extreme negativism (an apparently motiveless resistance to all instructions or maintenance of a rigid posture against attempts to be moved) or mutism

(4) peculiarities of voluntary movement as evidenced by posturing (voluntary assumption of inappropriate or bizarre postures), stereotyped movements, prominent mannerisms, or prominent grimacing

(5) Echolalia or echopraxia

Diagnostic Criteria for Schizophrenia, Undifferentiated Type

A type of Schizophrenia in which symptoms that meet Criterion A are present, but the criteria are not met for the Paranoid, Disorganized, or Catatonic Type.

Diagnostic Criteria for Schizoaffective Disorder

A. An uninterrupted period of illness during which, at some time, there is either a Major Depressive Episode, a Manic Episode, or a Mixed Episode concurrent with symptoms that meet Criterion A for Schizophrenia.
   Note: The Major Depressive Episode must include Criterion A1: depressed mood.

B. During the same period of illness, there have been delusions or hallucinations for at least 2 weeks in the absence of prominent mood symptoms.

C. Symptoms that meet criteria for a mood episode are present for a substantial portion of the total duration of the active and residual periods of the illness.

D. The disturbance is not due to the direct physiological effects of a substance (eg, a drug of abuse, a medication) or a general medical condition.

Specify type:

Bipolar Type: if the disturbance includes a Manic or a Mixed Episode (or a Manic or a Mixed Episode and Major Depressive Episodes).

Depressive Type: if the disturbance only includes Major Depressive Episodes.

Diagnostic Criteria for Schizophreniform Disorder

A. Criteria A, D, and E of Schizophrenia are met.

B. An episode of the disorder (including prodromal, active, and residual phases) lasts at least 1 month but less than 6 months.

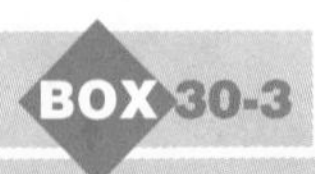

Personal Accounts

Clients with schizophrenia have much to teach their health care providers about their illness. If we listen, we can take steps to improve the quality of psychiatric-mental health care.

One former client, Lovejoy, describes her many years, starting at age 17, as a chronically mentally ill person with schizophrenia. She describes the years of hospitalization, day treatment, foster care, medications, shock treatment, and eventually, chemical dependency treatment. She learned about her illness and identified four stages in its progression:

1. Feeling estranged from herself—The surroundings appear more sharply defined, her voice echoes a bit, and she feels uncomfortable around other people.
2. Everything appearing clouded—Confusion and fear are increased, she takes control of life by organizing, she senses greater meaning in songs, she notices others looking and laughing at her, and she misinterprets others' actions.
3. Believing that others are making her crazy—she ascribes blame to others for causing terrible things to happen to her, notices increased sound levels, and has a heightened sensitivity to the looks of others.
4. Chaos—she sees, hears, and believes unusual things; she fails to question beliefs and acts on them.[4]

In one study, clients identified four major sources of stress in coping with schizophrenia:

1. Altered perceptions—Visual stimuli may appear brighter and sharper, auditory stimuli may appear louder, and the sensations change unpredictably.
2. Cognitive confusion—They feel bewildered and disoriented, their minds "go blank," and they are unable to control their ideas.
3. Attentional deficit—Problems of attention and concentration occur, such as mind "wandering," and feelings of being "captured" by a stimulus instead of choosing what to attend to.
4. Impaired identity—They lack a sense of where their bodies and selves end and the rest of the world begins.[1] This identity impairment is explained by Leete, one former client with schizophrenia:

> My identity began to fragment and seemed to blend with my environment. Rather than just enjoying the wind, for instance, I thought I had merged with it. I had to stare at the sun to appreciate its warmth[3] (p 487).

One researcher interviewed 30 newly rehospitalized people with long-term schizophrenia and found that between hospitalizations, they had lived an inadequate level of subsistence and a stigmatized lifestyle filled with crisis-precipitating events. Their problems with role transition, living arrangements, financial worries, and other people were important factors in their inability to remain living in the community. The clients also expressed that they wanted companionship, associates, or a friend.[2]

The hopelessness of the years in psychiatric hospitals, says Lovejoy, years of being treated as a child, seeing other clients abused, and wishing for death, was turned around by one hope-inspiring psychiatrist who believed she could recover. In time, she became aware of prodromal signs of her illness and how to guard against her symptoms. For example, she discovered that her symptoms were most likely to occur when she was overly tired or in contact with large groups of people with whom she was uncomfortable. She learned to secure more quiet time and sleep, take in a low-sugar diet, attend to her physical health needs, and seek out emphatic individuals who listened to and acknowledged her feelings and reminded her of things she could do to regain control.[4]

Lovejoy learned a way to judge whether an experience was real or a hallucination; she would examine her surroundings to determine whether they appeared different, and if so, she concluded that the voice or sight was not real. To counteract hallucinations, she learned to warm and relax her feet and legs ("grounding" techniques), studied hatha-yoga, and began a high-protein, low-carbohydrate diet to decrease her mood swings and increase her energy.[4]

Keeping a journal, writing and repeating positive self-statements to dissolve the deprecating voices, engaging in physical exercise, and eventually, developing a trusting attitude toward people-

continued

BOX 30-3 (Continued)

and a spiritual relationship with God "as I understand God to be" were the steps she took to her own recovery:

> When I waited for a miracle drug or magic therapy, I did not change—I stagnated. When I believed there was no hope for me, I found no avenues for change. When I distrusted all and feared being hurt, I acted unlovable and was disliked or at best ignored by others. Giving up distrust was the focus of my effort for many, many years[4] (p 812).

Hope, she says, gives one courage to try, change, and trust, which are essential elements in recovery from a major mental illness.

References

1. Hatfield AB: Patients' Accounts of Stress and Coping in Schizophrenia. Hosp Community Psychiatry 40 (11): 1141–1145, 1989
2. Hicks MB: A Community Sojourn From the Perspective of One Who Relapsed. Issues in Mental Health Nursing 10: 137–147, 1989
3. Leete E: The Treatment of Schizophrenia: A Patient's Perspective. Hosp Community Psychiatry 38 (5): 486–491, 1987
4. Lovejoy M: Recovering From Schizophrenia: A Personal Odyssey. Hosp Community Psychiatry 35 (8): 809–812, 1984
5. Myers DM: Aunt Janet's Sick Spells: A Lay Look at Schizophrenia. J Psychosoc Nurs 32 (9): 45–46, 1994

cal theories and psychosocial theories. Biological theories clearly predominate today. A biopsychosocial model of schizophrenia has been proposed to incorporate all relevant data from the biological and psychosocial approaches. The view that schizophrenia is a collection of disorders rather than a single disorder implies a variety or combination of etiologies.

Biological Theories

Various structural and functional abnormalities have been identified in schizophrenics. These biological abnormalities are thought to be the basis of deviations in information processing, attention, perception, cognition, and affective functioning.[48] According to the biological theories, the etiology of schizophrenia is related to organic or physiological factors. These biological theories are discussed according to genetic, biochemical, and neuroanatomical influences.

Genetic Influences. There is evidence of a genetic factor in the development of schizophrenia. A higher incidence of schizophrenia occurs in the relatives of people with schizophrenia than in the general population. It has also been demonstrated that the closer the family relationship, the higher the incidence of schizophrenia in the relatives. For example, if a man is known to have schizophrenia, the chance that his son will also develop schizophrenia is much greater than the chance that his nephew will do so. Nevertheless, the risk will be greater for the man's son and his nephew than for the general population. Children with one schizophrenic parent are 10% to 16% more likely to develop schizophrenia than is the general population.[37]

Genetic influences in the development of schizophrenia have been demonstrated through the study of twins. Studies of twins have shown that if one monozygotic (so-called identical) twin becomes schizophrenic, the incidence for the other twin is significantly higher than it is for dizygotic (so-called fraternal) twins. Also, the incidence of schizophrenia in the children of schizophrenic mothers when the children were adopted away in the first few weeks of life equals the rate that would have been expected had they been reared by their biological mothers. The incidence of schizophrenia in children of nonschizophrenic mothers adopted away early in life equals the incidence (about 1%) seen in the general population.

The mode of inheritance in schizophrenia has not been established; opinion is divided between competing monogenic and polygenic theories. One hypothesis, the single major locus theory, posits that there is a susceptibility gene of major effect but with reduced penetrance or modifying genes. Another possibility is that schizophrenia is a genetically heterogeneous group of disorders. A third possibility, the polygenic hypothesis, is that schizophrenia is the result of many genes interacting, none of which is potent enough to produce schizophrenia when acting individually.

Schizophrenia may occur through the interaction of a genetic susceptibility with some kind of environmental stress. The presence of a major gene for susceptibility to schizophrenia has not been supported in recent studies. Nevertheless, the genetic factors in schizophrenia have specificity, because they increase the risk of this disorder but not of other psychotic disorders. The "new genetics" of recombinant DNA technology may offer more useful information about the genetics of schizophrenia.

Neurochemical Influences. Much recent research has focused on the neurochemical influences on the development of schizophrenia. Through advanced tech-

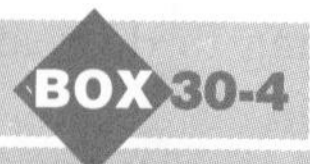

Historical Views of Schizophrenia

Some important figures in medical history have conceptualized, developed, and refined what today is known as schizophrenia.

Emil Kraepelin

At the end of the 19th century, Emil Kraepelin (1856–1926) differentiated a condition he called *dementia praecox.* This diagnosis implied a fatalistic prognosis, because dementia, Kraepelin believed, occurred precociously, or early in life, and followed a gradual but continuous downhill course leading to intellectual deterioration. Kraepelin attributed the etiology of this disorder to an endogenous factor, such as organic pathology or an error of metabolism, not to societal influences.

The identified symptoms of dementia praecox included hallucinations, delusions, disorders of thought and speech, poor insight and judgment, flat affect, and reduced attention to the outside world.

Eugen Bleuler

The Swiss psychiatrist Eugen Bleuler (1857–1930) renamed the syndrome *schizophrenia* to indicate the "splitting" of various mental functions. Bleuler classified the disorder's symptoms into two major categories:

1. Fundamental symptoms (also known as the "four As") that indicated the underlying process specific to schizophrenia:

Associative disturbance: thought disturbance

Affective disorder: a flat or blunted affect or one that is inappropriate or incongruous to the thought or situation

Autism: detachment from external reality and withdrawal into fantasies

Ambivalence: the simultaneous existence of opposing feelings, thoughts, and desires

2. Accessory symptoms, or symptoms that were frequently present but not specific to schizophrenia nor diagnostic of it, including hallucinations, delusions, and catatonic posturing

Sigmund Freud

Sigmund Freud (1855–1939) emphasized the importance of psychological factors in the etiology of schizophrenia. He described the process of the development of hallucinatory psychoses, which, he felt, originated from frightening and unbearable ideas. He coined the term *projection* and described it in relation to paranoid disturbances.

Adolf Meyer

Attention to the psychological factors in the development of schizophrenia was also advocated by Adolf Meyer (1866–1950), a Swiss-born and Swiss-educated psychiatrist who became a prominent medical authority in America. Meyer proposed that the longitudinal study of schizophrenic patients would offer insights into various etiological influences.

Carl Jung

Carl G. Jung (1875–1961) raised the idea of certain individuals' "predisposition" to emotional disturbance. He saw the schizophrenic patient as an "introvert" who directs a great deal of energy into himself. Jung also considered the possibility of a psychosomatic factor in operation in schizophrenia; he proposed that an emotional disorder could cause a metabolic disturbance and, eventually, physical brain damage in psychotic patients.

One of Jung's important concepts was the "collective unconscious," which stores the archetypes, or mythological images, of all people. Jung thought that the symptoms of schizophrenia were "reproductions of the archetypes deposited in our collective unconscious."

Harry Stack Sullivan

An American psychoanalyst, Harry Stack Sullivan (1892–1949) examined the impaired interpersonal relations, not the intrapsychic forces, that predominate in schizophrenia. He believed that children who became schizophrenic adults had undergone disturbed interpersonal relations with their parents and significant others. Sullivan's major life work was the psychotherapy of schizophrenia in which he interacted, not as an observer, but as a participant with the patient.

(From Arieti S: Interpretation of Schizophrenia, 2d ed. New York, Basic Books, 1974; Cancro R: Individual Psychotherapy in the Treatment of Chronic Schizophrenic Patients. Am J Psychother 37 (October): 493–501, 1983; and Goldstein WN: DSM-III and the Diagnosis of Schizophrenia. Am J Psychother 37 (April): 168–181, 1983.)

nologies, the brain's metabolic changes, blood flow, electrical activity, and neurochemistry can be studied with more precision than previously. For example, positron emission tomography (PET) produces slice images of radioisotope density, which have indicated relative metabolic underactivity of the frontal lobes of schizophrenics. They have shown decreased activity in the basal ganglia that can be reversed with neuroleptic treatment.[32]

Biochemical differences in the nervous system of the person with schizophrenia cause sensory information to be processed abnormally, resulting in disturbances of attention, inadequate social interaction, isolation, and hypersensitivity.

The symptoms of schizophrenia are related to dysregulation of one or more neurotransmitter systems.[60] Schizophrenic disorders are associated with a disturbance in the adrenergic systems of the brain. Dopamine, serotonin, norepinephrine, acetylcholine, cholecystokinin, glutamate, and gamma-aminobutyric acid are the neurotransmitters most commonly linked to schizophrenia.[30] An overactivity of dopamine or an insufficiency of norepinephrine at certain central synapses of the brain or an imbalance between the two substances could be among the biological factors present in schizophrenia. Some people with schizophrenia have a decreased number of serotonin receptors with increased levels of serotonin. Others demonstrate increased levels of norepinephrine in the brain, cerebrospinal fluid, and plasma.[37]

The dopamine theory of schizophrenia, that an excess of dopamine is responsible for the symptoms, is the major theory today. The positive behavioral effects resulting from the biochemical action of the antipsychotic medications also support this theory. The positive symptoms of schizophrenia are thought to be associated with disturbances of the mesolimbic dopaminergic system, while negative symptoms are thought to be associated with the mesocortical system.[60] Newest theories focus on the interaction of dopamine, serotonin, and other neurotransmitters.

The viral hypothesis of schizophrenia suggests that exposure to a virus in utero is a risk factor for the development of schizophrenia. An immunological theory of schizophrenia continues to be studied.

Psychopathological research has attempted to link schizophrenia to certain patterns of hemispheric brain dysfunction. These studies have suggested left hemisphere overactivation and consequent temporal abnormalities and delays in processing sensory information. Hallucinations have been correlated with accelerated glucose metabolism in the left temporal lobe. The PET scans show a relative decrease in metabolic activity in the frontal lobes with a low metabolic rate in the basal ganglia, which is raised with neuroleptic medication.[37] Electroencephalography has shown increased delta activity in the frontal lobes, corresponding to decreased glucose and blood flow activity.[37]

Other pathophysiological findings in schizophrenia include dysfunctions of eye movements; impaired modulation of stimulus input, allowing too much information to reach higher brain centers; laterality differences, in which the left hemisphere may be less efficient than the right; impaired selective attention; and directed attention in the form of vigilance.

Neuroanatomical Theories. Computed tomography and magnetic resonance imaging (MRI) have demonstrated structural abnormalities, including enlarged lateral ventricles, enlarged third ventricles, asymmetries, and cortical atrophy. These abnormalities appear to be present from the earliest stages of the illness and may be related to the symptoms of impaired motivation, socialization, and complex problem solving. Studies of twins suggest that the observed structural abnormalities are due to acquired rather than to genetic factors. Results of a recent study replicate the findings of third ventricular enlargement in some schizophrenic clients. There is a high correlation between lateral and third ventricular size, suggesting a pathological process affecting both structures.[57]

Neuropathological studies indicate a slightly decreased volume of the putamen, substantia nigra, and various portions of the limbic system, especially the temporal lobe and hippocampus. Reduced numbers of neurons have been reported in several cortical areas. Frontal-lobe abnormalities have also been found with MRI, PET scanning, and neuropsychological testing; these abnormalities may account for some of the cognitive, attention, and affective symptoms of schizophrenia.

The current data reveal a complex picture of brain dysfunction in persons with schizophrenia that includes cerebral atrophy, enlargement of the ventricles of the brain, disturbances in cerebral metabolism and electrical activity, neurological soft signs, and a variety of neuropsychological deficits. These findings further support the belief that schizophrenia is not one disorder, but a group or collection of disorders.

The advances in methodological techniques to study all aspects of the brain and its functioning are helping scientists test their theories about schizophrenia more directly.

Psychosocial Theories

The psychosocial theories of schizophrenia focus on the intrapsychic and interpersonal dimensions of the client's development and life experiences.

Intrapsychic Influences. A person becomes schizophrenic, says one theorist, not because of what others did to him or her, but "because of what he does with what was done to him."[5] An intrapersonal approach to the etiology of schizophrenia is based on the theory that the personality is predisposed to break down under high levels of stress. Certain characteristics of the person (eg, hypersensitivity, increased anxiety, and social detachment) may, under extensive stress, escalate into suspicion, intolerable fears, withdrawal, and isolation.

The child who later becomes schizophrenic may be extremely sensitized to certain negative characteristics of a parent (eg, emotional detachment or hostility) and may incorporate these feelings into his or her own distorted self-image.[4] The person views himself or herself as a worthless, guilty, helpless person.

The person's social network, which is often diminished in schizophrenia, is an important determinant of whether he or she is accepted and supported or isolated and vulnerable to a schizophrenic episode.

Vulnerability. According to the vulnerability model, schizophrenia is characterized by vulnerability, not by continuous symptoms. Under the stress of biological and psychosocial factors, the person with schizophrenia succumbs to the disorder.[66] These stressors include the neurological dysfunction in schizophrenia, resulting in increased dopamine activity in the mesolimbic dopamine system; the psychobiological influences of the disease and perhaps substance abuse; and environmental and interpersonal stressors. Moderators, such as perceived social support, symptom management skills, and antipsychotic medication, protect the person with schizophrenia from the effects of stressors.[43]

Interpersonal Influences. An interpersonal view of schizophrenia is based on the premise that a person learns values, attitudes, and communication patterns through family and culture. Disordered communication and interaction may, therefore, be a learned phenomenon that may be unlearned through therapeutic intervention.

One aspect of disturbed communication is the lack of adequate feedback mechanisms. Normally, when two people communicate, one person sends a message to another, and the second person sends back a response that informs the first person of the effect of the initial message. Feedback and the correction of information, essential components of effective interpersonal interaction, are absent or defective in the communication patterns of the schizophrenic.[53]

In the 1960s and 1970s, a theory implicated ineffective family communication patterns in the etiology of schizophrenia. For historical purposes, those ideas are summarized here. Communication within the family of a schizophrenic client was perceived as indirect, unclear, incongruent, and growth impeding.[54] The communications of family members were thought of as discounted.

The old theory of *double-bind communication* was considered to be at the core of schizophrenic maladaptation. The double-bind phenomenon means that the child receives two opposing messages from the parent, both of which must be obeyed. For example, the parent holds out his or her arms and says, "Come here and give me a hug." When the child responds, the parent pushes the child away and says, "Why would I want to touch a bad boy like you?" The child is punished for expressing love for the parent *and* for not expressing it; there is no way out of the situation.[7]

Some families with a schizophrenic member were seen as severely *fused*, wherein the members never adequately separated or developed into individuals with their own viewpoints, thoughts, and feelings. Rather than having separate identities, members of such a family possess an *undifferentiated family ego mass*.[8] The member with the least amount of differentiation from the others is the one who may become psychotic.

In light of recent knowledge from biological studies of schizophrenia, these theories of family communication and interaction have been largely discounted.

Another interpersonal influence that has received attention and research efforts is that of *expressed emotion*. Expressed emotion has been defined as a measure of relatives' expressed attitudes about the client.[39] Three of the five expressed emotion scales—criticism, hostility, and emotional overinvolvement, called *high expressed emotion*—predict relapse in the 9 months following discharge from inpatient hospitalization. The other two expressed emotion scales—warmth and positive comments, called *low expressed emotion*—are family factors that may protect against relapse.

The findings of the last 35 years of research in expressed emotion indicate that family members with high expressed emotion, believing that the strange behavior of the person with schizophrenia is deliberate and malicious, are unsympathetic, critical, and hostile to the person. Conversely, family members with low expressed emotion tend to look at the behaviors of the schizophrenic as symptoms of an illness and therefore show greater acceptance toward the person.[10]

Rationale for this research lies in the belief that the client with a major psychiatric disorder, such as schizophrenia, has cognitive and biological dysfunctions that produce high vulnerability to socioenvironmental stressors and demands. The environment—whether family, milieu, or community—can either provide the client with stress or with protection and support.[39]

A spokesperson for the National Alliance for the Mentally Ill (NAMI) says that major mental illness is a family problem only in the sense that all family members are affected by the illness of one member.

She further asserts that family systems theory, as a blueprint for working with families dealing with a member with a brain disease, is "irrelevant, stigmatizing, and misleading."[14] On the other hand, those who find this theoretical approach useful in their work with schizophrenic clients and their families maintain that the family systems theory is a blanket concept for a number of applied theories of family intervention, focusing on specific behavior in the present and attending little or not at all to the problems' origins in the past.[26]

TYPES OF SCHIZOPHRENIA

The types of schizophrenia are defined according to predominant symptoms (see Box 30-2, p. 568). According to the DSM-IV,[1] these types include the following:

1. *Schizophrenia, disorganized type* (formerly called hebephrenic). The client demonstrates disorganized speech, which may be accompanied by silliness or laughter, disorganized behavior, and flat or inappropriate affect. The disorganized behavior may interfere with activities of daily living. Delusions are usually absent. Grimacing, mannerisms, and other odd behavior may be seen.
2. *Schizophrenia, catatonic type.* The client exhibits a marked psychomotor disturbance, such as motoric immobility, stupor, catalepsy (waxy flexibility), or excessive motor activity; extreme negativism, such as maintaining a rigid posture against attempts to be moved; mutism; peculiar voluntary movement, such as posturing, stereotyped movements, mannerisms, or grimacing; and echolalia or echopraxia.
3. *Schizophrenia, paranoid type.* The client is preoccupied with delusions of persecution, delusions of grandeur, ideas of reference, or frequent auditory hallucinations that involve persecutory or grandiose material or both. Delusions are usually organized around a coherent theme. Feelings of being persecuted or grandiose predispose the client to suicidal and violent behavior.
4. *Schizophrenia, undifferentiated type.* The client evidences psychotic symptoms, such as hallucinations and delusions, but does not meet the criteria of paranoid, catatonic, or disorganized types.
5. *Schizophrenia, residual type.* The client had at least one episode of schizophrenia in the past but at present has no prominent positive symptoms (hallucinations, delusions, disorganized speech or behavior). The client still shows signs of negative symptoms, such as withdrawal from others or flat affect, or weak positive symptoms, such as odd beliefs or eccentric behavior.[1]

Types I and II Schizophrenia

Type I schizophrenia, marked by positive symptoms, such as hallucinations and delusions, responds to neuroleptic medication and may be associated with increased numbers of dopamine receptors in the brain. Type I schizophrenia is characterized by an acute onset of symptoms, absence of intellectual deficits, a normal brain structure, dysfunctional dopamine metabolism, a good neuroleptic treatment response, and a better prognosis than Type II schizophrenia.[16,37]

Type II schizophrenia, marked by negative symptoms, such as avolition, flat affect, social withdrawal, and decreased motor activity, has been linked to viral infections and abnormalities in cholecystokinin. Type II schizophrenia is characterized by a slow onset of psychotic symptoms, intellectual decay, enlarged ventricles, and a nonpositive response to typical neuroleptic medication.[16,37] Negative symptoms do respond to the novel, atypical antipsychotic medications, such as clozapine and risperidone.

◆ Schizoaffective and Schizophreniform Disorders

Closely related to schizophrenia are two other disorders, schizoaffective disorder and schizophreniform disorder.

In *schizoaffective disorder,* the client experiences a mood episode and the active-phase symptoms of schizophrenia together. The disturbance is preceded or followed by a period of delusions or hallucinations without prominant mood symptoms.[1]

Schizophreniform disorder is characterized by symptoms similar to schizohrenia but of shorter duration, lasting 1 to 6 months. The client may not show a decline in functioning as seen in schizophrenia.[1]

Application of the Nursing Process to the Client With a Schizophrenic Disorder

The steps of the nursing process—assessment, nursing diagnosis, planning, intervention, and evaluation—are applied to the client with schizophrenia and to the client's family.

ASSESSMENT

Nursing assessment and diagnosis of the client with a schizophrenic disorder are complex processes. Chapter 8, Assessment and Nursing Diagnosis, offers guidelines for gathering assessment data about clients. From the foundation of client data and nursing diagnoses, treatment goals and interventions are derived. Specific nursing approaches, such as openness, honesty, cultural appreciation, and acceptance of the unique properties of the client, are essential and common to all comprehensive assessments and plans of care.

Positive and Negative Symptoms

Characteristic symptoms of schizophrenia are classified in two broad categories—positive and negative symptoms. The *positive symptoms* denote an excess or distortion of normal functions, such as distorted perception (hallucinations), distorted thinking (delusions), distorted language and communication (disorganized speech), and distorted behavior (bizarre or disorganized behavior).[1]

Negative or *defect symptoms* represent a diminution or loss of normal functions. These include restricted emotional expression (affective flattening); restricted fluent and productive thought and speech (alogia), formerly called "poverty of thought"; loss of interest and pleasure (anhedonia); social withdrawal; and restricted initiation of goal-directed behavior (avolition).[1,16,45]

The positive symptoms of schizophrenia seem related to chemical imbalance in the brain and tend to respond to psychopharmacological agents. The negative symptoms seem related to structural changes in the brain. They do not improve with medication alone but require psychosocial, environmental, and rehabilitative interventions, such as helping the client develop personal, social, and vocational skills.[22] Newer medications, however, such as clozapine and risperidone, do affect the negative symptoms.

Nursing assessment and analysis of the client who exhibits behaviors of the schizophrenic disorders address the following major areas:

1. Thought disturbances
2. Affect disturbances
3. Social or behavioral disturbances

Thought Disturbances

Thought disturbances are generally considered the primary characteristic of schizophrenia. The client gives evidence of "loose associations" or disconnectedness of thought through verbal patterns. Because speech is the only means through which one person can understand another person's thoughts, the nurse must be attuned to the client's communication to assess *disorganized speech.*[1]

While listening to the client speak, the nurse may realize that the thoughts are not following each other logically. Instead, the thinking may be chaotic, disorganized, and confusing. The listener feels ill at ease, unable to comprehend what is being said, and unable to take part in the conversation. At times when the client becomes more anxious, thinking and speech become increasingly illogical. The uncomfortable feeling experienced by the nurse who is trying to establish communication with this client is difficult to describe; it is, however, a readily identifiable and diagnostically important feeling once it has been experienced.

The client with schizophrenia may experience *delusions,* or fixed, false beliefs that cannot be corrected by reasoning. They usually involve a misinterpretation of experiences or perceptions.[1] The content of delusions may be persecutory, grandiose, religious, somatic, or referential.[1] The client with paranoid schizophrenia generally has *persecutory delusions.* The person thinks that others are planning to harm him or her in some fashion; that he or she is being spied on, tormented, followed, or subjected to ridicule[1]; or that creatures from other planets are controlling his or her mind or have taken over his or her body. The client with paranoid schizophrenia may have *grandiose delusions,* that is, that he or she is Jesus Christ, the Virgin Mary, Napoleon, or some other important, famous, or historically significant person (Box 30-5).

These words of a client with schizophrenia demonstrate grandiose delusions:

> I felt that I had power to determine the weather, which responded to my inner moods, and even to control the movement of the sun in relation to other astronomical bodies.[63]

To identify a delusion, the nurse must first understand the beliefs characteristic of a culture, because a delusion is a belief that is not in keeping with the beliefs accepted by a person's culture. For example, in the United States, we would consider it delusional for a person to believe that semen could wander up into a man's head and cause his brain to deteriorate, yet this belief is culturally acceptable in parts of India.

In referential delusions, the client believes that certain gestures, words in newspapers, lyrics of songs, or other environmental cues are specifically directed at him or her.[1]

Clients with schizophrenia may experience *hallucinations,* or false sensory perceptions (without external stimuli), or sensory perceptions that do not exist in reality, such as seeing visions or hearing voices (Box 30-6, p. 577). A client may hear voices, such as the voice of God, the devil, or a close relative, that are perceived as distinct from his or her own thoughts. The hallucination may be experienced as two or more voices that keep up a running commentary on the client's behavior or thoughts.[1] The voice is frequently one that berates or condemns for past and present evils but may be a comforting or pleasant experience. *Auditory hallucinations* are the most common form of hallucinations; *vi-*

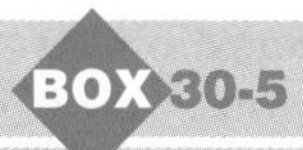

Therapeutic Dialogue: Gathering Information About the Client's Perceptions

Nurse: (Seated at table near client, looking directly at her.) You were telling me, Mrs. D, about how you came to this hospital.

Client: I know why I came here. (Throws her head back, stiffens her neck, and grips the arms of her chair.) I have a calling.

Nurse: A calling? What kind of calling?

Client: To help my friends. (Expansive, sweeping gesture of her hand towards the others in the room.)

Nurse: Who do you think called you, Mrs. D? (Questioning tone of voice; maintaining eye contact.)

Client: (Winks one eye and hunches forward as though sharing a secret.) The Master Doctor, the Big Physician.

Nurse: Do you mean God? (Straightforward, inquiring facial expression and voice.)

Client: Of course I mean God. (Impatient tone of voice, frowning, stands up and shouts.) Who else would I mean?

Discussion

Often the nurse wants to gather information regarding the client's perception about, and events surrounding, relapse and admission to the psychiatric unit. At times, the client's perception is at odds with the reality-based facts of the situation.

Mrs. D believes that she has been chosen as a special person and has received this "calling" to come into the hospital to help other people. The nurse, in interacting with Mrs. D, is asking her for clarification about this "calling," which the client believes has come from God.

The nurse neither agrees nor disagrees with Mrs. D about the truth of her beliefs. Such agreement or attempts to disprove her beliefs usually reinforce or strengthen the delusional material of the client. Instead, the nurse gathers information in a nonthreatening, supportive manner and communicates acceptance of Mrs. D as a valuable human being. A subsequent nursing goal will focus on the clarification of reality with the client.

sual hallucinations are the second most common. Visual hallucinations are likely to be threatening, frightening monsters or scenes but may be otherwise. Although hallucinations involving the other senses (gustatory, tactile, olfactory) do occur, they are less common.

Hallucinations, like dreams, reflect primary process or primitive mechanisms. The content of the hallucination reveals information about areas of conflict and personal importance to the client. The theoretical formulations of Sullivan and Arieti and classical psychoanalysts view hallucinations as adaptive mechanisms.[67]

The view that hallucinations evolve from good (ie, supportive and nurturing) to bad (ie, condemning and hostile) is not universally accepted. Other patterns of hallucinations, such as voices representing opposing perspectives—one less healthy and one more healthy—often occur. When investigating the content of a client's hallucinations, the nurse should assess for alternative (opposing) voices, especially when command hallucinations urge suicide or homicide. These alternative voices may provide a valuable treatment ally, the drive toward health and life.[67]

Hallucinations may be part of a religious experience in certain cultures. A question that must be asked is whether the hallucination is appropriate or even expected within the cultural framework. For example, a person's role in society (eg, a medicine man or an artist) may necessitate or involve some symptoms that appear to be schizophrenic.

Magical thinking is seen in a client believes that his

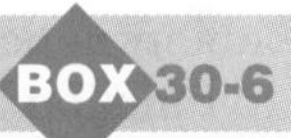

Hallucinations and Delusions: How Do They Develop?

A well-known theorist and writer about schizophrenia, Silvano Arieti, has proposed that hallucinatory voices occur only in particular situations, that is, when the client expects to hear them. The client, for example, perceives hostility, expects to hear the neighbors talking about him or her, is in a "listening" attitude, and then experiences the hallucination (hears them talking).

Another example of this phenomenon occurs in ideas of reference. The client thinks that people are laughing at him or her, hears laughing and giggling, and looks at people and sees them smiling. They may not be smiling; the client may have misinterpreted their facial expressions. If they are smiling, it may be for reasons that have nothing to do with the client.

The goal in treating such clients says Arieti, is to help them recognize that they see or hear people laughing at them when they expect to. Next, clients must recognize that they feel people *should* laugh at them because they are "laughable" individuals. They hear laughing because they think people should laugh at them; that is, "what he thinks of himself has become the cause of his symptom."

The return to reality is slow because the client's reality is sad and worsened by vulnerability. Therapists must be careful to promote the client's return by improving the reality. Eventually, the client moves toward mastery of his or her situation, no longer the victim of external forces.

or her thoughts or wishes can control other people or events. This form of primary process, or primitive, thinking is part of the normal development of preschool children, as suggested by a child skipping down the sidewalk and chanting, "Step on a crack, break your mother's back." Its presence in an adult who believes that he or she can manipulate the actions of others through mind control, however, is neither acceptable nor appropriate behavior in American society.

The client with schizophrenia may have minimal or seemingly no awareness of the environment, wandering around as though in foreign surroundings or in a dream world. This lack of regard for personal well-being is an important safety-related factor when implementing nursing care. The client may step in the path of oncoming traffic or perform other potentially dangerous acts, while giving the impression of being oblivious to the obvious danger.

Clients with schizophrenia may also experience feelings of *depersonalization*, for example, a man who feels that his body belongs to another person or that he is somehow removed from his body. He may believe that his spirit is hovering above his body and watching its movements and behavior with detachment.

The client with schizophrenia may attempt to communicate with others through *symbolism*. Symbolic words and actions can be viewed as a part of disordered thinking. Language may be private and idiosyncratic. The client may create new words, called *neologisms*, which have a private meaning and purpose. The client may use *cryptic language*, which means speaking in an abbreviated fashion; for example, he or she may speak aloud only every fourth, or sixth, or ninth word of each thought.

Illusions may be another sign of the client's thought disorder. An *illusion* is a misinterpretation of a real sensory experience. An example is the experience of seeing a shadow in the room when awakening in the middle of the night and immediately concluding that a robber has broken into the house. Schizophrenic clients are often disturbed and frightened by illusions.

Affect Disturbances

Schizophrenic disorders are marked by an absence of affect or flat, blunted, or inappropriate affect. Affective flattening is characterized by the client's face appearing immobile and unresponsive, with poor eye contact and no body language.[1] The range of emotional expressiveness is reduced. The client's apparent lack of emotional expression may make the nurse feel like he or she is trying to communicate with something inanimate. The client's affect may also seem inappropriate in relation to the conversation or the context of the situation (eg, the client who laughs and smiles in response to hearing sad news).

The client's apathy or seeming absence of caring

about himself or herself may depress and anger the nurse. Again, the nurse must examine the client's affective state in relation to the cultural context and the severity of the illness. A client exhibiting inappropriate affect used these words to explain his experience:

> Half the time I am talking about one thing and thinking about half a dozen other things at the same time. It must look queer to people when I laugh about something that has got nothing to do with what I am talking about, but they don't know what's going on inside and how much of it is running around in my head.[63]

Social or Behavioral Disturbances

The client with a schizophrenic disorder may retreat from interpersonal contact, appearing aloof, uninterested in others, and content with inner fantasies. A pronounced fear of others and of himself or herself prevents the client from making contact or responding to the social overtures of others. The client may fear harm from other people or fear a lack of self-control that may bring harm to others.

Social communication is either lacking or directed toward private, idiosyncratic goals. Rather than using language and nonverbal communication to establish rapport with other people and to derive pleasure from those relationships, the schizophrenic client uses communicative efforts as a means of self-stimulation or reinforcement of preoccupying fantasies.

The client may exhibit grossly disorganized behavior, from extreme silliness to unpredictable agitation. He or she may be unable to perform activities of daily living and may appear disheveled and wearing unusual dress, such as multiple layers of clothing.[1]

Catatonic motor behaviors may be seen, including extreme unawareness of the environment (catatonic stupor), resistance to efforts to be moved from a rigid posture (catatonic rigidity), bizarre psotures (posturing), or purposeless and excessive motor activity (catatonic excitement).[1]

The client may show signs of extreme dependency or helplessness. This behavior is often aversive to people who value independence and assertiveness and may elicit anger and frustration in even the most conscientious and self-aware mental health professionals. Impulsive, bizarre, or otherwise uninhibited behavior, such as masturbation in public, gesturing, or posturing, may also be signs of the behavioral disturbances of schizophrenia.

The client with schizophrenia may have concerns about sexual identity. Inadequate social skills, withdrawal, and isolation contribute to a lack of sexual partners. In psychiatric hospitals, where sexual activities are generally discouraged or prohibited, clients encounter medical, social, and cultural obstacles to their sexual expression (Box 30-7).

Assessing the client's ability to perform self-care and activities of daily living, to function in the work setting, and to respond appropriately to personal physical needs is critical. At times, a client may be unaware of safety needs and the need for food, water, rest, and activity. Disordered water balance characterized by compulsion to drink, polydipsia, disturbed gait, slurred speech, confusion, disorientation, and agitated behavior may occur.[51]

The client's role in the family and community and the availability and responsiveness of a support system are important variables in the assessment process. The eventual level of adaptation is strongly influenced by the presence of supportive, caring significant others. The absence of a support system reinforces a lifetime of failure and rejection and may offer the client little hope for a satisfying future.

The nurse needs to assess the client's relationships with the significant figures in his or her life. From these observations and objective descriptions of family and community interaction, the nurse will formulate treatment goals and interventions for and with the client and the people who are important to him or her.

Relapse Symptoms

Relapse symptoms typically appear in this order: disrupted sleep cycle; significant mood changes, most often depression; decreased appetite; and somatic complaints, such as headache, malaise, and constipation. During relapse, clients often become resistive and ambivalent, isolative, and withdrawn. They pace relentlessly and are preoccupied with psychotic symptoms.[48]

Other Unique Characteristics

In addition to these behaviors, nurses will identify many other behaviors and needs. No symptom picture characteristic of a psychiatric disturbance is ever the same in two clients. Because every person is different and has unique distinguishing characteristics, no one will ever appear "just like all the others"—whether emotionally disturbed or healthy and adapting. Individualization and objectivity are key words in any nursing assessment and analysis.

NURSING DIAGNOSIS

Formulating medical or nursing diagnoses of schizophrenia relies on an accurate history and clinical assessment. Following analysis of assessment data, nurses identify nursing diagnoses for the client with schizophrenia.

Nursing diagnoses that are appropriate to guide the planning and implementation of nursing care of the client with schizophrenia include the following:

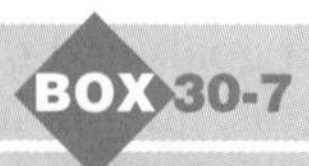

Schizophrenia and Sexuality

Historical views have held that schizophrenia was caused by hormonal changes or immature psychosexual development and that it caused deterioration of moral inhibitions. Although unfounded, these views may still influence the mental health professional's approach to the sexual needs of schizophrenic clients. Schizophrenia, however, does seem to affect sexual behavior; for example, some schizophrenic clients can become preoccupied with sex in distorted and bizarre ways, although there is little evidence of acting out these ideas.

Mental health directly affects sexual functioning. Behaviors associated with schizophrenia may distort a person's sexual self-concept, alter the physiological sexual response cycle, and interfere with sexual relationships and feelings of sexual pleasure. For example, research shows that schizophrenic men engage in autoerotic sexual activity (masturbation) two to three times more often than men in the general population. This may be a way of coping with stress associated with the disorder or of validating the reality of their existence. It also may stem from a lack of opportunity for sexual contacts or from interpersonal deficits. Schizophrenic men and women express guilt about their sexual preoccupation, an area of self-concept that is amenable to nursing intervention.

Neuroleptic medication changes sexual functioning by suppressing sexual behavior produced by the blocking of dopaminergic neurotransmission. These changes are thought to be one of the major reasons why many clients do not take their psychotropic medication as prescribed. Sexual dysfunction associated with neuroleptic medication regimens are reported more often in men than in women and include erectile and ejaculatory disturbances. Although changes in libido have also been reported, these have not been carefully studied. Sexual dysfunction related to pharmacotherapy may be perceived by the client as more disabling than the mental illness itself. Giving "drug holidays," changing the medication, and reducing dosages may help diminish sexual dysfunction and increase client compliance with pharmacotherapy.

Before helping a schizophrenic client deal with sexual problems, nurses must evaluate their own attitudes, values, beliefs, and biases. Talking honestly with colleagues in an accepting atmosphere about one's perceptions, rehearsing client education approaches, and anticipating client questions and needs are helpful ways to begin to meet the generally unrecognized sexual needs of schizophrenic clients.

Nurses and other health care professionals are often viewed as sex educators by clients and families. Sex education for schizophrenic clients, whether individually or in group settings, must include attention to social skill development, use of clear language, appropriate teaching methods, coverage of pertinent content, group reactions and interactions, and referrals as needed. Helping clients become comfortable with their sexuality is the goal of these nursing interventions.

(From Jacobs P, Bobek SC: Sexual Needs of the Schizophrenic Client. Perspect Psychiat Care 27 (1): 15–20, 1991.)

1. Sensory/Perceptual Alterations, auditory or visual, related to withdrawal into the self; panic level of anxiety, evidenced by poor concentration, rapid mood swings, disordered thought sequencing, and inappropriate responses
2. Altered Thought Processes related to low self-esteem, repressed fears, inability to trust, possible hereditary factor, panic level of anxiety, evidenced by hypervigilance, altered attention span, distractibility, inability to concentrate, commands, obsessions, and impaired ability to make decisions, problem solve, reason, calculate, abstract, or conceptualize
3. Social Isolation related to fear of interpersonal closeness, lack of trust, regression to earlier level of development, delusional thinking evidenced by sad, dull affect, inappropriate or immature interests and activities for developmental age or stage, preoccupation with own thoughts, repetitive and meaningless actions, isolating behavior
4. Risk for Violence: Self-directed or directed at others related to catatonic excitement, hallucinatory commands, panic level of anxiety, rage reaction evidenced by increased pacing; overt and aggressive acts; goal-directed destruction of objects in the environment; self-destructive behavior or aggressive suicidal acts; hostile, threatening verbalizations; increased motor activity; excitement; agitation; and irritability
5. Impaired Verbal Communication related to disordered, unrealistic thinking, regression, withdrawal, panic level of anxiety evidenced by loose association of ideas; use of clang association; word salad, neologisms, and echolalia; verbalizations reflecting concrete thinking; and poor eye contact
6. Bathing/Hygiene and Dressing/Grooming Self Care Deficit related to perceptual or cognitive impairment, withdrawal evidenced by impaired ability to perform hygiene tasks, dress, groom, maintain appearance at satisfactory level, toilet, and eat
7. Altered Family Processes related to presence of long-term mental illness in family member evidenced by alteration in family's goals and plans, social activities, and daily activities according to the mentally disordered member

PLANNING

Preparation of the client's treatment plan is a collaborative effort of the mental health team, which includes the client and the client's family. Flexibility and creativity are essential ingredients in the continuous processes of planning, evaluating, and replanning treatment efforts. No single treatment modality will effect the desired behavioral changes for all clients. Holistic nursing care aims to help clients achieve maximum health potential by defining client goals and outcomes based on individual needs, strengths, and limitations.[48]

Although preoccupation with fantasies, poor reality testing, and symbolic forms of communication are characteristic of schizophrenia, each client exhibits specific disturbances that require individualized nursing approaches. Some psychiatric inpatient facilities may prepare standardized nursing care plans or treatment plans that offer general principles of care; these standard plans then require individualization in nursing diagnoses, specific client outcomes, and interventions for the client.

More commonly today, treatment settings are relying on the use of clinical pathways to monitor the client's progress. Table 30-1 is an example of a clinical pathway designed to streamline care of a client with schizophrenia.

Goal Setting

The major goals for the schizophrenic client include the following:

1. Promoting trust
2. Establishing a nonthreatening environment
3. Encouraging satisfactory social interaction
4. Increasing self-esteem
5. Validating perceptions
6. Clarifying and reinforcing reality
7. Promoting physical safety
8. Encouraging independent behavior
9. Attending physical needs
10. Reducing psychotic symptoms through psychopharmacotherapeutic agents
11. Coordinating treatment and education with the client's family or significant others

Client outcomes are more specific than goals and are measurable, attainable, realistic, time-oriented, and client-focused (Nursing Care Plan 30-1, p. 582).

Discharge Plans

Discharge planning begins at the time of the client's admission to the psychiatric inpatient unit. Many schizophrenic clients suffer not only the long-term effects of their disorder, but also what is called the "Rip Van Winkle syndrome;" that is, they awaken from a long sleep to find a world with changed technologies, cultural values, and economics. It is a frightening world for discharged clients who may have been comfortable in the protected hospital environment.

To prepare for discharge into the community, social skills, work or job skills, self-confidence in dealing with problems, and involvement in the outside community need to be fostered. For example, before discharge from a psychiatric facility, the long-term client must learn, prac-

(text continues on page 585)

Table 30-1 Clinical Pathway: Schizophrenic disorder (295.1x, catatonic 295.2x, delusional 297.10, brief reactive psychosis 298.80)

Patient Name: ____________ **Case Manager:** ____________ **Physician:** ____________ **Medical Record #** ____________
Admit date: ____________ Expected LOS: ____________ UR days certified: ____________ Discharge Date: ________
Actual LOS: ____________

Day/Date:	0–8 Hours	8–24 Hours	Day 2	Day 3	Day 4	Day 5
ASSESSMENTS & EVALUATIONS	Nursing Assessment Nutritional screening, wt Admit note, Precautions	H & P, Social HX, RT/TA; Dr. Initial TX Plan/Admit Note Prec. Eval. AIMS Scale	Precaution Evaluation Document sleep patterns Observe/document nonverbal behavior	Psych Eval done Social Hx done Precaution Evaluation	Assess readiness for discharge	Assess for goals achieved
PROCEDURES	Lab ordered-Admit profile UA, UDS, UCG, EKG, Other:	Lab done: UA, UDS, UCG, EKG Other:	Lab results checked Abnormals called to Dr.	Physician progress note r/t abnormal lab values		
CONSULTS	IT ordered Y/N FT ordered Y/N GT ordered Y/N	GT started Psych Testing Order Y/N	Schedule MTP meeting	IT started, FT started Psych Testing Done Home Contract		Psych Testing results
TREATMENT PLANNING	N1: ______ Axis III ______		RT/TA started School started	Master TX Plan Update/Revise, RT/TA		
INTERVENTIONS	Assess S/H or Aggr. monitor anxiety stimulus	Monitor sleep pattern, orient X 4	Encourage group interaction	Give honest and consistent feedback	Encourage oral hygiene, adeq. fluid intake 2000 ml	Assess client support network, outpt resources
MEDICATIONS	Meds ordered, Inf. Con.	Assess for EPS	Drug interaction √'d, Dr. signs Inf. Con. √ for EPS	Meds evaluated/ readjusted Assess for EPS	Observe/document response to Rx, √ for EPS	Discharge instructions for medication self-admin
LEVEL	Level ordered		Re-evaluate	Re-evaluate	Re-evaluate consider PHP	Re-evaluate
TEACHING	Patient Rights Orient to Unit	Orient to Program	Goals setting, relaxation techniques	Meds reinforced; Altered perceptions as symptom	Coping skills for unusual perceptions	Teach family S/S of Rx non-compliance
NUTRITION/ DIET	Type: ______	Chart daily intake	Chart daily intake	Chart daily intake	Chart daily intake	Chart daily intake
CARE CONTINUUM	Initial D/C Plans	Placement Search Outcome survey		Discharge Plan updated/rev		After care plan written Outcome survey
PATIENT OUTCOMES	Controls violent impulses	ADLS w/assist, oriented ×3	Tolerates peer interaction	Improve insight	Uses adaptive coping skills	Goal directed interactions

Strategic Clinical Systems, Inc., 3715 Mission Ct., Granbury, TX 76049 (817) 326-4239. PsychPaths™, Darla Belt, RN & Vickie Pflueger, RNC—Authors

(Key: EKG = electrocardiogram; FT = family therapy; GT = group therapy; H & P = history and physical; IT = individual therapy; MTP = master treatment plan; RT/TA = recreational therapy/therapeutic activities; S/H = suicide/homicide precautions; S/S = signs and symptoms; Signs Inf Con = signs informed consent; TX = treatment; UA = urinalysis; UDS = urine drug screen; UCG = urine test for pregnancy; √ for EPS = check for extrapyramidal symptoms.)

Nursing Care Plan 30-1

A Client With Paranoid Schizophrenia

Alice McGuire, RN, C, Nurse Manager, Adult Acute Division, Terrell State Hospital, Texas Department of Mental Health and Mental Retardation, Terrell, Texas.

Mr. Robert L is a 34-year-old man who has been readmitted to the state hospital for the sixth time after being picked up by police when he refused to leave someone's property where he had taken up residence.

Mr. L stated that he had to live out in the country because of the "contamination" of the air and water in the city. He told the police that the water was contaminated by the government and that he had to leave his mother's home and live on his own because the world was ending. He was easily agitated and rambling about the end of the world. He said that, through the television wires, he had overheard the government plotting to kill all citizens.

On admission, Mr. L was disheveled, unshaven, dressed in several layers of seasonally inappropriate clothing, and had a strong body odor and matted hair. He refused to eat anything except foods with thick skins, such as bananas, peanuts, and oranges, and would only drink distilled water. He said that all other food and drink were contaminated.

His mother, with whom he has lived all his life, stated that following his last discharge from the hospital, Mr. L took his antipsychotic medication haloperidol [Haldol] for about 3 months and was doing fairly well. Then he had a brief flu episode during which he did not take his Haldol. When the flu symptoms abated, he told her he "didn't need the medicine anymore." During the next few weeks, he began to pace, stopped bathing and eating except for certain foods, and was not sleeping well. One morning, Mr. L was gone. His mother notified the police but heard nothing about his whereabouts until he was readmitted to the hospital and called her to come and get him out.

Nursing Diagnosis

Altered Thought Processes related to inability to distinguish reality from fears and beliefs

Outcome

Client will communicate and behave in a manner that is compatible with living in a community.

Intervention	Rationale
Accept client's delusions without agreeing or disagreeing with them.	Trust begins to develop when the client feels that he and his beliefs are accepted.
Establish a consistent routine; prepare client for daily events.	Specific instructions about what to expect and what will be expected of him decrease client's suspiciousness and paranoia.
Provide consistency of staff members.	Contact with staff who are known to him helps to diminish client's fears and build trust.
Orient the client to reality, and engage him in reality-based conversation.	Reality orientation explains and reinforces to client what is happening around him to counteract his fears.

Evaluation

Client interacts with others in a way that does not interfere with ability to live in a community setting.

Nursing Diagnosis

Bathing/Hygiene and Dressing/Grooming Self Care Deficits

continued

Nursing Care Plan 30-1 (Continued)

Outcome

Client will bathe and dress in clean clothes, eat and drink adequately, and care for bodily needs appropriately.

Intervention	**Rationale**
Perform physical assessment. Assist client with bathing, dressing, eating, toileting as needed.	Inattention to physical needs and living out-of-doors may have led to multiple health problems, including malnutrition, dehydration, skin ulcers, tics, and lacerations that require prompt treatment.
Allow extra privacy and sufficient time to carry out any idiosyncratic routines, such as blessing the water before bathing.	Client's delusions may require that he perform certain activities to control his fears; these should be permitted to prevent escalating anxiety.
Accommodate client's delusional food requests.	Supplying the food client agrees to eat ensures that he receives at least some nutrients.
Do not argue about client's beliefs that food or fluids are poisoned.	Arguing or disagreeing with the client only strengthens the delusion.
Encourage client to eat with others in dining room.	Bringing food to the client apart from other clients may increase his suspiciousness that food is poisoned.
Encourage family to bring food to client if possible.	Client may not include his family in delusion and may accept food from them.
Monitor food and fluid intake closely.	Monitoring ensures that intake is sufficient to meet physiological needs.
Monitor laboratory results, such as electrolytes and white blood counts.	Because client is unable to meet his physical needs, nurses assume the responsibility for health assessment and monitoring.
Establish a normal routine of sleep and awake periods for client; encourage him to get up in the morning and stay out of bed during the day.	The client with schizophrenia tends to spend the majority of time in bed. Helping him establish a sleep–wake routine promotes physical and mental health.
Teach client and mother about his illness, symptom awareness, how to recognize his own symptoms, desired and side effects of his medication, how to diminish side effects, the importance of following his medication regimen, and not stopping his medication suddenly.	Client and significant others need information about the mental illness and its treatment; abruptly stopping the medication causes side effects to increase.

Evaluation

Client exhibits normal sleep–wake, eating, toileting, and bathing patterns of behavior.

Nursing Diagnosis

Social Isolation related to suspicious fears about others.

Outcome

Client will interact with and live around others without becoming threatening to them.

continued

Nursing Care Plan 30-1 (Continued)

Intervention	Rationale
Provide consistent staff to work with client.	Consistency reduces the client's anxiety.
Initiate contact with client, explaining expectations, orienting to reality, giving positive reinforcement, and pointing out when interaction with another is going positively.	Client with schizophrenia is unlikely to initiate interpersonal contact; therefore, nurse and other care providers must promote interaction.
Explore client's interests, and discuss how to fill his days with structure and activities.	Client is unlikely to know how to structure his time.
Explore community resources to meet client's educational and social needs.	Mental health caregivers must assist client in locating needed services.
Introduce client to support groups through Alliance for the Mentally Ill, local Mental Health Associations, mental health care services, 12-step programs, churches.	Support groups are useful in promoting a sense of belonging for the client and helping him meet his social needs.

Evaluation

Client actively participates in the community, whatever the scope of his community, and spontaneously interacts with others.

Nursing Diagnosis

Risk for Violence: self-directed or directed at others related to fear of environment and others

Outcome

Client will not injure self or others.

Intervention	Rationale
Always approach the person while talking to him.	Approaching the client without warning could frighten him.
Keep distance between client and nurse; never invade personal space without permission; ask permission before touching him.	Client has fears about harm from others; keeping a distance and asking permission convey respect for the client and his beliefs.
Watch for signs of escalation, such as talking to self, pacing, or hostile, angry expressions while pacing or talking to self.	Optimal intervention involves assessing and intervening in escalating behavior before it erupts into violence.
Help the client de-escalate by approaching calmly and discussing what you observe; ask what's bothering him and whether the voices are telling him to do something.	A calm demeanor defuses the situation and helps the client to remain calm. Asking the client to describe his experiences gives nurses information on which to plan interventions.
Offer a calm, quiet environment and antipsychotic medication before violent behavior surfaces.	Providing a nonstimulating environment helps the client de-escalate; antipsychotic medication helps manage psychotic symptoms of delusional, paranoid thinking.

Evaluation

Client demonstrates no aggressive, violent outbursts.

tice, and be tested in the basic, practical aspects of daily living, such as how to ride a bus, shop for groceries, apply for a job, cook a meal, and take medication (see Chapter 45, Community Support and Rehabilitation).

Community involvement means that the client should become familiar with his or her future landlord and employer. These individuals will play a significant role in the client's adjustment to life outside the hospital. Employers and landlords must know the discharged client as a person and must realize the need for direct and constructive feedback. The person with schizophrenia is not a fragile or helpless person and should not be treated as such. A continuous crisis telephone line to the client's former psychiatric-mental health care providers also helps smooth discharge to family and community.

Community Care

Community centers have not replaced the state hospital system in treating the chronically mentally ill. Instead, deinstitutionalization has led to reinstitutionalization of long-term psychiatric clients in jails, nursing homes, and shelters and on the streets.[37] The problems of people with schizophrenia are complex. For example, one study of chronic schizophrenic outpatients in a community support program documented lifetime histories of substance abuse in 43 of 60 subjects.[33]

Community support programs promote continuity of care through intensive case management. These programs are primarily intended to maintain seriously dysfunctional clients with histories of repeated psychiatric hospitalizations within the community. They do so by stabilizing the clients' behavioral and social functioning in the community, reducing the need for rehospitalization, and improving the self-assessed quality of their lives.[33]

Elderly clients with schizophrenia and other long-term mental disorders have special needs in the community. These needs include accurate physical and psychiatric assessment and management, pharmacological monitoring, housing, clothing, food, rehabilitation, and community support.[52]

INTERVENTION

Certain personal characteristics are considered necessary when working therapeutically with a client with schizophrenia. The mental health professional needs to be straightforward, hopeful, and accepting and must hold unconditional regard for the dignity of another human being—even when that person is severely withdrawn and regressed.[4] This mandate includes, for example, demonstrating respect for the client's desire for silence so that the nonverbal communication becomes a shared experience.

Factors Influencing Recovery

Recovery from any severe mental illness is an illusive concept. It is described as a way of living a hopeful, satisfying life and contributing to society within the limitations imposed by the illness.[62] The following factors have been identified by former mental health clients as important to their success in recovery:

1. Medication
2. Self-control or self-monitoring of symptoms
3. Community support and mental health services
4. Vocational activity
5. Spirituality
6. Mutual aid groups and supportive friends
7. Significant others
8. Knowledge and acceptance of the illness[62]

Intervening in the Client's Thought Disturbance

Searching for Meaning. When confronted with the client's symbolic words, actions, or other examples of disordered thinking that may seem almost impossible to understand, the nurse must remember that it does have meaning to the client. The nurse listens for the themes, searches for the meaning in communication, and reflects that back to the client. The client's verbal and nonverbal behaviors cannot be dismissed as senseless or as gibberish.

The client's rhyming communication may also give clues to the nurse about thoughts and feelings, as in the following example:

Mary Mary dictionary
blowing smoking
not even caring.

In these words, the client, Mary, conveys to the nurse several possible routes to explore. Is she feeling apathetic ("not even caring") or angry ("blowing" or "smoking")? Is there a meaning to "Mary dictionary"? The nurse listens to these unusual forms of communication and attempts to decode the communication and determine, through validation, what meanings they hold for the client.

Reinforcing Reality. Much of the nurse's work with the client with schizophrenia will focus on clarifying reality and validating perceptions. This is accomplished by describing real events or circumstances to the client and by involving the client in conversations or activities that focus on the here and now.

When dealing with the client who has feelings of depersonalization, the nurse will need to state what he or she sees as a fact (eg, that one part of the client's body is not dead, that the client has not become an inanimate object) but will also need to avoid getting involved in an argument. No one can argue away feelings of depersonalization, hallucinations, or any other psychotic symptom, such as reality impairment. Nevertheless, psychiatric-mental health professionals should state the facts as they see them to the client in a simple, concise, and nonthreatening manner.

After stating these facts, the nurse attempts to bring the client back into contact with reality by involvement in some reality-oriented activity. Perhaps the nurse could talk with the client about a picture in a magazine and attempt to kindle interest in this concrete topic. Involving the client in a physical activity, such as taking a walk and conversing about the scenery along the way, may be therapeutic. These are reality-oriented activities that the nurse may use in day-to-day contact with clients.

The client who is overcome by the idea that he or she is living in an unreal environment should not be left alone for long periods. Staying with the client is an essential step in reinforcing reality, because the nurse signifies a major link with the real world. Allowing the client to remain isolated may encourage increased involvement in or preoccupation with fantasies. Again, engaging the client in reality-oriented activities and conversations is a helpful intervention.

Promoting Clarification. The client with a confused sense of identity will require much clarification from the nurse. In conversations, the nurse must help the client realize what he or she said or did as distinct from what others said or did. When ambiguous and confusing topics arise, the nurse must stop the conversation and request clarification from the client. Because the client may say, "you know what I mean," the nurse must ask first for clarification. Obtaining information directly from the client is the only sure way to understand the message being conveyed.

The loose associations of the client with schizophrenia are extremely difficult to understand. Pretending to understand a line of thought only widens the gap between client and nurse. The most helpful approach to what may seem like incoherent rambling is to ask clarifying questions. Perhaps the nurse may determine a recurrent idea or theme in the speech and further pursue its meaning for the client. The nurse and other psychiatric-mental health caregivers are healthy role models for the client when they communicate in a clear and concise manner.

Intervening in Hallucinations. The client who is hallucinating is preoccupied and frightened; leaving the person alone only deepens preoccupation and fear. The nurse's presence is a reassuring force that helps calm fears.

The nurse must remember that the hallucination is real to the client. When working with the hallucinating client, the nurse communicates concern that the client is upset or bothered by the things he or she hears or sees. At the same time, the nurse makes it clear to the client that he or she does not see or hear the hallucinations being described.

The nurse must never agree with a client about hearing the voices or sharing any hallucinatory experience. Because it is the mental health professional's function to serve as the healthy role model for the client, the nurse cannot reinforce the reality impairment. It is also not beneficial to argue about whether or not the hallucination or delusion is real. Rather than engage in activities that strengthen the client's withdrawal, the nurse encourages the client to regain contact with reality by gently introducing conversation or activities focused on the here and now (Box 30-8). In addition, active mental work, rather than passive mental activity, and activity involving a verbal response, rather than nonverbal activity, have been effective.[67]

It has been suggested that the voices are heard in specific situations when the client expects to hear them. This expectation causes the client to develop a "listening attitude," especially in times of stress.[4] The nurse may help the client actively defend against the hallucination, first by discovering the relationship between feelings (anxiety) and the "listening attitude." The nurse then disrupts the process of falling into the next stage of experiencing the voices. The nurse administers antipsychotic medication, discussed later in this chapter, to interrupt the client's hallucinatory experience. Offering competing stimuli, redirecting attention, and providing client and family education about hallucinatory experiences, including clear, reassuring explanations that the hallucinations are symptoms of the illness, are essential nursing interventions.

Research findings demonstrate that clients with schizophrenia can be taught to monitor early nonpsychotic symptom indicators effectively, which improves functioning and may prevent hospitalization.[23] A self-regulation model proposes that clients monitor their symptoms that signal exacerbation of illness and take actions to manage their illness. Self-regulatory approaches can help clients monitor themselves (or have another person help monitor them) for prodromal symptoms, such as affective signals; learn from other people with schizophrenia; initiate specific actions; and prevent relapse.

To help a client self-regulate or self-control hallucinations, the nurse can teach the client the following:

1. Recognizing the anxiety that precipitates hallucinations
2. Using other ways to cope with anxiety
3. Using "dismissal intervention" (ie, telling the voices to go away)
4. Developing coping strategies, such as jogging, seeking the company of others, telephoning, playing sports and games, and using relaxation techniques

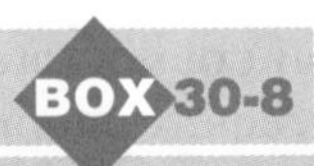

Therapeutic Dialogue: Dealing With Hallucinations

Nurse: What has been troubling you, Jeff? (Sitting with the client, trying to establish eye contact.)

Client: I hear voices. (Looking down at the floor, shoulders hunched forward.) They are punishing me and want me to repent.

Nurse: Do you want to share with me your thoughts on what you believe you heard? (Leaning toward client, arms and hands open and resting on lap.)

Client: (Sitting very quietly, brow furrowed, staring at his hands.) There were two men—one was 62 and one was 42. The 42-year-old was good. His face was in stone on the floor. When you went by he went into your mind. It was like a strong wind. (Pauses, looks at the nurse's face.) You really don't want to hear this.

Nurse: (Softly, maintaining eye contact.) You don't think I want to hear about these "voices," Jeff?

Client: Two weeks after I was discharged from this hospital, I was walking down this road—the voices started, then the wind telling me to kill myself for my repentance. (Stands up, begins to pace back and forth in front of the couch, his eyes cast downward.)

Nurse: (Still seated, looking up at the client as he paces.) Do the wind and noises bother you a lot, Jeff?

Client: Yes, and its' always at 6 o'clock. (Walks away from the nurse.)

DISCUSSION

Communicating verbally and nonverbally with the client who experiences hallucinations requires skilled use of therapeutic techniques and willingness to hear what the client has to tell.

Jeff is open in expressing the torment he is experiencing from the punishing "voices." Many clients lack the trust, reality contact, or verbal skills needed to share these hallucinatory events with psychiatric-mental health care providers.

The nurse verbalizes concern for Jeff and offers him the opportunity to share or withhold information about "what he believes he hears." In discussing hallucinatory material, the nurse demonstrates acceptance of the client's hallucination as a "real" event to him. At the same time, the nurse neither agrees with the client nor tries to dissuade him or convince him that the "voices" are not really occurring. For the client, the "voices" are present, and they are likely to be a source of anxiety, fear, and agitation.

A strong theme of guilt, repentance, and punishment is evident in Jeff's conversation. The nurse has not yet begun to explore the sources of these feelings of worthlessness and blame nor the possible ways to intervene with Jeff to reduce his unpleasant, and perhaps unbearable, feelings.

This interaction represents one aspect of the process of establishing trust and building rapport with the client.

5. Using competing stimuli (eg, music and others' or own voice to overcome auditory hallucinations and visual stimuli to overcome visual hallucinations)[67]

Intervening in the Client's Affect Disturbance

Role Modeling. The nurse models appropriateness of affect by displaying a somber facial expression when discussing a serious topic or a joyful expression when engaging in a happy or pleasant topic of conversation. Using body language to convey a mood appropriate to the thought is one aspect of the nurse's repertoire of communication skills.

Developing Tolerance. Bizarre or inappropriate client behavior or affect should not be reinforced by a nurse's smile, nod, anger, or laughter. Nurses and other mental health caregivers may, at times, feel disgust or amusement at the client's behavior. It is often difficult to admit negative feelings to oneself, especially while trying to be therapeutic. Nevertheless, the therapeutic self is primarily a person of honesty, and insights about one's feelings must be acknowledged openly before they can be faced. It is particularly important to deal honestly with feelings because the client with schizophrenia may have learned to discount his or her own feelings. During interactions with psychiatric-mental health staff, the client may communicate that he or she perceives certain feelings as "dangerous." Feelings should be examined in a supportive, open environment.

Promoting Hope. Nurses and other psychiatric caregivers are pivotal in helping clients develop hope through the following:

1. Relationships built on rapport, communication, and trust
2. Facilitation of successful experiences
3. Association of the client with a successful role model with schizophrenia
4. Strategies to manage the illness, including symptom and medication management
5. Education for clients and the community[31]

Managing Stress. Stress-management strategies are useful to promote mental health in healthy or mentally ill individuals. One program teaches stress management techniques, including breathing and relaxation exercises, visualization, aerobic exercise, and nutritional measures, to clients with schizophrenia. Clients participate in and learned these techniques with minimal adaptation.[61]

Intervening in the Client's Social or Behavioral Disturbances

Promoting Safety. Because the client with schizophrenia may be unable to monitor physical health needs, the nurse must assume that responsibility until the client progresses to the point of self-care. Clients with disordered water balance require monitoring of electrolyte levels, supervision, education and self-monitoring, and milieu management to ensure their safety.[51]

During severe catatonic excitement or stupor, the client requires close supervision and intervention to prevent harm to self or others. Potential risks include malnutrition, self-inflicted wounds, fever, and exhaustion.[1]

Clients with schizophrenia are at risk for suicide. As many as 25% to 50% of clients with schizophrenia attempt suicide at some point in their lives. Refer to Chapter 42, Suicide, for information about interventions to safeguard the suicidal client.

Developing Trust. The development of a trusting relationship is basic to nursing care approaches to the schizophrenic client. The nurse–client relationship assists clients to develop trust and open communication.[48]

Nurses and other psychiatric-mental health professionals must show interest in and accept the total person who is the client. Although this goal is partly accomplished by means of the nurse's words, it is also heavily influenced by nonverbal behavior. The nurse's nonjudgmental attitude and genuineness cannot be manufactured. A genuine desire to offer assistance will be perceived accurately by the client, who will begin to view the nurse as a person who is helpful and sincere.

Through the nurse's body language, facial expression, eye contact, tone of voice, and verbalizations, the client receives messages about the nurse's trustworthiness. The client, in turn, responds to these messages. Because it is likely that the interpersonal experiences of the client with schizophrenia have been unsuccessful or unsatisfying, he or she may be unwilling to take risks in encounters with another person. Therefore, the client's response to a nurse, even if the nurse is warm, open, and genuine, may be reticent. Establishing rapport with the client may not be easy, but it is essential. Gradually, as a result of continued, consistent, and pleasant interpersonal experiences, the client's level of trust in another person should increase. The nurse slowly breaks through the wall of isolation and assumes more and more significance for the client.

At this point, the nurse may begin to introduce other people into the client's experiences. Hopefully, the client will transfer some of his or her trust in the nurse to another person and then to a third person until he or she has learned meaningful ways to interact with a larger sphere of people. If the initial interpersonal contact with the nurse is pleasant and rewarding, the client will be more inclined to risk opening up to others.

On the other hand, if the nurse does not regard the client positively and feels fear, repulsion, and hopelessness, the client will sense this attitude. Sometimes, the client's perceptions are so painfully acute that he or she will overtly respond to whatever he or she senses in the other person—the "vibes" he or she receives from the person. The nurse in this situation may be saying all the correct words but will not establish a therapeutic rapport if sincerity is lacking. In fact, between verbal and nonverbal behavior, the most important factor in dealing with the psychiatric client is probably nonverbal communication. The goal is to combine verbal and nonverbal communication skills to deal effectively and therapeutically with clients.

Approaching the Client. Because the client tends to withdraw from others, the nurse needs to make the initial approach. Waiting for the client to make the first contact is fruitless, because he or she typically lacks the self-confidence necessary to initiate contact with another person. Remembering that the client is likely to be frightened of others, the nurse approaches in a nonthreatening way. The nurse is encouraged to sit near the client (without crowding or impinging on personal space—some clients fear harm from close contact with others) and to speak in a soothing voice. Both of these approaches demonstrate to the client that the nurse is interested but willing to advance slowly and respond to cues.

A close interpersonal relationship may develop in the therapeutic environment. Hopefully, the client learns that other people can care for, not just take care of, him or her.[3]

Dealing With Hostility. The need to deal with hostility may arise because of the nature of the client's projection and fear of rejection. Hostility may be disguised as extreme passivity, testing behaviors, or projection.[3] The nurse should not overwhelm the client with too much talk or closeness. Although touch is an important therapeutic technique, it must be used judiciously; indiscriminate touch can be frightening to the client. For example, the paranoid schizophrenic client who thinks that he or she can be destroyed by someone's touch will become very agitated if touched by psychiatric caregivers (see Chapter 31, Aggressive and Violent Behavior).

Encouraging Self-Care. Encouraging the client's self-care skills and rewarding or reinforcing participation in activities of daily living promote independent behavior. The client may need the opportunity to experience small successes for a period of time. As the client is able to tolerate and accept more responsibility, he or she is given more opportunities.

Preventing Relapse. Many individuals with schizophrenia are able to monitor their symptoms of an impending relapse. For some, these may include symptoms of dysphoria, such as decreased appetite and difficulty sleeping and concentrating. For others, mild psychotic symptoms occur more frequently as signs of relapse. A recent study found that most clients with schizophrenia are able to monitor their relapse symptoms, including identifying the feelings and behaviors associated with getting worse, identifying *triggering* situations in which distress increases, and actively self-monitoring to detect early signs of relapse.[6]

Noncompliance with medication and alcohol and drug abuse are commonly related to the frequency of rehospitalization. Client education about the importance of following medication regimens and abstaining from alcohol and other substances has been shown to lengthen the time between hospitalizations.[25]

One psychiatric program schedules brief, planned admissions for clients with long-term, persistent, disabling mental illness. The purpose of this brief admission is to help clients maintain an optimal level of functioning and prevent decompensation. Clients participating in the program attend therapy, relaxation, didactic or information, and medication education groups.[38]

Psychiatric Rehabilitation

The field of psychiatric rehabilitation is founded on the belief that people with schizophrenia or any severe mental illness are key in designing their own plan for rehabilitation. Its aim is to increase the functioning of people with psychiatric disabilities and their satisfaction with their lives, with the least amount of professional intervention.[44] The following are basic principles of psychiatric rehabilitation:

1. Improve the competencies of people with psychiatric disabilities
2. Target behavioral improvements according to need
3. Work toward eventual independence of consumers of mental health services
4. Develop consumer life skills and environmental support
5. Rely on hope as an essential aspect of recovery
6. Use an eclectic approach to accomplish goals[44]

Working With the Client's Family

The challenges and problems faced by the family with a schizophrenic member are immense. The schizophrenic client's failure to care for personal needs, difficulty managing money, social withdrawal, strange personal habits, suicide threats, and interference with the family's work, school, and social schedules and the family's fear for the safety of the schizophrenic and other family members are genuine and realistic concerns.[63] The family's physical and psychological resources often deteriorate so much that the individual members' well-being and the stability of the family are threatened. Some members experience chronic sorrow related to their unending caregiving responsibilities.[19]

Family members have their own needs. These include the need to be part of the decision-making process (about public policies affecting care of people with schizophrenia and individualized treatment planning for the client), access to appropriate help in crises, information about useful resources, and access to respite care.

Family members need to be seen as individuals with valuable knowledge of and experience in coping with schizophrenia. They need helpful advice on practical management issues of living with schizophrenia and on formulating realistic goals for their member with schizophrenia.

Any therapeutic work with the client with schizophrenia must also be undertaken with the client's family. Supportive measures can enlarge the client's and family's social sphere, raise their level of interpersonal functioning, and increase their ability to become aware of feelings and learn to handle them effectively. The success of any treatment plan depends in large part on the mental health team's ability to effect change in the client together with his or her family and significant others, not merely as a separate entity.

In response to their dissatisfaction with care and treatment programs, family members of persons with schizophrenia have formed numerous advocate and support groups, many of which are affiliated with NAMI, founded in 1971. These consumer advocacy groups have emerged around the country in response to the family's need to be involved and to function collaboratively in the treatment of the mentally ill family member. Nationally, NAMI lobbies for funding to improve treatment and support research in schizophrenia and other serious mental illnesses.[22] An account of one family's work to help their son with schizophrenia and the help they received from NAMI is presented in Box 30-9.

Couples therapy groups for married clients with schizophrenia or parents groups for parents of young, unmarried clients with schizophrenia offer problem-solving skills and provide outside contacts for family members. If the client is not to return home following inpatient or residential treatment, he or she may be discharged to a group home or some alternative living arrangement. Plans for this move to a new living situation need to be worked out in detail long before the client is ready to leave the psychiatric facility. Needs of caregivers of clients with schizophrenia at home often go unmet—particularly information and social support needs. Psychosocial intervention, such as health education and family stress management, can help reduce the incidence of relapse and promote mental health of family members. When community psychiatric nurses use psychosocial intervention to intervene with families, family members are much more satisfied with service provided and report that their own minor mental health problems improve.[10]

As a result of deinstitutionalization of psychiatric clients from inpatient treatment facilities, the burden of providing community care has increasingly fallen on the shoulders of clients' families.[49] Family members perceive the difficulty of their burden in part according to the severity of the client's symptoms and whether the client resides with them. Coping abilities and social support are identifed as two of the most important factors that reduce family members' stress.[59]

Client and Family Education

Within recent years, families of people with mental illness have begun to be recognized as people with strengths and resources who are instrumental in their ill member's care and recovery.[21,59] This view has improved collaboration between mental health professionals and families.

Psychoeducation refers to interventions that emphasize coping skills and information about the illness and its management. Current approaches to family psychoeducational intervention may be based on a crisis intervention model, ongoing relatives' groups, survival skills for relatives and ongoing family therapy, family behavioral model, or client and family educational approach. These psychoeducational programs have demonstrated effectiveness in reducing relapse rates.[59] Psychoeducational family programs, based on the concept of expressed emotion, have been effective in decreasing relapse, especially when the client is taking medication.[37]

Families caring for a schizophrenic member at home must adapt to an extremely difficult situation. Their greatest need is education about schizophrenia. Specifically, educational programs should include the following information: diagnosis, etiology, symptomatology, course and prognosis, medication therapy, and management of the disorder (Box 30-10, p. 593).[10]

The optimal approach to the client's family is to view the family not as a source of pathology, but as a means of restoration to health.[5] Psychiatric-mental health professionals work with family members to help them add understanding to their personal concern, to explore the client's areas of vulnerability, and to learn to clarify and respond to the client's communications. The goal is to reintegrate the client into the family whenever possible.

Therapies

Individual Psychotherapy. The client with a schizophrenic disorder has difficulty relating to others; these difficulties are reflected in behaviors such as anxiety in interpersonal contacts, mistrust, fear, and misinterpretation of others' behavior. The therapist tries to counteract the client's anxiety, offer warmth and reassurance, and remove the fear "almost automatically

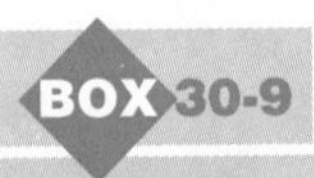

A Family's View of Chronic Mental Illness

Herbert J. Barr, Past President, Alliance for the Mentally Ill, Los Angeles, California

The nightmare started as we were preparing for the holidays. A telephone call from someone out of state said, "Come pick up your son." We had no idea what was to come or how it would affect our lives. Our son had been off at college. He had been on the Dean's list, had 4 years of undergraduate studies, and was pursuing a degree in pharmacology. What we found was a sick, withdrawn, almost catatonic son, who was eventually diagnosed as schizophrenic, sometimes paranoid, sometimes with depression, and at times suicidal.

At first, he required acute care in the county mental health system. He improved to the point of being warehoused in a board-and-care facility. He continued to improve and was able to get a job with an understanding large aerospace company. He lived independently in his own apartment, but this did not last very long. He decompensated and went through several cycles: the need for acute care, stabilization, and again the need for acute care. He has recently progressed from a skilled nursing facility to a transitional living facility where he is learning to live more independently. We hope that he will progress to a satellite apartment, with the possibility that he may become capable of performing nonstressful productive vocational activities and that his quality of life will improve.

What have we learned? Our son is ill. His illness is probably not due to any one of many stressful and traumatic childhood or growing-up experiences. The stresses he had may not have affected others, but for him, they were too much. We now know that he was probably vulnerable to the illness due to genetic, biochemical, or biological factors that are showing up in research. Stress will provoke or exacerbate the attacks or crises. Safe, commonplace things that we take for granted—decision making, meeting new people, dealing with problems and disappointments—are crisis-inducing experiences for those who are sensitive to stress and cannot cope in a stressful environment.

What are our frustrations? The foremost is that he may never achieve a reasonable level of happiness and the enjoyment of life that everyone strives for and that parents universally want for their children. Next is the frustration that there is not enough research to help the professionals learn how to diagnose, treat, cure, or prevent these chronic mental illnesses, primarily schizophrenia and the affective disorders. The Diagnostic and Statistical Manual of Mental Disorders is still a crude shotgun when aimed at understanding the subtleties of brain disorders. Next is the lack of an effective public mental illness care system. The present system's modality is governed by a shortage of tax dollars, inadequate and inhumane legal criteria for involuntary treatment, and lack of community based, low-cost housing for those who do not require expensive full-time care in state mental hospitals. Finally, the frustration that hurts the most—because it is solvable through education and understanding of professional caregivers—is the stigma.

In the 1950s, theories were proposed that serious mental illnesses were caused by double-bind communication or bad parenting. Throughout the history of these serious illnesses, this concept had not surfaced. Witchcraft and other religious reasons had been cited, yes, but not bad parenting. Today, the originators of that theory and modern researchers have repudiated the theory, but the stigma lingers on—primarily in older texts from the 1950s and in practitioners trained during that time.

The consequence of that lingering stigma is that if you believe it, you prejudge the parents as a malevolent influence. You will not want to involve them in the treatment. They are blamed and shut out. Stigma also says that a mentally ill person is somehow "bad" and only needs to "shape up." The political and societal consequence of stigma is not wanting to fund and care for those who are seriously mentally ill. State mental hospitals were almost emptied in the 1960s, with no provisions for local community care and housing; the present homeless population, many of whom are chronically mentally ill, is an outgrowth of that stigma.

Modern teaching and education are slowly correcting the problem of stigma, but treatment and long-term housing for the chronically mentally ill are dismally poor.

One of the best things that has happened to us as a family with an ill member is hearing about the National Alliance for the Mentally Ill (NAMI). It is

continued

BOX 30-9 (Continued)

a family support group organized to help family members understand and cope with the chronic mental illnesses and advocate for more research and better care and housing. Many communities have affiliates of NAMI. Families can write to the National Alliance for the Mentally Ill, 2101 Wilson Boulevard, Suite 302, Arlington, VA 22201, or call (703) 524-7600 or (800) 950-NAMI, for information.

It was only after we became active in NAMI that we began to understand the illness and how better to help our son. At first, caregivers would not talk to us, but this situation is now improving. Many now speak at our NAMI meetings, and they talk to us as caring parents. Through advocacy efforts and fund-raising for research NAMI also helps the caregivers. We now appreciate that in our family, we have been spared the heartache and grief of other families in which the mental illness was more severe, perhaps complicated with concurrent substance abuse or involvement in the criminal justice system. It is difficult enough to know that your family member has a serious mental illness, but when he or she is also involved with alcohol or drugs, the problems are much more severe, and there are very few, if any, provisions for concurrent treatment. This is only one hole in the care system. Likewise, it is painful to see a mentally ill family member, in a marginally acute state and very vulnerable, thrown in jail with criminally inclined people.

As family members who care about our ill one, we are advocating more appropriate legislation that will guarantee mentally ill people the treatment they need, rather than allowing them to remain homeless and live on the streets, with all the horrors that involves.

Finally, because too many families have been denied information by many government agencies and medical practitioners regarding the location, condition, or medication of an ill family member, we are advocating that the laws of confidentiality, although reasonable for people capable of informed consent, be modified for those who are too ill to make judgments about their own health and welfare.

With approximately one-third of schizophrenics recovering to a normal life with or without treatment and one-third requiring institutionalization, the remaining one-third of the population present a serious issue to the family and to the client. Should the ill family member stay at home or seek care as an independent adult? Parents receive mixed signals from professionals. We are chastised by some for not keeping our ill family member at home, but we are advised by others that it is best for the ill family member to develop his or her own coping skills. Many families keep their ill one at home, at great emotional and physical cost to the ill person and the rest of the family. Each family has to decide for itself. Our family would dearly love to see our son stay home in a nice, warm, clean room of his own, but that could lead to a great shock and upheaval when we are no longer here to take care of him. As parents, we would have failed to prepare him for the fundamental task of taking care of himself. As a result, we advocate that the public mental health system be improved to the point that it is adequate, humane, and available for all those who are dependent on it. It has to be a public system, because the average family cannot purchase group insurance to cover a lifetime of need, and whatever financial resources the average family possesses will evaporate after a few months or a year of private care. What happens then?

We would not be a caring family if we settled for less than what we are doing for our ill family member. We need to help the professionals discover better cures, and we need the support and understanding of the caregivers, because it is *our* loved one who is ill.

aroused by interpersonal contact."[5] The client and therapist must first learn to know, trust, and not be afraid of each other.

The principles of psychotherapy for the schizophrenic client are as follows:

1. Stimulate very little or no anxiety, and diminish the anxiety already present in the client.
2. Prevent the client from returning to a premorbid (prepsychotic) state, which would promote continued vulnerability for psychosis.
3. Achieve and maintain a state of "delicate balance" prior to the client's independence from treatment because of continued poor tolerance for frustration, discomfort, and anxiety.
4. Use a therapeutic approach by which the client moves toward gradual and progressive self-acceptance.[5]

Successful individual psychotherapists with schizophrenic clients demonstrate certain process and personal attributes, including honesty, hopefulness, commitment to the client and his or her welfare, flexibility, and tolerance for uncertainty and ambiguity.

The important commonalities in different effective

BOX 30-10

The Moller/Wer Model of Simultaneous Client and Family Education About Schizophrenia

In 1985, two clinical nurse specialists with advanced knowledge of neuroanatomy, physiology, biochemistry, therapeutic nutrition, psychopharmacology, diagnosis and etiology of schizophrenia, and healthy coping techniques began teaching a course about schizophrenia to conjoint groups of families and their relatives with schizophrenia.

The leaders, Moller and Wer, were knowledgeable in group theory and process (participants share through self-disclosure and role playing during classes), family development (multigenerational families attend classes), and principles of adult education. The course is termed health education, rather than psychoeducation, which they believe further stigmatizes and discriminates against the mentally ill.

Hallucinations or flat affect, says Moller, happen to people when they have a disease that affects the brain; discounting or ignoring hallucinations and delusions will not make them go away. Further, clients conclude that they are "just not doing something right and feel more hopeless."

The content for this and other client education courses for people with schizophrenia includes information about schizophrenia, medication and side effects, importance of physical self-care, management of social stigma, social and communication skills training, recognition and labeling of feelings, family support and response to mental illness, anticipation and management of future episodes of illness and crisis, and community resources.

Moller and Wer find that, armed with knowledge and understanding about schizophrenia, family members and clients experience less guilt and fear of the unknown; begin to trust, accept, and respect themselves; and begin to work with the health care system.

(From Moller MD, Wer JE: Simultaneous Patient/Family Education regarding Schizophrenia: The Nebraska Model. Archives of Psychiatric Nursing III (6): 332–337, 1989.)

psychotherapies may be therapists' attitudes and attributes rather than their theoretical beliefs. At present, there is little support for the use of insight-oriented or exploration-based psychotherapy with schizophrenic clients.[37]

Group Therapy. Various forms of group therapy may be used as a psychosocial form of treatment for psychotic clients in mental health facilities. Communication with the psychotic person, in group and other kinds of therapies, is usually concrete, brief, and direct.

Behavior Therapy. In a behavioral approach, the client with schizophrenia is seen as an individual with specific and measurable problems.[35] These problems are then treated by certain behavioral interventions, such as positive and negative reinforcement. In recent years, the focus of treatment has shifted from attempts to alleviate the schizophrenic disorder itself with different forms of psychotherapy to programs designed to improve the client's symptom management, social adaptation, vocational functioning, and subjective well-being.

Milieu Therapy. In inpatient settings, milieu therapy is a multidisciplinary team effort to treat clients with schizophrenia. The psychiatric-mental health staff must feel free to talk openly about clients, families, events, and their own feelings about their work. The overall milieu attitude reflects the therapeutic effectiveness of the environment that has been designed for clients. Client or ward government activities may offer opportunities for clients to participate in decision making relevant to their living situation.

An optimal milieu provides structure, routine expectations, education, and safety.[48] Keeping in mind that the client's judgment may be impaired will alert the nurse to important safety needs. Due to poor reality contact, the client may place himself or herself in potentially dangerous situations indoors and outdoors. Nursing responsibility dictates that the environment must be safety oriented and that care providers must attend to the client in a conscientious manner. If left alone, the client may neglect basic physical needs. The nurse, therefore, assumes the responsibility for physical health when the client is unable to meet his or her own needs. The nurse must observe the client carefully and frequently for signs of possible illness, unmet physical needs, and medication effects and side effects and intervene promptly and appropriately.

In a therapeutic milieu, clients are encouraged to share internal experiences, allowing nurses to interrupt hallucinations with music, simple games, and one-to-one interaction. Clients are also encouraged to use "open-door seclusion" in their rooms to escape overload of sensory stimulation from the television, peers, and conversations.[48]

Current treatment approaches view the family as the treatment team's ally and the client's most valuable support system. Treatment should support the family in dealing with the illness and its effects. Therapeutic interventions provide needed structure, distance, and stimulus control. Help to families should recognize the long-term nature of schizophrenia and their caregiving burden.[19,59]

Treatment goals include providing education for clients and family, maintaining alliances with families and community caregivers, and maximizing adaptation in relationships, self-care, and vocational pursuits.

Rehabilitative and Activities Therapies. Participation in a variety of social, activities, and rehabilitative therapies improves the client's social and recreational skills and self-esteem.

Psychopharmacotherapy. Adherence to medication regimens is the most effective way to prevent relapse of psychotic symptoms in clients with schizophrenia.[6,25] The nurse administering antipsychotic medication must be knowledgeable about the drug's action, use, usual dosage, desired therapeutic effects, route of administration, side effects, contraindications, and nursing implications. The nurse must also teach the client and family about the medication's action, use, dosage, desired effects, side effects, and needed interventions in case of an adverse reaction (Box 30-11).

Psychopharmacotherapy has moved from the status of an adjunct to psychological therapies to the dominant form of treatment for psychiatric disorders. Psychotropic drugs are useful in preventing relapse and hospital readmissions for a many psychiatric clients.[25]

Antipsychotics. Antipsychotic medications treat a wide range of symptoms effectively. The older medications, such as fluphenazine and haldoperidol, are effective in treating the positive symptoms of schizophrenia, such as hallucinations and delusions. The newer, atypical antipsychotic medications, such as clozapine and risperidone, treat the negative symptoms, such as apathy, avolition, and social withdrawal.

Administration of antipsychotic medication is an essential part of a comprehensive treatment program for the client with schizophrenia, although other interventions are useful and necessary for optimal functioning. The antipsychotic medications control some symptoms of the schizophrenic psychoses, such as withdrawal, aggression, extreme anxiety, hallucinations, and delusions. The client who receives antipsychotic medication often becomes more amenable to the various forms of social, recreational, and rehabilitative therapies. The choice of any psychotropic medication depends on its effectiveness and safety for the client. Most clients with schizophrenia are helped by antipsychotic medications; others may not experience the desired effects.

The side effects of antipsychotic medications are distressing and harmful. The nurse carefully observes the client for any of the following side effects: extrapyramidal effects (including tardive dyskinesia [TD]), autonomic effects, metabolic and endocrine effects, hypersensitivity reactions, and sedative effects. More serious is the development of neuroleptic malignant syndrome. (For a thorough review of the actions, therapeutic effects and side effects, and nursing implications of the antipsychotic medications, see Chapter 20, Psychopharmacology.)

After several months of treatment with antipsychotic medications, TD can occur and is often irreversible. At least one-third of clients with schizophrenia treated with antipsychotic medications develop the symptoms of TD—uncontrollable lip-smacking, writhing movements, neck twisting, tongue and chewing movements, and restlessness.

To decrease the incidence of TD, psychoactive medication is administered in reduced amounts, either through low-dosage treatment or intermittent or targeted medication treatment.[56] Intermittent medication administration involves episodic, rather than continuous, use of medication for symptom reduction in some clients with schizophrenia who do not need medication continuously. This method of medication administration requires the identification of prodromal symptoms (eg, feeling tense and nervous or experiencing difficulty sleeping or decreased enjoyment) and the early resumption of medication before the client becomes so disturbed as to require hospitalization.

Other extrapyramidal effects include muscle spasms and fatigue, akathisia, and the pseudoparkinsonian symptoms of rigidity, masklike facies, and stiff gait. These symptoms are understandably frightening to clients and families and require support and education.

In the past, although antipsychotic medications had a dramatic effect on the majority of clients with

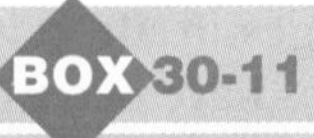

BOX 30-11

Medication Teaching About Atypical Antipsychotics

Clozaril (clozapine) and Risperdal (risperidone) are newer antipsychotic medications that are called atypical because they are unlike the older medications that were prescribed to reduce symptoms such as hallucinations.

The intended effects of the atypical antipsychotic medications are to eliminate or reduce your symptoms of hallucinations and paranoia (thinking that other people are trying to harm you). The medication helps you in these ways: to have more energy; to have fewer misperceptions about what is happening around you; to feel less paranoid and more like being around people (that is, not like keeping yourself isolated from others).

Side effects of these atypical antipsychotic medications include drowsiness and a drop in blood pressure, especially when getting up from a chair or bed (orthostatic hypotension). Both of these side effects are more likely to occur when you first start taking the medication and will usually disappear as your body adjusts to the medication. As long as these side effects persist, do not operate heavy equipment, do not drive, and stand up slowly from a seated or lying position. Some people who take an atypical antipsychotic medication have increased salivation and some feel nervous to the point of keeping them up at night. If this happens, notify your doctor or nurse practitioner.

Sometimes people have relapses or periods when their symptoms return. This may even occur when you are taking your medication regularly. You may feel more uncomfortable around people or think that they are talking about you. Talk with your doctor about these symptoms and continue to take your medication regularly. Never stop your medication all of a sudden.

Clozaril is taken 2 or 3 times a day: Risperdal is usually taken twice a day. When you take Clozaril, you must have a blood test every week to watch your white blood cell count. A serious side effect of Clozaril is that it can cause agranulocytosis, which is a dangerously low white blood cell count. The weekly blood test will tell your doctor and nurse that the white blood cells are not too low. Taking Risperdol does not require blood tests.

schizophrenia, some individuals receive little if any benefit from these drugs. Now, however, clozapine, an atypical antipsychotic medication, has been useful in treating clients who received little benefit from typical neuroleptics.

In 1989, the Food and Drug Administration announced its approval of clozapine to treat severe schizophrenia in clients who failed to respond to other available medications.[12,65] Clozapine, a dibenzodiazepine, offers antipsychotic efficacy without the associated extrapyramidal effects.[42] Clinical trials have shown that it may even ameliorate the symptoms of TD. Originally clozapine was released with its own client monitoring system in place, which added significantly to the cost (about $9,000 per year), but after 1 year of complaints and outcry from consumer advocacy groups, the manufacturer agreed to allow other blood monitoring systems to take effect.[24] Clozapine is indicated for clients with treatment-resistant schizophrenia. Clients with severe TD and extrapyramidal sensitivity also may benefit from a trial of clozapine.[24] Families of clients taking clozapine have reported remarkable, positive changes in their ill member; improved family relationships; and increased ability of the ill member to participate in social activities.[41]

Nursing interventions for a client receiving clozapine include continuous assessment and attentive interpersonal contact during the 7- to 10-day wash-out, or medication-free, period before beginning and during medication administration; baseline and comparative behavioral data collection; use of room restriction or quiet time if needed; observation for seizures and agranulocytosis; and extensive client and family education. The nurse also must monitor weekly hematological studies and report and document any drop in white blood cell count.[24] (An estimated 1%–2% of clients receiving clozapine therapy will develop agranulocytosis, which can be reversed if detected early.[47])

Risperidone is a new, atypical antipsychotic medication used to treat psychotic disorders. It has broad therapeutic effects, resulting in improvements in positive and negative symptoms of schizophrenia and reduced extrapyramidal and dyskinetic side effects. Anxiety, somnolence, dizziness, constipation, nausea, rhinitis, rash, and tachycardia are the most commonly reported side effects of risperidone.[28] While clozapine is restricted to clients who are treatment resistant or cannot tolerate other antipsychotics, risperidone is approved as a first-line drug. Other new antipsychotics are under development and testing, including olanzapine and ziprasidone.

Medication management is imprecise and at times, faulty. Clients sometimes complain that health care professionals often fail to recognize extrapyramidal effects and when clients report them, tend to interpret them as elevated anxiety and increase psychotropic medication dosage in response.[37] One study of clients' attitudes toward treatment demonstrated that clients perceive medication as a positive force in their lives, second in importance only to family support; they also identified medication as the most valuable treatment in their recovery.[13]

Public Education

The public's stigmatized views of, and misinformation about, mental illness have been documented since the 1950s. Recently one state surveyed its citizens about their beliefs about serious mental illness and undertook a program of public education about mental illness and its treatment. They found that the educational efforts did not significantly improve the misinformation and negative attitudes about people with mental illness.[20] Perhaps destigmatizing mental illness must begin with very young people. Stigma continues to be a major deterrent to the availability of community support programs for people with severe mental illness, such as schizophrenia.

EVALUATION

The success of any treatment program is measured not only by how many clients are discharged from the program, but by the availability of community support services and aftercare resources and by the local community's tolerance of behavioral difference. Schizophrenic clients who are ready for discharge and community living need to know that they will not be abandoned, will be helped to succeed in the community, and have the confidence of care providers in the ability to succeed.

Evaluating the effectiveness of nursing interventions requires reassessment to determine what therapeutic results or gains have occurred. Have specific nursing interventions affected a specific disturbed behavior of the client? What changes in affect, thinking, or social and family relationships have occurred?

The evaluation process is continuous. By constantly examining changes in the client's behavior, the nurse has the opportunity to change and strengthen certain aspects of the treatment plan.

Humanistic influences that reflect on the care of the mentally disturbed include the voiced rights of psychiatric clients, a multidimensional understanding of behavior, respect for the basic worth and dignity of each client, and community education that promotes acceptance and tolerance of the mentally ill. Similarly, more humanistic forms of treatment, such as open-door policies and client government, are common therapeutic modalities. Evaluation of these modalities and their benefit to schizophrenic clients may encourage us to examine and critique the philosophy and practices of our own psychiatric-mental health setting.

◆ The Nurse's Feelings and Attitudes

The nurse's feelings deserve, but rarely receive, considerable attention. Working with the schizophrenic client, the nurse is confronted with a wide range of unusual, and sometimes threatening, client behaviors. The nurse must, in the face of "madness," remain sane and secure—essential ingredients in therapeutic effectiveness—while not being aloof or emotionally distant.

Working with a client who is in poor contact with reality is often frustrating and may be frightening for the nurse. The client's delusions or hallucinations are at a very primitive level and may be likened to nightmares. Some of the nurse's own most basic fears may be put into words or acted out by the client with a schizophrenic disorder.

Nurses and other mental health professionals are encouraged to become involved with their clients as an essential part of the therapeutic process. The client with schizophrenia, however, may elicit great anxiety or other disturbing feelings in the nurse. Seeing a person who is severely regressed, withdrawn, and apathetic is a tragic experience for any of us. Applying therapeutic skills to the care of this client may be an overwhelming and emotionally draining task. Although nurses need to maintain and convey hope for the client's improvement, they may feel distraught over the difficulties inherent in that responsibility. Feelings of guilt about "not getting through" or "not doing enough" may arise and further complicate the therapeutic assignment.

Recognizing the reality of the client's disorder and treatment possibilities will help the nurse set realistic goals with the client. Professional supervision and involvement in support groups with colleagues will help the nurse keep a balanced view of the client's needs and gains. Nurses must cultivate close, rewarding relationships with family and friends as part of the process of personal growth and self-renewal and to ensure their own therapeutic effectiveness.

Human involvement and caring are prerequisites to therapeutic intervention. The nurse's caring manner demonstrates to the client that he or she is accepted and respected as a fellow human being. With time, the client will see that he or she is not viewed as hopeless, but as a person of dignity and worthy of respect.

The client with schizophrenia may be particularly sensitive to others' feelings and be able to see through facades; he or she may arouse strong feelings of anxiety, anger, and depression in mental health professionals. The intensity of the relationship with a schizophrenic client often brings to the surface interpersonal and emotional issues for the nurse. The nurse needs to address these issues to prevent them from hindering therapeutic effectiveness.

◆ Chapter Summary

This chapter has presented an overview of the schizophrenic disorders and the application of the nursing process to the client with a schizophrenic disorder. Chapter highlights include the following:

1. Because it affects an estimated 1% of the population and its onset occurs during adolescence and young adulthood, schizophrenic disorders are common and tragic mental illnesses.
2. The biological theories of the etiology of schizophrenia are built on data that support genetic, biochemical, immunological, or structural influences on the client and his or her behavior.
3. The psychosocial theories of the etiology of schizophrenia focus on the intrapersonal and interpersonal factors that lead to its development.
4. The five types of schizophrenia—disorganized, catatonic, paranoid, undifferentiated, and residual—are explained in terms of their operational criteria, and DSM-IV proposed subtypes are discussed.
5. Assessment and nursing diagnosis of the client are approached by examining the three major areas of thought, affect, and social and behavioral disturbances.
6. The foundation of an accurate assessment is a nonjudgmental attitude and careful, objective observation and description of client behaviors.
7. The psychiatric-mental health nurse is involved in treatment planning as a collaborative effort with other members of the mental health team, which includes the client and family or significant others.
8. Specific goals and outcomes are set for and with the client and family to intervene in the present behavior and to begin preparation for discharge to the community.
9. The nurse is encouraged to be consistent and genuine when dealing with the schizophrenic client.
10. The educational approach to clients with schizophrenia and their families uses skills workshops, family support and problem-solving sessions, and medication to increase the intervals between rehospitalizations and to promote optimal adaptation.
11. The nurse must acknowledge and deal with his or her own feelings while working with the schizophrenic client, because they are an important part of the therapeutic process.
12. Individual, group, and family therapy; the behavioristic approach; milieu therapy; rehabilitative and activities therapies; and psychopharmacotherapy are useful treatment modalities.
13. Nurses and other psychiatric professionals should work toward advocacy efforts to ensure a range of appropriate and available services for clients and families.
14. Evaluation of nursing intervention is the continuous process of examination and assessment of the therapeutic effectiveness of each specific intervention.

Critical Thinking Questions

1. *When you encounter a person with schizophrenia, you may find yourself reacting to many factors of which you may not be aware. What are some of these factors?*
2. *Identify your feelings about the person and about caring for him or her.*
3. *Reread the story of Mr. Robert L. in Nursing Care Plan 30-1. How much hope do you feel for Mr. L?*
4. *In your opinion, what will it take for Mr. L.'s life to improve significantly?*

Review Questions

1. Which of the following is known about schizophrenia?
   A. It is a single disease.
   B. It occurs only in certain cultures.

C. Medication can manage the symptoms of the disorder.
D. Positive symptoms include social withdrawal, apathy, and avolition.

2. The subtypes of schizophrenia include
   A. catatonic, which is marked by a psychomotor disturbance.
   B. disorganized, which is marked by prominent delusions.
   C. undifferentiated, which is marked by delusions, command hallucinations, and ideas of reference
   D. paranoid, which is marked by disorganized behavior and speech.
3. Clients with schizophrenia may help prevent relapse by all of the following interventions *except*
   A. self-monitoring symptoms, such as decreased appetite, difficulty sleeping, or mild psychotic symptoms.
   B. identifying triggering situations that bring about increased distress.
   C. using alcohol and other drugs to treat the uncomfortable symptoms of schizophrenia.
   D. following medication regimens even when they "feel good."
4. To work effectively with the families of clients with schizophrenia, the nurse should do all of the following *except*
   A. recognize and acknowledge the caregiving burden.
   B. prepare the treatment plan for the client without the family's input.
   C. provide education about the illness, relapse prevention, symptom monitoring, and medication management.
   D. provide resources to meet needs during crises, for respite care, and affiliation with support groups.
5. The atypical antipsychotic medications, such as risperidone, target the symptoms of
   A. hallucinations and magical thinking.
   B. delusions and illusions.
   C. apathy and avolition.
   D. disorganized speech and behavior.
6. Extrapyramidal side effects of antipsychotic medication include all of the following *except*
   A. agranulocytosis.
   B. masklike facial expression.
   C. muscle rigidity.
   D. akathisia.

◆ References

1. American Psychiatric Association: Diagnostic and Statistical Manual of Mental Disorders, 4th ed. Washington, DC, American Psychiatric Association, 1994
2. Andreasen NC, Carpenter WT: Diagnosis and Classification of Schizophrenia. Schizophr Bull 19 (2): 199–214, 1993
3. Arieti S: Interpretation of Schizophrenia, 2d ed. New York, Basic Books, 1974
4. Arieti S: Psychotherapy of Schizophrenia. In West LJ, Flinn DE (eds): Treatment of Schizophrenia: Progress and Prospects, pp 115–130. New York, Grune & Stratton, 1976
5. Arieti S: Psychotherapy of Schizophrenia: New or Revised Procedures. Am J Psychother 34 (October): 464–476, 1980
6. Baker C: The Development of the Self-Care Ability to Detect Early Signs of Relapse Among Individuals Who Have Schizophrenia. Archives of Psychiatric Nursing IX (5): 261–268, 1995
7. Bateson G, et al: Toward a Theory of Schizophrenia. In Jackson DD (ed): Communication, Family, and Marriage, pp 31–54. Palo Alto, CA, Science and Behavior Books, 1968
8. Bowen M: Family Psychotherapy. In Howells JL (ed): Theory and Practice of Family Psychiatry, pp 843–862. New York, Brunner/Mazel, 1971
9. Brooker C: A New Role for the Community Psychiatric Nurse in Working With Families Caring for a Relative With Schizophrenia. Int J Soc Psychiatry 36 (3): 216–224, 1990
10. Brooker C: The Health Education Needs of Families Caring for a Schizophrenic Relative and the Potential Role for Community Psychiatric Nurses. J Adv Nurs 15: 1092–1098, 1990
11. Brundage BE: What I Wanted to Know But Was Afraid to Ask. Schizophr Bull [Special Issue, Schizophrenia: The Experiences of Patients and Families]: 32–34, 1987
12. Carpenter WT, Conley RR, Buchanan RW, Breier A, Tamminga CA: Patient Response and Resource Managment: Another View of Clozapine Treatment of Schizophrenia. Am J Psychiatry 152 (6): 827–832, 1995
13. Chapman T: The Nurse's Role in Neuroleptic Medications. J Psychosoc Nurs 29 (6): 6–8, 1991
14. Conn VS: Commentary: The Case Against Family Systems Theory. Journal of Child and Adolescent Psychiatric and Mental Health Nursing 3 (1): 29–33, 1990
15. Davis JO, Phelps JA, Bracha HS: Prenatal Development of Monozygotic Twins and Concordance for Schizophrenia. Schizophr Bull 21 (3): 357–366, 1995
16. Dingemans PM: The Brief Psychiatric Rating Scale (BPRS) and the Nurses' Observation Scale for Inpatient Evaluation (NOSIE) in the Evaluation of Positive and Negative Symptoms. J Clin Psychol 46 (2): 168–174, 1990
17. Domenici N, Griffin-Francell C: Role of Family Education. J Clin Psychiatry 54 (35): 31–34, 1993
18. DuVal M: Giving Love ... and Schizophrenia. Schizophr Bull [Special Issue, Schizophrenia: The Experience of Patients and Families]: 8–13, 1987
19. Eakes GG: Chronic Sorrow: The Lived Experience of Parents of Chronically Mentally Ill Individuals. Archives of Psychiatric Nursing IX (2): 77–84, 1995
20. Fraser ME: Educating the Public About Mental Illness: What Will It Take to Get the Job Done? Innovations and

Research in Clinical Services, Community Support, and Rehabilitation 3 (3): 29–31, 1994
21. Gamble C, Midence K: Schizophrenia Family Work: Mental Health Nurses Delivering an Innovative Service. J Psychosoc Nurs 32 (10):13–16, 1994.
22. Gomez GE, Gomez EA: Chronic Schizophrenia: The Major Mental Health Problem of the Century. Perspect Psychiatr Care 27 (1): 7–9, 1991
23. Hamera EK, Peterson KA, Handley SM, et al: Patient Self-Regulation and Functioning in Schizophrenia. Hosp Community Psychiatry 42 (6): 630–631, 1991
24. Hamilton D: Clozapine: A New Antipsychotic Drug. Archives of Psychiatric Nursing IV (4): 278–281, 1990
25. Haywood TW, Kravitz HM, Grossman LS, Cavanaugh JL, Davis JM, Lewis DA: Predicting the "Revolving Door" Phenomenon Among Patients with Schizophrenic, Schizoaffective,and Affective Disorders. Am J Psychiatry 152 (6): 856–861, 1995
26. Hirschmann M: Commentary: The Case for Family Systems Theory. Journal of Child and Adolescent Psychiatric and Mental Helath Nursing 3 (1): 29–33, 1990
27. Houghton JF: Maintaining Mental Health in a Turbulent World. Schizophr Bull [Special Issue, Schizophrenia: The Experience of Patients and Families]: 17–21, 1987
28. Judd LL, Rapaport M: A New Antipsychotic Medication for the Treatemnt of Schizophrenia. Innovations and Research in Clinical Services, Community Support, and Rehabilitation 3 (1): 1–7, 1994
29. Kanba S, et al: Selective Enlargement of the Third Ventricle Found in Chronic Schizophrenia. Psychiatry Res 21: 49–53, 1987
30. Kaplan HI, Sadock BJ: Synopsis of Psychiatry, 7th ed. Baltimore, Williams & Wilkins, 1994
31. Kirkpatrick H, Landeen J, Byrne C, Woodside H, Pawlick J, Bernardo A: Hope and Schizophrenia: Clinicians Identify Hope-Instilling Strategies. J Psychosoc Nurs 33 (6): 15–19, 1995
32. Kishimoto H, et al: Three Subtypes of Chronic Schizophrenia Identified Using ^{11}C-Glucose Positron Emission Tomography. Psychiatry Res 21: 285–292, 1987
33. Kivlahan DR, Heiman JR, Wright RC, et al: Treatment Cost and Rehospitalization Rate in Schizophrenic Outpatients With a History of Substance Abuse. Hosp Community Psychiatry 42 (6): 609–614, 1991
34. Lanquetot R: Confessions of the Daughter of a Schizophrenic. Schizophr Bull [Special Issue, Schizophrenia: The Experiences of Patients and Families]: 57–61, 1987
35. Liberman RP: Behavior Therapy for Schizophrenia. In West LJ, Flinn DE (eds): Treatment of Schizophrenia: Progress and Prospects, pp 175–206. New York, Grune & Stratton, 1976
36. Littrell KH, Freeman LY: Maximizing Psychosocial Interventions. Journal of the American Psychiatric Nurses Association 1 (6): 214–218, 1995
37. Malone JA: Schizophrenia Research Update: Implications for Nursing. J Psychosoc Nurs 28 (8): 4–6, 8–9, 1990
38. Merchant DJ, Henfling PA: Scheduled Brief Admissions: Patient "Tuneups." J Psychosoc Nurs 32 (12): 7–10, 1994
39. Mintz LI, et al: Expressed Emotion: A Call for Partnership Among Relatives, Patients, and Professionals. Schizophr Bull 13 (2): 227–235, 1987
40. Moller MD, Wer JE: Simultaneous Patient/Family Education Regarding Schizophrenia: The Nebraska Model. Archives of Psychiatric Nursing III (6): 332–337, 1989
41. Najarian SP: Family Experience With Positive Client Response to Clozapine. Archives of Psychiatric Nursing IX (1): 11–21, 1995
42. Nordstrom A, Farde L, Nyberg S, Karlsson P, Halldin C, Sedvall G: D1, D2, and 5-HT2 Receptor Occupancy in Relation to Clozapine Serum Concentration: A PET Study of Schizophrenic Patients. Am J Psychiatry 152 (10): 1444–1449, 1995
43. O'Connor FW: A Vulnerability-Stess Framework for Evaluating Clinical Interventions in Schizophrenia. Image: Journal of Nursing Scholarship 26 (3, Fall): 231–237, 1994
44. Palmer-Erbs VK, Anthony WA: Incorporating Psychiatric Rehabilitation Principles Into Mental Health Nursing: An Oportunity to Develop a Full Partnership Among Nurses, Consumers, and Families. J Psychosoc Nurs 33 (3): 36–44, 1995
45. Peralta V, Cuesta MJ: Negative Symptoms in Schizophrenia: A Confirmatory Factor Analysis of Competing Models. Am J Psychiatry 152 (10): 1450–1457, 1995
46. Perry W, Moore D, Braff D: Gender Differences of Thought Disturbance Measures Among Schizophrenic Patients. Am J Psychiatry 152 (9): 1298–1301, 1995
47. Piercy BP: Making the Best of It. Schizophr Bull [Special Issue, Schizophrenia: The Experiences of Patients and Families]: 62–64, 1987
48. Puskar KR, McAdam D, Burkhart-Morgan CE, et al: Psychiatric Nursing Management of Medication-Free Psychotic Patients. Archives of Psychiatric Nursing IV (2): 78–86, 1990
49. Reinhard SC: Perspectives on the Family's Caregiving Experience in Mental Illness. Image: Journal of Nursing Scholarship 26 (1): 70–74, 1994
50. Reiss D, Plomin R, Hetherington M: Genetics and Psychiatry: An Unheralded Window on the Environment. Am J Psychiatry 148 (3): 283–291, 1991
51. Ribble DJ, Thelander B: Patients With Disordered Water Balance: Innovative Psychiatric Nursing Intervention Strategies. J Psychosoc Nurs 32 (10): 35–42, 1994
52. Ricci MS: The New After-care Clinic: Treating Individuals Rather Than Masses. J Psychosoc Nurs 28 (8): 18–21, 1990
53. Ruesch J: Synopsis of the Theory of Human Communication. In Howells JG (ed): Theory and Practice of Family Psychiatry, pp 227–266. New York, Brunner/Mazel, 1971
54. Satir V: Peoplemaking. Palo Alto, CA, Science and Behavior Books, 1972
55. Schizophrenia: The Experiences of Patients and Families. Schizophr Bull [Special Issue NIMH, US Department of Health and Human Services], Rockville MD, 1987
56. Schooler NR, Levine J: Strategies for Enhancing Drug Therapy of Schizophrenia. Am J Psychother 37 (October): 521–532, 1983
57. Schwarzkopf SB, Olson SC, Coffman JA, et al: Third and Lateral Ventricular Volumes in Schizophrenia: Support

for Progressive Enlargement of Both Structures. Psychopharmacol Bull 26 (3): 385–391, 1990

58. Serper MR, Alpert M, Richardson NA, Dickson S, Allen MH, Werner A: Clinical Effects of Recent Cocaine Use on Patients With Acute Schizophrenia. Am J Psychiatry 152 (10): 1464–1469, 1995
59. Solomon P, Draine J: Subjective Burden Among Family Members of Mentally Ill Adults: Relation to Stress, Coping, and Adaptation. Am J Orthopsychiatry 65 (3): 419–427, 1995
60. Spitzer VM: Biological Aspects of Schizophrenia. Journal of the American Psychiatric Nurses Association 1 (6): 204–207, 1995
61. Starkey D, Deleone H, Flannery RB: Stress Management for Psychiatric Patients in a State Hospital Setting. Am J Orthopsychiatry 65 (3): 446–450, 1995
62. Sullivan WP: A Long and Winding Road: The Process of Recovery from Severe Mental Illness. Innovations and Research in Clinical Services, Community Support, and Rehabilitation 3 (3): 19–27, 1994
63. Torrey EF: Surviving Schizophrenia: A Family Manual, rev ed. New York, Harper & Row, 1988
64. Tugrel KC: Pharmacological Treatment of Schizophrenia: A Review. Journal of the American Psychiatric Nurses Association 1 (6): 208–213, 1995
65. U.S. Department of Health and Human Services: HHS News October: 3, 1989
66. Wasylenki DA: Psychotherapy of Schizophrenia Revisited. Hosp Community Psychiatry 43: 123–127, 1992
67. Williams CA: Perspectives on the Hallucinatory Process. Issues in Mental Health Nursing 10: 99–119, 1989

Aggressive and Violent Behavior

Bonnie Louise Rickelman

31

Growing up often means facing the anguished isolation of no longer belonging as we wander in exile through a strange world that makes no sense. Each of us must make his or her separate way through an indifferent, unfamiliar landscape, in which good is not necessarily rewarded, nor evil punished. Adding to the confusion, we find ourselves or others graced with unearned love and happiness or burdened with "undeserved" calamity and pain.

Sheldon Kapp, **An End to Innocence: Facing Life**

Daily observations and media stories document that violence, pervasive in American society, is a key public health issue. More health care professionals working in inpatient hospital settings, outpatient clinics, forensic facilities, and even general practice settings are treating clients for whom violent behavior is the primary reason for therapy.[30] By 2010, an estimated 25% increase in admissions of violent clients to specialty mental health facilities will occur.[44] Furthermore, many clients with chronic mental illness remain institutionalized because of their assaultive behavior. Violence results in personal injury, lost productivity, lost time, lawsuits, negative milieu and staff morale, and staff turnover.[32,49]

Exposure to aggressive and violent behavior by clients is common for nurses and other mental health workers. To prevent or minimize exposure to violent behavior, nurses must have a pertinent knowledge base for assessing people at risk for aggressive and violent behaviors and applying therapeutic intervention skills as they intervene to prevent or manage aggressive episodes. Although incidences of violence and repeat violence can never be predicted with certainty, certain congruent findings across disciplines regarding biological, psychological, and social risk factors can be used to develop assessment protocols and design prevention and intervention strategies. Knowledge of known risk factors for potential violence should be incorporated into basic and inservice education of all health care providers and professional staff.

In this chapter, aggressive and violent behavior are discussed in terms of adults who have been diagnosed with mental illness and who are receiving care in a mental health facility. Certain terms that are relevant to a conceptual understanding of aggression are defined, and current perspectives regarding psychobiological, social, and environmental determinents of aggressive behaviors in adult clients with a diagnosis of mental illness are discussed. Emphasis is given to the essential components of the nursing process in addressing aggressive and violent behaviors, namely client assessment, diagnosis, goals and outcomes, interventions, and evaluation. In addition, pertinent case material and nursing care plan guidelines are presented.

Learning Objectives

On completion of the chapter, you should be able to accomplish the following:

1. *Define the broad range of responses constituting aggressive behavior, including pertinent hostility-related variables and violence.*
2. *Discuss client profiles of violence in terms of psychiatric diagnosis, arrests for violent crimes, inpatient factors and staff–client interaction, outpatient factors, urban versus rural residence, families with a violence-prone member who is mentally ill, and comparison with the general population.*
3. *Discuss the psychological, neurobiological, social, and environmental or situational determinents of aggression in terms of pertinent theory and research findings.*
4. *Apply nursing care guidelines to assess, diagnose, establish client outcome goals, intervene, and evaluate nursing care and client outcomes.*
5. *Verbalize awareness of own feelings and attitudes when interacting with a client who is exhibiting aggressive or violent behavior.*
6. *Discuss relevant cultural and legal issues regarding the treatment of aggressive and violent clients.*

◆ Aggression, Hostility-Related Variables, and Violence

AGGRESSION

Although definitions of aggression often differ across disciplines and among various reported studies, aggressive behavior generally includes abusive language, violent threats of harm, physical assault to self or others, and damage to property.[141] As a behavior, aggression can be analyzed and understood not only in terms of negative appraisals and attitudes toward self, others, the world, and the future,[7] but also in relation to the emotions that may or may not accompany it, such as the hostility-related variables of anger, suspiciousness, irritability, and impulsivity.

HOSTILITY-RELATED VARIABLES

Hostility-related variables are emotions, attitudes, and behaviors that occur with regularity and predictability in aggressive and violence-prone individuals.[15] Hostility-related emotions encompass anger, irritability, and resentment and have been linked with aggressive behaviors and with the potential to develop certain medical conditions, such as essential hypertension, cardiovascular hyperreactivity, and atherosclerotic heart disease.[12,25,75,111,112]

Hostility-related attitudes are persistent negative views of others and the world. These views encompass cynicism, mistrust, suspiciousness, and a readiness to look at everyday life events and the actions of others in the worst light.[15] Hostility-related behavior is a logical outgrowth of the hostility-related emotions and attitudes that are present prior to the behavior and are associated with a predilection for aggression. Hostility-related behavior, sometimes called *expressive hostility,* can be observed in facial expressions; body language; verbalizations; gestures; overt acts against self, other people, or property; or any combination of these.

Anger and impulsivity play pivotal roles in an individual's march toward aggressive or violent behavior and are singled out of hostility-related emotions for discussion here. Anger is an emotion that often results when an individual's expectations are not met. These expectations may be of oneself, another person or people, an organization (including the government), or a life event. Anger can be a positive emotion when it motivates a person to change through the use of various strategies, services, and educational opportunities. Anger can also motivate more mature individuals to organize and help institute constructive change when this would be beneficial or when injustices prevail. Anger loses its constructiveness when it turns inward; when it flails ineffectively at others with little or no cause; when it bullies others with less strength, power, or resources; when it harms or hurts the self or others physically or emotionally; and when its expression is out of control. The ways an individual deals with anger tend to persist with time. If the person whose anger results in destructiveness is not motivated to change or if help that the person may seek is not available or is poorly administered, the anger, with all of its negative consequences to self and others, is likely to persist.

Impulsivity is a mode of interacting manifested by acts performed with little or no regard for the consequences.[79] Relevant to clinical practice, impulsivity is viewed as a symptom of an underlying disorder or as a pervasive personality trait.[5,36] *Impulse control disorders* are generally characterized by three criteria: 1) an inability to control an impulse to behave in a manner that is viewed as harmful to oneself or to others; 2) a sense of increasing tension (increased feelings of pressure, discomfort, or energy) prior to acting on the impulse, which may or may not be premeditated or consciously resisted; and 3) a sense of excitement, gratification, and tension release during the act.[11] Individuals typically experience some degree of regret or remorse following the act, although regret or remorse is often transient due to a tendency to rationalize the behavior.

The following possible etiological factors associated with impulsive behavior have been identified: a life pattern of impulsive behavior, nervous system abnormalities, anxiety, life crisis, and sexual and aggressive drives. Characteristics of impulsiveness include unpredictable behavior, threats toward others, irresponsible acts, low frustration tolerance, poor problem-solving skills, disturbed interpersonal relationships, restlessness, and general disregard for social rules and customs.[79]

VIOLENCE

Violence is a form of aggression that includes the following:

- Threats, including verbal or written statements that imply harm to a person or property (sexual harrassment is included)
- Physical assault (including sexual assault) with or without a weapon that results in actual physical harm, such as bruises and lacerations, or death
- Damage to property[142]

Acts of aggression that are violent are the primary focus for legal assessment of dangerousness in all clinical and forensic settings.[6] Dangerousness includes actions that have a high risk of being harmful or injurious to self or others. The *intent* to harm another person is an important criterion when evaluating and differentiating situations of accidental harm or injury as opposed to situations in which harm is done intentionally to other people or property.[6]

◆ Aggressive and Violent Client Behaviors Associated With Psychiatric Diagnoses

Incidents reflecting the range of aggressive behavior, including physical violence, occur in all clinical diagnostic categories and are not exclusively manifested by individuals diagnosed with a mental disorder. The *Diagnostic and Statistical Manual of Mental Disorders IV* classification system provides for the possibility of multiple disorders that carry the potential for aggressive behavior.[4] Examples of psychiatric diagnoses and common patterns of aggression or violence are listed in Table 31-1.

Numerous studies have attempted to find an association between clients' diagnoses and risk of assaultive incidents in psychiatric hospitals. However, because a diagnosis is a longitudinal label that represents varying behavioral characteristics and clients with the same diagnosis or multiple diagnoses vary in their types of behavior, diagnosis is viewed by some researchers as an unreliable predictor of the type of aggressive or violent incident of which individual clients might be vulnerable.[61] Nevertheless, a longstanding debate about the relationship between serious mental illness and incidence of violence in the following groups has been rekindled by recent research studies: individuals who have been arrested; psychiatric inpatients; psychiatric outpatients; families with a seriously mentally ill member; and the general population in the community.[17,132]

CLIENT ARREST PROFILES

Most studies since the 1960s indicate that people who have been hospitalized primarily in public psychiatric facilities tend to have postdischarge arrest rates that are higher than those for the general population.[55,57,64,66,122,123,131,132] In addition, higher levels of arrests for violent behavior

Table 31-1

Psychiatric Diagnoses and Patterns of Aggression or Violence

- **Intermittent explosive disorder:** Explosive outbursts of anger that are out of proportion to any provocation or precipitating psychosocial stressor may result in serious assaultive acts or destruction of property; generalized impulsivity or aggressiveness may be present between explosive episodes.
- **Conduct disorder (children):** Aggressive conduct threatens or causes physical harm to other people or animals.
- **Oppositional defiant disorder:** Hostility directed at adults or peers, primarily by deliberately annoying others or by verbal aggression.
- **Attention deficit-hyperactivity disorder:** predominantly hyperactive-impulsive type: The client displays low frustration tolerance; has temper outbursts; interrupts or intrudes on others; is bossy; insists that requests be met; and displays oppositional behavior.
- **Antisocial personality disorder (adults):** Adults with antisocial personalities are impulsive, inclined to seek constant excitement, feel little or no guilt, and form few affectional bonds with others. Violence can be a way of getting what they want.
- **Paranoid personality disorder:** Paranoid people are suspicious and guarded and may present a facade of self-sufficiency that disguises underlying feelings of inadequacy. These individuals may be belligerent and intimidating and always ready to attack preemptively to avoid perceived humiliation or conspiracy, and tend to insist that their victims get what they deserve.
- **Personality change due to a general medical condition, such as head injury:** Irritability and aggression commonly increase after traumatic brain injury.
- **Dementia:** Dementia is characterized by generalized irritability and low frustration tolerance, confusion, destructive attempts at self-protection.
- **Substance-related disorders** (eg, alcohol, amphetamines, cocaine, hallucinogens, inhalants): Aggressive episodes are frequently due to the direct physiological effects of a substance (eg, a drug of abuse or a medication).
- **Schizophrenia, paranoid type:** Persecutory themes may predispose the individual to suicidal behavior, and a combination of persecutory and grandiose delusions with anger may predispose to violence.
- **Bipolar disorders I and II (especially manic episodes):** These disorders are characterized by irritability, agitation, and episodic antisocial behavior with interpersonal or occupational difficulties.
- **Post-traumatic stress disorder:** These clients display irritability or outbursts of anger and hypervigilance.
- **Dissociative identity disorder:** Self-mutiliation, suicidal, and aggressive behavior may occur.
- **Delusional disorder, persecutory type:** Individuals with persecutory delusions (eg, of being conspired against, cheated, spied on, maliciously maligned, poisoned or drugged) are often resentful and angry and may use violence against those they believe are threatening are harmful to them.

(From DSM-IV. Washington, DC, The American Psychiatric Association, 1994)

have been found for individuals with antisocial personality, paranoid schizophrenia, and substance abuse disorders.[92]

In a recent study of 172 state hospital inpatients, investigators examined associations between a history of violent crime, substance abuse, and four types of major psychopathology—schizophrenia, schizoaffective disorder, and bipolar and unipolar affective disorders.[45] Results indicated that clients with schizoaffective disorder had been arrested for violent crimes significantly more often than clients in the other diagnostic groups. Similar findings occurred for psychotic clients compared with nonpsychotic clients, clients who had paranoid schizophrenia compared with those who had schizophrenia without paranoid features, and clients who had coexisting substance abuse compared with those with no history of substance abuse. In addition, findings revealed that clients from racial minority groups and male clients were more likely than white and female clients to have an arrest record for violent crime. Similarly, a Swedish study of 644 individuals with schizophrenia who were followed for 15 years postdisharge from an initial psychiatric hospitalization revealed that these people committed four times more violent offenses than did a normal control group.[65]

INPATIENT PROFILES: SALIENT FACTORS IN AGGRESSIVE AND VIOLENT EPISODES

In a review of 75 psychiatric hospital incident reports exploring behavior patterns of clients immediately prior to the incidents, a study found the following:

1. Most incidents occurred during clients' first week of hospitalization and declined steadily thereafter.
2. The rate of incidents was significantly higher for male clients between the ages of 26 and 35 and for female clients between the ages of 36 and 45.
3. The type of incidents differed significantly between male and female clients (eg, physical altercations, assaults, and destructive behavior were higher among male clients, whereas suicide attempts were higher among female clients).
4. The most common diagnoses were schizophrenia, substance abuse, or major depression.
5. Clients with schizophrenia evidenced an increased risk of committing assault.[61]

The researchers concluded that client behavior patterns may be valuable for predicting the type of aggressive incident and for intervening to prevent further incidents.[61]

A series of studies exploring aggression and violence by people with a mental illness found that in contrast to nonviolent inpatients who primarily had a characteristic interaction style of accommodation, violent inpatients primarily manifested an exploitative, coercive interaction style (ie, using others for self-gain).[86-91] A coercive interaction style was identified as a primary precursor to the use of aggression and violence by people with mental illness. Previous research has documented patterns of coercion, power, and control in families of antisocial children and bullying patterns in young children that continued into adulthood.[98,100] Power and control patterns have been further substantiated in domestic violence and sexual assault research.[105]

Staff–Client Interaction

Additional research reveals the importance of interpersonal and situational factors as precursors of violent incidents on psychiatric units, particularly the influence of staff–client interaction.[140] Two types of antecedent events have been linked with escalating client violence. First are occasions when clients are angered or frustrated by the behavior of other clients, such as disputes over cigarettes or food, or by staff behavior that in the process of caring for the client, may intrude on or frustrate the client.[1] Examples of such staff behavior include preventing the client from leaving the ward,[19] disputes over medication, general enforcement of rules or denial of requests,[110] physically restraining or guiding the client, taking something from the client, or simply requesting the client to do or refrain from doing something.[139] An escalation of aggressive client behavior may be avoided if the nurse and other staff can influence the client's appraisal of the interaction. The staff's behavior or verbal requests should be explained and justified to the client whenever possible so that the client has the opportunity to view staff behavior as purposefully helpful and well intended rather than arbitrary or punitive.[139]

The second type of antecedent event that is associated with client violence in psychiatric units is that of being ignored by staff.[28,139] Some staff may avoid seriously disturbed clients because interaction with such clients is considered stressful.[28] However, such clients may become aggressive to gain staff attention.[20]

Client Background: Rural Versus Urban

Some evidence indicates that the level of violence that occurs in inpatient settings may be influenced by clients having lived in a rural versus an urban setting prior to hospitalization. While research findings are relatively sparse regarding profiles of rural mental health services and clientele, one study of the profiles of 609 clients admitted to Arkansas State Hospital, with equivalent numbers from rural and urban areas, indicated that clients from rural areas (nearly one-half) were more likely than those from urban areas (39%) to be aggressive and destructive, even after controlling for age, gender, race, educational level, diagnosis, legal status, and substance abuse.[22] However, more violence-prone clients from rural areas abused substances prior to admission than did those from urban areas. Numerous barriers may impede the delivery of mental health services to the seriously mentally ill who live in rural areas, resulting in a greater severity of illness threshold and an increased rate of violence for those who enter the system and are hospitalized.[22] The delays in initiation of treatment and the fact that rural clients may be more likely to be separated from family and other social support networks when hospitalized may contribute to the increased rate of violence among rural versus urban clients, at least in this study.

OUTPATIENT PROFILES

Recent studies reveal that about 30% of male and female psychiatric clients with a history of violent behavior exhibit violent behavior again within 1 year of discharge.[54,55,85] In one study, a history of medication noncompliance by outpatients was strongly correlated with higher levels of hostility and rehospitalization. Of the outpatients who were rated as destructive and assaultive 71% reported problems with medication compliance, while only 17% of outpatients with behaviors other than assault and destruction reported such problems. The use of time during outpatient clinic visits to help clients understand their medications, the importance of compliance, and the consequences of noncompliance cannot be overemphasized. Proper referral and involvement of family and significant others are crucial in detering recidivism.

FAMILIES WITH A VIOLENCE-PRONE MENTALLY ILL MEMBER

The National Alliance for the Mentally Ill has conducted extensive surveys of families in which a family member had been diagnosed with a serious mental illness, such as schizophrenia, biopolar disorder, or major depression. In one survey of 1,401 families, findings indicated that 10.6% of the seriously mentally ill individuals had physically harmed another person, while 12.2% had threatened harm.[118] In addition, gender differences were found among those who threatened harm (24.9% of men and 12.5% of women), but interestingly, no gender difference was found among those who harmed another person (11.9% of men and 9.5% of women).[118] Two other studies have revealed that among clients who had physically attacked someone within the previous 2 weeks of admission to a psychiatric hospital, family members had been the object of their attacks 65% of the time in the earlier study[126] and 56% of the time in the more recent study.[120]

VIOLENCE IN THE GENERAL POPULATION VERSUS THE SERIOUSLY MENTALLY ILL IN THE COMMUNITY

The Epidemiologic Catchment Area (ECA) surveys between 1980 and 1983 were conducted by the National Institute of Mental Health in five sites: New Haven, Connecticut; Eastern Baltimore; St. Louis; Durham, North Carolina; and Los Angeles. The purpose of the ECA surveys was to assess violent behavior among individuals with serious mental illness using the following criteria: hitting or throwing things at one's wife, husband, or partner; hitting one's child hard enough to cause bruises or inury; physically fighting with others; and using a weapon such as a stick, knife, or gun in a fight.[9,122] A methodological limitation of this study is that no attempt was made to differentiate the severity of these acts of aggression. Findings indicated that when compared with individuals with no psychiatric disorder, seriously mentally ill individuals who live in the community report more incidents of violence in the past year, more use of weapons in fights, and more violence-related drug and alcohol dependence and abuse.[122]

While the majority of individuals with serious mental illness are no more violent or dangerous than members of the population in general, evidence supports an increased risk of violence among a subgroup of mentally ill individuals who have a history of violent behavior and substance abuse and noncompliance with medications when compared with the general population.[92,132]

◆ Determinants of Aggression

Violent and aggressive behaviors have multiple determinants, including psychological, biological, sociocultural, and environmental factors. The relative contribution of each of these determinants is an ongoing issue in professional debate and research studies.

PSYCHOLOGICAL THEORIES

Freud's drive theory postulated that all individuals have a reservoir of aggressive energy that sometimes overflows and is released, but others discount an aggressive drive or instinct in favor of more cognitive and social theories for explaining aggression and violent behavior. The classic frustration-aggression theory proposes that as individuals become more frustrated (ie, are blocked or interrupted in their goal-directed behavior), the probability of manifesting aggressive behavior increases. Other intrapersonal influences that have been linked with a lack of impulse control and violent behavior include temperament; cognitive appraisal; various medical and neurobiological conditions, including imbalances in neurotransmitter systems; and dual diagnoses, such as mental illness and substance abuse.[33,46,92]

Temperament Theory

Recently, researchers have shown an increasing interest in *temperament,* defined as constitutional or biologically based personality dispositions that are partly inherited, evident early in life, and somewhat stable across situations and over time.[2] Three personality dimensions are believed to be shaped by temperament: negative emotionality, positive emotionality, and constraint.[2]

Negative emotionality can be classified on a continuum from intense distress to calm stability. Most commonly discussed is the "difficult" temperament manifested by irregularity in biological functions; behavioral inhibition, including shyness and the tendency to become fearful in and to withdraw from new or novel situations; slow adaptability; and an intense and negative mood.[52,76] For example, on the first day of preschool, the child who is behaviorally inhibited will stand silently, while the uninhibited child will freely explore the environment and interact with others.

Positive emotionality is viewed as an "easy" temperament manifested by regular biological functions, a positive and active engagement with people, seeking out new situations, positive adaptation, agreeableness, and a mild and generally positive mood. Temperament is thought to continue throughout the lifespan, and while most studies have focused on infants and children, some researchers have examined adults and found that adults at risk for adjustment problems had experienced difficult temperaments as preschoolers.[18,43]

Individuals high in *constraint* are generally conscientious, cautious, deliberative, reliable, responsible, hardworking, well organized, and self-controlled. Those who are low in constraint are impulsive, careless, and respond to their immediate wants rather than establishing and working toward long-range goals.

Environment can be an important mitigator of temperament. Personality at any age reflects the interplay of temperament and experience related to the demands, expectations, and opportunities of the environment. While parenting can influence a child's personality, a child's temperament can influence parenting. A distress-prone child who is irritable and complaining may elicit more parental criticism. Experiences of emotional or physical trauma in childhood may increase negative emotionality, inhibit capacity for pleasure (positive emotionality), and decrease capacity for control and emotional regulation (constraint).[2] While negative emotionality may be difficult to change, individuals who experience negative emotionality can be encouraged to become more positive thinkers and to gain confidence and more positive emotional experiences if strongly motivated and helped to achieve some experience and success in these endeavors.

Cognitive Theory

A cognitive model explains how one's attributions, appraisals, expectancies, and self-talk mediate between stimuli and aggressive reactions. Attributions are attitudes, beliefs, and appraisals used to explain events that happen to people.[137] Appraisals of events are highly individualistic. Certain ways of interpreting situations and events produce an aggressive disposition and expectations that result in negative self-fulfilling prophecies. The role of attributions in anger arousal has been proposed as follows: 1) Events are perceived as aversive based on expectations of an event and the appraisal of the event's meaning. 2) When individuals expect a certain outcome and receive a different one, they appraise the extent to which the unwanted outcome is provocative (eg, frustrating, threatening), which influences the level of anger arousal and the resulting behavior. 3) When individuals appraise an impending event as aversive and anger inducing, it is likely that they will react with anger when the event occurs.

Expectations and appraisals are also influenced by the kind of self-talk they use.[7,97] Such self-talk has been called *automatic thoughts*[7] or *private speech*.[97] For example, suppose two people are served the wrong order in a restaurant. Person A may think "These things always happen to me" or "Waiters are dumb" and reacts angrily by cursing and shouting at the waiter. On the other hand, person B may think, "Mistakes sometimes happen—no big deal" and reacts calmly by stating the error to the waiter and asking that it be corrected. Person A likely perceives the mistake as aversive or catastrophic in some way, whereas person B does not. While the situation is the same, the self-talk is different, and the perceptions and emotional outcomes are different.

NEUROBIOLOGICAL THEORIES

Garza-Trevino's review of the literature from 1977 to 1993 regarding the neurobiological components of aggression reveals that essentially four kinds of studies have been used: 1) electroencephalogram (EEG) recordings of aggression in animal models during electrical stimulation of selected areas in the brain; 2) EEG studies of human brains; 3) neuroimaging studies of human brains using computerized axial tomography, magnetic resonance imaging, and positron emission tomography to detect brain abnormalities in abnormally aggressive subjects; and 4) studies of the type and prevalence of psychological deficits among mentally ill clients who are repeatedly violent.[37]

The overlapping, sharing, and coexistence of many functions in numerous areas of the brain make its study complex. Brain neuroimaging studies indicate that aggressive behavior is associated with deficits or damage to the portions of the brain located in the limbic structures and frontal and temporal lobes. Limbic tumors often result in personality changes, with irritability as a predominant symptom. Tumors may irritate neurologic mechanisms for aggression or destroy inhibitory mechanisms for aggression. Rabies, encephalitis, and types of brain injury that damage portions of the limbic system or the frontal lobe are associated with loss of impulse control. It is believed that connections between the amygdaloid complex and the hypothalamus and between the hippocampal cortex and frontal lobes modulate the control and expression of aggressive behavior.[37] Compulsive aggressive behavior has been reported in clients with lesions in the hypothalamic, orbitofrontal, anterior cingulate, and temporal areas of the brain.[99,130,134]

When the complex functions housed in the frontal lobe are examined, it becomes apparent what serious disorders may occur when these functions are disrupted. Self-disciplinary functions, including the abilities to resist distraction, inhibit inappropriate behavior, and exert social control, are located in the frontal lobe, as is the ability to judge or weigh the merits of behavior. A change in personality and the onset of impulsive behavior are often early signs of a lesion in the frontal lobe. The *orbitofrontal syndrome* (damage to specific areas of the frontal lobe) is associated with such behavioral excesses as impulsivity, disinhibition, hyperactivity, distractibility, and mood lability, as is often seen with frontal lobe tumors or injury. Outbursts of rage and violent behavior can occur after damage to the inferior orbital surface of the frontal lobe and anterior temporal lobes. Uncontrollable aggression also may occur with damage to other cortical and subcortical structures.[143]

Debate continues on the issue of whether intermittant explosive reactions may result from undetected temporal lobe epilepsy (TLE). Some experts believe that people with TLE are easily provoked to violence by feelings of injustice in the periods between seizures (interictal periods). The *interictal behavioral syndrome theory* views such violence as a result of changes in the sensitivity of the limbic system and brain stem due to repeated uncontrolled electrical discharges—a phenomenon known as *kindling*.[128]

Because schizophrenic syndromes seem to be related to multiple neurobiological factors, some researchers speculate that clients with schizophrenia who are violent may have a disorder of the dominant temporal lobe involving the amygdaloid nuclei.[37] This is a compelling hypothesis in view of the fact that people with temporal lobe lesions often manifest aggressive symptoms, and people with schizophrenia have a higher than average incidence of epilepsy.[39] However, some neuropsychological studies reveal that schizophrenic individuals who are violent seem to have a scattered pattern of brain pathology involving both hemispheres.[38,57,136] In addition, more violent than nonviolent schizophrenic individuals seem to have such deficits as poor visual-spatial orientation, astereognosis, and tandem walk, which may imply deficits in integrative sensory functions and motor coordination.

Client profile data linked with biologically based aggression reveal that aggressive incidents are usually sudden and relatively unprovoked. Furthermore, clients whose aggression is biologically based seem to move quickly from calm to rage to calm, and they typically show remorse.[21]

Neurotransmitter Dysregulation

Linnoila and Virkkunen[68] coined the term *low serotonin syndrome* to specify conditions characterized by episodes of mood changes, impulsive behavior, or both. Several studies have found a low concentration of 5-hydroxyindoleacetic acid (5-HIAA), a metabolite of serotonin, in the cerebrospinal fluid (CSF) of clients with chronic schizophrenia who had attempted suicide.[96,135] One study was conducted of three groups of clients: clients with schizophrenia who attempted suicide, nonsuicidal clients with schizophrenia, and a control group of normal subjects. This study found that of the three groups, the clients who attempted suicide had the lowest CSF levels of 5-HIAA.[135]

Other researchers who studied healthy subjects have found a link between increased monoamine oxidase (MAO) activity in the brain and increaed total scores on the Buss and Durkee Aggression Inventory[13] and increased scores on the negativism and verbal aggression scales.[14] Such findings indicate that MAO activity may be linked to the behavioral expression of aggression; MAO metabolizes serotonin and thus contributes to decreased serotonin levels in the brain.

Substance Abuse

Alcohol intoxication is a frequent contributor to episodes of violent behavior.[59,60] Research suggests that alcohol abusers have a neurological defect in serotonin turnover, and this defect may be inherited.[69] For instance, a study of 21 arsonists revealed that 19 had significantly lower mean levels of CSF 5-HIAA and a history of paternal alcoholism.[69] The low levels of 5-HIAA may lead to alterations in normal day–night activity rhythm and ultimately to dysphoria. While the use of alcohol may provide a false and temporary relief from dysphoria, eventually the serotonergic deficit is exacerbated, thus increasing the individual's potential for violent behavior. Other substances that are often implicated in violent episodes include amphetamines, cocaine, hallucinogens, barbiturates, and prolonged use of benzodiazepines.

SOCIOCULTURAL FACTORS

Social learning theory is often applied to explain aggressive behavior that is learned from exposure to aggressive models or as the result of random positive reinforcement of direct experience.[73] Exposure to aggressive models may occur in the family; a subculture, such as gangs; or in media, such as television, movies, and video games. Some researchers and theorists believe that television, video, and movie violence portrays how coercive behavior can result in obtaining material rewards, social recognition, or successful retaliation against enemies; in essence, the media glorification of violence teaches people how to aggress.[58]

Stressors such as parental rejection and coercive family processes (eg, physical or sexual abuse) have been linked with the development of antisocial behavior and violence in children, although a direct cause and effect relationship does not exist. Acts of violence are often precipitated by intense family quarrels and social situations that threaten self-esteem. Subcultures, such as gangs, may promote violent crime as a means of achieving recognition and status. Aggressive sports and war may also lead to imitation of aggressive behavior.

Interpersonal and social contexts are important factors in assessing risk for violence in people with mental illness. In a study of 169 people with serious mental illness and 59 of their significant others, researchers investigated the relationship between violent acts and threats by people with serious mental illness, the size and composition of their social networks, and type of social support received.[31] Findings revealed that individuals with a diagnosis of schizophrenia were more likely to commit violent acts than were respondents with other diagnoses but were not more likely than others to threaten violence.[31] Individuals who were more likely to engage in violent threats and acts were financially dependent on family members and perceived hostitily from others. Most of the targets of violence were relatives, particularly mothers living with an adult offspring with schizophrenia. While most respondents who were violent perceived others as threatening, they did not view themselves as threatening in return. The researchers concluded that mothers who live with an adult offspring with schizophrenia may be at increased risk for a violent attack.[31] In addition, violence by people with psychiatric disorders may be linked to their experience of being threatened by others.[31] These conclusions support earlier findings that a significant degree of dependency exists on the part of the abuser and the abused.[101] The role of dependency (physical, emotional, and financial) requires further study.

ENVIRONMENTAL AND SITUATIONAL FACTORS

Dehospitalization or deinstitutionalization has resulted in thousands of people being displaced from sheltered inpatient settings of state hospitals to outpatient mental health facilities that are often understaffed and underskilled in supervising or managing aggressive behaviors of previously hospitalized clients. Some clinicians prefer the term "dehospitalization" rather than "deinstitutionalization" to emphasize the need for a supportive social network after discharge.[67] Dehospitalized and unsupervised clients in the community may become involved in antisocial acts and violence. The number of people who are homeless and living and sleeping on streets, in parks, and in shelters is estimated to be 600,000.[127] It is also estimated that one third of homeless, single adults suffer from severe mental illnesses, such as schizophrenia or manic depressive disorder. If untreated, these "disorders fog thought, sap motivation, and can turn emotions into engines of terror, rage, or despair. Severe mental illnesses and their attendant disabilities may be life-long and recurring, with symptoms waxing and waning. They affect virtually every aspect of life."[127] The lack of adequate nutrition; higher incidence of drug, alcohol, and physical abuse; and increased severity of disease can affect the mental ablities of the homeless.[50] Poor housing, crowded slums, low levels of education, and unemployment may contribute to the spectrum of aggressive responses.

Situations in which the likelihood of aggression is increased because of the structure of social systems have been observed in animal and human studies.[80] For instance, when animals meet for the first time, they often aggress against one another until hierarchies are established. Similar human responses may occur among families or organizations in which structural variables and expectations either shift often or remain unidentified. In residential homes and inpatient psychiatric facilities, administrators and staff should be aware that changes in personnel, staff responsibilities, living rules, and client privileges may be interpreted as threats and may increase the risk of aggressive outbursts among clients.[80] Minimizing disruptions and changes that clients may view as negative and providing thoughtful support during changes that affect clients could help deter or avoid instances of client anger and aggression.

Application of The Nursing Process to Aggressive and Violent Behavior

ASSESSMENT

Assessing for Dangerous Behavior

Watching for behavioral cues and listening carefully for the feeling tone or latent communication of a client enables the nurse to prevent angry and hostile feelings from escalating into dangerous actions. Some indicators of potentially violent or dangerous behavior include the following:[78]

1. *Thinking and perception:* Hallucinations or delusions that threaten the client with harm or command the client to harm (eg, a wife becomes convinced that her husband is trying to kill her)
2. *Motor activity:* Increased psychomotor agitation, which is often a signal that the client cannot tolerate physical closeness or that an alternative outlet for preventing rising tension is unavailable to the client for whatever reason (eg, a client begins to pace the hall rapidly)
3. *Mood or affect:* Increased intensity of affect or verbalizations or a noticeable change in the manner in which a client expresses wants and needs (eg, a client's angry tone of voice gets louder as he states he wants the staff to let him out of the hospital)
4. *Physical state:* Organic states in which the client may

be unable to communicate a warning, such as beginnings of seizures, delirium, or brain lesions

5. *Context:* A history of violent outbursts against self or others, which may include repeated criminal behavior or suicide attempts (eg, a client is known to have engaged in physical fights with other clients and staff on previous admission) and use of alcohol, other addictive drugs, or hallucinogenic drugs that remove control from behavior

In studies of predictors of violence, client characteristics have been the primary focus. In addition to the client profiles previously discussed, what kinds of client responses should alert nurses and other clinicians? Some experts believe that concern about the following types of clients is warranted: those who lack perspective regarding their anger (eg, they are not aware that their anger may reflect their own appraisals and tendency to misinterpret life events); those who continually want to hurt specific others, even if plans to do so are unspecified; those with a history of episodic aggression; and those who do not verbally communicate their anger to others.[80] The first three types of clients are considered high risk for violence because they may be less concerned about possible consequences of aggessive behavior and tend not to consider alternative ways of dealing with anger. The fourth type of client may be highly dependent on the person toward whom they are angry and may manifest unpredictable outbursts of anger.

Some studies indicate that the best single predictor of violence is a history of violence.[23,83] In clinical settings, nurses must obtain an accurate history of incidents of aggression from the client and the client's family, friends, or significant others. How the client manages aggressive feelings in the present is usually expressive of how the client has handled these feelings in the past. During initial interviews, or whenever the nurse suspects the possibility of suicidal or homicidal behavior, the nurse should ask, "Do you feel like hurting yourself or anyone else?" Experts agree that doing so will not suggest ideas of violence to the client. Rather, asking the question directly promotes a healthy role model of verbalization and alternative problem-solving in place of acting-out behavior.[125]

Most studies of acutely disturbed clients who are evaluated shortly before or during hospitalization suggest that clinical variables rather than demographic variables are the better predictors of violence.[83,84] For instance, in a study of 330 newly admitted clients with a variety of diagnoses, researchers examined the relationship between acute psychopathology and short-term risk for violence.[83] While symptom patterns varied across diagnoses, incidents of assault occurred more frequently by clients who were diagnosed with schizophrenia, mania, or organic psychotic conditions. In addition, higher levels of hostile-suspciousness, agitation-excitement, and thinking disturbance generally characterized the violence-prone clients.[83] As noted previously, other client characteristics as predictors of potential violence include client verbal aggression,[23] escalating anxiety,[110] substance abuse,[23] severe pathology, and acute stage of psychotic illness.[107]

Selected Tools for Measuring Aggressive or Violent Behaviors

Careful assessment is essential to evaluate and manage adequately the risk of aggressive behavior and to develop and implement an appropriate treatment plan. Clinicians in different clinical sites may use different measuring tools for assessing aggressive behavior, and in some instances, a comprehensive battery of measures may be used. The following are examples of some of the more commonly used measurements of psychological and environmental determinants of aggressive behavior:

1. The Overt Aggression Scale (OAS)[145] is designed to document client behaviors and staff interventions that occur during an aggressive episode in a clinical area. The OAS has been used to document patterns of aggression for individuals and groups to justify the use of medication and to provide data for comparison of clinical facilities in terms of the use of seclusion, restraints, and prn medications.[32]
2. A general psychopathology inventory includes the Minnesota Multiphasic Personality Inventory (MMPI); a depression measure (eg, Beck Depression Inventory); a measure of assertiveness or coping strategies (eg, Assertiveness-Aggressiveness Inventory; Revised Ways of Coping checklist); an index of drug or alcohol abuse (eg, Michigan Alcohol Screening Test); and specific measures of angry, violent, and abusive behavior (eg, Index of Spouse Abuse; Spielberger State-Trait Anger Expression Inventory). Although lengthy, the MMPI has a number of subscales relevant to various subtypes of anger and hostility (eg, overcontrolled hostility); validity scales to measure the subject's test-taking attitudes and response styles, such as defensiveness, lying, and minimization; and anger dyscontrol issues, such as paranoia, anxiety, depression, and general personality features.[73]
3. The Brief Anger-Aggression Questionnaire (BAAQ), derived from the Buss-Durkee Hostility Inventory, is a six-item measure designed for the rapid assessment and identification of generalized irritability and a tendency to act in an aggressive and violent manner.[74] The BAAQ can be administered in about 1 minute and has normative data for distinguishing domestically violent and generally assaul-

tive men. Another advantage of the BAAQ is that there are two forms of the instrument, one that allows direct assessment of the client and another that allows an independent rating of the client by a spouse, friend, or relative (BAAQ-O).[73,74]

NURSING DIAGNOSIS

Nurses are encouraged to use standardized lists of nursing diagnoses, such as those specified by the North American Nursing Diagnosis Association, to select those relevant to the client.[94] Data gathered during assessment, including specific risk factors and defining client characteristics, lead to the formulation of specific diagnoses and a relevant nursing care plan. Desired outcome standards, specific client outcomes, and relevant nursing interventions are identified for each nursing diagnosis, and such information is written on the care plan. The nursing diagnosis that is primarily relevant to potentially aggressive and violent clients and that is emphasized in this chapter is Risk for Violence: Self-directed or directed at others.[133] Guidelines for formulating a nursing care plan for clients at high risk for violence, including relevant assessment criteria, client outcome goals, and nursing interventions, are presented in Nursing Care Plan 31-1.

CLIENT OUTCOMES AND GOALS

How the nurse assesses the multiple factors involved in the client's expression of anger, hostility, and aggressive feelings with potential for violence determines goals for client outcomes and how appropriate interventions are planned. The ultimate goals are to improve the client's health outcomes and health status.

Measurement criteria for expected client outcomes specify that the outcomes are derived from the diagnoses; are client centered, therapeutically sound, realistic to the client's present and potential capabilities, attainable, and cost-effective; are documented as measureable goals; are developed collaboratively by the nurse, client, the client's significant others and other team members when possible; estimate a time frame for attainment; provide direction for continuity of care; are based on a sound scientific knowledge base in mental health care; and are a record of change in the client's health status.[3]

PLANNING

Clinical Pathways

With increasing emphasis on managed care and case management health care delivery models, *clinical pathways* provide case management plans that contain vital information needed to attain quality, cost-effective client care.[34] Common elements of a critical pathway include nursing diagnoses, standard client outcomes, resource utilization, and the critical events or interventions that assist the client toward specific outcomes within a designated length of stay.[34] Length of stay is usually allotted by diagnosis-related groups and the current institutional length of stay and input from physicians. A maximum of three or four key nursing diagnoses are specified "to prevent cluttering and maintain a realistic plan of care."[34] Client outcomes that are realistic, attainable, and client centered are identified for each nursing diagnosis. Key interventions or critical events are then specified as client care guidelines.

Variances are identified as any deviation from the pathway that occurs whenever client care or outcomes are not the same as what was predicted.[140] Variances can include clients, caregivers, and systems of care.

The development of clinical pathways is a multidisciplinary process, involving coordinated efforts of clinical nurses, nurse managers, nurse administrators, nurse educators, clinical nurse specialists, physicians, and other health professionals. While current literature regarding specific clinical pathways for clients in psychiatric treatment is sparse, it is anticipated that this type of care planning will become more prevalent within the growing managed care focus for mental health care delivery.

Discharge Planning

While hospitalization may continue to seem most appropriate for clients who are deemed dangerous to self and others, decreased length of hospital stay due to efforts at cost containment seem inevitable.[24] Early discharge of violent or potentially violent individuals is a growing and urgent concern, not only of health professionals, but of families and the general populace. The shift to outpatient case management mandates development of realignment strategies to fit inpatient education and treatment into an implemented plan of care that reinforces and maintains continuity of treatment when the client is discharged. Some strategies for achieving such continuity of care include the following:

1. Designing a "seamless" care delivery system in which nurses create a comprehensive client database that the hospital and community care systems can use to articulate care services based on client needs. Treatment protocols can be designed so that inpatient interventions, such as cognitive therapy or anger-management groups, can be continued in community outpatient settings. Discharge planning for clients who have been violent may involve intensive case management and strong linkages and coordination with community centers that provide mental health services; substance abuse treatment;

Nursing Care Plan 31-1

The Client at Risk for Violence

Nursing Diagnosis

Risk for Violence: Self-directed or directed at others

Outcome

Client will maintain self-control, thereby avoiding harm to self or others.

Intervention	Rationale
Assess for history of violent behavior and early signs of anger, hostility, or aggressive behavior.	History of violent behavior is often predictive of subsequent violence, and prevention of escalation of anger, hostility, or aggressive behavior is an essential safety measure.
Reduce environmental stimulation by maintaining low lighting and noise level in an area with few people.	Environmental stimuli may increase agitation and promote loss of control in form of aggressive behavior.
Remove potentially dangerous objects (sharp objects, belts, glass items, and drugs).	External control of environment prevents impulsive actions when client lacks internal controls.
Convey attitude of caring and concern toward client.	Caring attitude will promote feelings of trust and client self-worth.
Approach client in calm, nonthreatening manner, and speak in soft, even tone of voice.	The nurse's calm attitude and demeanor provides client with feelings of safety and security and models positive behavior.
Discuss behavioral expectations and consequences.	This informs client of behaviors that are acceptable and not acceptable by societal norms and promotes client's choice of responding in more adaptive ways.
Offer opportunity for client to express concerns and to talk about events, thoughts, and feelings (especially anger) that may have triggered current reaction.	This expression allows client to confront unresolved issues and gain self-awareness about own behavior.
Help client consider ways in which pent-up tension can be used constructively, thereby averting aggressive responses.	Activities that require physical exertion are helpful in reducing pent-up tension.
Obtain a behavioral contract from client that he or she will not harm self or others.	Encourages client to share in responsibility for self-control.
Inform client that staff will intervene if additional safety measures are needed to protect client and others (eg, tranquilizing medication, restraints, isolation, suicide precautions).	This provides control boundaries for client and promotes a feeling of safety and security.

Evaluation

Client does not engage in violent behavior and demonstrates strategies to prevent escalation.

social service agencies, such as public health agencies; probation and other criminal justice departments; and welfare services. If clients have exhausted their previous supports, new support systems must be developed. Families may be frightened of a client returning home if incidents of hostile and aggressive behavior were traumatic, and family members have not worked through their feelings.[78] Staff in community centers must be trained in the same systematic and thorough manner as institutional staff in managing violent behavior to protect the client and others.[24]

2. Creating a comprehensive, computerized client database that can be quickly accessed by caregivers in inpatient or outpatient mental health service sites.[24] Nurses in hospitals can organize pertinent observa-

tional data and interactional incidents into useful client assessment data. For example, for the potentially violent client, such data might include any behavioral patterns typical of the client escalating into violence and any particular interventions that were successful in helping the client reorganize or regain self-control.
3. Collecting outcome data.[24] In the ever-changing health care system, nurses must document client outcomes related to nursing interventions, including what client symptoms improved and to what extent. Close monitoring of medication effects and client compliance with the treatment plan is essential.

Recent research findings indicate that intensive case management programs are effective in reducing clients' dangerousness in the community.[29] To date, outcome studies of violence reduction as related to case management have been few, but findings are optimistic for the case managment approach. For instance, one study of New York State's intensive case management program indicates that case management for 5,121 adult clients who received services through the program between 1989 and 1992 successfully reduced clients' dangerousness in the community in terms of measures of harmful behavior, antisocial behavior, and alcohol and drug abuse.[109] Another study of 229 adult offenders released from the Harris County, Texas, criminal justice system with intensive case managment follow-up found that 75% of the clients had no arrests within 1 year; 92% did not return to state prison; and 80% of the case management program participants who were on parole had no parole violations.[95]

INTERVENTION

It is the responsibility of mental health care facilities to provide information regarding intervention strategies with aggressive clients. It is incumbant on every employee who works with these special individuals to be knowledgeable about guidelines and strategies for intervention and to be able to exercise them at a moment's notice. Rehearsal of specific strategies and techniques in a nonstress environment is essential for smooth and coordinated execution.

The principles of *safety* and *least restrictive environment* must be carefully weighed by nurses and other mental health care professionals while caring for aggressive and assaultive clients. It is extremely important that staff maintain attitudes of caring, concern, and nonauthoritarianism, while setting appropriate limits to demonstrate social norms within the milieu.[125] While this balance is often difficult to achieve, it is essential to prevent violent behavior, especially on inpatient units. Even a floridly psychotic client whose tension increases prior to violence may respond positively to nonprovocative, nonjudgmental interpersonal contact and expressions of concern and caring, particularly by one who has established good rapport and trust during earlier contacts with the client.

Self-Awareness by the Nurse

Nurses should be aware of their own feelings about aggressive and violent behavior and in particular about specific violent clients so they do not act on any negative feelings. In the face of aggressive or assaultive behavior, a universal response is fear. Feeling fear and understanding what it signals can direct a nurse to action. Possible outcomes of this experience of fear include countertransference reaction due to angry feelings, leading to limit setting without talking-through behavior; anxiety reaction due to helpless feelings, leading to flight from the situation; or therapeutic reaction, leading to self-awareness through exploration of own thoughts, feelings, and behavior. In addition, nurses and other staff members should monitor the milieu in terms of staff dynamics or conflicts that may interfere with appropriate client care in the management of violence.

Types of Intervention Strategies

When interacting with clients who are aggressive and violent (or potentially so), the three types of intervention strategies include verbal, pharmacological (medications), and physical (seclusion and restraint). These interventions may be used separately or in combination according to protocols in given treatment settings.

Safety Guidelines

When interacting with angry and potentially aggressive clients, staff should be concerned for their own safety and the safety of the client and others. Some general guidelines for safety awareness include the following:

- Position yourself just outside the client's personal space (slightly out of arm's reach).
- If possible, stand on the client's nondominant side (usually the side a wristwatch is worn).
- Keep the client in visual range.
- Make sure the door of a room is readily accessible.
- Avoid letting the client come between you and the door.
- Retreat from the situation and summon help if the client's aggression has escalated to violence.
- Avoid dealing unaided with a violent client.[16,63]

Verbal Interventions to Prevent an Escalation of Aggression

Verbal intervention is emphasized when interacting with aggressive clients at all levels of escalation, but it is generally most useful with milder levels of aggression.

Verbal intervention can prevent an escalation of the client's aggressive behavior.

People want to be listened to and understood. When interacting with an angry client, the nurse can reduce the client's defensiveness by attending to what the client is saying with empathy and genuine concern and by focusing on the feeling and content of what the client has said. For example,[78] a client says, "I've been in this *@$!*?! hospital for 3 days, and no one will go to my house and get my clothes. I'm being held against my will, and I'm going to sue everyone on this unit." The nurse might respond as follows: "I hear how frustrated you are to be here and not have your own clothes. Let's talk about how we can help you get your clothes." Such a response from the nurse demonstrates interest, direct attention to the client's concern, and a willingness to work with the client. Such a response will likely defuse at least some of the client's anger.

A nurse who has previously established a therapeutic relationship and a sense of trust with a client may intervene to prevent the outbreak of aggression by talking with the client on a one-to-one basis. During this time, the nurse can validate assumptions about what the client is experiencing in terms of feelings and intentions. The nurse encourages the client to describe and clarify the present experience to increase the client's awareness of problematic feelings and what triggers them. The nurse then explores with the client ways to express and act on feelings in a constructive, socially acceptable manner and hopefully to experience a sense of acomplishment in doing so.

The Prevention and Management of Aggressive Behavior program developed by the human resources division of the Texas Department of Mental Health and Mental Retardation emphasizes three phases of verbal intervention in preventing the escalation of aggressive behavior, as follows: 1) making contact; 2) discovering the source of distress; and 3) assisting the person with alternative behaviors and problem solving.[48] These verbal intervention strategies are discussed below and selectively applied to the following case example:

> Dan G., 45 years old, is an inpatient in detoxification for alcohol abuse. He has a history of excessive drinking of alcohol and aggressive behavior in the form of property damage (eg, kicking in walls, smashing windows) when he experiences disappointment and frustration. It has been 4 days since his admission, and he has been compliant with treatment regimens. However, the nurse notices that Dan has gone into the day room and is pacing back and forth, pounding his right fist into the palm of his left hand. Several other clients are watching television in the day room. The nurse recognizes Dan's behavior as potentially volatile. What interventions can the nurse use to prevent the escalation of Dan's agitated and seemingly angry behavior?

Step 1: Making contact: It is important to appear calm and in control when approaching any client and to speak in a normal tone of voice in a nonprovocative, nonjudgmental manner. Be alert to the person's verbal and nonverbal behavior that indicates how the person may be feeling. Based on your observations, ask yourself what the person might be feeling. State to the person what you see him or her doing behaviorally and how you think he or she might be feeling, and then check out your understanding with the person,[48] as in the following example:

Nurse: Dan, I see you pacing and hitting your fist into your hand. You seem angry. Are you angry?

Client: You're *@#?$! right!

Step 2: Discovering the source of distress: Attempt to discover the person's concern. Respond to the person with empathy, interest, and a willingness to help. During this time, try to validate assumptions about what the person is experiencing in terms of feelings and intentions and the antecedent events. Encourage the client to describe and clarify the present experience to increase his or her awareness of problematic feelings and what triggers them. Use open-ended questions, such as who, what, when, where, and how rather than closed-ended yes or no questions. Open-ended questions elicit more meaningful description. Yes or no questions are useful when specific information is requested, such as "Are you feeling pain?" However, a series of yes or no questions can seem like an interrogation. Avoid using "why" questions, because these may seem accusatory rather than empathetic and may put the person on the defensive. When the person responds, listen and paraphrase (do not parrot) the person's feelings and the source or reasons given for feelings; ask if your understanding is correct,[48] as in the following example:

Nurse: I can see that you are angry, Dan. What happened?

Client: Aw, *$!@#!, I missed my wife's phone call while I was in group therapy, and now she's not home; I don't know when I'll get to talk to her.

Nurse: You're disappointed not to have received your wife's call as expected?

Client: Yeah. It makes me *#$@#! mad!

Step 3: Focus on the client's competency and alternative problem solving: Too often we are aware of only the deficit side of various disturbing behaviors and affect of an angry person rather than the person's competency to prevent anger escalation by maintaining control and rebuilding constructive functioning.[113] If possible, talk with the person about his or her ideas regarding a plan of action that would help deal with the situation. This affirms the person's competency and provides information for further problem solving. It is useful to discuss the following: What does the person want? What has the person tried in the past to get what he or she wants? How well did it work?[48] Recognizing what has been tried and how well it worked can help the individual avoid repeating ineffective behavior and make more adaptive choices. For example, the therapeutic dialogue in Box 31-1 turns a client's angry outburst into an opportunity for reflection and communication.

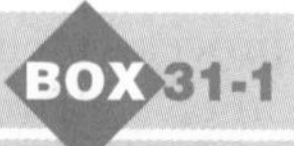

Therapeutic Dialogue With an Angry Client

Nurse: Dan, sometimes when people's expectations are not met, they feel frustrated and angry, much like you do now. What do you want to happen so that you can feel better?

Client: I'd like to talk to my wife *now*!

Nurse: Since you said that your wife is not home now, what other plans can you make to talk to her? *(Encouraging alternative problem-solving.)*

Client: I guess I can call her later. *(Alternative problem-solving.)*

Nurse: That's right, you can. Do you feel OK with that plan? *(Positive validation.)*

Client: Yeah.

Nurse: In the past, when you have felt disappointed and angry, what have you done to deal with those feelings? *(Discover past coping methods.)*

Client: I've lost my temper a lot of times and done some crazy things.

Nurse: What do you mean by crazy things? *(Get pertinent description.)*

Client: I lose my temper easy, even when I'm not drinking. I've put holes in the wall with my feet and fists, wrecked the apartment.

Nurse: What have been the consequences of such actions for you? *(Facilitate self-awareness.)*

Client: Nothing but trouble. My wife may leave me. I know I have to stop drinking and start thinking about things differently. The anger management group is helping, I think.

Nurse: Yes, you've been willing to talk about and understand your angry feelings rather than to act on them in aggressive ways. *(Compliment client for positive behavior).*

Client: Yeah, thanks. I guess I'm getting there.

Nurse: What are some other positive activities you can do to work off some steam when you're feeling tense and angry? *(Alternatives to violent behavior.)*

Client: I like to shoot baskets, play racquetball, work on my car.

Nurse: Would you like to shoot some baskets during recreation time?

Client: Sure, why not.

Limit Setting

Continual assessment of the client's tone and signs of anxiety or fear that could escalate into angry, hostile feelings and behaviors is essential in preventing violence in mental health settings. The nurse must recognize warning signs of impending aggression or violence that have preceded violence in clients in the past. A client may have manifested a specific pattern of behavior or speech before a violent episode, such as pacing in front of the nursing station with clenched fists, repeating the same word or phrase, or some other behavior. Loss of control associated wth aggression and violence damages self-esteem and interpersonal relationships.[125] The nurse must have a keen sense of detecting a client's desire for control and must be able to set limits without being punitive. It is usually reassuring to clients to know that they will not be allowed to be destructive to self, others, or property. If the client tries to engage the nurse in a power struggle, the nurse can tell the client that he or she is not interested in a power struggle but would like to see the client remain in control. The nurse can also compliment clients on whatever degree of control they can maintain. Saying "Aren't you proud of yourself?" rather than the more common "I'm so proud of you!" focuses the client on pride in his own behavior rather than that of pleasing another person.

Limit setting has been defined as a process through

which someone in authority determines temporary and artificial ego boundaries for another person.[72] The nurse often must remind clients of the boundaries of acceptable behavior and set limits on those behaviors. However, as discussed previously, the staff must explain to clients in a therapeutic, caring manner the need for the application of limits to avoid escalation of aggressive behavior. If appraised positively by clients, limit setting can be viewed as providing protection and security for the client and others, help decrease the client's anxiety, and help the client view his or her environment more realistically. Knowing established limits gives the client a framework within which to function more freely and adequately, maintain self-esteem, learn new behaviors, and gain new self-awareness. The following are some useful steps and techniques when communicating with potentially aggressive clients and setting limits:[72]

1. *Assess the need for limit-setting.* Attempt to understand what the client is experiencing. Use knowledge, understanding, and rational interpretation of the dynamics of the client's behavior to assess whether limits are needed.
2. *Describe the client's unacceptable behavior; communicate expected behavior; and give alternatives.* Prior to setting a limit, the nurse should remind the client that his or her behavior is inappropriate or unacceptable, state the expected behavior in the particular situation, and offer some acceptable substitute behaviors, such as walking with the nurse, talking about feelings and thoughts, or participating in recreational therapy. Clients can usually save face when they are given a choice of more constructive alternatives than their intended violent behavior. The point is to use simple, straightforward explanations and to offer such clients some constructive channels for their pent-up emotions and energy.
3. *State the limit.* When the need for the limit has been identified and stating the expected behavior did not elicit the necessary behavior, then the nurse should inform the client exactly what the consequence or limit is. State the limit as a matter of fact, not as advice, bribery, or punishment. The limit tells the client specifically what he or she is to do or not do in the situation.
4. *Help the client understand the reason for the limit* and the consequences if he or she tests the limit or continues inappropriate behavior. The explanation of consequences is of therapeutic value, because it gives the client a sense of responsbility for the outcomes or results of his or her behavior.
5. *Enforce the limit.* The limit must be reasonable and one that can be realistically and uniformly enforced. If there is no way to enforce the limit, then not only is there no point in setting it, but such failure undermines the entire process, including the credibility of the nurse or other staff members. Applying limits uniformly means that all clients are expected to adhere to certain standards of behavior; certain antisocial behaviors are not ignored or condoned in some clients but strictly prohibited in others. Injustices tend to incite anger in most people in any setting and may kindle the flames of anger in a setting in which control, anger, and violence are prominant and urgent concerns. When a client tests a limit, he or she usually experiences some anxiety, and having staff respond in a predictable manner to ensure the safety and protection of the client and others provides security and confidence on which the client can lean and count for support and strength. A useful anagram to remember when communicating with potentially violent clients is a four-step process known as *DISC: D*—describe client behavior; *I*—indicate desired behavior; *S*—specify nurses' actions; and *C*—confront with positive or negative consequences.[10]

Intervention With Medication

If the client's aggression escalates and the client does not respond to verbal intervention, the nurse is encouraged to use medication as prescribed to calm the client. While no medication has been approved by the Food and Drug Administration specifically for treating aggression, several classes of psychotropic medications, such as antipsychotics, lithium, antidepressants, sedatives, anxiolytics, anticonvulsants, opiate antagonists, and beta-blockers, have been used for managing acute aggressive episodes and chronic aggressive behavior.[21] The client's behavior and responses must be observed and carefully documented prior to and following the initiation of the medication regimen. Evaluation of the appropriateness of a specific medication for an individual will be the basis for continuing the medication, stopping it, or changing to another drug. Medications may not be an advisable if the assaultive client is believed to be under the influence of an unknown drug. See Table 31-2 for examples of medications used to treat aggressive behavior.

Antipsychotics are the most commonly used drugs for treating aggression that results from acute psychoses (such as violent responses to delusional threats). It is typically the sedative effects rather than the antipsychotic properties of neuroleptics that decrease aggression.[21] Some studies indicate that antipsychotics are often ineffective, seriously compromise clients' quality of life, and essentially place clients in chemical restraints when used to treat cases of chronic aggression, especially episodes caused by brain trauma.[144] *Rapid tranquillization* is used in some instances of aggressive and violent client behavior.[140] Research findings reveal that haloperidol and diazepam (a benzodiazepine) are the most commonly used *prn (as needed)* drugs to achieve sedation and calmness.[102] In addition, when clients receive this medication combination, nursing staff report a significant reduction in clients' aggressive disturbance within 30 minutes, a *calm settle* within one hour, and infrequent need for a second injection.[102] Such prn medication has been described as the filling of the sandwich of nursing interventions, with other interventions such as talking to or distracting the client being used before and after the medication.[82]

Studies have revealed that *lithium* is effective in diminishing aggression, irritability, manipulation, and persecutory delusions secondary to mania, as well as hostile behaviors secondary to other biological etiologies.[21,56] Lithium is also known to siginificantly diminish aggression and self-injurious behavior in children with conduct disorders, head-injured adults, selected prison inmates, schizophrenic adults, or adults with personality disorders.[21,145] However, some studies have shown that lithium paradoxically increases the frequency of aggressive behaviors in individuals with temporal lobe epilepsy.[108] Another noteworthy caution is that lithium, in combination with either the older tricyclic antidepressants, such as imipramine, or with the newer serotonin selective antidepressants, such as fluoxetine, may actually induce or exacerbatie mania or a manic episode in individuals with bipolar disorder.[56]

Antidepressants have also been used to control aggressive behavior. Biological studies suggest that impulsive, aggressive, and self-destructive behaviors of personality disordered clients arise from an abnormality in CNS serotonergic functioning, and that medications with serotonergic-enhancing properties, such as sertraline, provide effective treatment.[53] In addition, studies have reported the effectiveness of amitriptyline in the treatment of clients with severe brain injury,[124] and trazadone in the treatment of aggression secondary to organic mental disorders.[103]

Sedatives and anxiolytics, such as the benzodiazepines, barbiturates, and related drugs such as chloral hydrate diminish aggression through sedation of clients who are assaultive and unresponsive to verbal persuasion and commands or gentle physical guidance. In general, these drugs are recommended for short-term use only during periods of current assaultive outbursts.[21] There has been some controversy in the literature about whether prolonged administration of benzodiazepines may actually increase clients' aggression via a disinhibiting effect, and thus it is recommended that these medications not be used on a long-term basis with individuals manifesting chronic aggression.[21,26] Once again, careful observation and documentation of behavior is needed.

A nonbenzodiazepine anxiolytic, *buspirone,* has shown usefulness in treating aggessive, hostile behaviors that covary with anxiety and depression, although studies of the efficacy of buspirone for aggression management are relatively new.[21] Initial studies indicate that buspirone is effective in decreasing aggression and agitation in clients with head injury, dementia, and developmental disability, although further study is needed to validate these findings.[116,145] Unlike the benzodiazepines, buspirone does not have the effects of sedation, muscle relaxation, or anticonvulsant activity.[56]

Anticonvulsants, such as *carbamazepine,* have also been effective in managing aggressive behaviors in psychiatric clients, especially those with abnormal EEGs,[119,143] and in decreasing hostile behavior associated with dementia.[42,62] However, clinicians should be aware of several potentially serious side effects of carbamazapine, especially bone marrow suppression (including aplastic anemia) and hepatotoxicity.[21] In addition, *valproic acid* has reportedly been used successfully in suppressing the manifestations of irritability and aggression that commonly increase after traumatic brain injury (Case Study 31-1).[41] Potential common side effects of valproic acid include gastrointestinal upset, appetite stimulation and weight gain.

In several case studies and clinical trials, *beta blockers* have been found to diminish aggressive behavior in both children and adults.[21] While most studies have focused on the use of propranolol, other beta blockers, such as nadolol, pindolol, and metoprolol are also known to lessen aggressive behavior.[145] Noteworthy side effects include hypotension, bradycardia, and rarely, depression.[21]

Seclusion and Restraint. Therapeutic and ethical issues arise regarding the use of seclusion and restraint procedures. Such procedures often require physical force, increasing the risk of injury to both clients and staff. Some experts believe that seclusion and restraint do not teach clients coping skills that will help them avoid future aggression, but instead, may foster distrust and dislike between clients and staff.[21] In addition, with current staffing cut backs, decreased length of stay, and budgetary belt tightening due to the growth of managed care, some inpatient psychiatric units are no longer able to place clients on constant watch or on one-to-one observation at the first sign or hint of suicidal/homicidal ideation. Instead, greater use is being made of less restrictive forms of isolation, i.e. placing clients in the quiet room without using restraints or even using the quiet room with the door open so the stimuli is reduced and isolation is minimal.

The purposes of seclusion and restraint are containment of injurious actions, isolation to reduce difficult interpersonal interactions, and decreased sensory input to relieve sensory overload.[115] In general, seclusion and physical restraint should be used only when all other

(text continues on page 620)

Table 31-2

Examples of Medications Used to Treat Aggressive Behavior

Types of Medication	Dosage Range	Indications	Cautions
ANTIPSYCHOTICS			
Haloperidol (Haldol)	0.5–5 mg orally two to three times daily; adjust as necessary Maximum—100 mg/d Acute psychosis: 2–5 mg IM, may repeat at 1-h intervals or every 4 to 6 hours if symptoms are under control	Active psychosis: thought disorder, dangerous and destructive behavior, agitation, hostility, paranoia	Tolerance to sedative effects: akathesia mistaken for increased agitation
Chlorpromazine (Thorazine)	Psychosis: 10–25 mg two to four times daily Increase dose by 20–50 mg daily, every 3 to 4 d as necessary Maximum—1500 mg/d	See above	Orthostatic hypotension
Clozapine (Clozaril)	300–900 mg daily	Clients with schizophrenia who cannot tolerate or fail to respond adequately to standard antipsychotic agents	Dose-related seizures; leukopenia and agranulocytosis Clozapine discontinued if WBC < 2,000/mm or granulocytes < 1,000/mm
Risperidone (Risperdal)	3–6 mg/d (elderly should start off slowly)	Delusions, hallucinations, depression, apathy	Insomnia, agitation, increased anxiety, headache, extrapyramidal reactions (eg, tremors, dystonia, oculogyric crisis)
SEDATIVES AND HYPNOTICS			
Benzodiazepines (eg, Lorazepam [Ativan])	1–10 mg/d Anxiety: 2–3 mg two or three times daily Insomnia: 2–4 mg at bedtime, total daily dosage should not exceed 10 mg	Acute agitation, aggression, insomnia	Paradoxical rage; tolerance to sedative effect
Chloral hydrate	Sedative: 250 mg three times daily Hypnotic: 500–1,000 mg 15–30 min before bedtime, total daily dosage should not exceed 2,000 mg	Used primarily as a bedtime sedative in sufficient dosage to induce sleep; may be used prn to achieve sedation in agitated clients	Tolerance to sedative effect
Diphenhydramine (Benadryl)	25–50 mg/4 to 6h; daily dosage should not exceed 300 mg	Central antimuscarinic effects (antiparkinson action)	Hemolytic anemia; reduced white blood cell count; blood platelet destruction
Clonazepam (Klonopin)	Initially 0.5 mg three times daily; may be increased by 0.5–1.0 mg every 3 d Maximum dose—20 mg	Aggression and anxiety	Hyperactivity
Buspirone (BuSpar)	20–60 mg/d in divided doses; should not exceed 60 mg	Chronic aggression (eg, head injury and dementia), aggression related to anxiety	Paradoxical aggressiveness

ANTIDEPRESSANTS			
TRICYCLICS			
Amitriptyline (Elavil)	Initially 25 mg two to four times daily; may be increased cautiously as needed and tolerated by 10–25 mg daily at 1-wk intervals; not to exceed 150 mg/d[71]	Recent severe head injury in which agitation has not responded to behavioral techniques[93]	Orthostatic hypotension, cardiac arrythmias, seizures
Trazodone (Desyrel)	50 mg three times a day, may be increased by 50 mg daily at intervals of 3 or 4 d as needed; not to exceed 400 mg daily	Depression (with or without anxiety)	Confusion, muscle tremors; excitement; priapism in men
SERETONIN-SELECTIVE RE-UPTAKE INHIBITORS (SSRIs)			
Fluoxetine (Prozac)	Initially 20 mg daily; if no improvement after 3 wk of treatment, dose may be increased by 20 mg/d as needed; not to exceed 80 mg/d	Irritability, aggression, and brain injury	Drug-induced seizures (0.2%); serum sickness-like syndrome (2%–3%)
Sertraline (Zoloft)	50 mg daily; may increase at weekly intervals up to a maximum of 200 mg/d	Personality disordered clients with impulsive aggression	Headaches, nausea, diarrhea, insomnia, and male sexual dysfunction
ANTIMANIC			
Lithium	300–1,200 mg/d Therapeutic plasma levels—0.6–1.0 mEq/L	Impulsive aggression; aggression and irritability related to mania; useful with prison populations or mentally retarded clients	Monitor plasma levels; potential fatal toxicity; leukocytosis; hypothyroidism; diabetes insipidus-like syndrome
ANTICONVULSANTS			
Carbamazepine (Tegretol)	100–200 mg/12 h; may be increased at weekly intervals by 200 mg daily as needed; not to exceed 1,200 mg daily	Irritability and aggression related to complex seizure disorders and other organic brain disorders	Bone marrow suppression, hemotologic abnormalities, hepatoxicity
Valproic acid (Depakene)	Initially, 15 mg/kg every 24 h; dose increased cautiously by 5–10 mg/kg per 24 h every 7 d as needed; usual dose from 1,000–1,600 mg in divided doses; not to exceed 60 mg/kg daily	Episodic explosiveness related to brain injury	Bizzare behavior, hallucinations; drug-induced hepatitis with jaundice; pancreatitis
BETA BLOCKERS			
Propanolol (Inderal)	20 mg 3 times daily or 60 mg every 3 to 4 d to maximum dose of 640 mg/d	Chronic or recurrent aggression related to organic brain disorders or injuries; irritability and aggression not directly related to psychotic ideation; hypertension	Onset of action, 4–6 wk; aggravation of arterial insufficiency; bronchospasm; hyperglycemia; hypoglycemia; insomnia; nightmares Clients with bronchial asthma; chronic pulmonary obstructive disease; insulin-dependent diabetes; cardiac disease; severe peripheral vascular disease; severe renal disease; and hyperthyroidism excluded
Pindolol (Visken)	10–60 mg 2 times daily	See above	
Metoprolal (Lopressor)	100–450 mg 1–2 times daily	See above	

Case Study

Episodic Explosiveness Related to Brain Injury Treated Successfully With Valproic Acid

Mr A., 18 years old, suffered a severe closed head injury in an automobile accident in which he was not wearing a seat belt. A computed tomography (CT) scan of the head in the emergency room revealed multiple shear hemorrhages and contusions and diffuse edema of the brain. While these abnormalities were no longer visible on the CT scan 1 week after admission, Mr. A. remained comatose for 8 days, recovering neurological functioning gradually over a period of months. Residual symptoms included some memory impairment, shortened attention span, and spasticity of the left leg. In addition, Mr. A. began having episodes of violent explosiveness and was initially treated with phenytoin 600 mg/d with no benefit. The phenytoin was discontinued, and he was given amitriptyline 100 mg/d, which worsened his explosive temper. The amitriptyline was discontinued, and he was referred to a psychiatrist whom he told "My problem is it doesn't take much to tick me off. I just snap, and later, I regret it." He described being "ticked off" as "getting mad and hitting things." He had struck fellow clients in the face during his rehabilitation and in anger had slammed his fist through the wall and door of his bedroom. He had also assaulted his family members and girlfriend. Mr. A.'s mother confirmed that his violent behavior had its onset following his head injury and that "He explodes at the least little thing" about once a week. Mr. A.'s psychiatrist prescribed valproic acid at 250 mg three times per day. After 6 weeks of treatment with valproic acid, Mr. A. had had no repeat episodes of explosive violence. Mr. A.'s psychiatrist notes, however, that since no EEG was done, it is possible that the valproate was treating a seizure disorder.

Questions for Discussion

1. What other antiseizure medication may be prescribed by the physician to treat assaultiveness associated with brain seizure activity?
2. What other types of treatment or support services and nursing interventions may be of benefit to Mr. A. and his family?

(Source: Geracioti TD: Valproic Acid Treatment of Episodic Explosiveness Related to Brain Injury. Letters to the Editor. J Clin Psychiatry 55(9): 416–417, 1994)

interventions fail to curb the client's aggressive behavior and the client is deemed dangerous to self or others. In 1982, the Supreme Court ruled in the case of *Youngberg v. Romeo* that Mr. Romeo, a violent, profoundly mentally retarded man who was institutionalized, could be deprived of his liberty in terms of being restrained if it could be justified to protect himself or others. The court allowed such justification to be based on professional clinical judgment and professional standards of care and practice.[125] According to guidelines established by a Task Force of the American Psychiatric Association, indications for emergency use of seclusion and restraint are as follows:

1. To prevent imminent harm to the client and others, if other means are not effective or appropriate.
2. To prevent serious disruption of the treatment program or significant damage to the environment.
3. As part of an ongoing behavior treatment program.
4. At the client's request (for seclusion).[125]

As noted above, violence need not actually occur for the emergency use of seclusion and restraint. Imminent violence, in which it is apparent that a client is on the verge of exploding, or a case in which the client's past pattern of escalation to violence is known, may also justify the use of seclusion and restraint. The decision regarding whether seclusion, restraint, or involuntary medication is used should be based on a careful clinical assessment of the individual needs and status of the client. Box 31-2 presents a summary of guidelines for the seclusion and restraint of violent clients.[125]

While the Task Force of the American Psychiatric Association did not recommend specific strategies of intervention with violent clients, it did state that seclusion and restraint should be viewed as analogous to cardiopulmonary resuscitation in mental health institutions and should provide the following:

1. Written specific guidelines and a manual for the use of intervention procedures
2. Approval of the guidelines by hospital administration, attorneys, and the state
3. Education of the staff regarding the guildelines and actual rehearsal of the techniques
4. Revisions of the guidelines based on identification of problems using staff feedback[125]

When a client's behavior is so unsafe or out of control that a decision is made to use seclusion and restraint, a clinical staff member who acts as the team leader directs the actions of everyone else according to established and practiced routines.[125] Ideally, a team of four staff members should assemble behind the team leader as the client is approached. All staff should appear calm, helpful, and nonprovocative. If possible, another staff member should be appointed to clear the area of other clients and to observe and monitor the procedure. The leader informs the client what is occurring and why, keeping verbalizations concise and matter-of-fact. For example, the leader may say to a client, "Mr. Jones, it is necessary to place you in the quiet room until you feel calmer and more in control." The client may be asked to walk quietly with or without staff assistance. If the client refuses, each of the team members will be assigned a limb to hold and transport the client to the seclusion room or to apply restraints.

Common types of mechanical restraint include wrist and ankle cuffs, sheet restraints, and camisoles (straitjackets). Prevention of behavior requiring restraint is a key nursing action, and if restraint is necessary, all other attempted interventions must be documented as having failed to help the client maintain control. Restraining elderly clients requires extra consideration because of the problems that immobilization and osteoporosis present to the elderly. A combination of geri-chair, sheet restraint, vest posey, leather cuffs, and periodic seclusion has been used successfully in a geropsychiatric unit as an alternative to traditional four-point restraint and continuous seclusion.[121]

The decision to terminate the use of seclusion rooms or restraints must be based on objective criteria, rather than on the arbitrary feeling states of the nursing staff.[78] Criteria for release from seclusion or restraint may be categorized as follows:

1. *Decreased psychomotor agitation,* as evidenced by decreased restlessness, lowered blood pressure, and pulse rate
2. *Stabilization of mood,* as evidenced by absence of physical threats, lowered anxiety level, consistency of verbal and nonverbal behavior, and feelings of trust in staff
3. *Cognitive processes,* as evidenced by signs of insight and ability to look at precipitating incident in an objective manner, increased ability to concentrate, and improved reality testing[115]

Once a violent client episode has occurred on the unit, the staff should discuss it among themselves to identify the effectiveness of strategies used in intervention and the need for possible revision of strategies or guidelines; the episode should also be discussed with the client. Discussion centers on what happened, what would have prevented it, the rationale for seclusion or restraint (if used), and the reactions of the client and staff members. Most clients tend to have negative reactions to being restrained and secluded, although some recognize the link between their out-of-control behavior and the need for this type of intervention.[125] It is also important to talk about the violent episode with other clients on the unit so they will understand the reason for the seclusion and restraint and to allay their anxiety about the possibility of being restrained or secluded without apparent reason (Case Study 31-2).

Behavior Therapy

A fundamental expectation in mental health treatment settings is that clients will act or behave in socially appropriate ways. In some settings, special programs of behavioral treatment of violent behavior are planned and conducted by clinical staff who are skilled in behavioral analysis and therapy and who adhere to standardized policies and review processes to prevent inappropriate treatment or abuse of clients.[125]

A behavioral therapy program requires that target behaviors must be clearly stated. Terminology should be specific. For instance, general terms, such as assaultive or violent, should be avoided; terms that describe specific behaviors should be used instead, such as pushing, shoving, hitting, pulling hair, and throwing chairs. In addition, the consequences of specific behavior must be clearly specified.[125]

The consequences include a broad range of limit-setting and behavioral management techniques, ranging from behavioral contracts, token economies, and other means of positive reinforcement to more restrictive procedures, such as seclusionary time out.[21,125] Typically, treatment is initiated with a behavioral contract,

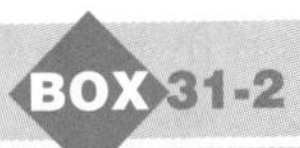

Guidelines for Seclusion and Restraint of Violent Clients

- This is indicated to prevent harm to client or others if other methods are not effective.
- It shall not be used as punishment or for the convenience of staff or other clients.
- The medical and psychiatric status of the client (eg, drug overdose, medical disease, self-mutilation) must be considered.
- Adequate staff (at least four must be present for implementation).
- Once decision is made to use seclusion, the procedure and reasons should be explained to the client, and the client should be given opportunity to comply by walking to seclusion room.
- If client does not comply, each staff member should grasp a limb and bring client safely backward to the floor.
- Restraint devices are applied, or client is carried to seclusion room by staff.
- Client should remain in seclusion only with clothing items that do not pose a safety hazard. Any belts, pins, watches, and other dangerous objects are removed and documented on a checklist.
- Physician sees client for first episode, preferably within 1 hour and definitely within 3 hours and writes specific order for the seclusion, including reasons for implementation, time, date, and maximum time authorized.
- Should the physician's order expire before the client can be released, an extension must be obtained.
- Physician is contacted for new orders for subsequent seclusions.
- Physician must see a client in seclusion or restraint at least every 12 hours.
- Nursing staff is to be present outside seclusion room door at all times to monitor the client for any self-abusive or continued aggressive or agitated behaviors.
- Nursing staff should observe client every 15 minutes and document observations.
- Meals (with plastic spoon only), fluids, and toileting should be provided with caution.
- With four-point restraints, each limb should be released or restraint loosened every 15 minutes.
- Client should be gradually released from seclusion and restraint.
- When the client appears calm and ready to process the situation, the nurse may attempt to counsel with the client. Prior to release, the client should be calm, in control, and agreeable to reenter the regular unit.
- On release, personal effects are returned, and the client is escorted to the regular unit.
- Each decision, observation, measurement, and care must be documented in detail in the client's record or log.
- Staff and clients should discuss each seclusion or restraint after each episode.

(Adapted and reprinted with permission from Tardiff KJ: Violence. In Talbot JA, Hales RE, Yudofsky SC (eds): Textbook of Psychiatry. Washington, DC, The American Psychiatric Press, 1988)

Case Study

When Behavior is Out of Control

Joe K. was admitted for the first time to the psychiatric inpatient unit at a local general hospital. He was a freshman at the community college, living at home, when his parents noticed increasingly bizarre behavior. The incident precipitating hospitalization occurred at the dinner table when Joe rambled on and on praying before the evening meal. When his 14-year-old sister made a sarcastic remark interrupting him, he attempted to choke her, saying that she was "possessed by Satan." Attempts by his parents to calm him after physically pulling him away from his sister were futile, and he began threatening them also. His parents called the police, who took Joe, accompanied by his father, to the emergency room and finally to the hospital unit for inpatient treatment.

Joe was given antipsychotic medication in the emergency room and was quietly mumbling to himself when he arrived on the unit 1 hour later. Joe was shown to his room by a nurse and introduced to a roommate, who was listening to rock music on his radio. The nurse said she would leave and return in a few minutes with a unit handbook and would do Joe's admission interview at that time.

When the nurse returned with the admission packet, she witnessed Joe being held by his father to prevent him from leaving the room. Joe began yelling threats; the nurse called for assistance, and when three more staff responded, Joe was carried to the seclusion room. Joe's father remained in the room, crying. The nurse obtained an order for seclusion and antipsychotic medication. As she gave Joe the medication, she explained that she knew Joe was frightened and needed to regain control of his behavior. She further explained that Joe was now in a hospital and could not leave at present.

Questions for Discussion

1. What needs does Joe's family have at this time, and how might they best be met?
2. In what way might the presence of a roommate have affected Joe's response?
3. What factors influence a decision to place a client in a particular room on admission?
4. What indicators of dangerous behavior did Joe exhibit? (Consider thinking and perception, motor activity, mood or affect, physical state, and context.)
5. What could the nurse have done differently initially?
6. What verbal interventions would have been useful in interacting with Joe?
7. What is legally involved when a client is placed in seclusion?
8. Suggest possible reactions to Joe by the staff and other clients based on his behavior on admission.
9. Formulate a nursing care plan for Joe based on identified client outcomes, Joe's competencies, and the nursing interventions to assist him to reach the desired outcomes.

(Adapted and reprinted with permission from McElvain MS: Suspiciousness and Aggression: The Delusional and Acting-Out Disorders, p. 509. In Johnson B (ed): Adaptation and Growth: Psychiatric-Metnal Health Nursing, 3rd ed. Philadelphia; JB Lippincott, 1993)

a positive reinforcement, or self-controlled time out. These techniques are demonstrably successful with most clients. However, for a few clients, more restrictive procedures, such as restraint or seclusion, may be used if the client manifests extremely violent behavior. A *behavioral contract* or *no-harm contract* is a statement signed by the client that he or she will not harm self or others. Such a contract encourages the client to share in the responsibility for self-control.

A three-step *token economy* is probably the most commonly used behavioral management strategy in which positive interpersonal and self-care behaviors that are to be reinforced are identified; the number of tokens received for each target behavior and rules for token exchange are established; and contingency guidelines are specified to describe if–then relationships between response and consequence.[125] Desired behavior results in receipt of tokens, while undesired behavior can result in the loss of tokens. Token economies are most effective when tokens can be exchanged for goods or privileges that the client values. Goods and privileges vary based on age, gender, interests and desires of clients, and type and intensity of symptoms the client manifests. Research indicates that reinforcing clients' positive social behaviors can proactively diminish hostile and aggressive responses on inpatient units.[21] Inpatient units that have implemented token economies have significantly fewer aggressive episodes than more traditional settings.[21]

Time out is a behavioral strategy to remove clients who are exhibiting socially inappropriate behavior from overstimulating and often reinforcing situations.[21] Time out is most successful with clients who experience loss of social contact as a negative consequence. For instance, if a client's aggressive behavior appears to be escalating, the nurse may offer medication as prescribed or prompt the client to enter the "quiet room" for a few minutes until the client regains a calmer and more self-controlled demeanor. When the client feels he or she is ready to leave the quiet room, he or she can inform the nurse and return to his or her unit. Some quiet rooms are locked, and others are not, depending on the hospital philosophy and the degree of client control lost. Some clients actually request self-controlled time out, which is a less restrictive alternative to seclusion and restraint and involves less humiliation and risk of injury. Such a request is viewed positively, because it shows some insight and awareness on the client's part and responsibility in requesting help to prevent possible escalation.

Cognitive Interventions

In collaboration with clients, nurses can plan and implement cognitive strategies to assist clients to strengthen their abilities to deal with stressors in more constructive ways. Cognitive therapy is a brief, directive, collaborative form of psychotherapy that is useful in assisting clients to confront their dysfunctional and irrational thinking, test the reality of their thinking and behavior, and learn to use more positive and assertive responses in interactions with others.[7,138]

The "guided discovery" technique is one form of cognitive retraining that has been successful with depressed clients and those with anger-control problems.[104,106] Both types of clients tend to have a negative bias in their thinking and view aggressive behavior (either toward self or others) as their only option in dealing with life's problems. Specific learning experiences are designed to teach clients how to recognize the connection between their thoughts, feelings, and behaviors; identify their automatic negative thinking and replace it with more positive thinking; and identify dysfunctional expectations and appraisals, substituting more reality-based interpretations.[7]

Additional opportunities for self-improvement may be available through psychoeducational programs and other cognitive-behavioral approaches pertinent for clients who manifest dysfunctional anger, hostility, impulse-control problems, aggression, and violence. The goals of such psychoeducational programs are to "1) increase the patient's self-awareness, appreciation, and accountability for own acts; 2) enhance the client's ability to identify and manage the attitudes and emotions that are associated with violent behavior; 3) decrease social isolation and provide a supportive milieu for change; 4) decrease hostile-dependent relationships, in those cases in which they exist; and 5) develop nonviolent and constructive conflict resolution skills."[73]

A key cognitive-behavioral treatment program for assaultive individuals is anger-management training. In this program, clients are taught anger cues and dynamics, behavioral and physiological signals related to anger arousal, signs of impending loss of control, and rechanneling aggressive responses in the early stages of arousal.[73] Clients are also taught to differentiate acceptable emotional responses (anger, frustration, fear) from inappropriate and destructive behavioral responses (verbal abuse, physical assault).

Anger responses in assaultive individuals are often experienced as automatic or reflexive reactions that are deeply ingrained, often from being used so often in previous confrontive episodes. Less anger is aroused if a person can define a situation as a problem that calls for a solution rather than as a threat that calls for an attack. The further a person has progressed into a provocation sequence, the less likely the person is to initiate anger control.[97] Defining a situation as a problem and seeking a solution is not a skill that is easily mastered. Assisting the client to shift to a cognitive, problem-solving mode often de-escalates angry feelings and allows the client to examine antecedent events and consider specific alternative ways of viewing the situation and responding. If a client can experience some success in using cognitive problem-solving methods rather than emotional reactionary responses, he or she may begin to take pride in new ways of coping with anger. In problem-solving skills training, clients are taught to be aware of others' points of view and to anticipate and understand the consequences of their own emotional and behavioral responses.

Group and Family Therapy

Group therapy may be a desirable treatment modality with clients who use angry or antisocial behaviors, because they can receive feedback from other group members regarding their interactive style. Problem solving among peers and peer pressure for socially acceptable behavior may often be more helpful to such clients than one-to-one therapy. In addition, when clients' aggressive and violent behavior is specific to or exacerbated by interactions with their families or significant others, family therapy may be indicated. Family members or significant others can also be educated about anger deceleration and problem-solving strategies pertinent to their own and to the client's responses.

The decision tree depicted in Figure 31-1 provides an example of the options relevant to pharmacotherapeutic, cognitive-behavioral, and group or family interventions designed to foster prosocial (antiassaultive) client outcomes.[21]

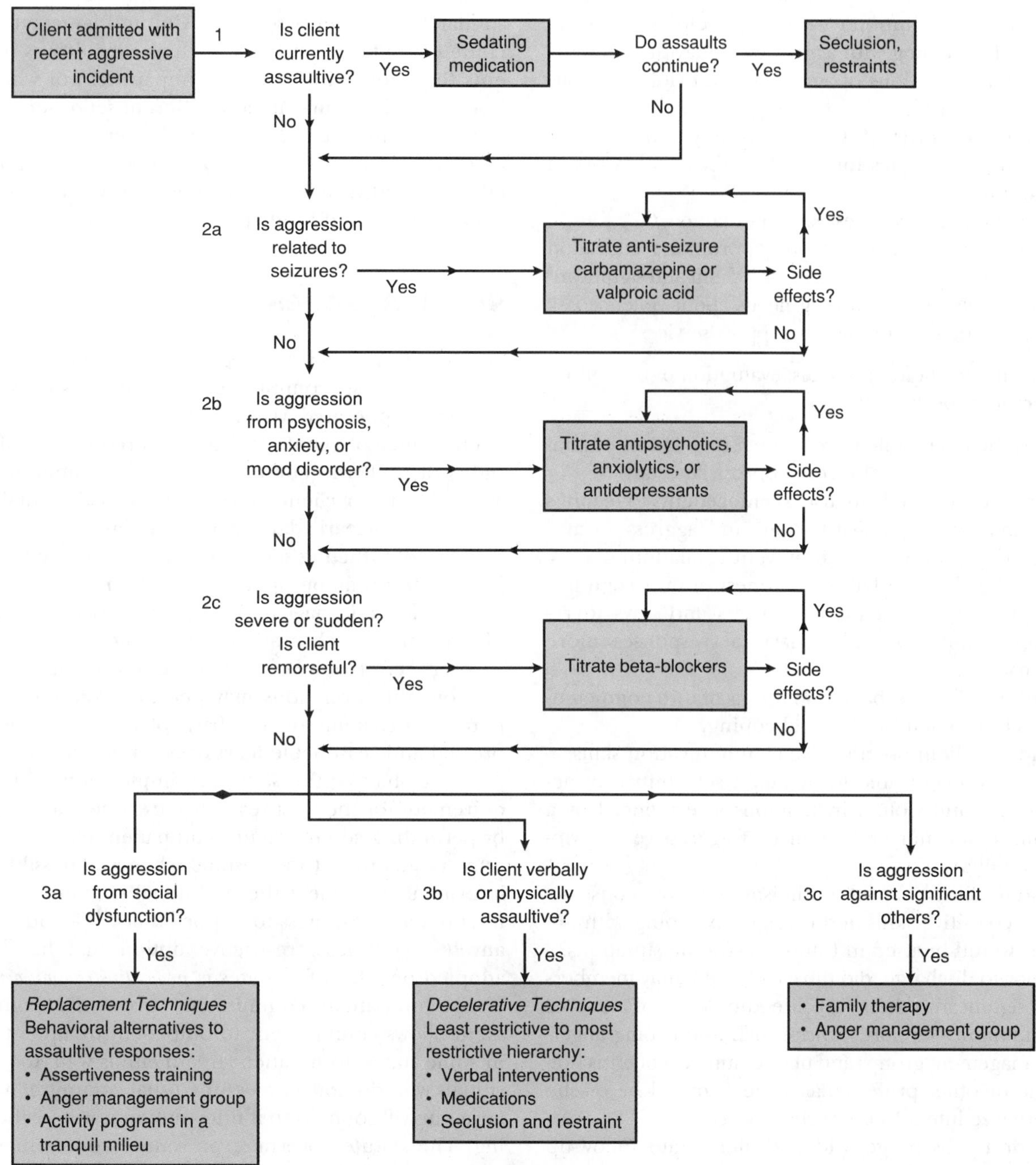

Figure 31-1. Decision tree for selecting intervention strategies for aggressive clients based on biological, interpersonal, and environmental factors. (Adapted with permission from Corrigan PW, Yudofsky SC, Silver JM: Pharmacological and Behavioral Treatment for Aggressive Psychiatric Inpatients. Hospital & Community Psychiatry 44 (2): 131, 1993.)

EVALUATION

A close examination of nursing and client efforts is needed to determine whether client goals and behavior outcomes were met and to decide what additional therapeutic interventions might be more effective in reinforcing clients' efforts in exerting internal control of aggressive and violent inclinations. Evaluation of nursing interventions relative to a range of aggressive and violent behavior considers the following factors:

1. Was an escalation of aggressive and violent behavior prevented, although emotions may have been intense?[78]

2. Was everyone's safety maintained?[78]
3. Were the institution's written guidelines and strategies for dealing with aggressive behavior followed?
4. Did manifestations of aggressive and violent behavior decrease?[78]
5. Did the client (and nurse) learn any new problem-solving techniques for handling these behaviors in the future?[78]
6. Was the client's self-esteem maintained?[78]
7. Were steps taken to provide appropriate education and discharge information to the client and significant others relevant to learning needs about violence risk assessment and community support services?

Specific to client outcomes, evaluation of the following factors is pertinent:

1. Was the client able to report feelings of loss of control and ask for help from appropriate staff?
2. Was the client able to discuss antecedents to feelings of anxiety, anger, frustration, and aggression and describe positive ways to prevent escalation?
3. Did the client verbalize awareness of own cognitive appraisals of precipitating events and ways to reframe thoughts and behavioral responses more constructively?
4. Did the client verbalize awareness of own competencies in problem solving and coping?
5. Did the client use assertive communication skills?
6. Was the client able to maintain self-control of aggressive and violent inclinations as evidenced by a calm demeanor and absence of aggressive and violent behavior?
7. Did the client express optimism that more constructive cognitive skills and changes in coping with anger would be used in future frustrating situations?
8. Prior to discharge, did the client and family members or significant others verbalize knowledge of available community support services, such as on-going anger-management groups and phone numbers of crisis hotline or other professionals if needed; did he or she verbalize intent to use such resources?
9. Prior to discharge, did the client state follow-up appointment information, such as date, time, and location?

◆ Cultural Issues

Although most traditional mental health programs are staffed by white, middle-class workers, clients who are likely to be arrested for violent behavior generally do not share this demographic profile; they may feel disenfranchised and choose not to use such mental health services.[29] To provide relevant mental health services for these clients, mental health delivery systems should employ case managers who are culturally similar to the clients served.[29] Cultural issues may include other factors as well, such as subcultures of clients (eg, those with a hearing impairment or who are homosexual and may need a different set of social services and supports). Clients will be served best when caregivers at all levels are concerned, caring, knowledgeable individuals who represent diverse cultures, backgrounds, and lifestyles.

◆ Legal Issues

Four primary legal issues regarding violent behavior include involuntary commitment to mental hospitals, protection of potential victims of a client's aggression, maintenance of clients' rights, and preservation of the rights of staff. In general, involuntary commitment is allowed only for clients who are diagnosed mentally ill and who are clearly dangerous to themselves or others in terms of inflicting serious physical injury. States vary in the interpretation of anticipated harm. Rigorous interpretation criteria may include anticipated harm as "imminent," "a clear and present danger," or require an overt act of violence within the past month.[129] Less rigorous interpretations may permit involuntary commitment of clients on the basis of threats or the expressed and reasonable fears of potential victims.

About half of the states are implementing the requirement for the least restrictive treatment alternative by permitting commitment to outpatient treatment settings rather than to a hospital whenever possible for individuals who meet the traditional commitment criteria of dangerousness to self or others.[114] Another relatively recent least restrictive option that has been adopted only by a few states is *preventive commitment.*[114] Unlike outpatient commitment, preventive commitment allows commitment to outpatient treatment and in some states, to inpatient treatment as well, for individuals who do not yet meet the usual commitment criteria but will soon do so if intervention is not forthcoming. The statute governing preventive commitment is called a *predicted deterioration* standard.[114] For instance, Hawaii and North Carolina allow outpatient commitment to prevent a relapse or deterioration toward imminent dangerousness for people who have previously been dangerous to self or others as a result of a severe mental disorder.[40,47] It is likely that preventive commitment statutes were enacted to address several concerns, including the increasing number of homeless people with mental disorders who could not be hospitalized under more rigorous commitment criteria, concerns among mental health professionals regarding "overlegalization" of the mental health care system, and pressure by advocacy groups, especially the National Alli-

31-3 Case Study

The Violent Plumber

Mr. P. is a 46-year-old unemployed plumber who appears at the emergency room stating, "I don't want to hurt nobody." In the assessment interview, Mr. P. reveals that he has recently been having nightmares in which he is shooting his wife or running her over with his car. Six months ago, he lost his job due to employee cutbacks. He began drinking and beating his wife, who left him 3 months ago for another man. Since then, Mr. P. has been irritable, involved in numerous barroom fights, and has occasional blackouts. He believes that the only option he has for reducing his misery is to kill his wife and perhaps the other man. He is not certain where his wife is living, but he thinks he can easily find her. Being a hunter, he has several guns and rifles at home with ammunition, and he fears that he may use them to kill his wife.

Mr. P.'s history reveals that he has never before seen a psychiatrist or been in a hospital for psychiatric treatment. He has never been arrested, although he does have a lifelong history of impulsive and somewhat dangerous behavior. As a child, he was often truant, began smoking and drinking at an early age, and was suspended during his junior year of high school. While he received an honorable discharge from the Army, he was involved in incidents of drunken driving, vandalism, and being absent without leave that resulted in numerous fines and reduction in rank. He settled down after getting married and a steady job, but would occasionally go on a drinking binge, complete with rowdiness and barroom fighting in which he broke the noses of several people. He has not experienced the desire to kill anyone until now.

Mr. P. seeks assistance now because he feels that he is losing control and may actually stalk and kill his wife. He has been drinking about a fifth of bourbon daily for the past month. During the assessment interview, he does not appear intoxicated, has a clear sensorium, and is not impaired on the mental status testing. He is cooperative with the consultant interviewer but adamantly refuses hospitalization with such comments as "I'd rather kill myself; I came here for help and you want to put me in jail." He promises not to harm his wife and to keep any outpatient appointments that the consultant deems appropriate.

Mr P.'s psychiatric diagnosis is as follows:

Axis I: Impulse control disorder (not otherwise specified); adjustment disorder with disturbance of conduct
Axis II: None
Axis III: None
Axis IV: Stress (severe): Loss of job, marital separation.
Axis V: Highest level of functioning currently (poor: some danger of hurting self or others)

Questions for Discussion

1. What risk factors put Mr. P. at high risk for violent behavior (apply Nursing Care Plan 31-1)?
2. What defining characteristics are relevant to Mr. P.'s potential for violence (apply Nursing Care Plan 31-1)?
3. Is Mr. P. currently dangerous? (Cite the rationale for your answer.)
4. What steps should be taken to ensure the safety of Mr. P.'s wife and the man with whom she is currently involved?
5. Do the factors of the case warrant Mr. P.'s involuntary hospitalization?
6. What client outcome goals and nursing interventions, including the discharge planning, are appropriate for Mr. P. in the event that he is hospitalized?
7. Is preventive commitment an alternative to involuntary hospitalization for Mr. P.?
8. What client outcome goals, treatment, and support services are appropriate for Mr. P. in the event that he is referred for outpatient treatment?

(Adapted and printed with permission from Clarkin J: The Case of the Violent Plumber. In Perry S, Frances A, Clarkin J: (eds): A DSM Casebook of Treatment Selection, pp. 278–279. New York, Brunner/Mazel, 1990.)

ance for the Mentally Ill, which favors less strict commitment standards.[114]

Another least restrictive treatment option is *conditional release,* currently available in about 40 states.[114] Conditional release requires continued supervision of a person following discharge from a hospital. The hospital or a court in criminal cases informs the client of the release conditions (for example, attending group therapy or reporting to a clinic for medication supervision). If the client violates the conditions of release, immediate rehospitalization may result or in some cases, may follow a court hearing. Conditional release tests the individual's ability to function in the community (supposedly under supervision) and frees up hospital beds.[114]

Regarding confidentiality and duty to warn, *The Principles of Medical Ethics* states that a "physician shall safeguard client confidence within the constraints of the law." An exception to this was legally enforced by the Tarasoff decision (Tarasoff versus Regents of University of California, 1974), which states that "protective privilege ends where public peril begins."[8] As a result of this decision, any clear threats by psychiatric clients to harm specific people is reportable. Psychotherapists and other mental health care providers must warn authorities (specified by law) and potential victims of possible dangerous actions of their clients.[129] If possible, the client should be included in the decision to warn, which may strengthen the therapeutic alliance and improve the client's relationship with the person threatened[129] (see Case Study 31-3, p. 627).

Regarding the rights of clients within hospitals and clinics, voluntary clients may refuse any treatment, although they may be asked to leave. In most states, involuntary clients have a right to refuse antipsychotic drugs unless they are found incompetent. In any case, medications can be administered legally by qualified personnel in an emergency (ie, client is dangerous to self or others).

Clients and staff in mental hospitals and clinics have a right to be free from violent assault, but this is usually weighed against the right of clients to be free of unnecessary medication and seclusion. If violent clients, hospitalized or not, have made clear threats to harm specific people, psychotherapists and other direct mental health care providers can be held responsible if potential victims are not warned.[129] While staff members may fear legal liability for whatever approach they take, personal injury and legal damages are likely to be lower if they opt for preventing violence.[129]

◆ Chapter Summary

This chapter has included a discussion of research-based profiles and etiologies of aggressive and violent behaviors of adult individuals with mental illness and ways to intervene therapeutically to prevent or manage the escalation of such behaviors in psychiatric treatment settings. Chapter highlights include the following:

1. Aggression encompasses a broad range of behaviors from abusive language to violent threats of harm and actual physical assault or damage to property that is preceded or accompanied by such hostility-related variables as anger, impulsivity, and persistent negative views of self, others, or the world in general.
2. Although the range of aggressive behaviors, including violence, occurs in all clinical diagnostic categories, certain subgroups of psychiatric diagnoses have been linked with violent behavior, such as antisocial personality disorder, paranoid schizophrenia, schizoaffective disorder, bipolar disorder, and substance abuse disorder.
3. Common client behavioral patterns as risk factors or predictors of violence on inpatient units have been identified as hyperactive, verbally loud and abusive, hostile, angry, escalating anxiety or fear, withdrawn, isolated, confused, hallucinating, or delusional.
4. Antecedent events that have been linked with client violence on inpatient units are argumentative interactions with other clients and with staff, whose behavior in the process of caring for the client is interpreted by the client as intrusive and frustrating or indifferent.
5. Theories and research-based findings regarding the determinents of aggressive and violent behavior point to such biopsychosocial factors as neurobiological deficits or injuries in the limbic system or frontal or temproal lobes of the brain; neurotransmitter dysregulation; substance abuse; temperament; a tendency toward negative appraisals and attitudes toward self, others, and the world; various sociocultural stressors, such as parental rejection and abuse or coercive family processes; and the impact of dehospitalization, homelessness, and untreated mental illness.
6. When developing a nursing care plan for the client who is at high risk for aggressive and violent behavior, the nurse gathers information risk factors and client characteristics, such as a history of aggressive or violent behavior and substance abuse; factors associated with increasing anxiety levels, agitation, and inclinations toward violence; cognitive awareness (or lack thereof) regarding appraisals of life events and aggressive responses; inability to generate alternative problem solving; and inability to communicate angry feelings.
7. When planning therapeutic interventions, the nurse and client choose desired client outcomes based on the client's needs and ability to maintain self-control of aggressive and violent inclinations.
8. Three types of intervention strategies include verbal, pharmacotherapeutic, and physical (seclusion and restraint), which may be used separately or in combination as indicated by client needs and treatment setting protocols with adherence to the principles of safety and least restrictive environment.
9. Prevention of violent behavior through de-escalating rising feelings and supporting the client who attempts to control violent inclinations in socially acceptable ways are preferable to applying seclusion and restraint.

These should be used only when all other interventions fail to prevent a client's violent behavior, and the client is deemed dangerous to self or others.

10. Therapeutic strategies with reported success in helping clients toward greater self-awareness and positive management of anger dyscontrol include behavior modification, cognitive therapy, and anger-management groups.
11. Discharge planning should incorporate client and family or significant other education based on an assessment of learning needs regarding the risks and characteristics of violent behavior, de-escalation strategies, and community support resources. In addition, pertinent nursing care plan information regarding the client should be communicated to appropriate referral agencies to ensure continuity of care, effective monitoring, and support.
12. Evaluation requires a close examination of client and nursing efforts to determine whether client goals and behavior outcomes were met and to decide what additional therapeutic interventions might be more effective in reinforcing clients' efforts in exerting internal control of aggressive and violent inclinations.

Critical Thinking Questions

1. *Is temperament a result of innate traits or interpersonal and situational influences or a combination of all?*
2. *Recent research indicates that spanking may foster aggression in children.*[117] *What is your opinion? Cite your rationale.*
3. *Is limit setting appropriate for all clients who are potentially violent?*
4. *Have you observed situations in which limit setting was applied with therapeutic caring and explanation versus punitive authoritarianism? What were the results of each?*
5. *What are some other strategies for nurses to use when interacting with clients who have a coercive interaction style?*
6. *What increased client safety concerns occur in hospitals due to reduced staff availability?*
7. *With staff shortages, have there been significant increases in clients' acting on suicidal or homicidal ideation?*
8. *In your clinical experiences in psychiatric settings, have you observed the application of the kinds of interventions for assaultive clients as diagrammed in the decision tree (Fig. 31-1)?*
9. *What adaptations or modifications would you suggest in the decision tree in terms of nursing care of assaultive clients?*

Review Questions

1. According to recent research studies, which of the following risk factors is the *best* predictor of violent behavior?
   A. Argumentative personality style
   B. A history of violent behavior
   C. Decreased brain serotonin
   D. Negative thinking
2. Which of the following statements regarding the cognitive theory of anger arousal is false?
   A. Individuals' anger arousal is influenced by their negative perceptions and appraisals of self, other people, and the world.
   B. Individuals who interpret certain situations and events as aversive and anger inducing tend to react with anger when the event occurs.
   C. Individuals' appraisals of events are unrelated to their expectations about the events.
   D. The kind of self-talk that individuals use influences their expectations and appraisals of events that happen to them.
3. Which of the following events on a psychiatric unit are most likely to precipitate an episode of aggressive or violent behavior in a violence-prone client, Mr. A.?
   1. A psychiatric technician asks Mr. A. if he would like to have some juice during snack time.
   2. The nurse notices Mr. A. frowning, cursing, and pacing up and down the hall, and she asks him if he is feeling upset about something.
   3. Mr. A.'s therapist has just seen him and told him that since he did not attend the group therapy sessions as prescribed, he did not earn privileges to go bowling with the rest of the clients.
   4. Another client on the unit picked up Mr. A's pack of cigarettes and said that they were his.

   A. 1, 2
   B. 1, 4
   C. 2, 3
   D. 3, 4
4. Which of the following statements about the emergency use of seclusion and restraint is false?
   A. Violent behavior must be demonstrated by a client before selcusion and restraint can be implemented by professional staff.
   B. Specific written guidelines and a manual for the use of intervention procedures should be available in mental health institutions.
   C. Justification for the emergency use of seclusion and restraint is legally based on professional clinical judgment and professional standards of care.
   D. A professional nurse can act as the leader

to direct the actions of a team of staff in implementing emergency seclusion and restraint procedures for a client whose behavior is violent and out of control.

5. Which of the following medications is most commonly used to treat aggressive behavior resulting from acute psychoses?
   - A. Diazepam
   - B. Haloperidol
   - C. Lithium
   - D. Fluoxetine
6. Which type of intervention is appropriately used by the nurse in interacting with aggressive clients at all levels of escalation?
   - A. Administration of sedating medication
   - B. Seclusion and restraint
   - C. Time out
   - D. Talking with the client to discover the source of distress and alternatives to violent behavior
7. Some states allow a client to be committed to outpatient treatment instead of involuntary hospitalization under the predicted deterioration standard and preventive commitment. The primary purpose of preventive commitment is to
   - A. prevent the occurrence of mental illness.
   - B. free up hospital beds.
   - C. prevent relapse or deterioration toward imminent dangerousness for mentally ill individuals who have previously been dangerous to self or others.
   - D. prevent relapse or deterioration toward imminent dangerousness for individuals who have criminal records and have served jail or prison time but who have no record of mental illness.
8. All of the following statements reflect outcome goals of anger-management training for violence-prone clients, except which one?
   - A. Gaining awareness of one's own thoughts, feelings, and behaviors that are related to anger arousal
   - B. Rechanneling aggressive responses in the later stages of anger arousal
   - C. Reappraising certain arousal situations as a problem that calls for a solution rather than as a threat that calls for an attack
   - D. Gaining awareness of others' points of view and the consequences of one's own emotional and behavioral responses
9. Which of the following statements is false regarding legalities of treating violent clients within hospitals and clinics?
   - A. Although involuntary clients may refuse antipsychotic medication, such medications may be administered by the nurse as prescribed if the client is dangerous to self or others.
   - B. Involuntary commitment criteria and interpretation vary among the states.
   - C. If violent clients, hospitalized or not, make clear threats to harm specific people, the mental health care provider who hears such a threat cannot be held responsible if potential victims are not warned and are harmed.
   - D. Some advocacy groups favor less strict commitment standards.
10. Which of the following conditions has been consistently linked with medication noncompliance among discharged, previously violent clients?
   - A. Substance abuse
   - B. Broodiness
   - C. Feelings of resentment
   - D. Coercive interaction style

◆ References

1. Aiken G: Assaults on Staff in a Locked Ward: Prediction and Consequences. Med Sci Law 24: 199–207, 1984
2. Allen JG: Temperament: The Biological Shaper of Personality. The Menninger Letter 2 (10), 4–5, 1994
3. American Nurses' Association, American Psychiatric Nurses Association, Association of Child and Adolescent Psychiatric Nurses, and Society for Education and Research in Psychiatric-Mental Health Nursing: Statement on Psychiatric-Mental Health Nursing Practice and Standards of Psychiatric-Mental Health Nursing Practice. Washington, DC, American Nurses Publishing, 1994
4. American Psychiatric Association: Diagnostic and Statistical Manual of Mental Disorders, 4th ed. Washington, DC, American Psychiatric Association, 1994
5. Apter A, van Praag HM, Plutchick R, Sevy S, Korn M, Brown SL: Inter-relationships Among Anxiety, Aggression, Impulsivity, and Mood: A Serotonergically Linked Cluster? Psychiatry Res 32: 191–199, 1990
6. Baron RA: Aggression. In Kaplan HI, Saddock BJ (eds): Comprehensive Textbook of Psychiatry IV, pp 213–226. Baltimore, Williams & Wilkins, 1985
7. Beck AT: Cognitive Therapy and the Emotional Disorders. New York, International Universities, 1976
8. Bernal y Del Rio V: Psychiatric Ethics and Confidentiality. In Kaplan HI, Saddock BJ (eds): Comprehensive Textbook of Psychiatry, p 2003. Baltimore, Williams & Wilkins, 1985
9. Betemps EJ, Ragiel C: Psychiatric Epidemiology: Facts and Myths on Mental Health and Illness. J Psychosoc Nurs 32 (5): 23–28, 1994
10. Blair DT: Assaultive Behavior: Does Provocation Begin in the Front Office? J Psychosoc Nurs Ment Health Serv 29: 21–26, 1991

11. Booth GK: Disorders of impulse control. In Goldman HH (ed): Review of General Psychiatry, 2d ed, pp 381–389. Norwalk, CT, Appleton & Lange, 1988
12. Burns JW, Friedman R, Katkin ES: Anger Expression, Hostility, Anxiety, and Patterns of Cardiac Reactivity to Stress. Behavioral Medicine 18: 71–78, 1992
13. Buss AH, Durkee A: The Aggression Questionnaire. Journal of Personaliaty and Social Psychology 63(3), 452-459, 1992
14. Castrogiovanni P, Capone MR, Maremmani I, Marazziti D: Platelet Serotonergic Markers and Aggressive Behavior in Healthy Subjects. Neuropsychobiology 29 (3): 105–107, 1994
15. Cates DS, Houston BK, Vavak DR, Crawford MH, Uttley M: Heritability of Hostility-Related Emotions, Attitudes, and Behaviors. J Behav Med 16 (4): 237–256, 1993
16. Cembrowicz S, Ritter S: Attacks on doctors and nurses. In Shepherd J (ed): Violence in Health Care : A Practical Guide to Coping With Violence and Caring for Victims, pp 13–41. New York, Oxford University Press, 1994
17. Chaiken J, Chaiken M, Rhodes W: Predicting Violent Behavior and Classifying Violent Offenders. In Reiss AJ, Roth JA (eds): Understanding and Preventing Violence: Consequences and Control, vol 4, pp 217–295. Washington, DC, National Academy Press, 1994
18. Chess S, Thomas A: The New York Longitudinal Study (NYLS): The Young Adult Periods. Can J Psychiatry 35: 557–561, 1990
19. Convey J: A Record of Violence. Nursing Times 82 (46): 36–38, 1986
20. Cooper AJ, Medonca JD: A Prospective Study of Patient Assaults on Nurses in a Provincial Psychiatric Hospital in Canada. Acta Psychiatr Scand 84: 163–166, 1991
21. Corrigan PW, Yudofsky SC, Sliver JM: Pharmacological and Behavioral Treatment for Aggressive Psychiatric Inpatients. Hosp Community Psychiatry 44 (2): 125–133, 1993
22. Cuffel BJ: Violent and Destructive Behavior Among the Severely Mentally Ill in Rural Areas: Evidence From Arkansas' Community Mental Health System. Community Ment Health J 30: 495–504, 1994
23. Davis D: Violence by Psychiatric Inpatients: A Review. Hosp Community Psychiatry 42 (6): 585–590, 1991
24. Delaney K, Ulsafer-Van Lanen J, Pitula CR, Johnson ME: Seven Days and Counting: How Inpatient Nurses Might Adjust Their Practice to Brief Hospitalization. J Psychosoc Nurs 33 (8): 36–40, 1995
25. Dembroski TM, Costa PT: Coronary Prone Behaior: Components of the Type A Pattern and Hostility. J Pers 55: 211–235, 1987
26. Dietch JT, Jennings RK: Aggressive Dyscontrol in Patients Treated With Benzodiazepines. J Clin Psychiatry 49: 184–189, 1988
27. Doenges M, Townsend MC, Moorhouse MF: Psychiatric Care Plans: Guidelines for Planning and Documneting Care, 2d ed. Philadelphia, FA Davis, 1995
28. Drinkwater J: Violence in Psychiatric Hospitals. In Feldman P (ed): Developments in the Study of Criminal Behavior, vol 2, Violence. Chichester, John Wiley, 1982
29. Dvoskin JA, Steadman HJ: Using Intensive Case Management to Reduce Violence by Mentally Ill Persons in the Community. Hosp Community Psychiatry 45 (7): 679–684, 1994
30. Eichelman B: Toward a Rational Pharmacotherapy for Aggressive and Violent Behavior. Hosp Community Psychiatry 39 (1): 31–39, 1988
31. Estroff SE, Zimmer C, Lachicotte W, Benoit J: The Influence of Social Networks and Social Support on Violence by Persons With Serious Mental Illness. Hosp Community Psychiatry 45 (7): 669–678, 1994
32. Fagan-Pryor EC, Femea P, Haber LC: Congruence Between Aggresive Behavior and Type of Intervention as Rated by Nursing Personnel. Issues in Mental Health Nursing 15: 187–199, 1994
33. Fagan J, Wexler S: Family Origins of Violent Delinquents. Criminology 25: 643–649, 1987
34. Ferguson LE: Steps to Developing a Critical Pathway. Nursing Administration Quarterly 17 (3): 58–62, 1993
35. Fortinash KM, Holoday-Worret PA: Psychiatric Nursing Care Plans, 2d ed, St. Louis, CV Mosby, 1995
36. Gallop R, McCay E, Esplen MJ: The Conceptualization of Impulsivity for Psychiatric Nursing Practice. Archives of Psychiatric Nursing 6 (6): 366–373, 1992
37. Garza-Trevino ES: Neurobiological Factors in Aggressive Behaviors. Hosp Community Psychiatry 45 (7): 690–699, 1994
38. Garza-Trevino ES, Volkow ND, Cancro R, et al: Neurobiology of schizophrenic syndromes. Hosp Community Psychiatry 41: 971–980, 1990
39. Garza-Trevio ES, Hollister LE: Psychiatric Manifestations of Complex Partial Seizures. In Garza-Trevino ES (ed): Medical Psychiatry: Theory and Practice, vol l. River Edge, NJ, World Scientific, 1989
40. General Statutes of North Carolina, sec 122C-271 (a) (1), 1989
41. Geracioti TD: Valproic Acid Treatment of Episodic Explosiveness Related to Brain Injury. J Clin Psychiatry 55: 9, 1994
42. Gleason RP, Schneider LS: Carbamazepine Treatment of Agitation in Alzheimer's Outpatients Refractory to Neuroleptics. J Clin Psychiatry 51: 115–118, 1990
43. Goldsmith HH, Rothbart MK: Contemporary Instruments for Assessing Early Temperament by Questionnaire and in the Laboratory. In Strelau J, Angleiter A (eds): Explorations in Temperament, pp 249–272. London, Plenum Press, 1991
44. Goldsmith HF, Manderscheid RW, Henderson MJ, Sacks AJ: Projections of Inpatient Specialty Mental Health Organizations: 1990 to 2010. Hosp Community Psychiatry 44 (5): 478–483, 1993
45. Grossman LS, Haywood TW, Cavanaugh JL, Davis JM, Lewis DA: State Psychiatric Hospital Patients With Past Arrests for Violent Crimes. Psychiatric Services 46 (8): 790–795, 1995
46. Grosz DE, Lipschitz DS, Eldar S, Finkelstein G, Blackwood N, Gervino-Rosen G, Faedda GL, Poutchik R: Correlates of Violence Risk in Hospitalized Adolescents. Compr Psychiatry 35 (4): 296–300, 1994
47. Hawaii Revised Statutes, sec 334–121, 1985
48. Human Resources Development: Prevention and Man-

agement of Aggressive Behavior: Lesson Plan on Communication, pp 2–15. Austin, TX, The Texas Department of Mental Health and Mental Retardation, 1991

49. Hunter M, Carmetl H: The Cost of Staff Injuries for Inpatient Violence. Hosp Community Psychiatry 43 (6): 586–588, 1992
50. Jackson M, McSwane D: Homelessness as a Determinant of Health. Public Health Nurs 9 (3): 185–192, 1992
51. Janssen Pharmaceutica: Risperdal: Questions and Answers. Titusville, NJ, Smith Kline Beecham Pharmaceuticals, 1994
52. Kagan J: Unstable Ideas: Termperament, Cognition, and Self. Cambridge, MA, Harvard University Press, 1989
53. Kavoussi RJ, Liu J, Coccaro EF: An Open Trial of Sertraline in Personality Disordered Patients With Impulsive Aggression. J Clin Psychiatry 55 (4): 137–141, 1994
54. Klassen D, O'Connor WA: Demographic and Case History Variables in Risk Assessment. In Monahan J, Steadman HJ (eds): Violence and Mental Disorder: Developments in Risk Assessment. Chicago, University of Chicago Press, 1994
55. Klassen D, O'Connor WA: Assessing the Risk of Violence in Released Mental Patients: A Cross-validation Study. Psychological Asessment. J Consult Clin Psychol 1: 75–81, 1990
56. Koda-Kimble MA, Young LY: Applied Therapeutics: The Clinical Use of Drugs. Vancouver, Washington, Applied Therapeutics, 1993
57. Krakowski MI, Volavka J: Schizophrenic Violence and Psychopathology, in Brizer DA, Crawner ML (eds): Current Approaches to the Prediction of Violence. Washington, DC, American Psychiatric Press, 1989
58. Lande RG: The Viodo Violence Debate. Hosp Community Psychiatry 44 (4): 347–351, 1993
59. Lau MA, Pihl RO: Alcohol and the Taylor Aggression Paradigm: A Repeated Measures Study. J Stud Alcohol 55: 701–706, 1994
60. Lau MA, Pihl RO, Peterson JB: Provocation, Acute Alcohol Intoxication, Cognitive Performance, and Aggression. J Abnorm Psychol 104 (1): 150–155, 1995
61. Lee HK, Villar O, Juthani N, Bluestone H: Characteristics and Behavior of Patients Involved in Psychiatric Ward Incidents. Hosp Community Psychiatry 40 (12): 1295–1297, 1989
62. Leibovici A, Tariot PN: Carbamazepine Treatment of Agitation Associated With Dementia. Journal of Geriatric Psychiatry and Neurology l: 110–112, 1988
63. Levy R, Goldman B: Emergency psychiatry. In Goldman HH (ed): Review of General Psychiatry, 3rd ed, pp 470–476. Norwalk, CT, Appleton & Lange, 1992
64. Lidz CW, Mulvey EP, Gardner WP: The Accuracy of Predictions of Violence to Others. JAMA 269: 1007–1011, 1993
65. Lindquist P, Allebeck P: Schizophrenia and Crime: A Longitudinal Follow-up of 644 Schizophrenics in Stockholm. Br J Psychiatry 157: 345–350, 1990
66. Link BG, Andrews H, Cullen FT: The Violent and Illegal Behavior of Mental Patients Reconsidered. American Sociological Review 57: 275–292, 1992
67. Linn L: Clinical Manifestations of Psychiatric Disorders. In Kaplan HI, Saddock BJ (eds): Comprehensive Textbook of Psychiatry IV, p 582. Baltimore, Williams & Wilkins, 1985
68. Linnoila VM, Virkkunen M: Aggression, Suicidality, and Serontonin. J Clin Psychiatry 53: 46–51, 1992
69. Linnoila VM, DeJong J, Virkkunen M: Family History of Alcoholism in Violent Offenders and Impulsive Fire Setters. Arch Gen Psychiatry 46: 613–616, 1989
70. Littrell K: Clozaril: Guide to Clozaril Therapy. East Hanover, NJ, Sandoz Pharmaceuticals, 1994
71. Long JW: The Essential Guide to Prescription Drugs. New York, Harper Perennial, 1991
72. Lyon G: Limit Setting as a Therapeutic Tool. In Backer G, et al (eds): Psychiatric-Mental Health Nursing, 3rd ed, pp 181–193. Monterey, CA, Wadsworth Health Science division, 1985
73. Maiuro RD: Intermittent Explosive Disorder. In Dunner DL (ed): Current Psychiatric Therapy, pp 482–489. Philadelphia, WB Saunders, 1993
74. Maiuro RD, Vitaliano PP, Cahn TC: A Brief Measure of the Assessment of Anger and Aggression. Journal of Interpersonal Violence 2: 166–178, 1987
75. Matthews KA: Coronary Heart Diseae and Type A Behaviors: Update on and Alternative to the Booth-Kewley and Friedman (1987) Quantitative Review. Psychol Bull 104: 373–380, 1988
76. McClowry SG: Temperament Theory and Research. Image 24 (4): 319–326, 1992
77. McDonald JM: Crime and Mental Disorder: An Epidemiological Approach. Crime and Justice: An Annual Review of Research 4: 145–189, 1991
78. McElvain MS: Suspiciousness and Agression: The Delusional and Acting Out Disorders, pp 495–515. In Johnson BS (ed): Adaptation and Growth: Psychiatric-Mental Health Nursing, 3rd ed. Philadelphia, JB Lippincott, 1993
79. McFarland G, Wasli E: Nursing Diagnosis and Process in Psychiatric Mental Health Nursing. St. Louis, JB Lippincott, 1986
80. McGuire MT, Troisi A: Aggression. In Kaplan HI, Saddock BJ (eds): Comprehensive Textbook of Psychiatry, vol 5, pp 271–282. Baltimore: Williams & Wilkins, 1989
81. McKenry LM, Salerno E: Pharmacology in Nursing. St. Louis, Mosby-Year Book, 1995
82. McLaren S, Browne FW, Taylor PJ: A Study of Psychotropic Medication Given *as Required* in a Regional Secure Unit. Br J Psychiatry 156: 732–735, 1990
83. McNiel DE, Binder RI: The Relationship Between Acute Psychiatric Symptoms, Diagonosis and Short-term Risk of Violence. Hosp Community Psychiatry 45 (2): 133–137, 1994
84. McNiel DE, Binder RI, Greenfield TK: Predictors of Violence in Civilly Committed Acute Psychiatric Patients. Am J psychiatry 145: 965–978, 1988
85. Monahan J: Mental Disorder and Violent Behavior. Am Psychol 47: 511–521, 1992
86. Morrison EF: Theoretical Modeling to Predict Violence in Hospitalized Psychiatric Patients. Res Nurs Health 12: 31–40, 1989
87. Morrison EF: Violent Psychiatric Inpatients in a Public

Hospital. Scholarly Inquiry of Nursing Practice 4 (1): 65–82, 1990

88. Morrison EF: A Coercive Interactional Style as an Antecedent to Aggression in Psychiatric Patients. Res Nurs Health 15: 421–431, 1992
89. Morrison EF: The Violence Scale: The Measurement of Aggression and Violence in Psychiatric Inpatients. Int J Nurs Stud 30 (1): 51–64, 1993
90. Morrison EF: Toward a Better Understanding of Violence: Debunking the Myths. Archives of Psychiatric Nursing 8: 328–335, 1993
91. Morrison EF: The Evolution of a Concept: Aggression and Violence in Psychiatric Settings. Archives of Psychiatric Nursing 7 (4): 245–253, 1994
92. Mulvey EP: Assessing the Evidence of a Link Between Mental Illness and Violence. Hosp Community Psychiatry 45 (7): 663–668, 1994
93. Mysiw WS, Jackson RD, Corrigan JD: Amitryptyline for Post-traumatic Agitation. Am J Phys Med Rehab 67 (1): 29–33, 1988
94. North American Nursing Diagnosis Association: NANDA Nursing Diagnoses: Definitions and Classification 1993–1994. Philadelphia, The Association, 1994
95. Nancy H: Project Action: Program Evaluation. Presented at a Solutions 2000 conference, Houston, Sept. 30, 1992
96. Ninan PT, van Kammen DP, Scheinin M, et al: CSF 5-Hyroxyindolacetic Acid Levels in Suicidal Schizophrenic Patients. Am J Psychiatry 141: 566–569, 1984
97. Novaco RW: Anger Control: The Development and Evaluation of an Experimental Treatment. Lexington, MA, Lexington Books, 1976
98. Olweus D: Bully/Victim Problems Among School Children: Basic Facts and Effects of a School-Based Intervention Program. In Pepler D, Rubin K (eds): The Development and Treatment of Childhood Aggression, pp 411–488. Hillsdale, NJ, Erlbaum, 1991
99. Paradis CM, Horn L, Lazar RM, Schwartz DW: Brain Dysfunction and Violent Behavior in a Man With a Congential Subarachnoid Cyst. Hosp Community Psychiatry 45 (7): 714–718, 1994
100. Patterson GR: A Social Learning Approach: Coercive Family Processes. Eugene, OR, Castalia Press, 1982
101. Pillemer K, Frankel S: Domestic Violence Against the Elderly. In Rosenberg ML, Fenley MA (eds): Violence in America: A Public Health Approach, pp 158–183. New York, Oxford University Press, 1991
102. Pilowsky LS, Ring H, Shine PJ, et al: Rapid Tranquilization: A Survey of Emergency Prescribing in a General Psychiatric Hospital. Br J Psychiatry 160: 831–835, 1992
103. Pinner E, Rich CL: Effects of Trazadone on Aggressive Behavior in Seven Patients With Organic Mental Disorders. Am J Psychiatry 145: 1295–1296, 1988
104. Reeder DM: Cognitive Therapy of Anger Management: Theoretical and Practical Considerations. Archives of Psychiatric Nursing 5 (3): 147–150, 1991
105. Reiss AJ, Roth A: Understanding and Preventing Violence. Washington, DC, National Academy Press, 1993
106. Rickelman BL, Houfek J: Toward an Interactional Model of Suicidal Behaviors: Cognitive Rigidity, Attributional Style, Stress, Hopelessness, and Depression. Archives of Psychiatric Nursing 9 (3): 158–168, 1995
107. Rossi AM, Jacogs M, Monteleone M, Olsen R, Surber RW, Winkler EL, Wommack A: Characteristics of Psychiatric Patients who Engage in Assaultive or Other Fear-Inducing Behaviors. J Nerv Ment Disease 173 (3): 154–160, 1986
108. Schiff HB, Sabin TD, Geller A, et al: Lithium in Aggressive Behavior. Am J Psychiatry 138: 1346–1348, 1982
109. Sheila A, Joseph GR, Felton H, et al: Adult Intensive Case Mangement Evaluation. Albany, New York State Office of Mental Health, June 30: 1992
110. Sheridan M, Henrion R, Robinson L, & Baxter V: Precipitants of Violence in a Psychiatric Inpatient Setting. Hosp Community Psychiatry 41 (7): 776–780, 1990
111. Siegman AW, Dembroski TM, Ringel N: Components of Hostility and the Severity of Coronary Artery Disease. Psychosom Med 49: 127–133, 1987
112. Siegman AW: Cardiovascular Consequences of Expressing, Experiencing, and Repressing Anger. J Behav Med 16 (6): 539–569, 1993
113. Simms C: How to Unmask the Angry Patient. Am J Nurs April: 37–40, 1995
114. Slobogin C: Involuntary Community Treatment of People Who Are Violent and Mentally Ill: A Legal Analysis. Hosp Community Psychiatry 45 (7): 685–689, 1994
115. Soloff PM, Gutheil TG, Wexler DB: Seclusion and Restraint in 1985: A Review and Update. Hosp Community Psychiatry 36 (6): 652–657, 1985
116. Stanislav SW, Fabre T, Crismon ML, Childs A: Buspirone's Efficacy in Organic-Induced Aggression. J Clin Psychopharmacol 14 (2): 126–130, 1994
117. Strassberg Z, et al: Spanking in the Home and Children's Subsequent Aggression Toward Kindergarten Peers. Development and Psychopathology 6 (3): 445–461, 1994
118. Steinwachs DM, Kasper JD, Skinner EA: Family Perspectives on Meeting the Needs for Care of Severely Mentally Ill Relatives: A National Survey. Arlington, VA, National Alliance for the Mentally Ill, 1992
119. Stone JL, McDaniel KD, Hughes JR, et al: Episodic Dyscontrol Disorder and Proxymal EEG Abnormalities: Successful Treatment With Carbamazepine. Biological Psychiatry 21: 208–212, 1986
120. Straznickas KA, McNeil DE, Binder RL: Violence Toward Family Caregivers by Mentally Ill Relatives. Hosp Community Psychiatry 44: 385–387, 1993
121. Strome TM: Restraining the Elderly. J Psychosoc Nurs Ment Health Serv 26: 18–21, 1988
122. Swanson JW, Holzer CE, Ganju VK, et al: Violence and Psychiatric Disorder in the Community: Evidence From the Epidemiologic Catchment Area Surveys. Hosp Community Psychiatry 41 (7): 761–770, 1990
123. Swanson JW: Mental Disorder, Substance Abuse, and Community Violence, in Monahan J, Steadman HF (eds): Violence and Mental Disorders: Developments in Risk Assessment. Chicago, University of Chicago Press, 1994
124. Szlabowicz JW, Stewart JT: Amitryptyline Treatment of Agitation Associated With Anoxic Encephalopathy. Arch Phys Med Rehabil 71: 612–613, 1990
125. Tardiff K: Violence. In Talbot JA, Hales RE, Yudofsky SC

(eds): Textbook of Psychiatry, pp 1037–1057. Washington, DC, The American Psychiatric Press, 1988

126. Tardiff K: Characteristics of Assaultive Patients in Private Hospitals. Am J Psychiatry 141: 1232–1235, 1984

127. Task Force on Homelessness and Severe Mental Illness: Outcasts on Mainstreet. Report of the Task Force on Homelessness and Severe Mental Illness. Rockville, MD, National Institute of Mental Health, 1992

128. The Harvard Mental Health Letter: Violence and violent patients: Part I. 7 (12): 1–4, Boston: The Harvard Medical School, 1991

129. The Harvard Mental Health Newsletter: Violence and violent patients: Part II. 8 (1): 1–4, Boston: The Harvard Medical School, 1991

130. Tonkonogy TM: Violence and Temporal Lobe Lesion: Head CT and MRI Data. Journal of Neuropsychiatry 3: 189–196, 1991

131. Torrey EF, Steiber J, Ezekiel J: Criminalizing the Seriously Mentally Ill: The Abuse of Jails as Mental Hospitals. Washington, DC, National Allieance for the Mentally Ill and Public Citizen's Health Research Group, 1992

132. Torrey EF: Violent Behavior by Individuals With Serious Mental Illness. Hosp Community Psychaitry 45 (7): 653–662, 1994

133. Townsend MC: Nursing Diagnoses in Psychiatric Nursing: A Pocket Guide for Care Plan Construction, 3rd ed. Philadelphia, FA Davis, 1994

134. Valzelli L: Psychobiolgy of Aggression. New York, Raven, 1981

135. Van Praag HM: CSF 5-HIAA and Suicide in Nondepressed Schizophrenics. Lancet 2: 977–978, 1983

136. Volkow ND, Tancredi L: Neural Substrates of Violent Behavior: A Preliminary Study With Positron Emission Tomography. Br J Psychiatry 151: 668–673, 1987

137. Weiner B: An Attributional Theory of Motivation and Emotion. New York, Springer-Verlag, 1986

138. Wesorick B: Standards of Nursing Care: A Model for Clinical Practice pp 283–284. Philadelphia, JB Lippincott, 1990

139. Whittington R: Violence in Psychiatric Hospitals. In Wykes T (ed): Violence and Health Care Professionals, pp 23–43. New York, Chapman and Hall, 1994

140. Windle P: Critical Pathways: An Integrated Documentation Tool. Nursing Management 25 (9): 80F–80L, 1994

141. Wykes T (ed): Violence and Health Care Professionals. New York, Chapman & Hall, 1994

142. Yatham LN, McHale PA: Carbamazepine in the Treatment of Aggression: A Case Report and Review of the Literature. Acta Psychiatr Scand 24: 188–190, 1988

143. Yudofsky SC, Silver J, Yudofsky B: Organic Personality Disorder, Explosive Type. In Karuso TB (ed): Treatment of Psychiatric Disorders. Washington, DC, American Psychiatric Press, 1989

144. Yudofsky SC, Silver J, Schneider SE: Pharmacologic Treatment of Aggression. Psychiatric Annals 17: 397–407, 1987

145. Yudofsky SC, Silver J, Jackson W, et al: The Overt Aggression Scale for the Objective Rating of Verbal and Physical Aggression. Am J Psychiatry 143: 35–39, 1986

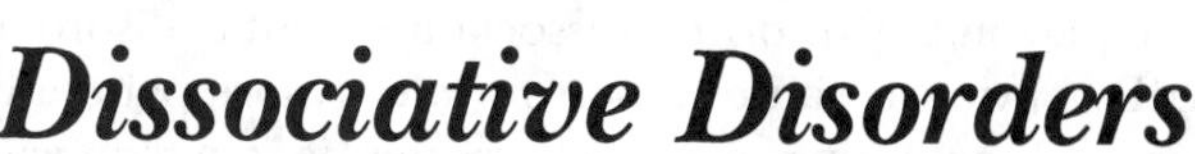

Dissociative Disorders

Jan Dalsheimer

32

What have I learned? You can use my body and shatter my mind. But my soul lives on. I will survive.

Karen G., incest survivor

This chapter addresses disturbances in self-concept known as dissociative disorders. Dissociation *is a method of coping with an experience that would otherwise be overwhelming. It helps people to deal with trauma, especially repetitive trauma, from which they could not escape. Because they physically could not get away, they found a way to escape, or separate, from the event by "running away" from it in their mind.[15] Ultimately, though, in response to severe acute or chronic trauma, dissociation may become a regular part of the person's functioning and may result in depression, low self-esteem, and self-defeating and self-destructive behaviors.*

Dissociation leading to impairment in functioning requires treatment. The degree of disruption of the self and the intensity and types of interventions vary in the dissociative disorders. The four types of currently recognized dissociative disorders are described, and etiology is discussed in this chapter. The nursing process is explored, with particular attention to interventions and milieu management. Addictions commonly associated with dissociative disorders are discussed and cultural considerations presented.

Learning Objectives

On completion of this chapter, you should be able to accomplish the following:

1. *Define dissociation.*
2. *Differentiate the four types of dissociative disorders.*
3. *Describe the etiology of dissociative disorders.*
4. *Apply the nursing process to clients with dissociative disorders.*
5. *Describe treatment modalities for dissociative disorders.*
6. *Describe addictions commonly associated with dissociative disorders.*
7. *Understand cultural considerations applicable to the care of clients with dissociative disorders.*

◆ The Concept of Dissociation

Dissociation refers to the absence from conscious awareness of some ordinarily familiar information, emotion, or mental function.[18] In other words, a person may not be able to bring to consciousness certain mental processes, but they are still present in the person's behavior or feelings. People may not remember their identity and travel far away from home (dissociative fugue), they may lose their memory (dissociative amnesia), they may take on two or more identities or personalities (dissociative identity disorder), or they may feel that they are not in touch with their body (depersonalization disorder).

However, dissociation is not always a pathological state. Everyone forgets things now and then. We all daydream (and some daydream more than others), and sometimes we drive a car so automatically that we forget traveling a familiar route. On the Dissociative Experience Scale administered by Ross, Joshi, and Currie (1990), 29% of the general population reported that in almost one-third of their conversations, they did not hear part or all of what was said.[18] Also, in some cultures voluntary experiences of trance or meditation are accepted practices and should not be considered a psychiatric disorder.

When is dissociation a problem? Because mild states do not usually cause a person much difficulty in everyday functioning, dissociation can be conceptualized as being on a continuum (Fig. 32-1). Formerly called multiple personality disorder, dissociative identity disorder (DID) obviously causes a person much more pain and impairs functioning to a much greater degree than will daydreaming. Everyday functioning deteriorates as the continuum is viewed from left to right.

◆ Definitions of Dissociative Disorders

The Diagnostic and Statistical Manual of Mental Disorders, fourth edition (DSM-IV), defines dissociative disorders as "a disruption in the usually integrated functions of consciousness, memory, identity, or perception of the environment. The disturbance may be sudden or gradual, transient or chronic"[1] (p 477).

Four disorders are included in this definition:

1. In *depersonalization disorder,* people feel that they are outside of their mind or body, much like an observer (Case Study 32-1).
2. *Dissociative amnesia* is characterized by loss of memory that is not organic and that involves an inability to recall events or facts too extensive to be labeled as mere forgetfulness.
3. *Dissociative fugue* involves sudden travel away from home coupled with an inability to remember the past and confusion about identity or the adoption of a new identity.
4. In *dissociative identity disorder,* the person acquires two or more identities or personality states (*alters*)

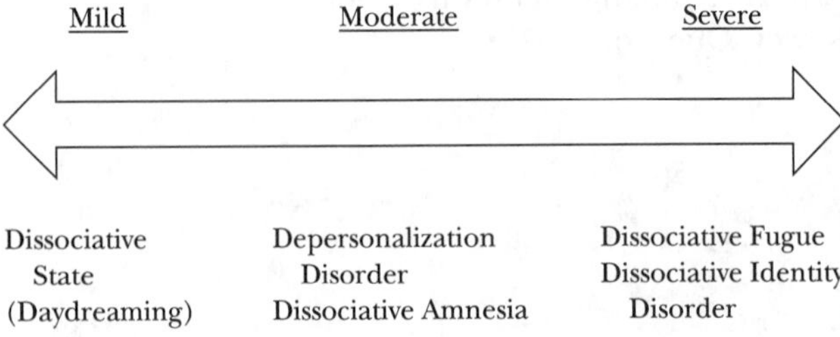

Figure 32-1. A Continuum of Dissociation

32-1 Case Study

A Client With Depersonalization Disorder

A 20-year-old male college student, John, sought psychiatric consultation because he was worried that he might be "going insane." For the last 2 years he had experienced increasingly frequent episodes of feeling "outside" himself. These episodes were accompanied by a sense of "deadness" in his body. In addition, during these periods, he was uncertain of his balance and frequently stumbled into furniture. This behavior was more likely to occur in public, especially if he was somewhat anxious. During these episodes, he felt a lack of natural control of his body and his thoughts seemed "foggy."

John's subjective sense of lack of control was especially troublesome, and he would fight it by shaking his head and saying "stop" to himself. This would momentarily clear his mind and restore his sense of autonomy but only temporarily; the feelings of "deadness" and of being outside himself would return. Gradually, over several hours, the unpleasant experiences would fade. The client was anxious, however, about their return, and he found them increasing in both frequency and duration.

John's grades actually improved over a 6-month period, because he was spending more time studying than had previously been the case. His girlfriend tired of listening to his symptoms and began dating other men. Although John was discouraged by his symptoms, he slept well at night, had noted no change in appetite, and had experienced no problem with concentration. He felt neither tired nor "edgy" because of his worry.

Because a cousin had been hospitalized for many years with severe mental illness, John had begun to wonder if he might face a similar fate and sought reassurance on the matter.

Questions for Discussion

1. What are possible factors related to the development of John's depersonalization disorder?
2. How would you evaluate and reassure John, considering his fears of severe mental illness?

(Used with permission. From Spitzer, RL, Gibbon, M, Skodol, AE, Williams, JBW, First, MB (eds): DSM-IV Casebook. Washington, DC, American Psychiatric Press, 1994)

that take control of behavior. As with amnesia, this disorder involves an inability to recall important personal information that is too extensive in nature to be labeled as forgetfulness.

Box 32-1 outlines DSM-IV criteria for these four disorders. The DSM-IV also includes a fifth category, *dissociative disorder not otherwise specified.* The disorders in this category have a dissociative symptom as a primary feature but do not meet the criteria for any of the four dissociative disorders. Examples of disorders in this category include brainwashing, loss of consciousness not attributable to a medical condition, and trance disorder. In this definition, the trance disorder is not a normal part of a broadly accepted collective cultural or religious practice.

◆ Etiology

BIOLOGICAL FACTORS

Dissociative symptoms can be induced by various substances or by a medical condition. For example, amnesia may be caused by a seizure disorder or by prolonged use of alcohol. It is important, then, for clients to be thoroughly evaluated medically before definitively diagnosing dissociative disorder as psychological in origin.

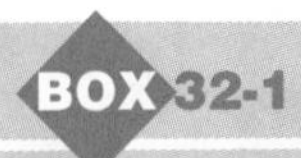

DSM-IV Diagnostic Criteria for Depersonalization Disorder

A. Persistent or recurrent experiences of feeling detached from, and as if one is an outside observer of, one's mental processes or body (eg, feeling like one is in a dream).
B. During the depersonalization experience, reality testing remains intact.
C. The depersonalization causes clinically significant distress or impairment in social, occupational, or other important areas of functioning.
D. The depersonalization experience does not occur exclusively during the course of another mental disorder and is not due to the direct physiological effects of a substance (eg, a drug of abuse, a medication) or a general medical condition (eg, temporal lobe epilepsy).

DISSOCIATIVE AMNESIA

A. The predominant disturbance is one or more episodes of inability to recall important personal information, usually of a traumatic or stressful nature, that is too extensive to be explained by ordinary forgetfulness.
B. The disturbance does not occur exclusively during the course of Dissociative Identity Disorder, Dissociative Fugue, Posttraumatic Stress Disorder, Acute Stress Disorder, or Somatization Disorder and is not due to the direct physiological effects of a substance (eg, a drug of abuse, a medication) or a neurological or other general medical condition (eg, Amnestic Disorder Due to Head Trauma).
C. The symptoms cause clinically significant distress or impairment in social, occupational, or other important areas of functioning.

DISSOCIATIVE FUGUE

A. The predominant disturbance is sudden, unexpected travel away from home or one's customary place of work, with inability to recall one's past.
B. Confusion about personal identity or assumption of a new identity (partial or complete).
C. The disturbance does not occur exclusively during the course of dissociative identity disorder and is not due to the direct physiological effects of a substance (eg, a drug of abuse, a medication) or a general medical condition (eg, temporal lobe epilepsy).
D. The symptoms cause clinically significant distress or impairment in social, occupational, or other important areas of functioning.

DISSOCIATIVE IDENTITY DISORDER

A. The presence of two or more distinct identities or personality states (each with its own relatively enduring pattern of perceiving, relating to, and thinking about the environment and self).
B. At least two of these identities or personality states recurrently take control of the person's behavior.
C. Inability to recall important personal information that is too extensive to be explained by ordinary forgetfulness.
D. The disturbance is not due to the direct physiological effects of a substance (eg, blackouts or chaotic behavior during Alcohol Intoxication) or a general medical condition (eg, complex partial seizures). **Note:** In children, the symptoms are not attributable to imaginary playmates or other fantasy play.

People with dissociative amnesia, depersonalization disorder, and dissociative identity disorder (DID) appear to be particularly susceptible to being hypnotized when tested for this capacity. Clients with depersonalization disorder and DID also seem to have a high capacity to dissociate.[1] This ability to dissociate is believed to be originated, in part, by having the biological capacity to perform this function when subjected to repeated stress.[6,9]

PSYCHOSOCIAL FACTORS

Dissociative disorders not caused by substances or medical conditions are believed to be primarily psychological in origin.[18] These illnesses allow a person to avoid anxiety while providing a way for some needs to be met. In other words, using the defense mechanism *repression* helps a person not only survive trauma, but also function to a degree (Case Studies 32-2 and 32-3). Abused people, as those with DID, are especially prone to using dissociation to defend against feeling the pain of remembering what has been done to them.

◆ Cultural Considerations in Diagnosing Dissociative Disorders

Cultural considerations regarding dissociative disorders include the acknowledgment that trance states are seen in cultures in Indonesia, Malaysia, the Arctic, India, and Latin America. These trance states are seen or induced as part of a system of spiritual beliefs. In dissociative trance, there is a narrowing of awareness of the person's

Case Study

A Client With Dissociative Amnesia

A 18-year-old man, Sam, was brought to a hospital emergency room by the Coast Guard. He appeared exhausted and showed evidence of overexposure to the sun. He named the date incorrectly, and it was difficult to get him to focus on specific questions. With encouragement, however, he was able to supply some facts. He remembered sailing with friends off the Florida coast when they encountered bad weather. The client was unable to recall any following events and did not know what had happened to his friends. He had to be reminded several times that he was now in a hospital and seemed surprised every time he was told.

Other than being exhausted, Sam was in good physical condition. After sleeping 6 hours, he remembered where he was and that he had fallen asleep after being interviewed. He still could not recall the events of the sailing trip, although he knew he was a student and had a good relationship with his family and friends. He had no psychiatric history and denied abuse of alcohol or other drugs.

Because of his good physical condition, Sam was considered to be a candidate for a sodium amytal ("truth serum") interview in which he would be prompted to remember the sailing events. He subsequently revealed that when bad weather erupted, he secured himself to the boat. His friends did not do this and were washed overboard. For 3 days, Sam had existed on a small supply of food until he was picked up by the Coast Guard. He never saw his friends again.

Questions for Discussion

1. How was Sam's amnesia a "survival mechanism"?
2. What kind of treatment will Sam need now that he has regained his memory?

(Used with permission. From Spitzer, RL, Gibbon, M, Skodol, AE, Williams, JBW, First, MB (eds): DSM-IV Casebook. Washington, DC, American Psychiatric Press, 1994)

Case Study

A Client With Dissociative Fugue

The client is a 42-year-old man who was brought to the emergency room by the police. He was involved in a fight at the diner where he is employed. When questioned, he gave his name as Burt Tate, but he had no identification. He had come to town several weeks earlier but could not recall where he had worked or lived prior to this time.

When asked, the client accurately related the current date and named the town. The fact that he could not recall his past life did not appear to cause him distress. He had no physical abnormalities nor was there evidence of alcohol or other drug abuse.

The police found that Mr. Tate met the description of a missing man, a Mr. Saunders, who had disappeared 1 month before from a city 200 miles away. Mrs. Saunders confirmed the identity of her husband. She explained that for 18 months before his disappearance, Mr. Saunders, who was a middle-level manager at a large manufacturing company, had been having considerable difficulty at work. He had been passed over for a promotion, and his supervisor had been very critical of his work. Several of his staff had left the company for other jobs, and the client found it impossible to meet production goals.

Work stress made him very difficult to live with at home. Previously an easy going, gregarious person, he became withdrawn and critical of his wife and children. Immediately preceding his disappearance, he had had a violent argument with his 18-year-old son. The son had called him a "failure" and stormed out of the house to live with some friends who had an apartment. Two days after this argument the client disappeared.

When brought into the room where his wife was waiting, Mr. Saunders stated that he did not recognize her. He appeared noticeably anxious.

Questions for Discussion

1. Why is this case diagnosed as dissociative fugue instead of DID?
2. How would you help Mr. Saunders reunite with his wife and children?

(Used with permission. From Spitzer, RL, Gibbon, M, Skodol, AE, Williams, JBW, First, MB (eds): DSM-IV Casebook. Washington, DC, American Psychiatric Press, 1994)

immediate surroundings. There may also be stereotyped behaviors or movements that are beyond the person's control. "Possession trance" in these cultures involves acquiring a new identity that is attributed to the influence of a spirit, power, deity, or other person. For diagnostic purposes, an individual must be experiencing dysfunction and stress, and the behaviors noted must not be a normal part of a broadly accepted collective cultural or religious practice.[1]

Research has shown that DID can be misdiagnosed in the Hispanic population because "ataque de nervios" or "Puerto Rican syndrome" is accepted as a diagnosis for this group, yet it has symptoms similar to DID. Amnesia is a predominant symptom of "ataque" and is often a culturally acceptable reaction to stress within the Hispanic community (Case Study 32-4).

◆ Addictions and Dissociative Disorders

Experts on dissociative disorders have found that there is a link between addictive behaviors, particularly eating disorders, and dissociative disorders.[16,4] Some eating disordered clients report trancelike experiences during episodes of binge eating or purging. Some feel "unreal" when binge eating.[4]

Case Study

Dissociative Identity Disorder With Cross-Cultural Issues

Mrs. C, a 40-year-old divorced Hispanic woman, contacted a Hispanic clinic in Connecticut at the suggestion of her previous psychiatrist in Puerto Rico. For 18 years, Mrs. C's diagnoses had included depression, schizophrenia, post-traumatic stress disorder, schizoaffective disorder, and hysterical personality. Antipsychotic and antidepressant medications had provided no relief. A complete history revealed that Mrs. C had been both severely physically and sexually abused by her parents. She had been married twice, and both husbands were physically and emotionally abusive to her.

Mrs. C's episodes of "ataque" included experiencing auditory and visual hallucinations, with the voices originating both from herself and from "spirits." She further described the voices as being command voices that were telling her to harm herself. Amnesia, rapid mood swings, and "out of body experiences" were syndromes that she had experienced since childhood. She sometimes referred to herself by another name during therapy sessions and did not remember previous sessions.

For 1 year in this current therapy, Mrs. C began to display different alternate personalities. In examining the total picture of her symptoms, Mrs. C was accurately diagnosed as having dissociative identity disorder. Separate symptoms over the years had complicated a diagnosis for Mrs. C, and cultural acceptance of "ataque" had been a complicating factor.

Questions for Discussion

1. What individual symptoms, when evaluated collectively, indicated that Mrs. C has dissociative identity disorder?
2. How do certain symptoms or syndromes come to be more acceptable in some cultures than in others?

(Used with permission. From Spitzer, RL, Gibbon, M, Skodol, AE, Williams, JBW, First, MB (eds): DSM-IV Casebook. Washington, DC, American Psychiatric Press, 1994)

Clients with DID who have an additional diagnosis of eating disorder may develop the eating dysfunction as a coping mechanism to handle abuse. Binge eating can be seen as a form of self-medication, a way of comforting oneself and escaping frightening feelings. Some anorectic clients were told that they are not worthy to eat and adopt starvation as a punishing technique.[4]

When a client with an eating disorder presents for treatment, it is wise to assess for symptoms of a dissociative disorder. Presence of atypical eating behaviors, such as the onset of anorexia and bulimia later in life, combined with a history of multiple symptoms and previous treatment failures could signal dissociative disorder. In this case, the dissociative disorder should be the focus of primary treatment with the eating disorder considered secondary.[16]

Chemically dependent clients may also use their substance of choice to deal with dissociative symptoms. In one study of 100 people with serious chemical dependency problems, 39 were found to have a dissociative disorder, and 43 reported childhood abuse. Because substance abuse can be the cause rather than the result of dissociative symptoms, the researcher emphasizes that the study needs to be replicated. Given the results of this study, the preliminary findings indicate that further investigation is warranted.[23]

THE ROLE OF FAMILY DYNAMICS

The concept of "self psychology" supports the importance of a parent's "mirroring" a child's budding self-esteem. For a child to become a mentally healthy adult, a parent must confirm and admire the child's specialness in the first few years of life. Later, in a functional relationship with the parent, the child uses the parent(s) as an idealizing self-object, meaning that the child views the parent as a source of strength, care, and calmness. This foundation will then enable the child to grow into an adult who has high self-esteem and self-confidence.[14]

A healthy family system allows open communication among family members, including the expression of negative and positive feelings. Tough questions are answered honestly, and family secrets, such as alcohol abuse, are discouraged. While family members may share some common qualities, there is respect for individual differences. The need to control relationships is low.[7]

Conversely, abusive family systems are rigid, closed, and may lead to the development of DID. Power and control issues are priorities in this family system, and power is often used abusively to maintain control. Change and diversity are rarely permitted. The following beliefs are commonly held:

- People are basically bad and must be continually controlled to make them good.
- Children are bad if they express any needs that are in opposition to those of the abuser.
- Severe punishment is the best method to control a bad child.
- Survival for children depends on absolute obedience to the abusers.
- Children have no rights.
- Children are objects to be used for the pleasure and benefit of others in the family.[7]

Physical and sexual abuse are common in families that hold these beliefs. The abused child may be told by the abuser that if he or she tells another family member what is going on, that person will die. The abused child then feels responsible for the life of the potentially threatened member. Oddly enough, the child may form an attachment to the abuser, because there is no one else to whom to turn for protection. Instead of having a healthy role model to internalize, the child will internalize the characteristics of the person who is available—the abuser. The child's "mirror" will be the abuser, and his or her emotional "attachment" will be out of a desperate attempt to survive. The only calming experience the child will have is the protection that DID provides.[2] The development of personality fragments or "alters" will provide the child with a buffer for not feeling the overwhelming trauma. For example, generating an alter will help a child emotionally remain in her family without conscious awareness of repeated abuse so that she will not have to feel the pain of being betrayed by someone on whom she is dependent[13] (Case Study 32-5).

The diagnosis of DID is made three to nine times more frequently in adult females than in adult males. Women tend to have more "alters" than do men; women average 15 or more personality fragments, while men average eight.[1] Although child abuse in boys is certainly prevalent and must always be considered, abuse toward girls has historically been more evident.

◆ Repressed Memories: Are They Real?

The dramatic rise in reported cases of DID in the United States has caused the diagnosis to come under question. While some professionals believe that the disorder appears more prevalent because more awareness has been promoted, others assert that this syndrome has been overdiagnosed in people who are highly suggestible.[1]

University of Washington researcher Elizabeth Loftus, an experimental psychologist, asserts that there is no scientific evidence that long-forgotten memories can be suddenly remembered. Loftus does not dispute that many people are abused as children or that they may try to avoid the memories as adults. She contends, though, that there is no evidence to support that memories can be completely repressed and then remembered later in life in complete detail. Loftus and other therapists are concerned that if a client cannot remember abuse, some therapists will "suggest" it until the person does "remember." Loftus believes that memories become distorted and cannot be recalled in their original form.[21]

Supporting this position, David Holmes of the University of Kansas reviewed 60 years of research and found no controlled studies showing that an event can be accurately recalled after years of repression. Also, studies of children who have experienced murder of their parents and other horrific events show that these children are continually flooded with pangs of emotion about the incidents. In other words, the children do remember.[17]

Other therapists, such as Helen R. Friedman, a clinical psychologist in St. Louis who claims to have a high number of clients with DID, argue that when one sees the symptoms of DID and the presence of "alters," the validity of the diagnosis cannot be questioned.[24]

Far from seeking out or encouraging abuse disclosures, many therapists state that when they began treating survivors of devastating childhood trauma, they often did not believe what they were hearing and did not understand the symptoms that they were witnessing. Instead, they tried to diagnose these clients with "acceptable" diagnoses, such as borderline, schizophrenia, and hysteria. The therapists were resistant to admitting that the clients were in terrible emotional shape because of the things that had been done to them.

Case Study

A Client With Dissociative Identity Disorder

Mary K is a 35-year-old social worker who was referred to a psychiatrist for treatment associated with chronic pain. During her evaluation, the client reported the strange observation that on many occasions when she returned home from work, the gas tank of the car was nearly full, yet when she got into the car to go to work the next day, it was half empty. She began to keep track of the odometer and discovered that on many nights, 50 to 100 miles would be put on the car overnight. The client, however, had no memory of driving it anywhere. Further questioning revealed that she had gaps in her memory for large parts of her childhood.

After several months of hypnosis for pain control, the explanation for the lost time emerged. One day while the client was under hypnosis, the physician again asked about the lost time. Suddenly a different voice responded, "It's about time you knew about me." The personality (alter) with a slightly different name, Marian, now spoke and described the drives that she took at night to "work out problems." As the physician got to know Marian, it was apparent that she was as abrupt and hostile as Mary was compliant and concerned about others. Marian considered Mary to be rather pathetic and far too interested in pleasing. She said that "worrying about anyone but yourself is a waste of time."

In the course of therapy, six other personalities emerged. The memories that finally surfaced were those of physical and sexual abuse by Mary's father and Mary's guilt about not having protected other children in the family from such abuse. After 4 years of psychotherapy, Mary gradually integrated parts of her multiple personalities.

Questions for Discussion

1. What other signs of dissociative identity disorder should be monitored in Mary's daily life?
2. What is the role of psychiatric nursing for the long-term course of her therapy?

(Used with permission. From Spitzer, RL, Gibbon, M, Skodol, AE, Williams, JBW, First, MB (eds): DSM-IV Casebook. Washington, DC, American Psychiatric Press, 1994)

Colin Ross, MD, a leading researcher and writer on DID, states that working with severely abused clients and listening to their stories is like watching hours of atrocity films. Therapists treating DID clients agree that the impossible-to-fake agony of these people is the most powerful evidence for the truth of their experiences. Is every detail that a client describes true? Ross, who estimates that approximately 5% of clients on adult psychiatric inpatient units have DID,[22] believes that it is not an error to maintain some skepticism when hearing terrifying stories of abuse, particularly satanic ritual abuse. Other therapists treating DID might also agree that every detail of what a client recounts does not have to be believed. What becomes most important, however, is believing in the abuse itself and in the client's pain and suffering.[29]

THE ROLE OF RITUAL ABUSE

Ritual abuse is a severe form of abuse in which a child is repeatedly physically and sexually abused in ceremonies by an organized group of perpetrators. Such groups may be pseudoreligious (as in satanic cults), or they may not associate themselves with a religious belief. The abuse in ritual abuse is frequently violent and may involve threats of death or the witnessing of death of other victims, both human and animal.[10]

Although it is sometimes difficult for a therapist or

nursing staff to believe the stories of horror that a client may begin to remember, it is wise for professionals to be alert to the self-protective countertransference dynamics that may be evoked as information is presented by the client. Many stories are difficult to hear and therefore hard to believe. While accounts of ritual abuse have been doubted, some therapists point to comparable stories related independently by people who are geographically and personally unrelated.[28]

The uniqueness of ritual abuse that causes it to differ from other settings of extreme abuse is the presence of structured alters that the cult has established in the child to serve particular cult functions. These functions usually lie outside the awareness of the child's core (or "host") personality. Unless the person seeks therapy later in adulthood for help with breaking free from the cult, he or she will usually maintain lifelong ties. Examples of cult functions that the individual will be programmed to perform are maintaining contact with the cult and reporting information, self-injuring if the ties to the cult are broken, and disrupting the therapeutic process that could lead to the client breaking free of the cult. The challenge for the therapist and nursing staff is to form a therapeutic alliance with the client's alters so that the client will have a reasonable chance to make healthy, self-protective choices.[12]

◆ Treatment Modalities

INDIVIDUAL THERAPY

Because the onset of dissociative amnesia and dissociative fugue is often acute, supporting the client in talking about recent events may prompt rapid recovery of memory. If talking alone is not effective, hypnosis may be helpful to prompt the client to reveal events and feelings and ultimately assist in restoring the person's memory. A sodium amytal ("truth serum") interview may also be an effective approach if conducted soon after the onset of the amnesia. Supporting the client with depersonalization disorder to talk about antecedent events surrounding the client's feelings of anxiety and then planning behavioral techniques to cope with stressful situations are effective treatment strategies.

Because of the extreme severity of DID, only psychotherapists who are trained in working with these clients should provide individual therapy. Initially these individuals can be fascinating to work with, but they can also become overwhelming as personality fragments (alters) appear. Untrained therapists may find themselves having intense countertransference reactions, either wanting to overprotect the client or wanting to flee from the client. Advanced Practice Nurses may have occasion to work in therapy with DID clients, while generalist nurses will need specialized knowledge in milieu management (Nursing Care Plan 32-1).

GROUP THERAPY

While group therapy may be helpful for people with a dissociative process that is less severe than DID, the value of group therapy must be carefully assessed for DID clients. Group work may be too intense and threatening for these clients, and the type of group should be evaluated carefully. Generally, a highly structured group with a clear focus and time frame seems to be most useful.

As clients with dissociative disorder progress in their recovery, a 12-step group may be a helpful adjunct to individual therapy when their work includes recovery from addictions. However, because 12-step programs promote belief in a higher power, it is important that the client not feel overwhelmed or threatened by this concept.

PHARMACOTHERAPY

Psychotropic medication is not a primary treatment for dissociative disorders.[3] Antianxiety medications, such as lorazepam, however, may be helpful for short-term management of severe anxiety. Antidepressant medication may also be indicated, but clients should be evaluated on an individual basis for necessity and category of drug. With DID clients, it is not uncommon for the different alters to report conflicting responses and side effects to the same medication. Also, for DID clients who hear voices, antipsychotic medications are generally ineffective.

ART THERAPY

Art therapy is a helpful adjunct when well timed and led by a trained professional who has knowledge of dissociative disorders. Art therapy encourages clients to tell their stories in a nonthreatening way; it is a safe alternative to acting out feelings destructively and a means to erode denial gently. Art may often present the whole picture of a client long before the client's consciousness can grasp what has happened in the past. For DID clients, art can also be a useful tool for promoting integration of alters. The different personalities can participate in a common activity and contribute toward a collective whole.[11]

MILIEU MANAGEMENT

Clients with dissociative disorders may be hospitalized in psychiatric inpatient units when their symptoms interfere grossly with daily functioning, when they are out of touch with reality, or when they are a danger to self or others.

Nursing Care Plan 32-1

Dissociative Identity Disorder

Susan, a 20-year-old part-time college student, was admitted to a psychiatric unit for evaluation of suicidal ideations. A psychological history revealed that she had attempted suicide by cutting her wrists two years ago. As a child, Susan had been physically and sexually abused by several male family members for approximately seven years. Susan first sought psychiatric treatment at age 17 and had been diagnosed as having Major Depression with Borderline Personality Disorder. Separate trials with several antidepressant medications failed to provide relief from her symptoms, which included self-destructive thoughts, feelings of hopelessness, and occasional mood swings.

During this hospitalization, Susan admitted to hearing voices and having an imaginary companion who had "tried to protect her" since childhood. As her treatment increased, she began to exhibit different child-like behaviors and trance-like positions. Susan's subjective distress also increased, and she began saying, "I just want to die." Further therapy revealed that Susan had two alternate personalities, "Betty" and "Barb." Barb was the older of the two "alters" and tried to protect Betty, the abused child.

Nursing Diagnosis

Risk for Self-Mutilation related to emerging memories of abuse

Outcome

Client will remain physically safe.

Intervention	Rationale
Negotiate a "no harm" contract with client. All "alters" should be included in the contract and held accountable.	Agreement with "no harm" contract increases client safety and responsibility for self.
Help client identify coping mechanisms and activities she enjoys, and encourage her to use them when she considers self-harm.	Coping mechanisms and enjoyable activities can be calming and avert self-harm crisis.
Encourage client to identify at least one "safe" person per shift that she can turn to for support.	Availability of one "safe" person promotes client's sense of security and responsibility.

Evaluation

Client complies with "no harm" contrast and remains physically safe.

Nursing Diagnosis

Personal Identity Disturbance related to presence of multiple alters

Outcome

Client will learn to maintain the healthy, adult part of the self.

Intervention	Rationale
Orient client using physical means; light areas if dark, ask client to keep eyes open and hold eye contact, reposition client, ask her to walk and observe surroundings.	Orientation measures can break the dissociative state by focusing client on physical reality. Senses connect client to the "here and now."

continued

Nursing Care Plan 32-1 (Continued)

Intervention	Rationale
Orient client verbally; call by her legal name, not an "alter," identify yourself and the place, day, and date if needed, ask her to look in a mirror to see that she is an adult, if measure is not too alarming.	"Grounding" techniques remind clients that they are in the present and are safe and adult.
Support client's therapy program.	Therapy moves client toward personality integration.

Evaluation

Emergence of alters decreases and client becomes more integrated.

All disciplines that work with clients with dissociative disorder will be responsible for effective milieu management, but no other discipline will be involved as much as nursing. Staff nurses set the tone of the unit and see that guidelines are upheld. Some of these guidelines follow:

- Involvement in the unit and following rules for appropriate behavior should be expected of dissociative disorder clients. This expectation conveys a sense of self-responsibility and ultimately empowerment as the client learns coping skills.
- Staff should convey that impulses related to violent and self-injurious behavior need to be verbalized rather than acted out. This includes contracting with the client for safety.[26] Physical restraints should be used only as a last resort due to their traumatic nature.
- Consistency in treatment issues must be upheld among the staff. Because of their histories of mistreatment and abuse, it is not uncommon for clients with DID to try to split the staff into "good" people and "bad" people. Testing staff to determine trustworthiness and reliability also should be expected.[6]

Other issues to address regarding DID clients follow:

- DID clients will not easily accept new staff members or new peers.[26] People new to the milieu should allow the client physical and psychological space to allow her or him to determine closeness.
- Staff should use touch judiciously with DID clients and always ask if a gesture of touch is acceptable to the client. Because the client may have an exaggerated startle response, never touch the person from behind where the movement cannot be seen. The best guideline is not to touch the client unless there is sound therapeutic rationale for doing so and the client's permission has been obtained. Knowing which personality is giving permission is important to predict the response.[6]

Application of the Nursing Process to the Client With a Dissociative Disorder

ASSESSMENT

Behavior

Assessment of the client's behavior requires astute attention to multiple details, as in the following questions:

- Does the client exhibit inconsistencies in physical behaviors, such as switching right or left handedness; voice changes; or marked differences in clothing and hair styles on different occasions? These behaviors can indicate the presence of more than one personality.
- What is the client's sleeping pattern? Are nightmares present, and if so, what is their content? Are there any other disturbances in sleep?
- Has the client ever found herself at a place, unable to remember how she got there? This behavior indicates a "blackout," which, in the absence of other dissociative disorder symptoms, could indicate alcohol abuse.
- Has the client written notes or created artwork of which she has no memory?
- What is the client's eating pattern? Does she overeat or undereat, get rid of food by purging, or use alcohol or other drugs? How much does she use?

Thought and Perception

Assessment of the client's thoughts and perceptions provides essential information about past and present experiences. What is the client's earliest childhood memory? If the client reveals having an abusive childhood, the type of abuse, how long the abuse occurred, and the number of people involved should be ascertained. While DID is not usually diagnosed until adulthood, alters that emerge during therapy may be as young as 5 years old.[26] The following questions are helpful to assess thought and perception:

- Did the client ever have an imaginary childhood friend? If so, what was the nature of the relationship? Does the client still have conversations with this friend?
- Does the client have gaps in memory? Are there periods that cannot be remembered?
- Is the client sometimes accused of lying but does not think she has lied?
- Does the client sometimes feel as if she is standing outside herself as if watching another person?
- Does the client ever "space out" or go to a safe place in the mind to escape from a stressful situation? Is this deliberate, or does it seem to be something over which the client has no control?
- Does the client hear voices? Are the voices familiar or unfamiliar? What is the content that the voices are conveying? What is the age(s) of the voices? Do the voices have names? Does the client communicate with them?[8]
- Does the client refer to herself as "we" rather than "I"?
- Does the client exhibit rapid changes in mood and thought process during one interview?[26]
- Does the client express psychophysiological complaints, such as severe headaches, chest pain, or a fluctuation in pain threshold?

Assessment of Dissociative Disorders in Children

Diagnosing DID in children may be more difficult than in adolescents and adults, because the symptoms may be more subtle. Dissociation, however, can present in various forms. Amnesia may be present for information that most children would readily remember, such as their homeroom teacher and best friend's name, favorite activities, or important events. Pathological lying tends to be universal as the child tries to cover up not knowing certain information. Trancelike states that appear as dreamy or "spacy" may label the child as having attention problems in school. Often these children lag behind in class, still working on the last activity when the other students have moved on to other work. Difficulty concentrating is common as are auditory hallucinations that present as critical voices. The voice may sound like the abuser's voice. Behavioral problems may include aggression coupled with anger, self-injurious behaviors, and sexual acting out. Sleep disturbance and intermittent depression are common.[20]

Several assessment instruments are available to measure symptoms of pathology in children. Some depend on feedback from the parent or other caregiver, and some involve direct feedback from the child. However, no behavior or symptom rating can be used to assess for dissociative pathology on an ongoing basis. The instruments, while helpful, have their limitations.[19]

Examples of two standardized instruments most frequently used to measure the impact of sexual abuse on children are the Child Behavior Check List and the Louisville Behavior Checklist. Because these instruments are completed by the parents, information of a child's unusual behavior to which a caregiver may be sensitive could be revealed. An obvious disadvantage is that if the parent completing the instrument is the perpetrator, responses may be distorted. Another test, used by nurse-researchers, is the Traumatic Events Drawing Series, which evaluates stress responses of children to sexual abuse. Completed by the child, it is thought to be highly effective for examining the effects of sexual abuse. The Child Abuse and Trauma Questionnaire has five scales that measure physical abuse or punishment, psychological abuse, sexual abuse, neglect, and negative home atmosphere. It is completed by the child and considered to have good reliability. A drawback, however, is that there is latitude for a wide variety of interpretations of answers. For example, what might be considered abuse in one family or culture may not be considered abuse in another setting.[19]

NURSING DIAGNOSIS

Possible nursing diagnoses for a client with a dissociative disorder include the following:

- Personal Identity Disturbance related to multiple alters or amnesia for legal name and identity
- Risk for Self-Mutilation related to emerging memories of abuse
- Anxiety related to fragmented identity and nonintegrated self
- Chronic Low Self Esteem related to history of prolonged abuse
- Powerlessness, severe, related to being physically and emotionally controlled by others
- Ineffective Individual Coping related to possible substance abuse or eating disorders
- Sensory/Perceptual Alterations related to hearing voices of alters
- Body Image Disturbance related to history of physical or sexual abuse
- Sleep Pattern Disturbance related to nightmares or insomnia
- Altered Role Performance related to amnesia and resulting adoption of false identity and related to

inability to maintain employment, school work, or stable relationships
- Spiritual Distress related to satanic cult abuse and resulting conflict regarding religious issues

PLANNING

Throughout the process of the client's recovery, the treatment team must maintain a sense of collaboration and congruency to provide a milieu of safety and consistency. As much as possible, the client should be included in the treatment planning to foster the development of empowerment and self-responsibility.

Goals for the client with DID include expression and healing of feelings, reintegration of the self as much as possible, and learning new coping skills to deal with maladaptive behaviors. An important long-term goal is for the client to feel in control of his or her emotions.

In individual therapy, the client is supported in recalling early memories to produce "abreactions," that is, feelings associated with the traumatic events.[26] Talking with a therapist in a safe environment may help the client regress to the earlier, painful time, or hypnosis may be useful in bringing about regression. Working through the original feelings with a trusting person in a safe environment can help the client reintegrate the self. The therapist may find it necessary to work with all of the alters as different people in therapy for them to accept each other. Since integration of the personalities may not be possible, the client should be helped to acquire new coping skills to deal with maladaptive behaviors.

New coping skills that are important to discharge planning and may be practiced while the client is still in the hospital include calling a friend on the telephone to talk about feelings of anxiety or to focus on topics that decrease anxiety; using self-talk that reassures the client of safety; engaging in moderate exercise; and focusing on a favorite activity, such as painting, reading, singing, or watching a relaxing video.[5]

INTERVENTION

Nurses design care plans for dissociative disorder clients based on their individual needs. Nursing interventions for dissociative disorder clients include the following:

- Educating the client about the recovery process. Clients may have idealistic fantasies that the treatment team can give them a "quick fix." Clients need to know that they will need to uncover painful feelings and memories to begin recovery.
- Providing a safe, nonjudgmental environment to encourage the client to diminish defensive responses
- Monitoring the client's pace in uncovering memories. Moving too fast may be seen behaviorally in attempts at self-mutilation, symptoms of psychosis, and increased incidences of dissociation.
- Assisting the client in learning "grounding" techniques. These concrete techniques bring the client into the present and remind her that she is a safe adult (see Nursing Care Plan 32-1).
- Helping the client identify times when strong emotions begin to be overwhelming. Journaling antecedent events and developing a concrete plan for managing emotions are helpful strategies. An example of this intervention is found in Nursing Care Plan 32-1.
- Assisting the client in planning for discharge from the hospital. A measure that the client can use is compiling a list of people who can be contacted for support as needed. These people may include family members, friends, members of 12-step groups, and people staffing "hotlines." Lists should be posted where the client can see them, reminding him or her of options and lending a sense of control. Identifying safe places and comforting activities when feeling stressed will help the client continue to gain a feeling of self-responsibility and control.[5]

EVALUATION

How will nurses know whether the plan of care for the dissociative disorder client is effective? What will signs of recovery look like? Just as illness is a matter of degree, so too is recovery. Generally, a recovering client will slowly begin to trust people worth trusting. He or she will have personal boundaries and begin to trust feelings. The client will begin to try new activities with less fear and will be able to use new coping strategies to deal with anxiety some of the time. People reminiscent of the abuser will begin to remind him or her less of that person. The client will sleep better at night and will have times of contentment during the day.

◆ The Nurse's Feelings and Attitudes

Nurses who work with clients with dissociative disorder, especially those with DID, need much collaboration and support. How do nurses work with clients who have had unspeakable horrors done to them and still maintain some kind of psychological balance? Nurses must be able to process with each other honestly. Rotating the days of intense time spent with clients may help. Being able to say, "I'm dealing with some problems at home today. It would be helpful if I could be the medication nurse today" and knowing that nonjudgmental support will be offered are important. Believing in the team's approach and its consistency in treatment is vital to individual and group morale. When consistency is not present on a unit treating clients with dissociative disorder, staff splitting by clients and dysfunctional communication may be rampant.

A nurse's attitude toward DID clients may quickly become negative if she or he does not have a life outside of work. Replenishing oneself is important to maintain optimism in the face of client trauma. A support group is helpful, as are hobbies and other relaxing activities. Spiritual or religious beliefs may be uplifting when the burden of work becomes heavy.

◆ Chapter Summary

This chapter has presented the concept of dissociative disorder, with particular attention given to dissociative identity disorder. Major points include the following:

1. Dissociative disorders are usually caused by trauma. The individual attempts to deal with this trauma by escaping into the mind. Behaviors of the person, however, are dysfunctional.
2. Types of dissociative disorders include depersonalization disorder, dissociative amnesia, dissociative fugue, and dissociative identity disorder (DID, formerly called multiple personality disorder). The most severe of the dissociative disorders is DID.
3. The role of family dynamics is important in laying the foundation for DID. Prolonged physical or sexual abuse is a common factor in all cases of the disorder. Ritual abuse may be part of the history of some clients.
4. Although abuse usually begins in a person's childhood, DID is often not diagnosed until adulthood; DID is diagnosed three to nine times more frequently in women than in men.
5. Cultural considerations should be examined when diagnosing a dissociative disorder. Group and religious norms and the person's degree of functioning should be explored.
6. Treatment modalities for dissociative disorders may include individual and group therapy, art therapy, and milieu management.
7. The nursing assessment for DID should include detailed questions about the client's family history and the client's present level of functioning. The total client picture must be considered, because many clients with DID have been misdiagnosed, as symptoms were treated independently.
8. Nursing diagnoses include attention to the client's safety, level of anxiety, coping mechanisms, self-esteem, role performance, and multiple personality fragments.
9. Planning the client's treatment involves collaboration with the client and other disciplines. Goals include assisting the client with learning new coping strategies and in DID, reintegrating the client's personality as much as possible.
10. Interventions for DID clients include providing a consistent milieu for client safety, holding the client responsible for the behaviors of all alters teaching the client "grounding" techniques, and providing the client with opportunities to practice new coping strategies prior to discharge.
11. Recovery may be evaluated by the client's functional level. Recovery from DID is a lifelong process, and subtle, rather than dramatic, changes occur.
12. Working with clients with DID is exhausting and rewarding. Nurses must be aware of their own needs and maintain their own mental health.

Critical Thinking Questions

1. *What purposes are served by the development of symptoms of depersonalization?*
2. *Prior to your psychiatric nursing experience, what did you believe about the occurrence of DID (formerly called multiple personality disorder)? How have your views changed?*
3. *Imagine yourself as a student pursuing a postgraduate degree to please your parents, who place a great deal of importance on academic achievement. You have been experiencing symptoms that have been diagnosed as depersonalization disorder. Describe the symptoms you are experiencing and explain the possible underlying cause for them.*

Review Questions

1. Which of the following treatment modalities appears to be most appropriate for the client with DID?
   A. Antidepressant medication
   B. Group therapy
   C. Individual psychotherapy
   D. All of the above
2. Dissociative fugue has as its major symptom which of the following?
   A. Sudden travel away from home or place of work
   B. Several personality alters
   C. A feeling of being out of touch with one's body
   D. A positive blood alcohol level
3. Primary etiology for the dissociative disorders appears to be
   A. an identified defective gene.
   B. ineffective parenting.
   C. stresses of western culture.
   D. severe stress or trauma.

4. Define dissociation.
5. A childhood background of severe emotional or physical abuse may lead to the development of
   A. dissociative fugue.
   B. dissociative amnesia.
   C. DID.
   D. depersonalization disorder.
6. Which of the following symptoms may indicate that a client has DID?
   A. Rapid mood swings
   B. Depression that is responsive to antidepressant medication
   C. Gaps in memory that are easily retrieved
   D. All of the above
7. List two addictions that may be present in clients with dissociative disorders.
8. Milieu management on a psychiatric unit treating dissociative disorder clients will include
   A. contracting with clients for personal safety.
   B. providing consistent therapeutic treatment by all of the disciplines.
   C. being cautious regarding the use of physical touch.
   D. All of the above
9. The effectiveness of nursing interventions for dissociative disorder clients can be evaluated by
   A. the complete absence of symptoms.
   B. the client's feelings of contentment with self and life.
   C. being able to cope without support.
   D. rarely feeling afraid.

◆ References

1. American Psychiatric Association: Diagnostic and Statistical Manual of Mental Disorders, 4th ed. Washington, DC, American Psychiatric Association, 1994
2. Barach P: Multiple Personality Disorder as Attachment Disorder. Dissociation 4: 117–123, 1991
3. Barach PM: ISSD Guidelines for Treating Dissociative Identity Disorder: Multiple Personality Disorder in Adults. Skokie, IL, ISSD, 1994
4. Barber LC: Eating Disorders and MPD. Multiple Facets. The Journal of the Dissociative Disorders Foundation January–March: 7, 1991
5. Benham E: Coping Strategies: A Psychoeducational Approach to Post-traumatic Symptomatology. J Psychosoc Nurs Ment Health Serv 33 (6): 30–35, 1995
6. Braun BG: Issues in the Psychotherapy of Multiple Personality Disorder. Braun BG (ed): Treatment of Multiple Personality Disorder, pp 3–28. Washington, DC, American Psychiatric Press, 1986
7. Bryant D, Kessler J, Shirar L: The Family Inside: Working With the Multiple. New York, WW Norton, 1992
8. Curtain SL: Recognizing Multiple Personality Disorder. J Psychosoc Nurs Ment Health Serv 31 (2): 29–33, 1993
9. Fink D: The Comorbidity of Multiple Personality Disorder and DSM-III-R Axis II Disorders. Psychiatr Clin North Am 14 (3): 547–566, 1991
10. Fraser GA: Satanic Ritual Abuse: A Cause of Multiple Personality Disorder. Journal of Child and Youth Care 55–66, 1990
11. Frye B, Gannon L: The Use, Misuse, and Abuse of Art With Dissociative/Multiple Personality Disorder Patients. Dissociation 6 (2–3): 188–192, 1993
12. Gould C, Cozolino L: Ritual Abuse, Multiplicity, and Mind-Control. Journal of Psychology and Theology 20 (3): 194–196, 1992
13. Kluft RP: Clinical Presentations of Multiple Personality Disorder. Psychiatr Clin North Am 14 (3): 605–629, 1991
14. Kohut H: The Restoration of the Self. New York, International Universities Press, 1977
15. Lefkof GD: Common Questions Asked About Multiple Personality Disorder and Dissociation. Multiple Facets: The Journal of the Dissociative Disorders Foundation 5–21, 1992–1993
16. Levin AP, Kahan M, Lamm JB, Spauster E: Multiple Personality in Eating Disorder Patients. International Journal of Eating Disorders 13 (2): 235–239, 1993
17. Loftus EF: You Must Remember This . . . or Do You? How Real Are Repressed Memories? The Washington Post June 27: C1–C2, 1993
18. Maxmen JS, Ward JG: Essential Psychopathology and Its Treatment, 2d ed. New York, WW Norton, 1995
19. Pinegar C: Screening for Dissociative Disorders in Children and Adolescents. Journal of Child and Adolescent Psychiatric Nursing 8 (1): 5–14, 1995
20. Putnam FW: Dissociative Disorders in Children and Adolescents. Psychiatr Clin North Am 14 (3): 519–531, 1991
21. Roan S: Researchers Argue Validity of "Repressed Memory" Recall. Saint Paul Pioneer Press August 29: 1993
22. Ross CA, Anderson G, Fleisher WP, Norton GR: The Frequency of Multiple Personality Disorder Among Psychiatric Inpatients. Am J Psychiatry 148 (12): 1717–1720, 1991
23. Ross CA, Kronson J, Koensgen S, Barkman K, Clark P, Rockman G: Dissociative Comorbidity in 100 Chemically Dependent Patients. Hosp Community Psychiatry 43 (8): 840–842, 1992
24. Sileo CC: Multiple Personalities: The Experts Are Split. Insight October 25: 18–22, 1993
25. Spitzer RL, Gibbon M, Skodol AE, Williams JBW, First MB (eds): DSM-IV Case Book. Washington, DC, American Psychiatric Press, 1994
26. Stafford LL: Dissociation and Multiple Personality Disorder: A Challenge for Psychosocial Nurses. J Psychosoc Nurs Ment Health Serv 31 (1): 15–20, 1993
27. Steinberg M: Transcultural Issues in Psychiatry: The Ataque and Multiple Personality Disorder. Dissociation 3 (1): 31–33, 1990
28. Van Benschoten SC: Multiple Personality Disorder and Satanic Ritual Abuse: The Issue of Credibility. Dissociation 3 (1): 22–29, 1990
29. Wylie MS: The Shadow of a Doubt. Networker September–October: 18–29, 70, 1993

Application of the Nursing Process to Addictions

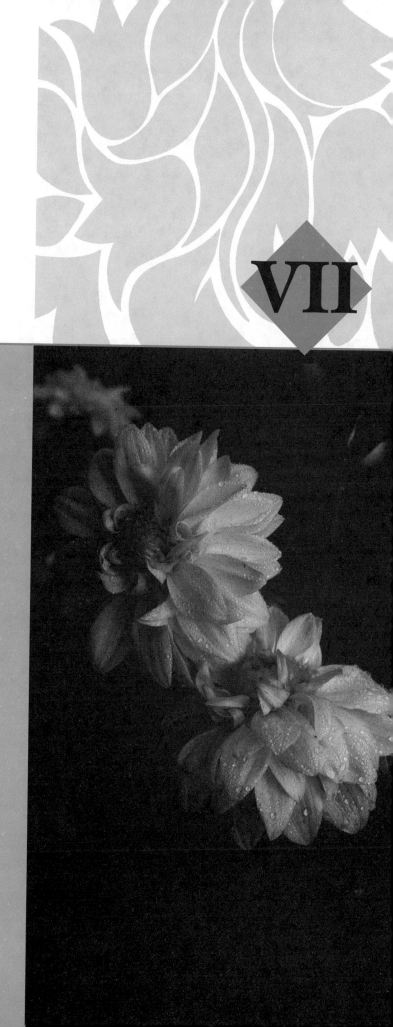

VII

Substance Abuse and Dependency

Barbara A. Thurston

33

O God that men should put an enemy in their mouths to steal away their brains: that we should with joy, pleasance, revel and applause, transform ourselves into beasts.

William Shakespeare,
Othello

This chapter discusses the abuse of substances that affect the central nervous system (CNS) and examines the physical and behavioral changes that occur in people who abuse and eventually become dependent on such substances. These substances are classified as drugs. The generic meaning of the term drug, *which includes ethyl alcohol (ethanol), applies throughout this chapter. Because alcohol is socially acceptable, it frequently does not elicit as forceful a relationship to drug classification as illegal drugs, such as heroin or cocaine, or even prescription drugs, such as barbiturates or amphetamines. Nevertheless, alcohol, by its properties and actions, is a drug that can be abused and needs to be treated as such.*

All drugs of abuse and dependency have certain factors in common, and certain factors are specific to each drug. This chapter addresses the commonalities of substance abuse and dependency and the factors particular to each drug classification. Wherever possible, the emphasis is on the common concepts. This generic concept embraces the idea that the problem of abuse or dependency and manifestations resulting from the problem may differ. For example, the manifestations of dependence on heroin differ from those of dependence on alcohol, but the core problem remains the same: the abuse of or dependence on a substance. People who abuse or become dependent on substances are impaired physically, socially, and psychologically at some time during their disorder. The behaviors manifested by people abusing drugs are not tolerated or accepted in most cultures. Prolonged abuse of or dependency on drugs and the concomitant adverse behavioral changes that affect the person's life and well-being usually culminate in a self-destructive course unless the substance use is discontinued or the lifestyle is altered. Ultimately, drug-dependent people must learn to adapt to the stresses of life with means other than the drug abuse. This chapter examines systems of classification and various concepts related to the etiology and dynamics of substance abuse and dependency. A focus is on the application of the nursing process to people who abuse or are dependent on drugs.

Learning Objectives

On completion of this chapter, you should be able to accomplish the following:

1. *Discuss the application of Selye's theory of stress and adaptation to the problems of substance abuse and dependency.*
2. *Define substance abuse and dependency, and explain current diagnostic categorization.*
3. *Differentiate among various types of substance abuse and dependency disorders.*
4. *Discuss the common etiological concepts related to substance abuse and dependency.*
5. *Discuss the incidence and significance of substance abuse and dependency.*
6. *Describe the dynamics, physical effects, behavioral changes, medical consequences, social and family problems, and specific characteristics of abuse or dependency on alcohol, sedatives, hypnotics, anxiolytics, narcotics, cocaine, amphetamine and similarly acting sympathomimetics, hallucinogens, and cannabis.*
7. *Apply the components of the nursing process to the client who abuses or is dependent on substances.*
8. *Recognize your own feelings and attitudes toward substance abuse and dependency disorders.*
9. *Explain the importance of recognition, intervention, rehabilitation, and prevention in the chemically impaired professional.*
10. *Recognize the importance of prevention in substance abuse and dependency as a physiopsychosocial problem on the continuum of human development from the unborn child to the elderly adult.*

◆ Stress and Adaptation and Substance Abuse

Hans Selye's stress adaptation syndrome may be applied to problems of substance abuse and dependency, with implications for the treatment and rehabilitation of drug-dependent people. (See Chapter 1, Introduction to Psychiatric-Mental Health Nursing, for a full discussion of Selye's theory of stress and adaptation.)

STRESS ADAPTATION SYNDROME

Stress, says Selye, is "the nonspecific response of the body to any demand made upon it."[59,60] Clearly, the source of the stress and the pleasantness or unpleasantness of the agent or situation of stress do not matter. What does matter is the intensity of the demand for adaptation or readjustment. Stressors, or stress-producing factors, differ in various situations and in the responses they elicit from people. Stressors may originate from physical, chemical, physiological, biological, and emotional sources and from the internal or external environment. Selye's *general adaptation syndrome* is composed of the following three stages:

1. *Alarm stage.* The body recognizes the internal or external stress that affects its physiological homeostasis and then prepares to resist by means of "fight or flight."
2. *Stage of resistance.* The body uses the defense mechanisms of fight or flight to repair the damage it suffered or to adapt to the stressor. If the body is unable to adapt, it will enter the third stage; if the person adapts to the stressor, the third stage is prevented.
3. *Stage of exhaustion.* If this stage of fatigue continues, physical or emotional diseases of adaptation (migraine headache, mental disorder) may occur. If this stage is not reversed, the body will be unable

to adapt and will become exhausted; death will ensue.[59,60]

Fight or Flight Mechanisms

Selye emphasizes the importance of making good use of adaptation energy to prevent the diseases of adaptation. The defense mechanisms of fight or flight may be applied to interpersonal relationships and to physiological problems. That is, a person may manage interpersonal stress by running away from or passively waiting out a situation that cannot be changed. The choice of the proper defense needs to be tailored to each situation. To remember how to use these adaptation mechanisms wisely to achieve goals, particularly when events threaten equanimity or cause concern or doubt, Selye created the following jingle:

> Fight for your highest attainable aim.
> But never put up resistance in vain.[60]

The process of reflection and choice of an appropriate response for the situation and circumstances may appear simple, but it is a complex task. Selye believes that each person has to live life as innate freedom of choice directs.[59,60]

DRUG DEPENDENCE AS A MEANS OF COPING

The general adaptation syndrome and proper choice of adaptation methods can be applied to the issues of substance abuse and dependency: Drug use, abuse, and dependency serve a purpose for the chemical-dependent person. There are legitimate reasons for the use of many drugs. Ethyl alcohol is a drug and a legal substance with approved recreational and social use. Many people drink alcoholic beverages without encountering problems. Some drugs, such as narcotics and sedative-hypnotics, are controlled substances and are used for medical purposes to alleviate physical pain and emotional suffering. When taken as prescribed under medical supervision, these drugs may be used to diminish stress without the serious adverse consequences of abuse and dependency.

For the person who abuses or is dependent on substances, the drugs have become a way of coping or adapting to any of life's stressors. In other words, drugs are a way of life for this person.

The person may use drugs to relieve anxiety or unpleasant feelings of any kind, to experience and increase pleasant or "high" sensations, to sustain a world of daydreams or an existence beyond the bounds of reality, and to express or repress feelings of joy, love, anger, or hate. Drugs not only do things *to* people who take them, they also do things *for* people who take them. Thus, it is important to understand what these substances do for people to effect primary prevention of chemical dependence and to help people adapt to or cope with stress in a more effective, healthy manner.

Substance abuse and dependence cuts across all socioeconomic and cultural groups and all ages. The reasons for misuse of, abuse of, and dependence on drugs generally include an attempt to adapt to stress. Ironically, the process becomes a vicious cycle, because the method of adapting to life's stressors becomes another stressor and eventually a disease of dependency. There is no single etiological concept to explain the cause of substance-related disorders (see Etiological Factors). Biological, social, and psychological factors are considered to have a part in the cause. Although the cause is multifunctional, using substances as a coping mechanism for stress must also be considered as a factor in the development of the disease process (Fig. 33-1).

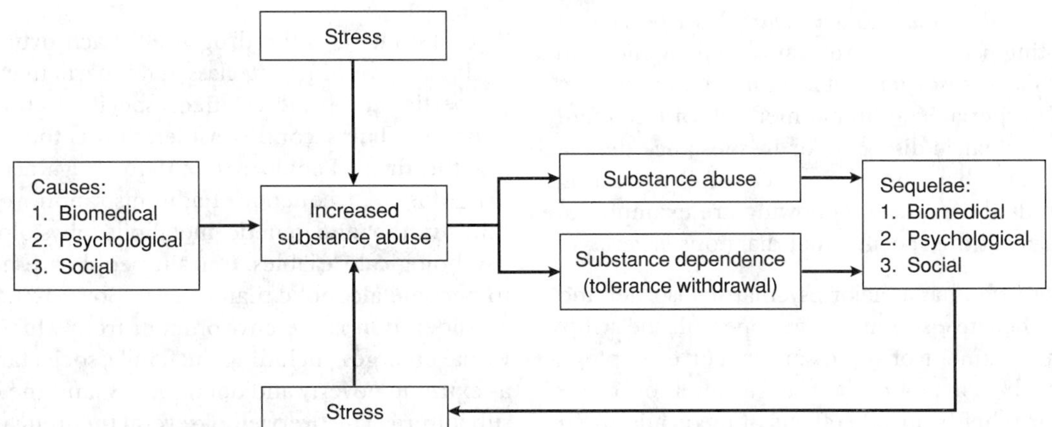

Figure 33-1. A conceptual model of substance abuse. (From Clark, HW, et al: Substance Related Disorders: Alcohol and Drugs, in Goldman, H.: Review of General Psychiatry, Appleton and Lange, CT, 1995.)

The use of drugs as a coping mechanism destroys or diminishes a person's ability to master life's events. Letting go of substance abuse as a method of adaptation and learning healthy methods of adaptation may result in successful recovery from chemical dependence.

◆ Defining Substance Abuse and Dependency

The fourth edition of the Diagnostic and Statistical Manual of Mental Disorders (DSM-IV) classifies the use of substances as substance-related disorders. This classification includes disorders related to drugs of abuse and the side effects of medications or exposure to a toxin. The use of the term substance in the criteria can indicate a drug of abuse, a medication, or a toxin. The substance-related disorders are divided into two categories:

1. Substance use disorders, which include substance dependence and substance abuse (Box 33-1)
2. Substance-induced disorder

The category of substance-induced disorders describes the mental disorders caused by the substance. The substance may cause more than one syndrome (Table 33-1). Some symptoms are similar; others are different. For example, symptoms of withdrawal from alcohol and withdrawal from sedative-hypnotics are similar, but symptoms of opioid withdrawal differ. The symptoms of delirium are the same for any mental cognitive disorder regardless of etiology, but delirium associated with drugs has a specific cause that must be incorporated into the client's plan of care.

DUAL DIAGNOSIS

The terms *dual diagnosis* and *comorbidity* describe a client with coexisting psychoactive substance dependency and major psychiatric disorder that are unrelated and meet the DSM-IV criteria. Traditional methods of treatment for major psychiatric disorders or in substance dependence programs have not been successful in treating clients with dual diagnoses. Following are examples of clients who meet the specific dual diagnosis criteria:

1. The client who has a major psychiatric disorder and uses psychoactive substances to cope with the symptoms or treatment of the disorder. For example, a client with schizophrenia uses alcohol or other drugs for relief from side effects of medications. (If this client did not meet the criteria for substance dependency, then treatment for the psychiatric illness would relieve both problems, and treatment and rehabilitation would focus primarily on the major psychiatric disorder.)
2. The client who has psychoactive dependency disorder and presents psychiatric symptoms as a result of intoxication or withdrawal or other effects of the psychoactive substance used. For example, a client has a psychotic episode produced by the use of amphetamines. (The treatment for substance abuse would alleviate the symptoms; treatment and rehabilitation would focus on substance dependence.)
3. The client with a dual diagnosis of two basically unrelated psychiatric disorders that may interact to exacerbate each other. For example, a client has bipolar disorder and alcohol dependence. (Treatment and rehabilitation need to address the bipolar disorder and substance dependency.)

Research on identification, treatment, and rehabilitation of clients with dual diagnoses is needed. In one state, 30% to 40% of the outpatient and 60% to 80% of the inpatient population among the chronically mentally ill are dually diagnosed with addictive and nonaddictive psychiatric disorders.[23] A specific program for clients with dual diagnosis has been created in that state. The National Institute of Mental Health has granted funds to a number of states for projects related to clients with dual diagnosis.

◆ Etiological Factors

No single theoretical concept explains the etiology of substance abuse and dependency. The etiological factors are complex and varied.

THE DRUG, THE ENVIRONMENT, AND THE INDIVIDUAL

The Drug

The first factor is the drug itself. Each drug class and each drug within that class have particular chemical properties and produce effects specific to the chemical structure. The second consideration is the person taking the drug. People respond to drugs according to drug dosage, frequency of administration, route of administration, and genetic, metabolic, physiological, and psychological variables. Certain people are more likely to become alcoholic than others (Box 33-2). The third consideration is the environment from which the individual emerges, including the family; social factors, such as extreme poverty and delinquency; and the culture or subculture. The overview of several theoretical concepts postulated to explain the nature and cause of substance abuse and dependency includes some concepts specific to the drugs of abuse (eg, the disease concept of alco-

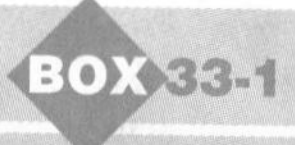

DSM-IV Diagnostic Criteria for Substance Dependence

A maladaptive pattern of substance use, leading to clinically significant impairment or distress, as manifested by three (or more) of the following, occurring at any time in the same 12-month period:

(1) tolerance, as defined by either of the following:
  (a) a need for markedly increased amounts of the substance to achieve intoxication or desired effect
  (b) markedly diminished effect with continued use of the same amount of the substance
(2) withdrawal, as manifested by either of the following:
  (a) the characteristic withdrawal syndrome for the substance
  (b) the same (or a closely related) substance is taken to relieve or avoid withdrawal symptoms
(3) the substance is often taken in larger amounts or over a longer period than was intended
(4) there is a persistent desire or unsuccessful efforts to cut down or control substance use
(5) a great deal of time is spent in activities necessary to obtain the substance, (eg, visiting multiple doctors or driving long distances), use the substance (eg, chain-smoking), or recover from its effects
(6) important social, occupational, or recreational activities are given up or reduced because of substance use
(7) the substance use is continued despite knowledge of having a persistent or recurrent physical or psychological problem that is likely to have been caused or exacerbated by the substance (eg, current cocaine use despite recognition of cocaine-induced depression, or continued drinking despite recognition that an ulcer was made worse by alcohol consumption)

CRITERIA FOR SUBSTANCE ABUSE

A. A maladaptive pattern of substance use leading to clinically significant impairment or distress, as manifested by one (or more) of the following, occurring within a 12-month period:
  (1) recurrent substance use resulting in a failure to fulfill major role obligations at work, school, or home (eg, repeated absences or poor work performance related to substance use; substance-related absences, suspensions, or expulsions from school; neglect of children or household)
  (2) recurrent substance use in situations in which it is physically hazardous (eg, driving an automobile or operating a machine when impaired by substance use)
  (3) recurrent substance-related legal problems (eg, arrests for substance-related disorderly conduct)
  (4) continued substance use despite having persistent or recurrent social or interpersonal problems caused or exacerbated by the effects of the substance (eg, arguments with spouse about consequences of intoxication, physical fights)

B. The symptoms have never met the criteria for Substance Dependence for this class of substance.

CRITERIA FOR SUBSTANCE WITHDRAWAL

A. The development of a substance-specific syndrome due to the cessation of (or reduction in) substance use that has been heavy and prolonged.

B. The substance-specific syndrome causes clinically significant distress or impairment in social, occupational, or other important areas of functioning.

C. The symptoms are not due to a general medical condition and are not better accounted for by another mental disorder.

CRITERIA FOR SUBSTANCE INTOXICATION

A. The development of a reversible substance-specific syndrome due to recent ingestion of (or exposure to) a substance. **Note:** Different substances may produce similar or identical syndromes.

B. Clinically significant maladaptive behavioral or psychological changes that are due to the effect of the substance on the central nervous system (eg, belligerence, mood lability, cognitive impairment, impaired judgment, impaired social or occupational functioning) and develop during or shortly after use of the substance.

C. The symptoms are not due to a general medical condition and are not better accounted for by another mental disorder.

Table 33-1

Substance-Induced Disorders

Substance-Induced Mental Disorders	Barbiturate and Similar-Acting Sedatives			Amphetamine and Similar-Acting Sympathomimetics	PCP	Hallucinogens	Cannabis
	Alcohol	*Hypnotics*	*Opioids*				
Intoxication	×	×	×	×	×	×	×
Withdrawal	×	×	×	×			
Intoxication delirium	×	×	×	×	×	×	×
Withdrawal delirium	×	×					
Dementia	×	×					
Amnestic disorder	×	×					
Psychotic disorders	×	×	×	×	×	×	×
Mood disorders	×	×	×	×	×	×	×
Anxiety disorders	×	×		×	×	×	×
Sexual dysfunctions	×	×	×	×			
Sleep disorders	×	×	×	×			

holism) and other concepts with more general application (eg, the learning theory). The etiological concept may be reflected in the treatment and rehabilitation process. For example, those who embrace the disease concept of alcoholism will strongly advise abstinence to treat alcoholism. On the other hand, proponents of learning theory may believe that a person's behavior may be modified or changed and that social or recreational drinking may be resumed.

Social or Environmental Factors

The social conditions or environment from which a person emerges may contribute to or predispose to substance abuse and dependency. For example, a high incidence of abuse of opioid derivatives, such as heroin, occurs in poverty-stricken areas of large cities. The abuse of cocaine and hallucinogens is associated with subculture groups and those seeking mystical experiences. Cocaine abuse also is high in the upper economic bracket and among entertainers and athletes.[4]

Personality Factors

A review of research studies has not substantiated that one personality type is associated with substance abuse and dependency.[4,37,70] Instead, there is wide variation in personality types, including people from all social, cultural, and economic backgrounds.[97] Personality disorders, however, may be intensified by abuse of or dependence on substances, especially in the antisocial personality.[4,37] Depressed people and those with affective disorders may abuse substances to treat symptoms related to their disorder.[4] Although research does not support the concept of an addictive personality type, some factors are important to those seeking to understand, prevent, and treat substance abuse. Most of the differences between people who abuse alcohol and those who abuse other drugs seem to reflect age, sex, race, socioeconomic status, and the use of legal or illegal drugs, rather than intrapsychic dynamics. A common factor in all forms of substance abuse and dependence is a negative self-concept, marked by a sense of failure, inadequacy, guilt, shame, loneliness, and despair.[37]

Self-Destructive Phenomenon

People who abuse and become dependent on substances do so despite severe physical, psychological, and social consequences. This lack of concern for one's own well-being has led to the view of drug dependency as a self-destructive phenomenon.[97] It is also difficult to estimate with certainty the incidence of intentional suicide by drug overdose. The risk of suicide is high in people who abuse substances, in sober and intoxicated states.[4,50,66]

Ethnic and Cultural Factors

Substance abuse and dependency are found in all cultures and ethnic groups. There are variations, however, in the incidence and prevalence of the problem, the drug preferred, and the aspects of treatment, prevention, and rehabilitation. For example, a low incidence of alcoholism but a high incidence of opiate dependency is reported in the Asian culture and population.[4,31,69] Researchers attribute the low incidence of alcoholism to a possible genetic intolerance to alcohol, manifested by unpleasant physical symptoms when even small amounts of alcohol are ingested.[31,69] There is also a low incidence of alcohol dependency in the American Jewish population but a high incidence in the Native American and Irish populations and relatively high in-

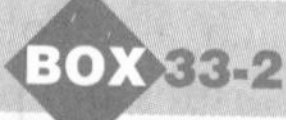

At Risk for Alcoholism

There is a wealth of evidence that one of the greatest risk factors for becoming an alcoholic is to be the son, daughter, or sibling of an alcoholic. Research indicates that both genetics and environment are involved in the development of alcoholism and alcohol abuse.

Adoption studies have identified two types of alcoholism: type 1 (milieu-limited) and type 2 (male-limited). Milieu-limited alcoholism is influenced by genetic predisposition and environmental factors. Male-limited alcoholism is highly heritable and influenced very little by the environment.

Evidence of the importance of factors other than familial ones comes from a recent study that discovered a steady increase in frequency of alcoholism and a decrease in the age of onset in comparing different age cohorts. Younger cohorts had a higher prevalence of alcoholism than older ones, and they became alcohol-dependent earlier. These secular trends, which are seen in the general populations as well as in the relatives of alcoholics, suggest that broad social factors are influencing the risk for alcoholism.

The interaction of genetics and environment is a fundamentally important issue in the development of alcoholism, and future research on alcoholism will focus more on this interaction.

(From Seventh Special Report to the US Congress on Alcohol and Health. US Department of Health and Human Services, January 1990)

cidence in Scandinavian and German populations. The reasons for these phenomena are related to cultural drinking habits and accepted use of alcohol.[69] Since the 1950s, research related to cultural aspects of alcohol abuse and dependency has increased. The importance of ethnic factors and cultural diversity and their effect on substance abuse and dependency are now being emphasized. Knowledge acquired through study and research has special application in drug prevention and treatment programs.

Learning Theory

The learning theory concept, involving a conditioned response mechanism, has been applied to substance abuse and dependency. For example, the drug use may initially produce pleasant physical responses, desired social consequences, increased feelings of self-confidence, or relief from tension or anxiety. The conditioned response is always positive in the beginning; however, even after severe negative consequences occur, the repetitive or learned behavior continues, although the initial reasons for the behavior are no longer in operation.[36,37,69]

Biological Theory

There is a high incidence of alcohol abuse and dependency (alcoholism) in children and family members of alcoholics. Several research studies have suggested a possible inherited predisposition to alcoholism.[4,30,31,70] Studies of twins with a family history of alcoholism have yielded interesting results. Monozygotic twins (those who share the same genetic material) are more concordant for alcoholism than are dizogotic twins (those who have the same genetic material as siblings). Adoptive studies examine data of children born to alcoholic parents but separated after birth from their natural parents and raised by nonalcoholic foster parents. These studies indicate that these children are particularly susceptible to becoming alcoholic.[4,30,31]

Researchers are investigating what genetic characteristics may place a person at risk for alcoholism. In addition, brain-wave studies have revealed peculiar and apparently genetically based electrical phenomena in the brains of people at risk for alcoholism.

A family history of alcoholism does not necessarily indicate that alcoholism is genetic. Consider that most children are raised by their biological parents and that social, cultural, and psychological factors within the family environment have profound influence on the behavior of children. The question is whether the familial aspect of alcoholism comes from a learned pattern of behavior, rather than from a genetic predisposition to alcoholism.[30,31] There may be a nonfamilial and a familial type of alcoholism. There is no direct evidence that narcotic addiction is genetically transmitted.[32] Nevertheless, researchers are conducting psychobiological studies in an attempt to identify a common link or aspect of drug addiction. There has been an increase in polydrug users; that is, people who take various substances, including alcohol, with no specific drug of choice.[4,37]

Disease Concept of Alcoholism

Viewing alcoholism as a disease rather than as a moral problem originated with the work of E. M. Jellinek. A pioneer in the study of alcoholism, Jellinek classified alcoholics into five categories. The disease concept he proposed was based on the statistical analysis of a survey of 2,000 alcoholic men. The classes or types of alcoholics that he identified, however, were not meant to reflect theories of the cause or nature of alcoholism.[33,34]

The concept of alcoholism as a disease has had a great effect on the acceptance of alcoholism as an illness or process outside the control of the afflicted person.

Jellinek's disease concept, labeled by some as the *traditional model of alcoholism,* has been challenged by a more recent concept of alcohol dependence as a behavioral disorder with adverse health effects. This latter concept has been called the *multivariant concept of alcoholism.*[53] Most authorities in the field of alcohol abuse continue to view the disease concept of alcoholism as the more valid approach to treatment and eventual recovery.

More recently, authorities have concluded that alcoholism, like hypertension, diabetes, and coronary artery disease, is a disease with a biological basis in which a genetic predisposition is activated by environmental factors. Alcoholism is not an infectious disease or a disease in which cells multiply wildly. Rather, in alcohol dependence, biology and behavior interact in complex ways. Alcohol-dependent people may experience predictable withdrawal syndromes, severe physical effects resulting from abstinence, and intense, overwhelming compulsions to drink. Withdrawal and craving may contribute to the development of impaired control over drinking. In addition, alcohol-dependent people develop a tolerance to alcohol.[33]

INCIDENCE AND SIGNIFICANCE OF SUBSTANCE ABUSE AND DEPENDENCY

The drug of abuse is a main consideration when examining the incidence and significance of substance abuse and dependency. For example, of the many people who use alcohol, a legal substance socially approved for recreational use, about 1 in 10 experience abuse or dependency. In contrast, the users of heroin, an illegal substance, have a higher incidence of dependency. Also, abuse or dependency occurs more quickly with narcotics than with alcohol.[4,15]

The culture or social status from which the drug user comes also has an impact on the incidence of substance abuse. Teenagers may experiment with a variety of drugs, including heroin, cocaine, stimulants, alcohol, sedative-hypnotics, phencyclidine, or almost any substance available. During the Vietnam war, servicemen used and abused heroin and cannabis in large quantities with a resulting high incidence of abuse and dependency. When returning to the United States, some were able to stop using heroin completely or changed the drug of abuse.[4]

The type of drug used by low-income urban men or women may be different from that used by suburban middle-income men or women. Because of class distinctions and social variables, the latter group may choose a prescription or legal drug, such as alcohol. Frequently, entertainment or sports celebrities and people of high economic status are associated with cocaine abuse or dependency.[29]

Age, sex, culture, and social setting affect the incidence and significance of drug abuse. Other considerations include the drug's availability and cost, peer pressure, and the drug-oriented American culture, which extols the use of alcohol and prescription drugs for relief of tension and pain. To counteract this prevalence of substance abuse, health professionals in all fields are uniting to combat abuse and dependency problems in psychological, physiological, and social areas through treatment, research, and prevention.

◆ Dynamics of Substance Abuse and Dependency

This section describes major substances, specific diagnostic criteria, and particular physical, behavioral, and familial consequences.

ALCOHOL ABUSE AND DEPENDENCY

Alcohol abuse and dependency are among the most serious public health problems in the United States. The incidence of alcohol-related accidents resulting in fatalities or in permanent disabilities is enormous. The social impact of the disorder on family members, especially on children, is devastating. Many American adolescents are affected by destructive drinking patterns or suffer alcoholism themselves; many children are born with abnormalities or suffer from fetal alcohol syndrome (Box 33-3; Fig. 33-2).

Nature of Alcohol

The substance commonly referred to as *alcohol* is ethyl alcohol (C_2H_5OH), also known chemically as *ethanol* and sometimes abbreviated as ETOH.[37] It is a legal chemical substance or drug; that is, the commercial distribution of alcohol-containing beverages differs from the regulation and sale of other classes of drugs.

Ethyl alcohol has pharmacological properties that produce mind- and mood-altering effects. It is a CNS depressant similar to barbiturates and ether.[17] Chloral hydrate and paraldehyde are sedative-hypnotic drugs derived from ethyl alcohol. Chloral hydrate is used to induce sleep; paraldehyde was used in the medical management of alcohol withdrawal symptoms before the introduction of modern tranquilizers.

Most drugs that affect the CNS have a use in medicine, but ethyl alcohol is not commonly used as a drug in medical treatment. In contrast to other drugs, which

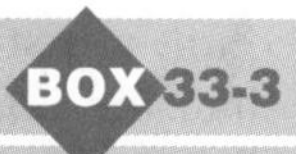

Magnitude of the Problem of Alcoholism

The abuse of licit and illicit drugs represents a major public health problem in the United States. Abuse of alcohol and other drugs has been associated with many problems (see Fig. 33-2), costing Americans an estimated $144.1 billion annually.

Federal survey data estimate that 11.4 million Americans aged 12 and older used illegal drugs in 1992, continuing a steady decline from a peak of 24 million in 1979. Findings from the 1992 National Household Survey found the following about specific drugs:

- **Illegal Drugs.** Since 1979, overall rates of current use (defined as use within the last 30 days) have dropped in all age groups, except those aged 35 and older, whose use of drugs has remained level. This has resulted in a general shift in the age distribution of illegal drug users.
- **Cocaine.** The number of cocaine users decreased 31% from 1.9 million users in 1991 to 1.3 million in 1992. This is down from a peak of 5.8 million in 1985. The number of occasional users (defined as those who used the drug in 1992 but less often than monthly) also continued a sharp decline from 4.3 million in 1991 to 3.4 million in 1992. This is down from a peak of 8.6 million in 1985. Frequent use of cocaine (defined as use on a weekly basis) remained unchanged between 1991 and 1992. In fact, no significant change has occurred in this number since it was first estimated in 1985.
- **Marijuana.** This is the most common illegal drug—used by 78% of all illegal drug users in 1992.
- **Other illegal drugs.** No major changes in the prevalence of the use of hallucinogens, such as lysergic acid diethylamide (LSD) and phencyclidine (PCP), between 1991 and 1992. The survey estimates that approximately 1.8 million Americans have used heroin at least once. However, the data on these categories are somewhat unreliable, as these users are less likely to be contacted and reported in a household survey.
- **Alcohol.** In 1992, approximately 98 million persons over the age of 12. This number is down from an estimated high of 106 million drinkers in 1988. The number of heavy drinkers (defined as having five or more drinks per occasion on 5 or more days in the past month) has remained steady at an estimated 9 million people.

(From Technologies for Understanding and Preventing Substance Abuse and Addiction, OTA-EHR-597, US Congress, Office of Technology Assessment, Washington, DC; US Government Printing Office, September, 1994)

produce their effects from small quantities, alcohol usually requires large quantities used over a period of time to cause physical dependence.

Alcohol-containing beverages include beer, wine, and distilled spirits. The alcohol content of a beverage is expressed as *proof,* that is, the concentration of ethyl alcohol. In the United States, proof is twice the ethanol concentration: 100 proof is 50% ethyl alcohol, and 80 proof is 40% ethyl alcohol.

Ethyl alcohol is a CNS depressant, as are the sedative-hypnotics, antianxiety drugs, and general anesthetics. These drugs cause the following pattern of effects as the dose of the drug is increased: sedation, impaired mental and motor functioning, deepening stupor with a decrease in stimulation response (including painful stimulus response), coma, and eventually death from respiratory and circulatory collapse.[16,17,37]

Alcohol often is erroneously considered a stimulant. The reason for this misconception is that after drinking alcoholic beverages, some people may become more

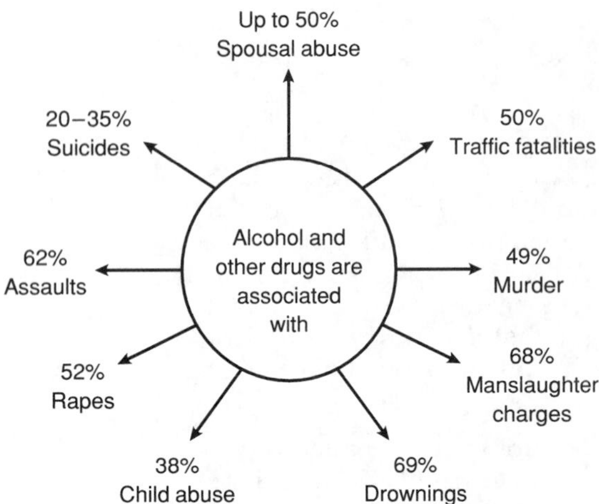

Figure 33-2. Association of alcohol and other drugs with problems. (Source: Office of Substance Abuse Prevention, 1991.)

talkative or hyperactive, euphoric, self-confident, or aggressive. This behavior has been attributed to the disinhibiting effect produced by a low dose.[16,17,37]

Alcohol Concentration in the Body

The physical and behavioral manifestations of the effects of alcohol on the CNS are related to the level of alcohol in the blood, the concentration of alcohol in the brain, and other contributing factors. The blood level of alcohol is expressed in the number of milligrams of alcohol per milliliter of blood.[37]

Blood alcohol level is determined by a laboratory blood test to measure the degree of alcohol (ethanol) intoxication. It may be used in medicolegal procedures to rule out intoxication in a person who is comatose. The degree of intoxication also may be measured by a Breathalyzer.

Alcohol concentration in the blood depends on the rate of absorption, transportation to the CNS, redistribution to other parts of the body, metabolism, and elimination. Alcohol is absorbed through the mouth, stomach, and small intestine. It is absorbed unchanged into the blood and circulates throughout the body, including the brain; it also crosses the placenta into the fetal circulation. Intoxication occurs when the circulating alcohol interferes with the normal functioning of brain nerve cells.[17,37]

The rate of absorption into the blood varies with the following factors:

1. Substances in the beverage, such as the carbonation (CO_2) in champagne, increase absorption.
2. The rate of alcohol ingestion can affect the rate of absorption. Drinking alcoholic beverages slowly over a long period may slow absorption and allow for metabolism of alcohol by the liver. Because the body metabolizes alcohol at a steady rate, when a person drinks faster than the body can metabolize the alcohol, it accumulates in the blood.
3. The rate of drinking may vary, but alcohol leaves the body at a fixed rate.[17,37]

Oxidation, which occurs mainly in the liver, eliminates 90% of the alcohol absorbed by the body. The other 10% is eliminated unchanged through breath, sweat, urine, and other body fluids. The healthy liver metabolizes approximately 1 oz of alcohol per hour; the excess alcohol that the liver cannot metabolize continues to circulate in the blood. Food in the stomach (especially fatty food) slows absorption, whereas an empty stomach increases absorption. The drinker's emotional state may also affect absorption of alcohol. For example, stress, fear, anger, and fatigue may increase or decrease absorption. The drinker's body size affects the concentration of alcohol in the blood. The same amount of alcohol ingested by a 100-lb person and a 200-lb person will result in greater blood alcohol concentration in the lighter person, because the heavier person has more blood volume in which the alcohol is diluted. A person's body chemistry and cultural influences may also alter the behavioral effects of alcohol.[17,37]

Tolerance

Prolonged heavy drinking results in physical and behavioral tolerance. Physical tolerance, or tissue adaptation, means that changes occur in the cells of the nervous system so that more drug is required to achieve the desired effect. When physical tolerance develops, the person may experience withdrawal or abstinence syndrome after cessation or a decrease in alcohol consumption. Physical tolerance to alcohol never reaches the high-dose tolerance of the opiates. Cross-tolerance to sedative-hypnotics and other CNS depressants also occurs.[17,37]

Behavioral tolerance to alcohol is manifested by the ability to mask the behavioral effects, for example, the acquired ability not to slur words, to walk straight, and to function in ways that would not be possible in a nondependent person. The drinking history of alcoholics frequently reveals the ability to increase tolerance and maintain this increase for a long time, perhaps several years. Frequently, this increased tolerance is followed by an irreversible drop in tolerance; the person becomes intoxicated with smaller amounts of alcohol.[16,37]

Blackout

Persistent heavy drinking frequently results in the chemically induced alcoholic blackout. This is not the same as passing out, which is defined as a loss of consciousness. During a blackout, the person appears to function normally while drinking but later is unable to remember what occurred. The blackout may last a few hours or several hours. The person may come out of the blackout period and wonder, "Where did I leave my car last night?" He or she may wake up in a strange city not remembering leaving home and wonder, "How did I get here?" or "Was I with someone?" These blackouts may be a symptom of alcohol abuse and dependency.[16,37]

Alcohol-Induced Disorders

Intoxication

Intoxication occurs after drinking alcohol and is evidenced in behavior such as fighting, impaired judgment, interference with social or occupational functioning, or other maladaptive behavior. Physiological signs, such as slurred speech, incoordination, unsteady gait, nystagmus, and flushed face, may accompany intoxication. Psychological signs also may be observed, such as mood changes, irritability, talkativeness, or impaired attention.

Alcohol Withdrawal

Alcohol withdrawal, or abstinence syndrome, occurs after reduction in or cessation of prolonged heavy drinking. A coarse tremor of hand, tongue, and eyelids may occur, as may nausea and vomiting, general malaise or weakness, autonomic nervous system hyperactivity (eg, increased blood pressure and pulse), anxiety, a depressed or irritable mood, and orthostatic hypotension. Sleep disturbances, insomnia, and nightmares may also occur during withdrawal.

Alcohol Withdrawal Delirium

Alcohol withdrawal delirium, called *delirium tremens,* is the most serious form of withdrawal syndrome. It occurs after cessation of or reduction in prolonged heavy drinking and can occur as long as 1 week after cessation of drinking. Symptoms include clouding of consciousness (unawareness of environment); inability to shift, focus, and sustain attention to stimuli in the environment; misinterpretations, illusions, or hallucinations that are usually visual and vivid; incoherent speech; insomnia or daytime drowsiness; increased or decreased psychomotor activity; frequent agitation; and increased blood pressure, sweating, and temperature. Seizures may also occur as a result of alcohol withdrawal. If untreated, this syndrome can cause serious medical complications, such as fluid and electrolyte imbalance, pneumonia, and dehydration.

Alcoholic Hallucinosis

Alcoholic hallucinosis usually occurs within 48 hours after cessation of or reduction in drinking. Vivid, perhaps threatening, auditory hallucinations may develop, but clouding of the consciousness does not occur. The person's response to the hallucinations is typically anxiety or fear. Auditory hallucinations are usually experienced as voices but may be experienced as hissing or buzzing sounds.

Alcoholic Amnestic Disorder

The alcoholic amnestic disorder results from heavy, prolonged drinking and is thought to be related to poor nutritional intake. If the disorder is related to thiamine deficiency, it is known as *Wernicke-Korsakoff syndrome.* Amnesia consists of impairment in the ability to learn new information (short-term memory) and to recall remote information (long-term memory). Other neurological signs, such as neuropathy, unsteady gait, or myopathy, may be present.

Alcoholic Dementia

Alcoholic dementia is associated with prolonged, chronic alcohol dependence. Signs of dementia include loss of intellectual ability that is severe enough to interfere with social or occupational functioning and impairment in memory, abstract thinking, and judgment. The degree of impairment may range from mild to severe and may include permanent brain damage.

Medical Consequences

Heavy consumption of alcohol can adversely affect almost every body system. Various medical conditions may alert the nurse to the early recognition of alcohol abuse problems.

Gastrointestinal problems occur as a result of the irritating effects of alcohol on the gastrointestinal tract, resulting in gastritis or gastric ulcers. Acute or chronic pancreatitis may occur. Esophagitis may result from the direct toxic effects of alcohol on the esophageal mucosa, increased acid production in the stomach, or frequent vomiting. Alcohol cardiomyopathy results from the direct toxic effects of the substance and malnutrition.[16,37]

The liver is highly susceptible to the damaging effects of alcohol because it is the primary organ that metabolizes alcohol. Alcohol is toxic to the liver regardless of the person's nutritional status.[37] Alcohol liver disease has been divided into three major types. In fatty liver, deposits of fats (triglycerides) build up in the normal liver cells. This condition is reversible. Alcoholic hepatitis is a more serious condition, involving inflammation and necrosis of the liver cells. This condition is also frequently reversible. Cirrhosis of the liver, the most serious condition, is irreversible. In cirrhosis, the liver cells are destroyed and replaced by scar tissue. About 90% of deaths from cirrhosis of the liver are associated with chronic alcoholism.[6] A high risk of cancer, especially of the mouth, pharynx, larynx, esophagus, pancreas, cardia of the stomach, and colon, is also associated with alcoholism.[16,37]

ABUSE OF CONTROLLED SUBSTANCES

Drugs other than alcohol are regulated by the Controlled Substance Act (Title II, Comprehensive Drug Abuse Prevention and Control Act of 1970, Public Law 91-513), promulgated to decrease the illegal use and abuse of drugs in the United States. Box 33-4 gives some pharmacological and slang terms for commonly abused controlled substances, and Box 33-5 lists some street terms associated with substance abuse and dependency.

Barbiturates and Similar Sedative-Hypnotic Drugs

The barbiturates and other CNS depressants are called *sedative-hypnotics* and *anxiolytics*. The main difference between a sedative drug and a hypnotic drug is the degree of sedation produced compared with the antianxiety-producing effects.[17] The barbiturates are the most common drugs of abuse after alcohol in the United States.

Effects

The barbiturates and similarly acting drugs are capable of producing intoxication withdrawal and physical and psychological dependence and tolerance. The route of administration may be oral or parenteral (ie, intravenous or intramuscular). Basically, the organs with greater blood flow absorb the drug first. Most commonly used barbiturates are metabolized by the liver; some (eg, phenobarbital) are not metabolized and are excreted unchanged by the kidneys.[17,37] Because barbiturates cross the placental barrier, the fetus of a drug-dependent mother may experience physical dependence. Physical withdrawal symptoms may occur in the infant up to 7 days after delivery and may include high-pitched cry, tremors, restlessness, disturbed sleep, increased reflex action, hyperphagia, diarrhea, vomiting, and major motor seizures.[37]

Barbiturates and alcohol produce cross-tolerance and when taken together, will increase absorption and produce additive depression of the CNS. Because of this, people have taken barbiturate overdoses while intoxicated with alcohol, perhaps unaware of the additive effects of alcohol and the sedative-hypnotics.

Patterns of Abuse

Barbiturates are frequently used by people who abuse or are dependent on drugs to relieve or counteract the effects of other drugs. For example, barbiturates may be used to relieve symptoms of heroin withdrawal. The person may be unaware that cross-tolerance does not occur between opiates and barbiturates and may think that because tolerance to heroin is high, tolerance to barbiturates will be high also; as a result, the person may unintentionally overdose on barbiturates. Heroin addicts may substitute barbiturates for heroin when heroin is unattainable and because there is no cross-tolerance, may develop physical dependence on both drugs.[37] Barbiturates also may be taken to relieve the anxiety related to flashbacks from lysergic acid diethylamine (LSD) abuse or to counteract the symptoms of anxiety, paranoia, and depression due to excessive use of amphetamines.[4,37]

People may abuse barbiturates and sedative-hypnotics or anxiolytics for the many reasons that people abuse alcohol, including relief of anxiety and disinhibiting effects. Some may believe the barbiturates are less detectable than alcohol or find the taste of alcohol unpleasant. Many people combine or alternate alcohol with the barbiturates or similarly acting sedative-hypnotics.[37] The behavioral differences that may occur in intoxication are usually due to the personality of the user or the social setting in which intoxication occurs; for example, violence or aggressive behavior may be more readily exhibited in social settings where alcohol is consumed.[4,37] Two general patterns of abuse and dependency are seen for this class of drugs:

1. People who obtain the drug through legal means, such as prescriptions for medical problems, find the drug useful to relieve anxiety; they increase dosage and frequency of consumption. This pattern is often found in people from middle-class backgrounds and in 30- to 60-year-old women.
2. People who illegally obtain the drug are frequently in their late teens or early 20s and use the drugs to get high or get relief from the stimulant effects of the amphetamines.[4]

Sedative-, Hypnotic-, or Anxiolytic-Induced Disorders

Intoxication. Intoxication occurs after a recent ingestion of sedatives, hypnotics, or anxiolytics. Signs and symptoms of this class of substance are similar to those of alcohol intoxication.

Withdrawal. Withdrawal occurs hours to several days after decrease in or cessation of prolonged heavy use of the barbiturate or similarly acting sedative-hypnotic agent. Signs and symptoms of withdrawal are similar to those of alcohol withdrawal. They do not necessarily follow a specific sequence, and their severity depends on individual differences, doses, and duration of use. Abrupt withdrawal from these drugs is not recommended; detoxification should take place in a medical setting.

Withdrawal Delirium. Withdrawal signs and symptoms from the barbiturates are the same as those of alcoholic withdrawal delirium and usually occur within 1 week after cessation or reduction of the drug. Some people experience delirium without seizures, some experience seizures only, and some exhibit both.[16] This condition

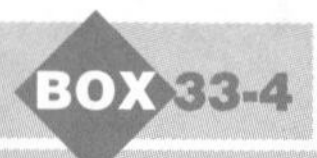

Pharmacological and Slang Terms for Commonly Abused Controlled Substances

SUBSTANCE	GENERIC AND TRADE NAME	STREET OR SLANG NAME
Barbiturates	Amobarbital (Amytal) Pentobarbital (Nembutal) Phenobarbital (Luminal) Secobarbital (Seconal)	Candies, Peanuts, Blue Dots, Softballs, Secies, Red Bullets, Yellow Bullets, Seggies, Blue Bullets, Blue Heaven, Goofballs, Phennies, Barbs, Blockbusters, Bluebirds, Blue Devils, Blues, Christmas Trees, Downers, Green Dragons, Mexican Reds, Nebbies, Nimbles, Pajaro Rojo, Pink Ladies, Pinks, Rainbows, Reds and Blues, Red Birds, Red Devils, Reds Sleeping Pills, Stumblers, Yellow Jackets, Yellows
Opiates		
Morphine		
Heroin	Diacetylmorphine	Cube, First Line, Goma, Morf, Morfina, Morpho, Mud Big H, Boy, Caballo, Chiva, Crap, Estuff, H, Heroina, Hombre, Doogie, Dogie, Brown Sugar, Horse, Junk, Mexican Mud, Scag, Smack, Stuff, Thing
CNS Stimulants		
Amphetamine	Amphetamine (Benzedrine) Methamphetamine (Desoxyn, Methedrine) Dextroamphetamine (Dexedrine)	White Crosses, Footballs, Uppers, Pep Pills, Hearts, Wake-Ups, Beanies, Roses, Dexies, Whites, Oranges, Blackbird, Black Cadillacs, Crystals, Beans, Ice, Glass, Quartz, Crank, Bombidos, Lightning, Meth, Nuggets, Dynamites, Splash, Sparkle Plenties, Speed, Marathons, Bennies, Black Beauties, Black Mollies, Rosas, Copilots, Crossroads, Decies, Double Cross, Minibennies, Uppers, Thrusters, Truck Drivers
Cocaine		Coke, Cecil, Coconut, Corrine, Bernice, Join, Sniff, Bernies, Rock, Frisky Powder, Incentive, Dream, Gold Dust, StarDust, Paradise, Carry Notion, Heaven Dust, Uptown, Toot, Blow, C, Coca, Crack, Flake, Girl, Heaven, Dust, Lady Mujer, Nose Candy, Perico, Polvo Blanco, Rock, Snow, White
Hallucinogens	Lysergic acid diethylamine (LSD)	Sugar Cubes, Big D, Ghost, LSD Hawk 25, Beast Coffee, Blue Heaven, Orange Mushrooms, Mellow Yellowies, Chocolate Chips, Trips, Acid, Blotter Acid, California Sunshine, Haze, Microdots, Paper Acid, Purple Haze, Sunshine Wedges, Window Panes
Cannabis		
Marijuana		Pot, Dope, Hemp, Weed, Herb, Panamanian Gold, Mary Jane, Zacatecas Purple, Mexican Green, Broccoli, Bush, Gage, Dry High, Greta, Yesea Sweet Honey, Acapulco Gold, Cannabis, Colombian, Ganga, Grass, Griffa, Hemp, Herb, J, Jay, Joint, Mota, Mutah, Panama Red, Reefer, Sativa, Smoke, Stick, Tea, Weed, Yerba
Hashish		Goma de Mota, Hash, Soles

BOX 33-5

Street Terms Associated with Substance Abuse and Dependency

Artillery	Equipment used for injecting drugs
Blasted	High on drugs
Booting	Intravenous injection of a drug by drawing blood into the syringe a number of times
Boxed	In jail
Chipping	Using heroin infrequently
Clean	Not using drugs
Connection	A person from whom drugs can be bought
Crash	Coming down from drugs
Dealer	One who sells drugs
Dirty	Using or holding narcotics
Dirty urine	Urine testing positive for an illegal drug
Fix	To inject oneself with heroin
Hustling	Obtaining money for drugs by illegal nonviolent means (eg, pimping, prostitution, shoplifting)
Mainlining	Injecting drugs into veins
Pusher	One who sells drugs
Rush	Intense, immediate euphoric feeling after intravenous injection of heroin or cocaine or freebasing cocaine
Run	Binge-type drug use (frequently with cocaine) lasting until the drug is depleted or person is exhausted
Wasted	Stuporous or comatose from a drug

is a medical emergency requiring hospitalization and medical intervention.

Amnestic Disorder. Amnestic disorder occurs after prolonged heavy use of barbiturates or similarly acting sedative-hypnotics. Predominant signs and symptoms are impaired short-term memory (inability to learn new information) and long-term memory (inability to remember learned information). Full recovery from this disorder is possible.

Medical Consequences. Severe complications may result from intravenous barbiturate use. Inadvertently injecting the drug into subcutaneous tissue may cause cellulitis, in which subcutaneous tissues become swollen, inflamed, and painful. Vascular complications occur if the drug is accidentally injected into an artery; these may result in the loss of a hand or fingers. The intravenous user may also suffer other medical complications from self-injections, particularly serum hepatitis, endocarditis, pneumonia, tetanus, and other bacterial infections. Also, syphilis or malaria may result, as may allergic reactions to substances that may have been added to the drug.

Barbiturates are frequently used in suicides; more than 15,000 deaths secondary to barbiturate poisoning are reported yearly. The extent to which these deaths are attributable to accidental or intentional suicide is difficult to ascertain. People rarely use only one sedative-hypnotic drug; most use a variety of these drugs and alcohol. In detoxification, it is crucial to assess whether the person used alcohol, other drugs concurrently with alcohol, or other drugs without alcohol.

The Opiates

The opiates are narcotics or drugs that produce depressant effects on the CNS. Included in this definition are opium and derivatives of opium, such as morphine, codeine, and heroin and synthetically produced drugs, such as meperidine and methadone.[4,37]

The pharmacologically active ingredients of opium are the alkaloids, the most common of which are morphine and codeine. The opiates may be taken orally or rectally or may be smoked, but usually they are injected intramuscularly or intravenously.

Effects

Essentially CNS depressants, the opiates produce analgesia, mood changes, and sedation; depress respirations; and inhibit coughing. They are effective pain relief medications. The physiological actions of heroin are similar to morphine, but heroin is four or five times more potent than morphine.[57] The body metabolizes heroin and morphine similarly. Heroin is converted into morphine, metabolized primarily in the liver, with end products secreted through urine and bile.[57] Tolerance to the opiates develops rapidly, and physical dependence occurs after a brief period of use.

Patterns of Abuse

Opiate abusers may be separated into two classes: street abusers and those who obtain opiates from medical sources. The latter generally are an older, middle-class, well-established group; the street abusers obtain opiates from illegal sources.[57]

The street abuser tends to be a young man. The person begins using opiates occasionally but progresses to daily use and quickly develops dependence and tolerance. Frequently, there is a history of delinquent or antisocial behavior. The drug's illegal status brings legal problems. There is a high incidence of death in this group due to suicide, homicide, accidents, and diseases, such as infections and tuberculosis. The mortality rate is about 5 to 10 people per 1,000 opiate users.[57]

Medical abusers tend to be women from a middle-class environment or those with pain syndromes who misuse their prescribed drugs and often misuse other drugs as well. Two high-risk groups for this type of abuse are people with pain syndromes and health care workers, especially physicians and nurses.[57] Opioid abuse and dependency is usually preceded by a period of polydrug use, which continues after opioid use is acquired.[4]

Opioid-Induced Disorders

Intoxication. Opiate intoxication is marked by pupillary constriction, drowsiness, slurred speech, impaired attention or memory, euphoria, dysphoria, apathy, and psychomotor retardation. Problems in social or occupational functioning and impaired judgment may result in maladaptive behavior.

Opioid Withdrawal. After cessation or reduction of prolonged heavy opioid use, withdrawal symptoms may include tearing, runny nose, dilated pupils, gooseflesh (piloerection), sweating, diarrhea, yawning, mild hypertension, tachycardia, fever, and insomnia. Accompanying symptoms may be irritability, depression, restlessness, tremor, weakness, nausea, vomiting, and muscle and joint pains. All of these symptoms may resemble flu symptoms. Duration of the withdrawal period depends on the specific drug. Withdrawal symptoms may elicit a great deal of discomfort but are usually not life-threatening unless the person has a concurrent serious medical problem, such as cardiac disease.

Medical Consequences. Prolonged opiate use often results in decreased motivation to engage in high-quality life experiences, personal and social deterioration that usually involves problems with police and law enforcement agencies, and family and interpersonal problems.[57] Serious medical problems may result from drug overdose, additives in the street drugs, poor nutrition and health, and infections due to unsterile needles and equipment used in self-injection. Some common problems encountered are abscesses and infections of skin and muscle, tetanus, malaria, liver disease, hepatitis, HIV, gastric ulcers, endocarditis, heart arrhythmias, anemia, infections of bones and joints, pneumonia, tuberculosis, lung abscesses, and kidney failure caused by infections of additives in street drug mixtures. Sexual function problems may occur secondary to low testosterone levels during chronic opiate use. In addition, serious emotional problems, such as depression, may result from opioid abuse.[57]

Amphetamines and Cocaine: Central Nervous System Stimulants

Stimulants act directly on the CNS. The person taking stimulants becomes more talkative and active and has an increased sense of well-being, self-confidence, and alertness. Stimulants are frequently used to decrease appetite, reduce fatigue, and combat mild depression. A common stimulant is caffeine, an ingredient in coffee, tea, and soft drinks.

Amphetamine is the prototype for this class of drug and other chemically related drugs with similar pharmacological properties.[4,37] Cocaine, also a stimulant, is classified as a narcotic and falls under the Controlled Substances Act.

Effects of Amphetamines and Similarly Acting Sympathomimetics

This category includes all substituted phenylethylamine structures, such as amphetamine and methamphetamine (or *speed*), substances with different chemical structures but amphetamine-like actions, and some substances used as diet pills. These substances may be taken orally or intravenously.[4] Tolerance develops within hours to days, and there is cross-tolerance to most stimulants. It is not known whether this tolerance is related to cocaine.[57]

A crystallized form of methamphetamine known as *crystal, ice, glass,* or *quartz* (because it resembles transparent crystals) recently has appeared on the drug scene. It can be taken orally, inhaled, injected, or smoked. When smoked, the drug produces a high in a few seconds, which may last up to 24 hours. As with other CNS stimulants, ice can have serious adverse effects, including acute psychosis, severe paranoia, hallucinations, and violent behavior. These effects may last from a few days to weeks or even months. A person can quickly become addicted after using it just a few times. More research is needed to determine long-term effects.

Patterns of Amphetamine Abuse

Abusers of amphetamine generally can be classified into medical abusers and street abusers.[57] Medical abusers may obtain these drugs to aid in weight loss or to treat fatigue. Students may use them to help stay awake when studying for examinations; truck drivers may use them to stay awake during long distance driving. After the medication is discontinued, fatigue results, and need for sleep leads to an increased dose, eventually leading to chronic use.

Street abusers use amphetamine or similar drugs to get high or achieve an altered state of consciousness. The drug may be used alone or with depressant drugs. Another pattern is using the substance in runs; that is, taking the drug around the clock for 2 or even 4 days, usually intravenously.[57]

Amphetamine- and Similar Sympathomimetic-Induced Disorders

Intoxication. Physical symptoms of amphetamine intoxication include increased heart rate and blood pressure, dilated pupils, perspiration, chills, nausea, and vomiting. Psychological symptoms include psychomotor agitation, elation, grandiosity, talkativeness, loquacity, and hypervigilance. People intoxicated with amphetamine display maladaptive behavior, such as fighting, interference in social and occupational functioning, and impaired judgment.

Delirium. Symptoms of amphetamine delirium usually occur within 1 hour of oral intake or immediately after the intravenous injection and subside within 6 hours. Symptoms include hallucinations (visual, tactile, and olfactory), labile affect, and violent, aggressive behavior.

Delusional Disorder. Prolonged, chronic use of moderate to high doses of amphetamine may result in a delusional disorder. Symptoms include persecutory delusions, ideas of reference, aggressiveness, hostility, anxiety, and psychomotor agitation. The delusional person may experience distortion of body image or tactile hallucinations, such as feeling bugs crawling under the skin. The delusional disorder may last for 1 week or longer, even for as long as 1 year.

Withdrawal. Amphetamine withdrawal follows prolonged use with abrupt cessation or reduction in use. Symptoms include dysphoric mood (eg, depression, irritability, anxiety), fatigue, disturbed sleep, and increased dreaming. Dysphoric mood is the main feature of this disorder; if it is severe, agitation or suicidal ideation may occur. The sleep disturbance is related to an increase in rapid eye movement sleep and may persist for weeks. The withdrawal syndrome occurs within 3 days of cessation or reduction in the use of the substance and peaks in 2 or 4 days. Depression and irritability, however, may continue for months.

Medical Consequences. The medical consequences of abuse of amphetamine and similar drugs are those associated with overdose. Problems such as tetanus, hepatitis, abscesses, and infections may also result from the complications of self-injection. Cerebrovascular accident may result from strong contractions of blood vessels caused by stimulants; the increase in blood pressure may cause intracranial hemorrhage.[57]

Effects of Cocaine

Cocaine is an akaloid obtained from the coca plant (*Erythroxylum coca*), which grows in South America. It is a white, odorless, fluffy powder that looks like snow, giving the substance one of its street names. It may be taken by sniffing through the nose (snorting), where it is absorbed through the nasal mucous membranes. Cocaine can be absorbed from all mucous surfaces, including the gums or mucous lining of the mouth, rectal and vaginal mucosa, and abrasions of the skin surface. All of these routes can be used. Cocaine may be injected intravenously (mainlining), mixed in the same syringe with heroin (a speedball), or smoked (freebasing). Because cocaine hydrochloride decomposes at high temperature, *freebase* is the term used when the cocaine alkaloid is freed from the hydrochloride salt. Some users have kits to perform this process. In the United States, cocaine freebase for smoking is sold in *crack* or *rock* form. Crack appears to be the most addictive form of cocaine.[4,29,37]

Smoking cocaine is an efficient way of delivering the drug in a concentrated form to the brain. The alveoli of the lung offer a large area for absorption of the chemical substance. The appeal of smoking to users is the rapid circulation time from the lungs to the brain—about 6 to 8 seconds—whereas circulation from arm to the brain takes about 16 seconds. Cocaine is metabolized by plasma enzymes and the liver and excreted in the urine.[4,29,57]

Research has shown that cocaine acts directly on the brain's pleasure centers, brain structures that, when stimulated, produce an intense desire to experience the pleasurable effects again and again. This causes changes in the brain activity and by allowing the neurotransmitter dopamine to remain active longer than normal, triggers an intense craving for more of the drug.

Cocaine-Induced Disorders

Intoxication. Cocaine intoxication is marked by maladaptive behavioral effects, such as fighting and impaired judgment and problems in occupational or social functioning. Physical and psychological symptoms occur within minutes to 1 hour of taking the drug. The psychological symptoms include an increased sense of well-being and confidence, increased awareness of sensory input, psychomotor agitation, elation, talkativeness, pacing, and pressured speech. Physical symptoms are increased heart rate, dilated pupils, increased blood pressure, sweating, chills, nausea, and vomiting. Cocaine use, especially by intravenous injection, causes a characteristic *rush* or feeling of increased self-confidence and well-being. A severely intoxicated person may experience confusion, incoherent speech, anxiety, paranoid thoughts, headache, and palpitations. Following the physical effects, the user is likely to feel anxious, tremulous, irritable, depressed, and fatigued. In this state, known as *crashing,* the user craves more cocaine for relief of these unpleasant symptoms. Recovery from intoxication occurs in 24 hours.

Delirium. The symptoms of cocaine delirium usually occur within 1 hour of use (immediately when the substance is taken by intravenous injection) and subside within 6 hours. Symptoms include labile affect, violent aggressive behavior, and tactile and olfactory hallucinations.

Delusional Disorder. An organic delusional syndrome occurs soon after use of the drug. Symptoms include rapid development of persecutory delusions, distortion of body image, and misperception of faces. Persecutory delusions may lead to aggressive or violent behavior; tactile hallucinations, such as the feeling of insects crawling on the skin (formication), also occur.

Cocaine Withdrawal. Cocaine withdrawal follows abrupt cessation or reduction in prolonged (several days or longer) use. Symptoms include a dysphoric mood (eg, depression, irritability, anxiety) along with fatigue, psychomotor agitation, and insomnia or hypersomnia. Paranoid and suicidal thoughts may occur; suicide is a major concern of withdrawal. Symptoms last for more than 24 hours after cessation of drug use.

Medical Consequences. During cocaine intoxication, a person may experience formication.[4] Severe skin ulcerations may result from the user's attempts to dig out the "insects." Overdose can produce cardiac arrhythmias, convulsions, and respiratory depression.[37] Repeated heavy use by snorting the drug can cause tissue ulcerations in the nasal septum.[37] Cocaine use can produce a paranoid psychosis similar to paranoid schizophrenia disorder. This may require prolonged treatment and the use of antipsychotic medication.[37]

Hallucinogens

Effects

Also called *psychomimetics,* hallucinogens alter mood and perception. Ingestion of these drugs results in alterations in time and space perception, illusions, hallucinations, and delusions. The character and intensity of these reactions depend on the drug dosage and the personality of the user. The results are unpredictable: A person may experience a high on one occasion and a "bad trip" on another.[16,37] The most potent and most common hallucinogenic drug is LSD. Lysergic acid comes from ergot, a fungus that spoils rye grain. It was converted to LSD by a Swiss chemist in 1943. The odorless, colorless, and tasteless drug is classified as a hallucinogenic drug because it produces hallucinations.[16]

The LSD trips start within one-half hour after taking the drug and last for varying lengths of time. It is uncertain how LSD acts on the nervous system, but it is so powerful that only small doses—100 to 250 μg—are needed. The drug in liquid form is usually placed on a sugar cube; it has also been put on chewing gum, cookies, and blotting paper.[17,37] The misuse of LSD seems to be decreasing, possibly because of the widespread knowledge that side effects, such as flashbacks and chromosomal damage, may result from LSD use.

Hallucinogen-Induced Disorders

Hallucinogen Hallucinosis. After drug ingestion, a hallucinogen hallucinosis may result. It is evidenced by perceptual changes, dilated pupils, increased heart rate, sweating, palpitations, blurred vision, tremors, and incoordination. Also present are maladaptive behavioral effects, such as severe anxiety or depression, fear of losing one's mind, ideas of reference, paranoid ideation, impaired judgment, and interference with social and occupational functioning. The perceptual changes, the main feature of the hallucinosis, occur in a state of wakefulness and alertness and include subjective intensification of perceptions, depersonalization, illusions, hallucinations, and synesthesias (eg, seeing noise). The hallucinations are often visual and colorful and contain geometric forms and patterns. The hallucinosis syndrome begins within 1 hour after ingestion and lasts for several hours. Individual variations of the experience are related to the user's personality, the setting, and the user's expectations. Euphoria is common. The person is usually aware that the changes in perception are due to the hallucinogen, although in some instances, the person fears loss of sanity and believes this will be a permanent state.

Hallucinogen Delusional Disorder. The use of hallucinogens may result in an organic delusional disorder that exists beyond the period of the direct effects of the substance, lasting longer than 24 hours after cessation of use. The perceptual changes of hallucinogen hallucinosis occur, but the individual believes that these misperceptions and thoughts are based on reality.

Hallucinogen Mood Disorder. An organic mood syndrome caused by hallucinogen ingestion may result in a disturbance in mood, often a depressed mood accompanied by feelings of guilt, fearfulness, and restlessness. The person may be talkative and unable to sleep. The disorder may last for a brief or a prolonged time and may be difficult to differentiate from a mood disorder.

Medical Consequences. Flashbacks, recurrences of hallucinations when the drug is no longer being used, may occur weeks or months after stoppage of drug use.[37] People who have abused hallucinogens for a prolonged period are more likely to experience flashbacks. The episodes cause anxiety and the fear of going crazy. Physical dependence on hallucinogens does not develop. Tolerance develops and disappears quickly. Psychological dependence occurs in some people after chronic use. These people are known as *acid heads,* implying a personality change as a result of long-term hallucinogen use. The person becomes more passive and introspective and may lose the ability to concentrate.[16,37] Research has investigated the possibility of hallucinogen-induced chromosome damage that produces congenital malformations, but this has not been confirmed. Medical problems are related to self-injury during periods of impaired judgment or delusions.

Cannabis

Effects

Cannabis sativa comes from the hemp plant, which is grown in warm climates and from which marijuana and hashish are derived. Tetrahydrocannabinol (THC) is the active ingredient in marijuana and hashish. Marijuana consists of dried plant buds and leaves and contains less THC than hashish, which is derived from the resin of the plant flowers.[17,37]

The most predominant effects of cannabis are euphoria and altered level of consciousness without hallucinations. The drug can be smoked or eaten. The metabolites are excreted in feces and urine.[57]

During the 1960s, marijuana was popular and used for antiestablishment protest. Presently, use conforms to no specific social group, although many users are teenagers and young adults.[4,77]

Cannabis-Induced Disorders

Intoxication. Cannabis intoxication is marked by increased heart rate, conjunctival injection (bloodshot eyes), increased appetite (often for sweets or junk food), dry mouth, the psychological symptoms of euphoria, subjective intensification of perceptions, sensation of slowed time, and apathy. Maladaptive behavioral effects may include impaired judgment, interference with social or occupational functioning, panic attacks, suspiciousness, paranoid ideation, or excessive anxiety.

Cannabis Delusional Disorder. This delusional syndrome may occur with persecutory delusions during an episode of intoxication or immediately following use of cannabis. This disturbance does not usually last longer than 6 hours after cessation of use.

Medical Consequences. Marijuana smoke has an irritating effect on the lungs and may result in acute or chronic bronchitis and sinusitis in heavy smokers. Increased heart rate and decreased strength of cardiac contractions invariably result from marijuana use, bringing dangerous consequences to people with heart conditions. Research has indicated impairment in sperm production and chromosomal damage, but results have not been conclusive. There is also controversy concerning a causal link between marijuana use and brain damage. There is a theory that marijuana use leads to abuse of more potent drugs, although this has not been substantiated.[69]

PRENATAL ALCOHOL AND DRUG ABUSE

Prenatal drug use has profound effects on the mother, her baby, and ultimately, society. The number of women of childbearing age who use and are dependent on cocaine, alcohol, heroin, and other drugs that affect the CNS has increased dramatically. Drugs that affect the CNS cross the placenta into the fetal circulation. The exposed fetus is at a high risk for various medical, developmental, and behavioral problems (Boxes 33-6 and 33-7).

Many drug-dependent pregnant women use various chemical substances in combination with alcohol. For example, a woman's drug of choice may be cocaine, but after the euphoria of the desired effect wears off, she will experience unpleasant feelings of depression, nervousness, jitteriness, tense muscles, insomnia, and cocaine crash. She may use a CNS depressant, such as heroin, barbiturates, or alcohol, to relieve these symptoms. Such polydrug abuse puts the woman and fetus at increased risk.

A woman using harmful substances may not know that she is pregnant. In most instances, the drug-dependent mother-to-be is unable to stop using drugs on her own. Not even the new life within her can deter her from her addictions. Without help, her condition and that of her fetus is perilous. And even with intervention, the mother and fetus continue to be at risk for serious problems that may have lifelong consequences. Women who use alcohol and drugs during pregnancy come from all social situations, from the affluent to the severely impoverished. They may be street wise or homemakers, employed in a variety of jobs, have a professional career, or be on welfare. Many women are in drug-related and male relationships that involve violence. Many have been abandoned by their male partner or family. Some live in shelters or drug ghettos near crack houses; others live in suburbs or in high-income residential areas. Many have had their children taken from them and placed in protective foster care; some may lack even the most basic skills necessary to be parents. Some women may use drugs in a small circle of friends as a recreational process and think they can take or leave the drug alone whenever they choose. For

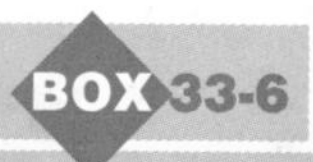

BOX 33-6

Effects of Prenatal Alcohol Use: A First-Person Account

Alcohol is a teratogenic drug; that is, when taken during pregnancy, it can cause adverse effects in the fetus. Many alcohol-related birth defects have been associated with alcohol use during pregnancy. The most clearly defined effect on the fetus is a specific pattern of neonatal defects called fetal alcohol syndrome (FAS). Fetal alcohol syndrome is manifested by a group of congenital birth defects including the following:

1. Prenatal and postnatal growth deficiency
2. A particular pattern of facial malformations, including a small head circumference, flattened midface, sunken nasal bridge, and a flattened and elongated philtrum (the groove between the nose and upper lip)
3. Central nervous system dysfunction
4. Varying degrees of major organ system malfunction

The following statement was written by Maureen, an 18-year-old in her first semester of college. Maureen is unique, not in her aspirations, but in her survival of physical and emotional trauma. She was born addicted to drugs. It would be inappropriate to assume that most people triumph over such afflictions, but Maureen is atypical in her coping ability and in her development of positive self-direction. Her social awareness, in combination with her internal and external support systems, created an accepting individual with significant tolerance for social ignorance. Maureen writes:

> Years ago my brother and I were born fifteen minutes apart. Not knowing what to expect, just like all other newborns, we had our first reality of life. We had to deal with withdrawal from drugs. Our biological parents were dependent upon drugs. On arrival into the world we were faced with going without the drugs which we were hooked on for nine months while inside of her womb. The painful struggle for the body was hard and long. After seeing adults who must be hospitalized for being so sick with pain, can you even imagine the pain your child and my brother and I went through? No, we don't remember, no child will because they have no knowledge, but it is extremely hard and upsetting to know that our parents put us through this by their unnecessary and selfish acts. My brother is quite healthy, but I had to have surgery right after birth to disconnect my cranial plates. I lost 50% of my hearing and am blind in one eye from hypertension. A shunt has been put in my spine to catch the overflow of spinal fluid and I still have arthritis in my hands that I was born with.
>
> It has been a life-long struggle for me to stay away from prescription drugs, because anything I take can cause blindness in my other eye. If you have any "smarts," stay away from drugs and alcohol while you're pregnant. The choice is yours, but just remember, your irresponsible acts can cause death or permanent damage to your unborn child.
>
> So Mommy, please let me breathe, think, and look like you when I come into that wonderful world.
>
> —Maureen

some, only when they become pregnant do they realize they are unable to stop using the drug.

Some people may not understand how a woman who is pregnant cannot stop using a drug that may severely damage her fetus and ruin her own health, family relationships, and ability to work; consume her income; and in many instances, involve her in illegal activities. The nurse must understand that the psychological craving to obtain the desired euphoric effects and to eliminate the dysphoric aspects of abstinence from the drug motivates the woman to continue to use the drugs regardless of the devastating consequences; she is drug dependent (see Box 33-7).

Serious legal and ethical questions arise concerning the rights of the mother versus the rights of the unborn child. Some authorities believe that the mother should be held legally responsible for endangering the life of her unborn child, but health professionals recognize the woman and fetus as victims of a disease. The American Nurses Association opposes the criminal prosecution of the drug-dependent mother and supports early detection of women at risk and rapid treatment of affected mothers and infants (see Case Study 33-2, p. 690).

Application of the Nursing Process to Substance Abuse and Dependency Disorders

The discussion of the use of the nursing process with clients who evidence disorders of substance abuse and dependency focuses on general concepts applicable in all areas of practice. Although the issue of rehabilitation is addressed in relation to psychiatric inpatient settings, nurses encounter problems of substance abuse and dependence in all areas of nursing.

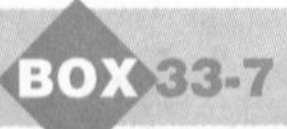

Cocaine Babies

There has been a rapid growth in the use of cocaine by pregnant women. The following overview depicts the possible devastating consequences that may occur in cocaine-affected pregnancies.

MATERNAL COMPLICATIONS

- Spontaneous abortions
- Higher incidence of abruptio placentae with increased stillbirth
- Increased cocaine-induced uterine contractibility
- Tachycardia, arrhythmias, angina
- Increased rate of premature births
- Seizures
- Cerebral vascular accidents
- Hypertension
- Anorexia resulting in weight loss
- Respiratory lung damage if cocaine is smoked
- HIV virus if used intravenously

EFFECTS ON THE FETUS

- Cerebral artery injury and infarction
- Acute hypertension
- Low birth weight
- Intrauterine growth retardation
- Decreased head circumference
- Decreased length
- Skull defects
- Increased cardiac anomalies
- HIV if used intravenously

EFFECTS ON THE NEWBORN

- Increased rate of sudden infant death syndrome
- Abnormalities on the Brazelton Neonatal Behavioral Assessment Scale
- Poor suck and swallow pattern
- Fine motor tremors of hands, arms, legs
- Unusual response to stimuli
- Vomiting, poor feeding
- Weak pull-to-sit development
- Irritability, difficulty sleeping
- Intolerance to cuddling
- Difficult to comfort
- Seizures in babies whose mothers use cocaine while breastfeeding

MOTHER–INFANT BONDING

Infants exposed to cocaine may be unable to bond with their mothers. To form attachment, the newborn and mother bond through an interactive process. The infant responds to the mother's eye contact, speaking, cuddling, talking and grasping. The infant who is unresponsive to these behavioral cues from the mother may produce feelings of frustration, anger, and inadequacy in the mother. This in turn may create a pattern of the mother's negative response to the infant and put the infant in danger of physical and emotional abuse.

ASSESSMENT

The Nurse's Attitude and Feelings

The nurse's attitude toward the client with substance abuse or dependency is a crucial component of the interview process. Clients with substance abuse problems are often sensitive to and perceptive of the attitudes and mannerisms of nurses and other health team members. The initial approach to interviewing a client needs to be nonjudgmental and objective. It is not unusual for the nurse to want to rescue the client; therefore, it is important to become aware of this possible reaction. The nurse's personal value system, unpleasant contact with people who abuse substances, and possible personal history of abuse or dependency may arouse judgmental feelings or attitudes toward the client. (Box 33-8 provides information on health professionals who have substance abuse problems.)

A therapeutic nurse possesses adequate knowledge about the substance abuse or dependency disorder and approaches the client with compassion and gentle firmness. During the interview, the nurse should avoid using words or terms that may be interpreted by the client as offensive, such as *drunk, addict, alcoholic,* and *boozer.* Rather, the nurse uses terms with a less negative connotation that convey the appropriate meaning, such as *alcohol use, feeling good,* and *feeling high.* The recovery process is another factor that may affect attitudes. Frequently, nurses and other health team members see more initial failures than successes. Relapse and return to drug use after treatment is not uncommon. Nevertheless, recovery does occur in many instances, and those who work in the area of substance abuse and dependence need to develop an attitude of hope. Feelings of hopelessness in the

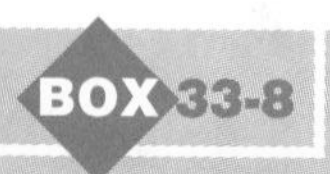

Update on Impaired Professionals

Suzanne Stanton RN., C., B.S., NCAC II Central & Western New York Coordinator Committee for Physicians' Health Medical Society of the State of New York Syracuse Regional Office, Syracuse, N.Y.

Treatment of chemical dependence and mental illness in the health care professional, particularly physicians and nurses, is a crucial issue in health care, because of the potential harm to clients if these diseases go untreated. Substance abuse and the ensuing mental illness that result in the loss of personal well-being seriously compromise the delivery of safe, quality health care to the public. Alcoholism and other drug addictions and some forms of mental illness are amenable to treatment; those affected should have the opportunity to obtain treatment and rehabilitation before action on licensure by the State Health Department. Because these diseases are progressive and lead to physical and mental deterioration, early detection and treatment are the primary goals of the American Medical Association (AMA) and American Nurses Association (ANA).

Impairment as defined by the AMA occurs when the physician is unable to practice medicine with reasonable skill and safety because of mental illness or excessive use or abuse of drugs, including alcohol. According to the ANA, nursing practice is impaired when the individual is unable to meet the requirements of the professional code of ethics and standards of practice because cognitive, interpersonal, or psychomotor behaviors are affected by conditions of the individual in interaction with the environment. These factors include psychiatric illness, excessive alcohol or drug use, or addiction. The Medical Society of New York State distinguishes between troubled and impaired. Within this context, physicians are described as troubled when their chemical dependence or mental illness has produced personal, family, or other interpersonal distress but has not yet affected the medical practice. It is important to intervene before a client is injured.

How many physicians are impaired? The most conservative statement is that no one knows. Reliable data are not available; however, medical societies are collecting data through computers, and soon more valid statistics will be available concerning those who are in treatment. Until the medical community becomes sophisticated enough, trusting enough of the programs in place for treatment, and makes referrals to these programs, many physicians will go untreated. However, a plausible estimate is that 3% of all physicians at some time in their career are impaired as a result of drugs or alcohol abuse; others estimate it at 5%. Others feel that the figure might be as high as 18%. In the general population, the figure is 10%, and there is no reason to think that this figure is lower in medical practitioners. There is some rationale to think it might be higher due to the vulnerability of this group and the easy access to drugs in the workplace. Of the cases seen in treatment, approximately 80% are treated for alcohol or drug abuse and 10% for senility; the others are treated for mental illness.

The degree of impairment in nurses continues to be unclear. Research data on the prevalence of chemical dependence and psychiatric illness in professionals are not readily compiled. However, many state programs are becoming computer literate and are beginning to track people who come under their auspices. The emergence of employee assistance programs and nurse advocacy or network programs is facilitating early treatment for nurses and preventing impairment in the workplace, thus allowing nurses to be rehabilitated without infringing on their practice and license. According to the Office of Professional Discipline (OPD) in New York State, only one or two nurses are disciplined each year because of mental illness, and this is because their behavior in the workplace is bizarre, placing clients at risk. More directors of nursing are recognizing early symptoms and referring nurses for treatment rather than terminating.

The Professional Assistance Program (PAP) is an alternative to the OPD system in New York State. It is a voluntary program that allows licensed health care professionals to seek treatment for substance abuse and avoid disciplinary action providing there is no evidence of client harm. This law was established in 1987 and is called the Donovan Law. The PAP current case load is 399 as of January 1996. In 1994, the PAP case load was 67 nurses out of a total case intake of 82. That year 45 RN licenses were restored.

In New York State during 1994, the OPD disciplined 276 nurses and in 1995, 272. Approximately 30% of those were for drug and alcohol usage and were not eligible for the services of the PAP. Of those 276 and 272, approximately 60 nurses would have been prosecuted but instead sought the service of the PAP, voluntarily surrendered their license to seek treatment, were monitored by the PAP, and with evidence of solid recovery, had their license restored. Those who are followed by PAP have no record of client harm, but the potential for client harm exists because of their addictions.

continued

BOX 33-8 (Continued)

In 1995, the PAP had 86 intakes on health care professionals, and 67 of those were nurses. Eighty nurses' licenses were restored by PAP in 1995. At any one time, the PAP case load is comprised of 70% to 80% nurses. If we apply the increasing knowledge that is being gathered concerning adult children of alcoholics, we may consider that these percentages might be higher, because the oldest child in alcoholic families often chooses a helping profession as a career. This would apply to physicians, pharmacists, nurses, clergy, and social workers. The real answer to prevalency, therefore, lies in future research.

Physicians and nurses are at high risk to develop the disease of chemical dependency. The genetic factor cannot be emphasized enough. Many come from alcoholic families, and this predisposes them to the disease and makes them at risk if they decide to use. The mechanics of work in medicine and nursing are often stressful and demanding and often lacking in recognition of effect and accomplishment; relief drug usage may be sought and seen as temporarily effective.

In 1981, the ANA resolved to address health problems of nurses. The ANA was particularly concerned with the practice of nurses whose judgment was impaired by drugs, alcohol, or psychological dysfunction. A resolution was made for action on alcohol and drug abuse and psychological dysfunction in relation to the ANA Code for Nurses. This was an effort to show responsibility to society, to self-regulate the practice of its members, and to ensure quality in professional performance. This issue was emphasized heavily at the ANA convention in 1984. At the district and state levels, nurses have planned and put into place programs for peer assistance for impaired nurses. Treatment is tailored to meet individual needs of the impaired nurse. It may include inpatient, outpatient, detoxification, rehabilitation, psychiatric treatment, and participation in self-help groups. Confidentiality is critical to the program.

If the nurse does not cooperate with treatment recommendations and his or her practice places clients in jeopardy, the nurse may be referred to the Board of Regents or State Boards of Nurse Examiners for further investigation.

Chemical dependency is a complex, progressive, but treatable illness that has been largely ignored or denied in the female population as a whole and, more specifically, in the predominantly female profession of nursing. To prevent the progression of these diseases, we need to recognize early symptoms, gently confront the nurse in the presence of another nurse, and offer assistance into treatment. The nurses doing the confrontation must be firm, supportive, prepared for denial and hostility, and have a plan for rejection. Early symptoms may be any combination of the following:

1. Absent or late for work, especially following several days off (Note, however, that drug-addicted nurses may never be absent and may "hang around" when not on duty because the hospital is their source of supply.)
2. Odor of alcohol on the breath (Any nurse who would report for duty after drinking is assuming a terrible risk and in doing so is evidencing loss of control and need for the drug.)
3. Odor of mouthwash and breath mints, which may be used to mask the odor of alcohol
4. Fine tremors of the hands, occurring with withdrawal from the drug (The alcoholic nurse will sometimes begin to use tranquilizers to mask signs of withdrawal and thus may develop cross-dependency.)
5. Emotional lability, such as abrupt change from being irritable and tense to being mellow and calm, inappropriate anger or crying
6. Returning late from lunch breaks
7. Sleepiness or dozing off while on duty
8. Shunning interaction with others and tending to withdraw
9. Frequent trips to the bathroom, carrying handbag
10. Deterioration in personal appearance
11. Frequent bruises or cigarette burns, resulting from crashing into furniture or falling while intoxicated or dozing off with a lighted cigarette
12. Impaired job performance, with sloppy or illegible handwriting, errors in charting (eg, charting on the wrong chart), and errors in client care
13. Memory lapses or confusion or euphoric recall of events
14. Shunning of job assignments or job shrinkage and dropping out of professional activities

The nurse who is stealing drugs from the unit may exhibit the following:

1. Always volunteer to give medications
2. Medicate another nurse's client
3. Always use the maximum PRN dosage when other nurses use less, or use the maximum PRN dosage on one shift but not on another (The PRN medications afford the greatest opportunity for the nurse to supply his or her habit.)
4. Have responsibility for clients who complain that medication given on one shift is not as effective as on others or that they did not receive medication when the record shows they did

continued

BOX 33-8 (Continued)

5. Have frequent wastage, such as spillage of drugs or drawing blood into the syringe
6. Work on a unit where drugs are disappearing or seals have been broken

With treatment, physicians and nurses emerge with improved practice. They now are able to recognize early symptoms of chemical dependence and mental illness in their clients and are able to diagnose and treat more accurately. They are able to look beyond the presenting symptom for further evidence of alcoholism or other drug dependencies. Physicians begin to look at their prescribing practices and refrain from freely prescribing benzodiazepines and begin to recognize the need to refer their clients for treatment of chemical dependency. Thus, to salvage a career for these professionals means getting improved treatment for many others.

nurse or other health team workers are projected to the client; the reverse is also true.

Approaching the Client

Drug-dependent clients who are being interviewed may be embarrassed about their behavior or may display uncooperative behavior. One way for the nurse to encourage cooperation is by demonstrating acceptance and a matter-of-fact manner, one that shows concern and conveys the messages, "I care about your well-being" and "I know you are uncomfortable; I want to help you feel better."

The nurse maintains an empathetic approach during the interview and even though the client may be defensive or vague, does not respond with defensiveness or hostility. Questions should be formulated to elicit specific factual information and should be stated in such a way that they cannot be answered with evasive statements or generalities (Case Study 33-1). If the client diverts the conversation, the nurse brings it back to the facts being discussed.

A format for eliciting information in major areas of assessment is provided in Box 33-9. These guidelines are not meant to be all-encompassing. The examples of assessment data are not the only observations that may be noted; there will be others that are not listed on this assessment form.

Because denial is frequently used by the client who abuses or is dependent on substances, some of the information obtained during the interview may be of questionable validity. A more reliable history or a clearer validation of the information obtained about the substance abuse disorder may be established by interviewing a significant other (spouse, parent, adult, child, employer, roommate) in the client's life. Although this information may also be somewhat distorted due to the emotional involvement and denial system operating in the spouse or significant other, it may corroborate data about the client's substance use and harmful consequences. Another important reason for interviewing the significant others is to involve them in the beginning of the treatment and rehabilitation process.

Recognizing Emergency Conditions

Substance intoxication, overdose, severe alcohol and sedative-hypnotic withdrawal, withdrawal delirium, withdrawal seizures, and prolonged narcotic withdrawal may be life-threatening disorders that necessitate interruption of assessment for immediate intervention. The severity of withdrawal or abstinence syndrome depends on many factors, such as the type of drug used, the extent of the addiction, drug history, nutritional status, and status of fluid and electrolyte balance.[17,37,58] Major medical complications, to which the nurse must attend, also may exist.

Intoxication

All of the drugs discussed in this chapter may cause intoxication. If the intoxication is severe, symptoms may include lethargy and stupor, and an overdose of the drug may be a possibility. The intoxicated client may also demonstrate bizarre behavior, panic, fright, confusion, or physical problems, such as vomiting or pain.[4] The treatment measures for simple intoxication may consist of careful observation of symptoms, emotional support, and protection from physical injury until the drug has been metabolized. In most instances, intoxication resolves within a few to several hours.

Overdose

Drug overdose may be a severe medical problem necessitating critical care until the emergency situation is resolved. It occurs most frequency with alcohol, sedative-hypnotics, and narcotic drug use.[16,37]

Withdrawal Syndrome

Various medications are given for detoxification purposes and relief of withdrawal symptoms. The nurse should be knowledgeable about the drug or drugs ingested, dose, route of administration, reactions, and

33-1 **Case Study**

Assessing An Elderly Client's Substance Abuse

You are working in a Home Health Agency. Your first assignment of the day is to visit John. He has been referred to you as a mental health consultant. You have the following history before you enter his home:

John is 70 years old, widowed, and lives alone in subsidized housing. He has been receiving medical treatment for high blood pressure, heart disease, and type II diabetes. His medical problems have been controlled by medications. He has been seen weekly by the home health nurse for management of his health care.

On previous visits by the home health nurse, John was well groomed, his apartment was clean, and he was able to do light housekeeping and his own cooking. He expressed pride in his independence. He was usually in a friendly mood, sharing bits of information about his week and general topics of the day. Recently he appeared unkempt; his clothing was wrinkled and soiled. His hygiene was poor; body odor and the smell of urine were noted. The nurse also noted cigarette burns on John's pants. There were several beer cans in the trash beside the kitchen door. John was irritable and quick tempered. He stated he had been drinking "several" beers a day to help his appetite. He denied any sort of problems associated with drinking in his past. John admitted feeling lonely, bored, and depressed. He said he may have forgotten to take his medication once or twice, but there was nothing wrong with him.

Questions for Discussion

1. What would your priority assessment be in this situation?
2. What questions might you ask?
3. How would you discuss this situation with the primary nurse case manager?
4. What follow-up plan, if any, might you have?

possible effects and toxic effects of the drugs. Generally, the following drugs are used in the treatment of withdrawal syndrome:

1. The barbiturates are used primarily for barbiturate withdrawal.
2. Anxiolytics, such as chlordiazepoxide (Librium) or diazepam (Valium), are used for alcohol withdrawal.
3. Codeine, propoxyphene (Darvon), or other opiate-type drugs are given for relief of narcotic withdrawal symptoms; if these symptoms are severe, methadone or morphine may be used.
4. Anticonvulsant drugs, particularly phenytoin (Dilantin), are given for alcohol and sedative-hypnotic withdrawal seizures.
5. Thiamine is usually given in the alcohol withdrawal treatment phase to prevent Wernicke-Korsakoff syndrome. Multivitamins are frequently administered because of the typically poor nutritional status of the drug-dependent client.[7]

Recognizing Behavioral Defenses

Defense mechanisms are processes within the mind (ie, intrapsychic processes) that are usually unconscious and that relieve the client's emotional conflict and anxiety.[4]

Denial

Denial is the outstanding defense mechanism used by clients who abuse or are dependent on substances. It is especially profound in alcohol abuse and dependency.

Denial is an unconscious process used to protect against intolerable feelings, thoughts, wishes, needs, or external reality factors by blocking knowledge of these factors from conscious awareness.[25] Defense or coping mechanisms are used in normal ways to adapt to threatening situations, such as the normal grief process in terminal illness. The use of defense mechanisms becomes unhealthy when they are used inappropriately and when they interfere with healthy functioning. The

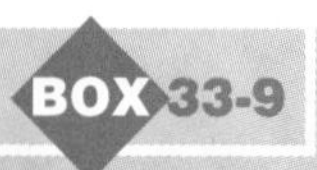

Assessment Guidelines

Demographic data:
Name:
Age:
Sex:
Ethnic group:
Marital status:
Religious affiliation:
Significant other:

What is the reason for coming to the hospital (eg, symptoms of withdrawal, marital-family crisis, work problems, referred by legal source, wants help to stop drinking or using drugs, medical problems)?

What is the motivation for treatment:	
General observations:	
Vital signs:	Blood pressure (hypotensive, hypertensive)
Pulse:	Rapid, regular, irregular
Temperature:	Elevated
Respirations:	Rapid, shallow, depressed
Appearance:	
Gait:	Unsteady, normal, weaving, shuffling
Eyes:	Conjunctival injection, bloodshot, dilated, pinpoint, normal pupils, lacrimation (tearing), vacant stare, poor eye contact, good eye contact
Skin:	Perspiration, cool, clammy, dry, bruises, needle tracks, scars, abrasions, gooseflesh, excoriations, reddened palms
Nose:	Running (rhinorrhea), congested, red
Presence of tremors:	Fine or coarse, slight-moderate or severe
Grooming:	Neat, unkempt, unshaven, odor (alcohol, foul)
Behavior:	
Speech:	Slurred, incoherent, loud, soft, normal, articulates clearly, monotone, hesitant, pressured, relevant, distractive
Attitude:	Quiet, calm, demanding, agitated, irritable, impatient, vague, withdrawn, suspicious, anxious, tearful, happy, silly
Dominant mood—Affect:	Euphoric, depressed, angry, sad, appropriate, inappropriate, normal
Sensorium:	Orientation to time, person, place; changes in memory
Perception:	The presence of illusions, hallucinations, delusions, hallucinosis
Potential for suicide:	Is the individual presently thinking about suicide? Is there a plan or a method to carry out that plan? Is there a history of previous suicide attempts or gestures? Were attempts in intoxicated state or sober state? Is there a family history of suicide? Is there a recent loss or anniversary of a loss? (Assess need for emergency consultation and intervention.)
Potential for violence:	Dose behavior indicate potential for violence (voice, manner, stance, verbal threats)? Assess need for consultation, emergency intervention if necessary. Ask if individual has a history of violence when taking substances or during withdrawal period.
Present drug history:	The areas that need specific assessment are the type of substance used, the amount taken, and the pattern of use.
Type:	Beer, wine, whiskey, cocaine, heroin, marijuana (cannabis), sedative-hypnotics, hallucinogens; one substance only, or a combination? This may mean combination within a class (ie, alcohol, beer, whiskey, and wine, or alcohol and sediative-hypnotics). It may be combinations in different classes (ie, heroin and alcohol and stimulants or narcotics and sedative-hypnotics). What is the predominant substance of choice? Does the individual use street drugs, prescription drugs?

continued

BOX 33-9 (Continued)

Amount: How much (approximate amount) does the individual drink? How many six packs, quarts, fifths? How much does he or she use, bags? What route (oral, intravenous, subcutaneous)? How many pills or hits daily?

Pattern of use: Does drinking occur daily, several times a week? Is it increased on weekends or only occur weekends? Do binge or episodic drinking or runs occur? Is he or she intoxicated daily? Has individual ever tried to control or cut down drinking or substance use? How?

When was last drink?
When was last drug dose? How was it taken?
What drugs are currently being taken?
Has individual developed tolerance? (explain)
When did it begin?
Has there been a change in tolerance?
Are withdrawal symptoms present?
Is there a history of withdrawal?
Is there a history of seizures?
Is there a history of hallucinations? (explain)
Is there a history of hallucinosis?
Was individual ever hospitalized? If yes, for what?
Are there any present medical problems?
Are there any chronic medical problems?
Is there a history of the following: liver disease, hepatitis, diabetes, heart disease, anemia, drug overdose?
Have there been any recent falls, injuries, accidents?
Is the individual taking any prescribed medication?
Has the individual any known allergies?
Drug history:
Has the individual ever stopped drinking or using drugs?
How long was the period of abstinence?
Why did the individual abstain; what was the motivation?
At what age did the individual start abusing or using substances?
At what age did the individual first begin having difficulty in life circumstances due to drug intake?
Has the individual ever been in treatment for drug abuse or dependency?
What type of treatment: detoxification, rehabilitation?
How many times in treatment for the above?
Is there a family history of alcohol abuse or dependency?
Is there a family history of other substance abuse or dependency?

Psychosocial history:

Conjugal: Married, separated, divorced, never married, widowed? What is spouse's reaction to client's abuse of substances? Does the spouse abuse substances? Is substance use causing marital conflicts?

Parenting: Are there children? How many, ages, and sex? Have children had school problems, health problems, or physical, emotional, sleeping problems?

Intrapersonal: What are the individual's leisure activities, hobbies? Has there been a change in participation in these activities? Has there been a change in friends or a loss of friendships? Do the social activities center on the substance use or abuse?

Occupation/employment: What is individual's occupation and present employment? How long in present employment? Has the individual ever missed work from alcohol or drug use? Has the individual abused substances while working? Is substance use jeopardizing work or business? How long has individual been employed?

continued

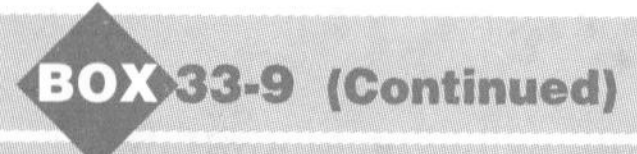

Finances and living conditions:	Approximate amount spent on substances. Source of income other than employment. Is the family suffering from less adequate housing or food due to substance abuse or purchases? What are present living conditions? Is individual living alone, in an apartment, own house, room; is there no address or no permanent living arrangement?
Legal problems:	Have there been any violations while intoxicated? Are any present legal offenses pending from substance abuse or dependency? Is present treatment court recommended?

person who abuses drugs often seems unaware of the apparent adverse psychological, social, and physical consequences of the excessive drug use. Frequently, the abuse or dependency disorder develops gradually, and denial and other defense mechanisms protect the individual from acknowledging the fact that the disorder is developing. This is especially true of alcoholism. Although denial can be found to some degree in all clients who abuse substances, it is most blatant in alcoholism and allows alcoholics literally to drink themselves to death. See Chapter 35, Codependency, for more information on enabling behavior.

People with alcohol abuse or dependence often cannot admit that alcohol is causing serious problems, so they continue drinking. One of the reasons for this denial in alcoholism is the blackouts that occur. The guilt feelings the person experiences as a result of drinking, the social stigma attached to the behavior or disorder, and the possibility of rejection by others foster the development of denial.[36] The family and significant others also contribute by denying that the drinking is a problem and by assuming caretaking or enabling roles rather than allowing the person to experience the serious consequences of the drinking behavior.

Projection

Projection is an unconscious mechanism whereby that which is emotionally unacceptable to the self is rejected and attributed to others.[25] Clients do not take responsibility for certain unacceptable behaviors and place their behavior outside of themselves, blaming other people, places, and things.

Rationalizing

Rationalizing is an unconscious mechanism by which the client justifies, by seemingly believable means, feelings, behaviors, or motives that would otherwise be intolerable.[25] For example, the client gives a reason for excessive use of a substance other than dependency. The drug use is not denied; an inaccurate, reasonable explanation is given instead.

Intellectualizing

Reasoning is used to defend against dealing with unconscious conflicts and their resulting stressful emotions.[25] Rather than discussing a personal awareness of an abuse or dependence problem, the client talks about the problem on an intellectual level, for example, analyzing the problem or giving theories related to the cause.

Minimizing

The client may admit to some drug abuse or dependence but makes it seem like a minor problem.

Diversion

The client may use certain tactics or techniques to change the subject to avoid the topic of abuse and dependency.

Anger

The client may express anger or displeasure in response to the subject of drug abuse or dependency. This reaction tends to induce the nurse or health care worker to change the subject, rather than confronting or dealing with the anger the discussion produces in the client.

The nurse recognizes that the denial process is a real phenomenon; that is, the client is not aware of the reality or extent of substance abuse or dependency disorder. Because the initial experience with the use of the drug was pleasurable and although the pleasant aspects of the experience have diminished and unfavorable consequences have developed, the search for recapturing the pleasure remains. The psychological compulsion to continue the drug use becomes so great that it becomes the priority in a dependent person's life.[36] What begins as a stress-relief or pleasure experience becomes the stressor. Denial helps drug-dependent clients maintain some sense of self-worth and remove themselves from the harmful consequences of behavior. In the process, however, clients become progressively out of touch with the reality of their situations.[36]

American society may contribute to this denial process because it promotes the use of substances, especially alcohol, for relief of stress and anxiety yet rejects the drug-dependent person as weak willed and amoral or as a "skid row bum." The drug user's significant others frequently overlook abuse or cover up the consequences of the behavior. In an effort to protect the person, they enable the harmful abuse to continue; this is the meaning of the term *enablers,* often used in the field of alcoholism.

Assessing Physical and Safety Needs

The physical needs of the client require constant assessment. The potential for infection is increased due to injuries, various medical consequences of the drugs, and factors that may result from substance-induced organic mental disorders. Table 33-2 provides a clinical pathway that includes the client's mental and physical needs.

The potential for physical injury is a serious problem. Ensuring safety and protecting the client from harm must be primary considerations. Substance-induced organic mental disorders present altered states of consciousness and impaired reality testing that will require vigilant assessment, thorough analysis, and appropriate nursing intervention.

Sleep disturbances are common, and conditions such as insomnia may result from withdrawal states, from the prolonged pattern of abuse or dependency, or from personal or family stress. Also, nightmares and increased dreaming may occur. Nursing measures to assess and alleviate sleep disturbances are undertaken; sedative-hypnotics are usually discouraged because of the abuse disorder.

Assessment and intervention must be individualized to deal with the feelings of anxiety stemming from underlying conflicts and other issues related to substance abuse or dependency and cessation of use.

Depression or feelings of profound sadness are related to decreased self-esteem because of substance abuse behavior or its familial, social, and legal consequences. These feelings require assessment and individualized treatment. Antidepressant medication may be used in conjunction with other supportive measures. The potential for suicide is a priority consideration and requires appropriate intervention (see Chapters 29, Depressive and Bipolar Disorders, and 42, Suicide).

Noncompliance with treatment is manifested in many ways, indicating a lack of motivation for treatment. It may be due to the denial syndrome and to a lack of understanding of the disorder. The nurse needs to be alert to these manifestations and help the client obtain insight into behavior.

NURSING DIAGNOSIS

Because of the wide range of physical and emotional needs of clients with substance abuse disorders, many of the accepted nursing diagnoses are appropriate guides for nursing care. Diagnoses applicable to the client's physical condition may include the following:

1. Fluid Volume Deficit
2. Altered Nutrition: Less than body requirements
3. Risk for Injury
4. Risk for Infection
5. Pain
6. Ineffective Airway Clearance
7. Impaired Skin Integrity
8. Sleep Pattern Disturbance
9. Constipation or Diarrhea
10. Self Care Deficit

Some diagnoses apply to the client's emotional state:

1. Ineffective Individual Coping
2. Ineffective Family Coping
3. Hopelessness
4. Self Esteem Disturbance
5. Altered Role Performance
6. Personal Identity Disturbance
7. Knowledge Deficit
8. Risk for Violence
9. Impaired Social Interaction
10. Spiritual Distress
11. Sensory/Perceptual Alterations
12. Altered Thought Processes
13. Altered Family Process: Alcoholism
14. Ineffective Denial

PLANNING

Developing therapeutic plans facilitates the client's participation in the treatment process and ultimate recovery. Individualized nursing assessment and intervention help the client achieve the desired behavioral outcomes that will aid in the restoration of emotional and physical well-being (Nursing Care Plan 33-1). Ultimately, the recovering client strives for increased satisfaction in a way of life free from mood- and mind-altering substances. Goal setting for clients who abuse or are dependent on substances includes the following elements:

1. Provision for physical requirements
2. Maintenance of emotional stability
3. Reduction and eventual resolution of the use of pathological defense mechanisms
4. Understanding and acceptance of the substance abuse or dependency disorder

(text continues on page 685)

Table 33-2 Clinical Pathway: Chemical Dependency, ETOH, Detox

Patient name: ______ **Case manager:** ______ **Physician:** ______ **Medical record #** ______
Admit date: ______ Expected LOS: ______ UR days certified: ______ Discharge date: ______ Actual LOS: ______

Day/Date:	0–8 Hours	8–24 Hours	Day 2	Day 3	Day 4	Day 5
ASSESSMENTS AND EVALUATIONS	Nursing Nutritional screen Admit note Precautions; V/S	H & P, Social HX, RT/TA; Dr. Initial TX Plan/Admit Note, V/S Prec. Eval.; AIMS Scale	Precaution Evaluation Nutritional Consult/Eval V/S	Psych Eval done Social Hx on chart Precaution eval.; V/S	Assess for readiness for discharge/change in level of care	Assess for goals achieved
PROCEDURES	Lab ordered-Admit profile UA, UDS, UCG, EKG, Other: PPD ordered	Lab done: Consider Ammonia level Other: PPD done	Lab results checked Abnormals called to Dr.	Follow-up for abnormal lab results; Read PPD-order CXR if needed		
CONSULTS	IT ordered: Y/N FT ordered: Y/N GT ordered: Y/N Psych Testing Order Y/N	GT started	Schedule MTP meeting	IT started, FT started, AIMS scale Psych Testing done Integrated summary done	AA referrals	Psych testing done
TREATMENT PLANNING	N1: Detox Potent.—Actual Axis III ______		School started (youth)	Master TX plan updated RT/TA entry	RT/TA started	
INTERVENTIONS	Assess safety needs	Avoid excessive stimuli	Monitor nutritional status	Effects of CD on body	Explore support system	Focus on strengths and accomplishments
MEDICATIONS	Meds ordered; informed consent		Drug interaction checked by Pharmacist/Dr. signs informed consent	Meds evaluated/ readjusted		Discharge instructions for medication self-admin
LEVEL	Level ordered		Re-evaluate	Re-evaluate for PHP	Re-evaluate for D/C	Re-evaluate
TEACHING	Patient Rights Orient to Unit	Orient to program	Medication teaching Nutritional goals	Meds reinforced; Positive coping skills	Stress reduction Relapse prevention	Promote self-reliance & diversional activities
NUTRITION AND DIET	Diet Ordered: ______	I&O, fluids	I&O, small frequent meals	Intake, Chg diet per lab	Weigh, chart daily intake	Diet D/C instruction
CARE CONTINUUM	Initial D/C Plans	Outcome survey	Support system	D/C Plan update/ revise	After care plan written	Outcome Survey
CLIENT OUTCOMES	No physical injury	Agitation decreased	Nutritional needs met	States CD effects on body	Verbalizes resources	Alternative coping skills

(Strategic Clinical Systems, Inc, 3715 Mission Ct., Granbury, TX 76049 (817) 326-4239; PsychPaths™ Darla Belt, RN, and Vickie Pflueger, RNC, Authors.

Key: AA = Alcoholics Anonymous; CD = chemical dependency; CxR = chest x-ray; D/C = discharge; EKG = electrocardiogram; FT = family therapy; GT = group therapy; H&P = history & physical exam; HX = history; I&O = intake and output; IT = individual therapy; MTP = master treatment plan; PHP = partial hospitalization program; PPD = skin test for tuberculosis; RT/TA = recreational therapy/therapeutic activities; TX = treatment; UA = urinalysis; UCG = urine pregnancy test; UDS = urine drug screen.)

Nursing Care Plan 33-1

A Client With Alcoholism

Sara was admitted voluntarily to the Chemical Dependency Unit. During the initial assessment, the nurse noted that Sara presented a well-groomed appearance although she looked 10 years older than her stated age of 34. She maintained good eye contact during the interview, and her speech was clear and appropriate. Her hands trembled as she reached out to shake the nurse's hand during the initial greeting; the handshake was weak and her skin moist to the touch. There were beads of perspiration on her upper lip and around her hairline, and her face was flushed. Her vital signs were blood pressure 148/90, pulse 92, and respiration 22. The nurse noted a faint odor of alcohol on her breath and an odor of heavy perfume in the room.

Sara stated that she decided to admit herself to the hospital after her husband "packed his bags and walked out." "He's hooked on Al-Anon and I'm left with the bills. I drink a lot on weekends but it's under control—still he never wants to go anywhere. So what else is there to do?"

Sara went on to say that she has been feeling very "down" the past few months. She denied suicidal ideation but reported a lack of energy and an overwhelming sense of failure, hopelessness, and apathy about the future.

Sara had been drinking for the past 15 years. She started drinking in high school and over the years smoked marijuana, used cocaine (snorted) and LSD, and smoked some opium. She denied IV drug use. She drinks every day and most heavily on weekends. She has taken sleeping pills in the past, remarking, "I don't sleep well; insomnia runs in my family. Also, tranquilizers take the edge off. I get the shakes sometimes, I haven't had any pills for a while. I'm out of touch with a source."

Sara eats very little, noting "I hate food." She smokes 1 pack of cigarettes and drinks 3 to 4 pots of coffee a day. Her usual diet consists of coffee, water, soda, salty and sugary foods. She "never eats a whole meal," and has been losing weight, but does not know how much.

She had one sibling, a twin sister who died in an alcohol-related automobile accident at age 30. She stated "I still miss her." Her mother died of breast cancer when the twin girls were 10 years old. Her father "took to drinking heavily" after her mother died. The girls were raised by her paternal grandparents. Her father died of cancer of the throat at age 57.

Sara has been married 14 years. She stated, "I live with him for financial reasons. He told me to get my act together or he's out the door. He leaves all this A.A. literature around, wants me to join a 'cult,' get brainwashed like him. Then we'd live happily ever after on spring water and lollypops."

Sara has no children and had one miscarriage 5 years ago. "I was taking a lot of 'coke' at the time. The doctor told me that was the reason, so we stopped doing drugs. We never go out now; we don't have any friends. My husband's too straight now for any fun."

Sara works as a secretary. She stated, "I hate my job. I don't want to go back to work but I probably will, I like the people I work with." There has been an increase in her workload recently. ("My boss is always on my case, I can't handle the extra work.")

Sara described herself as "loyal, honest, and a bit impulsive." In response to the question, "What do you like about yourself?" she said, "I don't know anything about myself I like. I'm shy. I lie around the house all day thinking about what I have to do. I don't know any way to make my life more worthwhile. I prefer to be alone, people get on my nerves. I like to be alone with my problems. I'm tired of people hounding me about my drinking. I talk easier after a few drinks and I like people more. My husband says I embarrass him and do and say things I don't remember. He makes things up. I'm happy playing my guitar and writing songs and poetry."

Nursing Diagnosis

Risk for Injury related to complications of withdrawal from alcohol

Outcome

Client will remain free from injury during withdrawal.

continued

Nursing Care Plan 33-1 (Continued)

Intervention	Rationale
Assess for symptoms of withdrawal (tremors, nausea, anxiety, increase in vital signs, seizures).	Physical signs and symptoms indicate status of withdrawal progression.
Document behaviors and stage of withdrawal.	Documentation is important for baseline and evaluation of increase or decrease in symptoms.
Monitor vital signs until stable.	Vital sign monitoring indicates the progression of withdrawal.
Maintain safe environment.	Reducing extaneous stimuli ensures physical and psychological safety.
Institute seizure precautions.	Seizure precautions help to protect client from injury.
Administer medications to relieve symptoms and prevent symptoms from worsening.	Administering prescribed medications treats and prevents withdrawal symptoms.
Reduce environmental stimuli to promote rest and sleep.	A quiet, nonstimulating environment helps calm the client.

Evaluation

Client remains free from injury during withdrawal from alcohol.

Nursing Diagnosis

Ineffective Denial related to a lifestyle of denial regarding negative aspects of alcohol and other drugs as destructive to self and relationships.

Outcome

Client will admit to alcohol and drug dependence and need for treatment.

Intervention	Rationale
Assess for clues of alcohol/drug use when denying the problem to help substantiate facts (eg, inconsistency of verbal/nonverbal statements, poor work performance, physical problems).	Assessment of clues indicating alcohol/drug use including feedback on inconsistencies, helps client acknowledge reality of the problem.
Help client identify times and situations related to alcohol/drug use and record in log or journal.	Journaling or recording helps client break through denial by looking at the facts and reality of the behavior.
Gently feedback the observed negative effects of alcohol/drug use to help client gain understanding and diminish denial.	Feedback provides reality of negative effects of substance use.
Provide with educational information about the addictive process of drugs/alcohol and its adverse consequences on the body, emotional well-being, and relationships; fetal alcohol syndrome and effects of substance use on fetus and infant (via film, discussions, written material).	Education increases awareness of deleterious effects of substances, assists in overcoming denial, provides knowledge of dependency.
Encourage client to attend therapeutic and self-help groups (A.A. and N.A.) to facilitate interactions between client and other recovering persons.	Identification with others with similar problems and confrontation by peers help clients acknowledge reality of maladaptive behaviors.
Teach client to replace alcohol/drug use with more functional, healthier activities (eg, hobbies, sports, music).	Client learns healthy methods for coping and stress reduction and identifies own positive resources.

continued

Nursing Care Plan 33-1 (Continued)

Evaluation

Client's behavior demonstrates decreased denial; client acknowledges alcohol and drug use and negative effects of use.

Nursing Diagnosis

Chronic Low-Self Esteem related to doubts and anxiety about self-worth and abilities

Outcome

Client will identify positive aspects of self and use coping methods to increase sense of self-worth.

Intervention	Rationale
Encourage client to verbalize feelings, including feelings of worthlessness.	Self-expression in a supportive environment allows the client to explore and work through feelings.
Encourage activities that promote positive thoughts and feelings about self.	Reinforcing activities reduces the likelihood of negative thinking and distressing feelings.
Help client identify, list, and discuss positive aspects of self.	The substance dependent person has difficulty recognizing positive self-attributes; these can be realistically examined with a supportive person.

Evaluation

Client reports a heightened sense of self-esteem.

Nursing Diagnosis

Altered Nutrition: less than body requirements, related to inadequate intake and loss of appetite secondary to alcohol consumption and increased caffeine intake

Outcome

Client will eat nutritionally balanced diet and eliminate or decrease intake of caffeine.

Intervention	Rationale
Collaborate with nutritionist and client on assessment of diet history and a nutritional plan or regimen.	Collaboration on these tasks determines adequacy of intake and increases client compliance.
Offer frequent, high protein foods and snacks.	This encourages balanced nutritional intake.
Teach client about need for nutritionally balanced foods including foods rich in B vitamins, and the addictive properties of caffeine.	Education about nutrition allows client to become responsible for own food selection.
Praise client for progress toward proper nutrition.	Positive feedback reinforces healthy behavior, builds confidence in client's ability to care for own health, and increases self-esteem.

Evaluation

Client reports intake of nutritionally balanced diet and decreased caffeine.

5. Identification with peers
6. Development of hope for recovery
7. Resocialization and increased interpersonal relationship skills
8. Development of increased self-worth and self-esteem
9. Establishment of alternative coping skills
10. Improvement of motivation to continue treatment and prevention of noncompliance
11. Involvement of family and significant others in the treatment and recovery process

INTERVENTION

The number of inpatient treatment programs for substance abuse disorders has decreased relative to cost-containment procedures and lack of reimbursement from medical insurance programs. Various types of treatment programs are available, including detoxification facilities, inpatient rehabilitation programs, outpatient programs, and private practice physician treatment. Table 33-3, Phases of Treatment of Alcoholism and Drug Abuse, identifies four sequential phases of treatment for alcohol and drug dependence. These phases need to be considered when treating clients' medical, social, and psychological needs. The clients will not always need to enter treatment in this sequence (ie, phase one followed by two, three, and four). Some clients may omit a phase; the needs of individual clients must be considered.

The Rehabilitation Process

The rehabilitation process usually focuses on the substance abuse or dependency disorder. The other problems that the client encounters, such as loss of job, marital conflicts, and legal problems, are often results of the drug abuse. Consequently, the client does not benefit from the resolution of these problems if the drug dependency continues. Conversely, many problems that stem directly from the drug use, such as physical illness or family or legal problems, diminish with rehabilitation and continued abstinence. Other significant problems—physical, emotional, and social—are treated concurrently with the substance abuse or dependency disorder.

The rehabilitation process generally involves detoxification, the restoration of physical and emotional stability, intervention methods to increase motivation to continue treatment, confrontation of the pathological defenses, intervention methods to increase self-esteem, facilitation of insight into problem areas, planning for discharge, and follow-up care.

An important aspect of the rehabilitation program is for the client to accept the responsibility for drug abuse or dependency and take the necessary actions toward recovery. Underlying the goal of discontinuing the substance use and maintaining abstinence is a change in the individual's behavior that will lead to a new lifestyle of greater personal enrichment.

Breaking Through Defenses

The breakdown of the pathological defense mechanisms manifested in the denial system is a gradual process. The nurse must recognize and understand the client's particular defensive maneuver. Gradually, the nurse assists the client to come face-to-face with the objective reality that is being denied. A consistent, persistent approach is necessary. This persistent stance of the nurse and other health team members conveys the message that there is never a valid reason for the client to use the substances of abuse and dependency. When the client focuses on other problems to the exclusion of the substance abuse or dependency problem, the nurse and treatment team refocus on the initial abuse or dependency problem. This approach assists the client to understand that other problems may be more effectively defined and resolved as a consequence of attacking the primary problem of substance abuse or dependence.

Understanding and Accepting the Disorder

The drug-dependent client needs to attain an intellectual comprehension of the disorder. One approach is to understand that it is an illness and not a moral problem. Educational material about the manifestations of substance abuse and clarification of misinformation assist in this process. An intellectual understanding helps the client accept the fact that the disorder is chronic and will not be cured. This requires acceptance of the disorder on an emotional level and recovery on a long-term, but day-by-day, basis. Most rehabilitation programs require abstinence as a prerequisite to recovery.

Identification With Peers

Peer group identification and confrontation of the abuse or dependence are powerful in recovery. Clients recognize and internalize the fact that they are not alone in their suffering, and they therefore receive emotional support and hope. The group also allows for confrontation by peers who attack pathological defense mechanisms and assist each other in the process of obtaining insight into behavior. The nurse may lead the group, encourage the client to attend the group, or discuss issues that may have surfaced after group attendance and participation.

Development of Hope

Clients enter the rehabilitation program with initial feelings of hopelessness, discouragement, and demoralization. They need to realize that escape from what

Table 33-3

Phases of Treatment of Alcoholism and Drug Abuse

Phase of Treatment	Typical Problems	Possible Solutions
Phase 1 (acute crisis)	Biomedical: gastrointestinal bleeding (eg, alcohol); angina (eg, cocaine); coma (eg, opioids)	Appropriate medical intervention, which may include hospitalization
	Psychologic: hallucinosis (eg, alcohol, LSD, or stimulants); paranoia (eg, PCP, marijuana stimulants, alcohol); suicidal ideation (eg, stimulants, alcohol, LSD)	Appropriate psychiatric intervention, which may include hospitalization
	Social: Family violence (eg, alcohol, stimulants, PCP)	Appropriate psychiatric intervention, which may include hospitalization, family therapy, home visit, domestic violence counseling
Phase 2 (withdrawal from substance abuse)	Biomedical: impending delirium tremens (eg, alcohol); impending seizures (eg, benzodiazepines); impending gastric distress ((eg, opioids)	Medical or social model detoxification; outpatient detoxification; appropriate medical intervention
	Psychologic: denial, worry about health; stressful life events	Counseling; brief individual or group therapy; AA/NA/CA
	Social: inadequate food and shelter, financial problems	Counseling; social services referral
Phase 3 (sequelae of substance abuse)	Biomedical: chronic medical problems; malnutrition	Appropriate medical intervention; vitamin supplements, proper diet, and exercise; disulfiram (alcohol); methadone (opioid); naltrexone (opioid)
	Psychologic: denial, depression; guilt stressful life events; craving for alcohol or drugs	Counseling; brief individual or group therapy; antidepressants; behavior modification techniques
	Social: family, housing, vocational, and legal problems; loneliness; unfilled leisure time	Counseling: social services referral; family therapy; recreational therapy; AA/NA/CA, Al-Anon or Alateen; halfway house
Phase 4	Biomedical: genetic factors	Counseling
	Psychologic: neurotic and personality disorders; major affective disorders; schizophrenia	Long-term group therapy; antidepressants; major tranquilizers; therapeutic communities; individual therapy
	Social: sociocultural and familial influences	Counseling

(Table from Clark HW et al: Substance Related Disorders: Alcohol and Drugs. In Goldman H (eds): Review of General Psychiatry. CT, Appleton and Lange, 1995.)

may be perceived as a hopeless situation is possible. Identification with others who have the same problems and with those who have recovered or are recovering is significant in initiating a feeling of hope. The positive attitude of the nurse and other mental health team members also instills hope in clients.

Resocialization

The drug user's life becomes drug centered, and in the process, the person becomes self-centered. Social skills may be diminished or lacking. It is a priority to assist the client to review and rebuild the capacity for establishing interpersonal relationships that the previously self-centered attitude has eroded.

Development of Self-Worth and Self-Esteem

Generally, self-esteem and self-worth increase with the client's ability to see the substance abuse problem as an illness. In addition, the client is helped by taking responsibility for making changes in attitudes and actions and for deriving satisfaction from achievements and relationships. The nurse also helps the client develop self-discipline. For example, the nurse may help the client organize and adhere to a daily routine, which may be difficult because of a previously chaotic lifestyle centered around substance abuse. The nurse expects and conveys the expectation that the client take an active part in the recovery program. Positive efforts to change are encouraged and supported. As the client experiences success, self-confidence, and self-esteem, hopefulness develops and alternatives to drugs are recognized. Motivation for recovery is enhanced as involvement in the program increases. Rehabilitation is a process that continues long after discharge from a treatment facility.

Other Important Therapies

Disulfiram (Antabuse) Treatment

The drug disulfiram (Antabuse) has been used in conjunction with other alcohol dependency treatment methods (see Table 33-4 for information on Antabuse and other therapeutic substances). The drug interferes with the metabolism to produce physical symptoms that may be severe, depending on individual variations and conditions. The general physical symptoms experienced by the client taking disulfiram after ingestion of even small amounts of alcohol include flushing of the skin, pounding headache, faintness, weakness, dizziness, nausea and vomiting, tachycardia, chest pain, shortness of breath, hypotension, blurred vision, and confusion.[16]

Disulfiram does not ensure sobriety or cure alcoholism. The chemotherapeutic purpose of the drug is to assist the client to control or to not act on the impulse to drink. The client understands that while taking the drug, these symptoms can occur after ingestion of alcohol. Therefore, the compulsion to drink during that time is lessened, and the client is free to concentrate on other areas of treatment. Because it takes several days for the drug to leave the body completely after use is discontinued, the client makes the decision to return to drinking on a conscious level rather than attributing it to an impulsive act. Most treatment programs offer disulfiram on a voluntary basis, and a written informed consent is usually required. The client must have full understanding of the drug's action and consequences. Candidates for this form of chemotherapy must be carefully screened by a physician and undergo baseline medical tests before the drug is administered.

The client must also understand that alcohol in any form (ie, in food, cough mixtures or other medications, and shaving lotions or other alcohol-containing substances applied to the skin) must be

Table 33-4

Medications to Treat Drug Dependency

Medication	Primary Therapeutic Category	Drug Addiction Treatment Mechanism	Response
FOR COCAINE			
Desipramine (Norpramin, others)	Antidepressant	Counters decreased norepinephrine transmission by blocking its reuptake	Decrease craving during withdrawal
Bromocriptine (Parlodel)	Dopamine receptor agonist for hyperprolactinemia	Counters decreased dopamine transmission by directly activating receptors	Decrease craving during withdrawal
Amantadine (Symmetrel, others)	Antiparkinson	Counters dopamine depletion by releasing stored reserves	Decrease craving during withdrawal
Phenylalanine and tyrosine	Amino acids; neurotransmitter precursors	Replete neurotransmitters, norepinephrine and dopamine	Decrease craving during withdrawal
FOR NARCOTICS			
Methadone (Dolophine, others)	Narcotic analgesic	Substitutes for heroin at narcotic receptors	Less euphoria, less frequent dosing, and not injectable
Clonidine (Catapres, others)	Antihypertensive	Inhibits central neural norepinephrine activity	Decrease discomfort during withdrawal
Naltrexone (Trexan)	Narcotic antagonist	Blocks response to narcotics by binding to the receptors	No euphoria from consumed narcotics
FOR ALCOHOL			
Disulfiram (Antabuse)	Interacts with alcohol	Interferes with alcohol metabolism	Distressing reaction to consumed alcohol
Diazepam (Valium, others)	Antianxiety	Substitutes for alcohol depressant effects on central nervous system	Reduce symptoms of withdrawal

(From Bender K: Psychiatric Medications. Newbury Park, CA, SAGE Publications, 1990)

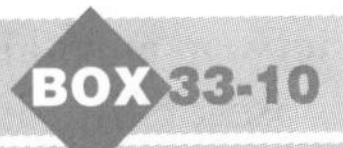

What is A.A.?

Alcoholics Anonymous (A.A.) is a program of recovery from the illness of alcoholism. It is an international fellowship of men and women who meet together to attain and maintain sobriety. It is nonprofessional, self-supporting, nondenominational, multiracial, apolitical, and almost omnipresent. There are no age or educational requirements. Membership is open to any alcoholic who wants to do something about his or her drinking problem.

WHAT DOES A.A. DO?

1. The A.A. members share their recovery experience with anyone seeking help with a drinking problem and give person-to-person service or sponsorship to the alcoholic coming to A.A. from a treatment or correctional facility or any other referral source.
2. The A.A. program, as set forth in the Twelve Steps to recovery, offers the alcoholic an opportunity to develop a satisfying way of life free from alcohol.
3. This program is discussed at the following A.A. group meetings:
   a. Open speaker meetings—open to alcoholics and nonalcoholics. (Attendance at an open A.A. meeting is the best way to learn what A.A. does and what it does not do.) At speaker meetings A.A. members tell their stories. They describe their experiences with alcohol, how they came to A.A. and how their lives have changed as a result of the A.A. experience
   b. Open discussion meetings—one member speaks briefly about his or her experience as an alcoholic and leads a discussion on a selected subject (guilt, resentments, self-pity) or on any subjects or drinking-related problems anyone brings up.
   c. Closed discussion meetings—same format as above.
   d. Closed Step meetings—discussion of one of the Twelve Steps.
   e. The A.A. members also take meetings into correctional and treatment facilities.
   f. The A.A. members may, in conjunction with court personnel, conduct meetings "about A.A." as a part of A.S.A.P. (Alchol Safety Action Programs) and D.W.I. (Driving While Intoxicated) programs. These meetings about A.A. are not to be confused with regular A.A. meetings.

WHAT A.A. DOES NOT DO

A.A. does not do the following:

1. Furnish initial motivation for alcoholics to recover
2. Solicit members
3. Engage in or sponsor research
4. Join councils of social agencies
5. Follow up or try to control its members
6. Make medical or psychological diagnoses or prognoses
7. Provide drying-out or nursing services, hospitalization, drugs, or any medical or psychiatric treatment
8. Offer spiritual or religious services
9. Engage in education about alcohol
10. Provide housing, food, clothing, jobs, money, or any other welfare or social services
11. Provide domestic or vocational counseling
12. Accept any money for its services, or any contributions from non-A.A. sources

The primary purpose of A.A. is to carry our message of recovery to the alcoholic seeking help. The primary purpose of any alcoholism treatment modality is to help the alcoholic attain and maintain sobriety. Therefore, regardless of the road we follow, we are all heading for the same destination—the rehabilitation of the alcoholic person. Together, we can do what neither of us could accomplish alone.

(From Information on Alcoholics Anonymous, New York, A.A. World Services)

avoided because the same reaction produced with the intake of ethyl alcohol will occur. A list of these substances is given to the client, along with a medical alert card or bracelet, when the client begins taking disulfiram.

Methadone Maintenance

Methadone maintenance is used in opiate dependence in conjunction with other treatment methods, although it is not a cure. Methadone is a longer acting narcotic that is substituted for the shorter acting opi-

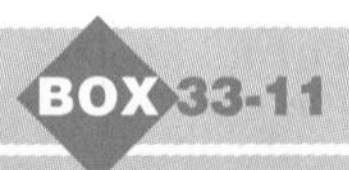

The Al-Anon Family

> The greatest fault of all is to be conscious of none.
> —Thomas Carlyle

Dear Friends,

Your faces are not known to me, yet I know we share the same burden, because in our humanity, we share the same struggle to come to wholeness, to know, accept and appreciate who we are, to take responsibility for our lives, and no matter what our calling is, to conduct our lives is such a way as to be a beacon of light.

Many years ago in search of a way to "save" my father from the scourge of alcoholism, I was introduced to the Twelve Steps of Alcoholics Anonymous through the Al-Anon program, a self-help support group for families and friends of alcoholics. In Al-Anon, I became conscious of my own weaknesses and shortcomings and experienced the humility to accept the fact that I was powerless over alcohol, that I could not make my father well or make well my husband who, I recognized from the knowledge and insight gained from the Al-Anon group, was in the early stages of alcoholism.

In Al-Anon I learned that the effects of alcoholism are pervasive; the entire family suffers; I learned that because of my Joan of Arc efforts to make things right, my continual failure to do so, my moldering sense of self-esteem in light of constant defeat, criticism, and confusion that I had become as sick as the alcoholic and that my life had become unmanageable. I came to believe that a Power greater than myself could restore me to sanity. I made a decision to turn my will and my life over to the care of God as I understood Him and in so doing embraced the Twelve-Step program.

Working the Twelve Steps, the constitution of all anonymous self-help groups, is not easy. It requires honesty and humility; it requires a commitment to grow in wholeness, to stay on the journey no matter what, and to trust that if we are faithful God will lead us to wellness, and to the peace and joy that comes when we accept the challenge "to grow," to take responsibility for our lives, and diligently work toward becoming the person we were created to be.

Growth requires change; it is often slow and sometimes painful; like the butterfly, we must gain strength from the struggle. The wisdom of the Al-Anon program, along with the dynamic interaction that happens in the honest and caring environment of a support group, has helped to give me the strength and the courage to undergo my own metamorphosis. Slowly I began to see that we change, our situation changes, as we become integrated, we become more secure and more loving and experience an inner harmony that affects all of our relationships. The family is the primary recipient of this blessed change in us.

Today there is more awareness than ever concerning alcoholism. What was once thought to be a disgrace is now known to be a disease, a disease of body, mind, and spirit. Tragically, my father died never knowing the serenity that can be found in Alcoholics Anonymous. Spiritually my husband was "reborn" and came to serenity through Alcoholics Anonymous. We have choices! Our choices make a difference!

Gratefully, JoAnn

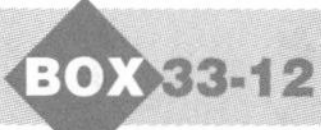

BOX 33-12 The Twelve Steps of Alcoholics Anonymous

1. Admitted we were powerless over alcohol—that our lives had become unmanageable
2. Came to believe that a Power greater than ourselves could restore us to sanity
3. Made a decision to turn our will and our lives over to the care of God as we understood him
4. Made a searching and fearless moral inventory of ourselves
5. Admitted to God, to ourselves, and to another human being the exact nature of our wrongs
6. Were entirely ready to have God remove all these defects of character
7. Humbly asked Him to remove our shortcomings
8. Made a list of all persons we had harmed, and became willing to make amends to them all
9. Made direct amends to such people wherever possible except when to do so would injure them or others
10. Continued to take a personal inventory and when we were wrong promptly admitted it
11. Sought through prayer and meditation to improve our conscious contact with God as we understood Him, praying only for knowledge of His will for us and the power to carry that out
12. Having had a spiritual awakening as the result of these steps, we tried to carry this message to alcoholics, and to practice these principles in all our affairs

ates, such as heroin. It has similar pharmacological properties as heroin, including addiction, sedation, and respiratory depression. It blocks the euphoric effects of heroin and other opiates, thereby preventing the impulsive use of heroin.[37,44] The purpose of a methadone maintenance program is to assist the client in developing a lifestyle free of street drugs. This enables improved family and social functioning and decreases or eliminates legal problems, traumatic injuries, and health problems associated with obtaining and abusing street drugs.[37] Methadone is administered in licensed clinics established to control its distribution and prevent its diversion for illegal use. The clinics maintain a careful screening process for candidates and have specific criteria for admission. Psychological and social rehabilitation of the client take place concurrently (see Table 33-3, p. 686).[37,44,74]

Drug-Free Communities

Drug-free communities are another approach to narcotic dependency treatment and rehabilitation. These therapeutic communities are usually long-term programs lasting up to 1 year. The client is removed from street culture and given a new identity within the group community. In this program, confrontation by group members and ex-addicts helps the client gain insight into problem areas and find more successful ways of coping with life situations and stresses.

33-2 Case Study

The Pregnant, Substance-Abusing Client: Ethical and Legal Considerations

You are assigned to care for a client on the psychiatric unit. You read the following history on her chart prior to interviewing her:

The client is 8 months pregnant with her fourth child. In a court appearance, she waived her right to an attorney and pleaded guilty to two counts of possession of crack-cocaine and one count each of disorderly conduct and possession of marijuana. She told the judge she had used cocaine recently. The presiding female judge gave the client the option to be sterilized after her child is born (have her fallopian tubes tied), be on probation for 2 years, and get counseling. If she did not accept this option she would be sentenced to 3 months in jail and a $950.00 fine.

The client chose the option rather than jail. The judge said that the sentence option was not punishment, but the judge believed the woman would not change her lifestyle unless drastic measures were taken.

Questions for Discussion

1. What is your opinion regarding the judge's decision and reasoning?
2. Discuss the reasons for your opinion.
3. What, if any, alternative options might be available?
4. One of the commonalities in substance-dependent individuals is low self-esteem. What are some interventions you would use to increase the client's self-worth?

Aversion Conditioning

Aversion conditioning is a behavioral approach related to the conditional response mechanism. The client may be taught not to drink by associating the sight, smell, and taste of alcohol with an unpleasant event, for example, a mild electric shock to the skin.

Other Modalities

Relaxation therapy is frequently used to teach clients methods to release tension, improve self-image, and relieve insomnia without drugs. Role playing includes rehearsed responses to specific situations, for example, when drinking or drug-taking opportunities may be encountered—and, it is hoped, refused—by the client. Social skills and responses to situations, such as job interviews, may be rehearsed to relieve anticipatory anxiety. Assertiveness training is another useful method to assist the client to meet dependency and interdependency needs and accept personal responsibility and satisfaction in achievements.

Self-Help Groups

The first, and perhaps the most influential, of substance abuse and dependency self-help groups is an organization called Alcoholics Anonymous (A.A.). This self-help program was founded in 1935 by two men, Dr. Bob, a surgeon, and Bill W, a New York stockbroker. At the time, these men were unable to obtain help for their alcoholism. They found that by sharing their life experiences with each other and identifying with each other in their common problem with alcohol, they were able to overcome their compulsion to drink. Al-Anon is a fellowship of spouses, relatives, and friends of alcoholics that started as an outgrowth of A.A. and is now a completely separate organization.(Boxes 33-10 and 33-11, pp. 688–689). Alateen is a component of Al-Anon, and the sponsor of Alateen is usually a member of Al-Anon; however, members of Alateen have separate groups and conduct their own meetings. Both groups follow the 12 steps of A.A. (Box 33-12).

Narcotics Anonymous (N.A.) is a fellowship of recovering addicts. It follows a program adapted from A.A.; that is, the 12 steps of A.A. are the basis of the program of recovery.[64] Although N.A. follows the same principles of recovery as its model, the concept has been broadened to include all mood-altering substances. There is also Cocaine Anonymous and Adult Children of Alcoholics, which is a component of Al-Anon.

EVALUATION

Evaluation is an ongoing component of the nursing process. The nurse continually assesses the degree to which interventions have been successful in assisting the client to resolve problems and meet short-term and long-term goals. The nurse reflects on questions related to the effectiveness of interventions. For example, why were interventions ineffective? Did the client's behavior change, and was the nurse able to foresee these changes? Evaluation applies to all steps of the nursing process, and modifications may be necessary because the changes reflect individual differences and responses to treatment. Individual treatment plans are initiated together with the client, family, and members of the multidisciplinary team caring for that client. Referrals for continuing care after discharge or a return to the facility for outpatient follow-up care are frequently arranged or advocated. Referrals to halfway houses may be arranged to facilitate readjustment to community and society for clients who require resocialization in a more structured environment. Continued participation in self-help groups is strongly recommended.

◆ Chapter Summary

This chapter has discussed the use of substances that affect the CNS and the physical and behavioral changes that occur in people who abuse or become dependent on these substances. The focus has been on commonalities of substance abuse and dependency and the specific factors particular to each drug classification. Major points of the chapter are as follows:

1. Selye's theoretical framework of the stress adaptation syndrome may be applied to the problem of substance abuse and dependency.
2. There is no single etiology of drug abuse and dependence. Rather, theories examine multiple factors, such as personality traits; genetic influences; social, cultural, ethnic, and environmental factors; and a self-destructive phenomenon.
3. Drug dependence may be viewed as a way of coping with life's stressors by people who abuse substances.
4. Substance use disorders are divided into the diagnoses of substance abuse and substance dependency.
5. Substance-induced organic mental disorders include intoxication, withdrawal, and delirium.
6. Each class of abused substances is described in terms of its effects, patterns of abuse, diagnostic criteria, organic mental disorders, and medical consequences.
7. A nonjudgmental, objective approach is essential for establishing rapport with clients who abuse substances.
8. Rehabilitation and eventual recovery are the focus of treatment planning and intervention with clients who abuse or are dependent on drugs.
9. Problems of substance abuse and dependency are encountered in all areas of nursing practice.

Critical Thinking Questions

1. *How do you think you would react if you observed a fellow student using drugs while working with you in the clinical area? What would you do?*
2. *How would you intervene with a client admitted with a DSM-IV diagnosis of cocaine dependence, and the client is 4 months pregnant?*
3. *What feelings and attitudes do you have that you consider would make a positive impact on your caring for a client with a substance-related disorder?*
4. *Are you aware of negative feelings and attitudes that might impede your therapeutic response to a client with a substance-abuse related disorder? How do you deal with your negative feelings and attitudes to establish a therapeutic relationship with the client?*

Review Questions

1. A 48-year-old man is admitted to the emergency room with the following symptoms: fever, 101.5°F; pulse, 104; respirations, 28; blood pressure, 178/94; profuse perspiration and tremulousness. The mental status examination reveals confusion, disorientation, visual hallucinations, and agitation. His neighbor who accompanied him to the emergency room states he stopped drinking 2 days ago after a long period of heavy daily intake of alcohol. What substance-induced disorder would the client be experiencing?
   - **A.** Wernicke-Korsakoff syndrome
   - **B.** Alcohol amnestic disorder
   - **C.** Alcohol withdrawal delirium
   - **D.** Substance-induced psychotic disorder
2. The 12-step program of AA (and other self help programs that follow the same 12 steps of AA) requires more than abstaining from alcohol. The program is a way of life for the recovering alcoholic. It effects changes in interpersonal behavior and continued participation in the program fellowship. Which of the following steps hastens the person's recovery by helping others to recover and expand the program message?
   - **A.** Tenth step
   - **B.** First step
   - **C.** Eighth step
   - **D.** Twelfth step
3. When assessing the client for possible substance abuse, which of the following would alert the nurse to possible opiate abuse?
   - **A.** Pupillary constriction
   - **B.** Liver disease
   - **C.** Reddened eyes
   - **D.** Tactile hallucinations
4. The coexistence of substance dependence and a major psychiatric disorder is termed
   - **A.** primary disorder.
   - **B.** addictive personality.
   - **C.** dual diagnosis.
   - **D.** substance psychosis.
5. During the initial interview, the nurse asks the client if he has ever experienced blackouts. Blackouts are
   - **A.** the denial of the unpleasant aspects of drinking and remembering only the pleasant experiences.
   - **B.** an inability to perform work requiring concentration.
   - **C.** permanent amnesia for events that occurred while intoxicated.
   - **D.** a state of unconsciousness from an overdose of alcohol.
6. Barbiturates and sedative hypnotics taken in combination with alcohol will
   - **A.** decrease the effectiveness of alcohol.
   - **B.** cause an increase in blood pressure.
   - **C.** produce hyperactivity, restlessness, tactile hallucinations.
   - **D.** potentiate the effects of alcohol.
7. Your client states he "snorts cocaine several times a day, spends all his earnings on ways to obtain it, and has been arrested once for threatening abusive behavior." He could be said to have which disorder?
   - **A.** Substance withdrawal
   - **B.** Withdrawal delirium
   - **C.** Substance dependence
   - **D.** Polysubstance abuse
8. What type of medication would you expect to see ordered in the treatment plan for a client being withdrawn from narcotics?
   - **A.** Barbiturates
   - **B.** Anxiolytics
   - **C.** Opiate-type drugs
   - **D.** Anticonvulsants
9. When the nurse does an initial admission interview on a client being admitted for detoxification, which of the following areas is critical to assess?
   - **A.** Reason for admission
   - **B.** A complete physical history
   - **C.** Type of drug(s) used
   - **D.** Family history
10. The nurse conducts an initial assessment for substance abuse or dependency to collect data on the
    - **A.** client's perception of the problem and coping mechanisms.
    - **B.** perpetuation of the problem through the enabling behaviors of the client's family.

C. client's pattern of drug use and the consequences of use.
D. family history of alcoholism.

◆ References

1. Aguilera D: Crisis Intervention, 7th ed. St. Louis, CV Mosby 1994
2. Ackerman R: Let Go and Grow: Recovery for Adult Children. Deerfield Beach, FL, Health Communications, 1987
3. Alexander D, O'Quinn-Larson L: When Nurses are Addicted to Drugs. Nursing 90 (August): 55–58, 1990
4. American Psychiatric Association: Diagnostic and Statistical Manual of Mental Disorders, 4th ed. Washington, DC, American Psychiatric Association, 1994
5. American Psychiatric Association: Practice Guidelines for the Treatment of Patients with Substance Use Disorders: Alcohol, Cocaine, Opioids. Am J Psychiatry 152 (11): 4–9, 1995
6. Antai-Otong D: Helping the Alcoholic Recover. Journal of Nursing 95 (8): 22–30, 1995
7. Bender K: Psychiatric Medications. Newbury Park, CA, Sage Publications, 1990
8. Bennett J, Scholler-Jaquish A: The Winner's Group: A Self Help Group for Homeless Chemically Dependent Persons. J Psychosoc Nurs 33 (4): 14–19, 1995
9. Black C: It Will Never Happen to Me! Denver, CO, M.A.C. Publications, 1990
10. Burk J, Sher K: Labeling the Child of an Alcoholic: Negative Stereotyping by Mental Health Professionals and Peers. J Stud Alcohol 51 (2): 156–163, 1990
11. Burkstein O: Treatment of Adolescent Alcohol Abuse and Dependence. Alcohol Health and Research World 18 (4): 296–301, 1994
12. Burns CM: Early Detection and Intervention for the Hidden Alcoholic: Assessment Guidelines for the Clinical Nurse Specialist. Clinical Nurse Specialist 8 (6): 296–303, 1994
13. Byrne M, Lerner H: Communicating With Addicted Women in Labor: MCN 17 (4): 198–203, 1992
14. Campinhe-Bacote J, Bragg E: Chemical Assessment in Maternity Care. MCN 18 (1): 24–28, 1993
15. Ciraulo D, Shader R (eds): Clinical Manual of Chemical Dependence. Washington, DC, American Psychiatric Press, 1991
16. Clark H, Kanas N, Smith D, Landry M: Substance-Related Disorders: Alcohol and Drugs. In Goldman H (ed): Review of General Psychiatry, 4th ed. Norwalk, CO, Appleton and Lange, 1995
17. Clark J, Queener S, Karb U: Pharmacologic Basis of Nursing Practice, 4th ed. St. Louis, CV Mosby, 1993
18. Clinebell H: Philosophical-Religious Factors in the Etiology and Treatment of Alcoholism. Journal of Ministry in Addiction and Recovery 1 (2): 29–46, 1994
19. Cowley D, Gordon C: Assessment of Family History of Alcoholism in Sons of Alcoholic Fathers. Journal of Addictive Diseases 14 (2): 75–81, 1995
20. Dixon L, McNary S, Lehman A: Substance Abuse and Family Relationships of Persons With Severe Mental Illness. Am J Psychiatry 152 (3): 456–458, 1995
21. Doenges M, Townsend M, Moorhouse M: Psychiatric Care Plans, 2d ed. Philadelphia, FA Davis, 1995
22. Dorris M: The Broken Cord. New York, Harper and Row, 1989
23. Drake R, Tegue G, Waeren SR: Dual Diagnosis: The New Hampshire Program. Addict Recovery (June): 35–39, 1990
24. Dube C, Lewis D: Medical Education in Alcohol and Other Drugs: Curriculum Development for Primary Care. Alcohol and Research World 18 (2): 146–153, 1994
25. Edgerton J, Campbell R (eds): American Psychiatric Glossary, 7th ed. Washington, DC, American Psychiatric Press, 1994
26. Endicott P, Watson B: Interventions to Improve A.M.A. Discharge Rate for Opiate-Addicted Patients. J Psychosoc Nurs 32 (8): 36–49, 1994
27. Fawcett C: The Substance Abusing Family. In Fawcett C (ed): Family Psychiatric Nursing. St. Louis, CV Mosby, 1995
28. Gerace L, Hughes T, Spunt J: Improving Nurses' Responses Toward Substance-Misusing Patients: A Clinical Evaluation Project. Archives of Psychiatric Nursing 14 (5): 286–294, 1994
29. Gold M: 800-Cocaine and the Crack Epidemic. Summit, NJ, The Pia Press, 1980
30. Goodwin DW: Alcoholism and Heredity. Arch Gen Psychiatry 36 (January): 57–61, 1979
31. Goodwin DW: Is Alcoholism Hereditary? New York, Oxford University Press, 1976
32. Gottheil E, Evans BD, Vereby K: Research Relating to Alcohol and Opiate Dependence. In Solomon J, Keeley KA, Wright J (eds): Perspectives on Alcohol and Drug Abuse: Similarities and Differences, pp 179–201. Boston, PSG, 1982
33. Jellinek EM: Disease Concept of Alcoholism. New Haven, United Printing Service, 1960
34. Jellinek EM: Phases of Alcohol Addiction. Quarterly Journal of Studies on Alcohol 13 (December): 673–684, 1952
35. Johnson B: Child, Adolescent and Family Psychiatric Nursing. Philadelphia, JB Lippincott, 1995
36. Johnson V: I'll Quit Tomorrow, rev. ed. New York, Harper & Row, 1980
37. Keltner N, Folks D: Psychotropic Drugs. St. Louis, CV Mosby, 1995
38. Killeen T, Brady K, Theuos A: Addiction Severity, Psychopathology and Treatment Compliance in Cocaine-Dependent Mothers. Journal of Addictive Disorders 14 (1): 75–85, 1995
39. Lewis K, Schmeder N, Bennett B: Maternal Drug Abuse and Its Effects on Young Children. MCN 27 (4): 198–203, 1992
40. Lindenberg C, Cendrop SC, Nenciol M, Adames Z: Substance Abuse Among Inner-City Hispanic Women: Exploring Resiliency. J Obstet Gynecol Neonatal Nurs 23 (7): 604–616, 1994

41. Luthar S, Walsh K: Treatment Needs of Drug-Addicted Mothers. Journal of Substance Abuse Treatment 12 (5): 341–348, 1995
42. Marron J: The Twelve Steps: A Pathway to Recovery. Primary Care Clinics in Office Practice 20 (1): 107–119, 1993
43. McFarland G, McFarland E: Nursing Diagnosis and Intervention, 2d ed. St. Louis, CV Mosby, 1995
44. McGonagle D: Methadone Anonymous: A 12-Step Program. J Psychosoc Nurs 32 (October): 5–12, 1994
45. Miller N: Pharmacotherapy is Alcoholism. Journal of Addictive Diseases 14 (1): 23–43, 1995
46. Miller W, C'DeBaca J: What Every Mental Health Professional Should Know About Alcohol. Journal of Substance Abuse and Treatment 12 (5): 355–365, 1995
47. Montgomery H, Miller W, Tonigan S: Does Alcoholics Anonymous Treatment Predict Treatment Outcome? Journal of Substance Abuse Treatment 12 (4): 241–246, 1995
48. Naegle M: The Need for Alcohol Abuse-Related Education in Nursing Curricula. Alcohol Health and Research World 18 (2): 154–157, 1994
49. Narcotics Anonymous. 4th Edition. World Service Office, Inc., Van Nuys, CA, 1987
50. National Institute on Alcohol and Alcoholism: Seventh Special Report to US Congress on Alcohol and Health from Secretary of Health and Human Services. Rockville, MD, National Institute on Alcohol Abuse and Alcoholism, 1990
51. Navarra T: Enabling Behavior: The Tender Trap. Am J Nursing 95 (1): 50–52, 1995
52. O'Connor S, Hasselbrock V, Bauer L: The Nervous System and Predisposition to Alcoholism. Alcohol Health and Research World 14 (2): 90–97, 1990
53. Pattison EM, Sobel MB, Sobel LC: Emerging Concepts of Alcohol Dependence. New York, Springer-Verlag, 1977
54. Psychotherapy and Pharmacotherapy for Ambulatory Cocaine Abusers. Capsules and Comments, Vol. 1 (3), (October-December) 51, 1994
55. Salaspuro, M.: Biological State Markers of Alcohol Abuse: Alcohol Health and Research World, Vol. 18 (2), 131-135, 1994
56. Schiaui R., Stimmel B., Madeli J., White D.: Chronic Alcoholism and Male Sexual Function. Am J Psychiatry 152:7, (July) 1045-1051, 1995
57. Schukit MA: Drug and Alcohol Abuse: A Clinical Guide to Diagnosis and Treatment. New York, Plenum Press, 1979
58. Schukit MA: The Disease Alcoholism. Postgrad Med 64 (December): 78-84, 1978
59. Selye H: The Stress of Life. New York, McGraw-Hill, 1956
60. Selye H: Stress without Distress. New York, New America Library, 1974
61. Starn J., Patterson K.,Bemis G., Castro O., Bemis P.: Can We Encourage Pregnant Substance Abusers to Seek Prenatal Care?. MCN: Am J of Maternal/Child Nursing, Vol 18 (3), (May/June), 148-152, 1993
62. Sullivan, E: Nursing Care of Clients with Substance Abuse. St. Louis, MO., Mosby, 1995
63. Sullivan E, Bissell L, Williams E.: Chemical Dependency in Nursing. Menlo Park, CA, Addison-Wesley, 1988
64. Sullivan E., Handley S., Connor H.: The Role of the Nurse in Primary Care: Managing Alcohol-Abusing Patients. Alcohol Health and Research World, Vol. 18 (2), 154-161, 1994
65. Sullivan J, Boudreaux M, Keller P: Can We Help the Substance Abusing Mother and Infant?. MCN 18 (3): 153–157, 1993
66. The National Nurses Society on Addictions: Position Paper: Peer Assistance: Perspectives on Addictions. Nursing 6 (1): 3–7, 1995
67. Tsai G, Gastfriend D, Coyle J: The Glutamatergic Basis of Human Alcoholism. Am J Psychiatry 152 (3): 332–339, 1995
68. Tsuang D, Cowley D, Ries R, Dunner D, Roy-Byrne P: The Effects of Substance Use Disorder on the Clinical Presentation of Anxiety and Depression in an Outpatient Psychiatric Clinic. J Clin Psychiatry 56 (December): 549–555, 1995
69. US Congress, Office of Technology Assessment: Technologies for the Understanding and Preventing Substance Abuse and Addiction, OTA-EHR-597. Washington, DC, U.S. Government Printing Office, September, 1994
70. Vaillant GF: The Natural History of Alcoholism. Cambridge, MA, Harvard University Press, 1983
71. Wallace J: Alcoholism: A New Light on the Disease. Newport, RI, Edgehill, 1985
72. Wallace J: Writings. Newport, RI, Edgehill, 1989
73. Woititz J: Adult Children of Alcoholism. Pompano Beach, FL, Health Communications, 1983
74. Woody G, McLeNan T, Luborsky L, O'Brien C: Psychotherapy in Community Methadone Programs: A Validation Study. Am J Psychiatry 152 (9): 1302–1308, 1995

Eating Disorders

Susan D. Decker

34

At age 13, I was totally immersed in self-starvation. Weighing less than 60 pounds . . . all the time I keep running into people who haven't seen me in a while. They all look shocked, they all say the same thing: "You're so thin! You don't look like yourself any more!" I thrive on their reactions. It's so reassuring to hear that I don't look like my supposed "self" anymore . . . Now, at age 30, I'm 5'5" and 120 pounds. Nicely "cured" of Anorexia Nervosa, right? I wish!

Annie Ciseaux, 1980

Mirror, mirror, on the wall.
Who's the fairest of us all?
Snow White

Many adolescent and young women in contemporary western society are overly concerned with weight and physical appearance. "Never too thin or too rich!" is a prevalent societal attitude. Two extreme manifestations of this concern with weight are anorexia nervosa and bulimia. Anorexia nervosa is a life-threatening condition characterized by an intense fear of becoming obese, emaciation, and disturbed body image. Many people with anorexia also engage in bulimia, a disorder characterized by binge eating and purging.

Why does a teenage girl determinedly starve herself when others view her as grotesquely thin? Why can't her parents make her eat? Why does a young woman ingest enormous amounts of food and furtively vomit? This chapter aims to help the reader understand the etiology and dynamics of eating disorders and use the nursing process effectively with anorectic and bulimic clients.

Eating disorders greatly challenge the nurse because of their complex psychosocial and physical problems. A sensitivity to the needs of clients with eating disorders helps the nurse intervene constructively with clients who resist help and willfully persist in self-destructive behaviors.

Learning Objectives

On completion of this chapter, you should be able to accomplish the following:

1. *Define the terms anorexia nervosa and bulimia.*
2. *Describe the incidence of eating disorders and the populations affected.*
3. *Describe the diagnostic criteria for anorexia nervosa and bulimia.*
4. *Discuss theories of the etiology of eating disorders.*
5. *Apply the nursing process in the care of clients with eating disorders.*
6. *Recognize your own feelings and attitudes toward clients with eating disorders.*

◆ Incidence of Eating Disorders

Anorexia nervosa and bulimia primarily affect adolescent and young women. Only 5% to 10% of all cases have been identified in young men.[3] The age at onset is usually 12 to 25 years; onset after age 30 is rare.[21] The manifestations of eating disorders do not necessarily disappear after young adulthood. A survey by the National Association of Anorexia Nervosa and Related Disorders indicates that among 1,400 anorectic and bulimic respondents, 5% were older than 60 years, 1.8% were older than 50 years, 2.7% were 40 to 49 years, and 20.5% were 30 to 39 years. The remaining respondents, 70%, were younger than 30 years.[6]

ANOREXIA NERVOSA

Anorectic clients in the United States commonly come from white, well-educated, middle- and upper-income families in which parents are overinvolved with and highly protective of children. Onset most commonly occurs between 12 and 18 years. Before the anorectic episode, clients typically are described as model children who are compliant, obedient, perfectionists, and want to please parents and teachers. They generally are high achievers in academic and athletic endeavors. Symptoms commonly begin following life changes, such as starting high school, moving to a new city or school, or going away to camp. Although families of anorectics at first appear loving and cohesive, unresolved and denied conflicts exist among family members. Sisters of anorectics also are at risk for developing an eating disorder.[15,36]

Although anorexia nervosa was described as early as the 17th century, health care professionals and the general public have become increasingly aware of eating disorders in recent years.[12] Anorexia nervosa may affect as many as 1 in 200 teenage girls, with mortality rates of 10% to 15%.[20,33] Incidence appears to be rising, although improved diagnosis and reporting may account for some of this increase. Many anorectic and bulimic clients never seek or receive treatment. One researcher reports that approximately 40% of anorectics recover spontaneously, 20% respond to treatment, and 40% become chronic.[21] An estimated 50% of anorectics also exhibit bulimic behavior.[9,29] Death from starvation, infection, or suicide occurs in up to 21% of cases.[26]

BULIMIA

The incidence of bulimia is much higher than that of anorexia nervosa. Recent studies estimate an incidence of 5% of young women.[23,29] Accurately determining the incidence of bulimia is particularly difficult because binging and purging generally are carried out secretly, and the person's weight may be relatively normal. The age of onset tends to be older for bulimia than for anorexia nervosa. The typical bulimic is a young, college-educated woman who achieves highly at work or school. Despite her achievements, she tends to be passive, dependent, and unassertive. Her family may be disorganized, noncohesive, in conflict, and characterized by confusing sex role expectations for women.[11,29] There commonly is a family history of affective disorders; some researchers have proposed that eating disorders are basically a form of depressive mood disorder.[42] Bulimic clients typically have difficulty with direct expression of feelings, are prone to impulsive behavior, and may have problems with alcohol and other substance abuse.[37]

◆ Definitions and Diagnostic Criteria

DEFINITIONS

Anorexia nervosa is characterized by a voluntary refusal to eat. In addition to psychological symptoms, there are multiple physiological consequences of starvation. The anorectic client has a distorted body image and to the bewilderment of others, views her emaciated body as fat. Although anorectics eat very little themselves, they typically are obsessed with food and cooking for others. Vigorous physical activity is often obsessively pursued to burn what the anorectic thinks are excess calories. Physiological changes resulting from extreme weight loss may include amenorrhea, lanugo hair, hypotension, bradycardia, hypothermia, constipation, polyuria, and electrolyte imbalances.

Bulimia is characterized by episodic, uncontrolled, rapid ingestion of large quantities of food. Bulimia may occur alone or in conjunction with the food-restricting behavior of anorexia nervosa. The bulimic client compensates for excessive food intake by self-induced vomiting, obsessive exercise, and laxative and diuretic use. The bulimic client may consume an incredible number of calories (an average of 3,415 calories per binge episode) in a short period, induce vomiting, and perhaps repeat this behavior several times a day.[35] The bulimic client may develop dental caries as a result of frequent contact of tooth enamel with food and acidic gastric fluids.[25] Other physiological complications may include electrocardiographic changes, parotid gland enlargement, esophagitis, gastric dilatation, menstrual irregularity, and electrolyte imbalances.[24,25]

DIAGNOSTIC CRITERIA

The Diagnostic and Statistical Manual of Mental Disorders, fourth edition (DSM-IV), criteria for anorexia and bulimia clearly delineate the clinical features of these disorders (Box 34-1). An area of some controversy is whether bulimia is really a separate clinical entity or more truly an extension or different expression of anorexia nervosa. Hilde Bruch, an authority on eating disorders, argues that bulimia is more accurately a symptomatic expression of anorexia nervosa.[7] Recent research that views eating disorders as existing on a spectrum supports Bruch's view.[2] Many people exhibit disordered eating patterns for many years—sometimes a lifetime.[2] Such people may fluctuate between food-restricting anorectic episodes and binge-purge episodes where weight may be low or relatively normal.

The DSM-IV clarifies the distinction between anorexia and bulimia. In the DSM-IV, binge eating and purging that occur concurrently with a diagnosis of anorexia nervosa is no longer given a separate diagnosis of bulimia nervosa but is subsumed as a subtype of anorexia nervosa.[1] Before the diagnosis of a primary eating disorder is made, other psychiatric diagnoses, such as depression or schizophrenia, and a physiological basis for anorexia must be ruled out.

◆ Etiological Theories

Multiple theories have been proposed to explain the development of eating disorders. Most experts agree that anorexia nervosa and bulimia develop from a complex interaction of individual, family, and sociocultural factors. Eating disorders can be best understood in terms of a multifactorial etiology. A vulnerable personality, sociocultural emphasis on slimness, family functioning style, a major life change or stressor, dieting, and the onset of puberty all may contribute to the development of eating disorders. Different theories of etiology, therefore, may add to the understanding of eating disorders.

PSYCHODYNAMIC THEORY

This theoretical viewpoint proposes that eating disorders stem from unresolved conflicts in early childhood. The tasks of trust, autonomy, and separation-individuation go unfulfilled, and the person remains in a dependent position. It is postulated that parents do not respond consistently to the child's cues for emotional and physical needs during infancy, resulting in feelings of ineffectiveness in the child. The child receives care, but everything is done in accordance with the mother's needs and feelings, not the child's demands.[7,8] During toddler years, the child's assertive, autonomous behavior is unrewarded, while clinging, dependent behavior is reinforced. Instead of becoming an independent, complete self, the child develops into an overly compliant person with a strong need to please others. Self-esteem becomes dependent on receiving approval from others, rather than on an internal sense of accomplishment and effectiveness. The child eventually is unable to recognize her own impulses, feelings, and needs. A crisis occurs at adolescence, when the child is unable to separate successfully from parents and engage in peer relationships.[7,8]

BIOLOGICAL THEORY

Although biological theories are controversial, proponents believe that eating disorders may originate from hypothalmic, hormonal, neurotransmitter, or biochemical disturbances. Studies of twins and sisters and daughters of people with eating disorders further suggest a

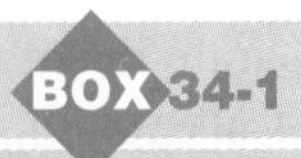

DSM-IV Diagnostic Criteria for Eating Disorders

DIAGNOSTIC CRITERIA FOR ANOREXIA NERVOSA

A. Refusal to maintain body weight at or above a minimally normal weight for age and height (eg, weight loss leading to maintenance of body weight less than 85% of that expected or failure to make expected weight gain during period of growth, leading to body weight less than 85% of that expected)
B. Intense fear of gaining weight or becoming fat, even though underweight
C. Disturbance in the way in which one's body weight or shape is experienced, undue influence of body weight or shape on self-evaluation, or denial of the seriousness of the current low body weight
D. In postmenarchial women, amenorrhea (ie, the absence of at least three consecutive menstrual cycles) (A woman is considered to have amenorrhea if her periods occur only following hormone, eg, estrogen, administration.)

Specify Type

Restricting type: During the current episode of anorexia nervosa, the person has not regularly engaged in binge eating or purging behavior (ie, self-induced vomiting or the misuse of laxatives, diuretics, or enemas).
Binge eating and purging type: During the current episode of anorexia nervosa, the person has regularly engaged in binge eating or purging behavior (ie, self-induced vomiting or the misuse of laxatives, diuretics or enemas)

DIAGNOSTIC CRITERIA FOR BULIMIA NERVOSA

A. Recurrent episodes of binge eating, characterized by both of the following:
   1. Eating in a discrete period of time (eg, within any 2-hour period) an amount of food that is definitely larger than most people would eat during a similar period of time and under similar circumstances
   2. A sense of lack of control over eating during the episode (eg, a feeling that one cannot stop eating or control what or how much one is eating)
B. Recurrent inappropriate compensatory behavior to prevent weight gain, such as self-induced vomiting; misuse of laxatives, diuretics, enemas, or other medications; fasting; or excessive exercise
C. Occurrence of binge eating and inappropriate compensatory behaviors at least twice a week for 3 months
D. Self-evaluation unduly influenced by body shape and weight
E. Disturbance not exclusive to episodes of anorexia nervosa

Specify Type

Purging type: During the current episode of bulimia nervosa, the person has regularly engaged in self-induced vomiting or the misuse of laxatives, diuretics, or enemas.
Nonpurging type: During the current episode of bulimia nervosa, the person has used other inappropriate compensatory behaviors, such as fasting or excessive exercise, but has not regularly engaged in self-induced vomiting or the misuse of laxatives, diuretics, or enemas.

(With permission from 4th ed, the Diagnostic Statistical Manual of Mental Disorders, Washington, DC, American Psychiatric Association, 1994.)

biological or genetic link.[27,41] Neuroendocrine abnormalities have been found in clients with eating disorders, but these are generally believed to be the result of extreme weight loss rather than the cause of the disorder. A state of malnutrition does affect the client's mental status and may play a role in the self-perpetuating nature of eating disorders.

Numerous studies have shown an association between depression and eating disorders, but it is difficult to determine whether affective disorders lead to eating disorders or vice versa. Antidepressant and antianxiety medications have been used effectively to treat bulimia.[14]

Recent studies from the National Institute of Mental Health suggest that anorexia, bulimia, and obsessive-compulsive disorders are associated with excessive levels of the brain hormone vasopressin. Vasopressin, which is released in response to physical and emotional stress, has been shown in studies with laboratory animals to prolong behaviors learned under conditioned circumstances. In the same way that animals injected with vasopressin retain learned associations longer, vasopressin may enhance the conditioned obsessive-compulsive cycle of vigorous dieting, exercise, binging, and purging in people with eating disorders.[18]

BEHAVIORAL AND SOCIOCULTURAL THEORIES

Supporters of behavioral theory argue that the client with an eating disorder initially may engage in dieting and gain approval for weight loss. As weight loss continues, this approval turns to concern. The client continues to receive attention around the issue of weight, thus reinforcing her maladaptive eating behavior.

Support for a sociocultural theory of eating disorders lies in the fact that anorexia nervosa is rarely found in countries with an inadequate food supply.[12] American culture has an abundance of food and places a heavy emphasis on physical attractiveness and slimness for women. This viewpoint explains an obsession with weight but does not explain why only some people go to extremes in the pursuit of thinness.

FAMILY SYSTEMS THEORY

Issues of control are central in families of clients with eating disorders. Families often consist of a passive father, a controlling mother, and an overly dependent child. The effects of a physically or emotionally absent father on a daughter are considerable. A father's lack of connectedness to his daughter may result in a neediness that is expressed through an eating disorder.[30] The family places a high value on achievement; the child feels obliged to satisfy parental standards. Minuchin identified four interaction patterns characteristic of families of anorectic children: enmeshment, overprotectiveness, rigidity, and lack of conflict resolution.[33,34]

Enmeshment

Enmeshment refers to a lack of clear boundaries between the parent and child subsystems and between individual family members. Members have failed to individuate, or adequately develop their own separate identities apart from the family identity. The enmeshed family speaks in terms of "we feel" and "we do." In healthy families, the parental subsystem functions as a unit distinct from the children to make decisions and meet adult needs. The enmeshed family often has an inappropriate alliance between a child and parent. The eating disorder may be a desperate attempt by the adolescent to separate herself from the family system, particularly from an overly dependent relationship with the mother.[39]

Overprotectiveness

Hypervigilance and overprotectiveness are common in families of anorectic clients. The overinvolvement of one or both parents makes it difficult for the child to learn to think, feel, and act autonomously. Although the parents usually love the child very much, they convey a lack of trust by not allowing the child to take appropriate risks. The child does not learn to trust the self and experiences a sense of personal ineffectiveness.

Rigidity and Conflict Avoidance

Families of anorectics have a low threshold for conflict. They believe that members are supposed to be happy and not have problems. Children may see very little conflict or expression of strong emotions between parents, because family norms discourage this behavior. The child does inevitably experience strong feelings and conflict; however, because these consistently are not validated, the child learns to doubt and deny her feelings, especially those of a "negative" nature. The family's politeness and superficial pleasantness interfere with the adolescent's need for autonomous expression of self. Rather than rebelling directly, the adolescent becomes more obsessive and perfectionistic in a search for love, approval, recognition, and reduced anxiety. Eventually, she desperately tries to establish her own identity by exacting tyrannical control over what she eats.

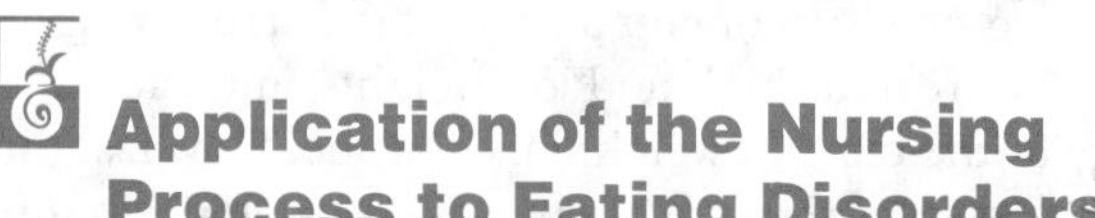

Application of the Nursing Process to Eating Disorders

ASSESSMENT

Because clients with eating disorders may be secretive and unwilling to portray themselves as having problems, the nurse must be skilled in eliciting feelings and thoughts; forming an alliance with the client is crucial.[28] A supportive but firm approach by the nurse is helpful in engaging the client in the therapeutic relationship. Knowledge of the diagnostic criteria and etiology of eating disorders guides the nurse in asking relevant questions (Box 34-2).

Assessment of the client with an eating disorder is complex. Clients with eating disorders may exhibit disturbance in nearly all of the 11 functional health patterns.[19]

Health Perception and Health Management Patterns

The client with an eating disorder frequently has an inaccurate perception of her health status. She often does not perceive herself as ill, even though others are alarmed by changes in her physical and mental health status. She frequently resists treatment and if a minor,

BOX 34-2

Quick Assessment Tool for Eating Disorders

	YES	NO
1. Do you spend most of your time thinking about food?	☐	☐
2. Do you panic if you gain a pound or two?	☐	☐
3. Do you ever eat uncontrollably?	☐	☐
4. Do you feel guilt and remorse after eating?	☐	☐
5. Do you ever fast or restrict your diet?	☐	☐
6. Do you vomit or use laxatives to control your weight?	☐	☐
7. Are your periods irregular, or have you stopped menstruating?	☐	☐
8. Do you have a strict exercise regimen?	☐	☐
9. Do you panic if you are unable to exercise as much as you'd like?	☐	☐

often receives treatment involuntarily through the actions of her parents. The nurse should explore issues with the client, such as how the client was referred to treatment.

Nutritional-Metabolic Pattern

Numerous disturbances exist in this pattern. The client has either a restricted food intake (anorexia) or an excessive food intake accompanied by purging (bulimia). The nurse needs to obtain an accurate current weight, history of previous high and low weights, and the chronology of the current weight loss episode. How fast did weight loss occur? Were there any associated circumstances, such as medical illness, psychiatric illness, situational crisis, or major life change? Because the client may be reluctant to reveal details about dieting or binge-purge behaviors, it is helpful to ask the client to describe food and fluid intake for a typical day. The nurse observes for clues of preoccupation with food. Does the client cook for others, hoard food, talk about food constantly, or have guilt associated with eating? Physical assessment may reveal numerous symptoms related to altered nutritional and metabolic status: fluid volume deficit (dehydration, poor skin turgor, hypotension), impaired skin integrity (dry skin, brittle hair and nails), hypokalemia (vomiting, using laxatives or diuretics), altered oral mucous membranes (dental caries, mouth sores, sore throat, esophageal inflammation), cardiac changes (arrhythmias, bradycardia), hypothermia (lowered core temperature and cold extremities), and fine, downy, lanugo hair (state of severe emaciation).

Elimination Pattern

Elimination disturbances occur in anorectic and bulimic clients. Constipation occurs as a result of restricted food intake, vomiting, and slowed gastrointestinal motility. Excessive laxative use causes diarrhea and loss of protein, fluid, and potassium in stools. Long-term laxative use may also lead to eventual reliance on laxatives for bowel elimination. Polyuria may be present in the client with severe weight loss.

Activity, Exercise, and Sleep-Rest Patterns

Clients with eating disorders typically are very active. They exercise compulsively, are restless, and frequently suffer from insomnia. Early morning awakening is common. A lowered pulse rate often occurs in response to excessive exercise and starvation. It is amazing to others that anorectic clients are able to engage in strenuous physical activity while consuming very few calories and appearing very frail. It is helpful to ask the client to describe her activity and sleep patterns for a typical day. In what kind of exercise does she engage? Is she involved in organized sports at school? Does she have difficulty sleeping? Is she often tired, or does she have a lot of energy?

Cognitive-Perceptual Pattern

Clients with eating disorders typically lack awareness of the connection between their eating behaviors and underlying feelings, needs, and conflicts. Presenting these clients with knowledge of eating disorders is a first step in helping them acknowledge that their behavior is maladaptive. These clients tend to exhibit intellectualization and all-or-none reasoning. They are more comfortable with abstract concepts than with recognizing and expressing feelings. Clients need to learn that strong feelings, especially those of a "negative" nature are acceptable and that one can experience and express strong feelings without losing control. These clients also tend to have perfectionistic personalities and to give up if something is not exactly right. They need to learn balance and moderation in thinking and behavior. They also tend to overgeneralize and believe that all of life's problems will be solved if enough weight is lost. The nurse might ask such questions as the following:

1. Would you describe yourself as a perfectionist?
2. Do you repeat things until you get them right?
3. Have you ever not been able to get something out of your mind?
4. Do you find yourself thinking about things over and over?
5. How do you feel if you lose control, such as getting very angry or eating too much?
6. What do you do if you feel you are losing control?
7. Have you ever had times when you have eaten uncontrollably? What did you feel, and what did you do?

Self-Perception and Self-Concept Patterns

Clients with eating disorders experience considerable anxiety about becoming obese. Anorectic clients have a distorted body image, seeing themselves as too fat even when others view them as alarmingly thin. They generally have low self-esteem even though they achieve well at school, sports, and work; they have unrealistically rigid and high expectations for themselves and look to others for approval. These clients perceive a lack of control over themselves and situations. They do not have the sense that their actions will significantly effect a desired outcome. To gain knowledge of the client's perceptual accuracy regarding body image, the nurse might ask the following questions:

1. What do you like the best about your body? What do you like the least?
2. If you could change how you look, how would you be different?

To explore self-esteem, the nurse might ask the following questions:

1. What do you like the best about yourself? What do you like the least?
2. How would you describe yourself to others?
3. How would others (family, friends) describe you?
4. What are your strengths and weaknesses?

Role-Relationship Pattern

Clients with eating disorders frequently become isolated from family and friends. They often exhibit immature interaction patterns and remain inappropriately dependent and childlike in their relationship with their parents, stop dating, and gradually abandon good friends. As the disorder persists, deficits in social skills increase. They often remain good students and spend much time alone studying. Isolation also may result from preoccupation with weight, food, and exercise. To assess roles and relationships, the nurse might ask the following questions:

1. How is your relationship with your parents?
2. How would you describe your family?
3. Do you have a lot of friends? Do you have a best friend?
4. What do you like to do with your friends?
5. What is school like?
6. Do you study a lot?
7. In what activities are you involved at school?
8. Do you feel pressure to do well in school, and if so, from whom?

Sexuality-Reproductive Pattern

As a result of excessive weight loss, reproductive hormones regress to prepubertal levels. Clients experience amenorrhea, breast atrophy, lanugo, and loss of axillary and pubic hair. Infertility accompanies amenorrhea, but this typically resolves once normal weight is regained and menses resume. Anorectic clients tend to be sexually inactive, while bulimic clients may exhibit impulsive sexual behaviors. The nurse might explore the following questions:

1. How do you feel about the body changes that occur at adolescence (eg, in females, breast development, menstruation, broadening of hips)?
2. Is dating something that you enjoy?
3. Have you had any sexual experiences?
4. How do you feel about the presence or lack of sexual experiences?

Coping-Stress Tolerance Pattern

Eating disorders are maladaptive attempts to meet life's demands, roles, and stresses. The client may exhibit the following difficulties in coping:

1. Inability to ask for help and nurturance
2. Inability to make decisions
3. Inability to meet role expectations of adolescence
4. Inability to express emotions
5. Perceived powerlessness

In addition to ineffective individual coping, family coping also may be compromised. Families may exhibit difficulties in expressing emotions, dealing with conflict, and facilitating autonomy of members. Issues of control commonly are present. To assess coping behaviors, the nurse might ask these questions:

1. How you make decisions about everyday things, like how to spend your free time? (For example, do you usually ask someone for advice or think things out for yourself?)
2. Is your life right now pretty much the way you want it? If not, what would you change? What can you do to make these changes?

3. What do you do to feel better when you are sad or upset?
4. Have you ever felt like hurting yourself when you are down?
5. Have you ever thought about committing suicide?
6. Have you ever used alcohol or drugs to feel better?
7. Have you ever stolen anything (eg, food or money)? If so, how do you feel about that?
8. Do you get along with your parents? What happens when you argue with them? What do you argue about? What happens when you talk to them about a problem or concern?
9. How do you get along with your siblings? Can you talk to them about your feelings and problems?
10. Do your friends help you out if you have a problem?

Value-Belief Pattern

Specific problems do not necessarily occur in this functional health pattern. Because the client generally has a low degree of self-knowledge and self-awareness, there may be a generalized deficit in clarity of value-belief patterns. In addition, eating disorders most often occur when the client is struggling to establish her own identity and formulate a philosophy about the meaning of existence. As trust develops between the nurse and client, it may be helpful for the client to explore the following issues:

1. What is important to me?
2. What do I care about?
3. What is the meaning of life?
4. Who am I?
5. What differences do I make?

NURSING DIAGNOSIS

Due to the multisystem nature of eating disorders, data analysis may suggest a large number of nursing diagnoses, including the following:

1. Altered Nutrition: Less than body requirements related to refusal to ingest or retain ingested food, physical exertion in excess of caloric intake
2. Self-Esteem Disturbance related to unrealistic expectations from self or others, lack of positive feedback, striving to please others to gain acceptance
3. Ineffective Individual Coping related to unmet developmental tasks (trust, autonomy), dysfunctional family system
4. Altered Family Processes related to enmeshed family system, ineffective communication patterns, denial of problems and conflicts, unresolved issues of control, inability to manage conflict
5. Fluid Volume Deficit related to diuretic or laxative abuse, vomiting, inability to concentrate urine
6. Constipation or Diarrhea related to refusal to ingest or retain ingested food, chronic laxative abuse
7. Altered Oral Mucous Membranes related to deficient nutritional status and frequent vomiting
8. Powerlessness related to deficiency in learning that one's actions can cause desired outcomes
9. Social Isolation related to fear of rejection, impaired age-appropriate social skills, preoccupation with obsessive thoughts and compulsive behaviors
10. Altered Sexuality Patterns related to impaired nutritional status, social isolation, low self-esteem
11. Decreased Cardiac Output related to hypokalemia, decreased blood volume
12. Altered Thought Processes related to all-or-none thinking, intellectualization, obsessions, overgeneralization, malnutrition
13. Risk for Injury related to excessive exercise and deficient nutritional status

PLANNING

Planning involves collaborating with the client and usually her family to formulate an appropriate approach to treatment and set goals. In many settings, the nurse, physician, psychotherapist, social worker, dietitian, and occupational therapist work together to formulate the treatment plan. Communication and consistency among members of the multidisciplinary team are critical. The primary nurse often coordinates client care among team members (Nursing Care Plan 34-1).

Client Outcomes

Short-term Goals. Short-term goals focus on decreasing anxiety, stopping weight loss, restoring the individual to an acceptable weight, and normalizing eating behaviors. Examples include the following:

1. Client will verbalize diminished fears and exhibit decreased anxiety regarding weight gain and loss of control.
2. Client will have adequate dietary intake to meet body requirements and maintain weight appropriate to age and height.
3. Client will not engage in binge eating or purging activities.
4. Client will maintain an appropriate activity level.

Long-Term Goals. Long-term goals focus on helping the client and, if possible, her family resolve the psychological issues that precipitated the eating disorder and to develop more constructive coping mechanisms. These may include the following:

1. Client will recognize and verbalize her emotions and needs.

Nursing Care Plan 34-1

A Client With an Eating Disorder: Anorexia Nervosa

Client Situation

A 15-year-old high school sophomore was referred to inpatient psychiatric care on a unit specializing in eating disorders. She is 5 ft 5 in tall and weighs 90 lb. She was treated by her family physician for the past 3 months for anorexia nervosa and has failed to gain any weight.

A physical examination revealed the following typical characteristics of a client with the diagnosis of anorexia nervosa: She has a cachexic body appearance with dry skin and dull, limp hair with evidence of lanugo growth on her trunk. Laboratory tests revealed evidence of mild anemia, elevated liver function tests, and electrocardiogram validation of sinus bradycardia. The client admits to amenorrhea for at least 4 months.

The client is still expressing an intense fear of gaining weight and reported to the admission nurse, "I'm still too fat; look at my thighs." Her parents report that she is an honor student in school and is involved in cross country running. They are quite upset and express disbelief that their daughter would have such a severe problem.

Nursing Diagnosis

Altered Nutrition: Less than body requirements related to reduced food intake and increased exercise to bring about weight loss

Outcome

Client will reach and maintain weight with minimum of 2 lb per week gain.

Intervention	Rationale
Institute behavior modification protocol for gradual weight gain.	Well-defined behavioral modification program will provide consistency, decrease power struggles, and enhance compliance.
Consult with dietician to provide nutritious foods with regard to client preferences.	Including client in meal planning will enhance client's sense of control.
Monitor vital signs, food and fluid intake, output, and weight. Weigh daily at same time & under same conditions.	Hypotension and bradycardia may occur as a result of starvation. Monitoring intake, output, and weight ensures client safety.
Supervise meals, and remain with client up to 1 hour after eating.	Direct observation will diminish client's opportunity to avoid eating, hoard or hide food, or vomit.
Monitor activity level to prevent excessive exercise. Focus exercise on physical/mental fitness, not weight reduction.	Client may engage in excessive exercise to burn calories. By focusing on physical fitness, the client may begin to associate exercise with health promotion goals, instead of weight loss.
Provide liquid diet via nasogastric or nasoduodenal tube if client is unwilling to maintain adequate oral intake.	Liquid diet will provide adequate nutrition and fluid when client is unwilling to eat and drink.
Use supportive, firm, nonjudgmental, matter-of-fact approach in regulating client's eating behavior.	A matter-of-fact approach is not viewed as punishment by the client and tends not to induce feelings of guilt. The client experiences feelings of acceptance.

Evaluation

Client returns to and maintains adequate weight for age and size.

continued

Nursing Care Plan 34-1 *(Continued)*

Nursing Diagnosis

Self Esteem Disturbance related to perfectionism, overdependence on appraisals and approval of others, and inadequate social skills

Outcome

Client will verbalize a realistic perception of her body, exhibit age-appropriate autonomy, and interact comfortably with peers.

Intervention	Rationale
Assist client to review her own and others' bodies realistically	External, objective feedback will help client attain a healthier more realistic body image.
Help client acknowledge relationship between overly high self-expections and feelings of inadequacy.	Realistic expectations of self will increase self-esteem.
Help client identify her strengths and resources.	Realistic positive reinforcement and feedback enhances client's self-esteem.
Encourage client to make decisions and choices for self.	Opportunities to practice independent functioning will lead to improved self-confidence and self-esteem.
Enhance client's communication and socialization skills through promotion of information, role-playing, and participation in group activities with peers.	Enhanced social skills will improve peer relationships and contribute to improved self-esteem.

Evaluation

Client demonstrates social interaction with peers and realistic perception and acceptance of own body.

Nursing Diagnosis

Altered Family Processes related to enmeshed family system, denial of problems and conflicts, unresolved control issues, and dysfunctional communication patterns

Outcome

Client's family will manage conflict constructively, encourage autonomy of all family members, and communicate directly with each other.

Intervention	Rationale
Encourage family members to identify and express conflicts openly.	Family members frequently need help to identify and express conflicts directly & constructively. Communicating assertively fosters individuality and personal efficacy among family members.
Encourage family members to speak for themselves by making "I," rather than "we," statements.	Enmeshed, overinvolved family members often speak for each other and need to learn to distinguish and be responsible for own feelings, words, and actions.
Explore with members ways to increase autonomy and decrease parental overinvolvement with children.	When parents become aware of and consciously work to decrease overinvolved behaviors, children can make decisions and accept responsibility for own behavior.
Role model direct, constructive communication patterns for family members.	Role modeling of open-communication provides an example and gives family members permission to express their thoughts and feelings openly.

Evaluation

Client's family encourages age-appropriate autonomy and open communication among members.

2. Client will exhibit a realistic thinking process and perception of her body.
3. Client will verbalize adequate self-esteem.
4. Client will perceive control over her actions.
5. Client will demonstrate age-appropriate autonomy.
6. Client will recognize maladaptive coping behaviors and demonstrate adaptive coping behaviors.
7. Family will demonstrate constructive communication patterns.
8. Family will manage conflict constructively.
9. Family process will assist members toward individuation.

INTERVENTION

The treatment of clients with eating disorders is a complex and frequently long process. Client improvement is often gradual and characterized by two steps forward and one back. Clients may resist treatment; the nurse is challenged to establish a relationship of open communication and trust.[13] Inpatient and outpatient treatment approaches generally include one or more of the following therapies: individual psychotherapy, behavior modification, group therapy, and family therapy. Recent research suggests that success is greatest with family therapy, moderate with intensive individual psychotherapy, and lowest with behavior therapy alone.[15] Different methods are effective for different clients and their families (Case Study 34-1).

Treatment Settings

Treatment of eating disorders occurs in outpatient and inpatient settings. Clients with anorexia nervosa are hospitalized more frequently than are those with bulimia. The primary reasons for hospitalizing anorectic clients are low weight, depressed mood, low serum potassium, lack of response to outpatient treatment, and family discouragement and demoralization. Reasons for inpatient treatment of bulimia include the client's desire for treatment, low weight, dangerously low potassium levels, or a diagnosis of maladaptive personality patterns, such as an impulse disorder or borderline personality.[2]

Because many clients with eating disorders never seek treatment, nurses commonly encounter the more severely ill clients in the hospital setting. Clients with eating disorders may be admitted to general psychiatric units or to units or facilities specializing in the treatment of eating disorders. Families are frequently frustrated, angry, and scared after months of trying to get the client to eat. Temporarily removing the client from the home may relieve the family's distress and set the stage for behavior changes in the client and her family.

Behavior Modification

Behavior modification programs generally are begun in an inpatient setting. Although programs vary, the client typically starts a program with no privileges. Privileges are gained in response to appropriate eating behaviors. A criticism sometimes aimed at behavior modification techniques is that the nurse manipulates and controls client behavior without dealing with underlying issues.[8] Several research studies conclude that behavior modification is useful to restore lost weight but inadequate to deal with psychological symptoms.[4,5] Behavior modification is generally used in conjunction with psychotherapy, however, and can be very helpful in meeting the goals of restoring weight and nutritional status.[22]

Establishing a contract that spells out the expected behaviors, rewards, privileges, and consequences of noncompliance may be useful in eliminating power struggles with the client.[28] If the client feels she contributes to the planning of rewards and privileges, she will perceive more control over her environment and body and more likely will adhere to the treatment regimen. All health team members must consistently carry out the terms of the contract.[38] Even though the client may rebel against contract terms, it reassures her to know that consistent limits are being maintained and that she can trust the staff to help her maintain control.

Hospitalized anorectic clients frequently express frustration with limitations placed on them in regard to exercise. Recent studies suggest that examining the type of exercise may help in setting sound guidelines for exercise protocols. Rigorous aerobic exercise is generally contraindicated when weight gain is a goal. Allowing the client to engage in moderate resistance training (eg, weight lifting), however, would increase the lean body mass as the client gains weight and minimize the gain in "fat weight," which is a great fear of the anorectic client. Developing a contract that allows the client to participate in exercise of this nature would acknowledge the benefits of exercise in a healthy lifestyle and enable the client to feel more in control and develop a more positive body image during the process of gaining weight.[32]

The nurse communicates caring to the client through a kind, firm, matter-of-fact approach; for example, "When you gain 5 pounds, you will earn privileges to participate in more activities. This is your choice." The nurse avoids offering punitive responses, arguing about limits, bribing, cajoling, and being excessively vigilant and overprotective. Through his or her interactions, the nurse conveys to the client, "You are a worthwhile person, and I care about you; I have expectations of you, and you are capable of meeting these expectations."

34-1 Case Study

Julie, An Adolescent With Anorexia

JULIE

Fifteen-year-old Julie, a sophomore in high school, 5 ft 8 in tall and 115 lb, was referred to the school nurse by a teacher who had heard Julie vomiting on several occasions in the bathroom. In talking with Julie, the nurse initially observed that her teeth were in very poor condition. When asked about the vomiting, Julie looked embarrassed but confided that she was worried about gaining weight and vomited when she ate too much. When asked how long she'd been vomiting, Julie reported that during the summer before her freshman year in high school, she went on a diet to lose weight. Several other girls whom she admired were on diets, and Julie, although not overweight, gradually ate less and less. Between July and December, her weight dropped from 114 to 87 lb. Julie stated that her parents didn't worry at first but eventually became upset about her weight loss. Julie recalls that they tried to bribe her with food and fought with each other about her refusal to eat. That whole period now seems somewhat unreal to her.

Right before Christmas in her freshman year, her mother took her to the family physician, who told Julie she would have to go into the hospital if she didn't eat. No other intervention occurred at this time. Julie was a "straight A" student; the idea of being hospitalized and missing school frightened her. She agreed to start eating and did so that day. She rapidly regained the lost weight by eating everthing she wanted. She couldn't remember exactly when the thought occurred to her that she could eat as much as she wanted without gaining weight if she could vomit. She soon learned that if she drank a lot of water after eating she could easily induce vomiting. With this discovery, she began eating larger amounts of food. So that her family wouldn't be suspicious that food was disappearing so quickly she began buying, and then stealing, candy and cookies from the grocery store and hiding them in her room. This behavior was still occurring, and Julie stated that her parents did not suspect she was doing this. She said that her parents were happy when she started eating, and they never talked about her weight loss again.

Julie told the school nurse that she sometimes wondered if she was crazy and that she was ashamed of her teeth. She wondered if vomiting had anything to do with dental decay, even though she brushed her teeth immediately after vomiting. The nurse provided Julie with some basic information about anorexia nervosa and bulimia. Julie didn't know that there was a name for what she was experiencing and was relieved to hear that others had the same problem. The nurse explained that there was an association between frequent eating, vomiting, and dental caries but that Julie should not blame herself. She didn't get anorexia and bulimia on purpose and couldn't have prevented it.

With Julie's permission, the nurse called her parents in for a conference. The nurse explained what Julie was going through and that she needed assistance to cope more effectively. Without blaming the family, the nurse explained that it would help Julie if all family members would meet with a counselor experienced in eating disorders. Julie's parents initially reacted by denying that Julie had a problem. They said that she did well in school, ate well, and everyone in their family had poor teeth. After hearing in more detail, however, about Julie's vomiting and stealing of food they agreed to attend a family session. The family did attend family therapy for 3 months. The school nurse continued to see Julie and to provide support.

During the next year, Julie's eating patterns were normal most of the time. She reported that she occasionally binged and purged when she was experiencing anxiety. Extensive dental reconstruction had been completed, however, and Julie did not want to ruin her teeth again. Even though she had more insight into why she developed an eating disorder, she continued to feel considerable shame and guilt about her previous eating behaviors and stealing.

Questions for Discussion

1. What is the relationship between the school system and the mental health system?
2. Was the intervention by the family physician appropriate? If not, how would you have modified this approach?
3. Was the intervention by the school nurse effective? What was effective? What would you have modified?
4. What are the goals of family therapy?
5. Formulate a nursing care plan for Julie beginning where the case study ends.

Individual Psychotherapy

Individual psychotherapy generally is part of inpatient and outpatient treatment protocols. Individual therapy is particularly helpful in assisting the client to establish more realistic thinking processes, increase self-esteem, establish a healthy sense of control, and express emotions and needs more directly.

Expression of Emotions and Needs. When working with clients with eating disorders, the nurse gives the client permission to discuss feelings. Because the client may be fearful that strong feelings will lead to loss of control, the nurse repeatedly helps her distinguish between feelings and behaviors. The nurse tells the client that it is normal to have strong feelings that we sometimes do not like. The nurse communicates that the client can be very angry at another person without being hurtful. As an adjunct therapy, assertiveness training also may help increase the client's ability to express feelings directly and constructively.

Realistic Thinking Processes. People with eating disorders tend to have perfectionistic personalities and to think in all-or-none terms. This kind of thinking helps to explain the characteristic extreme fear of becoming obese. For example, a client who eats two cookies might conclude, "I couldn't control myself; I might as well give up and eat the whole bag of cookies." The client has rigidly defined appropriate behaviors for herself in terms of "walking on a tightrope," with the need for constant vigilance to keep from falling off. The nurse can reassure the client that life is more like walking in a big meadow and that she can safely move in many directions. The nurse encourages the client to try out new behaviors, explaining that although this may be frightening, the client gradually will learn to be more confident about her behavioral choices in all areas, including eating.

Self-Esteem. Low self-esteem in clients with eating disorders is associated with overly high self-expectations, need for approval and acceptance from others, and possible deficiencies in social skills. The nurse helps the client see the association between overly high self-expectations and feelings of ineffectiveness and helps the client identify her positive attributes and achieve self-approval. Along with undergoing individual therapy, the client may improve her social skills by participating in group psychotherapy with clients with similar needs. Self-esteem can also be enhanced by successful participation with peers in activities such as recreational or occupational therapy.

Control and Autonomy. The client's perception of control and autonomy increases as she learns to express her emotions and needs more directly, think in a less rigid fashion, and establish more realistic self-expectations. The nurse encourages the client to assume responsibility for choices and decisions. For the client to take risks and grow, she must trust that the nurse cares about her well-being and will maintain appropriate limits. The nurse assures the client that she will learn to trust in her ability to exert appropriate behavioral controls and act autonomously.

Solution-Focused Brief Therapy

In response to increasing pressures to treat clients as cost-effectively as possible, solution-focused brief therapy reflects a paradigm shift away from pathology to one in which the clinician views clients as basically healthy, inherently resourceful, and able to solve their own problems. The clinician's role is to learn the client's unique view of her problem and what needs to be different as a result of treatment. Although this approach originated from economic pressures, it has many virtues. Rather than looking for causes and taking deep excursions into the past, clients are empowered to recognize and acknowledge their own abilities and resourcefulness.[31]

The two key techniques of solution-focused brief therapy are asking "the miracle question" and "searching for exceptions": "How would your life be different if your eating disorder were miraculously gone?" "What are the times like when you are managing your eating behavior more successfully?"

Family Therapy

Family therapy may occur in conjunction with inpatient treatment or entirely on an outpatient basis. Family therapy is particularly important when the client will be returning to the home. The nurse must not automatically assume that dysfunction exists in the family, however. Because families may already feel guilty, helpless, and frightened, the nurse should convey a supportive, nonblaming attitude. Family therapy focuses on fostering open, healthy interaction patterns among members. One innovative program uses family meal therapy as the primary technique in a multicomponent approach to changing eating behaviors.[17] Some family therapists find it helpful to focus on the four dysfunctional interaction patterns identified by Minuchin: enmeshment, overprotectiveness, rigidity, and lack of conflict resolution.[33]

Enmeshment and Overprotectiveness. Members of enmeshed families have failed to establish individual identities apart from a meshed family identity. Parents are typically overprotective and intrusive toward activities of their children. When working with these families, the nurse helps all members to make "I" statements instead of "we" statements; for example, "I feel sad" and "I am so angry!" as opposed to "We are all so upset!"

Members are encouraged to speak for themselves and not for each other.

Parents in enmeshed families frequently try to protect their children by speaking for them, as in "She feels happy most of the time." Members are not accustomed to identifying and expressing their own feelings and need frequent prompting from the nurse: "You look upset; what are you feeling right now?" Because enmeshed families typically have weak or inappropriate boundaries between generations, the nurse may ask siblings to sit together as a unit distinct from the parents. Such seating arrangements reinforce appropriate boundaries and help to disrupt dysfunctional alliances that may exist between a parent and child.

Conflict Avoidance and Rigidity. Families of clients with eating disorders tend to brush conflicts under the carpet. It may be an unspoken family rule that it is not acceptable to feel sad or upset or to have problems. The nurse helps family members bring existing conflicts to shared awareness. If members try to avoid or deny conflict, the nurse refocuses them on the conflictual issue. The nurse helps members to express their conflict constructively—without shouting, threatening, accusing, or demanding—so other family members can listen and respond.

Because the anorectic client may be accustomed to diverting parental conflict onto herself, the nurse keeps the parents talking to each other and instructs them not to involve the adolescent; for example, "Jane is not part of this conflict. This is between you and your wife. Keep talking to her, and don't involve Jane in it." Family members may have difficulty listening to each other's concerns and requests. The nurse models appropriate communication skills and helps members repattern their communications with each other.

Group Therapy

Clients with eating disorders also may benefit from group therapy. Groups may have specific therapeutic goals, such as fostering self-esteem or gaining insight into feelings and behavior. Groups also may be organized as primarily supportive or self-help groups. Members gain self-acceptance by sharing concerns with others and receiving constructive support and feedback from peers.[16,40]

EVALUATION

Evaluation of care for the client with eating disorders involves examining all phases of the nursing process. Did the nurse accurately and thoroughly assess the client's physiological, psychological, and social status? Were nursing diagnoses accurate and comprehensive? Evaluating the planning and implementation of care is an ongoing process. Daily evaluation of nursing care plans and client progress toward meeting goals results in modification of treatment approaches as indicated.

The nurse evaluates the client's physical and psychosocial responses to intervention. Desired physical outcomes include weight gain, normal laboratory values and vital signs, and return of secondary sexual characteristics and menstruation. Desired psychosocial outcomes include a realistic perception of body image, direct expression of feelings, improved self-esteem, a sense of control over self and environment, and constructive family process.

As a client recovers, she may feel guilty about and ashamed of her behavior while ill. Such feelings can persist long after normal weight is attained. The nurse reassures the client that she could not have prevented herself from becoming ill and that her behavior while ill was an ineffective attempt to cope with stressors. The nurse stresses that the client now has increased coping skills and will not need to resort to the immature responses she used previously.

The nurse also evaluates the family's interaction patterns. Desired outcomes are that family members communicate directly with each other and deal openly with conflicts and that parents relinquish previous patterns of overcontrol and overprotectiveness to allow the client an appropriate degree of autonomy. Even if these goals appear to be met, most clients require follow-up treatment to reinforce behavioral changes and prevent a return of disordered eating. Follow-up should span at least 4 years because of the high rate of relapse.

◆ Chapter Summary

This chapter has examined two eating disorders, anorexia nervosa and bulimia, that encompass a broad range of physiological, psychological, and social disruptions. The application of the nursing process to clients with these disorders is complex and challenging. Chapter highlights include the following:

1. Anorexia nervosa and bulimia primarily affect adolescent and young women.
2. Anorexia nervosa and bulimia have many etiological factors in common and may be viewed as existing along a single spectrum of eating disorders.
3. Although multiple theories exist, most experts agree that eating disorders develop from a complex interaction of individual, family, and sociocultural factors.
4. Clients with eating disorders exhibit disturbances in many or all of the functional health patterns.
5. Treatment of clients with eating disorders occurs in inpatient and outpatient settings and is a complex and often lengthy process.

6. Treatment approaches generally include a combination of individual psychotherapy, behavior modification, group therapy, family therapy, and solution-focused brief therapy.
7. Desired client outcomes include normalization of weight and eating patterns, improved self-esteem, and development of realistic thought processes, adaptive coping mechanisms, and constructive family processes.
8. Most clients require follow-up treatment to reinforce behavioral changes and prevent a return of disordered eating.

Critical Thinking Questions

1. *Briefly explain why anorexia nervosa and bulimia primarily affect adolescent and young women.*
2. *Describe the four interaction patterns characteristic in families of anorectic children: enmeshment, overprotectiveness, rigidity, and lack of conflict resolution.*
3. *Briefly explain how the functional health patterns may be helpful in assessing the client with an eating disorder.*

Review Questions

After returning to school last fall, 16-year-old Paula was referred to the school nurse by several teachers. She had had a noticeable weight loss over summer vacation, and faculty members were concerned that she was either ill or anorectic. Betty, the school nurse, arranged a health conference with Paula.

1. When considering a diagnosis of anorexia nervosa in Paula, which one of the following statements does not apply?
   A. It occurs in girls from 12 to 18 years of age.
   B. Fears of sexuality are often present.
   C. Clients are usually representative of middle to upper socioeconomic class.
   D. Fifteen percent of clients also exhibit bulimia.
2. The nurse contacts Paula's parents. They are surprised and describe Paula as
   A. hostile and dangerous.
   B. anxious and restive.
   C. devious and manipulative.
   D. a model child.
3. Paula is admitted to the adolescent unit for treatment of anorexia nervosa. Paula's primary nurse uses a "client contract" approach with her. This technique serves the important function of
   A. providing the client with a feeling of responsibility and control of her behavior.
   B. providing the therapist with a strategy for client compliance.
   C. allowing the client a tool to negotiate behavior.
   D. establishing an effective assessment tool.
4. An important distinction to make between anorectics and bulimics is that
   A. most bulimics do not have a distorted body image.
   B. bulimics do not use cathartics, diuretics, or laxatives.
   C. bulimics make no attempt at self-control.
   D. bulimics are not depressed or self-critical.
5. Some researchers postulate that eating disorders are primarily a form of
   A. depressive mood disorders.
   B. schizophrenic disorders.
   C. personality disorders.
   D. anxiety disorders.
6. The family system of the client with an eating disorder is likely to exhibit all of the following except
   A. ennmeshment.
   B. rigidity
   C. conflict avoidance.
   D. underprotectiveness.

◆ References

1. American Psychiatric Association: Diagnostic and Statistical Manual of Mental Disorders, 4th ed, rev. Washington, DC, American Psychiatric Association, 1994
2. Andersen AE: Anorexia Nervosa and Bulimia: A Spectrum of Eating Disorders. J Adolesc Health Care 4: 15–21, 1983
3. Andersen AE, Mickahide AD: Anorexia Nervosa in the Male: An Underdiagnosed Disorder. Psychosomatics 24: 1066, 1983
4. Bemis K: Current Approaches to the Etiology and Treatment of Anorexia Nervosa. Psychol Bull 85: 3, 593–617, 1978
5. Bhanji S, Thompson J: Operant Conditioning in the Treatment of Anorexia Nervosa: A Review and Retrospective Study of 11 Cases. Br J Psychiatry 124: 166–172, 1974
6. Brozan N: Anorexia: Not Just a Disease of the Young. The New York Times, July 18, 1983
7. Bruch H: Eating Disorders: Obesity, Anorexia and the Person Within. New York, Basic Books, 1973
8. Bruch H: Perils of Behavior Modification in the Treatment of Anorexia Nervosa. JAMA 230: 1419–1422, 1974
9. Casper R, Eckert E, Halmi K: Bulimia: Its Incidence and Clinical Symptoms in Patients With Anorexia Nervosa. Arch Gen Psychiatry 37: 1030–1035, 1980

10. Ciseaux A: Anorexia Nervosa: A View from the Mirror. Am J Nurs 80 (8): 1468–1470, 1980
11. Coburn J, Ganong L: Bulimic and Nonbulimic College Females' Perceptions of Family Adaptability and Family Cohesion. J Adv Nurs 14: 27–33, 1989
12. Crisp AH: Anorexia Nervosa: Let Me Be. London, Academic Press, 1980
13. Deering CG: Developing a Therapeutic Alliance With the Anorexia Nervosa Client. J Psychosoc Nurs Ment Health Serv 25 (3): 11–17, 1987
14. Dippel NM, Becknal BK: Bulimia. J Psychosoc Nurs Ment Health Serv 25 (9): 12–17, 1987
15. Doyen L: Primary Anorexia Nervosa: A Review and Critique of Selected Papers. J Psychosoc Nurs Ment Health Serv 20 (6): 12–18, 1982
16. Edmonds MS: Overcoming Eating Disorders: A Group Experience. J Psychosoc Nurs Ment Health Serv 24 (8): 19–25, 1986
17. Forisha B, Grothaus K, Luscombe R: Dinner Conversation: Meal Therapy to Differentiate Eating Behavior From Family Process. J Psychosoc Nurs Ment Health Serv 28 (11): 12–16, 1990
18. Freund K, Graham S, Lesky L, Moskowitz M: Detection of Bulimia in a Primary Care Setting. J Gen Intern Med 8: 236, 1993
19. Glezos S: Alcohol, Drug Abuse, and Mental Health. Administration News 18 (3): 9–11, 1992
20. Gordon M: Nursing Diagnosis: Process and Application, 2d ed. New York, McGraw-Hill, 1987
21. Halmi KA: Anorexia Nervosa: Demographic and Clinical Features in 94 Cases. Psychosom Med 36: 18–25, 1974
22. Halmi KA: Pragmatic Information on Eating Disorders. Psychiatric Clin North Am 5 (2): 371–377, 1982
23. Halmi KA, Powers P, Cunningham S: Treatment of Anorexia Nervosa With Behavior Modification. Arch Gen Psychiatry 32: 93–95, 1975
24. Hart K, Ollendick T: Prevalence of Bulimia in Working and University Women. Am J Psychiatry 142: 851–854, 1985
25. Hawkins RC: The Binge-Purge Syndrome. New York, Springer, 1984
26. Herzog DB, Copeland PM: Eating Disorders. N Engl J Med 313: 295–303, 1985
27. Kalucy RS, Crisp AH, Lacey JH, Harding B: Prevalence and Prognosis in Anorexia Nervosa. Aust N Z J Psychiatry 11: 251–257, 1977
28. Kaplan A, Garfinkel P (eds): Medical Issues and the Eating Disorders. New York, Brunner-Magel, 1993
29. Lam R, Goldner E, Solyom L, Remick R: A Controlled Study on Light Therapy for Bulimia Nervosa. Am J Psychiatry 151 (5): 744–750, 1994
30. Leitenberg H: Comparison of Cognitive-behavior Therapy and Desipramine of Bulimia Nervosa. Behav Res Ther 32 (1): 37–45, 1994
31. Lilly G, Sanders JB: Nursing Management of Anorexia Adolescents. J Psychosoc Nurs Ment Health Serv 25 (11): 30–33, 1987
32. Lipscomb P: Bulimia: Diagnosis and Management in the Primary Care Setting. J Fam Pract 24 (2): 187–194, 1987
33. Maine M: Father Hunger. Carlsbad, CA, Gurze, 1991
34. McFarland B: Brief Therapy and Eating Disorders. San Francisco, Jossey-Bass, 1995
35. Michielli D, Dunbar C, Kalinski M: Is Exercise Indicated for the Patient Diagnosed as Anorectic? J Psychosoc Nurs 32 (8): 33–35, 1994
36. Minuchin S: Families and Family Therapy. Cambridge, MA, Howard University Press, 1974
37. Minuchin S, Baker L, Rosman B, Liebman R, Milman L, Todd T: A Conceptual Model of Psychosomatic Illness in Children: Family Organization and Family Therapy. Arch Gen Psychiatry 32: 1031–1038, 1975
38. Mitchell J, Eckert E, Pyle R: Frequency and Duration of Binge-eating Episodes in Patients with Bulimia. Am J Psychiatry 138: 835–836, 1981
39. Moore J, Cowlman M: Anorexia Nervosa: The Patient, Her Family, and Key Family Therapy Interventions. J Psychosoc Nurs Ment Health Serv 19 (5): 9–14, 1981
40. Pyle R, Mitchell J, Eckert E: Bulimia: A Report of 34 Cases. J Clin Psychiatry 42: 60–64, 1981
41. Rock C, Curran-Celetano J: Nutritional Disorder of Anorexia Nervosa; A Review. International Journal of Eating Disorders 15 (1): 53–61, 1994
42. Schlemmer JK, Barnett PA: Management of Manipulative Behavior of Anorexia Nervosa Patients. J Psychosoc Nurs Ment Health Serv (November): 35–41, 1977
43. Sours JA: Starving to Death in a Sea of Objects. New York, Aronson, 1980
44. Staples NR, Schwartz M: Anorexia Nervosa Support Group: Providing Transitional Support. J Psychosoc Nurs Ment Health Serv 28 (2): 6–10, 1990
45. Strober M: A Controlled FAmily Study of Anorexia Nervosa: Evidence of Familial Aggregation and Lack of Shared Transmission With Affective Disorders. International Journal of Eating Disorders 9, 239, 1990
46. Swift W, Andrews D, Barklage N: The Relationship Between Affective Disorder and Eating Disorder: A Review of the Literature. Am J Psychiatry 143: 290–299, 1986
47. Telch C, Agras W: Obesity, Binge-Eating, and Psychopathology: Are They Related? International Journal of Eating Disorders 15 (1): 53–61, 1994
48. Welch S, Fairburn D: Sexual Abuse and Bulimia Nervosa; Three Integrated Case Control Comparisons. Am J Psychiatry 151 (3): 402–407, 1994
49. Zerbe K: The Body Betrayed: Women, Eating Disorders, and Treatment. Washington, DC, American Psychiatric Association Press, 1993

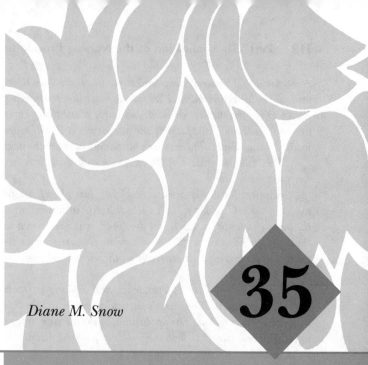

Codependency

Diane M. Snow

35

To "let go" does not mean to stop caring; it means I can't do it for someone else.
To "let go" is not to cut myself off; it's the realization I can't control another.
To "let go" is not to enable, but to allow learning from natural consequences.
To "let go" is to admit powerlessness, which means the outcome is not in my hands.
To "let go" is not to try to change or blame another; it's to make the most of myself.
To "let go" is not to care for, but to care about.
To "let go" is not to fix, but to be supportive.
To "let go" is not to judge, but to allow another to be a human being.
To "let go" is not to be in the middle arranging all the outcomes, but to allow others to affect their destinies.
To "let go" is not to be protective; it's to permit another to face reality.
To "let go" is not to deny, but to accept.
To "let go" is not to nag, scold, or argue, but instead to search out my own shortcomings and correct them.
To "let go" is not to adjust everything to my desires, but to take each day as it comes and cherish myself in it.
To "let go" is not to criticize and regulate anybody, but to try to become what I dream I can be.
To "let go" is not to regret the past, but to grow and live for the future.
To "let go" is to fear less and love more.

Anonymous

A mother of a 15-year-old boy bails him out of jail three times and allows his girlfriend and her baby to move into the family's house. One day, the mother sends her son a plane ticket home after he steals his grandfather's car and drives it 2,000 miles until it breaks down. The mother's husband leaves her the next day. This mother needs help to recognize and deal with her codependent behavior.

Codependency, *a disease involving loss of self, is an aspect of the addictive process in which living is masked, and the person's identity either is not developed or is not known to that person. For this mother, codependency represents her reactions to the present that are rooted in the unfinished business of her past.*[23]

This chapter defines codependency and explores its roots and manifestations. The nurse's particular propensity for this disorder is investigated. The application of the nursing process to codependent clients to help them recover from the disorder is discussed.

Learning Objectives

On completion of this chapter, you should be able to accomplish the following:

1. *Define the term codependency within a theoretical framework.*
2. *Trace the development of the concept of codependency as part of the addictive process.*
3. *Relate codependency to the caretaking aspects of the nursing profession.*
4. *Identify codependent behaviors of individuals, families, and organizations.*
5. *Apply the nursing process to a client with codependency.*
6. *Discuss the process of spiritual recovery from codependency.*

◆ Etiology and Theoretical Models of Codependency

Codependency is a progressive yet treatable illness characterized by self-defeating behaviors, distorted thinking, problems expressing feelings, and difficulty with relationships. Codependency begins in a person's family of origin, that is, the family in which one grows.

In a codependent family system, there may be an addict, a family member addicted to a substance (eg, alcohol or prescription or illicit drugs) or to a behavior (eg, gambling, sex, food, work, or spending). There may be a chronically mentally ill person, a physically ill person, or perhaps a person with a strongly moralistic orientation. The family may have rigid, unwritten rules that encourage dishonesty and manipulation within the family system and prevent normal development. For example, "Don't feel—just smile;" "Always be perfect;" "Don't embarrass the family;" "Loyalty is everything;" "Don't have fun;" or "Don't ask for help." There may be a role reversal in which a child is expected to assume an adult role (for example, as confidante of one or both parents or as caretaker of the house and younger children). There also may be rigid role orientation for family members, such as "scapegoat," "hero," "clown," or "lost child." Secrets abound in the family and prevent healthy communication and trust development. All these factors may combine to create an environment in which there is a high risk for codependency (Box 35-1).

◆ Contributing Factors

ABUSE

A common etiological factor in the development of codependency is abuse, whether physical, emotional, sexual, intellectual, spiritual, or religious. The traumas caused by physical, emotional, and sexual abuse are common factors in codependency (see Chapter 41, Violence Within the Family). In intellectual abuse, children are taught not to think for themselves; ideas and creativity are discouraged. Spiritual abuse may involve a constant parental message that all the child needs is the family and that believing in and relying on a Higher Power is wrong. In religious abuse, parents use religion to make the child conform by instilling guilt and shame.

In response to abuse, the child develops codependent patterns of coping in an attempt to escape pain

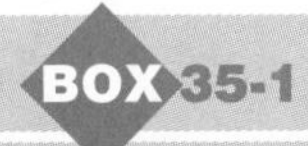

BOX 35-1

High Risk Groups for Codependency

- Spouses of addicts
- Practicing and recovering addicts
- Adult children and grandchildren of addicts
- Professionals who work in caretaker role
- Families with a secret or unresolved trauma
- Families that do not foster autonomy
- Families that reward helplessness
- Families with a chronically ill person
- Families with a fundamentalist and moralistic emphasis
- Children with workaholic parents, grandparents, or siblings
- Adult survivors of abuse (physical, sexual, emotional, spiritual, intellectual)

through controlling external factors or other people. The underlying message is, "If I hide from my pain, then maybe I won't ever have to feel my feelings." As a result, the child's feelings get submerged, and emotional development is arrested. Childhood patterns of survival behavior result in adult codependency. The cycle repeats itself through succeeding generations unless interrupted by an adult's recovery from this disease of the spirit.[23]

IMPAIRED GROWTH AND DEVELOPMENT

The child of a dysfunctional family has considerable difficulty progressing through the normal stages of growth and development. Based on Erikson's theory of growth and development, Friel's iceberg model demonstrates a deficit in interpersonal trust resulting in distrust and fear of abandonment (Fig. 35-1).

Shame, a sense of being flawed as a person, develops from the shaming messages given by caregivers that thwart the child's autonomy. Guilt replaces the initiative that normally develops, because the child takes responsibility for all the abuse and conflict within the family. Because the basic tasks of trust, autonomy, and initiative are not developed, the child approaches adolescence and young adulthood (the identity and intimacy stages of development) without the internal strengths necessary to master these stages. Thus, codependency symptoms result from the lack of identity and intimacy development and are rooted in shame, guilt, and fear of abandonment.[12]

It is not uncommon for the person to develop addictions (the icebergs of Friel's model) to deal with pain. For example, a person may use alcohol to feel more comfortable with himself or herself or may overeat because food is nurturing, always satisfying, and never demanding. Thus, a core of codependency underlies all addictions.

Children growing up in healthy families learn to see themselves as separate but still related to the family. When children are not encouraged to separate and become emancipated from the family as they approach adulthood, they learn that sameness and obedience are rewarded and that autonomy and individuality are not. In this environment, the child essentially never leaves home. The person may leave physically but not psychically, replaying the patterns ingrained from growing up in the family of origin in adult relationships.[23]

INEFFECTIVE BOUNDARIES

Another contributing factor to codependency is difficulty in negotiating boundaries, a problem that was reinforced in the dysfunctional family of origin. Instead of knowing where the self ends and others begin, the codependent person develops either an overly diffuse boundary that lets in people and information that are not in that person's best interests or a rigid boundary that does not permit anyone to enter. These boundary violations have serious consequences, yet the same behaviors are repeated while expecting different results.[21]

A person with a too-diffuse boundary may have grown up in an *enmeshed* family of origin that did not recognize and reward individuality. The adult child or codependent may have trouble saying "no" even when failure to do so is harmful to health or wellbeing. In contrast, a person with a too-rigid boundary may have grown up in a family of origin that did not respond to the child's needs. Perhaps the child felt abandoned by being constantly shifted between family members or by being sexually abused with no one to whom the child could turn to stop the abuse.

In family systems theory, Bowen speaks of the "togetherness force" in which a person's thoughts, feelings, and needs are determined by other people.[5] The concept of the *undifferentiated self* matches the concept of codependency in which people spend energy getting approval from others.[6] The concept may be viewed on a continuum from poorly differentiated to highly differentiated selves (Fig. 35-2), just as codependency can be viewed on a continuum.[10] How to maintain a unique separate identity while developing healthy relationships is a pivotal issue in codependency.

IMBALANCED INTERNAL EGO STATES

In transactional analysis theory, codependency is understood from the standpoint of three internal ego states: parent, adult, and child. The ideal configuration is a balance among all three states (Fig. 35-3).

Codependency, however, involves several possible patterns of imbalance. The inner child is the free creative spirit inside the person and the rebellious part of the person. Often, the inner parent has difficulty nurturing the inner child and is instead a shaming parent. The inner adult, the seat of logic and problem solving, wrongfully expects the inner child to have the answers and "drive the bus." The child is left in charge. Often, the rebellious, controlling child keeps the inner adult from making responsible decisions based on healthy, available choices.

For example, a woman who discovers that her boyfriend is being unfaithful continues to send him cards and letters, calls him every night, and waits for him to return to her. This is the way she reacted to her father, who abandoned her at age 4. She is repeating the past because she is unaware of the options and support available through her inner parent and inner adult. They

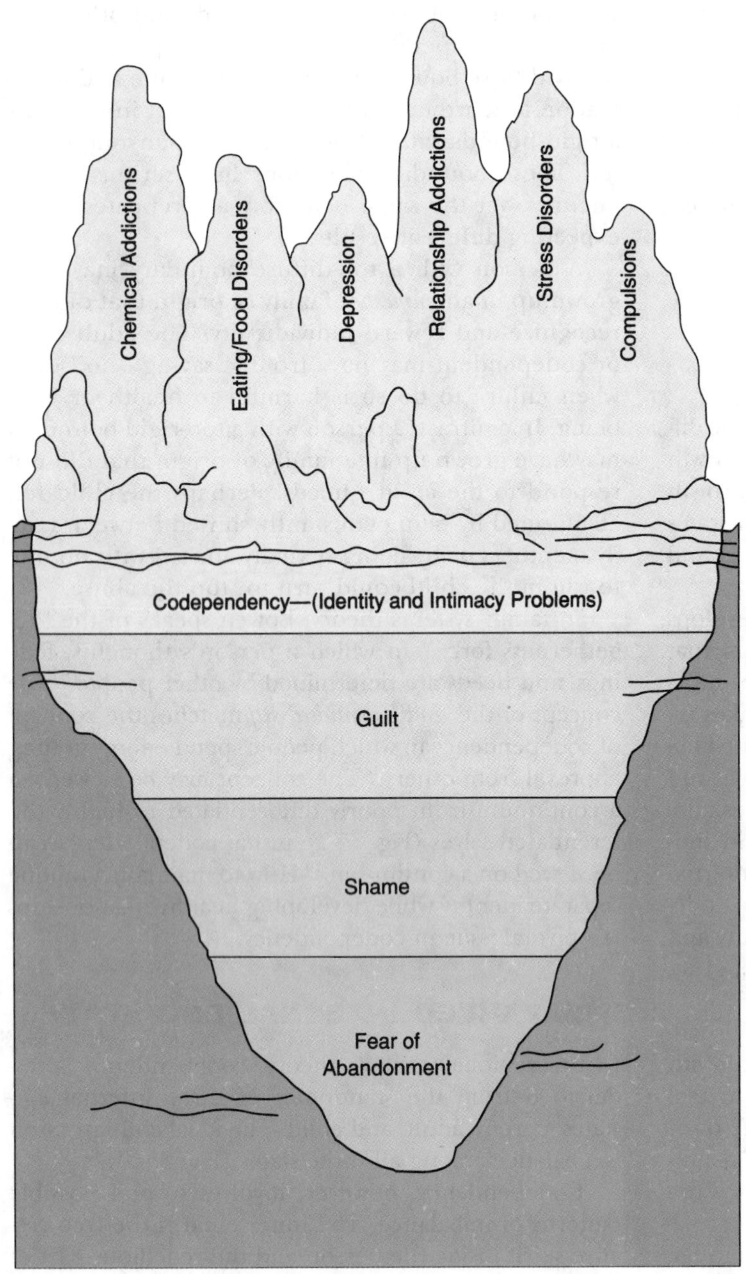

Figure 35-1. Unifying model of codependency and addictions. (From Friel J, Friel L: Adult children: Secrets of dysfunctional families. Deerfield Beach, FL, Health Communications, 1988)

have abandoned her, too. Using this metaphor of *the family within,* codependency can be understood as the lack of a strong ego system or identity. The rule is "just don't be."[23]

◆ Evolution of the Concept of Codependency

The concept of codependency began in the chemical dependency field when alcoholism was first understood as a family disease. At this time, the title *chief enabler* was given to the spouse, referring to the behaviors that keep the alcoholic drinking.[19] These behaviors include trying to control the alcoholic's drinking while picking up the pieces and rescuing the alcoholic from the consequences of his or her actions. The focus on changing the enabler's behavior was aimed at keeping the alcoholic from drinking. Codependency thus meant that the spouse was addicted to the alcoholic as much as the alcoholic was addicted to the alcohol. In this early view, codependency was considered to be the result of living with alcoholism, not a disease in itself.[19]

The concept of *coalcoholism* was identified when it

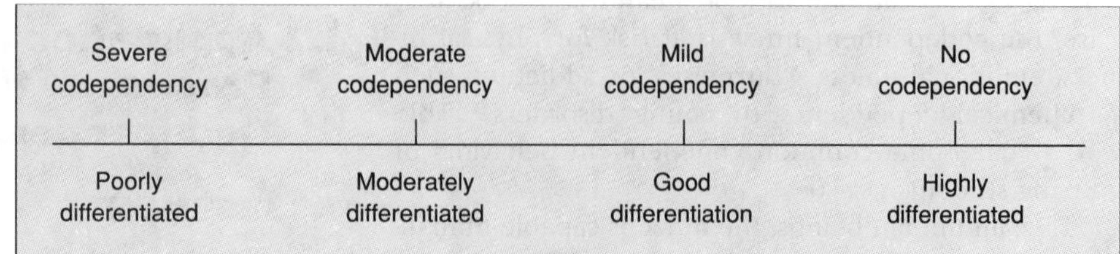

Figure 35-2. Continuum of differentiation and codependency

became clear that family members suffer from the disease of alcoholism and need help to recover from alcoholism as much as the alcoholic does. AlAnon, Alateen, and Alatot 12-step spiritual recovery programs and other treatment programs for family members serve this population.

With time, the term *codependency* evolved to describe a person in a relationship with any kind of addict, whether an alcoholic, gambler, anorectic, or sex addict. Common rescuing and controlling behaviors were identified in all such relationships. Eventually, it became apparent that codependency is a disease that affects the personality.[22]

Codependency results from living in a dysfunctional family—particularly an addictive, overly religious, or fundamentalist family or a family with a chronically ill member. Instead of learning to care for the self, the codependent person learns to care for and control others at expense of the self. In a dysfunctional family, the spouse and all family members—even the addict—are considered to have codependent symptoms. Physical complications abound in codependency; common problems include back problems, chronic headaches, ulcers, and hypertension. Codependency is considered an ultimately fatal disease if not treated.[19]

Codependency also can be understood as part of the addictive process at any level: individual, family, organization, and society. It is built on dishonesty and abnormal thought processes. For example, a dysfunctional organization can be described as codependent.[20] Chaos is familiar and feels normal to those from dysfunctional organizations. Blame, resentment, dishonesty, control, and manipulation are cornerstones of the dysfunctional organization. Attempts to control others and feelings increase at the same intensity as out-of-control feelings. There is little opportunity for personal growth, because the system demands compliance and lack of autonomy. It is a replay of family dysfunction, with many of the same roles assumed. The "hero," "scapegoat," "mascot," "lost child," "chief enabler," and "victim" all continue to play out their roles and keep the organization "sick."

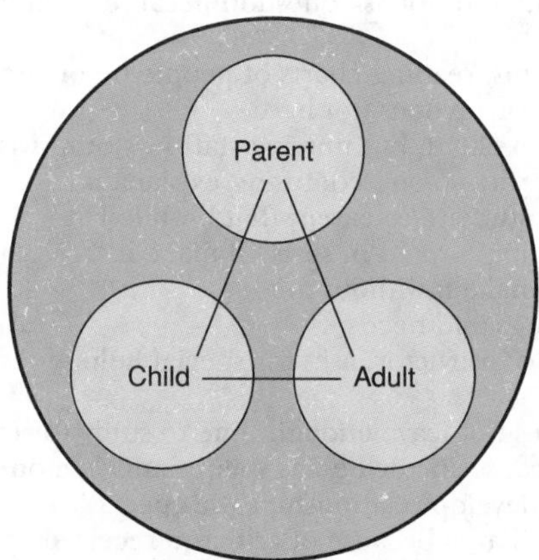

Figure 35-3. Model of the healthy family within. (From Subby R: Healing the family within. Deerfield Beach, FL, Health Communications, 1990)

◆ Nurses: At High Risk for Codependency

Nursing involves caring and helping clients attain higher levels of wellness in a mutually empowering relationship.[8] Many people who become nurses played a "fixer" role in their family of origin. Through caretaking behaviors, they tried to survive and control a chaotic or otherwise dysfunctional environment. It is not surprising that many are attracted to a work situation in which they can find some satisfaction using previously learned survival behaviors. For example, the nurse may feel that "If I can't change my family, maybe at least I can 'fix' my clients." They may take on the pain of others and overreact to situations.[1] Control and perfectionism dominate (eg, "I alone have the answers for the client").

What is lost in this codependent scenario is the nurse's self. The nurse's core identity is sacrificed for the client or the system through false feelings of duty. The client becomes overly dependent on the nurse instead of maintaining a sense of control and competence.[22] The nurse's self-worth comes from being needed by others.[14] The work setting may perceive the nurse's behavior as a sign of commitment and will often reward him or her for devotion "to the cause." The codependent nurse will view this recognition as a sign of his or her self-worth and may become frustrated, angry, and resentful if it is not continually reinforced.[8] Rather than serving as an example of good health and good self-care, the codependent nurse is at risk for physical illness, emotional illness, "burnout," or addiction, such as chemical dependency or eating disorders. Table 35-1 details some common codependent behaviors of nursing students.

Like all human beings, the nurse is capable of making mistakes and is not capable of controlling or "fixing" clients. All clients need to make their own choices; the nurse's best approach is to present available options and help the client and family deal with the decisions they make.

All nurses need accepting and nurturing support systems. They need a spiritual source of strength and courage to deal with the daily trials of their lives. Often they need intensive therapy for codependency as they begin to sort out the negative messages of their family of origin. It is then possible to have the energizing, spontaneous, free expression of true caring as nurses learn to set limits on responsibility without feeling guilty[16] and replace the "excitement" of codependency with a sense of peace of mind.[1]

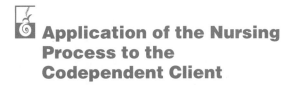

Application of the Nursing Process to the Codependent Client

ASSESSMENT

Codependency can be measured on a continuum from codependency and loss of identity to a strong sense of identity and capacity for intimacy.[23] Codependency manifests itself in all aspects of the client's life. It shows up in compulsive caretaking behaviors in which the client protects, takes care of, and controls others at his or her own expense.[3,18]

Life is driven by chaos, and crisis is created in an attempt to feel useful and needed. As a result, the client has difficulty accepting help from others and has poor self-care. The nurse can assess such behavior by asking the client, "What are you doing to help or 'fix' others that is keeping you from taking care of yourself?" A codependent client becomes resentful when others do not do what he or she has decided is best. The client

Table 35-1

Codependent Behaviors of Nursing Students Using Mellody's Core Symptoms

Symptom	Behavior
Difficulty experiencing appropriate levels of self-esteem	Overinvestment in family, grades, and being friend and "mother" of all
Difficulty setting functional boundaries	Exhausted, sleeping through class and conference because of taking care of friend or family member all night
	Late for examination because of lending car to a friend who promised to have it back on time but did not
	Angry with instructor for pushing him or her to take care of certain type of client
	Avoids responsibility; fearful; did not ask question because "you looked so busy and tired"
	Found in other clients' rooms, reading charts of people he or she knows
Difficulty owning own reality	Claims to have degrees she or he does not have
	Boasts about terrific job with client, but nursing staff says otherwise
	Late for clinical; gives long, drawn-out, confusing explanation
	Overinvolved with another student, to extent that both fail
	Denies that she or he is failing; says "I'm sure I'll make it"
Difficulty acknowledging and meeting own needs and wants	Says "My family could not make it without me"
	Uses logic that avoids feelings and needs
	Gives empty compliments to instructor, asks for special help; does so with each instructor
Difficulty experiencing and expressing reality moderately	Overdoes written work, does not leave enough time to study for examination
	Does not purchase text because she or he has spent family's money
	Says "I don't have time to develop relationships with peers"
	Expresses "hate" for clinical area because of criticism received

(Adapted from Mellody P: Facing Codependence: What It Is, Where It Comes From, How It Sabotages Our Lives. San Francisco, Harper & Row, 1989).

has difficulty identifying and expressing feelings.[23] When asked, "How do you feel?" he or she might respond "I don't know; how should I be feeling?"

The client has difficulty setting boundaries and often is overextended and overcommitted. His or her behaviors reflect the moods and reactions of others. The client constantly seeks approval, attempting to alleviate shame and low self-esteem through winning the approval of others.

Codependency involves control of others proportionate to the degree to which the client is out of control. He or she will do anything to control the uncontrollable, causing depression and negativity in a refusal to let go.[19] The client has difficulty with intimacy, fearing that others will discover the truth—that he or she is bad, unworthy, maybe even evil. Because the inner child has not been nurtured, the toxic shame of feeling flawed and unlovable runs rampant.

Just as addictions are denied, the client will deny the severity of the problem. When asked, "How much pain are you in?" the response is often, "I'll be okay as soon as I figure out how to help my spouse." When asked, "What can you do to take better care of yourself?" the response is often, "I thought I was doing just fine. Is there something wrong with me?"

The spiritual self is nonexistent, unable to be expressed when fear is the motivator. When asked, "What gives you a sense of purpose and meaning in your life?" the codependent response, "I just want to make other people happy," reflects a lack of spiritual perspective. The client has difficulty focusing on the here and now, expressing regret for the past and fear of the future.

NURSING DIAGNOSIS

There is no mental disorder listed in the Diagnostic and Statistical Manual, 4th edition (DSM-IV), for codependency; thus, it may go unrecognized as a major focus for treatment. Related DSM-IV diagnoses, in which codependency may be a significant problem to be addressed, include major depressive disorder, substance abuse and dependency, anorexia nervosa, bulimia nervosa, panic disorder, obsessive-compulsive disorder, generalized anxiety disorder, post-traumatic stress disorder, and personality disorders, such as dependent personality disorder and borderline personality disorder.

Some possible nursing diagnoses reflecting the patterns of behavior associated with codependency and the clinical judgment of the nurse include the following:

1. Ineffective Individual Coping related to lack of or distorted sense of self-identity (or lack of personal boundaries in the family), as evidenced by codependent relationships
2. Ineffective Family Coping related to enmeshed boundaries in the family, as evidenced by compulsive overcontrol in relationships
3. Chronic Low Self Esteem related to feelings of shame and guilt, as evidenced by an inability to express needs and feelings
4. Personal Identity Disturbance related to damaged boundary patterns, as evidenced by verbalized lack of self-knowledge and indecisiveness
5. Powerlessness related to perceived loss of control over self and environment, as evidenced by overcontrol in the work environment and poor self-care
6. Fear related to unresolved abandonment or abuse issues, as evidenced by superficial relationships, angry affect, and verbalized feelings of loss of control
7. Ineffective Denial related to lack of personal control, as evidenced by minimization of symptoms and inappropriate affect

Other possible nursing diagnoses include Spiritual Distress, Post-Trauma Response, Self Care Deficit, Altered Family Process: Alcoholism, and Risk for Violence: Self-directed or directed at others.

PLANNING

Long-term goals for recovery from codependency may include the following:

1. The client will express increased feelings of self-esteem.
2. The client will set healthy boundaries for the self.
3. The client will identify thoughts and feelings as his or her own.
4. The client will express a sense of internal motivation.
5. The client will be truthful and honest with self and others.
6. The client will be able to grieve for the past and learn to live in the present.
7. The client will be able to feel pain and move toward forgiveness of those who have hurt or abused him or her.
8. The client will have a solid support system of healthy relationships.
9. The client will find spiritual support and renewal through a relationship with a higher power.
10. The client will communicate clearly and directly (Nursing Care Plan 35-1).

Short-term goals include ensuring safety, admitting powerlessness and a need for help, recognizing and decreasing destructive behavior, managing anxiety, setting limits with others, gaining courage and strength to

Nursing Care Plan 35-1

The Codependent Client

Rachel is a 40-year-old woman who was admitted to an inpatient psychiatric facility for major depression. She is separated from her husband and has two daughters; her two sons died in a car accident. She describes her support system as her mother, sister, daughters, and two "best friends." She has juvenile diabetes and has not dealt with her anger about the limitations placed on her by her chronic illness.

Though separated, she is still in close communication with her husband, "for the sake of the girls." He continues to manipulate her and blame her for his problems and still manages to get her to give him money for his gambling addiction. She says she is "afraid she will not be able to make it alone."

Nursing Diagnosis

Chronic Low Self Esteem related to guilt and shame

Outcome

Client will verbalize positive self-statements and acknowledge personal needs and feelings.

Intervention	Rationale
Encourage the client to verbalize personal strengths and accomplishments.	Focusing on positive aspects of self provides a mechanism for changing the client's self-perspective from self-deprecation to a more realistic positive self-appraisal.
Teach client thought-stopping and reframing techniques to prevent dwelling on negative aspects of self.	Irrational beliefs and behaviors can be overcome by awareness of when negative thoughts occur and controlling them through distraction and relabeling.
Role play with client setting limits and saying "no" to her husband.	Healthy boundaries can be developed by experiencing actual successes in self-care through role playing.
Provide positive reinforcement for any attempts to self-care and constructive coping.	Reinforcing positive behavior increases likelihood that client will repeat positive behavior and feel empowered.
Discuss healthy decision-making strategies with client.	By learning to focus on one's own needs and feelings better decisions can be made.
Encourage client to access healthy support system for needed support.	Empowering a codependent client to receive and accept help will increase self-esteem.
Ask client to identify and verbalize feelings that are preventing her from taking charge of her life.	Helps the codependent client learn that her thoughts and feelings are valid, that she has worth and value, and can make choices that are healthy for her.

Evaluation

Client verbalizes less guilt and more positive self-statements.

change, developing trust in the therapeutic relationship, and accessing resources for support and recovery.

INTERVENTION

Recovery from codependency is a lifelong process of building intimacy with oneself and others. It involves a spiritual awakening of one's creative potential, becoming responsible to oneself and to others, and giving up feeling responsible for the feelings and actions of others. It is a change process that involves facing and feeling the pain rooted in childhood or other early experiences, examining the decisions made during this time, and making healthy changes based on available options that formerly were unknown.

The task of recovery is to increase self-nurturing

while replacing the core of shame with positive affirming messages to build self-esteem and healthy relationships. The nurse can use several strategies to help a client achieve these goals.

Teaching Self-Affirmation

Because codependency involves negative messages about the self that came from childhood experiences and results in feelings of inadequacy, replacing the negative messages with positive ones changes the cognitive mind-set to a positive mind-set. Self-affirmations are written positive messages about the self that are empowering.

For example, a client who has been shamed for having feelings may have such negative internal messages as, "I am not as valuable as everyone else;" "Everyone else deserves to be happy, but not me;" or "If people knew me, they wouldn't like me." In writing a self-affirmation, these negative messages are transformed into positive ones, such as "I am worthwhile;" "I am valuable;" "I deserve to be happy;" "I am a unique, special creation;" and "I can maintain healthy boundaries." The nurse instructs the client to write these messages and read them at least three times a day (Box 35-2).

Self-affirmation may be a useful intervention with groups as well. As group members repeat the messages out loud to one another or together as a group, codependent clients begin to hear the truth about their own value and worth.

BOX 35-2

Affirmations

I, ________________, have enough, do enough, and am enough.

I, ________________, am a worthwhile, capable, and lovable person.

I, ________________, can be successful in relationships.

I, ________________, can find the courage I need to change what I choose to change.

I, ________________, have the resources to make good choices.

I, ________________, can love and be loved.

I, ________________, can ask for what I want.

I, ________________, am a child of my Higher Power.

I, ________________, can forgive and be forgiven.

I, ________________, can find strength from my inner resources.

Use of Journaling as a Tool of Recovery

A codependent client has very little self-knowledge; thoughts, feelings, and needs are outside of awareness. Daily recording of thoughts, feelings, and needs in a notebook provides the client with helpful information about the self. It helps create ownership of personal needs and feelings, which in turn builds a sense of desperately needed identity. Journaling can be helpful to reflect on progress. The client may share the journal with the nurse or other caregiver or may keep it private. A client even may address a journal to a Higher Power.

Sharing Personal Experiences With the Client

A codependent client has a sense of uniqueness that says, "You could never understand me." This usually stems from the lack of trust and the resulting isolation in the dysfunctional family. Distorted thinking results, including the belief that "No one has ever experienced anything like this."

The nurse's self-disclosure may be a valuable therapeutic tool to demystify this sense of differentness. When the nurse shares a personal experience with the client in which a lesson or truth is made evident through the experience, the client can then begin to understand that his or her experience is universal to some degree.

Everyone has had painful experiences. It can be very healing and comforting for a client to hear a nurse share a story about an experience that brought about a change in the nurse's attitude or behavior. Nurses should use this kind of sharing only when they feel it will benefit the client's self-acceptance.

Involving the Client in a Spiritual Recovery Program

As in any addictive process, codependency entails a loss of spirituality. The creative self is unavailable in codependency as the client struggles to survive, unaware of all the available choices. Interventions to awaken the codependent client's spiritual nature include encouraging participation in a 12-step recovery program. A common prescription is to attend 90 meetings in 90 days. Codependency Anonymous is an ideal program (Box 35-3). Other options include AlAnon, if the client has an alcoholic family member or friend; Adult Children of Alcoholics, if he or she is from an alcoholic or other dysfunctional family; or other programs, such as Emotions Anonymous or Overeaters Anonymous.

Nurses who are involved in 12-step recovery themselves may want to share personal experience and rewards to help motivate and reassure the client. Groups are initially frightening to many clients who have iso-

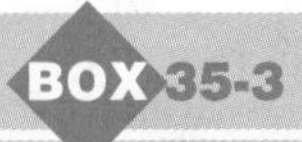

The 12 Steps of Codependents Anonymous

1. We admitted we were powerless over others, that our lives had become unmanageable.
2. We came to believe that a power greater than ourselves could restore us to sanity.
3. We made a decision to turn our will and our lives over to the care of God as we understood God.
4. We made a searching and fearless moral inventory of ourselves.
5. We admitted to God, to ourselves, and to another human being the exact nature of our wrongs.
6. We were entirely ready to have God remove all these defects of character.
7. We humbly asked God to remove our shortcomings.
8. We made a list of all people we had harmed and became willing to make amends to them all.
9. We made direct amends to such people whenever possible, except when to do so would injure them or others.
10. We continued to take personal inventory and when we were wrong, promptly admitted it.
11. We sought through prayer and meditation to improve our conscious contact with God as we understand God, praying only for knowledge of God's will for us and the power to carry that out.
12. Having had a spiritual awakening as the result of these steps, we tried to carry this message to other codependents and to practice these principles in all our affairs.

(Reprinted and adapted with the permission of A.A. World Services, Inc.)

lated themselves and were taught in their families of origin never to trust anyone outside the family. The nurse can reassure the client that trust will develop with time, as they practice reciprocal relationships with people who struggle with similar issues.[18]

Even if nurses are not involved in 12-step programs, they should attend at least one 12-step group meeting so that they can describe the format and significance of anonymity to clients. Moreover, familiarity with such 12-step slogans as "one day at a time," "let go and let God," and "easy does it" and with literature, such as daily devotion books, helps nurses connect with clients on a spiritual level. Encouraging other spiritual practices, such as prayer or meditation, will bring comfort and promote healing.

Helping the Client Grieve Over Past Losses

Family of origin experiences for the codependent client typically involve many losses. The client may describe such losses as the unavailability of an adult; the loss of a stable, secure home environment; the loss of freedom resulting from living in an unpredictable, unsafe environment; and even the loss of the dream of having a normal childhood and family.

The nurse can assist the client in beginning the grieving process by breaking through denial.[11] The nurse also can help the client recognize and accept the particular losses experienced. The client can describe, write about, and explore these losses and their impact. Working through the grieving process can be a way to focus on the present and the future, where choices remain.

Letting go means accepting memories of the past as real and important but deciding to live in the present. Ultimately, it means learning to forgive the self and others, a difficult yet important aspect of recovery from codependency.

Helping the Client Create a Healthy Inner Child

Maturation is deterred in the dysfunctional environment. Although the child may assume the role of parent in a type of role reversal, the child does not have adequate skills to perform this role. Childhood is thwarted as the child assumes parental responsibilities.

The codependent adult needs assistance to find the child inside who desperately needs to play and have fun, find comfort from the parent, and become the creative spirit within. To facilitate this search, the nurse can provide or encourage media for play, such as drawing materials, clay, sand, musical instruments, and other materials that invite the inner child to feel alive. The client then learns to nurture the inner child through his or her own inner parent, which also may not have been developed. Some codependent adults celebrate the birth of their inner child, so long hidden from awareness. Some self-help books may be helpful for codependent clients (Box 35-4).

Teaching Cognitive Methods to Deal With Shame Attacks

Shame is a constant companion of codependency. Shame attacks occur when a shaming message is triggered from earlier experiences. By externalizing the shame message, the client can begin to repattern unhealthy responses into healthy responses.[7] Steps of a shame reduction exercise include the following:

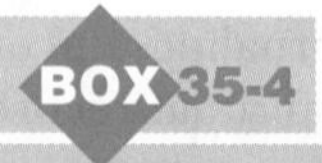

Suggested Book List for Caring and Coping for Yourself

Smith A: Overcoming Perfectionism. Deerfield Beach. FL, Health Communication. 1990

Beattie M: The Language of Letting Go: Daily Meditations for Codependents. New York, Prentice-Hall, 1990

Schaef AW: Meditations for Women Who Do Too Much. New York, Harper & Row, 1990

Evans P: The Verbally Abusive Relationship. How to Recognize It and Respond. Holbrook, MA: Bob Adams, 1992

Oldham JM, Morris LB: Personality Self-Portrait. Why You Think, Work, Love, and Act the Way You Do. New York, Bantam, 1990

Wilson SD: Released from Shame. Recovery for Adult Children of Dysfunctional Families. Downers Grove, IL, Intervarsity Press, 1990

Katherine A: Boundaries. Where You End and I Begin. Park Ridge, IL, Parkside Publishing, 1991

Kritzberg W: Healing Together. A Guide To Intimacy and Recovery for Co-Dependent Couples. Deerfield Beach, FL, Health Communications.

Michaelson PA: Secret Attachments. Exposing the Roots of Addictions & Compulsions. Naples, FL, First Prospect Books, 1993

Boynton MI, Dell M: Goodbye Mother Hello Woman. Reweaving the Daughter Mother Relationship. Oakland, CA, New Harbinger, 1995

Matsakis A: I Can't Get Over It. A Handbook for Trauma Surviviors. Oakland, CA, New Harbinger, 1992

Caplan S, Gordon L: Grief's Courageous Journey. A Workbook. Oakland, CA, New Harbinger, 1995

Schessinger L: Ten Stupid Things Women Do To Mess Up Their Lives. New York, HarperCollins, 1994

1. Identifying a recent overreaction to a situation and identifying thoughts, feelings, and behaviors surrounding this event
2. Listing all the bad things told to the inner self about this event and determining when this feeling of shame first occurred in earlier experiences
3. Arguing with the bad things and being positive
4. Honoring positive, affirming voices[7]

Helping the Client Develop Healthier Boundaries

Boundary issues are paramount in codependency. To identify boundaries—physical, sexual, emotional, spiritual, or relational—a client must be aware of self as separate from others.[13] A client's tolerance for boundary violations is high when abuse is part of his or her history. The nurse can ask the client, "How do you tell someone that they're too close or too distant?" The client can role play saying "no" to someone who is in his or her space.

Another codependent client may have rigid walls that prevent anyone from getting close.[15] The nurse can ask this client, "How do you protect yourself?" Empowerment begins when the client changes previous boundary patterns based solely on survival to new boundaries based on choice.

Encouraging Healthy Communication Patterns

In dysfunctional families, children are taught not to deal directly with anything. These children learn to lie, manipulate, and engage in passive-aggressive behavior to get their needs met. They also learn to isolate themselves rather than reach out for help.

A codependent adult can benefit from practicing listening skills, learning how to have healthy friendships, and expressing feelings openly and honestly. The client can be taught not to triangulate in relationships, that is, to work out problems directly with the person involved and not get hooked into others' problems. By saying something like, "I hope you can work the problem out with him," the nurse reinforces the message that clients are never responsible for anyone other than themselves.

Teaching Relaxation Techniques

The chronic stress in a dysfunctional family typically produces a highly stressed adult. The nurse can teach the client to use progressive relaxation, breathing techniques, self-hypnosis, and guided imagery techniques to achieve a state of relaxation conducive to recovery from codependency.

EVALUATION

As the client begins recovery from codependency, many changes become evident. The client should be cautioned that periodic slips are normal and do not mean failure. Relapse prevention for codependency involves recognizing places, people, and events that trigger codependent behaviors. For one client, it might be a telephone call from a person who also is codependent and who pulls the client into previous caretaking behaviors. The nurse should remind the recovering client to be gentle with himself or herself and not expect to be able to change everything at once.

Recovery also involves increased self-awareness. An expected outcome is that the client becomes more open and honest, expressing feelings and needs and recognizing ways to get these needs met. Giving up control means acknowledging that others are free to live their own lives but not at the expense of other people. The focus is on self-care and self-nurturing; resentment and blame are replaced with spiritual growth. A relationship with a higher power is often central to recovery. Release of the creative self occurs as the recovering codependent client develops and rewards the inner self. Life takes on new meaning through fellowship with others who are reaching new dimensions of their own spirituality.

◆ Chapter Summary

This chapter discusses codependency and its devastating effects on individuals and families. Chapter highlights include the following:

1. A disorder involving loss of self, codependency is an aspect of the addictive process in which living is masked, and the affected person's identity either is not developed or is unknown to the person.
2. Codependency begins in a person's family of origin. Abuse—physical, emotional, sexual, intellectual, spiritual, or religious—is a common etiological factor in the development of codependency.
3. In response to abuse, the child develops codependent patterns of coping in an attempt to escape pain through controlling external factors or other people. Childhood patterns of survival behavior result in adult codependency.
4. Difficulty in negotiating personal boundaries is a contributing factor to codependency.
5. In family systems theory, Bowen's concept of the undifferentiated self is closely linked with codependency; both are on a continuum.
6. In transactional analysis theory, codependency is understood from the standpoint of three internal ego states: parent, adult, and child. Whereas the ideal configuration is a balance among all three states, codependency involves several possible patterns of imbalance.
7. Nurses, many of whom played a "fixer" role in their family of origin, seem to be at particularly high risk for codependency.
8. Recovery from codependency is a lifelong process of building intimacy with oneself and others. Nursing interventions to facilitate this process may include teaching self-affirmation, sharing personal experiences with the client, teaching journaling, encouraging the client to join a 12-step spiritual recovery program, helping the client grieve over the past, helping the client create a healthy inner child, teaching cognitive methods to deal with shame attacks, helping the client develop healthier boundaries, encouraging healthy communication patterns, and teaching relaxation techniques.

Critical Thinking Questions

1. *Identify codependent behaviors you observe in your teachers, the other nurses and nursing students, your clients, and yourself.*
2. *Discuss interventions to change those codependent behaviors.*

Review Questions

1. Spiritual abuse can be a related factor in the development of codependency. Which of the following is an example of spiritual abuse?
   A. Mother constantly reminding a child of his or her overweight
   B. Father promising to take a child fishing but never carrying through with his promises
   C. Father insisting that the child does not need to believe in anything but the family
   D. Mother holding the child's hand in boiling water to "teach" consequences
2. Role reversal in the family of origin may cause an adult to
   A. "parent" everyone, looking for approval and recognition.
   B. play out the role of siblings instead of his or her own role.
   C. select partners who remind him or her of his or her parents.
   D. search for nurturing in healthy relationships.
3. Self-affirmation is one tool for healing from codependency. Which of the following meets all the criteria for a self-affirmation?
   A. "I am not going to answer the phone if it is my ex-boyfriend."
   B. "You are not going to interfere with my life anymore."
   C. "I will improve in my ability to set limits with people."
   D. "I choose healthy relationships for myself."
4. Katy, a psychiatric nursing student, finds working with the mentally ill to be draining and starts at-

tending Codependents Anonymous. She is told by a longstanding member that in this group, she may find

A. answers to her questions about her clients' problems.
B. people she can really help.
C. a place to refer her friends for their codependency problems.
D. spiritual support where she can share her own needs and feelings and learn to take better care of herself.

5. In a dysfunctional organization, there may be codependent behaviors that prevent the meeting of organizational goals. Rigid role behaviors may be obvious to the observer, such as
   A. a boss who plays the family hero role, refusing to delegate tasks and taking all the credit for the success of the company.
   B. a secretary who asks for help when she is stuck with a computer problem.
   C. a committee member who refuses to do her share of the tasks because she does not believe in the project.
   D. a staff nurse who volunteers to take care of the most difficult client despite staff criticism.
6. Which of the following is a goal for improving boundaries in codependency recovery?
   A. Mary will attend three group therapy sessions.
   B. Mary will verbalize two areas in her life in which she has felt successful.
   C. Mary will set limits with her mother when her mother demands that she not see the rest of the family.
   D. Mary will write a letter to inner child.
7. Mary is working on preventing relapse of her codependency. She identifies her friend Andrea as a trigger for her codependency. What advice would you give Mary?
   A. Talk to Andrea only about relationship problems.
   B. Set limits with Andrea, and remind her that you are going to take care of yourself no matter what.
   C. Encourage Andrea to listen but not give advice.
   D. Tell Andrea she needs to go to Codependency Anonymous with you.
8. What does the expression "Controlling increases as the person feels out of control" mean?
   A. The person tries to control external things, such as other people or organizations, proportionate to how out of control they feel on the inside.
   B. The person feels more in control when he or she takes charge of the things that are within his or her control.
   C. Control is in proportion to the need for control.
   D. The more a person controls his or her life, the more people and organizations they can take charge of.
9. George was the chief enabler for his friend Jeff's drinking. These behaviors might include which of the following?
   A. George confronted Jeff on the effects of his drinking on his relationships.
   B. George called every night to check to see if Jeff had gotten home safely and would go out looking for him if he did not find Jeff at home.
   C. George refused to go out drinking with Jeff despite Jeff's insistence.
   D. George called Alcoholics Anonymous when Jeff expressed his need to quit drinking.

◆ References

1. Armstrong J, Norris C: Codependence: A Nursing Issue. Focus on Critical Care 19: 2, 105–115, 1992
2. Beattie M: Beyond Codependency and Getting Better All the Time. New York, Harper/Hazelden, 1989
3. Beattie M: Codependent No More: How to Stop Controlling Others and Start Caring for Yourself. New York, Harper/Hazelden, 1987
4. Booth FL: When God Becomes a Drug: Breaking the Chains of Religious Addiction and Abuse. Los Angeles, Jeremy Tarcher, 1991
5. Bowen M: Family Therapy and Family Group Therapy. In Kaplan H, Saddock B (eds): Comprehensive Group Psychotherapy, pp 384–421. Baltimore, Williams and Wilkins, 1971
6. Bowen M: The Use of Family Theory in Clinical Practice. Comprehensive Psychiatry 7: 345–374, 1966
7. Bradshaw J: Healing the Shame that Binds You. Deerfield Beach, FL, Health Communications, 1988
8. Caffrey RA, Caffrey PA: Nursing: Caring or Codependent. Nursing Forum 29: 1, 12–17, 1994
9. Chappelle LS, Sorrentino EA: Assessing Co-dependency Issues Within a Nursing Environment. Nursing Management 24: 5, 40–44, 1993
10. Fagan-Pryor EC, Haber LC: Codependency: Another Name for Bowen's Undifferentiated Self. Perspect Psychiatr Care 28: 4, 24–27, 1992
11. Forward S: Toxic Parents: Overcoming Their Hurtful Legacy and Reclaiming Your Life. New York, Bantam Books, 1989
12. Friel J, Friel K: Adult Children: The Secrets of Dysfunctional Families. Deerfield Beach, FL, Health Communications, 1988
13. Katharine A: Boundaries: Where You End and I Begin. Park Ridge, IL, Parkside Publishing, 1991
14. Klebanoff NA: Codependency: Caring or Suicide for Nurses and Nursing? In Neil R, Watts R (eds): Caring and Nursing: Explorations in Feminist Perspectives, pp 151–161. New York, National League for Nursing, 1991

15. Mellody P: Facing Codependence: What It Is, Where It Comes From, How It Sabotages Our Lives. San Francisco, Harper & Row, 1989
16. Misiaszek C: Supervising the Codependent Nurse. Nursing Management 24: 2, 60–62, 1993
17. Navarra T: Enabling Behavior: The Tender Trap. Am J Nurs 95: 1, 50–52, 1995
18. Ryan J: Codependency in Nursing: Healing Wounds and Changing Patterns. Journal of Christian Nursing 8: 2, 10–16, 1991
19. Schaef AW: Codependence: Misunderstood, Mistreated. San Francisco, Harper & Row, 1986
20. Schaef AW: When Society Becomes an Addict. San Francisco, Harper & Row, 1987
21. Snow D: Caring for Yourself as Well as Your Patients. Imprint 40 (2), 59–61, 1993
22. St. Onge JL: Codependence: Addictive Relationships and HIV Care. Addictions Nursing Network 3: 1, 4–7, 1991
23. Subby R: Healing the Family Within. Deerfield Beach, FL, Health Communications, 1990
24. Woititz J: The Self-Sabotage Syndrome: Adult Children in the Workplace. Deerfield Beach, FL, Health Communications, 1989

Special Topics in Psychiatric-Mental Health Nursing

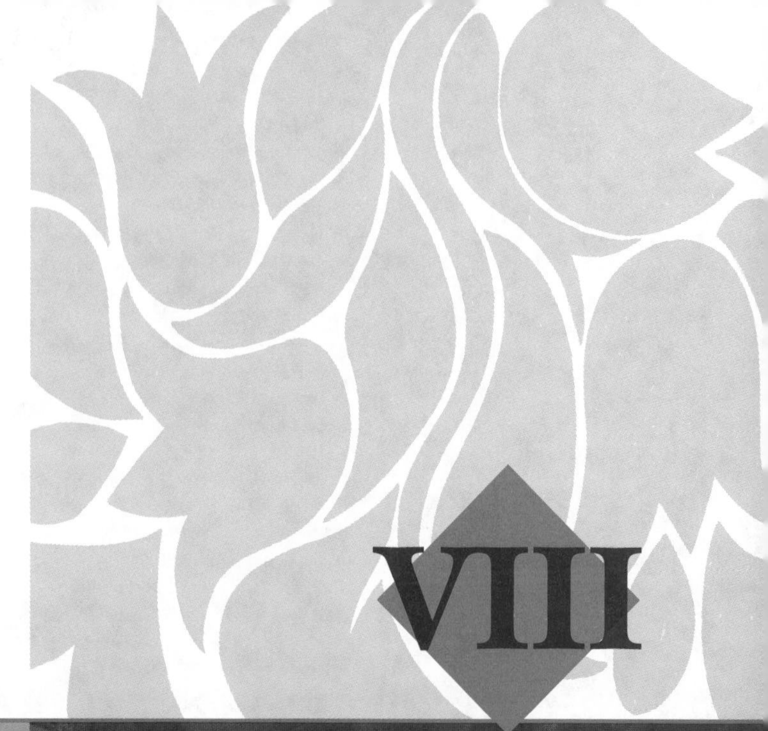

VIII

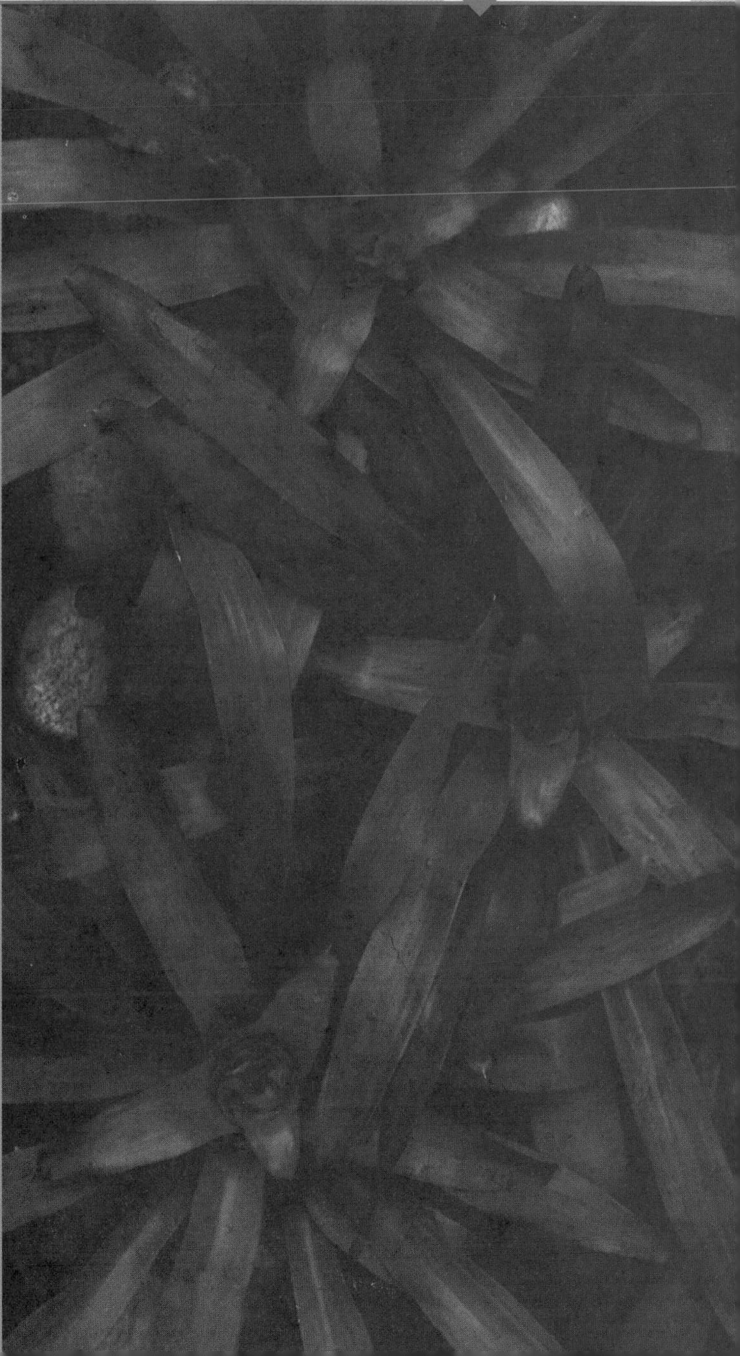

The Homeless Mentally Ill

Kay Peterson

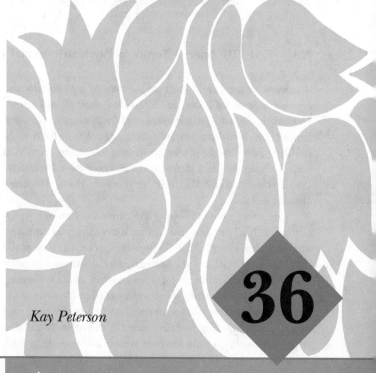

And homeless near a thousand homes I stood
And near a thousand tables pined and wanted food

William Wordsworth,
Guilt and Sorrow, *1791–1794*

A woman in her late 20s sits on the steps of a public library. Her many layers of clothes are soiled and smell of stale urine. Her hair is matted, her skin weathered. On the concrete around her feet are several overstuffed plastic bags. She appears to be counting the threads in her scarf, and she talks angrily to herself. Passersby divert their eyes to avoid their own discomfort. Who is this woman? Where is her family? Why is she here? What is her story?

This young woman is one of approximately 1 million homeless mentally ill people in the United States. She calls attention to homelessness because she, being among the many mentally ill, is the most visible of the homeless. Her situation represents a significant consequence of a complex set of social problems.

This chapter examines demographical characteristics of the homeless population, factors contributing to homelessness, and critical issues affecting homeless mentally ill people. It also discusses application of the nursing process when working with homeless mentally ill clients.

Learning Objectives

On completion of this chapter, you should be able to accomplish the following:

1. *Describe the historical factors leading to the rise in homelessness.*
2. *Identify and describe the homeless population.*
3. *Discuss factors that contribute to homelessness.*
4. *Discuss the effects of deinstitutionalization on the homeless mentally ill population.*
5. *Identify and discuss barriers that prevent access to care for homeless mentally ill people and measures to promote access to care.*
6. *Describe and discuss specific health care concerns of homeless mentally ill people.*
7. *Apply the nursing process to the care of homeless mentally ill clients:*

◆ Homelessness: A Historical Perspective

In 18th-century America, the philosophy of treating the mentally ill came from our European predecessors, some of whom believed that the mentally ill were possessed by the devil and, therefore, were to be feared. The end of the century brought a new era of "moral treatment," with the establishment of state mental asylums. Throughout the 19th and early 20th centuries, the approach kept evolving, albeit gradually, toward a model based on care and protection.

During the great depression of the 1930s, a surge in the number of homeless began as young men left their parents' homes seeking employment in other parts of the country. Following World War II, *skid rows* began to develop in major urban areas, populated primarily by middle-aged, unemployed, or underemployed white men, many of whom struggled with alcoholism and some of whom were disabled as a result of mental or physical problems.

A rise in the client census caused changes to occur in the mental health system. State hospitals found themselves increasingly unable to provide adequate care for the growing number of chronic clients. Institutional care began to deteriorate, and the care of the mentally ill became known as *warehousing.* Institutional nursing care of psychiatric clients became more and more challenging as nurses attempted to provide care with fewer resources than those available to nurses in the private sector. In the 1940s, media exposure increased public awareness of deplorable mental hospital conditions; in 1948, the National Institute of Mental Health was established.

Treatment changed significantly with the introduction of the first major tranquilizers in 1953. During the 1950s and 1960s, as the national conscience focused on the civil rights movement, the rights of the chronically mentally ill were also brought to the forefront, giving rise to the community mental health movement.[33] As social reform responded to deplorable hospital conditions, the movement toward deinstitutionalization began. The widespread transfer of former mental hospital clients to community-based care culminated in the Community Mental Health Act of 1963, which gave communities the primary responsibility for providing mental health treatment. During this time, the treatment community acknowledged a *social breakdown syndrome* associated with institutional living, marked by withdrawal, excessive dependency, and lack of initiative.[19]

Ideally, clients discharged from state institutions would live within family support systems. In reality, however, by the late 1960s, clients were being discharged to nursing homes, single-room occupancy dwellings, hotels, boarding houses, and available low-income housing units.[33] By the end of the 1970s, many of these deinstitutionalized people were counted among the ranks of the homeless.

The early 1980s brought a new type of homeless population no longer concentrated in skid rows but scattered throughout urban areas. This homeless population was younger and more economically destitute than before and included more women and children. Although the homeless population was still predominantly Caucasian, African Americans and Hispanics were over-represented.[24]

Throughout the 1980s and early 1990s, the federal government significantly decreased funding for low-income housing and reduced federal entitlements to the disabled, many of whom were mentally ill. The nation also faced a rising unemployment rate, rising inflation, and the consequences of persistent poverty and widespread family breakdown. In earlier times, extended families were more likely to take in disenfranchised members; traveler's aid was prevalent in many communities. A climate has developed of decreased tolerance for people on the social margins and outside the cultural mainstream. One consequence of such attitudes has been that chronically mentally ill people once more have become casualties of a well-intended system. Unfortunately, the criminal justice system and homeless shelters are often now the primary care providers for homeless mentally ill people.

◆ Who Are the Homeless?

Before defining any homeless population, it is important to consider some of the problems associated with studying homelessness. For example, studies have different operational definitions of homelessness. Most studies focus on people in shelters. As a result, many homeless people go uncounted, such as families doubling-up with other families in single-family dwellings, people displaced by domestic violence, runaways, and "invisible" homeless people who live on the streets, under bridges, or in homeless camps. Even in the shelters, difficulties in interviewing make the accuracy of data suspect.[1,31]

Every 10 years, the United States census attempts to document the number of homeless people in the nation. The data influence federal funding for urban and rural programs and policies regarding the homeless in many areas for the next 10 years. Based on 1990 census data and other studies, there may be as many as 3 million homeless people in the United States, representing approximately 1% of the total population.

In general, there are three defined categories of homeless: those who have suffered severe economic setbacks, thus experiencing the pervasive effects of poverty; those whose personal lives and decisions have been complicated by crisis or more likely a series of crises; and those who are seriously disabled with mental illness or substance abuse disorders and are without the social network to support them through such catastrophic illnesses. It is important to realize that these groups overlap.[1,11,25]

According to primarily shelter-based studies, the homeless population remains mainly Caucasian, although African Americans and Hispanics are overrepresented. Fewer than 50% of homeless people have high school diplomas. Most are long-term residents of the area in which they are now homeless, and the percentage of women is increasing in many urban areas.[14,21,27]

The homeless population encompasses a diverse array of people. There are the disabled or chronically ill whose benefits do not allow them permanent housing; elderly people on fixed incomes who have lost their family support; Vietnam veterans who cannot regain their place in society; runaways who have been rejected by their families; immigrants, both documented and undocumented; ex-prisoners who have "burned their bridges" with previous social supports; unemployed people; and underemployed people, who work but do not earn enough to pay for the costs of housing.

HOMELESS FAMILIES

Families are the fastest growing subpopulation among the ranks of the homeless. The typical homeless family consists of a single mother with two or three young children.[25] Children in these families commonly experience developmental delays, depression, anxiety, and learning difficulties. Their homelessness may be a source of shame.[23] Due to the lack of policies and programs that target prevention, homelessness is becoming intergenerational as more children grow up in a climate of poverty.

HOMELESS MENTALLY ILL PEOPLE

Most research findings agree that the homeless mentally ill account for one-third of the homeless population and that half of the total homeless population demonstrates symptoms of depression. Compared with the general population, the homeless are much more likely to have experienced psychiatric hospitalization.

Schizophrenia is the most common mental illness affecting homeless people. This disorder is most distressing to a person without support, lost and helpless in a bureaucratic mental health system.[7] The incidence of major affective disorders and alcoholism is also higher in the homeless than in the general population. Box 36-1 delineates frequently observed DSM-IV diagnoses among the homeless mentally ill population.

Because of changes in treatment philosophy and mental health laws, chronically mentally ill young adults, most of whom have had minimal hospitalizations, are now joining the ranks of the homeless. Treatment of this younger segment of the homeless mentally ill population follows a common pattern. They are generally referred to community treatment programs yet often do now follow through and thus decompensate, perhaps resulting in hospitalization. When hospitalized, they are often discharged before

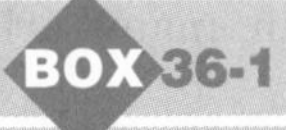

BOX 36-1 Common DSM-IV Diagnoses Observed in the Homeless Mentally Ill Population

Schizophrenia, Paranoid Type
Schizophrenia, Disorganized Type
Schizophrenia, Undifferentiated Type
Schizophrenia, Residual Type
Schizoaffective Disorder
Delusional Disorder
Psychotic Disorder NOS
Major Depressive Disorder
Bipolar I Disorder
Bipolar II Disorder
Obsessive-Compulsive Disorder
Posttraumatic Stress Disorder
Antisocial Personality Disorder
Borderline Personality Disorder
Personality Disorder NOS
Mental Retardation, unspecified
Alcohol Dependence
Alcohol-Related Disorder
Amphetamine Abuse
Hallucinogen-Induced Psychotic Disorder
Nicotine Dependence
Polysubstance Dependence

full remission occurs and return to stressful environments in which they cannot cope, thus starting the pattern over again. Many use alcohol or drugs to self-medicate their symptoms or to gain peer acceptance. Even homeless adolescents with no previous psychiatric diagnoses demonstrate high rates of depressive symptoms, suicidal thoughts and attempts, psychotic thought processes, and histories of dysfunctional and disruptive family life.[7,22,23,30]

Clearly, homelessness adversely affects mental health. People who become homeless due to economic stressors, domestic violence, or eviction are more prone to mental distress, substance abuse problems, and health concerns. This clinical picture may be complicated by loss of family or job and impaired intellectual functioning. These homeless people, who are not necessarily chronically mentally ill, may be brought to the attention of nurses by shelter staff because of behavioral characteristics associated with personality disorders. Such overly dependent, demanding, manipulative, or aggressive behaviors pose special challenges to the nurse who is also caring for the acutely psychotic or suicidal client.

◆ Factors Contributing to Homelessness in the Mentally Ill

There is no single cause of homelessness in mentally ill people. Generally, it is the final stage in a long series of crises, poor decision making, and missed opportunities. Common contributing factors include the lack of a comprehensive and effective mental health care system, the disabling functional deficits of chronic mental illness, substance abuse combined with severe mental illness, and the tendency for mentally ill people to pursue life goals in an unrealistic way.[20] These factors are addressed in other sections of this chapter. This section specifically addresses substance abuse, poverty, housing, and mobility in the homeless population.

SUBSTANCE ABUSE

Studies indicate that between 20% and 40% of homeless mentally ill people also have alcohol or substance abuse disorders.[12,25] Many mentally ill people, particularly young adults, misguidedly attempt to self-medicate psychiatric symptoms with street drugs or alcohol. The homeless person is at least three times more likely to have a primary diagnosis of alcoholism. While there are high rates of alcoholism in the general population, the drinking and drug use habits of the homeless person are far more visible than they are in the housed population. In general, health problems for virtually every disorder or disease, particularly liver disease, trauma, seizure disorders, and nutritional deficiencies, occur more often among the alcohol-abusing homeless than among the non–alcohol-abusing homeless.[4,34]

The introduction of crack cocaine onto the streets has changed the economic status of many people, including the homeless mentally ill. Many now spend their limited funds on this highly potent and rapidly addictive drug instead of on housing or even food. Many new drugs appear on the street each year, and others reemerge, such as LSD. Marketing of such drugs often targets such vulnerable populations as the homeless mentally ill.

Common psychosocial characteristics of homeless people with dual diagnoses (those with a mental illness and a substance abuse disorder) may include increased denial of illness, increased psychiatric symptoms, housing instability, family estrangement, higher rates of arrest, and a greater tendency toward suicidal thoughts and behaviors.[7,12,25]

POVERTY

In the United States, the gap between rich and poor continues to widen. For many, the margin between poverty and homelessness is quite narrow. The most seriously affected are people of color, children, and the elderly. High unemployment rates, cuts in funding for public assistance, and increased domestic violence all contribute to a cycle of poverty that promotes despair, poor self-esteem, and feelings of alienation. Homelessness is one visible consequence of this cycle.

Another compounding factor that increases homelessness is that a high percentage of the new jobs created in the 1980s and early 1990s pay minimum wage or only slightly higher. Many Americans in low-paying jobs may be only a few missed paychecks away from homelessness. Even those with better paying jobs are not immune.

INADEQUATE HOUSING

People with low incomes are paying more for housing. In the late 1980s, there were twice as many low-income families as there were available low-income housing units. There have been no significant improvements in the availability of low-income housing. The major victims of displacement due to eviction are the poor, the nonwhite, and the elderly.[11,21,25]

To accommodate the diverse functioning levels of the chronically mentally ill, a wide array of community housing is needed.[1,12,25] The process of establishing residential stability is difficult; moreover, the longer a mentally ill person has been homeless, the longer and more difficult that process may be.

HIGH MOBILITY

A phenomenon of restlessness affects many homeless mentally ill people. This may involve frequently moving in and out of homelessness or between residential and outpatient treatment facilities. Chronically mentally ill young adults struggling with the desire to obtain independence from their families may find a sense of autonomy in being homeless. However, this independence is complicated by lack of treatment, use of street drugs for self-medication, and inability to cope with mental illness.

Three interrelated types of mobility have been noted in homeless mentally ill people:

1. Episodic or intermittent movement in and out of homelessness
2. Seasonal-type movement within a geographically defined area
3. Migratory-type movement over wide geographical areas[1]

◆ Critical Issues Affecting the Homeless Mentally Ill

A homeless person incurs a loss far greater than simply a house; a sense of belonging and a psychological sense of a home are also lost. The process may begin with the loss of family ties, followed by the loss of friends, and finally the loss of community support. Chronic homelessness eventually occurs when support from the community is no longer available to prevent homelessness or to turn it around.[8] When attempting to cope with such losses, a person is likely to disaffiliate from conventional society and identify with a homeless culture. In this sense, acculturation is used as a survival mechanism.

EFFECTS OF DEINSTITUTIONALIZATION

Deinstitutionalization began as a positive process in support of mental clients' civil rights. The negative effects of deinstitutionalization come not from its intentions, but from the absence of community support, fragmentation of services, and lack of housing alternatives in the community. The homeless mentally ill population includes clients who have been discharged from psychiatric institutions and those who cannot be admitted because of changes in the commitment laws. These laws vary from state to state, but shared issues that have come to the forefront include the right to receive treatment, the right to refuse treatment, and the right to be treated in the least restrictive environment. However, the troublesome question arises whether the least restrictive setting is also the most therapeutic setting. Involuntary commitment now occurs only if a client is judged to be a danger to self or to others. In most states, if committed, the client must receive treatment and then be maintained in the least restrictive environment.

Deinstitutionalization has affected about 2 million seriously mentally ill people in the United States. Many times, those with financial resources do not suffer the negative effects as harshly as those who are without such resources. Deinstitutionalization is now not only a historical fact, but a philosophy and process that affects the entire mental health system.[1] The multiple effects of deinstitutionalization are listed in Box 36-2.

BARRIERS TO CARE

One of the first steps in promoting access to care for homeless mentally ill people is to identify the barriers to care, including the following:

1. Lack of insurance
2. Lack of transportation
3. Eligibility criteria, which may require an address
4. Loss of identification (a frequent requirement for accessing services)
5. Lack of knowledge of available services
6. Fear of having to leave, and possibly lose, possessions by attending clinic appointments

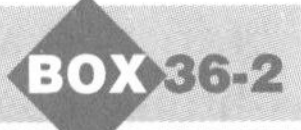

Problems of Deinstitutionalization

Deinstitutionalization has spawned some major problems:

1. There are at least twice as many seriously mentally ill persons living on streets and in shelters as there are in public mental hospitals.
2. There are increasing numbers of seriously mentally ill persons in the nation's jails and prisons.
3. Seriously mentally ill persons are regularly released from hospitals with little or no provision for aftercare or follow-up treatment.
4. Violent acts perpetuated by untreated mentally ill persons are increasing.
5. Housing and living conditions for mentally ill persons in the community are grossly inadequate.
6. Community mental health centers, originally funded to provide community care for the mentally ill so these persons would no longer have to go to state mental hospitals, are almost complete failures.
7. Laws designed to protect the rights of the seriously mentally ill primarily protect their right to remain mentally ill.
8. The majority of the mentally ill persons discharged from hospitals have been officially "lost."

(From Torrey EF: Nowhere to Go: The Tragic Odyssey of the Homeless Mentally Ill. New York, Harper & Row, 1988.)

7. Concern about missing meals
8. Fear of scrutiny by caregivers

Because of their inability to meet admission criteria or the need for an address, homeless mentally ill people may even be excluded from other homeless and community mental health programs. Also, clinician bias toward clients who respond more favorably to treatment may be an internal barrier to accessing care within the system.[19] Chronically mentally ill people routinely suffer from inconsistent treatment approaches, frequent medication changes, overmedication, and poor coordination of care, which has left them feeling justifiably distrustful of the system.

An internal psychological barrier in accessing care is the two-way process of withdrawal that may occur between the nurse and the client. When professional expectations do not balance with practice realities, the nurse may withdraw psychologically from the client. The effects of poverty and social isolation may promote a client's threatening and abusive behavior, further alienating the client from care providers.[8]

In an attempt to cope with this withdrawal process, nurses may focus on the physiological causes of the clinical situation, rather than examining their own feelings and attitudes. For example, a nurse may discuss only medications with a client; focus on legal issues, such as the right to refuse treatment; and blame external forces for feelings of frustration. Such withdrawal may be reversed by avoiding the all-or-nothing approach to treatment, thus giving the nurse and client more flexibility in devising a care plan and taking into account the client's adaptive abilities.[8]

The traditional health care delivery system does not usually reach the homeless population. Services that can improve access to health care include shelter-based clinics, clinical day programs, freestanding clinics specific to homeless people's needs, respite care services, mobile outreach units, and street outreach teams. Some of these services may be nurse managed, with others staffed by multidisciplinary teams.[13,25,26,28] Other access to care issues are specific to homeless families. For example, a family may have difficulty negotiating an unfamiliar health care system or because of the constraints of a shelter, may have difficulty maintaining records. Clinicians may fault parents for losing their child's immunization records. Sometimes simply because they are homeless, parents may fear being reported to protective agencies for child neglect or abuse.[3]

THE SHELTER SYSTEM

Shelters are a necessary stopgap to the problem of homelessness; however, they are not and never can be the solution. They have been given the impossible task of replacing the mental institutions in many urban settings. Shelters vary in capacity and services offered. Some shelters provide cots or beds; others may have only floor space available. Common services provided by shelters include meals, reading materials, and often laundry facilities and clothing. Some shelters even provide psychiatric and medical services.

Shelters commonly are staffed by both professional and nonprofessional volunteers. These staff members may need instruction in the areas of communicable disease, conflict resolution, seizure management, mental illness, substance abuse, and medication management.[4,15,28] These areas may offer nurses valuable opportunities to provide health education.

HEALTH CONCERNS

Compared with the general population, the chronically mentally ill have three times the disease morbidity and mortality rates; the homeless mentally ill have even higher rates. Chronic physical disorders commonly affecting homeless people include hypertension, diabetes, circulatory disorders, and peripheral vascular disease. These chronic disorders occur more frequently in the homeless population than in the general population. The average life expectancy of the homeless person is only slightly more than 50 years.[24] Other than mental illnesses, the most prevalent reported chronic disease of the homeless is hypertension. According to survey data, only half of homeless people with acute or chronic disease seek contact with a health care professional for their condition.[5] Health problems specific to urban homeless people are related to exposure, high population density, dependent positioning, as they are frequently on their feet most of the day, and poor ventilation. Other factors influence health conditions; however, these four are significant simply from the nature of homelessness. The recent rise in the tuberculosis rate is related to these factors.[4,6] Table 36-1 provides medication management suggestions that can assist the homeless person.

Thermoregulatory disorders, such as heat stroke and frostbite, are common. Secondary infections from infestation by lice, scabies, or insect bites occur in all seasons.[4] Underlying every acute and chronic illness is the poor nutritional state of most homeless people. Special challenges exist in the management of diabetes in an environment where dietary factors are, for the most part, out of the person's control.[34] Seizure disorders also are difficult to manage and may result in head injuries from falls. Trauma is a significant problem for urban homeless people; sexual assaults, stabbings, and head and eye injuries are common in most downtown areas. Because of their anonymity, homeless people are often victims of senseless crimes. In fact, the homeless mentally ill are the victims far more often than the perpetrators of such crimes.

Another significant health care concern is the increased risk of exposure to disease of younger homeless mentally ill people. Because of certain aspects of their illnesses, such as sexual acting out, poor impulse control, or hypersexuality associated with mania, they may participate in unprotected sexual practices. Substance abuse may involve sharing needles for intravenous drug use, thus increasing exposure to hepatitis, human immunodeficiency virus (HIV), and other diseases.[4,16,18]

Application of the Nursing Process to the Homeless Mentally Ill

ASSESSMENT

The Nurse's Attitudes

Stereotypes of the homeless may be the most pervasive barrier to providing care to this population. The homeless person, once stereotyped as a drunk, is now widely stigmatized as "crazy." To avoid this barrier and provide effective care, nurses need to examine the myths

Table 36-1

Medication Management Suggestions for the Homeless Person

Management Guidlines	Community Resources and Examples
When possible, simplify the dosage and times of medication.	Prescribing one or two pills every day or twice a day
Assist in locating a secure place to keep medications.	Helping to secure refrigeration or storage space
Provide client with suitable containers for medications on their person (if this is necessary) so that they do not make noise; rattling noises may identify person as a "target."	Providing Ziplock baggies or soft zippered storage bag
Provide written and verbal education to the client about medications, side effects, measures to control side effects.	Providing client and shelter personnel, case worker, or significant other with written medication information
Assist clients in obtaining adequate fluids, dietary needs, sun protection.	Mobilizing volunteer services, arranging for donations of sunscreen or water bottles
Establish a telephone resource for shelter and agency staff; provide answers to medication questions and concerns.	Being available for phone calls about unforseen side effects, prescription renewal procedures, lost or stolen medication

and stereotypes attached to homelessness and their own feelings and attitudes. It is not unusual for a nurse to feel uncomfortable and even fearful when beginning to work in homeless settings. Self-awareness of such attitudes and dealing with them are the prerequisites to effective nursing care of these clients.

Effects of Homelessness on Mental Health

Homeless people, with and without mental illness, are affected by the conditions in which they live each day. Box 36-3 lists common stressors that may influence the mental health of a homeless person.

Functional Abilities and Deficits

Homeless mentally ill clients are considered to be in a constant state of transition. Thus, their ability to function before, during, and after a crisis needs to be assessed. Such assessment factors should include the client's perceptions of the event, possible distortions in these perceptions, the presence or absence of situational supports, and the client's coping mechanisms. The nurse needs to assess the client's level of psychosocial rehabilitation potential, remembering that such potential may fluctuate from time to time and from situation to situation.[32]

Functional characteristics of the chronically mentally ill are often exaggerated in the homeless mentally ill population and may present special challenges when designing a treatment plan. Characteristics that the nurse should assess include the following:

1. Impairment in capacity to work
2. Difficulties with basic activities of daily living
3. Chronicity of treatment needs
4. Difficulty seeking out and enjoying leisure time
5. Difficulty relating to others effectively and appropriately
6. Lack of self-confidence and self-esteem
7. Strong dependency needs
8. Long-term effects from medications that limit motor capacity
9. Temporary episodes of acting out that interfere with interpersonal relationships
10. Lack of financial resources
11. Lack of motivation or self-direction toward defined goals

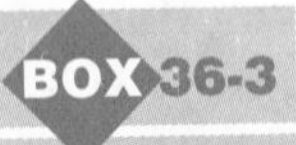

Stressors of Homelessness That Influence Mental Health

- The effect of constant vigilance for safety, resulting in lack of sound sleep, fearfulness, suspicion, and insecurity
- Social isolation, being shunned by others, or feelings of "invisibility"
- Use of drugs or alcohol in a futile attempt to create comfort or a sense of community
- Poor diet, which may contribute to biochemical imbalances and mood changes
- Susceptibility to physical illness
- Constant uncertainty and disruptions
- Lack of medical, psychiatric, or other needed assistance
- Pervasive sense of hopelessness and uncertainty

(From Haus A: Working with Homeless People. New York, Columbia University Press, 1988.)

Assessment Difficulties

Assessment of a homeless mentally ill client may present special challenges because of the lack of privacy and the high noise level in shelters. The distractions of the street may inhibit adequate assessment when outside the shelter. The client may not want to be identified with a psychiatric care provider and may agree to meet with the nurse only under pressure from shelter staff. The nurse must take time to consider and appreciate the impact on the client of having personal belongings inspected and perhaps being frisked for weapons or drugs before entering the shelter. Nursing Care Plan 36-1 describes one situation the nurse may encounter.

Mental Status

The nurse should proceed as far as possible with the mental status examination, including general appearance, mood, affect, sensorium, perception, thought content, orientation, memory, judgment, and insight. Family history, medical history, allergies, and previous psychiatric hospitalizations must also be assessed. While doing so, the nurse must keep in mind that the client's most pressing problem may be securing a place to stay that night and that the client's desire and ability to provide accurate information may be hindered.

Because homeless people have an increased likelihood of central nervous system impairment, a complete neuropsychiatric assessment may be indicated. Nursing assessment should include a careful history for head trauma and other organic damage, if possible contacting the family or health care agencies to obtain additional information. Screening may be indicated for sexually transmitted diseases, toxicology, risk factors for HIV, and with consent and pretest counseling, HIV blood testing.[17] Box 36-4 suggests measures that might facilitate communication with the homeless mentally ill client.

Nursing Care Plan 36-1

The Homeless Mentally Ill Client

A middle aged woman, Ms. N, came to the homeless shelter for the night. In the morning, the community health nurse making rounds at the shelter observed her to be sitting alone in a corner, mumbling to herself. She is disheveled, malodorous, infested and wearing multiple layers of clothing. She is clutching several bags of possessions, and the shelter staff report that she responded with anger when staff encourage her to use the showers.

The community health nurse initiates conversation with Ms. N, maintaining a comfortable personal space and ensuring eye level communication. The shelter staff further report that Ms. N has been coming to the shelter off and on for several months but has not been in for at least the past 3 weeks. They note that she has a known psychiatric history. After the community health nurse establishes a level of trust with Ms. N, Ms. N provides her with the name of mental health worker. The mental health worker reports that Ms. N has been hospitalized several times with a diagnosis of schizophrenia, disorganized type. She has not been keeping her clinic appointments at which she receives bimonthly injections of fluphenazine decanoate (Prolixin). The community health nurse initiates a nursing care plan and plans to follow up with the mental health center for further care.

Nursing Diagnosis

Social Isolation related to mistrust of others, lack of social supports

Outcome

Client will communicate desire to interact, identify socially inhibiting behaviors, and increase involvement with others.

Intervention	Rationale
Inform client of shelter resources; provide consistency in presence; tolerate isolating behaviors.	Information & acceptance precedes reduction in social isolation.
Reduce distracting stimuli: Decrease noise, number of people, other sensory distractions.	Ability to communicate with client is affected by client's ability to focus & understand.
Identify language or cultural barriers.	Language or cultural barriers affect client's ability to participate in interaction.
Tolerate and respect client's isolating behaviors.	This behavior is ego protecting for client.

Evaluation

Client increases amount of time tolerated in interactive activity.

Nursing Diagnosis

Powerlessness related to lack of control over environment

Outcome

Client will make reality-based decisions regarding care, environment, and future.

Intervention	Rationale
Provide available choices regarding environment.	Choice is the precursor to feeling control.
Support client's ability to make decisions; help client identify areas of life in which control exists.	Participating in control of one's environment increases self-esteem.
Include client in care planning and goal setting.	Involvement in planning reinforces self-esteem and ownership of the plan.

continued

Nursing Care Plan 36-1 (Continued)

Intervention	Rationale
Accept dependency of client if overwhelmed.	Acceptance of dependency allows client to mobilize resources and prepare for more independent functioning.

Evaluation

Client expresses a concrete goal or choice.

Nursing Diagnosis

Bathing/Grooming Self Care Deficit related to withdrawal and increased fears

Outcome

Client will identify personal care needs and measures to promote self-care.

Intervention	Rationale
Accept client and demonstrate acceptance regardless of status of personal hygiene.	Personal care requires a sense of security.
Inform client about available shower and laundry facilities.	Allowing client to make choice to use facilities increases sense of control.
Stay with client when attending to personal care needs and secure belongings if necessary.	Providing personal care may require skills training; securing belongings indicates respect for client.
Reward any steps taken toward self-care.	Reinforcement helps to ensure that the behavior continues.

Evaluation

Client tolerates shower and treatment for infestation.

NURSING DIAGNOSIS

Nursing diagnoses should be formulated cautiously. The psychiatric-mental health nurse must first be familiar with the norms and necessities of street life, because some unusual behaviors actually may be adaptive mechanisms. For example, clients may wear excessive clothing simply to prevent theft or to keep others from disturbing them. Likewise, clients may consciously exhibit bizarre behaviors to keep others away. Nursing diagnoses may address clients in relation to their illness, family, and community. Possible nursing diagnoses for a homeless mentally ill client include the following:

1. Altered Family Processes related to recent displacement
2. Social Isolation related to new onset of homelessness
3. Ineffective Individual Coping related to family disruption
4. Powerlessness related to lack of personal control over environment
5. Self Esteem Disturbance related to lack of family support
6. Social Isolation related to mistrust of others and lack of social support system
7. Risk for Infection related to congested environment and poorly ventilated shelter setting
8. Risk for Injury related to inability to maintain personal boundaries

Client Outcomes

When defining outcome criteria within the nursing process, the nurse must individualize to the client. Outcome criteria should be reasonable and attainable. For example, the outcome criteria for a particular client

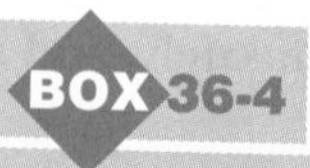

BOX 36-4

Suggestions for Communication With the Homeless Mentally Ill Client

1. Self-awareness
   - Be aware of your own feelings, fears, even your breathing.
2. Safe environment
   - Create a safety zone. Ensure that you and the client have a safe exit if either of you decide to leave.
   - Involve significant others in the communication process if it enhances the client's sense of security; involve others only after you have asked the client's permission.
   - Promote the client's sense of control and choice within his or her current environment; it may simply involve choosing where his or her bedroll may be or whether an injection should be given in the left or right side.
   - Be mindful and respectful of confidentiality issues.
   - Be sensitive to their possible feelings of not wanting to be identified with a psychiatric nurse or program; addressing basic needs or physical complaints may be a way of beginning an alliance.
3. Client assessment
   - Discuss client's basic needs.
   - Identify client's insights into his or her illness.
   - Be concrete in your interactions by avoiding metaphors.
   - Attempt to determine the client's level of cognitive functioning.
4. Special considerations
   - If a client is experiencing psychotic symptoms, let him or her know that you are not afraid and that your presence is not intrusive or demanding.
   - If a client is responding to internal stimuli, it may be helpful to ask if you could have his or her attention for a little while.
   - If a client is delusional, let him or her know that you have some sensitivity and understanding of the situation (or your desire for understanding); attempt to connect with the symbolism of the delusion.
   - If a client is paranoid, it may be helpful to sit side by side, rather than in front of him or her; it is possible to identify with the feeling more than the content of the paranoia and let the client know that you understand that feeling.
   - If you feel a client is suicidal, be direct in your concern and your questions in assessing for suicidality.
5. Conclusion
   - Summarize with the client, express your observations of the situation, and seek client feedback regarding your observations.

may be that the client controls paranoid thoughts long enough to spend a complete night in a shelter.

Other examples of measurable outcomes might include demonstrating an increase in appropriate independent functioning, increasing contact with case management services, or increasing use of clinic services. The nurse must be willing to evaluate outcomes in terms of small successes.

The nurse should not necessarily designate the end of homelessness as an outcome criterion; episodic homelessness should not be seen as a failure. The chronically mentally ill client may move in and out of homelessness as a part of a lengthy adjustment process to residential stability.

Goals

When planning for any treatment program, the nurse must recognize the realities of available local resources, the client's perception of needs, the conditions under which the client must operate as a homeless mentally ill person, and the nature and symptomatology of the client's mental illness. Another important consideration is that with time, the shelter lifestyle may have become the most important organizing factor in the client's life, providing much needed structure and support. Preparing for a new life typically produces anxiety and may even cause decompensation. Despite reality-based and reasonable goals, the nurse may have to function without a tangible treatment outcome.

In the process of goal-setting, the nurse should also be an instrumental change agent in planning for community needs. E. Fuller Torrey has described six crucial components for community planning:

1. Seriously mentally ill people must get first priority for public psychiatric services.
2. Psychiatric professionals must be expected to treat people with serious mental illnesses.

3. Government responsibility for seriously mentally ill people must be fixed at the state and local level.
4. Housing for seriously mentally ill people must be improved in quantity and quality.
5. Laws regarding mentally ill people must be amended to ensure that those who need treatment can be treated.
6. Research on the causes, treatment, and rehabilitation of serious mental illness must be increased substantially.[33]

INTERVENTION

Alliance

A homeless mentally ill client may distrust anyone representing the mental health system. Thus, the nurse must initiate the helping relationship in a nonthreatening manner, giving the client as much control as possible. The nurse needs to avoid attitudes of wanting to "fix" the client's problems. Nurses need to act as advocates for their clients, while knowing their own limits. Making quick referrals before building trust with the client should be avoided.

The nurse may need to postpone intervention for the most disturbing symptoms and perhaps even the discussion of interventions to avoid creating a negative therapeutic experience for the client (Case Study 36-1). Discussing medical conditions before psychiatric problems may help build the client's trust in the nurse and improve the nurse–client relationship. Alliance can develop as the client experiences a consistent and nonjudgmental attitude from the nurse toward the client's symptomatology.

Medication Management

A homeless mentally ill client has special medication management needs. Many medications have sedating effects that place the client in danger. Because homeless people must stay constantly vigilant for safety reasons, they cannot afford the risk of drowsiness. Carrying medications also increases the risk of assault and robbery, because almost any medication has street value. Clients also should be cautioned against combining medications with alcohol or other drugs.

The nurse should provide specific instructions to a client taking certain medications. For instance, a client taking lithium must be instructed to maintain an adequate fluid intake, which may be difficult depending on the availability of water in the client's environment; a client taking a phenothiazine needs to know the importance of extra sun protection to prevent sunburn, which may be difficult during summer. Nurses should involve clients in medication management. The clients can determine when they have access to their medication, how they can carry the medication safely, and the particular risk factors in daily life.

Education

A homeless client needs information to promote health and to access and use pertinent health care resources. Client education may include such topics as personal hygiene, dealing with infestation, thermoregulatory disorders, cancer risks, respiratory problems, sexually transmitted diseases, and substance abuse issues.[4,9] The client also needs education regarding the nature of mental illness; symptoms that can be expected; the side effects, risks, and benefits of prescribed medications; and the complexities of the mental health system.

Case Management

Case management is the key intervention that provides a connection between the client and the community. The nurse case manager is responsible for coordinating services to ensure that the client receives the structure and support needed to achieve and maintain optimal functioning. Case management encompasses health teaching, crisis intervention, symptom monitoring, assistance with federal entitlements, assistance with transportation, money management, and consumer advocacy.[2,25] For some homeless clients, the case management relationship may exist on a short-term basis; with others, the relationship may be extended for years, long after the client is domiciled. Case management responsibilities may not be transferred to a community agency for several reasons: The community agency may not be able to handle the increased case load; the nurse case manager may have difficulty trusting the effectiveness of the community agency in taking over the responsibility of case management; or the client may not be willing to interrupt the case management relationship with the nurse.[29]

Political Involvement and Advocacy

Nursing responsibilities involve interventions in the lives of homeless mentally ill clients and in the community. Nurses should be knowledgeable about governmental influences on health care and be willing to testify from knowledge and experience on the effects of homelessness. The nurse must go beyond bandaging symptoms of homelessness to address the structural problems of society. They must influence policies regarding health care of the homeless mentally ill, employment, housing, and the effects of poverty on the health status of all citizens.[10,11,21] Nurses can stay informed on such policies by using informational resources, such as those listed in Table 36-2.

Case Study

Mr. C

Mr. C is a 43-year old man who initially was referred to the psychiatric nurse in the homeless program by a police officer. He had been seen repeatedly in a public park apparently talking and singing to trees. The nurse made numerous visits to the park to establish alliance, gain assessment data, and establish a plan congruent with the client's goals. Mr. C was disheveled, emaciated, withdrawn, and actively hallucinating. Over a 2-week period, Mr. C was brought food, water, and clothing. He began to reveal more and more information as his basic needs were met and trust grew. He related a 12-year history of psychiatric illness; he also had begun to drink heavily as a way of self-medicating his psychotic symptoms. He revealed that he is divorced and has two children whom he has not seen in many years. He related that he has been homeless for approximately 10 years. During this time, he has had five psychiatric hospitalizations, all on an involuntary commitment basis. He worked as a salesman in a department store, but as his psychotic illness exacerbated and his drinking worsened, he was unable to hold down a job. Thus, in approximately 2 years, he lost his wife, his children, his friends, his job, and his mental health.

Following each hospitalization, Mr. C would attend outpatient clinics for a short time, miss his appointment, stop taking his medication, and then quickly decompensate, resulting in another hospitalization. He would return to the park, which was now his source of familiarity, comfort, and communication. He stated, "I'd talk to the trees, and they'd talk to me. At first I thought someone was putting on a picture show for me, and I kept looking for the hidden camera; then the devil showed up, and the more I talked, the madder he got. I began to see death walking the streets. I saw what I guess was a guy walking down the street, but to me it was death looking for me."

A comprehensive case management program was established for Mr. C. This included initial application for Social Security benefits, assessment for housing alternatives, a complete physical examination, and a referral for employment in a sheltered work setting. Mr. C was seen in the homeless psychiatric clinic for several visits before he was willing to approach the subject of medication and treatment. However, as alliance with the clinic staff grew, Mr. C decided to return to his medication regimen. He stated, "Somehow the medication made me lose my desire to return to the park, but you have to understand it is still home to me."

During 2 years of working with Mr. C, efforts were made to promote his insight and acceptance into his illness. He would attribute pride as the major reason that he quit taking his medication. He stated, "I wanted so badly to be normal like everyone else, and taking medication meant I wasn't. Now I feel like I've got something to lose if I quit taking my medication." As he achieved more stability, his goals changed as well. He stated, "I got to where I wanted more than what I had, and the help I needed was there." He began telephone sales in a sheltered work setting and became very successful in this endeavor. As expected, his self-esteem increased. He began to support himself financially and maintain his own small apartment. He stated, "It's okay now. I can accept my illness because now I have a place to stay and to keep my medications so no one is watching me take them. There are a lot of people like me who want to change but just don't know how."

Questions for Discussion

1. What factors contributed to Mr. C becoming homeless?
2. What characteristics in the nurse's approach to Mr. C facilitated his participation in his treatment plan?
3. What potential problems should be anticipated in Mr. C's ongoing care, and what measures should be included in his treatment plan to address these problems?

Rationale

The nurse must keep in mind the fundamental basis and principles behind his or her actions and goals. It is too easy to become lost in the busy work of one's tasks and forget the true task at hand. When considering interventions within the care plan, the nurse should examine the reasoning for such interventions. This is an appropriate application of theory to practice.

EVALUATION

Reviewing the effects of the nursing care plan is an integral part of the nursing process. Without this eval-

Table 36-2

Informational Resources on Homelessness

Name of Resource	Summary of Services
Community for Creative Non-Violence National Volunteer Clearinghouse for the Homeless 425 Mitch Snyder, Northwest Washington, DC 20001 202–393–1909	Provides information on grassroots organization of homeless projects, funding, services, multiple homeless issues
National Alliance for the Mentally Ill 200 N. Glebe Road, Suite 1015 Arlington, VA 22203–3754 800–950–6264	Provides support to families living with mental illness, education, advocacy for services, support for research, and a toll-free help line
The National Coalition for the Homeless 1612 K, Northwest, Suite 1004 Washington, DC 20006 202–775–1322	Uses education, advocacy, grassroots organizing toward housing, jobs, health care issues; provides a legislative telephone hotline
The National Mental Health Association 1021 Prince Street Alexandria, VA 22314 703–684–7722	Provides education advocacy for public policy, support services for consumers
Policy Research Associates, Inc The National Resource Center on Homelessness and Mental Illness 262 Delaware Avenue Delmar, NY 12054 800–444–7415	Clearinghouse for publications, bibliographies on subjects pertinent to issues of homelessness and mental illness
John Snow, Inc. Bureau Primary Health Care for the Homeless 210 Lincoln Street Boston, MA 02111 617–482–9485	Provides training and services to grantees of Health Care for the Homeless project, a quarterly newsletter, and a directory of programs

uative process, there is no learning or improvement. To measure the effects, behavioral criteria are defined. For example, such measures might include number of times target activities are accomplished, the amount of time spent on a target activity, the degree of insight gained by the client, or the number of symptoms that were relieved by the care plan. It is also important to reevaluate care plans in terms of new barriers to care that may have arisen or to clarify nursing diagnoses.

When qualitatively evaluating services, the nurse should perform an overall review of the program's characteristics. Such criteria would describe a quality program that is capable, comprehensive, continuous, individualized, willing and tolerant, flexible, and meaningful to the client. Nurses must continue their pioneering efforts in caring for this vulnerable population.

◆ Chapter Summary

This chapter has focused on homeless mentally ill clients. A historical perspective, a demographic description of the population, and some of the problems associated with homeless research were outlined. Factors contributing to homelessness were discussed, including substance abuse, poverty, housing, and mobility patterns among the homeless mentally ill. Issues specific to the homeless mentally ill include the ongoing effects of deinstitutionalization, the impact of loss on the person, ensuring access to care, the shelter system, and health care concerns. The nursing process has been applied to the homeless mentally ill population. Chapter highlights include the following:

1. The homeless population is heterogeneous and encompasses the young, the elderly, families with children, victims of domestic violence, runaways, veterans, ex-prisoners, immigrants, and the mentally ill. Families are the most rapidly growing segment of this population.
2. There is no single reason for becoming homeless. Homelessness is a result of a series of crises, lack of community and family support, poor decision making, external economic issues, and missed opportu-

nities, with the impact of these losses having physical and psychological effects.

3. Legal and ethical issues related to homeless mentally ill people are pertinent in light of the ongoing effects of deinstitutionalization. There is a need for an ongoing review of alternatives in community care; nurses should play a vital role in this process.
4. Homeless mentally ill people are at increased risk for acute and chronic illnesses. Their access to health care may be limited by attitudes of care providers, symptoms of mental illness, and the complexities of a bureaucratic mental health system.
5. Shelters and programs for the homeless are essential, but they do not offer the solution to the deeper structural problems of poverty, inadequate housing, and prejudice toward the mentally ill.
6. The process of returning from homelessness to the community is a complex and anxiety-producing experience for the chronically mentally ill person who has been on the street for any length of time.
7. The role of the nurse is crucial in identifying, assessing, and providing quality care to those who are so alienated in the margins of society that they are incapable of using the traditional mental health system.

Critical Thinking Questions

1. *When you see a mentally ill homeless person on the street, what are your initial reactions (attitudes, fears, judgments, stereotypes)? On what do you believe your reactions are based?*
2. *If you have personally known someone who is or has been homeless, how has it changed your feelings toward other homeless people?*
3. *If you were to lose your income and residence today, becoming immediately homeless, what three belongings would you take with you to a shelter? Remember, you must carry these items with you and be accountable for them 24 hours a day.*
4. *If you could rewrite history, how would you change the deinstitutionalization movement to prevent the increase in homelessness that has occurred?*

Review Questions

1. What are problems inherent in studies that attempt to count the homeless?
2. How has the composition of the homeless population changed in the last 20 years?
3. What components would be included in a comprehensive health teaching program for a homeless mentally ill group?
4. Of what should the nurse be aware when establishing client outcomes for a homeless mentally ill client?
5. How do environmental factors influence medication management with the homeless mentally ill client?
6. Which of the following would likely be a barrier preventing a homeless mentally ill person from seeking or maintaining services?
   - **A.** Acuity of symptoms
   - **B.** Family history of disease
   - **C.** Clinic eligibility criteria
   - **D.** Length of time of homelessness
7. Which of the following general factors would most contribute to health care concerns among the homeless population?
   - **A.** Dependent positioning, exposure, population density, poor ventilation
   - **B.** Dependent positioning, exposure, inadequate hygiene, poor ventilation
   - **C.** Exposure, poor ventilation, drug abuse, irregular eating patterns
   - **D.** Dependent positioning, exposure, anonymity, population density

◆ References

1. Bachrach LL: What We Know About Homelessness Among Mentally Ill Persons: An Analytical Review and Commentary. Hosp Community Psychiatry 43 (5): 453–464, 1992
2. Bawden EL: Reaching Out to the Chronically Mentally Ill Homeless. J Psychosoc Nurs 28 (3): 7–13, 1990
3. Berne AS, Dato C, Mason DJ, Rafferty M: A Nursing Model for Addressing the Health Needs of Homeless Families. Image Journal of Nursing Scholarship 22 (3): 8–13, 1990
4. Blakeney BA: Health Care and Homeless People. In Schutt RK, Garrett GR (eds): Responding to the Homeless: Policy and Practice, pp 163–190. New York, Plenum Press, 1992
5. Brickner PW, Scharer LK, Conanan B, Elvy A, Savarese M: Health Care of Homeless People. New York, Springer, 1985
6. Brudney K: Homelessness and TB: A Study in Failure. Journal of Law and Medical Ethics 21: 360–367, 1993
7. Caton CLM, Shrout PE, Eagle PF, Opler LA, Felix A, Dominguez B: Risk Factors for Homelessness Among Schizophrenic Men: A Case-Control Study. Am J Public Health 84 (2): 265–270, 1994
8. Chafetz L: Withdrawal From the Homeless Mentally Ill. Community Ment Health J 26 (5): 449–461, 1990
9. Cipollitti J: Teaching Health Care to the Homeless. Rock-

ville, MD, Department of Health and Human Services Division of Nursing, 1990

10. Cohen CI: Poverty and the Course of Schizophrenia: Implications for Research and Policy. Hosp Community Psychiatry 44: 951–958, 1993
11. Cohen CI, Thompson KS: Homeless Mentally Ill or Mentally Ill Homeless? Am J Psychiatry 149 (6): 816–823, 1992
12. Drake RE, Osher FC, Wallach MA: Homelessness and Dual Diagnosis. Am Psychol November: 1149–1158, 1991
13. Goldfinger SM, Chafetz L: Developing a Better Service Delivery System for the Homeless Mentally Ill. In Lamb HR (ed): The Homeless Mentally Ill, pp 91–107. Washington, DC, American Psychiatric Association, 1984
14. Harris M, Bachrach LL: Perspectives on Homeless Mentally Ill Women. Hosp Community Psychiatry 41 (23): 253–254, 1990
15. Haus A (ed): Working With Homeless People. New York, Columbia University, 1988
16. Kalichman SC, Sikkema KJ,Kelly JA, Bulto M: Use of Brief Behavioral Skills Intervention to Prevent HIV Infection Among Chronic Mentally Ill Adults. Psychiatric Services 46(3): 275–280, 1995
17. Kass F, Silver JM: Neuropsychiatry and the Homeless. Journal of Neuropsychology 2 (1): 15–18, 1990
18. Katz RC, Watts C, Santman J: AIDS Knowledge and High Risk Behaviors in the Chronically Mentally Ill. Community Ment Health J 30: 395–402, 1994
19. Lamb HR: Deinstitutionalization in the Homeless Mentally Ill. In Lamb HR (ed): The Homeless Mentally Ill. Washington, DC, American Psychiatric Association, 1984
20. Lamb HR, Lamb DM: Factors Contributing to Homelessness Among the Chronically and Severely Mentally Ill. Hosp Community Psychiatry 41 (3): 301–305, 1990
21. Milburn N, D'Ercole A: Homeless Women: Moving Toward a Comprehensive Model. Am Psychol November: 1161–1169, 1991
22. Mundy P, Robertson M, Robertson J, Greenblatt M: The Prevalence of Psychotic Symptoms in Homeless Adolescents. J Am Acad Child Adolesc Psychiatry 29 (5): 724–731, 1990
23. Rafferty Y, Shinn M: The Impact of Homelessness on Children. Am Psychol November: 1170–1179, 1991
24. Rossi PH: The Old Homeless and the New Homelessness in Historical Perspective. Am Psychol 45 (8): 954–959, 1990
25. Schutt RK, Garrett GR (eds): Responding to the Homeless: Policy and Practice. New York, Plenum Press, 1992
26. Slagg NB, Lyons JS, Cook JA, Wasmer DJ, Ruth A: A Profile of Clients Served by a Mobile Outreach Program for Homeless Mentally Ill Persons. Hosp Community Psychiatry. 45 (11): 1139–1140, 1994
27. Smith EM, North CS: Not All Homeless Women Are Alike: Effects of Motherhood and the Presence of Children. Community Ment Health J 30: 601–610, 1994
28. Stefl M (ed): Helping Homeless People With Alcohol and Other Drug Problems: A Guide for Service Providers. Rockville, MD, R.O.W. Sciences, 1992
29. Susser E, Goldfinger SM, White A: Some Clinical Approaches to the Homeless Mentally ill. Community Ment Health J 26 (5): 463–480, 1990
30. Susser ES, Lin SP, Conover SA, Struening EL: Childhood Antecedents of Homelessness in Psychiatric Patients. Am J Psychiatry 148 (8): 1026–1030, 1991
31. Taylor C: On the Conduct of Homelessness Research: Lessons From a Qualitative Study of Women Diagnosed with Chronic Mental Illness. Issues in Mental Health Nursing 14: 425–432, 1993
32. Thompson J, Strand K: Psychiatric Nursing in a Psychosocial Setting. J Psychosoc Nurs 32: 25–29, 1994
33. Torrey EF: Nowhere to Go: The Tragic Odyssey of the Homeless Mentally Ill. New York, Harper & Row, 1988
34. Wiecha JL, Dwyer JT, Dunn-Strohecker M: Nutrition and Health Services Needs Among the Homeless. Public Health Reports 106 (4): 364–373, 1991

Mental Retardation

Peggy J. Drapo
Linda Fischer

37

To change and to improve are two different things.

German proverb

This chapter focuses on the definitions, causes, and descriptions of mental retardation. The many causes and manifestations of mental retardation can lead to misunderstanding and often to poorly planned care. The chapter defines mental retardation, discusses the varied aspects of daily living and associated problems for mentally retarded people, and explains how to apply the nursing process to the care of the retarded. A greater awareness of the causes of mental retardation will strengthen the nurse's interest in preventive efforts.

No one chapter in any book can teach all there is to know about mental retardation; it is a nursing specialty in its own right. Another aim of this chapter, therefore, is to stimulate nursing interest in the field and encourage nurses to become instrumental in demystifying the problems of mental retardation for the public.

Learning Objectives

On completion of this chapter, you should be able to accomplish the following:

1. *Define the term mental retardation as defined by the American Association of Mental Retardation (AAMR).*
2. *Identify levels of mental retardation as described by Stanford-Binet, Cattell, and Wechsler.*
3. *Discuss the incidence of and significant issues related to mental retardation.*
4. *Identify the leading causes of mental retardation.*
5. *Discuss how the birth of a child with a mental or physical disorder affects family relationships.*
6. *Apply the nursing process to the care of a family with a child who is retarded and to the care of a child or adult who is retarded.*
7. *Recognize the role of the nurse advocate in the care of clients with mental retardation and related physical disabilities.*

◆ Defining Mental Retardation

In 1992, the main professional organization in the field of mental retardation, the AAMR, published the following new definition of mental retardation[2]:

> Mental retardation refers to substantial limitations in present functioning. It is manifested by significantly sub-average intellectual function, existing concurrently with related limitations in two or more of the following applicable adaptive skill areas: communication, self care, home living, social skills, community use, self direction, health and safety, functional academics, leisure, and work. Mental retardation manifests before age 18.

When applying this definition, the following four assumptions must be used:

1. Valid assessment considers cultural and linguistic diversity and differences in communication and behavioral factors.
2. The limitations in adaptive skills occur within the context of community environments typical of the individual's age peers and is indexed to the person's individualized need for supports.
3. Specific adaptive limitations often coexist with strengths in other adaptive skills or personal capabilities.
4. With appropriate supports for a sustained period, the life functioning of the person with mental retardation will generally improve.

The new definition uses a cutoff intelligence quotient (IQ) score for mental retardation of 70 to 75 or less, based on assessment using state-of-the-art clinical expertise and judgment to diagnose and classify the person's disability and degree of supports needed. These are now subclassified into *support systems* needed (ie, intermittent, limited, extensive, and pervasive).[2,28] These data should be reviewed by a multidisciplinary team and validated with additional evaluative information.

Although the AAMR no longer uses the following subclassifications, the Diagnostic and Statistical Manual of Mental Disorders, fourth edition (DSM-IV) continues to use the subcategory levels and lists the following IQ levels: mild mental retardation, 50–55 to 70–75; moderate retardation, 35–40 to 50–55; severe retardation, 20–25 to 35–40; and profound retardation, 20 to 25 or below. Mental retardation, severity unspecified, is a label used when there is a strong indication that the person is retarded, but the person is untestable because of impairment or is noncooperative, as in the case of infants.[3] This discussion uses the DSM-IV levels when appropriate (Box 37-1).

CLASSIFICATION

Labeling is a difficult and serious responsibility in the field of mental retardation. Systems of labeling vary, and the danger in attaching labels is that they may affect the care, treatment, and education of retarded people. Parameters for classification should take into consideration the other complex factors that often surround the diagnosis of mental retardation.[5]

Controversy arises related to educational placement of minority children who are poor achievers and often are from financially disadvantaged environments.[30] In this case, labeling takes on a negative connotation, because a disproportionate number of these children may now be classified as mentally retarded using AAMR's new criterion IQ of 75.

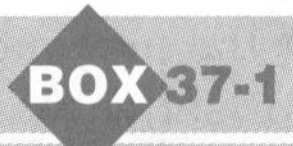

DSM-IV Diagnostic Criteria for Mental Retardation

A. Significantly subaverage intellectual functioning: an IQ of approximately 70 or below on an individually administered IQ test (for infants, a clinical judgment of significantly subaverage intellectual functioning)
B. Concurrent deficits or impairments in present adaptive functioning (ie, the person's effectiveness in meeting the standards expected for his or her age by his or her cultural group) in at least two of the following areas: communication, self-care, home living, social/interpersonal skills, use of community resources, self-direction, functional academic skills, work, leisure, health, and safety
C. The onset is before age 18 years

Mild Mental Retardation: IQ level 50–55 to approximately 70
Moderate Mental Retardation: IQ level 35–40 to 50–55
Severe Mental Retardation: IQ level 20–25 to 35–40
Profound Mental Retardation: IQ level below 20 or 25
Mental Retardation, Severity Unspecified: when there is strong presumption of Mental Retardation but the person's intelligence is untestable by standard tests

Testing

Determining subaverage intellectual functioning requires instruments that are reliable for measuring different items and factors of intelligence. Instruments used most frequently for testing intellectual function are listed in Box 37-2.

The assessment of a person for intellectual functioning must now equally include the area of adaptive skills. The 10 adaptive skill categories are communication, self-care, home living, social skills, community use, self-direction, health and safety, functional academics, leisure, and work.[2] Adaptive skills may now be measured with a variety of instruments. Some of these are also listed in Box 37-2.

Assessments are conducted only by qualified professionals and must include the use of a second person as a rater so that averages may be obtained. Case histories must be reviewed periodically, interviews held with significant others, observations made in the person's normal surroundings, and interviews or interactions with the client conducted in a social setting.

Consent for such assessments must be given by the client or the parents, and they have a right to participate in such assessments and appeal placement or program decisions. An individual may also refuse to be assessed and remove themselves from the diagnosis process and any consideration for services.[2]

Ranges of IQ generally suggest a level of adaptability. For example, mildly retarded people may be able to learn academic skills up to sixth-grade level during school-age years and are capable of social and vocational adequacy in adulthood if given opportunities and instruction (Table 37-1).

What happens to the person with an IQ score within one standard deviation below the mean, such as people with an IQ of 84 to 68 who from 1959 to 1973 were placed in the classification of borderline mental retardation? In 1973, this classification was eliminated by the AAMR. People with scores in this range were declassified as mentally retarded, and many lost services in the school system. The new definition will now bring some of these people back into the system. Because educational services are directed to those with moderate to severe handicaps, severely retarded students leaving school can choose from several support programs; those who are less retarded have fewer options. These people either drop out of school or enter the adult world without direction or adequate support programs. Better vocational and life training programs should be developed so that those who have not been classified in school as handicapped can become contributing members of society and realize their full potential.[33]

INCIDENCE AND SIGNIFICANCE OF THE PROBLEM

The incidence of mental retardation in the United States was previously thought to be 2.68%, about 6.5 million people. The new AAMR definition, however, raises that number dramatically. The proportion of the

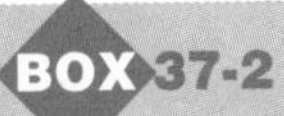

BOX 37-2

Tools for Assessing Intellectual Functioning and Adaptive Skills

INTELLECTUAL FUNCTIONING ASSESSMENT TESTS

Children

Weschler Intelligence Scale for Children III (1981)
Weschler Preschool and Primary Scale of Intelligence—Revised (1991)
Kaufman Assessment Battery for Children (1983)

Adults

Stanford-Binet Intelligence Scale
Weschler Adult Scale—Revised (1981)

ADAPTIVE FUNCTIONING ASSESSMENT TESTS

Children

Revised Vineland Adaptive Behavior Scales
Scales of Independent Behavior
School Edition of the Adaptive Behavior Scales

Adults

AAMD (American Association of Mental Deficiency) Adaptive Behavior Scales

population falling below the new cutoff of an IQ of 75 is now 5.48% on the normal curve. Every year, more than 125,000 infants are born who will be diagnosed as mentally retarded at some point in their developmental history. One in 10 people in America will have a mentally retarded person in his or her immediate family.[2]

Caring for the person who is retarded usually involves caring for other developmental disabilities. The nurse who chooses to work in the field of mental retardation also must be able to care for people with a spectrum of impairments.[24] Nevertheless, all nurses should know the basics of care for people with mental retardation, because these people are living longer, and normalization efforts are bringing them out of institutions and into the mainstream of society. Increasing numbers of retarded people are receiving care in the home with the help of outreach professionals.[10]

For nurses, preventing mental retardation is of prime importance. The goals of the nurse should be to promote preventive efforts and to prevent other problems resulting from mental retardation when it has occurred. This necessitates first recognizing the causes and manifestations of retardation. Since the 1980s, 40% of all children in the United States have been deemed at risk because they live below the poverty level.[32]

Every outreach and education team should include a nurse who is knowledgeable about mental retardation and the commonly associated physical disabilities. Every newborn nursery nurse, pediatric nurse, and public health nurse should be able to perform an assessment that will discern mental disabilities, be skilled and comfortable teaching and listening to families, recognize risk factors, and assist families to find resources. One concern of obstetrical and nursery nurses is the

Table 37-1

Impact of Retardation Levels on Daily Living

Mildly Retarded People	Moderately Retarded People	Severely Retarded People	Profoundly Retarded People
May learn academic skills up to sixth-grade level Capable of independent self-care and home maintenance Capable of vocational adequacy if given opportunities and instruction	Can learn basics of self-care in childhood Gain functional academic skills to grade-school level As adults, may be able to work in an unskilled or semiskilled occupation	Need controlled environments to learn self-care and communication skills May be able to work in a sheltered workshop vocation Need daily living assistance	Need daily care and supervision throughout life span May exhibit some motor and speech development

short stay in the hospital for mothers and newborns. Many newborns go home before adequate neurological and genetic assessments can be made. Therefore, many are in danger of missing an early screening and diagnosis of a condition that was not readily apparent the first day or two after birth.

Legislation

Probably because of the growing interest in the rights of members of society who are mentally or physically handicapped, the federal government has tried to ensure through laws interventions that society has neglected to do by itself. Recent legislation, such as Public Law 94-142, the Education of All Handicapped Children Act of 1977 and the Developmentally Disabled Assistance and Bill of Rights Act of 1975 (Public law 94-103), shows a trend toward more humane treatment of people with disabilities.

Public Law 94-142 ensures that extensive child identification procedures will be carried out to find children who are handicapped and in need of education. The parents are assured of full service and are assured that the programs will be maintained. Within these programs, children are entitled to free appropriate public education at no cost to the parents or guardians in the least restrictive environment and with nondiscriminatory testing and evaluation.

Public Law 94-103 is a bill of similar language that details the rights of the developmentally disabled for services, treatment, and habilitation in institutions and other residential programs.[7]

The success of this and other legislation that has been passed depends on appropriate funding, social incentives, and administrative action. Interest in legislation that affects clients who are retarded and their families should be a nursing concern.

Parents who are more informed about the rights of their children and advocates who are willing to lobby for the rights of retarded human beings have brought many positive changes to our courts of law. In 1973, the AAMR issued position papers of clients' basic rights that led to testing in courts. These rights include the following:

1. Freedom of choice within the client's ability and within the limitations that are placed on all people in the society
2. The right to live in the least restrictive environment that is individually appropriate
3. The right to be gainfully employed with fair pay and fair working conditions
4. The right to be part of a family
5. The right to marry and have a family as appropriate for the individual's ability to be responsible
6. The right to have freedom of movement and not be interned without just cause and due process of law[5]

One bill with interesting implications for nursing is Public Law 99-457, The Education for the Handicapped Act Amendments of 1986. The intent of the law is for families to take an active part in providing early intervention for their child with a disability. Due to many other health-related needs of children with disabilities such as mental retardation, families will benefit by having a nurse as a case manager because of the nurse's education and experience in working with children and adults with developmental conditions.[10]

Further extensions of the basic rights state that the client has the right to publicly supported and administered comprehensive habilitative programs and services designed to minimize handicaps. Another basic right is to have available publicly supported and administered programs of training and education, which may include, but are not restricted to, basic academic and interpersonal skills.[5]

At present, deinstitutionalization is a result of 20 years of discussion and litigation. Normalization, or social role volarization as it is now called, is a widely accepted concept in the area of mental and physical disability. It ensures that the client will not be segregated from the general population and made more deviant by lack of basic skills and age-appropriate dress and activities. The realization of clients' legal rights to the least restrictive environment and to habilitation has led to differing opinions among organizations and parents. Some see large state-run institutions as "warehousing" of the retarded and physically disabled and press for community group homes or foster homes as the only acceptable living arrangement outside of clients' own families. Others see the institution as a secure and permanent home with decent food, medical services, and physical comforts. Many states are witnessing a backlash by families who are discontented with the movement of their children out of the institutions against their wishes. These parents and some mental retardation experts see a need for both types of living arrangements.[31] Perhaps state institutions, with all of the expertise available to the community and with sound governmental backing, should become centers of research and advocacy. Certainly nursing and medical schools should take advantage of such places to develop clinical learning experiences for students. These environments offer rich experiences that provide valuable information and skills related to the needs of people who are mentally retarded and developmentally disabled.[8,18]

Today, even advocates for institutional placement believe that community placement has merit, and most large facilities are involved in placing people in the community. Community living is an ideal situation for all human beings, but placement into communities of people who are retarded, especially those who have been institutionalized for a long time, must be carefully planned and evaluated. A community not willing to accept a community group home for the mentally retarded creates an environment not unlike a state-run facility on the outskirts of town, isolated and stereotyped.[4] Movement of these people into the community is a responsibility for the case manager, who must ensure that the clients' behavioral skills are adequate for the community's demands and expectations. Lack of adequate preparation will lead to disappointment and failure for the client. The goal should be to remove barriers, not ignore them. Legislation can help create change, but to create improvement requires a change in the general public's values as well (Box 37-3).

ETIOLOGY

The causes of mental retardation are multiple. The etiology of mental retardation arises from two main sources: genetic and acquired factors. A survey of the list of factors causing or contributing to mental retardation is of interest to nurses in all fields of specialization.

Genetic Factors

The genetic code for each individual is carried in the nucleus of our cells by 46 chromosomes (22 pairs of autosomes and two sex chromosomes). Each pair of chromosomes is a certain length and carries pieces of the genetic code that is unique from that of any other pair.

Several types of chromosomal abnormalities, including changes in structure and changes in genes, can result in disabilities such as mental retardation. Changes or abnormalities in chromosomal structure can be caused by breakage; a piece may break off, become lost, attach itself in a new location, or attach itself to another chromosome. Because the chromosomal breakage involves the loss or rearrangement of genetic material, the individual chromosomal arrangement is changed. Changes in genes, also called genetic aberration, are

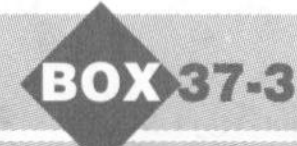

37-3

Values Clarification: Self-Assessment

Mental retardation and physical disability raise significant ethical and moral concerns. The present fiscal and political atmosphere forces nurses to reexamine feelings about human services. The issue of the right to health care will be a central theme in government over the next decade. Nurses need to evaluate their own feelings in regard to several factors that customarily have been linked with retardation. Some self-directed questions nurses might ask themselves follow:

1. Would I welcome a group of people who are retarded moving into our neighborhood, attending my family's church, using our community park, or eating in the restaurant where we eat?
2. How do I feel about my tax dollars being used to provide needed human services for people with mental retardation?
3. Do I believe that people who are mentally retarded belong in state-managed institutions or that families should be provided services and assistance when caring for their child or adult at home?
4. Could I support a couple who elect to abort a fetus having a known genetic condition that may lead to mental retardation or physical disability?
5. How do I really feel about costly technology being used to preserve the life of an infant born with genetic problems leading to a diagnosis of mental retardation? How do I feel about the effect of this care on insurance rates? How do I feel about the use of this technology when the family is indigent or uninsured?
6. Do I support preventive programs designed to provide assistance to children or pregnant women who are at high risk (ie, poverty, cultural diversity, physical, mental, or drug abuse, single-parent families)?
7. In light of limited educational funding, how do I feel about funding the support of programs for the gifted and talented and for those with mental retardation? What are my priorities for funding school programs?

chemical in nature. With genetic aberration, there is no noticeable change in the karyotype. To visualize chromosomes for study, a cytogenetic laboratory technician, using an electron microscope, enlarges a cell from blood or skin samples during the metaphase stage of cell division, photographs it, and then cuts and pastes these enlarged pictures of the chromosomes, matching pairs together. This procedure is called karyotyping. A *karyotype* is a picture of the composite of chromosomes matched in an order based on length, position of centromere, and banding (Fig. 37-1). In the banding process, dye is applied to the cells, and the dye is absorbed by deoxyribonucleic acid (DNA). Bands of DNA material are visible in the photographs and can be matched to bands on homologous chromosomes. Each pair of chromosomes has a unique banding pattern that is characteristic for humans (Fig. 37-2). A broken piece of chromosome without a centromere can reattach and heal on the same chromosome, translocate to another chromosome and attach itself, or become lost. The resulting problems are either an inheritance of too many genes, as in translocation, or the loss of the genes. The problem to the fetus depends on the quality and quantity of the genetic material. The karyotype illustrates these problems and enables scientists to see abnormal chromosomes more readily.

A recent development by image enhancement experts is the Genetiscan Digital Karyotype system. The technician directs the system using digital technology to classify each of the chromosomes and arrange them into karyotypes. After scanning and organizing the chromosomes, the system produces a high-resolution image of the karyotype that allows great accuracy in detecting small abnormalities, such as very small deletions and additions of chromosomal materials. The chromosomal image is then stored in the computer; it can be easily retrieved for further study, which may be screened directly on the monitor. After completing all desired procedures, the technician can create a laser-printed copy of the karyotype complete with all computer enhancements. This machine takes about one-half the time needed by the labor intensive hand karyotyping method.

As previously stated, there are normally 46 chromosomes in a human cell. To prepare a karyotype, one begins with the longest pairs of autosomes, starting with pair number one and proceeding to the smallest number 22. Two sex chromosomes are located at the bottom of the karyotype. A karyotype for a female will show two X chromosomes (XX); for a male, there is an X and a Y (see Fig. 37-1).

Normally, the centriole found in the cell cytoplasm migrates to the outside edge of the cell during cell division and forms spindle fibers that attach to the centromere of each of the 46 chromosomes. The fibers pull the replicated DNA (chromatids) apart. When the chromatids become separated, two new cells are formed, each containing half (23) of the complement of chromosomes. Sometimes this cell division process goes awry: One of the duplicated chromatids may not separate, resulting in one cell lacking chromosome material and the other cell containing both chromatids. This may occur with any of the 22 autosomes or with the sex chromosomes and is called nondisjunction (Fig. 37-3). In Down syndrome, chromosome 21 undergoes nondisjunction; the germ cell (ovum) contains 24 chromosomes instead of 23. If this cell is fertilized by a sperm containing 23 chromosomes, the resulting zygote has 47 chromosomes—22 pairs of autosomes, one extra chromosome 21, and two sex chromosomes. The consequences of this nondisjunction are an altered appearance and physical condition of the infant and retardation. Another dysfunction of cell division that may cause Down syndrome characteristics may be the result of *mosaicism.* Mosaic patterns occur when the individual has two cell lines, a normal cell line of 46 chromosomes and a cell line of 47 chromosomes. These individuals follow their own idiosyncratic pattern of developmental progress.[15]

A third way in which Down syndrome is sometimes transmitted is by *translocation* (Fig. 37-4, p. 752). A piece of a chromosome 21 breaks off and attaches to another chromosome, such as 15. If, during oogenesis, the normal chromosome 21 and chromosome 15 with the translocated 21 piece are grouped in the same ovum and fertilized, the result is two normal 21 autosomes, one from each parent, and two 15 autosomes, one of which contains extra 21 material.

Another disorder resulting from nondisjunction is Turner syndrome (XO). This is a situation in which one of the X chromosomes is missing due to nondisjunction (Fig. 37-5, p. 752). If the ovum containing no X chromosome is fertilized by sperm with the Y chromosome, the zygote is not viable. However, if the sperm contains an X chromosome and fertilizes the egg containing no X chromosome, the resulting individual has 45 instead of 46 chromosomes and has the physical characteristics of a girl but is usually sterile. Secondary sex characteristics develop poorly at puberty. Approximately 20% of people with Turner syndrome are mentally retarded.

Another condition called *polysomy of X* from nondisjunction of the X chromosome (three or more X chromosomes per cell) results in individuals having female sex characteristics. Although this condition is commonly called "super female," the result is not accentuated femaleness, but rather mental retardation and behavior problems.

People who have Klinefelter syndrome (multiple X and Y chromosomes) as a result of nondisjunction exhibit a masculine appearance because of the presence

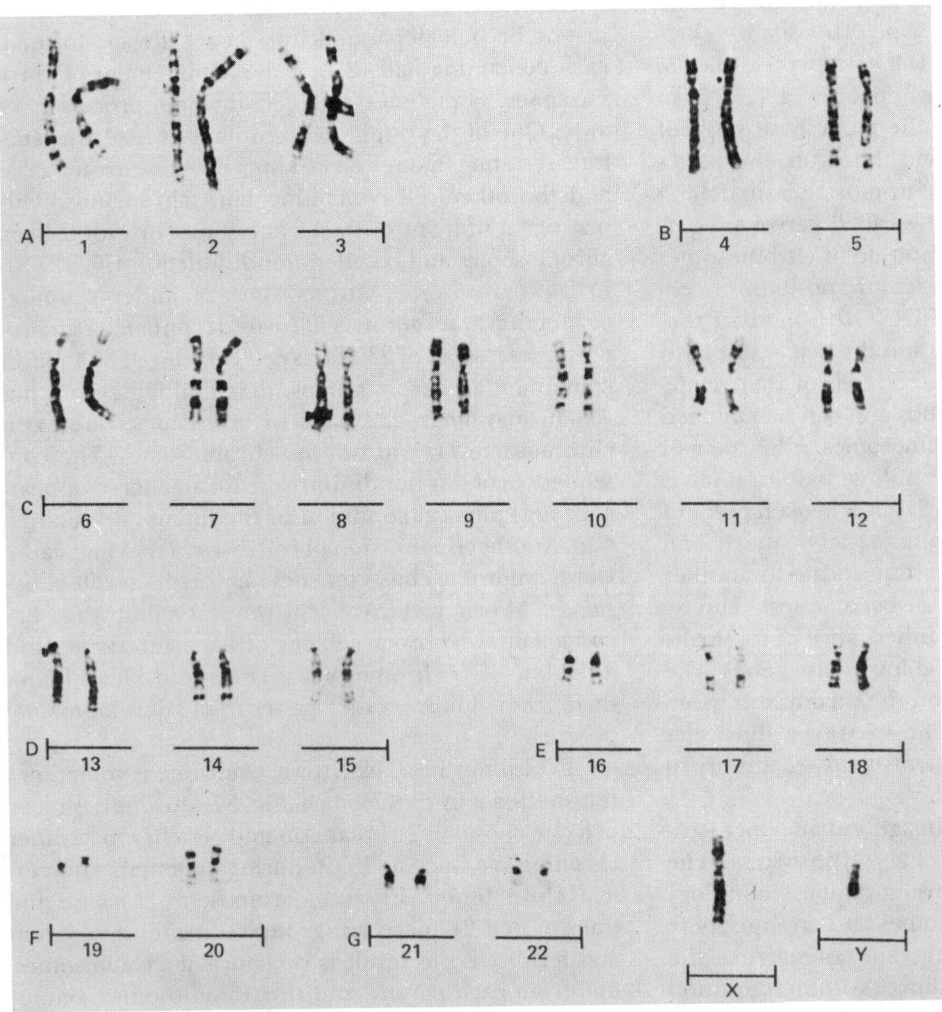

Figure 37-1. Photograph of a normal male karyotype.

of a Y chromosome, but the problem results from one or more extra X chromosomes (Fig. 37-6, p. 753). At puberty, female sexual characteristics develop. The male gonads are underdeveloped and sterile. Mental retardation and behavioral problems usually occur. Males also may be born with an XYY anomaly. This condition may produce a dull mentality, usually in the 80 to 95 IQ range. Internal and external genitalia are often affected, and the individual is usually quite tall. Some studies indicate that the aggressiveness attributed to these males with an XYY anomaly is related to their height acquired early in childhood, which resulted in teasing by peers. Other studies attempt to link their behavior with significant psychological differences.

Genetic diseases may be inherited in the same way eye color or hair color are inherited. Chromosomal differences remain the problem, but these differences are chemical or submicroscopic in nature. Some of these differences at the cellular level cause genetic disorders of metabolism.

Hereditary degenerative diseases and endocrine disorders also may cause mental retardation. One endocrine disorder that causes mental retardation is a deficiency of the thyroid hormone, leading to cretinism, a failure to develop physically and mentally.

Some of the previous conditions are transmitted in a dominant or recessive fashion. An abnormal recessive gene will not be expressed if paired with a normal dominant gene. If, however, the abnormal recessive gene is paired with an abnormal recessive gene from the other parent, the trait or disorder will occur. A dominant gene will produce its effect whether its homologous allele is dominant or recessive (Fig. 37-7, p. 754).

Dominantly inherited genetic disorders are said to be milder than those due to recessive or X-linked genes. Mental retardation resulting from a dominantly inherited disorder is usually mild; recessive disorders are more serious (Fig. 37-8, p. 754). Phenylketonuria is such a disorder. Profound retardation often occurs with inborn errors of metabolism. These errors may appear on the X chromosome also. The Lesch-Nyhan syndrome, for instance, will cause profound retardation. Many disorders and traits

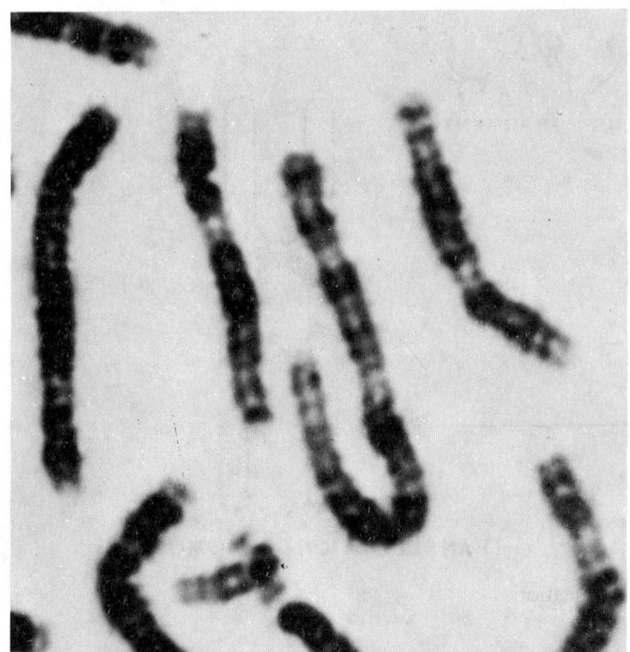

Figure 37-2. Enlarged photograph of chromosomes showing banding technique.

result from altered genes in the X chromosome, but the mode of inheritance of each one is slightly different.

Advanced technology now enables geneticists to visualize the cytogenetic cause of fragile X syndrome, which they had been observing in clients for some time. Through examination of chromosomes isolated from white blood cells, the defective site is now more clearly visible at the end of one of the long arms of the X chromosome. Fragile X syndrome accounts for a significant amount of mental retardation in newborns in the United States, second only to Down syndrome. It produces disabilities ranging from learning disabilities to mental retardation. Other physical anomalies of this syndrome are listed in the physical assessment checklist.

Because the defective site is on the X chromosome, females (who normally inherit an X from each parent) are less affected than males. When one has two like chromosomes, both carry the same type of genetic material. The nonaffected chromosome will cover most of the effects of the defect on the other one, but the female is a carrier of this condition.

Males, however, receive an X from the mother and a Y from the father. If the X chromosome that the male has received from the mother has the defect on it, the Y chromosome, which carries different genetic material than the X chromosome, is not able to provide a backup for the faulty X chromosome. However, the condition is perplexing in that not all of the females escape the effects, and about 20% of the males who inherit the defective X are unaffected. Carrier females may have normal intelligence or are less retarded. Normal brothers may carry the gene and be able to transmit the condition to their offspring.[11,29]

Acquired Factors

Acquired mental retardation involves prenatal, perinatal, and postnatal factors. Prenatal factors include infections, irradiation, toxins, drugs, and unknown causes. Perinatally, one of the most common causes of mental retardation is prematurity. Other factors are anoxia, brain damage, and infection caused by intrauterine disorders or abnormal labor and delivery. Postnatal conditions include childhood diseases, accidents, infection, anoxia, poisoning, hormonal problems, and environmental factors.

Birth defects, such as cerebral palsy, deafness, and blindness, may lead to sensory deprivation and result in

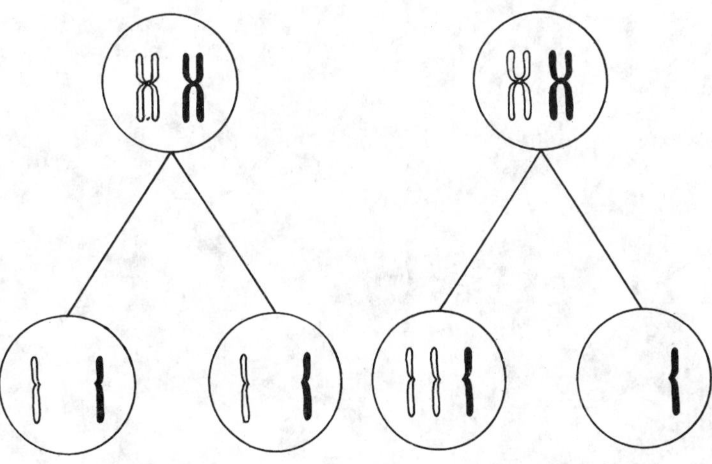

Figure 37-3. Normal cell division and nondisjunction.

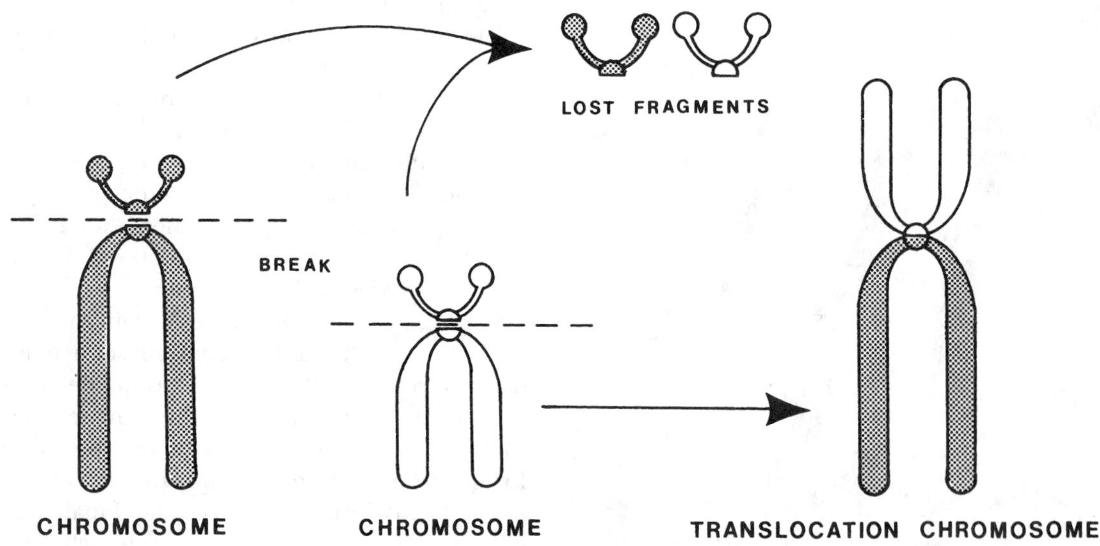

Figure 37-4. Translocation.

mental retardation. Early childhood intervention is of great importance in preventing retardation resulting from these problems and is discussed in more detail later in the chapter.

Psychiatric disorders may retard learning progress because of problematic behavioral activity. Child abuse may cause mental retardation through trauma or deprivation.

Prevention of mental retardation begins as early as family planning and continues throughout the devel-

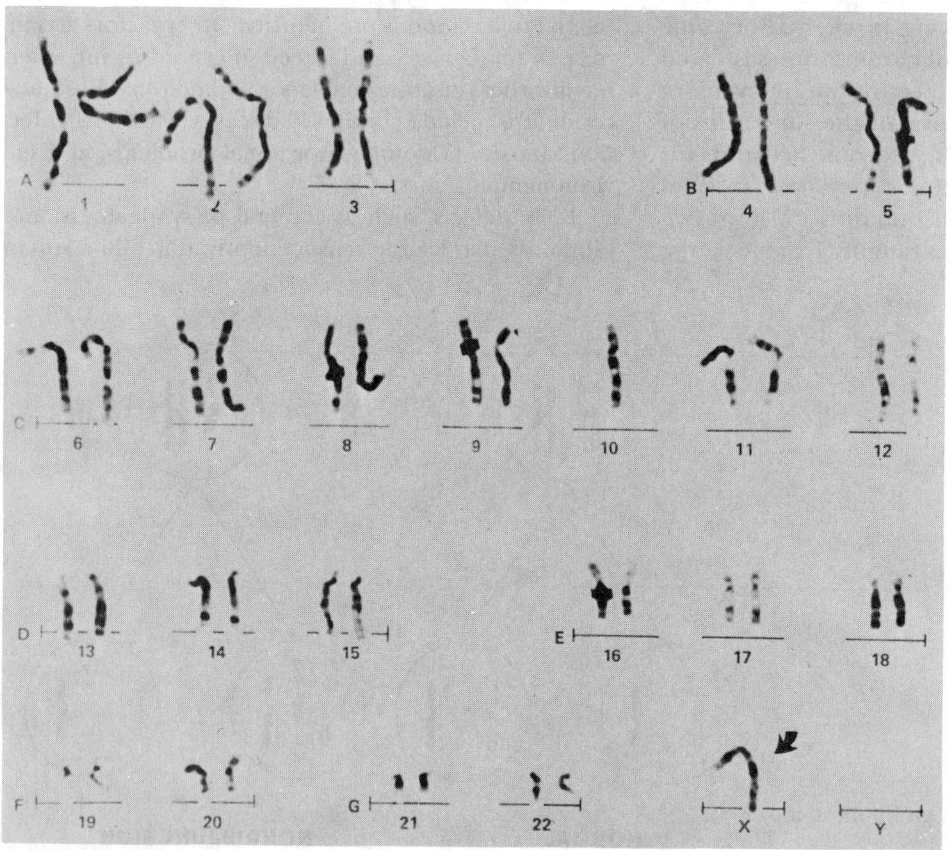

Figure 37-5. Photograph of karyotype of Turner syndrome.

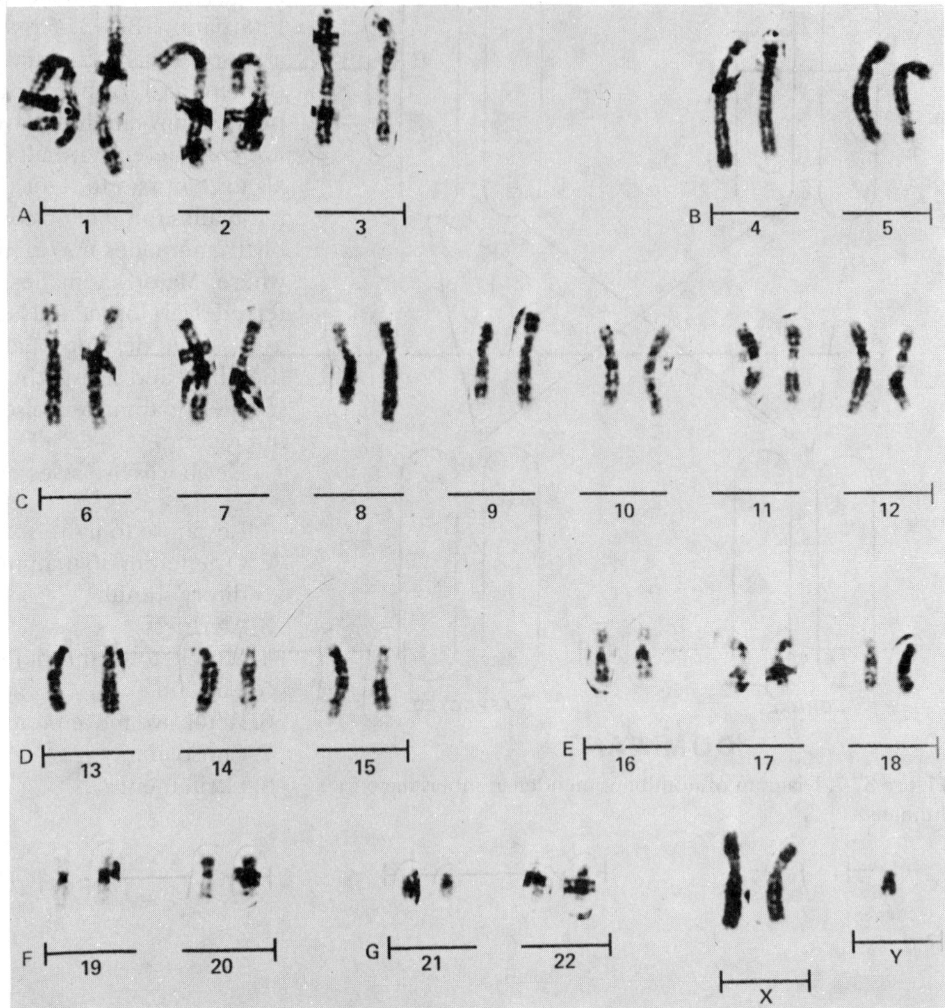

Figure 37-6. Photograph of karyotype of Klinefelter syndrome.

opmental years. The nursing process is a tool in these preventive efforts.

Application of the Nursing Process to Clients with Mental Retardation

Nurse educators need to enrich the existing curriculum with courses and practice opportunities related to genetics. This education should begin in ADN (Associate Degree Nursing) programs and continue through the mobility structure of BSN (Bachelor of Science in Nursing) and MSN (Master of Science in Nursing) preparation. Just as physicians are held accountable for the identification of genetic problems, nurses are also challenged to keep abreast of new genetic discoveries to expand the practice into the 21st century.[21] An understanding of genetics is critical for making an accurate physical assessment and planning client care that includes the needs of all members of the family. This section outlines some ways the nursing process is used to promote optimal wellness of mentally retarded clients (Box 37-4).

ASSESSMENT

During infancy and early childhood, developmental screening is of primary importance in finding children at risk for mental retardation. All systems need to be assessed, particularly the neurological, muscular, and skeletal systems.

The family planning stage is not too early to begin preventive nursing. Nurses who have the opportunity to work with families may begin assessing risk factors at this time. A good way to start a risk factor history is through a pedigree chart, a diagram in which family health or genetics is arranged in graphic form for easy visualization.

Knowledge of growth and development is necessary

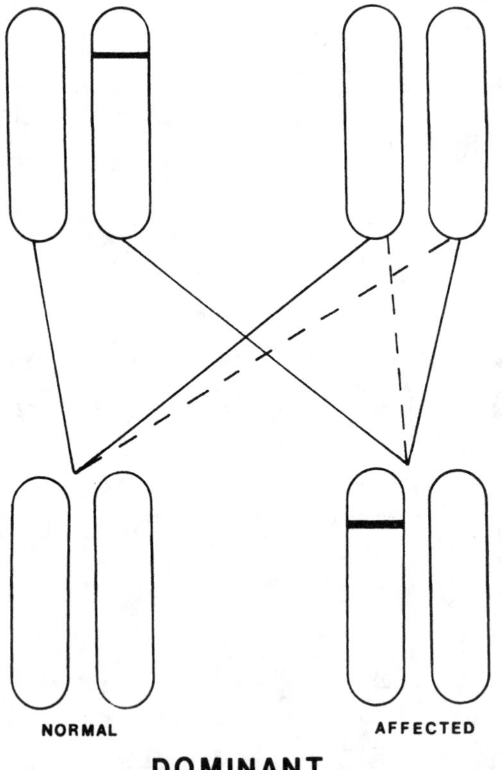

Figure 37-7. Diagram of dominant mendelian inheritance in humans.

for screening infants and children for signs of mental retardation. Box 37-5 is a beginning point for the nurse assessor. It can be a guide to normal growth and development and to the recognition of deviations from the norm. Many children have some of these deviations and are considered normal. Genetic counseling professionals urge nurses to refer clients with two or more minor anomalies for genetic counseling, because several small birth anomalies may signify a more major defect elsewhere. Major anomalies, of course, always must be referred. Developmental lags should be carefully followed as the child develops. Early intervention is important to the child and assists the parent in providing care. Assessment parameters also must include social and peer interaction.

Newborns are assessed in the following areas:

1. Response to light, sound, and pinprick
2. Orientation to inanimate and animate visual and auditory stimuli
3. Alertness
4. Muscle tone and pulling to sit
5. Cuddling
6. Defensive movements
7. Consolability
8. Excitement

(text continues on page 759)

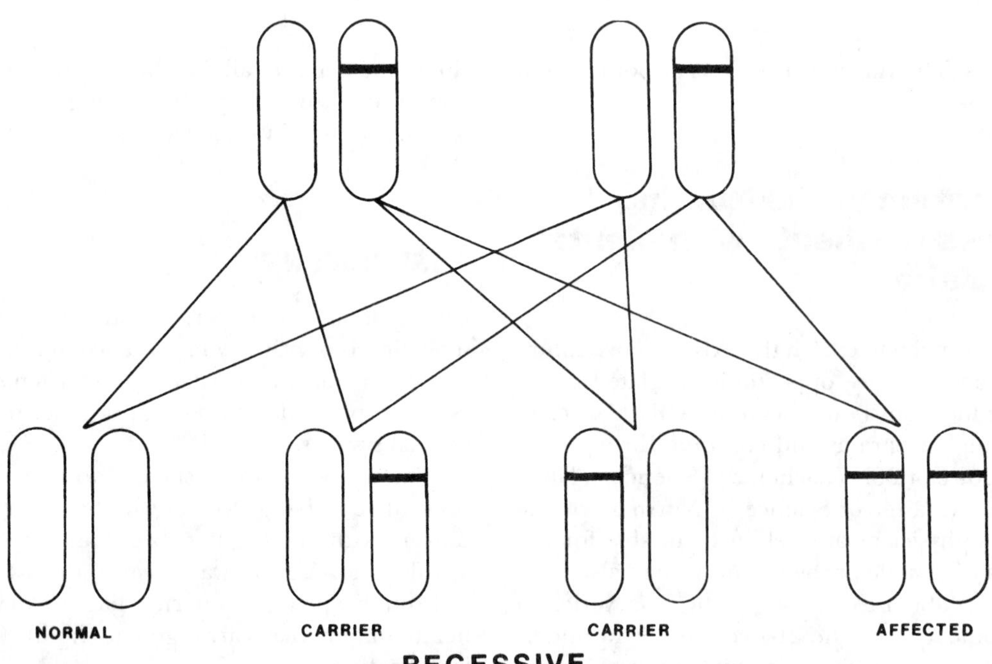

Figure 37-8. Diagram of recessive mendelian inheritance in humans.

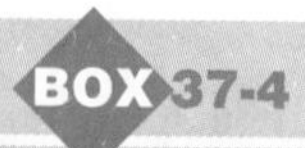

Nursing Process Guidelines

PRECONCEPTUAL PERIOD

Assessment and Analysis

Subjective Data

Nutritional interview—Lack of protein may be a risk factor. Check the mother's weight, and counsel her if she is below 50 kg.

History of disease or illness—Does the mother have a history of diabetes mellitus, cardiac disease, or chronic renal problems?

Reproductive history—Interview for miscarriages, abortions, previous premature deliveries, a history of delivery of an infant with congenital abnormalities. These are increased risks for the next pregnancy.

Family history (include genetic)—The easiest form is a pedigree chart. A history of retardation among family members, particularly males, may indicate fragile X syndrome.

Age of mother—very young mothers (younger than 16) have higher risk for translocation types of Down syndrome. Older mothers (over 35) have higher incidence of trisomy 21 (Down) syndrome.

Education of parents—Assess social and behavioral areas and formal education.

Objective Data

Results of nutrition testing and metabolic workups
Evaluation of pedigree information
Results of testing that rates adaptive behavior of an adult and examines risk factors prior to conception

Planning and Intervention

Goals are established with the client, and preoutcomes are defined that are measurable and time specific. Depending on the results of the assessment, the nurse may plan education and referral.

PRENATAL PERIOD

Assessment and Analysis

Subjective Data

Complaints of maternal infections, rubella, toxemia
Use of drugs
Exposure to radiation
Diet history
Financial status of parents
History of psychiatric problems
Is this child wanted?

Objective Data

Study laboratory work for results of the following:

Infections—Maternal infections may cause malformations, low birth weight baby, or prematurity.

Toxemia—It may result in poorly perfused placenta and poor fetal growth.

Polyhydramnios—It may indicate intestinal obstruction or the possibility that the fetus is unable to swallow.

Oligohydramnios—Urinary tract malformation is possible.

Amniocentesis—Results may indicate a genetic problem.

Sonogram—Results will provide information on placement of placenta, size of child, and developmental disability.

Maternal psychosis—A suicide threat is a potential danger for the mother. The fetus is also at risk for harm.

Planning and Intervention

The assessment parameters may indicate nursing care needs. At-risk individuals may need counseling, psychotherapy, and, possibly termination of pregnancy.

Evaluation

Look at the results of the laboratory work following birth to determine if nursing care was given correctly for each situation. What were the results of cord blood tests? What care is being given to the child as a result of a low Apgar score? Is the recovery of the mother following a normal process? If not, what nursing care is being carried out to assist her?

PERINATAL PERIOD

Assessment and Analysis

Subjective Data

When did labor start? This is important because of trauma damage resulting from long labor.

Last meal eaten—This is important to anesthesiologist for prevention of aspiration of stomach contents.

Previous prenatal care—Lack of previous medical care may be a risk factor, because these mothers have not been evaluated for problem areas.

continued

BOX 37-4 (Continued)

Objective Data

Monitor for complications. Areas to evaluate include hemorrhage, dystocia, trauma, placental damage, cesarean section, prematurity, or postmaturity.

Planning and Intervention

Fetal presentation
Maternal-infant condition
Assist with procedures for birth
Newborn Apgar score
Newborn care
Notification of nursery if problems are expected
Orders for special laboratory work if needed
As risk factors warrant, laboratory work may include the following:

Nutrition education
Referral to appropriate agency for financial assistance
Diet therapy
Genetic counseling
Birth control information and assistance
Family life education

Evaluation

This area is important in prevention.
Follow-up is a major step in the accountability of nursing care. Areas that will enhance evaluation procedures are as follows:

Follow-up visits
Physical assessments (ongoing) for weight gain
Nutritional follow-up
Family interview

Babies are at risk if parents have one or more risk factors that are not corrected. Are predicted outcomes achieved by the client? If not, the plan may need revision.

POSTNATAL–EARLY CHILDHOOD PERIOD

Assessment and Analysis

Subjective Data

Pitch and quality of the child's cry may indicate, in some cases, problem areas. Observe interaction of mother with infant.

Objective Data

Assessment throughout the child's developmental period must include the following factors; they should be carefully recorded by maternity, pediatric, or public health nurses for future use:

Apgar scores
Gestational age
Head size
Weight and length
Trauma
Infection
Neurological assessment results
Physical evaluation for birth defects
Maternal depression
Signs of child neglect or abuse
Prolonged separation from child

Planning and Intervention

Report any abnormalities to physician; parents and child may be referred to genetic counseling
Support parents if defect is found
Make other referrals as needed
Sensory stimulation may be needed for delayed infant
Behavior modification for client if needed
Parent education

Evaluation

Ongoing monthly physical and developmental checks are desirable if the child is at risk. These are performed at 6 months, 1 year, 18 months, and 24 months of age. A behavior problem checklist is valuable to maintain and should be followed up in progress notes. Child's cognitive level should be tested early. Language skills and achievement test reports will indicate if the individual program plan is adequate.

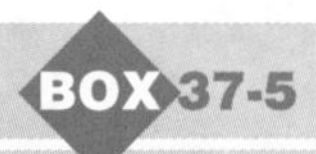

Physical Assessment: Checklist for Developmental Defects

HEAD

Size—Normal range for males is approximately 34.5 cm at birth, 49 cm at 2 years.

Normal range for females is approximately 34 cm at birth, 48 cm at 2 years.

Microcephaly—limited brain size two standard deviations below norm; brain tissue may be abnormal.

Hydrocephaly—increase in amount of cerebrospinal fluid; brain size may be normal or smaller than average; head size increases due to increased fluid.

The size of head is extremely important because the first 2 years of a child's life is vital for brain growth. A larger than normal head, sometimes by as much as two standard deviations, is found in fragile X syndrome.

Shape—should be normocephalic; abnormal findings may be in these areas:

- Prominent forehead as found in Hurler syndrome and fragile X syndrome
- Premature closing of suture lines, giving rise to oxycephaly, scaphocephaly, plagiocephaly, trigonocephaly
- Late closure of fontanels; most will be closed by 9 to 19 months. Late closure could indicate cretinism, Down syndrome, rickets, osteogenesis imperfecta, hydrocephalus, or syphilis; mean anterior fontanel diameter 2.1 cm, two standard deviations above or below (0.6 and 3.6 cm, respectively) are important; posterior fontanels rarely exceed measurements of 0.5 cm.

Face

Observe for spacing of features, symmetry, and signs of paralysis; width of a newborn face is approximately 8 cm; children with fragile X syndrome have long, thin faces and midface hypoplasia.

Eyes

Eyes are the same level and normally spaced

Hypertelorism refers to wide-spaced orbits, frequently associated with some syndromes of mental retardation; mean distance between inner canthi for term infant is 2 cm; 3 cm is judged as hypertelorism.

Hypotelorism is abnormally close-set eyes; this may indicate lack of nasal bridge or trigonocephaly.

Microphthalmia may indicate encephalo-ophthalmic dysplasia, toxoplasmosis, or retrolental fibroplasia.

Protruding supraorbital ridge is found in mucopolysaccharidosis and Marfan syndrome.

Ptosis of lids is caused by some neurological problems; sometimes it is an inherited trait; family history is important.

Slanting of eyes downward may indicate Treacher Collins syndrome; upward slant may be Down syndrome.

Epicanthal folds may be present in some normal children; most will disappear by 10 years of age; may be present as a result of Down syndrome, glycogen storage disease, renal agenesis, or hypercalcemia.

Eye lashes that are very bushy may indicate some syndrome disorders, such as Hurler syndrome; if absent on inner two-thirds, may indicate Treacher Collins syndrome.

Eyebrows that grow together in center may indicate a genetic syndrome, such as the Cornelia de Lange syndrome.

Permanent color of iris will be established in all children by 1 year; pinkish coloration may indicate albinism; light or white speckling (Brushfield spots) is often found in children with Down syndrome.

Absent red reflex in lens may indicate cataracts; these can be due to many problems leading to mental retardation; a dislocated lens may be the result of Marfan syndrome or homocystinuria.

Ears

Normally, the upper part of the pinna should meet an imaginary horizontal line that is drawn from the lateral aspect of the eye straight backward. This will indicate if the ear is normally positioned or low set. The rotation of the ear is also important. A vertical line is drawn from inner edge of the lobe of the ear straight up crossing the horizontal line. The measurement should not be more than a 10-degree an-

continued

BOX 37-5 (Continued)

gle. Abnormally shaped ears are also found in various disorders and should be reported. See if both ears are at the same level. Are they flat or protruding? Are they bigger or smaller than normal? Check the size and completeness of ear lobes. Check for sinuses or tags of skin on the ear. Children with fragile X syndrome have longer ears, often by two standard deviations, and are often posteriorly rotated. The ears are soft due to cartilge hypoplasia.

Nose

The nose should be at the middle and upper part of face. In many syndromes, the nose is shaped differently than the normal nose. In some cases, it is broad and flat, small and turned up. Notice if the nose is straight. Are the nares symmetrical? Palpate to examine bone and cartilage. Transilluminate with a flashlight on one nare, and look into the other to determine if perforation of the spectum exists.

Mouth

Is the mouth symmetrical? Are there clefts in the lip or palate? Drooling starts about 3 months and continues until the child learns to swallow saliva at about 9 to 12 months. Examine the palate for a gentle slope. Report a high arched palate. If a notch is noted at the junction of the soft and hard palate, report this because it may cause future speech difficulty. The lower jaw that is excessively small or large may indicate genetic problems that warrant further evaluation. Teeth that are delayed past 1 year of age may be a result of cretinism. Gums that have a black line along the margin may be a sign of metal poisoning. Do not confuse this with the normal dark pigmented coloration on the gums of African American children. A prominent jaw is found in people with fragile X syndrome.

The tongue that seems large for the mouth may indicate Down syndrome, cretinism, or Hurler syndrome. Protrusion of the tongue is a common finding in mental retardation. Note the normal developmental sequence of feeding. The rooting reflex disappears by 3 months. Sucking-swallowing remains for 3 to 5 months. The gag reflex diminishes slightly after the child begins to chew or at about 7 months. The bite reflex disappears at about 3 to 5 months. Lip closure begins at about 6 to 8 months.

Hair

Normally, head hair should begin high over the forehead. Some syndromes have hair growth low on the forehead, such as Hurler syndrome. Hair patterns found in Noonan and Turner syndromes allow growth of hair far down on the neck. Color is important. White hair may indicate albinism, and a white patch may be related to Waardenburg syndrome. One important factor in prevention is the color changes that occur in diets that are deficient in protein. These children may have red or greyish streaks in their hair. Hair whorls are usually located on the top at the back of the head. Number and location of whorls should be noted.

Neck

The average length of the trachea is 4 cm. An extra thick or a webbed neck may indicate Noonan or Turner syndrome. Extra skin folds at the back of the neck may indicate Down syndrome. Check for reflexes that should have disappeared earlier (primitive reflexes). These include a symmetrical tonic neck reflex or an asymmetrical tonic neck reflex, the startle reflex, or the tonic labyrinthine reflex. These will cause future problems, particularly in feeding the child.

CHEST

Any irregular shape of the chest should be reported. When the sternum protrudes from the chest wall, the child should be evaluated for syndromes such as Marfan or Morquio. Funnel chest is also found in Marfan syndrome. Spinal deformities may be a problem. A horizontal circumference of the thorax at the level of mammary glands with respiration is 34 to 35 cm.

ABDOMEN AND BACK

Note whether two arteries and one vein are present in umbilicus. Omphaloceles on the abdomen where the peritoneal contents bulge through a muscular defect are sometimes seen. It is important to know that up to one-half of these children have other associated defects. Distribution of hair that is not normal should be reported. A dimpling in the spine can be associated with spina bifida and should

continued

BOX 37-5 (Continued)

be evaluated. The spinal column and hips should be evaluated for defects. Many are related to genetic and developmental problems.

ARMS, LEGS, HANDS, AND FEET

The extremities are evaluated for deformities. Children with genetic problems often have defects of the extremities; for instance, in fragile X syndrome, the hands are often at least two standard deviations greater in length than normal. Hands are also soft, fleshy, and hyperextensible in this syndrome. Specific things to look for are number of fingers and toes, nail growth, any webbing of toes and fingers, and short fingers due to missing phalanges. Enlarged toes and fingers are also significant findings. A large space between the large toe and second toe is important. Any curving inward of small fingers (clinodactyly) should be reported. Fingers that override or cross over each other are sometimes seen in children with trisomy (18) syndrome. The thumb often has the appearance of another finger. Feet are rounded on the bottom and are called "rocker bottom." Dermatoglyphics of hands and toes often vary in children with syndromes. Down syndrome, in particular, has very different patterns from the normal population. An increased carrying angle of the elbows should alert the nurse to the possibility of gonadal dysgenesis in both sexes.

GENITALIA

Examination of the genitalia in the developing child is important. In small children, abnormalities of the genitals may indicate problems with other developmental disabilities. In young males, abnormal genital enlargement is often the result of neurogenic or idiopathic sexual precocity or of fragile X syndrome, in which the testes are significantly enlarged after puberty. In older males, small genitals can be the result of Klinefelter syndrome or an endocrine disorder. Secondary sexual characteristics may be missing in young women with Turner syndrome.

9. Irritability
10. Activity
11. Tremulousness
12. Skin color changes
13. Startle behavior
14. Self-quieting
15. Hand-to-mouth movements
16. Smiling

Assessment of an infant's behavior using tools such as the Brazelton scale gives clues to probable developmental outcomes. Abnormalities are easily spotted when this tool is used to assess children at risk for retardation or disability.

Developmental Skills

Developmental skills assessment should continue as the child grows. A child normally progresses through an orderly, unique growth and development pattern within certain parameters defined as normal. Children who are retarded may miss or be delayed in achieving some stages of growth and development.

Nurses need to be aware that the family can be affected by many stressors related to a child's chronic illness or disability. Such stressors as illnesses, surgery and other medical treatments, discovery of new medical problems, behavior problems, the emotional consequences when a child is surpassed developmentally by siblings and peers, and the search for daycare and school services to meet the child's needs evoke a wide range of responses from family members.[14,16] The child who is retarded has the same needs as any child with a chronic illness or disability. If normalization is to succeed, the child must be helped to acquire as many skills as possible. The AAMR list of behavior skills follows and is addressed to nursing for this chapter.[2]

Self-Care Skills

The skill to eat in an acceptable manner must be developed if the child is to achieve autonomy. An assessment of eating ability is the forerunner of a program to upgrade a client's skills. Parents must have assistance and teaching to learn how to select the right foods for their child and techniques to feed children with developmental problems.[12,13] Chances to practice are important; as the client learns, the opportunity to eat in public is an effective training method. Other self-care skills are toileting, dressing, hygiene, and grooming. The nurse-case manager may need to call on a multidisciplinary team approach to assist (ie, occupational therapist, physical therapist, nutritional management team, specialists who design adaptive equipment, psychologists, and pharmacists).

Communication Skills

Language skills are crucial for all people. Speech is simply one form of language development. Language skills are still being learned as the retarded person grows to adulthood and becomes more independent. Reading and writing are other means of communication. Information skills about the environment also must be stressed. Many young adults learn to recognize and understand signs related to health and safety in the community. The ability to use a telephone, tell time, and use money are important. The client's motivation for and mastery of these skills must be assessed.

Some children do not have effective language skills because of their other disabilities. They may be able to use an electronic communication board. Assessing a child's ability to use such a board can be done by working with pictures and having the child point to the object named. If a child cannot use hands or arms but has head control, a pointer may be taped on a helmet. Pictures should be as similar as possible to the scenes in the child's environment. Communication boards using symbols that cannot be readily understood may be lost on the general public, although such boards provide a means of expression for the affected person and his or her family and therapists. Colored pictures or black and white pictures may present problems to children with perceptual motor difficulties. Assessing the child's perceptual skills is essential before attempting to use visual aids in health teaching. Problems with eye–hand coordination, figure-ground discrimination, position in space, spatial relations, or form constancy also can impair learning. Collaboration with an occupational therapist or a speech therapist may be helpful in this area. The Frostig Developmental Test of Visual Perception is a valuable assessment tool.

Home Living Skills

Home living skills relate to the client's home environment. When the child is growing toward adulthood, skills must be developed that will allow him or her to function as independently as possible. Doing laundry, cooking, budget keeping, practicing home safety, and keeping the environment clean are essential skills. These skills are also closely related to social skills and community use. Unless the person who is retarded can manage these activities, case managers should plan for someone to be provide the client with the proper level of support.

Community Skills

Assessing the child's use of the community assists the nurse in planning effective interventions. All children need stimulation suitable for their physical and emotional needs. Children need to learn skills to use community resources. This means using available transportation, using shopping centers, purchasing needed goods, locating and using health care and service providers, attending a church of choice, controlling self-gratification needs, obeying laws, and using appropriate social behavior. Case managers need to address the use of these skills, which are also closely related to health and safety, communication, and functional academic skills.

Self-Direction Skills

Individuals should be assessed for the ability to make choices, use time and follow a daily schedule, complete tasks for work or self-care, ask for and receive help when needed, and demonstrate self-advocacy and problem-solving abilities.

Health and Safety Skills

The individual should be assessed for the ability to fulfill health care needs. Does the client wash his or her hands before eating, after using the bathroom, and when preparing food? Does this person know safety measures to use in the home and in the community? Has the person been informed about sexuality, interacting with strangers, and having regular medical and dental checkups? Can the individual relate reasons for safety measures, such as prevention of accidents or illness?

Functional Academics Skills

Independent living requires skills related to writing, reading, practical mathematics, sexuality, and health. These skills will assist the individual in daily living situations at home and in the community. Teaching specific words to identify which restaurant toilets one can enter is necessary. Words related to safety and health with the use of printed signs may be helpful. Most book stores have bulletin board cutouts that are useful tools for health and safety and other concepts of behavioral skills, such as money management, traffic, and hygiene.

Leisure Skills

Leisure time planning is a skill that will promote a full and enjoyable life for any person. It is particularly a skill requirement for those with a diagnosis of mental retardation. The person's age, culture, and personal preference should be taken into consideration when planning leisure activities. Children learn to share, exchange, take turns, and decide when to begin or stop leisure activities based on learned behaviors. As the child grows to adulthood, appropriate social behaviors and interactions in public settings are critical. Without these behavior skills, it is difficult to be accepted.[9]

Work Skills

Skills that are necessary at home, in the community, and at play are integrated into the work situation. Job-related skills require knowledge of how to seek help or assistance as needed, follow a schedule, manage a pay check, complete a task, observe work safety, groom properly, use transportation to and from work, and display social skills with coworkers.

NURSING DIAGNOSIS

To develop nursing diagnoses for the mentally retarded client and family, the nurse should look for patterns in the assessment data, using subjective and objective clues. From these data, the nurse can make a judgment about an appropriate or probable diagnosis. Appropriate nursing diagnoses may include the following:

1. Dysfunctional Grieving
2. Ineffective Family Coping: Compromised or Disabling
3. Altered Family Process
4. Spiritual Distress
5. Social Isolation
6. Self Esteem Disturbance
7. Altered Role Performance
8. Anxiety
9. Altered Growth and Development
10. Impaired Swallowing
11. Toileting Self Care Deficit
12. Feeding Self Care Deficit
13. Bathing/Hygiene Self Care Deficit
14. Dressing/Grooming Self Care Deficit
15. Impaired Verbal Communication
16. Risk for Infection or Injury
17. Impaired Home Maintenance Management
18. Knowledge Deficit[19]

A diagnosis should have a response component and an etiology component. The response is the client's unhealthy or potentially unhealthy behavior observed by the nurse, and the etiology is the probable cause of that behavior. The client's goal should be related to the response component, while the nurse's interventions are designed to change the cause or etiology, thereby altering the client response. The etiology, therefore, must be one that can be modified or eliminated by nursing intervention. For instance, a diagnosis of Dressing/Grooming Self Care Deficit related to cerebral palsy is not amenable to nursing intervention because the nurse cannot change the etiology. Nursing Care Plan 37-1 demonstrates the correct nursing diagnosis for this case. Comparing the actual outcomes to predictable outcomes will assist the nurse to evaluate whether the process was successful.[34]

PLANNING

Effective planning calls on the nurse's communication and interpersonal skills. The family of a mentally retarded child may be at any point from shock to acceptance at the time of initial contact with the nurse. Initially, the nurse guides the family through the stages of shock, grief, anger, resentment, and finally, acceptance. Planning revolves around the nursing assessment and analysis or diagnosis of the assessment data. The nurse must determine whether the family needs counseling at this point or if they are ready to progress to the stage of securing help for the child.

During the child's infancy, the family needs to work with the nurse and other health care professionals to provide stimulation and activities that promote growth and development. Planning may include training for parents to learn handling and special techniques to enhance the child's physical and mental condition.

As the child becomes older, needs and goals of care change. Services that meet the changing needs and goals must be identified and secured. Long-range plans should be formulated so that the parents have a time frame to help them understand what is required of them as they plan for the child's future.

Issues such as employment needs of the parents, respite care, and long-term care resources should be discussed during the planning stage. The nurse considers the needs of siblings and helps the parents work through their feelings about siblings.

Plans may be needed to include visits to various agencies with which parents will deal during the child's development. The nurse who is not familiar with long-term care facilities should visit such an agency.

Legislation related to handicapped or mentally retarded people must also be understood for informed planning with the parents and client. Moral and ethical problems must be addressed by parents, nurses, and other health care providers. A sensitive interview offers insight into how the parents feel about these issues as they pertain to their child and his or her condition.

INTERVENTION

Nursing intervention is based on a careful and thorough assessment, thoughtful analysis of client and family data, and collaborative planning. Support of the family is critical. It begins with the birth of a child and continues throughout the lifespan. Nurses interact with the family in many ways, such as in a school situation, in which clients are screened for vision, hearing, health problems related to the disability or its complications, and physical assessments. Nurses are also interested in the person's need for vocational education, sex education and birth control measures, securing of resources, monitoring of ongoing health, and skills needed to live in the community, whether at home or in a group home. Nurses and other health care professionals strive to help the client develop and maintain a positive self-image.

Nursing Care Plan 37-1

Paul: Intermittent Support in Home Care

Assessment Data

Ten-year-old Paul and his family have recently moved to a moderately sized community of 70,000 people. Paul attended school for the first time in the fall. He had previously been home schooled by his mother because they lived in a rural area 75 miles from the nearest community.

Paul has a medical diagnosis of mild mental retardation (IQ 68, Axis II 317.0) and mild cerebral palsy with fine motor deficit in hands (Axis III 343.9). Paul is able to use his hands and arms for gross motor activities but is unable to button shirts and coats and cannot pull up the zipper on his pants. This caused Paul "embarrassment at school last semester."

Paul and his family have never had services for his disability. His mother refused to "put him through the trauma" of a 150-mile trip each day to a community center where services were available. Therefore, the family was unaware of available resources for Paul.

The opportunity to attend a summer camp was presented to the family by his teacher last semester. His mother stated that she thinks "it sounds like a great idea. Paul has missed the company of other children until now." Paul, however, refuses to consider the idea. "I won't go. People would say I'm a baby. I can't even go to the bathroom alone because I can't unzip my pants." His mother states, "I've been helping him dress since he was born. Since he started school, I can't get him to use clothes with velcro because none of the other boys dress like that."

Nursing Diagnosis

Dressing Self Care Deficit related to lack of knowledge of adaptive devices

Outcome

Paul will develop self-care skills in dressing through the use of adaptive devices.

Intervention	Rationale
Assess Paul's self-care skills.	Baseline assessment data provide information needed to determine which skills client possesses or needs.
Locate appropriate adaptive devices to overcome client's lack of motor skill.	Knowledge about adaptive devices and their use enable Paul and his family to move Paul toward greater independence in self-care.
Instruct Paul in the use of button hook for shirt and pants; use velcro-closing athletic shoes.	Instruction and practice with adaptive devices help Paul become skilled and comfortable in their use, resulting in increased independence.

Evaluation

Paul uses adaptive devices for dressing and attends summer camp.

Nursing Diagnosis

Self Esteem Disturbance related to feelings of inadequacy, rejection by peers, and self-isolation

Outcome

Paul will verbalize feelings of self-confidence as a result of skill development.

continued

Nursing Care Plan 37-1 *(Continued)*

Intervention	Rationale
Collaborate with other care providers (teacher, coach, physical and occupational therapists) to promote multiple skill development in all areas of Paul's life.	Successful accomplishment of skills promotes feelings of self-confidence and self-esteem.
Encourage Paul to master and complete his self-care and encourage parents to assist Paul in developing independence.	Mastery of skills fosters independence; independence promotes increased self-esteem.
Encourage Paul to participate in peer activities; work with Paul's peer group to acknowledge Paul's abilities.	Peer interaction reinforces self-esteem for a child; adults promote awareness among Paul's peer group related to his abilities (not disabilities).

Evaluation

Paul relates or displays evidence of increased self-worth.

Working With the Grieving Family

Grief presents symptoms that are psychological and somatic and can be elicited by loss. The birth of a child with a handicapping condition triggers the grief response because the parents' expectations of a normal child are now impossible. Without supportive intervention, a sense of helplessness, hopelessness, and despair may result. Often, parents and normal siblings react in this grieving process by wishing that the child were dead. Some families experience additional guilt reactions because of these feelings. Grieving must take place; it assists families to solve problems and look to the future.

How does the nurse support the family? One of the nurse's first responsibilities is guiding the family through decision-making processes related to issues such as whether they will allow corrective surgeries for some disability related to the child's diagnosis. Within the community are many sources of assistance for such decision making. The nurse should know how to put the family in touch with available resources.

It would be ideal if all families were able to keep their children who are handicapped at home—nurturing, loving, and accepting them and their disabilities. We know that this is not possible in some families. How can the nurse present reality to parents?

The nurse helps the parents deal with one issue at a time, one day at a time. Resources for each need can be found. The nurse also helps the parents think through the consequences of each major decision for the child and the other family members.

Crisis Intervention

During the family's *crisis period,* often soon after learning of the child's diagnosis, family members are likely to experience confusion, disorganization, helplessness, dependency, anguish, and anger. The child and family need immediate supportive intervention. The family must be given information on the child's developmental expectations and capabilities. Services for the child must be secured, and support groups for the parents must be located. A place in the family value system needs to be made for the child.

Crisis intervention is a supportive nursing intervention for the family of a child with mental retardation until the family is able to solve problems using their own strengths and abilities. During crisis periods in which families are unable to function in a healthy manner, nursing intervention may mean stepping in and giving direction to the family or simply listening to family members and helping them shape their thinking and behavior.

Meeting Developmental Needs

Problems that the retarded child will face begin in infancy and can best be appreciated by examining the normal needs of all children. If these needs are not met for some reason, the child has troubles. Retarded children are at greater risk of having unmet needs.

The retarded child's emotional, sensory, and motor needs are the same as those of other children. Meeting these needs may call on the creativity of the nurse. The child's emotional adjustment depends on provision of security through affection, acceptance, and approval. It also calls for understanding intrinsic behavior patterns as children grow and develop. In an encouraging atmosphere, when children are accepted developmentally and there is optimism regarding their developmental capacity, children are more likely to attain their fullest potential.[5]

Social development relates to children's acceptance of the society in which they live. Role models are parents, siblings, and friends. The parents' culture and values influence children. As children progress through the maturational process, they need to develop autonomy and independence. Peer relationships become important, and play provides opportunities to help them shape qualities and character. Sexual identification and interest in the self as a sexual person are lifetime experiences, the roots of which are in infancy.

Progressing through these normal patterns of growth and development is extremely difficult for the mentally retarded or handicapped child. Mentally retarded children need special services, which are sometimes difficult to find, to help them achieve some degree of autonomy and independence. The retarded child may grow to adulthood being regarded as the "eternal child" and never experience independence beyond the most basic skills of daily living. Only in the last decade has it become possible for mentally retarded people to be considered peers or functioning parts of the society in which they live.

As in the general population, the population of people who are retarded is growing older. This is in part due to the better medical services available today. As nurses, we need to be aware of the biopsychosocial needs of this aging population.

Teaching the Retarded Child

According to the AAMR, teaching methods should be socially valid and promote learning skills used in the child's normal environment. Rather than blocking out special times to teach, the skills should be taught in routine activities as the opportunity arises. This is called *integrated instruction* and works best with students who are mentally retarded.

One of the most pressing needs of parents is to learn techniques to teach their retarded child. Families should be taught positive reinforcement tools. These include using nutritious food rather than candy as a reward and providing feedback to the child about performance or behavior; social approval, such as verbal praise, attention, and affection; and tokens that can be redeemed for something desirable to the child as payment for good behavior. Other methods to influence the child's behavior are punishment, restriction from a desired event, or ignoring wrong behavior (ie, refusing to give reinforcing attention).

Methods that help the client establish a right way to perform an activity include modeling the desired behavior and allowing the client a time and place to practice. Self-help skills are divided into very basic early, intermediate, and advanced skills. *Basic readiness skills* include looking when called and following a simple command, whereas *basic motor skills* include holding and releasing objects and finger painting. Walking is also a basic motor activity goal, and drinking from a cup is a self-help goal. *Intermediate self-help skills* include threading a belt through loops or washing hands and brushing teeth. Examples of *advanced self-help skills* are tying shoes, bathing, and setting a table.

Before teaching parents to work with their retarded child, the nurse should explore the parents' expectations for the child's learning. Expectations that are too high risk frustration and failure; those that are too low slow the child's progress. The amount of assistance given to a child also should be discussed; parents must be careful not to do everything for the child. Learning to become independent depends largely on the family's allowing the child opportunities to plan and carry out some tasks alone. What kind of reward system will the parent choose to increase motivation? Praise, encouragement, and attention are excellent methods.

Providing Information

Nurses need to give information. Many available resources can provide teaching tools. If there is a university within close enough proximity, the nurse will have a ready source of information.

The ARC (formerly known as The Association for Retarded Citizens but renamed in 1992 to avoid the word "retarded") has 1,200 affiliated chapters in all 50 states. Its goals are broad. Experienced member parents strive to help new parents deal with problems. Membership includes interested professionals, community members, family members, friends of the family, and the clients themselves. The ARC educates families about services available for the child with disabilities. Advocacy—particularly self-advocacy—is a high priority. Prevention of mental retardation is also one of the major goals of the group. Additionally, the ARC follows and explains legislation to members. Members are asked to participate fully with legislators when the law affects the needs of the retarded.

The AAMR (formerly known as the American Association of Mental Deficiency, AAMD) is an organization of 9,000 interdisciplinary professionals serving people with mental retardation and other developmental disabilities through publications, conferences, and governmental liaison. The AAMR has state, regional, national, and international chapters and groups. Active nursing divisions in each chapter recently produced standards for the clinical nurse specialist in developmental disabilities and handicapping conditions, in conjunction with the American Association of University Affiliated Programs. A copy of the standards may be ordered through the Department of Health and Human Services, Public Health Service, Health Resources and Services Administration, Rockville, MD 20857.

Outreach teams are groups of professionals who work out of specialized centers, such as state schools, birth defect centers, and school districts. Their membership can include teachers, nurses, occupational therapists, physical therapists, speech therapists, and specially trained aides. These teams travel to the home to help family members give appropriate intervention to their handicapped children, assisting them to develop as normally as possible or helping them progress by formal assistance. Catalogs are available to assist clients who need adaptive devices. An example is Sammon's Catalog, Bissell Health Care Co., PO Box 386, Western Springs, IL 60558-0386 (1-800-323-5547).

Children with disabilities need many special services. Most communities have speech, hearing, physical therapy, and occupational therapy services in local or state agencies. Depending on the disability, professional interventions, such as dentistry, child psychology, psychiatric services, and social work, may be needed. Local school administration offices can provide the names of service centers in their area.

Respite Care

The family may need to use respite care in times of family crises, for vacations, or for shopping or appointments when both parents need to be away from the home. Respite care is a temporary separation of the child from the family either in the child's home or outside of the home. The time may be for as little as a few hours or as much as 30 or more days in some cases. Home health aides may perform this respite service in the home, or the child may be placed in an agency.

EVALUATION

Evaluation of the plan and interventions should be a responsibility of the total health team, including the client and family. Evaluation is an ongoing activity aimed at the next client goal. Another form of evaluation involves examining actual outcomes of the client at the end of a planned intervention of care. Accurate documentation enhances the evaluation process.

◆ Vulnerability of the Mentally Retarded Client to Mental Disorders

INCIDENCE

A *dual diagnosis* refers to the occurrence of mental disorders in people with mental retardation. The growing need for services to individuals with dual diagnosis remains largely unmet, and little research has been conducted on dual diagnosis.[27] However, we do know that everyone can experience stress and health problems, leading to emotional disorders, and the retarded person is at greater risk for these disorders. The trauma or congenital defect that led to a particular cerebral dysfunction may also cause hyperactivity. The child born with disability is certainly at higher risk for rejection by significant others. If normal children sometimes are unable to adjust to the environment in which they live, imagine the problems faced by a person who has no neighborhood peers nor even a sibling with similar problems. The personality traits that we find hard to accept in others, such as tension and anxiety, prevent retarded people from making friendships, further increasing their adjustment difficulties.

Studies of retarded people in institutions before 1960 found a 16% to 40% incidence of emotional disturbances. More recent studies indicate that among institutionalized children with Down syndrome, 56% display emotional disturbance at the time of their admission to an institution. In the child population, the rate is 14% to 18%; in the general adult population, it ranges up to 40%. These figures indicate that retarded people have an increased susceptibility to emotional disturbance.[6,23] In the noninstitutionalized population, between 20% and 35% are currently diagnosed with a dual diagnosis.[26]

DYNAMICS

It is difficult to define mental illnesses in mental retardation. Mental retardation may result from many causes and is associated with many physically handicapping conditions. Through the normal growth and developmental phases, children's needs change continually. Mentally retarded people are less able to relate to family and community in general. Causes of mental disorders in the retarded are hard to separate from those related to mental retardation. Mentally retarded children are, as a group, subject to a high incidence of behavioral and psychiatric disturbances, which often are not recognized and go untreated.[6,27]

THE NURSING PROCESS AND THE MENTALLY ILL RETARDED CHILD

Assessment and Nursing Diagnosis

In his classic work, Menolascino provided descriptions of psychotic reactions in the mentally retarded, which generally include bizarre gestures or postures, communication problems, lack of discrimination between inanimate and animate objects, and deviant affective expression. The child may not make eye contact with or relate to the examiner. Speech may be monotonous or echolalic or may involve various abnormal responses. Motor behavior is repetitive or preoccupied. Children also may engage in unusual motor activity, such as hand flapping or tiptoeing. Psychosis is a syndrome of behaviors that cannot be separated from the cause, age of onset, the child's inheritance, and the child's environment.[23]

Personality disorders produce behaviors characterized by inability to delay gratification, impulsiveness, irresponsibility, and failure to adjust socially by learning from previous interactions with others. These personality disorders are not considered related to the causes of mental retardation and are not found in the mentally retarded population in greater proportions than in the normal population. Several good assessment tools can be used for diagnosing, such as the Aberrant Behavior Check List and the AAMR Adaptive Behavior Scales.

A major problem involved with assessing a client with a dual diagnosis is that the presence of the mental retardation often overshadows the significance of a diagnosis of a mental health disorder. It is often difficult to discern what effect the cognitive deficiency plays in certain behaviors that are also often found in psychiatric disorders. Concern exists that an added diagnosis to the diagnosis already imposed on a person with mental retardation may further cause stigmatization.[2]

The most frequently reported types of mental illness in this population are schizophrenic disorders, organic brain disorders, adjustment disorders, personality disorders, and affective disorders. These main categories of disorders can be further subclassified.[2]

People with dual diagnosis frequently exhibit negative behaviors, such as head banging, violent aggression, smearing of feces, sleep disorders, chronic pacing, hand wringing, and screaming out at people or things who are not present.[17]

Planning and Intervention

In the past, it was not considered feasible to treat the retarded with psychotherapy because therapy required that the client have good verbal skills. More recent thinking has suggested that treating the client in a humane and accepting manner in therapy is more important than using techniques that require the client's sophisticated intellectual skills.

Planning should include the parents and the client when possible. The treatment of mentally ill retarded clients may require parent counseling, individual or group therapy, and drug therapy. Client–therapist contact may begin on a one-to-one basis and may then expand to include a therapy or activity group.

Play therapy is useful even for clients with limited verbal skills. Music therapy and recreational therapy can be planned around the client's needs. Through demonstration or modeling, the client may be shown certain behaviors that need to be corrected and then shown the correct behavior. Art therapy is another useful tool incorporating many different media of expression, such as clay, finger paints, and designing prints on fabric. As behavior improves, the client is gradually moved out of the therapy group and into a transitional group.

Evaluation

Nurses must be accountable for nursing care through carefully recorded plans, interventions, and reports of client progress. Plans should reflect how goals and objectives are evaluated. Videotapes and progress notes describing outcomes are methods of accomplishing this. Meticulous records documenting the client's behavior and legal consents are time consuming but worthwhile, particularly when the nurse has a large case load or long-term interaction with clients.

◆ The Nurse's Attitude

The nurse acting as a client advocate invests time, energy, and skills helping the client maintain health, prevent injury or illness, and live effectively within the environment (Box 37-6). The nurse's attitude sets the tone for client interaction and for movement toward achieving the goals of care.

Mentally retarded people are moving into the community in ever-increasing numbers, and nurses must be prepared to care for them. Retarded people are more like the general public than they are different from it, but sometimes the differences seem impenetrable barriers to achieving independence.

Professional development is the responsibility of the nurse. Basic curricula to help nurses meet their career needs are the responsibilities of nursing educational programs. Unfortunately, few programs give nursing students the opportunity to become directly involved with retarded clients in clinical settings.[8,18]

The enlightened nurse has a responsibility to promote public awareness of the needs and rights of the mentally retarded and the historical attitudes that have been detrimental to the handicapped. Ar-

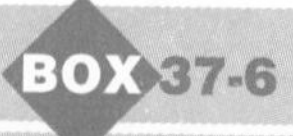

Client Advocacy for a Mentally Retarded Client: Annie

Annie was admitted to a state school for the mentally retarded when she was 15 years old. A combination of her behavior and size struck fear in the hearts of most of her caretakers and fellow residents. Annie was 5 ft, 7 in; weighed 240 lb; and was given to bouts of uncontrolled explosive anger without a stimulus.

She presented a real challenge to support personnel because of these sudden flareups, in which she often injured those around her. People who lived and worked with her believed her to be untruthful because she often stated that someone told her to behave badly. She talked to herself, ran away from the school, and soon learned to manipulate others fear of her reputation. Annie lived in a locked dorm with 15 to 20 girls. The dorm required more staff coverage, and very few staff liked to work on Annie's unit.

Annie was diagnosed as moderately retarded, with an IQ of 51. On admission, the only physical problems listed were obesity and periodic clonic-tonic seizures.

She had difficulty in describing symptoms leading to her behaviors, and at the time, little was known about dual diagnosis. It was unheard of to diagnose someone as depressed with mental retardation. Psychiatrists have only recently begun to learn how to treat retarded people with behavior found in psychiatric disorders.

Trial and error characterized her medical and health care regimen. None of these diagnoses and treatments led to change and often only worsened her behavior and demeanor.

Today it is known that Annie has schizoaffective disorder, Axis I, and moderate mental retardation, Axis II with an IQ of 51 (moderate). Her clonic-tonic seizures are controlled with valproic acid. Her blood levels are drawn quarterly and are 52 to 86 μg-mL (normal levels range from 50–100 μg-mL). She takes trifluoperazine (Stelazine, 15 mg qd), which has been quite effective.

Annie now sees a psychiatrist once a month and a psychologist and be1havior therapist daily. Slowly, she is overcoming years of learned behaviors related to misdiagnosis. Annie's new lifestyle includes living in an apartment on campus with a bedroom of her own, unlocked doors, and three housemates, all with dual diagnosis.

The nursing care plan for Annie stresses short-term goals that are designed to decrease acting on hallucinations and learning to test her reality within her ability to do so. She has lost 55 lb and is maintained on an 1,800 calorie diet. She participates in an exercise program, attends classes about self-medication, grooming, and hygiene, and is learning behavior skills for employment in the community vocational center. She has a long-term goal of moving to a community group home. Nurses collaborate with a multidisciplinary team to work with Annie and are assisting her to become a self-advocate. She is able to express her feelings in a positive way with encouragement from nursing. Annie is now 42 years old, and for the first time, she is making progress and enjoying her life, thanks to improved nursing care motivated by client advocacy.

chitectural barriers must be eliminated, and the need for recreational facilities must be demonstrated. Every nurse must share information and treatment ideas with clients, parents, other health professionals, and one another.

◆ Chapter Summary

This chapter has focused on a condition affecting about 5.48% of the population. Of the many causes of retardation, two main causes can be listed—genetic factors and acquired factors. The dynamics of the family into which a retarded child is born are complicated and often crisis laden. Some emphases of the chapter include the following:

1. Genetic factors may be chromosomal abnormalities, such as errors in numbers of the chromosomes (nondisjunction) or errors in the structure of the chromosome due to breakage or translocation.
2. According to the laws of mendelian inheritance, genetic disorders may be passed from generation to generation by traits found on the autosome or the sex chromosome in a dominant or recessive manner.
3. Acquired factors leading to mental retardation may occur prenatally, perinatally, or postnatally; these disorders may arise from trauma, disease, or infection of the woman during pregnancy or of the child following birth or from environmental problems, such as malnutrition, lead poisoning, or child abuse.
4. Usually, conditions more readily seen at birth causing multiple physical defects are the most difficult for parents.
5. Most mental retardation is mild and is usually not diagnosed until some time after birth when the child fails to develop academic skills.
6. Feelings such as guilt, depression, withdrawal, rejection, denial, and anger are normal following the birth of a retarded child, and the nurse must communicate effectively with the parents to help them work through these feelings.
7. When the family has progressed past the crisis stage and is more accepting of intervention for the retarded child, referrals are made to find sources of parent teaching and infant stimulation.
8. Normalization (or social role volarization, as it is now called) is a widely accepted concept in the area of mental and physical disability that ensures that the client will not be segregated from the general population and made more deviant by lack of basic skills and appropriate dress and activities for age.
9. The nurse becomes an advocate for the client and family; he or she directs the client and family to every resource that meets the needs of the client at each point in his or her life span and provides nursing care that accepts prevention, support, guidance, and teaching.
10. An advocate is also interested in the rights of the mentally retarded as citizens, including becoming involved in the legislative process and in ethical issues that affect clients.
11. Knowledge and experience help the nurse to dispel the false beliefs that many people still hold and that continue to separate the retarded from mainstream society.

Review Questions

1. In 1992, mental retardation was newly defined by the American Association of Mental Retardation as:
   - A. an intelligence quotient score of 70–75 or below.
   - B. a significantly sub-average intellectual function existing concurrently with limitations and in two or more applicable adaptive skill areas and manifested before age 18.
   - C. mild, moderate, severe, and profound levels.
   - D. intermittent, limited, extensive, and pervasive labels.
2. In order to identify sub-average intellectual functions, some reliable instruments that have been used to determine different factors of intelligence are:
   - A. the Stanford Binet, the Wechsler adult and/or pediatric scales, and the Kaufman Assessment Battery for Children.
   - B. echoencephalography and/or Computerized Axial Tomography.
   - C. the Bliss Symbolic System and the Vineland Social Maturity Test.
   - D. the Dubowitz Assessment Scale and the Ballard Score.
3. The increase in percentage of persons diagnosed with mental retardation has doubled in the last few years. This is a result of:
   - A. increased toxic materials released into the environment.
   - B. new technology available for diagnostic purposes (ie, genetic screening instruments).
   - C. the change in the definition of mental retardation.
   - D. Public Law 94-142, which assures that appropriate children will be mainstreamed into and tested by the public school system.
4. Multiple factors contribute to the etiology of mental retardation, such as genetic or acquired factors. Some acquired factors may occur as a result of postnatal conditions related to:
   - A. prematurity.
   - B. irradiation during pregnancy.
   - C. chromosomal aberrations.
   - D. childhood disease or accidents.
5. The role of the nurse advocate in caring for a person with mental retardation and related physical disabilities begins with assessment and results in appropriate interventions. Crisis intervention is most often necessary following:
   - A. parents receiving the diagnosis of the child's problems.
   - B. placing the child in a mainstreaming situation.
   - C. respite care.
   - D. outreach team interventions.

◆ References

1. Amado AR: Controversies Concerning the Deinstitutionalization and Community Integration Movement. In Heal W, Haney J, Amado A (eds): Integration of Developmentally Disabled Individuals Into the Community, 2d ed, pp 283–297. Baltimore, MD, Paul H. Brookes, 1988
2. American Association on Mental Retardation: Mental Retardation Definition, Classification and Systems of Support, 9th ed. Washington, DC, American Association on Mental Retardation, 1992
3. American Psychiatric Association: Diagnostic and Statistical Manual of Mental Disorders, 4th ed. Washington, DC, American Psychiatric Association, 1994
4. Anderson D, Jakin K, Hill B, Chen T: Social Integration of Older Persons With Mental Retardation in Residential Facilities. American Journal on Mental Retardation 96 (March): 448–501, 1992
5. Baroff S: Mental Retardation: Nature, Cause and Management, 2d ed. Washington DC, Hemisphere Publishing, 1986
6. Borthwick-Duffy SA, Eyman R: Who Are the Dually Diagnosed? American Journal on Mental Retardation 94 (May): 586–596, 1990
7. Braddock D: Federal Assistance for Mental Retardation and Developmental Disabilities II: The Modern Era. Ment Retard 24 (August): 209–218, 1986
8. Carmichael T, Urban R, Drapo P, Miller O: Developing Clinical Experience for Nursing Students in a Public Sector Setting. Ment Retard 31 (August): 252–255, 1993
9. Dattilo J, Schleien S: Understanding Leisure Services for Individuals With Mental Retardation. Ment Retard 32 (February): 53–59, 1994
10. Davis B, Steele S: Case Management for Young Children With Special Health Care Needs. Pediatr Nurs 17: 15–19, 1991
11. De La Cruz FT: Fragile X Syndrome. Am J Ment Defic 90 (September): 119–123, 1985
12. Drapo P: Feeding the Hospitalized Child With Special Needs. In Smith D, Nix C, Kemper J, Liquori R, Rollins J, Stevens N, Clutter L (eds): Comprehensive Child and Family Nursing Skills, pp 392–399. St. Louis, Mosby Year Book, 1991
13. Drapo P: Selecting Age Related Foods. In Smith D, Nix C, Kemper J, Liquori R, Rollins J, Stevens N, Clutter L (eds): Comprehensive Child and Family Nursing Skills, pp 371–379. St. Louis, Mosby Year Book, 1991
14. Dyson LL: Families of Young Children With Handicaps: Parental Stress and Family Functioning. American Journal on Mental Retardation 95 (May): 613–621, 1991
15. Fisher K, Koch R: Mental Development in Down Syndrome Mosaicism. American Journal on Mental Retardation 96 (November): 345–351, 1991
16. Fraley AM: Chronic Sorrow: A Parental Response. J Pediatr Nurs 5 (August): 268–273, 1990
17. Gabriel S: The Developmentally Disabled, Psychiatrically Impaired Client. J Psychosoc Nurs 32 (September): 35–39, 1994
18. Judkins BL, Coyner A, Harrison A: Education of Nurses in Mental Retardation: National Survey of National League for Nursing Accredited Baccalaureate Nursing Programs in the United States (HEW Special Training Grant 1D10 NU 02012-01). Unpublished manuscript, University of Utah, Salt Lake City, 1979
19. Lederer JR, Marculescue GL, Mocnik B, Seaby N: Care Planning Pocket Guide: A Nursing Diagnosis Approach, 4th ed. Fort Collins, CO, Addison-Wesley, 1991
20. MacMillan D, Greshom F, Siperstein G: Conceptual and Psychometric Concerns About the 1992 AAMR Definition of Mental Retardation. American Journal on Mental Retardation 98 (November): 325–335, 1993
21. McElhinney T, Lajkowicz C: The New Genetics and Nursing Education. Nursing and Health care 15 (December): 528–531, 1994
22. McKusic V, Froncomano C, Antonarokis S, Pearson P: Mendelian Inheritance in Man: A Catalog of Human Genes and Genetic Disorders, 11th ed. Baltimore, Johns Hopkins University Press, 1994
23. Menolascino FJ: Challenges in Mental Retardation: Progressive Ideology and Services. New York, Human Sciences Press, 1977
24. Moore MK: Who Is the Nurse Working With Individuals Called "Developmentally Disabled"? Michigan Nurse 61 (January): 8–9, 1988
25. Nehring WM: Historical Look at Nursing in the Field of Mental Retardation in the United States. Ment Retard 29 (October): 259–267, 1991
26. Parsons J, Hourcade J, Brimberry R: The Nature and Incidence of Mental Illness in Mentally Retarded Individuals. In Menolascino F, Starks J (eds): Handbook on Mental Illness in the Mentally Retarded, pp 3–44. New York, Plenum Press, 1990
27. Reiss S: Prevalence of Dual Diagnosis in Community-based Day Programs in the Chicago Metropolitan Area. American Journal on Mental Retardation 94 (May): 578–585, 1990
28. Reschly D: Adaptive Behavior. Tallahassee, FL, Department of Education, 1987
29. Rogers RC, Simensen RJ: Fragile X Syndrome: A Common Etiology of Mental Retardation. Ment Retard 91 (March): 445–449, 1987
30. Shapiro B: Normal and Abnormal Development: Mental Retardation. In Batshaw M, Perret Y (eds): Children With Disabilities: A Medical Primer, 3d ed. Baltimore, Paul H. Brookes, 1992
31. Spreat S, Telles JL, Conroy JW, Feinstein C, Colombatto JJ: Attitudes Toward Deinstitutionalization: National Survey of Families of Institutionalized Persons With Mental Retardation. Ment Retard 25 (October): 267–274, 1987
32. Texas Department of Mental Health and Mental Retardation: Strategic Plan Fiscal Years 1995–1999. Austin, TX, Texas Department of Mental Health and Mental Retardation, 1995
33. Zetlin A, Murtaugh M: Whatever Happened to Those With Borderline IQs? American Journal on Mental Retardation 94 (March): 463–569, 1990
34. Zigler SM, Vaughan-Wrobel BC, Erlen JA: Nursing Process, Nursing Diagnosis, Nursing Knowledge. Norwalk, CT, Appleton-Century-Crofts, 1986

Forensic Psychiatric Nursing

Cindy A. Peternelj-Taylor
Anita G. Hufft

38

For so many years I've stared alone,
At windows barred and walls of stone
Lost in the thought of reality,
That I was condemned from society. . . .
You talk about me behind my back,
In fear if I hear you, I may attack.
You say you've put me, in my place,
You've given me a label, that's hard to erase. . . .
Don't judge me, for mistakes I've made,
Don't run or hide or be afraid!
Try something different, try being nice
I did my time, I paid my price!

Anonymous,
Life Goes On

As a specialty area of psychiatric nursing practice, forensic psychiatric nursing is emerging as one of the most exciting and challenging contemporary developments confronting the nursing profession. Nursing practice in this domain is accountable to the public and reflects the social and political convictions of the society at large.

This chapter provides a brief history of the evolution of forensic psychiatric nursing, a description of the population served by this specialty group of nurses, and the settings in which forensic psychiatric nurses are employed. The social and cultural factors contributing to incarceration and critical factors affecting those in custody are also explored. More importantly, however, this chapter outlines the tremendous opportunities that exist for nurses to demonstrate leadership in the provision of mental health care to the forensic client. Offenders present with extraordinarily varied and complex mental health needs; helping offenders to reach their potential is a challenging and rewarding nursing experience.

Learning Objectives

On completion of this chapter, you should be able to accomplish the following:

1. *Describe the historical evolution of the role of the nurse in providing nursing care in the forensic milieu.*
2. *Identify sociocultural and environmental factors contributing to the increase in the forensic population.*
3. *Identify and describe characteristics of the forensic population, addressing the implications for nursing care.*
4. *Describe and discuss health concerns specific to the forensic population.*
5. *Apply the nursing process when caring for a client in a forensic setting.*

◆ Defining Forensic Psychiatric Nursing

Although aspects of forensic psychiatric nursing have been documented in the literature for more than a decade,[1,8,18,52,63] forensic psychiatric nursing as a specialty is rapidly emerging in Britain, Canada, and the United States.[9,30,50] A recent survey by Scales and associates[57] found that nurses working in forensic settings or with clients who were offenders shared distinct and common concerns about legal, ethical, political, administrative, and professional issues. These concerns, and the professional nursing response dictated by them, have strengthened the designation of forensic nursing as a specialty. Forensic psychiatric nursing is slowly gaining momentum as a way to bridge the gap between the criminal justice system and the mental health system.[9,39,50]

Many terms have been used to describe nursing with forensic populations, and generally, they are linked to the setting in which the nurse is employed. Forensic nursing, jail nursing, correctional nursing, and forensic psychiatric nursing are these terms. At one time, forensic nursing simply referred to "the application of psychiatric knowledge to the provision of mental health care to the mentally disordered offender"[52] (p 26). More recently, Scales and associates[57] defined the forensic nurse "as one who practices in a facility or program where the primary mission is the evaluation and treatment of mentally ill offenders" (p 40). In an attempt to clarify the scope of forensic nursing practice, the International Association of Forensic Nurses, founded in 1992, has defined the role of the forensic nurse more globally to include nurses working with victims, perpetrators, and their families.[38] See Box 38-1 for additional resources about forensic nursing.

For the purposes of this chapter, the forensic psychiatric nurse is one who integrates psychiatric mental health nursing philosophy and practice within a sociocultural context that includes the criminal justice system to provide comprehensive care to individual clients, their families, and communities. As crime and violence continue to escalate in society, all psychiatric nurses, regardless of setting, will need forensic knowledge and skills. Crime is an issue that transcends individual and family boundaries and must be viewed as a societal problem. Therefore, principles of psychiatric nursing are applicable to any setting in which criminal behavior and mental health problems occur.[7,10,39,23]

◆ Historical Highlights

Until the late 1960s, care for the mentally ill in prisons was generally nonexistent, and few nurses were employed by correctional systems.[25,50,62] A shortage of staff to evaluate and supervise behavior of the mentally ill offender was compounded by an absence of educational programs appropriate for those with mental or emotional disabilities. Health care officers, unprepared to practice professional nursing, carried out a wide range of duties, such as medication administration to control rather than treat the client. Any psychiatric services that were available focused on diagnosis, not treatment.[5,62]

It was not until the late 1960s that the mental health needs of the incarcerated individual began to be explored from a social and political perspective that was open to penal reform. During the 1970s, interest in ensuring adequate health care for inmates was growing. Solutions included implementation of specific programs for drug abuse, introduction of medical students to prisons and jails, and development of standards. Pro-

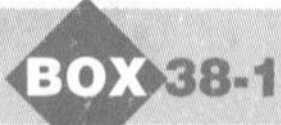

Additional Resources

1. *Standards for Nursing Practice in Correctional Facilities*
   Available from: American Nurses Association
   600 Marilyn Ave SW
   Washington, DC 20024-2571
   (202) 554-4444
   Fax: (202) 554-2262
2. International Association of Forensic Nurses
   Information available from: Debi Maines
   IAFN National Office
   6900 Thorofare, NJ 08086-9447
   (609) 848-8356 ext. 339
   Fax: (609) 848-5274
   Email: iafn@slackinc.com

grams met with varying degrees of success, and their shortcomings were attributed primarily to insufficient funding. In 1975, the Law Enforcement Assistance Administration provided a grant to the American Medical Association to develop health care delivery systems for correctional settings.[5] By 1981, many changes occurred: Model health care delivery systems were designed, health care standards were developed, literature on correctional health care emerged, training programs were delivered, conferences were convened, and an accreditation system spread throughout the United States.[4]

Following many years of unresolved debate regarding the care and treatment of the mentally ill in the Canadian correctional system, the Chalke report, published in 1972, recommended that the federal correctional system develop a unified psychiatric service that was sensitive to the needs of the forensic population and comparable to the community standard. Specialized psychiatric-mental health services are available in each of the five penitentiary regions of Canada. Health care centers exist in all of the provincial correctional facilities, and most often, psychiatric services are under contract with local mental health resources. However, longstanding discrepancies surrounding the delivery of mental health care to offenders within the correctional service of Canada continue to challenge authorities to provide services and programs that best suit the needs of forensic clients.[13,15,25,62]

CONTINUUM OF FORENSIC SETTINGS

Today, the settings in which forensic psychiatric nursing occurs are many and varied. This diversity includes a continuum of controlled environments that may be a part of the mental health system, the criminal justice system, or both. Great variations exist not only between countries, but also within countries. Nurses may be employees of highly specialized, secure mental health facilities, or more commonly, mental health services may be offered from hospitals or small health care centers within a correctional institution. Forensic settings include hospitals for the "criminally insane," state psychiatric hospitals, and locked units in general hospitals; however, the traditional practice site has been jails and prisons (state, regional, provincial, and federal).[3,9,19,34,37,50,53]

◆ Factors Contributing to Incarceration

Currently, the United States has the highest rate of incarceration in the western world. In 1994, the Department of Justice reported that nearly 1 million men and women were incarcerated in state and federal prisons.[14] Many factors contribute to the burgeoning forensic population, including increased rates of incarceration for illegal drug-related activities, increased interpersonal and urban violence, anticrime legislation, poor economic conditions and associated homelessness, and perhaps most tragically, the failure of deinstitutionalization.[30,36,50,56]

DEINSTITUTIONALIZATION

For many seriously and persistently mentally ill individuals, the realities of deinstitutionalization are unduly painful. Reeder and Meldman[54] conclude that "the jail has become the mental hospital that can't say no" (p 41). The phenomenon of the "criminalization of the mentally ill''[11] is a direct result of the deinstitutionalization movement that began in the 1950s, reached its peak in the 1970s, and continues today. Unfortunately, the ongoing lack of community-based services relevant to the needs of the chronically mentally ill client has resulted in a fragmented mental health care system. Many individuals are unable to access appropriate treatment and ultimately experience the ''revolving door syndrome'' that includes the courts, jails, and prisons.[8,11,28,30,42,64]

HOMELESSNESS

Coupled with deinstitutionalization is the problem of homelessness. The chronically mentally ill account for approximately one-third of the homeless population. These individuals are especially vulnerable to the influence of, and exploitation by, criminals and drug abusers. Their vulnerability to stress, lack of structure and support systems, constant exposure to the elements, and persistently poor decision making contribute to episodes with the criminal justice system.[58]

◆ Characteristics of the Forensic Client

Forensic clients present with complex and multifaceted issues, further complicated by the environmental and social factors unique to the forensic milieu. Factors to be taken into account when working with the forensic population include prevalence of mental disorder, cultural and demographic variations, and the needs of special at-risk groups, including women.[15,19,37]

The forensic clientele, as a group, demonstrate poor judgment, limited reasoning abilities, and a history of not learning from past mistakes.[19,30] There is also an exceptionally high level of substance abuse; drug offenders accounted for 61% of sentenced inmates in Federal prisons in 1993.[44] However, the inaccurate caricature of the mentally ill offender as a crazed psychotic killer has adversely influenced effective treatment planning for the forensic population. Depending on the setting, jurisdiction, geographical location, and facilities available, the population may include suspects or those convicted of a crime, those who are sentenced or unsentenced, those who are not guilty by reason of insanity or incompetent to stand trial, and those not criminally responsible due to mental disorder. As a result of this wide variation, nurses need to be informed regarding the laws and legal provisions governing the jurisdiction in which they find themselves.

THE MENTALLY ILL OFFENDER

For nurses working within the field of forensic psychiatric nursing, the predominant client group is the mentally disordered offender. A review of the research suggests that in any prison or jail population, at least 6% to 15% of those incarcerated will be designated as mentally disordered and require services usually associated with severe or chronic mental illness. As a rule, Diagnostic and Statistical Manual of Mental Disorders, fourth edition, diagnoses are easily identified; schizophrenia, mood disorders, and organic syndromes with psychotic features are common.[5,9,15,32] Psychotic presentations are often complicated by the coexistence of personality disorder and substance abuse. Many of these individuals self-medicate with drugs and alcohol.[32,49,50] Nurses need to be alert to assessing substance abuse in the forensic clients, because many clients continue to abuse illegal substances while incarcerated.

The young age of most of the mentally ill in prisons presents a set of characteristics distinct from other settings and contributes to the special nature of forensic psychiatric nursing. This subgroup is characterized by a tendency to be involved in illicit drug use, have a history of dropping out of treatment, be more violent, and resist viewing themselves as mentally ill [32](Case Study 38-1).

THE VIOLENT OFFENDER

In forensic settings, nurses work with clients with a proven capacity for violence, and although staff injuries are rare, violence is generally considered an occupational hazard.[30,49,53] Psychiatric clients in the prison setting often display maladaptive and inappropriate behavior, along with potential for dangerous and violent acts.

Studies of violence among prison inmates reveal two major categories of violent offenders–those with expressive violence and those with instrumental violence. *Expressive violence* involves interpersonal altercations, usually with people who are known to the assailant and are of similar age, ethnicity, and cultural background. Acts of *instrumental violence* are premeditated and unusually motive driven, committed to acquire property or for economic gain, and usually involve people who are unknown to each other and have dissimilar backgrounds. A third type of violence emerging from the forensic literature is gang violence, which is associated with group membership and is committed for retaliation or revenge.[35,59,65] Group alliances lead to gang violence, and typical victims, or those who are particularly vulnerable or at risk, are sexual offenders, those who have offended against children, and those with mental illness and or physical and mental handicaps.

Case Study

A Forensic Client

Tracy Edmonds, RN, Staff Nurse, Regional Psychiatric Centre, Correctional Service of Canada, Saskatoon, Saskatchewan

GH, 42 years old, has had a long history of antisocial acting-out behavior, coupled with longstanding difficulties in getting along with people. He had a troubled childhood. His father was an alcoholic who was often verbally and physically abusive. He had many difficulties with schoolwork and had to repeat grade four. At age 11, the courts ordered him to spend time in a closed custody facility for juveniles, because his parents were unable to provide the supervision he required. His initial feelings of loss and rejection were quickly replaced with feelings of anger and hatred. Reports indicated that he had a "short fuse" and often responded to others in a physically aggressive manner.

On release from the juvenile facility, he cut off all communication with family members and felt some satisfaction that he was inflicting his pain and loss on his family. He was bounced from foster home to foster home, primarily because of his acting-out behavior. His problems with school continued, and he eventually ran away to a large urban center far from his home. With no education and no job skills, he quickly found himself involved in criminal activities—robbery, drugs, and prostitution. He blamed the world for all his pain and suffering, lashing out at anyone who tried to get close to him. He experienced a great sadness, but could not cry.

In his late teens, he found himself in an experimental treatment group, following an involuntary admission to a psychiatric facility. The material presented in this group was far beyond his level of comprehension, and his feelings of powerlessness were soon replaced with a controlling coping style. He believed that if he could control everyone, then everything would be okay.

Following treatment, he further isolated himself from others. He would not let anyone get close to him for fear of getting hurt again. He began to drink heavily and do drugs as a way of numbing and self-medicating his depressive symptoms. His thoughts became more and more irrational, and he believed that the only way of dealing with his feelings of vulnerability was to hurt others before they could hurt him.

By age 20, his longstanding difficulties in getting along with others, coupled with a serious substance abuse problem, culminated in an indefinite sentence for a murder of which he had no recollection. Initially, he had no feelings about serving time for the rest of his life. Two years passed before he began to question his future; by then, he had abused alcohol, marijuana, cocaine, LSD, morphine, and opiates. For the next 13 years of his life, he was an angry and hateful man. He made numerous suicide and self-mutilation attempts and is constantly reminded by his scarred body. He lived one day at a time; his formula for success was morphine and opiates.

Drugs gave GH a sense of power and control. He sold drugs to make money in prison, which in turn gave him a sense of power. He was almost always "high" on something, which gave him a temporary sense of control over his emotions and environment. He began to realize that he had feelings of depression and turned to the health care center for prescribed antidepressants. When medication failed to "solve all his problems" he would turn to illicit substances for a temporary fix. He was in a vicious cycle of drugs, depression, and detoxification.

After serving 20 years in prison, GH states he has matured and is ready to lead a more prosocial lifestyle. He entered a specialized treatment program designed to deal with dual diagnosis and is beginning to deal with some of the feelings he has ignored for most of his life. He states that he will never be able to forgive himself for what he has done to himself and those around him, particularly the victim of his crime.

Questions for Discussion

1. What factors have contributed to his present circumstances?
2. What is his most immediate problem?
3. Is he a danger to himself or others? Why or why not?
4. In planning one-to-one therapy with GH, what issues or problems might the nurse encounter?

SPECIAL POPULATIONS

In general, special needs populations include women, the elderly, the culturally diverse, and more recently, clients with human immunodeficiency virus (HIV) or acquired immunodeficiency syndrome (AIDS). When working with these clients, mental health services must relate to the unique needs and concerns common to the population, in addition to the mission or mandate of the facility.[15,19]

Female Offenders

The most dramatic change in the forensic population is the increase in the number of women who are incarcerated. Trends among women offenders indicate increased incidence of those with personality disorders, substance abuse, and post-traumatic stress disorder. It is not unusual for these offenders to be victims and perpetrators of crime, often having experienced physical, emotional, and sexual abuse.[8,19,37]

The Elderly Offender

The "greying population" in many facilities has resulted in the need to make special adaptations to accommodate the growing number of elderly clients who find themselves in correctional settings. Elderly forensic clients in many ways are no different from their nonforensic counterparts and have many life issues (complicated by the correctional milieu) that need to be addressed. In addition to problems with mental health, the elderly are also more prone to the debilitating effects of chronic illness and as a rule, require more services for physical illnesses.[37]

HIV and AIDS

Issues raised by HIV and AIDS in the prison are not only controversial, but a challenge to the administrative and clinical management in forensic settings. The incidence of HIV and AIDS is higher in the correctional system than in the general public, primarily due to the high risk behaviors common to the forensic population. Tattooing, ear and body piercing, sexual activity, and intravenous drug use are common in the forensic milieu. Often, lower functioning clients have limited understanding of how to keep themselves safe and are vulnerable to exploitation by other, higher functioning clients. Availability of condoms, bleach, and needle exchange are recommended preventive measures; unfortunately, policies vary greatly in regard to these recommendations and are not the norm in many jurisdictions. Palliative care for clients with HIV and AIDS in the prison setting is a growing trend, particularly in areas where early release for compassionate reasons is prohibited.[16,37]

Cultural Minorities

Ethnic minorities may require special consideration in the forensic setting. Minority groups are disproportionately represented in most North American correctional facilities. Specific ethnic groups may predominate, and traditional psychiatric practices are often incompatible with cultural beliefs. Cultural implications need to be considered when providing mental health care.[8,19,37]

In many ways, the nature of client concerns in the correctional milieu are no different than those in more traditional health care settings. However, the impact of the controlled environment can create many barriers to care, and nurses must be cognizant of the problems unique to the clients with whom they are working.

◆ Effects of Incarceration on Mental Health

In addition to offenders who enter the correctional system with a mental disorder, forensic psychiatric nurses care for individuals who become mentally ill while incarcerated. The restrictive and punitive nature of most forensic settings presents a variety of stressors that demand more adaptation than many individuals can handle.[11,49]

Forensic clients, both with and without mental illness, are affected by the conditions in which they live every day. Creating a healing therapeutic environment in a forensic setting is a challenge to health care professionals and administrators. The physical setting, client population, and authoritarian interpersonal environment result in forensic settings being identified as the most extreme and stressful known to society.[30,53] Fletcher and associates[21] conclude that when these factors are taken into consideration, it is amazing to think that offenders can survive at all, let alone with their faculties intact. See Table 38-1 for a summary of stressors in the forensic setting.

Correctional facilities experience many challenges when caring for disadvantaged offenders. The chronically mentally ill, the mentally retarded, those with brain damage, or those lacking social skills or physical strength are cruelly abused by other inmates (especially among the male population) and endure torment, beatings, and sexual assault. The safety of these vulnerable populations presents ongoing dilemmas for prison administrators, who often find it necessary to confine individuals to segregation or protective custody units. Unfortunately, this can be counterproductive, leading to further decompensation of the client's mental illness.[13,49,50,64]

Table 38-1

Stressors to Mental Health in the Forensic Setting

Stressors That Affect the Client	Stressors That Affect the Nurse
Overcrowding	Actual or implied threats of violence
Double stigmatization	Constant barrage of swearing
Grief, isolation, loneliness	Need to be constantly on guard for manipulation
Gang violence	Dual responsibility of providing custody and caring
Inmate violence, stabbing, beating, sexual assault	Role confusion and ambiguity
	Professional isolation
Deteriorating living conditions	Stigma: "second class nurse"
Lack of privacy	Institutionalization
Forced isolation	
Protective custody	
Segregation	

◆ Role of the Nurse in the Forensic Setting

The priorities of the correctional system center on confinement and security, and these principles dictate the boundaries within which the forensic psychiatric nurse must function. Unlike nurses working in other settings, psychiatric nurses working in correctional institutions have two primary responsibilities: health care provider and correctional officer. Role ambiguity and role confusion between health care professionals and correctional officers are common in forensic environments, often the result of overlapping and conflicting expectations.[1,30,50] In 1985, the American Nurses Association[3] published *Standards of Nursing Practice in Correctional Facilities* in response to the growing number of nurses working in this specialty area.

Security standards must be maintained to provide a safe working environment for staff and clients, and much of the nurse's time is spent attending to issues related to the therapeutic milieu and security.[27,30,50,53] This dual responsibility, often referred to as custody and caring, can lead to increased self-esteem and accomplishment for the nurse who masters the inherent dilemmas between the two philosophies and achieves professional resolution and personal understanding. More commonly, however, nurses perceive this as a source of stress and role conflict.[27,30]

The correctional environment is not suited to all nurses, nor is it appropriate for all student nurse placements. Nurses working in correctional institutions must have good communication skills, be able to work within a team structure, and possess physical and psychological assessment skills. Furthermore, other essential attributes include professionalism, confidence, nonjudgmental attitudes, ability to work independently, decisiveness, and ability to work in a secure environment. Personal characteristics such as stability, integrity, assertiveness, maturity, and friendliness are viewed favorably by educational facilities and the correctional agencies.[18,45,49,52]

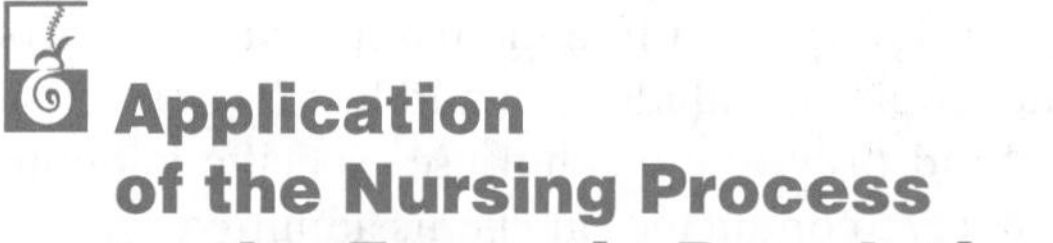

Application of the Nursing Process to the Forensic Population

The essence of nursing in the forensic setting is modified by the impact of the distinctive environment. Special adaptations are necessary to achieve professional standards and personal goals.[30,34,45,50]

ASSESSMENT

Regardless of the clinical practice setting, all forensic psychiatric nurses have a significant role to play in the observation and assessment of the forensic client.

The context of care can facilitate or hamper the nurse's ability to provide the necessary services for the mentally ill offender. Marx[40] reports that problems are related to assessing clients in isolation of their support systems, home environments, and daily routines, because in the forensic setting, the client is closely supervised, and behavior is restricted and mandated by the institutional policies. Assessment and diagnosis of the forensic client are further complicated by the physical environment and lack of privacy. Security concerns affect every aspect of nursing function in the practice of forensic nursing and can often complicate the creation of a therapeutic relationship.[9,33,61,66] Often interview rooms are completely glassed in to allow for maximum observation of the nurse who is conducting the assessment. These rooms are soundproof, but all can see inside, conflicting the right to privacy and confidentiality that is common to the psychiatric nurse–client relationship. Many clients may not want to be identified with the forensic psychiatric nurse because of the stigma associated with mental illness in prisons.[49,50] At times, correctional personnel are required to be present, and this further complicates the assessment process because clients are reluctant to disclose in front of security personnel.

Content of Assessment

In the correctional setting, mental health questions must be included as part of receiving, screening, and follow-up health history of every offender. Comprehensive assessments help to identify the needs of the client, particularly those in need of immediate care and treatment. Additionally, a separate mental health screening and evaluation process is performed on all admissions to mental health facilities or treatment centers to identify level of functioning and uncover less obvious mental conditions.[5]

Assessments in the forensic setting should include at the minimum a history of psychiatric illness, hospitalization and outpatient treatment, current psychotropic medication, suicidal ideation and history of suicidal behavior, and drug and alcohol use. Specific in-depth assessments are conducted on clients admitted for special programming, for example, sexual offenders, psychopathic offenders, and clients with anger management disorders or intermittent explosive disorder.[3,5,49,50]

Critical information needed for planning nursing care with the forensic client in a treatment setting often involves reviewing police reports, correctional files, and previous mental health records. Crime histories and history of aggression are essential components to the assessment of the offender.[23,37]

The most critical skill of the forensic psychiatric nurse is the ability to estimate the risk of violence in a client. Anticipatory planning and prevention are mediated through the teaching role of the nurse. The preventive role includes identifying risk factors for each client and developing an individualized care plan.[9]

Risk of Suicide in Forensic Settings

The incidence of self-violence and suicide in correctional settings is higher than that in the general population, with the suicide rate for people in custody at least six times that of the general population. The assessment of the high-risk client is not always easy because the staff-to-inmate ratio in many forensic settings, particularly within correctional facilities, prisons, and penitentiaries, does not allow for opportunities for observation by nursing staff. At times, correctional staff may be reluctant or skeptical of an inmate's presenting features, knowing of the tendency of inmates to feign general symptoms of illness to spend time in the less stressful environment of the hospital wing. However, strict guidelines for accurate and timely assessment of suicide risk are imperative. Unrestricted access to psychiatric care must be available for any offender presenting with suicidal ideation or at-risk behaviors.[10,29,60] A study conducted in New Zealand revealed a significant increase in suicide among the inmate population when unrestricted access to psychiatric hospitalization was abolished.[60]

Factors contributing to the significantly higher rate of suicide in the forensic population include history of a psychiatric illness, substance abuse, difficulties facing the crime and the length of the sentence, actual or perceived victimization by other offenders, inability to cope within a confined environment, and lack of communication with family.[10,29] Alexander-Rodriguez[1] reports that a correlation exists between increases in prison populations and increases in the rates of suicide. This is particularly noteworthy because of the overcrowding that is a growing reality in most forensic settings; it is not uncommon for facilities to house two or three individuals in rooms originally designed for a single person.[8,9] Green and associates[24] observed that regardless of the length of the sentence, the first 6 months after sentencing represent a particularly high-risk period.

Suicide (or attempted suicide) in the forensic setting must be followed by a full debriefing. Forensic psychiatric nurses have a role to play as facilitators and provide leadership for group processing of the event. This should include a meeting of all those who were on duty (or in the proximity during the incident) and at least one professional person removed from the incident. During this meeting, participants should be encouraged to describe their knowledge of the client and their feelings as they relate to the client's behavior. If the suicide occurred within a treatment or mental health facility, the other clients should also have the opportunity to debrief with the staff for therapeutic reasons and to prevent cluster suicides.[13] The staff and client debriefing should be done in a trusting, accepting environment. The objective of debriefing for staff is to allow them to grieve and reflect, to put the incident into perspective and continue with their work. This is also an opportunity to assess whether staff are able to cope with the incident and whether they are in need of individual counselling to resolve their feelings toward the client and perhaps toward suicide in prison in general.

NURSING DIAGNOSIS

As psychiatric clients, the forensic client falls into well-established categories of psychiatric disorders and nursing diagnoses. Common North American Nursing Diagnosis Association nursing diagnoses relevant to the forensic population are listed below:

- Ineffective Individual Coping
- Fear
- Dysfunctional Grieving
- Noncompliance
- Post-Trauma Response
- Chronic Low Self-Esteem
- Risk for Self-Mutilation
- Sleep Pattern Disturbance
- Sensory/Perceptual Alterations
- Impaired Social Interaction
- Social Isolation
- Risk for violence: Self-directed or directed at others

PLANNING

In planning, for any treatment program with forensic clients, the nurse must take into account the realities and limitations of the setting. Working knowledge of the operation of the correctional environment, the inmate subculture, and the culture of secure or controlled environments is essential to plan nursing care for this needy population.[50,63]

Planning short-term goals, which frequently involve completion of tasks and the practice of selected communication or self-care skills, must revolve around the mandatory regimens set up for the offender. In many settings, group therapy is in conflict with the work assignments mandated by the prison. The structured environment, which includes work details, lock-ups, formal counting of offenders, and endless security procedures, makes planning difficult. Nevertheless, it is important to set up manageable, feasible goals to achieve outcomes that bring the offender to a higher level of functioning, regardless of the environment. The challenge to the forensic nurse is to be sensitive to scheduled assignments that can be changed and those that cannot. Planning also requires attention to the processes that allow for continuity. It is not unusual for clients to be transferred from facility to facility, often without their health records. Whenever possible, planning should include the active participation of the client in the identification of realistic and attainable goals.

Long-term goals must be consistent with the reality of the client's circumstances. It is unrealistic to plan for re-entry to the community for a client with a life sentence. Often it is important to acknowledge that long-term goals, such as developing trusting relationships with peers and staff, may be totally unrealistic (Table 38-2).

INTERVENTION

Therapeutic Alliance

The trials and tribulations of forming therapeutic relationships with forensic clients are well known to forensic psychiatric nurses. Therapy issues with this population can be stressful and complicated. The cultural and ideological variations that exist between correctional personnel, inmates, and helping professionals must be considered and carried out when navigating the counseling role in forensic settings.[50,52,56] Recurring themes of power and control, trust building, and negotiating the relationship dominate therapeutic interventions in this setting.

Trust and rapport are generally deemed critical to the initiation and maintenance of a therapeutic relationship. However, clients in forensic settings have in varying degrees learned to adapt to an environment that rewards distrust, manipulation, and deceit.[2,50,56] Relationships are often dubious at best and easily broken. The nurse may be viewed as a confidante when requests are approved, or as a member of a much hated system

Table 38-2

Levels of Prevention in Forensic Settings

Primary Intervention	Secondary Intervention	Tertiary Intervention
Mental health promotion Classification of stressors Political involvement Appropriate referrals Provision of education and information Advocacy	Assessment, evaluation, diagnosis Crisis intervention Program planning and implementation Substance abuse treatment Sex offender treatment Aggressive behavior control Life and social skills training Acute inpatient psychiatric nursing Suicide prevention and management Psychotropic medication management Short-term therapy Counseling, psychotherapy	Case management After-care services Rehabilitation Vocational training Relapse prevention

if requests are denied.[13] Time, patience, and consistency are the key ingredients to the successful navigation of the therapeutic relationship with offender clients.[49,50,56]

The nature and boundaries of the professional nurse–client relationship are clearly an issue for forensic psychiatric nurses. All relationships have the potential for boundary violations; however, in the forensic setting, issues and problems surrounding transference and countertransference are an occupational hazard. Institutions are "ripe" for potential problems arising around issues of boundary violation and exploitation.[50,52]In the forensic setting, psychiatric nurses are always on guard for the meaning of communication and constantly questioning or validating the motives of the forensic client.

Often students and novice nurses have a hard time dealing with the sometimes sexually explicit remarks or compliments made by forensic clients, and instead of acknowledging the compliment or confronting the behavior, they withdraw. Nurses may be unsure how to respond to these "come ons." Allen and Bosta[2] observe that a simple "thank you" (generally accompanied by a blush) is not sufficient to get the message across to a client, and the offender will likely continue to express the compliment more often and in a more brazen manner. A more appropriate response stated in a matter-of-fact tone of voice is recommended: "Thank you for the compliment, but I would appreciate that from this point on, you keep your comments to yourself. Your remarks are irrelevant to my purpose with working with you."

Many clients have been incarcerated for long periods and have been in and out of foster homes or jails for a good part of their lives. As a result, forming relationships is difficult. Once a therapeutic relationship is established, clients often incorrectly perceive the nurse's warmth and concern as love and intimacy. When responding to compliments, a simple "thank you" may be misconstrued and interpreted as a sign that the nurse likes the attention and wants the client to continue. Additionally, no response or a silent response is interpreted as approval of the compliment or gesture. Any inappropriate responses by the client need to be confronted verbally "I'm not here to discuss my eyes, hair, or body," followed by documentation in the client's chart. Excessive familiarity is out of line, and clients generally are well aware of the rules but test them anyway, hoping to "catch" any unwary victim.[2,50,51,52]

Health Promotion

The belief that health care is a basic human right is critical to the forensic psychiatric nurse.[34] The scope of nursing practice includes health education and health promotion. Unfortunately, during times of fiscal restraint, nurses are increasingly preoccupied with acute care, with limited resources or time directed to the promotion of mental health. The needs of the target population, specifically the forensic client, need to be defined and delineated to provide a comprehensive mental health strategy in the forensic setting. Traditional mental health care has focused on highly specialized facilities, concentrating on a relatively narrow group of offenders.

Nurses in forensic settings are also responsible for mental health and wellness promotion. To promote health in the forensic setting, the nurse needs to be cognizant of the fact that by improving the opportunities for the highest level of physical, psychosocial, and social functioning, clients are in a "catch-22" position, because the skills to survive in prison are not the same as those required to survive on the street.[30]

General health promotion in correctional settings is an important vehicle for targeting specific mental health goals. Women offenders, in particular, are interested in their own health, and a discussion about contraception and birth control can be an opportunity to express feelings related to abuse, powerlessness, or social awkwardness. Because so many emotional issues are involved in the everyday experiences of offenders, the correctional setting is one in which all nurses and health care staff should either have psychiatric skills or have access to mentoring by other psychiatric-mental health nurses.

Stress management is not just a health promotion strategy in the correctional setting, it is a real life skill. Almost all inmates have poor coping skills and experience high levels of stress. Programs that promote adaptation and coping in selected situations may translate into life skills that allow for more effective rehabilitation.

Interdisciplinary Approach to Care

Teamwork is essential to working in forensic environments. Communication among nurses, other health care professionals, and the correctional personnel is vital to safe and professional practice.[50] Staff support and education is an important and often undervalued role of the forensic psychiatric nurse. The cross-training required of an interdisciplinary approach to forensic health treatment necessitates sharing knowledge of therapeutic modalities, while incorporating professional standards of practice.[22] Neither nurses nor other correctional employees acting on their own can resolve the complex issues confronting the needs of the forensic clientele.[50]

Many different health care providers staff the mental health services in prison settings, sometimes provided by contract and other times through a consulting arrangement. Regardless of the staffing arrangement, all members of the mental health care team work together as peers to deliver high-quality care consistent with the community standard. In correctional settings, the security personnel are also a part of the team, and information sharing is vital. Correctional personnel need to be informed when suicidal, homicidal, or out of control behavior is suspected or of concern.[56]

Nurses who work in this setting are challenged to participate in a creative delivery model that prioritizes client care, eliminating the importance of individual titles and professional boundary setting. Although the potential for territoriality is a reality, the most successful client outcomes are achieved when team members share a common philosophy—professionalism in providing security and quality health care to those in custody.[30]

Continuity of Care

Continuity of care is virtually nonexistent for offenders once they leave the forensic or treatment setting, and many mentally ill offenders experience high rates of recidivism, high symptom levels, and a poor quality of life.[32,37,53]

Little opportunity exists for long-term case management or discharge planning among clients who are eventually released from prison. The life skills learned to survive in prison may conflict with therapeutic goals. It is difficult to evaluate the progress of an individual client with a view of returning to the community if there are no opportunities to interact with that community.[17,30,41]

Dvoskin and Broaddus[20] have proposed a mental health care model for the efficient and systematic treatment of the mentally ill offender. This approach advocates a seamless continuum of services that includes the prison setting and satellite services within the community, linking correctional and parole staff with community mental health care providers. The underlying premise to this approach is that forensic settings are communities in which people live and work together under the influence of a variety of stressors. This program, designed to address stressors as challenges to community living, provides a framework that bridges the forensic and nonforensic setting. Components of this model include screening and referral, crisis beds, intermediate care (residential care), outpatient services, predischarge planning services, and postrelease services, including mental health, probation, and parole services. Such a system would be ideal for implementing continuity of care; unfortunately, funding and service restrictions make its implementation unlikely.

Advocacy and Political Action

The advocacy role in forensic psychiatric nursing is somewhat different from the role in other settings or in other nursing specialties, because the nurse embraces the destigmatization and decriminalization of the client group. Rehabilitation into the public arena is difficult, particularly due to the public and political antipathy toward offenders.

Traditional principles of advocacy involve informing clients of their choices and rights and then supporting the decision that the client makes. In any psychiatric setting, this standard is controversial; in the forensic setting, it is inflammatory. Client actions and communications are not privileged information, and advocacy standards demand that nurses be honest with clients regarding the fact that disclosure of medical records is a reality, and nurse testimony may be required in any court proceeding against the client. In forensic settings, "nurses in particular constantly 'walk the line' between the requirements of security, health care, and client advocacy"[50] (p 14).

Nurses need to acquaint themselves with policies that affect the forensic population and society as a whole. Supporting policy implementation that is based on well-designed research and questioning policy based on convenience or "conventional wisdom" are appropriate political roles for the nurse.[35]

EVALUATION

To assess the effectiveness of the nursing process in the forensic setting, the nurse must measure client behaviors that indicate resolution or change in the diagnostic criteria, specifically the signs and symptoms that indicated a psychiatric problem. Depending on the client's diagnosis and prognosis, the nurse learns to evaluate the client's outcome in terms of small successes, often "giant steps" for many clients. Change that leads the client to more effective problem solving, demonstrating the ability to reason and show good judgment or to comply with the rules of the institution is a form of success.[56]

Greenwood[26] observes that when measuring effectiveness of treatment outcomes in the forensic setting, the health care professional needs to be cognizant of the definition of forensic mental health treatment that is being used. The goal of mental health treatment is to address a mental disorder, whereas the goal of correctional treatment is to decrease the likelihood of recidivism. It is recognized that these terms are not mutually exclusive, but they do not always work in tandem. When evaluating the effectiveness of treatment, these definitions need to be taken into account. An individual may be dealing well with the mental health problem but may continue to break the law.

In one institution, a female offender was diagnosed with bipolar disorder, a nursing diagnosis of anxiety related to feelings of powerlessness, and inaccurate assessment of her potential to care for her infant. Once stabilized on medication, she entered into counseling with the psychiatric nurse, who developed an educative and cognitive therapy treatment program tailored to the client's needs. This approach included individual and group therapy to develop coping skills necessary on release. Measuring her behaviors and self-appraisal on release confirmed resolution of the problem of low self-esteem, but the woman was back in prison within 3 months as a result of writing bad checks.

The Nurse's Attitudes

Forensic psychiatric nurses care for a population that is frequently stigmatized and stereotyped. Negative attitudes held by nurses toward offender clients essentially inhibit the entire nurse–client relationship. Psychiatric-mental health nurses have traditionally based their nursing practice on the concept of caring. This commitment is not altered by the fact that the individuals receiving care are generally in correctional settings.[3,34]

When the client is a forensic client, the affective response of the nurse is often intensified and can be influenced by the client's mental health background and criminal history. Assessing and exploring common preconceptions, beliefs, and stereotypes (eg, "criminally insane,") help the forensic psychiatric nurse to decrease potential fears, anxieties, and negative attitudes. Participating in a tour, interacting with a client, or observing an experienced nurse in practice are ways to confront thoughts and feelings, verify reality, and overcome natural apprehension to working with the incarcerated client.[49,51]

Ongoing self-reflection and self-awareness on the part of the nurse are essential to successful adaptation to the realities of working with the forensic psychiatric client.[50] Being able to adopt the therapeutic role with forensic clients requires the nurse to "transcend judgmental and prejudicial attitudes toward those who have committed crimes against society"[30] (p 39).

◆ Survival of the Specialty and Professional Growth

Forensic psychiatric nursing is just beginning to emerge as a distinct and valued specialty. The visibility of forensic psychiatric nursing needs to be raised to expose the exciting and rewarding contributions that are made by nurses in forensic settings. Forensic psychiatric nurses need to be active in their practice settings, public lives, and professional organizations to educate others about the exciting developments occurring in forensic settings.[43,50,57] Forensic psychiatric nurses need to ask the following critical questions as they approach the next millenium:

1. What is the future role of the forensic psychiatric nurse?
2. How will the parameters of forensic psychiatric nursing be established?
3. What is the best way to care for the forensic population?

EDUCATION

Lynch[38,39] reports that forensic science is relevant to nursing curricula and that forensic nursing is the most important effort nurses can provide to break the cycle of interpersonal violence. Although there are limited educational opportunities for nurses interested in this specialty area, growing numbers of nurse educators are recognizing the need to include forensic psychiatric nursing content in the curricula of basic nursing education programs.[39,51,57] Peternelj-Taylor and Johnson[51] have examined issues related to the placement of nursing students in forensic psychiatric settings and have found that there are ample opportunities for role modeling by faculty and other professional nurses. Other critical factors to consider when planning for student placement in correctional facilities include the nature of the clinical setting, the amount of time spent in the facility, and the supervision received.

Continuing education and professional development efforts are necessary to provide nurses with ongoing specific and relevant information and are critical to the promotion and advancement of forensic psychiatric nursing as a specialty practice.

◆ Chapter Summary

This chapter has focused on the role of the nurse in providing mental health care to the forensic population. A historical perspective, a description of the population, and the settings in which forensic nurses are employed are identified and discussed. Factors contributing to the increase in the forensic population have been examined from a social and cultural perspective. The nursing process as applied to the care of the forensic client has identified the unique considerations and adaptations necessary in the forensic milieu. Chapter highlights include the following:

1. Forensic psychiatric nursing, often described as the last frontier for nursing, is emerging as a specialty area of the nursing profession. Forensic psychiatric nursing bridges the gap between the criminal justice system and the mental health care system.
2. The care and control of the criminal, the dangerous, and the mentally ill have historically plagued society. Deinstitutionalization, homelessness, in-

creased rates of incarceration for drug-related activities, interpersonal and domestic violence, and anticrime legislation have been attributed to the soaring forensic population.

3. The clients with whom forensic psychiatric nurses work present with extraordinarily varied and complex mental health needs. Clients are young and old, male and female, and often victims and perpetrators of crime. Issues surrounding the mentally ill offender, the substance abusing offender, and the violent offender have been discussed. Problems surrounding the care of special populations, including women, the elderly, ethnic minorities, and those with HIV or AIDS, have been identified.
4. Forensic settings include forensic psychiatric facilities, locked units of general hospitals, and state hospitals. However, the common practice sites are the jail and prison.
5. Legal and ethical issues related to the forensic client are pertinent to forensic psychiatric nursing, and nurses need to be familiar with relevant legislation governing the settings in which they are employed.
6. The application of the nursing process is a familiar role for the forensic nurse but is greatly influenced by the restrictiveness of the controlled environment.
7. Nurses as employees of public sector institutions are accountable to society and experience conflicting convictions as they struggle to balance the concepts of custody and caring.
8. Although the numerous dilemmas and challenges in practice are identified more easily than the rewards, forensic psychiatric nursing is a challenging and rewarding clinical experience.

Critical Thinking Questions

1. *What are the essential attributes necessary to manage the forensic psychiatric nursing role?*
2. *Hall*[28] *proposes that all space is regarded as potentially nurturing or potentially harmful. The forensic milieu is considered "lived space." Can this space lead to healing and personal growth, or does it simply reinforce the client as a criminal, an inmate? How will forensic psychiatric nurses create healing environments within the forensic milieu?*
3. *What does the current practice of incarcerating the mentally ill say about society?*

Review Questions

1. One universal characteristic common to forensic facilities is that they reflect
   - A. the latest health care technology.
   - B. the treatment needs of the population being served.
   - C. the social and political convictions of society.
   - D. the holistic needs of clients and family.
2. One of the largest changes in the composition of the forensic population is associated with
   - A. the mentally ill.
   - B. the amount of women.
   - C. the decrease in the elderly.
   - D. the even number of ethnic people.
3. A nurse is caring for a verbally aggressive forensic client who reminds her of an ex-boyfriend. At the end of the interview, she seeks out an experienced nurse colleague to explore her feelings about this client. The nurse's actions indicate
   - A. inability to cope with the forensic milieu.
   - B. the need for psychotherapy.
   - C. boundary exploitation.
   - D. appropriate self-awareness.
4. One example of the forensic psychiatric nurse's role in primary prevention is
   - A. conducting a relapse prevention group for sexual offenders.
   - B. applying principles of crisis intervention following a suicide attempt.
   - C. developing a medication management program for an offender with schizophrenia.
   - D. participating as a member of a multidisciplinary committee focusing on interpersonal violence.
5. Which of the following risk factors contribute to a higher rate of suicide in forensic populations?
   - A. History of psychiatric illness, difficulties facing the crime, perceived victimization by other offenders
   - B. Actual victimization by other offenders, lack of observation by nursing staff, ability to cope with a confined environment
   - C. Substance abuse, difficulties facing the length of the sentence, open communication with family members
   - D. Men older than 45 years, previous suicide attempts, acceptance of the crime

◆ References

1. Alexander-Rodriguez T: Prison Health—A Role for Professional Nursing. Nursing Outlook 31 (2): 115–118, 1983
2. Allen B, Bosta D: Games Criminals Play. Sacramento, Rae John Publishers, 1993
3. American Nurses Association: Standards of Nursing Practice in Correctional Facilities. Kansas City, MO, American Nurses Association, 1985
4. Anno BJ: The Role of Organized Medicine in Correctional Health Care. JAMA 247 (21): 2923–2925, 1982

5. Anno BJ: Prison health care: Guidelines for the management of an adequate delivery system. Chicago: National Commission on Correctional Health Care, 1991
6. Anonymous: Life Goes on. The John Howard Society of Saskatchewan Newsletter 3, 1995
7. Babich KS: Editorial: More Violence, More Need for Change. J Psychosoc Nurs 31 (4): 5, 1993
8. Bernier SL: Mental Health Issues and Nursing in Corrections. In McFarland GK, Thomas MD (eds): Psychiatric Mental Heath Nursing, pp 693–700. Philadelphia, JB Lippincott, 1991
9. Burrow S: An Outline of the Forensic Nursing Role. British Journal of Nursing 2 (18): 899–904, 1993
10. Burrow S: Suicide: The Crisis in the Prison Service. British Journal of Nursing 4 (4): 215–218, 1995
11. Canadian Nurses Association: Mental Health Care Reform: A Priority for Nurses. Ottawa, Canadian Nurses Association, 1991
12. Canadian Public Health Association: Violence in Society: A Public Health Perspective. Ottawa, Canadian Public Health Association, 1994
13. Conacher GN: Issues in Psychiatric Care Within a Prison Service. Canada's Mental Health 41 (1): 11–15, 1993
14. CorrectCare: Prison Population Reaches New Record. CorrectCare 8 (3): 1, 9, 1994
15. Correctional Service of Canada: Report of the Task Force on Mental Health. Ottawa, Minister of Supply and Services Canada, 1991
16. Correctional Service of Canada: HIV/AIDS in Prisons: Summary Report and Recommendations of the Expert Committee on AIDS and Prisons. Montreal, Minister of Supply and Service Canada, 1994
17. Crawford CA: Health Care Needs in Corrections: NIJ Responds. National Institute of Justice Journal 228: 31–38, 1994
18. Day RA: The Challenge: Health Care vs. Security. The Canadian Nurse 78 (7): 34–36, 1983
19. Dvoskin JA: The Structure of Correctional Mental Health Services. In Rosner R (ed): Principles and Practice of Forensic Psychiatry, pp 380–387. New York, Chapman & Hall, 1994
20. Dvoskin JA, Broaddus R: Creating a Mental Health Care Model. Corrections Today 55 (7): 114–115, 1993
21. Fletcher BR, Shaver LD, Moon D: Women Prisoners: A Forgotten Population. Westport, CT, Praeger Publications, 1993
22. Galindez EA: An Orientation Model for Correctional Health Nursing. Journal of Nursing Staff Development 6 (5): 225–228, 1990
23. Grant CA, Burgess AW, Hartman GR, Burgess AG, Shaw ER, MacFarland G: Juveniles Who Murder: Insights for Intervention. J Psychosoc Nurs 27 (12): 4–11, 1989
24. Green C, Andre G, Kendall K, Looman T, Polvi N: A Study of 133 Suicides Among Canadian Federal Prisoners. Forum on Corrections Research 4 (3): 17–19, 1992
25. Green CM, Menzies RPD, Naismith LJ: Psychiatry in the Canadian Correctional Service. Can J Psychiatry 36: 290–295, 1991
26. Greenwood A: Forensic Mental Health Treatment: Do We Really Know What We Are Talking About? Forum on Correctional Research 7 (3): 27–29, 1995
27. Gulotta KC: Factors Affecting Nursing Practice in a Correctional Health Care Setting. Journal of Prison and Jail Health 6 (1): 3–21, 1987
28. Hall BA: Use of Milieu Therapy: The Context of Environment as Therapeutic Practice for Psychiatric-Mental Health Nurses. In Anderson CA (ed): Psychiatric Nursing 1974 to 1994: A Report on the State of the Art, pp 46–56. St. Louis: Mosby-Year Book, 1995
29. Health Canada: Suicide in Canada. Ottawa, Minister of National Health and Welfare, 1994
30. Hufft AG, Fawkes LS: Federal Inmates: A Unique Psychiatric Nursing Challenge. Nurs Clin North Am 29 (1): 35–42, 1994
31. Jacobs C: "Three strikes" = 30 Years for Mentally Ill Man. NAMI Advocate 16 (5): 3, 12, 1995
32. Jemelka R, Trupin E, Chiles JA: The Mentally Ill in Prisons: A Review. Hosp Community Psychiatry 40: 481–485, 1989
33. Jones-Harris J: Innovative Roles: Nursing Care in Correctional Systems. Addictions Nursing Network 1 (1): 15–17, 1989
34. Kent-Wilkinson A: After the Crime, Before the Trial. The Canadian Nurse 89 (11): 23–26, 1993
35. Labecki LAS: Monitoring Hostility: Avoiding Prison Disturbances Through Environmental Scanning. Corrections Today 56 (5): 104–106, 1994
36. Lego SF: Review of the Book Live From Death Row. Journal of the American Psychiatric Nurses Association 1 (5): 171–174, 1995
37. Lloyd C: Forensic Psychiatry for Health Professionals. London, Chapman & Hall, 1995
38. Lynch VA: Forensic Nursing: Diversity in Practice. J Psychosoc Nurs 31 (11): 7–14, 1993
39. Lynch VA: Editorial: Forensic Nursing: What's New? J Psychosoc Nurs 33 (9): 6–8, 1995
40. Marx G: Prisons Try New Therapies to Treat Sex Offenders. CorrectCare 9 (1): 6, 1995
41. McDonald DC, Teitelbaum M: Managing Mentally Ill Offenders in the Community. Washington, DC, National Institute of Justice: NCJ145330, 1994
42. Milestone C: The Mentally Ill and the Criminal Justice System: Innovative Community-Based Programs. Ottawa, Minister of Supply and Services Canada, 1995
43. Morrison P, Burnard P: Aspects of Forensic Psychiatric Nursing. Brookfield, Averbury, 1992
44. National Criminal Justice Reference Service: Drugs and Crime Facts, 1994. Rockville, MD, ONDCP Drugs and Crime Clearinghouse, 1994
45. Niskala H: Competencies and Skills Required by Nurses Working in Forensic Areas. West J Nurs Res 8 (4): 400–413, 1986
46. Nussbaum D, Lang M, Repaci R: How Forensic Mental Health Staff Cope: Results of a Preliminary Study. Forum on Corrections Research 5 (1): 19–21, 1993
47. Osborne O: Public Sector Psychosocial Nursing. J Psychosoc Nurs 33 (8): 4–6, 1995
48. Peternelj-Taylor CA (Producer), Bulk F (Director): Psychiatric Nursing Practicum in Corrections [Video], 1994

(Available from Division of Audio Visual Services, University of Saskatchewan, 28 Campus Drive, Saskatoon, SK S7N 0X1.)

49. Peternelj-Taylor CA, Johnson RL (Producers), Bulk F (Director): Custody and Caring: A Challenge for Nursing [Video], 1993 (Available from Division of Audiovisual Services, University of Saskatchewan, 28 Campus Drive, Saskatoon, SK S7N 0X1.)
50. Peternelj-Taylor CA, Johnson RL: Serving Time: Psychiatric Mental Health Nursing in Corrections. J Psychosoc Nurs 33 (8): 12–19, 1995
51. Peternelj-Taylor CA, Johnson RL: Custody and Caring: A Unique Partnership in Psychiatric Nursing Education. Perspect Psychiatr Care In press
52. Petryshen P: Nursing the Mentally Ill Offender. The Canadian Nurse 77 (6): 26–28, 1981
53. Phillips RTM, Caplan C: Administrative and Staffing Problems for Psychiatric Services in Correctional and Forensic Settings. In Rosner R (ed): Principles and Practice of Forensic Psychiatry, pp 388–392. New York, Chapman & Hall, 1994
54. Reeder D, Meldman L: Conceptualizing Psychosocial Nursing in the Jail Setting. J Psychosoc Nurs 29 (8): 40–44, 1991
55. Rosenblatt A: Concepts of the Asylum in the Care of the Mentally Ill. Hosp Community Psychiatry 35: 244–250, 1984
56. Rynerson BC: Cops and Counsellors. J Psychosoc Nurs 27 (2): 12–17, 1989
57. Scales CJ, Mitchell JL, Smith RD: Survey Report on Forensic Nursing. J Psychosoc Nurs 31 (11): 39–44, 1993
58. Shenson D, Dubler N, Michaels D: Jails and Prisons: The New Asylums? Am J Public Health 80 (6): 655–656, 1990
59. Sigler RT: Gang Violence. Journal of Health Care for the Poor and Underserved 6 (2): 198–203, 1995
60. Skegg K, Cox B: Impact of Psychiatric Services on Prison Suicide. Lancet 338: 1436–1438, 1991
61. Skiles L, Hinson B: Occupational Burnout Among Correctional Health Workers: Perceived Levels of Stress and Support. American Association of Occupational Health Nursing Journal 37 (9): 374–378, 1989
62. Smale SL: Nursing Behind Bars: A Decade of Change. The Canadian Nurse 78 (7): 31–33, 1983
63. Stevens R: When Your Clients Are in Jail. Nursing Forum 28 (4): 5–8, 1993
64. Torrey EF, Stieber J, Ezekiel J, Wolfe SM, Sharfstein J, Noble JH, Flynn L: Criminalizing the Seriously Mentally Ill: The Abuse of Jails as Mental Hospitals. Innovations and Research 2 (1): 11–14, 1993
65. Visher CA: Understanding the Roots of Crime: The Project on Human Development in Chicago Neighborhoods. National Institute of Justice Journal 228: 9–15, 1994
66. Weinstein HC: Psychiatric Services in Jails and Prisons: Who Cares? Am J Psychiatry 146 (9): 1094–1095, 1989
67. Worth R A Model Prison. The Atlantic Monthly 276 (5): 38–44, 1995

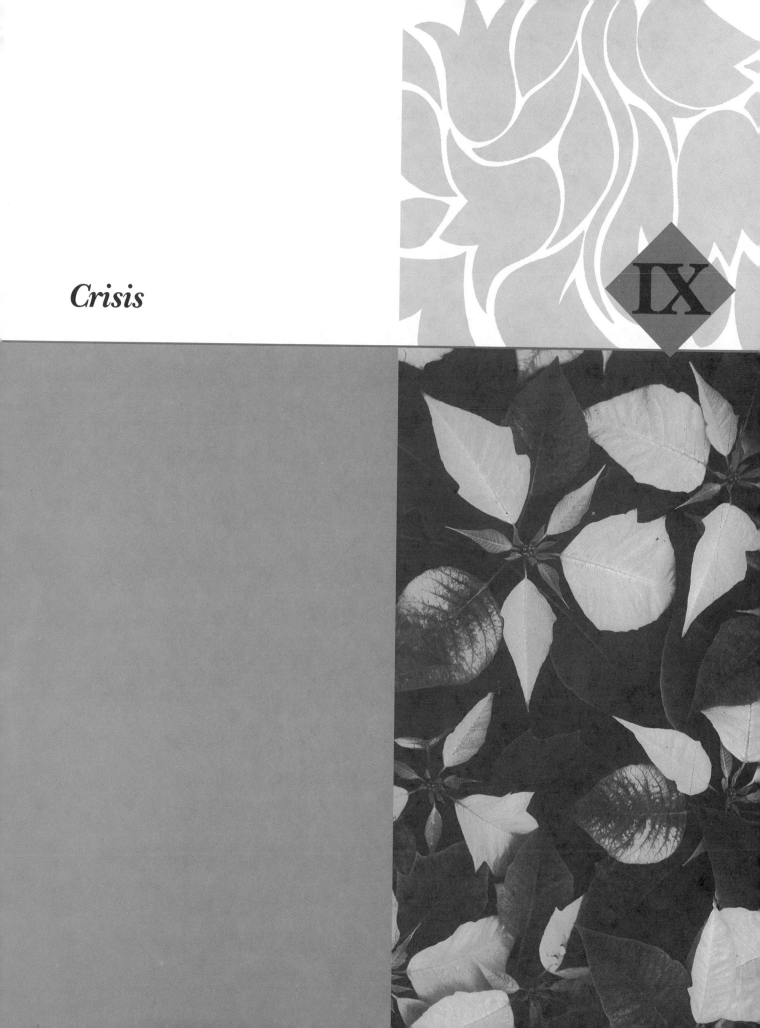

IX

Crisis

Crisis Theory and Intervention

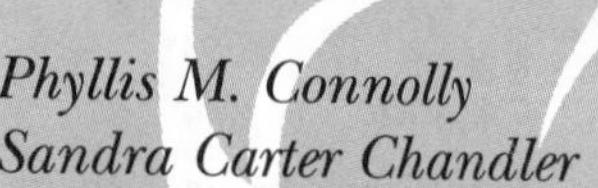

Phyllis M. Connolly
Sandra Carter Chandler

39

A small trouble is like a pebble. Hold it too close to your eyes, and it fills the whole world and puts it out of focus. Hold it at a proper viewing distance, and it can be examined and properly classified. Throw it at your feet, and it can be seen in its true setting, just one more tiny bump on the pathway to eternity.

Celia Luce

Crisis and stress are common words often used interchangeably; however, they are not synonymous. Everyone experiences stressful life events—a new career, prematurely gray hair, the loss of a friend, the acquisition of dentures, and so forth. As long as a person can cope with the stressful event and is not overwhelmed by it, it is not experienced as a crisis. On the other hand, any stressful event can precipitate a crisis, depending on the person's perceptions, coping skills, and available support systems. This chapter focuses on crisis theory and development of crises. It explores crisis intervention through the application of the nursing process to clients in crisis.

Learning Objectives

On completion of this chapter, you should be able to accomplish the following:

1. *Discuss the development of a crisis theory.*
2. *Describe the phases of a crisis.*
3. *Differentiate between maturational and situation crises.*
4. *Discuss the goals and methods of crisis intervention.*
5. *Contrast crisis intervention and traditional forms of therapy.*
6. *Apply the nursing process to a client or family in crisis.*
7. *Discuss the feelings and needs of the intervener in crisis.*
8. *Formulate a comprehensive nursing care plan for the client in crisis.*
9. *Discuss the process in critical incident stress debriefing.*
10. *Describe the application of crisis intervention to home care.*
11. *Discuss the role of crisis intervention as a component of case management, psychosocial rehabilitation, and managed care.*
12. *Discuss the need for culturally competent crisis intervention practice.*
13. *Discuss the use of the standards of psychiatric-mental health clinical nursing practice and the role of the nurse in crisis intervention.*
14. *Discuss the desired outcomes of crisis intervention.*

◆ Crisis Theory

Crisis means a turning point, whether in disease or another condition. In the Chinese language, two symbols communicate crisis: "danger" and "opportunity."

In times of crisis, a person is not sure what to do. Usual methods of problem solving are not effective or are unavailable. As anxiety and pain increase, the person becomes more willing to try new ways of problem solving. In this willingness lies the opportunity for growth. Good mental health is thought to be predominantly the result of a life history of successful crisis resolution.[17] Intervention during crisis has been found to reduce greatly the incidence and severity of mental disorders.

DEVELOPMENT OF CRISIS THEORY

Although people have been vulnerable to crisis since the beginning of human existence, crisis has been an issue of serious study only in the last 35 years. Caplan defines crisis as a threat to homeostasis. During crisis, an imbalance exists between the magnitude of the problem and the immediate resources available to deal with it. This imbalance results in confusion and disorganization.[10] The active crisis state is relatively short—approximately 4 to 6 weeks. No person can tolerate this level of anxiety and imbalance for very long. Quick, appropriate intervention is crucial for helping the person in crisis return to an optimal state of functioning.

Numerous researchers have contributed to the development of crisis theory. Lindeman studied the survivors and families of victims of the disastrous Coconut Grove nightclub fire in Boston in which many people died. Based on those observations and his study of other families who had lost a family member through death, Lindeman described the commonalities of the experience of crisis and bereavement.[25] From this classic study in 1944, some of the basic tenets of crisis theory were developed. Caplan, who has done the most extensive work on crisis theory, was influenced by the research and writings of Lindeman, Parad, Rapaport, Erikson, and others.

Crisis theory is derived from psychoanalytic theory and the work of ego psychologists. Ego psychology stresses the human ability to learn and grow throughout life.[21] Crisis theory is based on research on crisis in bereavement, the reactions of parents to a child born prematurely or with a birth defect, crisis of surgery, crisis experienced by Peace Corps volunteers, responses to the ordinary upsets of early married life, and crisis as a result of war.

Crisis theory emerged in an era of increased social consciousness. President John F. Kennedy passionately addressed the Congress and the nation about the need for a national health program with a new approach to mental illness. He maintained that the promotion of mental health was everyone's responsibility—government at every level, private foundations, and individual citizens. Congress directed the establishment of a Joint Commission on Mental Illness and Health. As a result of the work of this commission, funds were made available for a nationwide system of community mental health centers that emphasized prevention of emotional disorders.

WHAT HAPPENS IN A CRISIS

According to crisis theory, a person strives to maintain a constant state of emotional equilibrium. If a person is confronted with an overwhelming threat and is unable to cope, crisis ensues.

The state of disequilibrium known as crisis typically lasts 4 to 6 weeks. Because the crisis state is accompanied by high anxiety, the person will either adapt and return to the previous state of mental health, develop more constructive coping skills, or decompensate to a lower level of functioning.

Factors that influence the outcome of a crisis include the following:

1. the person's previous problem-solving experience
2. the way the person views the problem
3. the amount of help or hindrance from significant others[21]

Maladaptive crisis resolution increases the probability of unsuccessful resolution of future crises.

During a crisis, a person is more open to receiving professional help and learning new ways of problem solving, and is more likely to make changes in attitude and behavior in a short time. Crisis intervention focuses on the problem or stressor that precipitated the crisis state rather than on personality traits. The person in crisis is viewed as essentially normal, capable of problem solving and growth with assistance from others.[1,21]

PHASES OF A CRISIS

To understand how a crisis develops, it is necessary to examine the phases or steps that lead to an active crisis state. The first phase is an increase in anxiety in response to a traumatic event.[10] A person tries to use familiar coping mechanisms to resolve the feeling of increased anxiety. If coping mechanisms are effective, there is no crisis; if they are not effective, a person enters the second phase of crisis, marked by increased anxiety due to failure of usual coping mechanisms. In the third phase of crisis, anxiety continues to rise, and the person usually feels compelled to reach out for assistance. A person who is emotionally isolated before experiencing a traumatic event almost always will experience a crisis.

In the fourth phase, the active state of crisis, the person's inner resources and support systems are inadequate. The precipitating event is not resolved, and stress and anxiety mount to an intolerable level. The person in an active state of crisis demonstrates a short attention span, ruminates, and looks inward for possible reasons for the trauma and how it might have been changed or avoided. This rumination is accompanied by anguish, apprehension, and distress. Behavior becomes increasingly impulsive and unproductive. Relationships with others usually suffer. The person becomes less aware of the environment and begins to view others in terms of their ability to help solve the problem.

The high anxiety level may make people feel they are "losing their mind" or "going crazy."[23] Perceptive ability is greatly affected by anxiety, but this is not the same as psychosis. People in crisis often need this explanation and reassurance that when they feel less anxious, they will be able to think clearly again.

TYPES OF CRISES

There are two types of crises: *maturational*, precipitated by the normal stress of development, and *situational*, precipitated by a sudden traumatic event.

Maturational Crisis

Erikson identified specific periods in normal development when anxiety or stress increases and could precipitate a maturational crisis.[12] Some common events that may precipitate a crisis during the various developmental stages are being born, mastering control of body functions, starting school, experiencing puberty, leaving home, getting married, becoming a parent, losing physical youthfulness, and entering retirement.

A maturational, or developmental, crisis may occur at any transitional period in normal growth and development. Because each stage of development depends on the previous stage, the inability to master the tasks of one stage thwarts growth and development in subsequent stages. Why are these times considered a crisis for some and not for others? One explanation is that some people are unable to make the role changes necessary for the new maturational level. For instance, the birth of the first child brings numerous role changes for parents. Some are able to adapt and make the necessary role changes; others, because of emotional immaturity, marital discord, financial stress, or unmet dependency needs, may not be able to adapt readily to the new roles.

There are three main reasons why people may not be able to prevent a maturational crisis. First, they may not be able to visualize themselves in the new role because of inadequate role models. For example, a male child reared without the love and guidance of a father may have difficulty assuming the role of a loving, guiding, involved parent. Second, people may lack the interpersonal resources to make the appropriate and necessary changes. For example, a person may lack the flexibility to alter life goals to avoid a midlife crisis or may lack the communication skills needed to maintain a long-term relationship. Third, others may refuse to recognize the person's maturational role change. For instance, parents may fail to acknowledge their adolescent's movement toward adulthood and attempt to preserve the role of child, precipitating a crisis for the adolescent.

In each stage of development, a person needs nurturance from others to work through the risks of that stage and to obtain the necessary skills for the next stage.[21] With adequate social support from family and friends, increased anxiety and resultant energy can be channeled into constructive growth and feelings of accomplishment. Maturational crises are predictable and occur gradually; therefore, it is possible to prepare for these stressful transitional periods and prevent a crisis. Premarital counseling, preparation for parenting, and planning for retirement are examples of anticipatory guidance in crisis prevention.

Situational Crisis

A situational crisis is a response to a traumatic event that is usually sudden and unavoidable. When a stressful event threatens a person's physical, emotional, or social integrity, crisis is likely to result.

A situational crisis usually follows the loss of an established support. The usual ways of presenting the self are disrupted, which threatens the way people view themselves. From infancy on, each person develops an image of self through feedback received from important people in the environment. Later in development, people define themselves according to the various roles and the establishment of new role relationships. The threat or loss of a role viewed as necessary to maintain self-image usually will lead to a crisis state. The loss of a job, failure in academics, loss of a spouse, birth of a retarded child, or diagnosis of a chronic or terminal illness will affect the way people perceive themselves.[21] The most common response to a loss or deprivation is depression. The difficulty of dealing with a situational crisis is compounded when it occurs while the person is struggling with a developmental crisis. A client, J.R., related that on his 18th birthday, his father abruptly told him it was time for him to be out on his own. J.R. was unsure of where to go or what to do and felt hurt and abandoned. He packed his suitcase and went to Europe, where he spent the most miserable Christmas he could ever remember. Not long after that, his van exploded, resulting in a loss of most of his possessions and causing burns on his face and hands. He remembers wandering around in a daze without being able to think clearly. The American Embassy finally helped him get home. Possibly J.R. could have coped with the trauma of the fire if he had not been so vulnerable, struggling with his response to being forced to leave home.

BALANCING FACTORS IN A STRESSFUL EVENT

Certain balancing factors determine whether a person will enter a crisis state:

- how the person perceives the event
- experience with coping
- available coping mechanisms
- people who can be supportive to the person[1]

Figure 39-1 shows a paradigm devised by Aguilera and Messick to help the crisis intervener analyze and resolve a crisis situation.[1] The paradigm is a guide to help the intervener think clearly about the problem. People in crisis need assistance working through some of the feelings associated with what has happened to them.

◆ Crisis Intervention

The goal of crisis intervention is to assist the person in distress to resolve the immediate problem and regain emotional equilibrium. This problem solving hopefully will lead to enhanced coping ability to deal with future stressful events.

The role of the intervener is one of active participation with the person in solving the current problem. Because the crisis state is not an illness, the intervener does not take over and make decisions for the person unless the person is suicidal or homicidal.[21] Crisis intervention is a partnership. The underlying philosophy of crisis intervention is that with varying degrees of assistance, people can help themselves.[23] To maximize the opportunity for growth, the person must be actively involved in resolving the problem.

The intervener helps the person in crisis analyze the stressful event, encourages the expression of feelings, and affirms the right to those feelings no matter what they are. Methods of dealing with stress are explored, and the intervener reinforces the person's strengths and abilities. The person is encouraged to seek support from friends, family, and other resource groups in the community. Planning designed to avert possible future crises is accomplished through anticipatory guidance.[1]

CRISIS INTERVENTION VERSUS TRADITIONAL THERAPIES

The goal of traditional Freudian therapy is personality change. It emphasizes the client's past and the exploration of the subconscious. The Freudian therapist is usually nondirective, and therapy may last for years.[1] Brief psychotherapy attempts to remove the client's symptoms or prevent more severe neurotic or psychotic problems. Table 39-1 provides the reader with a comparison of crisis intervention with psychoanalysis and brief psychotherapy.

Crisis intervention, on the other hand, assists a client in resolving an immediate problem perceived by the client as overwhelming. Sometimes the crisis stirs up unresolved issues from the client's past. These issues are

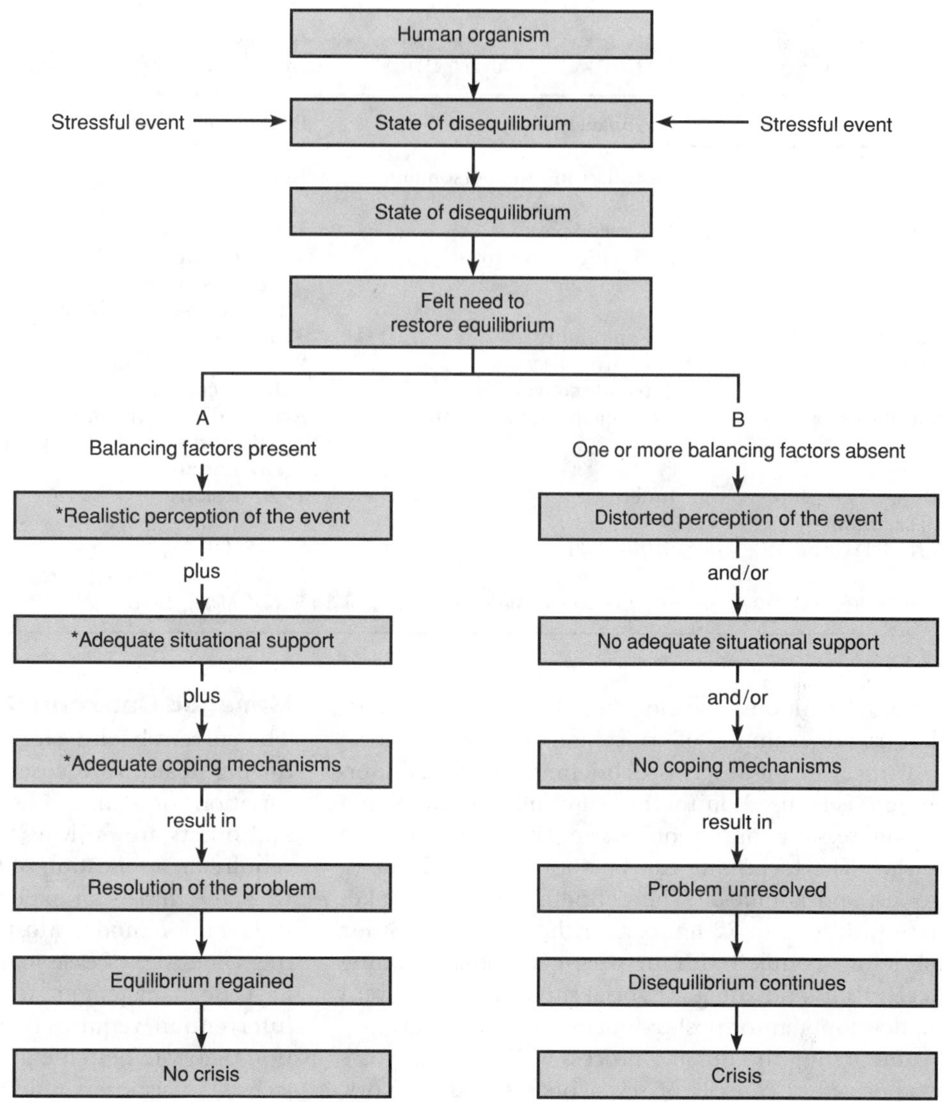

Figure 39-1. Paradigm: the effect of balancing factors in a stressful event. (From Aguilera DC: Crisis Intervention, 7th ed. St. Louis, CV Mosby, 1994.)

not confronted, however, until after the resolution of the crisis.

Crisis intervention emphasizes the healthy aspects, not the pathology, of the personality. There is no diagnosis of mental illness in crisis work. The client is evaluated in terms of ability to cope, existence of strengths and potentials, and ability to problem solve. The major focus on the therapeutic approach is the client's social structures, rather than the personality dynamics. It is assumed that the client will make appropriate decisions when given the necessary information and support. Crisis intervention requires a much more directive approach than traditional therapies.

CRITICAL INCIDENT STRESS DEBRIEFING

Critical incident stress debriefing, a type of crisis intervention, was reported by Jeffrey Mitchell[27] in a description of a program for emergency services personnel. Stress debriefing intervention facilitates effective coping. Critical incidents are any situation that occurs suddenly and unexpectedly, disrupts values and beliefs, and challenges basic assumptions of how the world operates.[27] There is a strong emotional reaction and a perception that the incident is life-threatening. Some examples include witnessing a violent act, sudden infant death, physical or psychological threats or losses, and unusual media events. Natural disasters, such as fires,

Table 39-1

Major Differences Between Psychoanalysis, Brief Psychotherapy, and Crisis Intervention Methodology

	Psychoanalysis	Brief Psychotherapy	Crisis Intervention
Goals of Therapy	Restructuring the personality	Removal of specific symptoms	Resolution of immediate crisis
Focus of Treatment	1. Genetic past 2. Freeing the unconscious	1. Genetic past as it relates to present situation 2. Repression of unconscious and restraining of drives	1. Genetic present 2. Restoration to level of functioning prior to crisis
Usual Activity of Therapist	1. Exploratory 2. Passive observer 3. Nondirective	1. Suppressive 2. Participant observer 3. Indirect	1. Suppressive 2. Active participant 3. Direct
Indications	Neurotic personality patterns	Acutely disruptive emotional pain and severely disruptive circumstances	Sudden loss of ability to cope with a life situation
Average Length of Treatment	Indefinite	1–20 sessions	1–6 sessions
Cost of Treatment	\$100–\$200	\$75–\$100	\$0–\$75/h

(From Aquiler, D.C. Crisis Intervention: Theory and Methodology 7th ed. St Louis, C.V. Mosby, 1994)

volcanic eruptions, earthquakes, hurricanes, and typhoons, are examples of critical incidents.

Critical incident stress debriefing, like crisis intervention, is focused on the here and now, is completed in one session, and requires an active role by the nurse.[30] The technique can be applied to individuals, groups, and families.[29] The debriefing generally takes place within 24 to 72 hours after the incident.[27] Stress debriefing, coupled with the person's adequate coping mechanisms and adequate social support, may prevent the development of post-traumatic stress disorder.[3]

Integrating the nursing process with debriefing crisis approaches consists of seven phases: introductory, fact, thought, reaction, symptom, teaching, and reentry phases.[30] The first five phases are part of the assessment process, the teaching and reentry phases are the intervention stage, and evaluation takes place at the end of the session.

CRISIS INTERVENTION AND COMMUNITY NURSING

As more health care is delivered in the community, crisis intervention theory provides an excellent framework for nursing practice.

Many home health care providers have programs for delivering psychiatric services in the home. According to Duffey and coworkers, "crisis intervention theory assists psychiatric nursing practitioners not only to determine if their patient is in crisis but also to predict the effect of that crisis on a patient's ability to function. Crisis intervention is a type of short term, cost effective therapy focusing on solving current problems" (p 23).[15]

Managed Care and Case Management

The current health care environment is focused on reducing health care costs and increasing quality. Many variations of managed health care are already in place, and others are evolving.[2] All systems of managed care require an application of the crisis intervention model; thus, the nurse can expect to practice within the crisis intervention model. Most managed care systems are using some type of case management model.

Case management, which is a delivery system and an intervention, requires that the nurse use crisis intervention theory to help the individual or family needing services.[12] Crisis intervention is an important component and congruent with the principles of psychiatric rehabilitation for nursing practice.[28]

CHARACTERISTICS OF THE CRISIS INTERVENER

To intervene in a crisis effectively, a therapist must demonstrate calmness and empathy. Because the person in crisis is often confused, the intervener must be able to identify the facts in a situation and think clearly to plan solutions to the problem.

The intervener must possess courage. The pain involved in a crisis is never pleasant. It is difficult to listen to the tragic things that happen to people; however, people in crisis need someone who will make the commitment to work with them until the problem is resolved, someone who can tolerate the uncomfortableness, sadness, and anger.

Culturally Competent Care

The intervener should be nonjudgmental and aware of different cultural values. There are different established patterns of response to death, illness, divorce, and pregnancy in various cultural, ethnic, and religious groups.[20] Crisis intervention is effective as long as the intervener does not impose a different lifestyle or value system on the client. For example, a very traditional Chinese American college student is in crisis because of failure in a course. The failure in this culture brings shame on the family and the student. Often the combination of shame, guilt, low self-esteem, and failure may precipitate a crisis for the student.[21] The crisis intervener from a traditional American background may not have the experience or knowledge regarding the significant meaning of the event (that is, the course failure). The intervener needs to be careful not to minimize the effect of the failure on the student because it might not seem to be a life-threatening danger for other students.

However, crisis intervention, with its focus on immediate problem solving, here and now, direct approach, avoidance of psychiatric diagnoses, health aspects, time limitations, and personal strengths, may be more acceptable to people from some ethnic groups and cultures than others.[19] Readers are encouraged to review Chapters 8 (Psychosociocultural Assessment and Nursing Diagnosis) and 10 (Sociocultural Aspects of Care) to ensure the provisions of culturally competent care.

Application of the Nursing Process to Crisis Intervention

ASSESSMENT

Assessment of the person in crisis is the most important, and often the most difficult, step of crisis intervention. First, the nurse must determine whether the client is really in a crisis state. Tears, anger, and being upset do not automatically mean that the person is overwhelmed.[1,3] If the client is experiencing great anxiety, having difficulty thinking clearly, and unable to identify solutions to the problem, then it is helpful to encourage the client to talk about the events that immediately preceded the distress.[1] This verbalization frequently calms the client and helps the nurse and client establish rapport, the beginning of a relationship (Box 39-1). The nurse must focus on the client's immediate problem, not on history. Usually when people in crisis reach out for help, the precipitating event has occurred within the previous 14 days, sometimes in the past 24 hours.[1]

The Client's Feelings

The nurse asks clients to describe the feelings they experience. By accepting the feelings without judgment, the nurse assists clients to accept their own feelings. The nurse naturally will feel some discomfort in the presence of a person in pain. The human inclination is to stop the person from crying and to stop talking about what is horrible and upsetting. By avoiding the topic of distress, the client at least appears to be in less pain. Nevertheless, it is beneficial for the person in crisis to express feelings and experience the pain or frustration. Therefore, the nurse must learn to tolerate these feelings of discomfort.

Usually, the nurse's increased anxiety stems from fear of saying the wrong thing or feeling inadequate to deal with the situation. The nurse must understand cognitively and emotionally that ultimately clients make their own decisions. In fact, it is not expedient for the nurse to have all the answers to a client's problems. For clients to grow, much of the work of problem solving must come first.

The Client's Perception of the Event

The nurse first determines the client's perception of the stressful event. How threatened is the client? Is the client realistic or distorting the meaning of the event?

The Client's Support Systems

After determining the client's perception of the event, the nurse focuses on who will be available to support the client. Questions such as the following can help identify the client's support systems: "Whom do you trust?" "Who is your best friend?" "Is there a member of your family with whom you are particularly close?" Children in a crisis situation can cope much better if they are with their parents.[21,26,33]

The nurse also should inquire into the client's religious beliefs. For many religious families, God is a source of comfort and strength. The client's or family's religious affiliation may be an excellent resource for support. It is best to have several supportive people involved with the client. Because a crisis period lasts for a brief time and the nurse will be involved only temporarily, the client needs others on whom to rely for continued support.

The Client's Coping Skills

To assess a client's coping skills, the nurse asks what the client does when a problem cannot be solved or how the client deals with anxiety or depression.[23] The nurse must encourage the client to describe coping methods as specifically as possible. The nurse then determines whether the client's coping mechanisms are adaptive or maladaptive. Is the client still functioning in a job? Is the client still attending school and fulfilling other roles, such as wife and mother? How are the client's significant others affected? Are they also upset?[1,3] They may need crisis counseling as well.

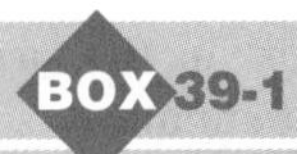

Therapeutic Dialogue: The Client in Crisis

Nurse: The nurse walks into the examining room and notices Mrs. A. has tears in her eyes. "Mrs. A. I'm going to pull up a chair. I can tell you are upset."

Client: "I don't know why—"

Nurse: "You must be feeling pretty miserable today. The spasms seem harder and more frequent."

Client: "I'm exhausted. The big muscle in my neck whips my head around so hard my neck pops." (Mrs. A. sobs)

Nurse: Squeezes her hand and waits.

Client: "I don't want to live this way anymore. When I look in the mirror, I don't recognize myself. I feel like an animal."

Nurse: "Because you can't stop your head from turning that makes you feel less than human?"

Client: "Yes."

Nurse: "I'm wondering if that makes you feel lonely too?"

Client: (angrily) "That is so frightening. No one knows what causes it. There's no cure and the treatment seems as bad as the problem. Having the muscles in my face temporarily paralyzed sounds bad too. What if I can't open my eyes? What if my arms and legs start jerking?"

Nurse: "You're going through a lot right now. The syndrome that you have affects the nerves that affect the muscles in the face and neck but not the rest of your body. I can see that you are absolutely miserable. I think Dr. M. can find a combination of medication to give you some relief."

Client: "I don't think I can stand it anymore."

Nurse: "Mrs. A. are you planning to do something to end your life?"

Client: "No, No!! I don't believe in it. I'm a Christian. I just don't want to be this way."

Nurse: "I'm glad you have strong faith. What about your family for support?"

Client: "I don't know what I would do without my husband. He tells me I would feel better if I would get out more. I don't feel comfortable. People can't help but stare at me. I can't eatwithout choking. I'm a mess. I'm surprised my husband hasn't left me."

Nurse: "How is your relationship with your husband?"

Client: "He has been very supportive. He arranges his work so that he can come for lunch every day."

Nurse: "What about your children?"

Client: "I'm fortunate they have also been supportive, but they both work and live away."

Nurse: "Friends?"

Client: "I have one friend that comes every week. She doesn't ask if she can come, she just says she's coming."

Nurse: "You have found that helpful?"

Client: "Yes, she just listens, and I can say whatever is on my mind. Oh, my minister comes by to visit too."

Nurse: "Mrs. A., you do have some things going for you. You have a supportive family, a good friend, and your minister. You have strong faith and you've mastered tough things before. Dr. M. and I are not going to give up. There has to be something that will give you some relief. Dr. M. will give you copies of the latest articles on treatment. I think the more you know will help you feel more in control."

Client: Nods.

Nurse: "I want you to come in more frequently for the next couple of weeks to assist in getting better control of the spasms. We are in this together. Also, there is an organization that supports research and sends out a newsletter. Let's talk about that a little later."

In this interview, the nurse did not take the client's first angry remark personally. The nurse allowed Mrs. A. to express her feelings even though it was hard to listen. Clients frequently lash out at nurses and physicians when the problem is not better and there is no cure. The client and family desperately need people that will not counter-attack but will "walk through" the pain with them. The nurse was able to assess Mrs. A.'s potential for suicide, which is low at this time. However, Mrs. A.'s perception of herself is damaged; therefore, frequent visits are essential to support her until the problem is in better control.

The Client's Potential for Self-Harm

Assessment of clients in crisis is not complete without asking if they are having thoughts of hurting themselves. Most clients will not volunteer this information but when asked, will readily talk about suicidal thoughts. Clients who have attempted suicide before or have decided how, when, and where to kill themselves need protection. The suicidal clients should not be left alone and needs an experienced therapist (see Chapter 42, Suicide).

NURSING DIAGNOSIS

A crisis or precrisis state is neither a psychiatric illness nor a prolonged, disabling condition. While gathering assessment data from the client and family members, the nurse begins to conceptualize the appropriate descriptions of the client's responses to health problems in terms of nursing diagnoses. Responses particularly evident in crisis are Ineffective Individual Coping, Anxiety, Altered Thought Processes and problem solving, Self Esteem Disturbance, Social Isolation, and Impaired Social Interaction. In addition, the client in crisis may be experiencing Powerlessness, Altered Parenting, Altered Role Performance, Sleep Pattern Disturbance, Impaired Verbal Communication, and Impaired Home Maintenance Management.

Possible nursing diagnoses for the client in crisis may include the following:

1. Anxiety related to situation and maturational crises, threat to self-concept, unmet needs, and traumatic event, as evidenced by restlessness, insomnia, verbalizations of fear of going crazy, feelings of inadequacy, fearlessness, and focus on self
2. Ineffective Individual Coping related to inadequate support systems, overwhelming problem, inadequate coping and personal vulnerability, as evidenced by inability to problem solve, altered societal participation, inappropriate use of defense mechanisms, inability to meet role expectations, and anxious mood
3. Altered Thought Processes related to situational and maturational crises, threat to self-concept, and high anxiety level, as evidenced by inability to problem solve or make decisions, inaccurate interpretation of the environment, egocentricity, altered attention span, easy distractibility, and inappropriate affect or thinking
4. Impaired Social Interaction related to self-concept disturbance and unmet dependency needs, as evidenced by verbalized or observed discomfort in social situations, verbalized or observed inability to receive or communicate a satisfying sense of belonging and caring, and dysfunctional interaction with peers, family, and others
5. Social Isolation related to high level of anxiety and possible regression, evidenced by absence of supportive significant others (family, friends, group), uncommunicative and withdrawn behavior, and preoccupation with own thoughts
6. Self Esteem Disturbance, Altered Role Performance related to perception of overwhelming problem, lack of support systems, and high anxiety level, as evidenced by self-destructive behavior, lack of responsibility for self-care, verbalization of sense of worthlessness, inability to recognize own accomplishments, and lack of appropriate behavior

PLANNING

No matter how critical the time factor, a plan is necessary. After collecting the data, the nurse obtains a specific statement of the problem from the client. To ensure the success of the plan, the client must be actively involved in planning solutions to the problem. A scenario illustrating inadequate client and family participation in planning follows:

> M. H. was hospitalized with a fractured hip. Due to her cardiac condition and the rehabilitation needed for her hip, she could no longer live safely alone in her home. Her son and daughter were both married, had their own families, and were employed full time.
>
> The daughter stated to the nurse, "I don't think we are going to be able to care for Mother at home." The nurse talked with M. H.'s doctor, and they called the social worker to find a nursing home placement for M. H.
>
> When M. H. learned of the plan, she refused to go to the nursing home. Her family was upset, and the nurse was irritated because she felt she had gone out of her way to be helpful.
>
> A difference in cultural values was part of this problem. In the nurse's family, moving into a nursing home was expected and accepted. In the client's family, it was neither. For a crisis to be resolved successfully, the solutions to the problem must be in keeping with the cultural values of the client.

The nurse should convey the attitude that the client will be able to work through the crisis and take charge of life again. Successful planning depends on thorough assessment and diagnosis of the client's level of functioning and dependency needs. A basic rule of thumb is not to do things for clients when they can do them and to do only what they cannot do for themselves. The more distraught and confused the client is, the more directive the nurse needs to be. Together, the nurse and client define a time frame and goals for crisis resolution.

Often in planning it is helpful for the intervener to outline the problem and available resources, using the paradigm of the balancing factors in a stressful event. By using the decision counseling approach, the intervener can clarify with the client the boundaries of the problem: What are the tentative solutions? Where will the solutions be tried? What is the time frame? Who will do what? Follow-up is critical and should be part of the initial plan. A sample clinical pathway is shown in Table 39-2.

Goal Setting for the Client in Crisis

The major goal of crisis intervention is to assist the client in reestablishing equilibrium. To reach that end, the following goals are set:

1. establishing a working relationship with the client
2. identifying the specific problem
3. reducing the distortion of the client's perception of the event
4. improving the client's self-esteem
5. decreasing the client's anxiety
6. promoting involvement of family and friends
7. reinforcing healthy coping mechanisms
8. validating the client's ability to solve the problem

It is sometimes difficult, but absolutely essential, for the nurse to accept that the goals of crisis intervention are different from the goals of other therapies. It is not the crisis intervener's task to deal with all the client's problems or to orchestrate major changes in the client's life.[1] Crisis intervention aims to assist the client in solving immediate problems that are so overwhelming that the client is unable to cope. Once the client has regained emotional equilibrium and is able to cope again, the work of crisis intervention has been accomplished. Nursing Care Plan 39-1 is a sample plan of care for a client in crisis.

INTERVENTION

Realizing the Potential for Growth

Nurturing, caring, listening, and willingness to help are powerful and saving forces for clients in crisis. In any crisis situation, the client faced with an overwhelming stressor has the potential to improve coping skills. Whether this possibility for growth is realized or not depends in part on the appropriateness of crisis intervention.

The nurse and client reexamine any feelings that might block adaptive coping. When a client has extremely negative feelings (for example, about mental illness or physical disabilities), it is particularly difficult to be faced with similar circumstances. The client must deal with those feelings to cope adequately with the crisis situation.

Learning to Ask for Help

In a crisis state, it is natural to feel isolated and withdrawn. Therefore, the client must be helped to communicate directly with significant others. In particular, a client who places a high value on independence may need assistance in recognizing interdependence as a healthy balance. Often, the client must be taught how to ask for help. The nurse can help demonstrate this skill to the client through role modeling.[26]

Using Adaptive Coping

The nurse also helps the client develop healthier coping skills. Helpful strategies may include open expression of feelings, progressive relaxation, physical exercise, and drinking warm milk or herbal tea to aid relaxation and sleep.[23]

Focusing on the Problem Resolution

As the crisis intervener, the nurse keeps the client focused on the problem and specific goals leading to its resolution. A high anxiety level may make it difficult for the client to focus on one issue, and direction may be needed to avoid fragmentation of the client's efforts. After the client has attempted some of the alternative solutions to the problem, the client and nurse evaluate their effectiveness and decide whether additional plans are needed. The nurse reinforces the client's abilities by reviewing the crisis event, coping ability, and any new methods of problem solving or coping that have been acquired.

Team Approach

A crisis team approach is sometimes used in short-term, inpatient psychiatric treatment facilities. The team may be composed of a psychiatrist, psychiatric-mental health nurse, psychologist, social worker, psychiatric aide, minister, and students in the mental health field. One clinician assumes the role of the primary person responsible for the management of a client; however, continuity of care must be built into the system because so many people are involved with the client. The crisis team meets daily to discuss the client's progress and make decisions about care. The psychiatrist outlines clinical indications for the client, and the other team members implement the plan and decide on time of discharge and method and frequency of follow-up. As in any crisis intervention mode, the goals must be kept clearly in mind, and as soon as they are reached, the client is discharged, even if it is on the day of admission.

The following scenario illustrates the team approach at work:

> A young woman, S.L., was admitted to a crisis unit following notification that her husband was reported missing in South Korea. The client had no relatives who could be supportive to her. She had not been able to eat or sleep for the last 3 days. Her only friend brought her to the hospital for admission. S.L. was becoming dehydrated; therefore, the physician ordered intravenous therapy and a mild sedative to be discontinued the following day. After the initial interview, the team met to discuss the areas in which S.L. needed assistance to facilitate coping with her distress.

Table 39-2 Clinical Pathway (Psychiatric): Crisis Stabilization

Patient Name: ____________ **Admission Date:** ___ **Time:** ____ **Physician:** ____ **MR#** ______

Case Manager: ____________ Discharge Date: ___ Time: ____ Disposition: ____________

LONG TERM GOAL: Patient will restore equilibrium, without catastrophe, at the same or better level of functioning than before crisis.

	Phase I—1st Contact Intake	Phase II—Problem Identification	Phase III—Plan for Problem Resolution	Phase IV—Action	Phase V—Stabilization
	0–30 minutes	*30 minutes–2 hours*	*2 hours–4 hours*	*4 hours–8 hours*	*8 hours–12 hours*
SHORT-TERM GOALS	Patient comes to the hospital for appointment.	Patient identifies a "workable" problem (something that can be changed).	Patient helps formulate plan of action to solve problem.	Patient takes action to solve the problem.	Patient acknowledges problem resolution.
ASSESSMENT	QMHP interview Does situation represent crisis Brief medical screening Physician evaluation DSM-IV Diagnosis Admit Note-TX plan	Suicide/homicide/detox danger/assaultive behavior Balancing factors (perception, social network, coping mechanisms) Why crisis today Medical HX/Physical Exam/Neuro Ck; Medication HX/Substance Abuse HX; Psychosocial HX—Lab Ordered Nursing Assessment/Nutrition	Prior coping mechanisms Why same approaches did not work this time Discourage client from blaming others Abnormal Lab reported to Dr.	Reaction to RX Strengths/Assets Family/Significant Others Other social network Re-assess for risk of danger	Response to interventions Knowledge of goal maintenance Knowledge of strategies for maintaining progress Commitment to discharge plan
INTERVENTIONS	Establish rapport Provide support Limit conversation no "telephone" therapy Patient Rights Financial Information Initial discharge plan	Avert catastrophe (suicide, homicide, family disintegration, assaultive behavior, dangerous withdrawal) Provide precautions if necessary Instill hope Expect crisis to be resolved Expect problems to be worked out Deal with feelings as they connect to problem Use rational exploration	Informed consent for RX Rx prescription/administration Evaluate med interactions Divert attacks by family on client's self-esteem Actively work toward problem resolution Help client identify steps to take toward problem resolution.	Show interest in non-problem aspects of life (hobbies, occupation, past accomplishments, etc) Raise & protect patient's self-esteem/self-image Enlarge & strengthen social network Support parent's self-image Assist, encourage client to take action for problem solving Help foster self-reliance Do not do for client what he can do for himself.	Assist client to write AfterCare Plan Give support—24 hr phone # Mobilize resources: family, friends Provide discharge instructions Establish resources: home health; MH clinic; social service agency; outpatient; partial hospitalization; intensive outpatient; crisis hotline.

Strategic Clinical Systems, Inc., 3715 Mission Ct., Granbury, TX 76049 (817) 326-4329. PsychPaths™ © Copyright 94

Darla Belt, RN & Vickie Pflueger, RNC—Authors.

Abbreviation Key:
HX = History; MR = Medical Record; RX = Medication; TX = Treatment; QMHP Interview = Qualified Mental Health Professional.

Reference: "Helping People in Crisis" by Douglas Puryear, M.D.

Nursing Care Plan 39-1

The Client in Crisis

Nursing Diagnosis

Ineffective Individual Coping related to inadequate support systems, perception of problem as overwhelming

Outcome

Client will identify steps to establish adequate support for self.

Intervention	Rationale
Provide verbal and nonverbal acceptance and support.	Acceptance and support validate client's value as person and increases self-esteem.
Encourage client to verbalize feelings related to current problems.	Verbalization will provide catharsis for client's pent-up emotions and objectify current situational stressors.
Assist client to identify priorities of problems to be solved.	Prioritizing provides client with sense of control and reinforces belief that solutions can be found.
Encourage client to review previous coping methods for past problems.	This reinforces client's sense of own ability as problem solver.
Help client generate several steps to increase current support systems.	Support systems are essential for assistance in crisis. Client-generated steps are usually more acceptable and help reinforce belief that client can take control.

Evaluation

Client seeks the support of significant others and uses adaptive coping skills during crisis.

Nursing Diagnosis

Anxiety related to situational and maturational crises, threat to self-concept as evidenced by restlessness, insomnia

Outcome

Client will use specific measures for anxiety relief.

Intervention	Rationale
Explain that client's current high level of anxiety is related to crisis situations.	Validation of reality of crisis situation will provide realistic framework for intervention
Teach client to identify symptoms of anxiety in self.	Correct labeling of symptoms as anxiety related will help reduce unrealistic fears about meaning of symptoms, such as "going crazy."
Teach client common coping measures useful for anxiety relief, such as exercise, talking with supportive person, treating oneself to an enjoyable experience, eating comforting foods.	Anxiety relief measures can be learned and will provide concrete tools for use when anxiety increases.

Evaluation

Client verbalizes reduction of anxiety experienced during crisis.

continued

Nursing Care Plan 39-1 *(Continued)*

Nursing Diagnosis

Self Esteem Disturbance related to divorce and school difficulties as evidenced by statement, "I feel like I'm a failure"

Outcome

Client will verbalize positive self-statements.

Intervention	Rationale
Help client view current feelings as related to crisis of divorce.	This will allow client to put into perspective the situation and recognize feelings as temporary.
Teach client that "all-or-nothing" thinking can be related to feelings of loss of self-esteem.	Reality of client's situation is that she is experiencing crisis of divorce and has received one failing grade. Neither of these situations mean that client is a failure.
Encourage client to list positive qualities about self as a person.	This validates and reinforces the client's self-esteem.

Evaluation

Client expresses positive assessment of own functioning and self-worth.

In the interview, the crisis team learned that S.L. was ordinarily independent, held a responsible job, and coped well with living alone in her husband's absence; however, S.L. was expecting her husband in 2 weeks. It was agreed that S.L. needed more people to be supportive for her to deal with this crisis. The nurse made plans to introduce S.L. to other clients who would be particularly supportive, and she encouraged S.L. to contact some of her coworkers. The minister investigated what community support was available. The social worker phoned the Red Cross to see if they could assist in communications with the government. In 3 days, S.L. was eating again and was able to sleep better. She had decided to move in with her friend temporarily. S.L. was discharged from the inpatient unit to outpatient status, where she was followed through four weekly appointments.

Crisis Groups

The goal of a crisis group is the same as that of individual crisis intervention: The members regain their precrisis functioning ability or develop an even higher level of ability to problem solve. Some clients find a crisis group more beneficial than one-to one therapy, particularly those who have difficulty with interpersonal relationships. Others who may benefit from a crisis group are those who have difficulty accepting information from psychiatric professionals or from people in positions of authority.

Advantages of a Crisis Group. In a crisis group, members feel less isolated and often make social contact with other members.[20] By seeing other people express their feelings, members realize that others have similar feelings and problems. Often, the reticent client can more easily express opinions and feelings after observing others in similar situations. Members offer each other suggestions for coping and solving problems, helping each other bolster members' self-esteem.

Disadvantages of a Crisis Group. The crisis group approach has some disadvantages. It is difficult to keep each client's crisis in focus in a group setting. Another problem is the destructive form of coping or maladaptive problem solving that may be suggested by group members. These problems point up the need for a trained crisis group leader.[1]

Format and Rules of the Group. Crisis groups usually are scheduled for $1\frac{1}{2}$ to 2 hours once a week for 6 weeks. Five to seven members are considered an ideal group size. Some crisis groups are homogeneous, with every member having a similar problem. For example, successful groups have been formed for divorced people, victims of incest, parents in crisis, homosexuals, cancer patients, and many other similar groupings. Some peer groups organized by lay people rather than professionally trained people also have been rather successful. The best known of these groups is probably Alcoholics Anonymous. In a heterogeneous group, the members have different problems, but all are in crisis. The group may be an open one, in which new members come in and others work through their problems and leave the group. This gives members an opportunity to deal with feelings about intrusion and separation. A closed group does not accept new members after it is formed and continues for a specified time.

Assessing members and clearly stating the purpose of a group are both crucial aspects of group formation.[34] The members must agree to the rules of the group, such as confidentiality, and must be able to accept other responsibilities required of group membership.

Families in Crisis

Seldom does a person live in total isolation. Usually a crisis occurs within a family constellation and affects all those in close contact with the client. It is not uncommon for parents to be struggling with midlife crisis at the same time their adolescent is struggling with establishing a separate identity.[1] People in crisis are either helped or hindered by those in their social network—friends, family, doctors, teachers, employer, and everyone else with whom the client routinely interacts.[1] The issues of crisis may be viewed within a social framework; until severed social relationships are reestablished, the crisis remains unresolved.

While working with families in crisis, the nurse determines which member of the family is most obviously upset in the crisis state. Different labels may be used: Who is the scapegoat? Who is the symptom bearer? Who is the identified client?[23] Next, the nurse identifies all members of the client's social resources that would be helpful to the client in crisis resolution. The nurse also explains the crisis to the person in crisis and explains how others can assist.

The intervener is directive in bringing together the client in crisis and all members of his or her social system for a conference. During the conference, all those involved in the crisis analyze the problem and its effect on each family member. Everyone is given an opportunity to voice comments or complaints. Available resources and possible solutions are discussed. By the end of the conference, the participants should develop a definite plan of action, including exactly who is to do what and when. The nurse should set up a follow-up meeting and help the group decide the time, place, participants, and purpose. The social system approach is effective in dealing with many-faceted crisis situations, such as family crisis.[18,26]

Frequently, the hospital scene is the scene of a family crisis:

> A 16-year-old boy was admitted to the hospital with the diagnosis of leukemia. Previously, he had been active in sports, and suddenly he was too tired to do anything but watch television. His father had recently died of a myocardial infarction. His mother refuses to allow her son to be informed about his illness and planned therapy.

Another admission may look like this:

> A 12-year-old girl has attempted suicide by taking an overdose of butalbital (Fiorinal). She has been living with her mother and step-father; however, she wants to live with her father and step-mother. The mother states that the child's father wants no communication or contact with the child. The mother told the student nurse, "Don't talk with my daughter about taking the pills. It just upsets her."

Case Study 39-1 explores the influence and effects of many people within and outside the family on the client in crisis.

EVALUATION

In the evaluation process, the nurse and client together evaluate whether the problem has been solved. Has the client regained equilibrium and usual level of functioning? It is important for the nurse to know when to let go of the client. Before dissolving the partnership, the nurse and client should engage in anticipatory planning to maximize the client's ability to avoid crisis responses in the future.[11] The client may need additional information about community services or community resources. After working through the crisis response, some clients are motivated to seek additional therapy to resolve old conflicts; referrals may be made.[1,21,23]

Outcomes

Within the managed health care environment and the total quality improvement model, client outcomes have great significance.[5,13,14] Additionally, the standards of psychiatric-mental health clinical nursing practice include outcome identification as one of the standards: "The psychiatric-mental health nurse identifies expected outcomes individualized to the client" (p 27).[3] The measurement criteria provide a framework for forming and evaluating the outcomes that result from applying crisis intervention theory and strategies. For example, one measurable outcome following interventions would be the length of time of the crisis—the target is 6 weeks. At the end of 6 weeks, the person's functioning level would be expected to be at the level of or higher than the precrisis state. Anxiety levels should be reduced; effective problem solving and adaptive coping skills should be present.

Standards of Psychiatric-Mental Health Clinical Nursing Practice

There is an excellent match between the use of crisis intervention theory and Standard of Care V-g. (Health Promotion and Health Maintenance), and with several of the Standards of Professional Performance (ie, Standard I, Quality of Care; Standard IV, Collegiality; Standard V, Ethics; Standard VI, Collaboration; Standard

39-1 Case Study

Assessing and Intervening With a Client in Crisis

Mrs. L, 36 years old, is a mother of two children (7 and 9 years old) and a full-time student in nursing school. One year before completing her nursing program, Mrs. L learned that her husband had been having an affair with a 20-year-old woman. He informed her that he was moving out and intended to live with the other woman.

Mrs. L came to the Community Mental Health Center for counseling because she was not maintaining a passing grade average and feared that she would not be able to remain in school. She was having difficulty coping with the abrupt changes in her personal life and the pressures of nursing school—and she desperately wanted to finish school.

Mrs. L felt alienated from everyone. Her parents, particularly her father, thought it must be her fault that her husband left. Her father remembered the trauma of his parents' divorce, and he did not want his grandchildren to grow up the way he did. Some of Mrs. L's friends were not able to spend much time with her. Her usual method of coping was to "work hard" and "stay as busy as possible." This coping tactic had not been useful for her lately because of her inability to concentrate, frequent crying spells, and insomnia. Mrs. L felt she was a failure as a woman and was concerned about her attractiveness to men.

The nurse, as crisis intervener, and Mrs. L agreed that the immediate problems were the impending divorce and staying in school. Financial options were explored, such as loans, scholarships, and working part time. Mrs. L was given permission and encouraged to get the help she needed. The nurse told her, "You have nothing to be ashamed of. You are having a difficult time as anyone would in your situation. Ask your teachers for the help you need." She was encouraged to reach out to some of her classmates for support.

An important point to consider when dealing with people who are getting a divorce is that often, the person's support system breaks down. Parents grieve the loss of their child's spouse and the family unit. Friends grieve as well; they will never interact as couples in quite the same way. Friends also experience fears and doubts about their own marriages. The person in crisis needs help in understanding the effects of the divorce on everyone. Through teaching direct communication and helping the client acknowledge with the parents and friends the natural sadness and loss, grieving is shared. It may be necessary to role play with the client how she might handle a difficult situation. For example, Mrs. L might role-play her encounter with her father. "Dad, I know you are very sad and hurt. This must bring back the feelings you had when your dad and mother got a divorce. I want you to know that I love you. That hasn't changed, and I need you to love me." If communication cannot be worked out with family and friends, the nurse must supply the emotional support to the client.

Other means of support should be explored, such as groups at the college's women's center. Mrs. L was able to work out better communication with her family and friends, which increased her feelings of being in control and increased her self-esteem. The children came into counseling for one session to work out communication problems within the family.

The nurse encouraged Mrs. L to make out a schedule for each day of the week and to include a treat every day—lunch with a friend, coffee in bed, and so forth. Mrs. L was frequently reminded to think highly of herself and to treat herself with respect. The nurse praised any efforts Mrs. L made to communicate with others and meet her own needs.

In dealing with her feelings about being a failure as a woman because her husband left to live with another woman, Mrs. L was helped to realize that for the last several years, she and her husband developed different goals that were in conflict. The reasons for the divorce, she began to understand, had nothing to do with her attractiveness as a woman.

After several weeks, Mrs. L was a member of a study group and was again making passing grades. She looked better and stated that she felt better. She was able to juggle care of her children, continue with school, work part-time, and socialize ocpcasionally with the help of classmates who were in similar circumstances. Mrs. L related that the divorce was the most painful experience of her life, but she was stronger than she ever thought possible and felt better able to cope with her present and future life.

Questions for Discussion

1. What does divorce mean in American society today? What are the cultural variations of the meaning of divorce?
2. Discuss the effects of divorce on family members and friends. Why is divorce such a devastating experience for most people?
3. What actions of friends and family might help the client avoid a crisis situation?
4. How could health care workers assist the client and her family?
5. Discuss therapeutic techniques to use when working with a client with a distorted perception of a stressful event.

VII, Research; and Standard VIII, Resource Utilization). Clearly, crisis intervention theory, with its roots in several different theoretical perspectives, is compatible with the phenomena of concern for psychiatric-mental health nursing and the focus on cost containment, outcomes, community-based care, and cultural diversity.[4]

THE NURSE'S FEELINGS AND ATTITUDES

The client facing an overwhelming threat needs assistance quickly. Nurses can, and must, provide effective crisis intervention. The nurse's first experiences in crisis intervention will not be easy or comfortable. Often, the novice needs assistance in determining the appropriate expectations for client and nurse.[9] Feelings of apprehension, frustration, anger, and wanting to escape from the situation are not uncommon. Even the most experienced crisis intervener needs a colleague or supervisor who will help discuss feelings, plan strategies, and offer support and encouragement.

Anyone who works with people in stressful situations needs to be aware of his or her own vulnerability to crisis.[10,26] Nurses who have learned to cope well with the inherent stress of the hospital setting have often created their own support system within the work environment. Debriefing after a particular traumatic event on the unit frequently brings some relief to the caregivers.[8,29,32] In one hospice unit, for example, the nurses meet together for a few minutes at the beginning and end of each shift to share what is going on with each other. Frequently, they bring food to share as well. When a nurse is having a difficult time, the others feel comfortable offering comfort as they would comfort a family member.[24] Support of this nature is advantageous, if not mandatory, in maintaining mental health.[1]

◆ Chapter Summary

This chapter has examined how clients and families respond when faced with an overwhelming stressor; it has also examined the therapeutic approach to help them avoid or grow from the crisis. The major points of the chapter are as follows:

1. Crisis theory evolved from the study of grief and bereavement by many researchers.
2. A client faced with an overwhelming threat tries to apply usual coping mechanisms; if they are unsuccessful in solving the problem, a mounting level of anxiety is experienced.
3. A crisis occurs when a client is unable to solve a problem that is perceived as overwhelming, when usual coping mechanisms fail to solve the problem, when perception of the event is distorted, and when the necessary support is not supplied.
4. A client experiencing a crisis is more open to learning new coping skills to deal with problems
5. The crisis client has the potential to develop more adaptive coping and healthier functioning capabilities after the crisis experience.
6. Maturational crises result from developmental changes and milestones, such as puberty, marriage, old age, and death of a loved one.
7. Situational crises result from a sudden, unexpected event, such as divorce, illness, injury, or loss of a job.
8. Crisis intervention is a thinking, directive, problem-solving approach that focuses only on the client's immediate problems.
9. Nurses are often the first health care professionals in contact with the client in crisis; therefore, they are uniquely positioned to intervene in crisis.
10. Any crisis intervener needs a colleague or supervisor to discuss feelings, plan approaches, and receive support and encouragement.
11. Critical incident stress debriefing is a form of crisis intervention.
12. Crisis intervention is an effective theory and model for home care nursing.
13. Crisis intervention is a component of case management, managed care systems, and psychosocial rehabilitation.
14. The crisis intervener needs to provide culturally competent care.
15. The standards of psychiatric-mental health clinical nursing practice provide a framework for the delivery of crisis intervention.
16. Client outcomes are a significant focus in the current cost-effective managed care system. Measurable outcomes of crisis intervention include functional level, anxiety, problem solving, coping skills, and time to resolution.

Review Questions

1. During the first phase of a crisis the nurse is likely to observe which of the following in the client:
   A. Increased levels of anxiety
   B. Effective problem solving
   C. Reaching out for help
   D. Short attention span and rumination
2. The nurse recognizes that the goal for crisis intervention is which one of the following?
   A. Resolution of long-term problems
   B. Gaining insight into past problems
   C. Reestabishment of precrisis level of functioning
3. The crisis that occurs as one grows older is called:
   A. Situational crisis
   B. Maturational crisis

C. Crisis of values
D. Crisis of spirit

4. The nurse utilizing the nursing process is most likely to identify which of the following nursing diagnoses:
   A. Ineffective individual coping related to inadequate support systems
   B. Impaired physical mobility related to neuromuscular impairment
   C. Anxiety related to situational crises
   D. Social isolation related to preoccupation with crisis event.
5. The nurse may evaluate the positive outcome for the nursing diagnosis of Altered Thought Process related to impaired ability to make decisions by which of the following:
   A. The client's report of a decrease in feelings of anxiety
   B. The client's use of the agreed upon coping (problem solving) strategies
   C. The client is able to give a realistic interpretation of the crisis event
   D. The client's recognition of personal capabilities.

◆ References

1. Aguilera DC: Crisis Intervention: Theory and Methodology, 7th ed. St. Louis, Mosby-Year Book, 1994
2. American Managed Behavioral Healthcare Association and National Association of State Mental Health Program Directors: Public mental health systems, medicaid restructuring and managed behavioral healthcare. Behavioral Healthcare Tomorrow September/October: 63–69. 1995
3. American Psychiatric Association: Diagnostic and Statistical Manual of Mental Disorders, 4th ed. Washington, DC, American Psychiatric Association, 1994
4. American Nurses Association: A Statement on Psychiatric-Mental Health Clinical Nursing Practice and Standards of Psychiatric-Mental Health Clinical Nursing Practice. Washington, DC, American Nurses Association, 1994
5. Bardadell J: Cost Effectiveness and Quality of Care Provided by Clinical Nurse Specialists. J Psychosoc Nurs 32 (3): 21–24, 1994
6. Bellak L, Small L: Emergency Psychotherapy and Brief Psychotherapy, 2nd ed. New York, Grune & Stratton, 1978
7. Bloom BL: Definitional Aspects of the Crisis Concept. In Parad H (ed): Crisis Intervention: Selected Readings, pp 303–311. New York, Family Service Association of America, 1973
8. Bultema J: The Healing Process for the Multidisciplinary Team: Recovering Post-inpatient Suicide. J Psychosoc Nurs 32 (2): 19–24, 1994
9. Burgess WA, Baldwin B: Crisis Intervention Theory and Practice: A Clinical Handbook. New York, Prentice Hall, 1981
10. Caplan G: Principles of Preventive Psychiatry. New York, Basic Books, 1964
11. Caplan G, Gruenbaum H: Perspectives on Primary Prevention. Arch Gen Psychiatry 17 (September): 333–345, 1967
12. Connolly P: What Does a Nurse Need to Know and Do to Maintain an Effective Case Management? J Psychosoc Nurs 30 (3): 35–39, 1992
13. Davis S, Greenly-Adams M: Integrating Patient Satisfaction With a Quality Improvement Program. J Nurs Adm 24 (12): 28–31, 1994
14. Donabedian A: The Role of Outcomes in Quality Assessment and Assurance. Quality Review Bulletin November: 356–360, 1992
15. Duffey J, Miller M, Parlocha P: Psychiatric Home Care: A Framework for Assessment and Intervention. Home Health Nurse 11 (2): 22–28, 1993
16. Eppard J, Anderson J: Emergency Psychiatric Assessment: The Nurse, Psychiatrist, and Counselor Roles During the Process. J Psychosoc Nurs 33 (10): 17–23, 1995
17. Erikson E: Childhood and Society, 2nd ed. New York, WW Norton, 1963
18. Fawcett C: Family Psychiatric Nursing. St. Louis, CV Mosby, 1993
19. Giglio J: The Impact of Patients' and Therapists' Religious Values on Psychotherapy. Hosp Community Psychiatry 44 (8): 768–771, 1993
20. Glenister DA: A therapeutic group for clients with acute mental health problems. J Adv Nurs 18 (12): 1968–1974, 1993
21. Godbey KL, Courage MM: Stress Management Program: Intervention in Nursing Student Performance Anxiety. Archives of Psychiatric Nursing 8 (3): 190–199, 1994
22. Goodman M, Brown J, Dietz P: Managing Managed Care: A Mental Health Practitioner's Survival Guide. Washington, DC, American Psychiatric Press, 1992
23. Hoff L: People in Crisis: Understanding and Helping. Menlo Park, CA, Addison-Wesley, 1989
24. Hoffman Y: Surviving a Child's Suicide. American Journal of Nursing, July 87: 955–956, 1987.
25. Lindeman E: Symptomology and Management of Acute Grief. Am J Psychiatry 101 (September): 141–148, 1944
26. Mandt KA: The Curriculum Revolution in Action: Nursing and Crisis Intervention for Victims of Family Violence. J Nurs Educ 32 (1): 44–46, 1993
27. Mitchell JT: When Disaster Strikes: The Critical Incident Stress Debriefing Process. Journal of Emergency Medical Services 8: 36–39, 1983
28. Palmer-Erbs V, Anthony E: Incorporating Psychiatric Rehabilitation Principles Into Psychiatric-Mental Health Nursing Practice: An Opportunity to Develop a Full Partnership Among Nurses, Consumers, and Families. J Psychosoc Nurs 33 (3): 36–44, 1995
29. Pickett M, Brennan Walsh AM, Greenburg HS, Licht L, Worrell Deignan J: Use of Debriefing Techniques to Prevent Compassion Fatigue in Research Teams. Nurs Res 43 (4): 250–252, 1994
30. Ragaisis KM: Critical Incident Stress Debriefing: A Family Nursing Intervention. Archives of Psychiatric Nursing 8 (1): 38–43, 1994
31. San Blise ML: Crisis Intervention: Aftershocks in the Quake Zone. J Psychosoc Nurs 32 (5): 29–30, 1994
32. Stanley SR: When the Disaster is Over: Helping the Healers to Mend. J Psychosoc Nurs 28 (5): 12–16, 1990
33. Ward P, Eck C, Sanquin T: Emergency Nursing at the Epicenter: The Loma Prieta Earthquake. Journal of Emergency Nursing 49 (July-August): 51–52, 1990
34. Yalom I: The Theory and Practice of Group Psychotherapy, 4th ed. New York, Basic Books, 1995

Rape and Sexual Assault

Sally Francis

The world breaks everyone and afterwards many are strong in the broken places.

Ernest Hemingway,
A Farewell to Arms

Rape is a crime of violence that touches everyone at some time in some way. In the United States, an estimated 1 in every 10 women is a victim of rape, and a rape occurs once every 6 minutes.[50] A victim and her family, friends, coworkers, and acquaintances must acknowledge and face their own fears of vulnerability, loss of control, perversion, bodily harm, and death. The hope in a crisis event that affects so many people is that all can become strong in the broken places and that psychiatric-mental health nurses will recognize and respond to the needs of the rape victim and her significant others during the mending and healing process.

This chapter discusses rape and sexual assault, its theoretical perspectives, the emotional effects and recovery, and interventions. The nursing process is discussed during the immediate or emergency phase, the intermediate phase, and the recovery phase of the rape crisis. Through the nursing process—assessment, nursing diagnosis, planning, intervention, and evaluation—individuals and families affected by rape or sexual assault can be assisted to cope and adapt.

Rape can and does occur with men as victims. Men raped by other men have been found to have long-term cases of depression, difficulties in peer relationships, and sexual dysfunction.[34] Men raped by women report sexual dysfunction and depression.[42] However, the overwhelming majority of rape victims are female. For this reason, this chapter focuses on the female rape victim. It is reasonable to assume that the nursing process as applied to women can also benefit male victims.

Learning Objectives

On completion of this chapter, you should be able to accomplish the following:

1. *Identify the typology of rape and sexual assault.*
2. *Define the term rape trauma syndrome, and discuss the behaviors of a victim during its acute, reorganization, and recovery phases.*
3. *Identify and define unresolved rape trauma and silent rape trauma.*
4. *Discuss primary motivating forces of the assailant in crimes of rape and sexual assault.*
5. *Discuss primary offender treatments.*
6. *Apply the nursing process to the care of the victim of rape or sexual assault.*
7. *Recognize and discuss feelings you have that may influence the therapeutic use of self with victims of rape and sexual assault.*

◆ Theoretical Perspectives of Rape and Sexual Assault

Rape and sexual assault can be viewed from historical, legal, psychological, and sociological perspectives. Until recent years, this overwhelming physical assault on women received very little research attention. Ancient Greek myths contain descriptions of rape that have persisted through the centuries. References to rape appear in literature from each era of civilization. Nevertheless, it was not until the early 1970s that researchers attempted to describe the victim and rapist in terms that could lead to intervention and influence the psychological impact of rape.

LEGAL PERSPECTIVE

Definition of Rape and Sexual Assault

Rape is a crime involving lack of consent, force or threat of force, and sexual penetration. Sexual assault refers to forcible sexual acts performed without the victim's consent and against his or her will. Rape is defined as a crime by the legal statutes of individual state governments.

The use of force is important in identifying rape or sexual assault. Rape and sexual assault are crimes of force and violence in which sex becomes the means of expressing violence, just as in a murder, a gun may become the means of expressing violence.

PSYCHOLOGICAL PERSPECTIVE

One of the most traumatizing aspects of rape or sexual assault involves the victims' feelings about being physically forced to do something against their will. The life-threatening nature of the crime, helplessness, loss of control, and experiencing of self as an object of rage all work together to produce overwhelming fear and stress for the victim. This experience has been described as the *rape trauma syndrome*.[3,4] This syndrome is viewed by some as a particular example of post-traumatic stress disorder as defined in the Diagnostic and Statistical Manual of Mental Disorders, fourth edition. This classification can be made when the following four conditions are met:

1. Existence of a recognizable stressor
2. Reexperience of the trauma, as evidenced by recurrent recollections of the event
3. Numbing of responsiveness or reduced involvement with the external world
4. Two additional symptoms, such as sleep disturbances, guilt about surviving or behaviors required for survival, memory impairment, difficulty concentrating, avoiding activities that arouse recollection of the traumatic event, and intensified symptoms on exposure to events that symbolize or resemble the event[18,25,26]

Regaining internal equilibrium and the ability to reorganize life into a meaningful and productive whole becomes the goal of intervention.

Types of Sexual Assault

Burgess and Holmstrom were the early researchers in the study of rape trauma syndrome.[6] Based on their study of 146 rape victims in the early 1970s, they identified four types of sexual assault: the blitz rape, confidence rape, accessory-to-sex with inability to consent, and the sex–stress situation. *Blitz rape* occurs when the victim does not know the rapist and is not aware of her vulnerability. Although blitz rape usually occurs in the victim's home, the rapist may attack suddenly in a parking lot, on the street, or in any place where the victim is isolated or helpless.

> I thought I was having a bad dream—that I was screaming. As I regained consciousness, I felt like I was moving up from a dark hole, screaming. It seemed like I slowly realized I wasn't dreaming. I was awake and screaming. A man was holding me down on the sofa where I had fallen asleep earlier in the evening. He had his hands on my face, pushing me down and trying to cover my mouth. He kept telling me to shut up, to stop screaming.

Confidence rape involves some interaction between the assailant and victim before the rape occurs. The rapist gains access to the victim by gaining her confidence in some way. For example, the man may ring a doorbell, ask to use the phone for some assistance, enter the woman's territory, and then rape her.

Accessory-to-sex describes sexual acts with a person who is unable to consent to sex. The inability to consent results from the victim's immature stage of personality or cognitive development, which prevents recognizing or understanding the overtures and sexual events. An example of the accessory-to-sex type of sexual assault would be a mentally retarded woman who is seduced by the promise of material goods in exchange for sexual activity.

Sex–stress situation refers to events arising after initial consent to sex is given. For example, a woman may agree to a sexual experience with a man who later becomes violent and physically abusive. She then withdraws her earlier consent, and he rapes her.

Date rape is similar to the sex–stress situation in that consent to be with the man has been given, but consent to sexual activity has not.[7,33]

In each of these situations, sexual acts are rapists' means for acting out their distorted perceptions. The woman becomes an object and experiences this objectification, powerlessness, and loss of self as a basic, consuming fear. The resultant trauma reaction of the victim—rape trauma syndrome—promotes self-preservation; it is a flight reaction when fight is not possible. Rape trauma syndrome identifies the psychological work in which the ego must engage to preserve its identity and integration.

SOCIOLOGICAL PERSPECTIVE

Myths About Rape

Although the motivation to rape arises from personality, societal attitudes influence the incidence, prevalence, and treatment of rape and sexual assault. The sociological perspective includes the myths that society holds about rape.[8,21,45] These myths and stereotypical views of rape define how a victim sees herself in relation to society, how society views the victim and the rapist, and the difficulty or ease with which a victim receives support from society. For example, a prevalent myth is that rape is motivated by sexual desire and that the woman who is raped must have "asked for it." Rapists are seen as exaggerations of the macho male. In fact, rape is not motivated by sexual desire but by a desire to do violence. Blaming the victim only adds to the violent assault on her self-integrity.

If the victim is a person who society believes would not "ask for it" (eg, a child or an elderly woman), the rapist is viewed as very sick. A young woman hitchhiking who is raped but not beaten by a driver who picks her up is frequently viewed with little sympathy; however, her fears, helplessness, and loss of control can be as traumatizing as those of a woman badly beaten in a blitz rape. Not infrequently, women who are raped share the myths of society. They experience self-blame and guilt and feel that they should have done something, or not done something, that could have prevented the assault.[32,49]

> A part of me was relieved when the police came that I looked so bad, that there was blood, that the door had been broken open, the house was torn up, and there were fingerprints. There couldn't be any doubt that something awful had happened to me.

Who Is to Blame?

Public education programs have made progress in changing society's attitudes about rape and sexual assault (Box 40-1). Nevertheless, rape continues to be one of the most frequently underreported crimes. In an attempt to understand public attitudes, several studies have examined how various segments of society attribute blame for the crime of rape.

In one study, four predominant causal attitudes toward rape were identified: blaming the victim, blaming the offender, blaming society, and blaming the situation.[51] Another study added ineffective law enforcement and judicial procedures as potential causes of rape.[15] The multidimensional nature of societal attitudes toward rape has been demonstrated by two studies in which victim blame, offender characteristics, situational characteristics, and societal blame emerged as factors in the development of these attitudes.[14,40] Other studies have identified differences between the sexes in attitudes toward rape.[14,15,40] Women tend to place greater blame on society for rape

BOX 40-1

Self-Assessment: Myths About Rape

1. Rape is a crime of passion. True False
2. In the acute phase of rape trauma syndrome, the victim is extremely vocal in expressions of distress with profuse crying and sobbing. True False
3. Unresolved rape trauma refers to a trauma that has never been discussed with anyone. True False
4. Assailants in rape and sexual assault are motivated by something about a woman that arouses their sexual interest. True False
5. All treatment programs for offenders are carried out in prison. True False
6. It is necessary to ask the victim a standard set of questions regarding the sexual assault to gain sufficient information to begin the nursing process. True False
7. "Blaming the victim" may be a useful tool to distance yourself from overwhelming feelings of fear, particularly when you realize that some victims are careless in their own personal safety habits. True False

Answers: 1. F; 2. F; 3. F; 4. F; 5. F; 6. F; 7. F.

and sexual assault. Clinical research, feminist writings, and popular literature have explored the socialization into sex roles and the role of violence in American society. In a society that encourages the treatment of women as sex objects and encourages violence, they argue that women cannot avoid attack.[8,9,53] What can change is who will be attacked.

Characteristics of Rapists

Who rapes and why? Groth, a leading researcher into rape offenders, concludes that rape is more than an illegal act or an extreme of cultural role behavior.[21,22] It is a sexual deviation wherein the offender's pathology becomes the etiology of the victim's trauma. Although similar acts may be performed, rapists are not alike. Rapists perform sexual acts in the service of nonsexual needs. It is through these needs, rather than through other behavioral characteristics, that rapists can be classified and described.

The *power rapist* wants to place a woman in a helpless, controlled situation where she cannot resist or refuse him. This situation provides the rapist with a reassuring sense of strength, mastery, security, and control, all of which compensate for his underlying feelings of inadequacy. Usually, the offender has no conscious intention to hurt his victim. His aim, rather, is to have complete control over her. Nevertheless, aggression may increase with time as the offender becomes repetitive and compulsive in his behavior and more desperate to achieve the feelings of power, control, and adequacy.

> He had a knife but he didn't use it. Thank God he didn't cut me. He used his fists instead and he pulled me around by my hair. All the time he was verbally abusive: called me names and told me if I did what he told me to, he wouldn't kill me. He made me get down on my hands and knees and crawl while he pulled me around by my hair. There was no way out of the room; he was in complete control. When the trial started, there were nine of us who had been raped by this one guy. It was amazing how much alike our stories were. He did the same things, used the same words. The most frightening part was that the police thought there were more; one woman was murdered.

The *anger rapist* uses sexual assault to express and discharge feelings of intense anger, frustration, and contempt. The sexual assault is an impulsive act of aggression to retaliate against a world for perceived wrongs. The assault is not compulsive; instead, it is characterized by more brutality and physical harm due to the expression of rage. The anger rapist derives satisfaction not from sexual gratification, but from the relief resulting from the discharge of anger and the degradation and humiliation of the victim.

The *sadistic rapist* finds pleasure in premeditated and ritualistic acts of violence, usually involving bondage and torture. The rapist's anger and need for control become sexualized through the intense pleasure derived from hurting, degrading, and frequently destroying the victim.

The *date rapist* is known to the victim, who has given consent to be with him. Frequently, rape by an acquaintance (following consent to share company but not sexual activity) is not reported. In a study of 71 self-disclosed college students who had raped, the significant influence came from the male's reference group (a supportive hypererotic male culture with peer-group pressure for sexual activity) and less from violence as a sexual stimulant. In date rape, the man fails to recognize or disregards the woman's rejection and continues to the coital experience. The coital experience, manifest and anticipated benefits, and the accompanying reaffirmation of self-worth as developed through the reference group appear to be the primary motivations.[7,24,33]

Treatment of Offenders

Treatment for sex offenders has gained support, because criminal prosecution does not completely prevent the offender from posing a continued threat to society.

Many offenders are back in their communities within 6 months to 4 years after conviction.[20] Early treatment is urged as an attempt to prevent deviant sexual activity from escalating into more violent activity. Treatment can occur in residential and community programs. Four basic approaches have been used: behavioral techniques, social skills training, psychodynamic techniques, and organic approaches.[20,31,35,40] Effective treatment of sex offenders described by McCarthy has four components:

1. Reduction in deviant arousal using aversive conditioning techniques
2. Sex education, assertiveness training, and competency training
3. Confrontation that causes offenders to empathize with victims, to label deviant behavior as inappropriate, and to apologize to victims
4. An appropriate adult sexual outlet[30]

The type of rape has implications for the treatment of the victim and offender. Anger rape is the most frequent type of rape; however, power rapists make up a larger population of incarcerated offenders. Conviction rates may be higher when there is more physical harm to introduce as evidence in court proceedings.[30] Just as the victim of an anger rapist is distressed by the physical abuse she suffered, the woman who was not outwardly harmed by a power rapist also has fears.[39] The victim of a power rapist may have recurring fears if the offender was not convicted, and she cannot be reassured by the knowledge that he is in prison. How victims cope and adapt to these overwhelming fears is discussed in the following section.

◆ Rape Trauma Syndrome

RAPE CRISIS

Rape crisis is the internal and external disequilibrium experienced by the victim of rape or sexual assault. The encounter with a life-threatening situation evokes extreme feelings of fear and vulnerability. The process of adaptation known as *rape trauma syndrome* involves becoming free from this fear, redefining feelings of vulnerability and helplessness, and regaining control and equilibrium in life. The clustering of symptoms in response to the trauma of rape appears to be fairly consistent. It occurs during an acute phase and a period of integration and resolution and constitutes a nursing diagnosis.[3,4,36]

ACUTE PHASE: DISORGANIZATION

The *disorganization phase* includes the rape victim's immediate expressed or controlled reactions, her physical reactions, and her emotional reactions to a life-threatening situation. In this phase, the prominent feelings are fright, anxiety, anger, and disbelief.[8] These feelings can be seen in an expressive response in which the victim actively displays and discusses feelings. Second guessing often occurs; for example, the victim asks herself "Did I do everything I should have to avoid this?" The second-guessing phenomenon of self-recrimination can be a source of guilt and in some instances can lead to severe depression. Self-blame also can be an adaptive coping process that allows the victim to identify changes she can make in the environment to increase feelings of control and mastery.

In a *controlled reaction,* the rape victim appears outwardly calm and composed. Although conventional wisdom might lead us to expect victims of rape or sexual assault to be crying, hysterical, or visibly upset in some manner, many women do not respond in these ways. A woman who has a controlled reaction to the rape has no less internal suffering and fear, just a different way of handling herself in the acute phase.

> I went next door to get my neighbor. I remember she said I seemed so calm while we waited for the police. Inside, I was shaking with relief to be with a safe person, but I didn't want to talk much until the police came. I think a shock reaction was setting in. By the time I got to the hospital, I was not so much calm as simply exhausted.

Physical reactions during the acute phase vary according to the injury incurred. Often, the woman is sore, which may be generalized as muscle tension eases or localized to parts of the body that were a focus of the assault. Sleep disturbances, eating pattern disturbances, and symptoms specific to the attack occur frequently.

> In the first days and weeks after the rape, I couldn't fall asleep until it was daylight. My scalp was sore for days and then just sometimes it seemed tender, even after the bruises were gone. I developed little rituals, patterns, for going to bed and for washing my hair. They provided some structure for my anxiety but didn't really take away the fear.

Emotional reactions to rape and sexual assault are primarily fear (ie, the fear of bodily harm, death, or mutilation), anger, humiliation, and self-blame. Frequently, the victim experiences heightened emotional reactions and overreactions in situations not related to the rape. Increased irritability, impatience, tearfulness, and anger can cause the victim to feel out of control and out of touch with herself. Incessant thoughts about the event and sudden memory flashes at unlikely and unexpected times add to the victim's feelings of loss of control during this initial phase.

> The first couple of weeks at work I was so busy, I didn't have much time to think about what had happened. Nights at home were the worst part. But there was one

> person at work that I just couldn't be around. He is a very nice, friendly person, but physically, he reminded me of the guy. Just his outgoing, friendly chatter would make me nervous, and I'd feel myself withdrawing and feeling threatened and vulnerable. It's an awful way to feel about someone who is just trying to be nice.

The length of the acute phase may vary from a few days to a few weeks. Often, the symptoms of this phase carry into long-term adjustment as post-traumatic stress syndrome.[12,46-48]

LONG-TERM PROCESS: REORGANIZATION

Reorganization refers to the adjustment and adaptation during the months following the rape or sexual assault. Of the 81 victims followed up 4 years after rape, Burgess and Holmstrom found that 74% felt recovered.[7] Half of these women felt recovered within months following the attack, and the other half said that it took years before they recovered. Some of the women (26%) did not yet feel recovered 4 years after the rape. Comparison of 35 rape victims with nonabused, matched control subjects found the victims to be significantly more depressed, more generally anxious, and more fearful than the control subjects, regardless of the number of years that had passed since the rape. The researchers concluded that sexually assaulted women have definite long-term psychological problems.[46] Two other studies found increased depression, substance abuse, anxiety disorders, and suicide in sexual assault victims.[47,48]

The period of reorganization involves regaining equilibrium in physical, psychological, social, and sexual lifestyles. The period of reorganization closely resembles the grief process described by Lindemann.[29] The process of regaining equilibrium is an interim period in which the victim appears to have adjusted and returns to the normal routines of life, school, or work.[6] This interim period is followed by a period of resolution in which feelings toward self and the rapist, feelings about sexuality, and feelings of loss are gradually assimilated. Issues important to the rape victim during the reorganization process include the following:

1. Regaining a feeling of physical well-being and safety
2. Working through fears and phobias
3. Coming to terms with losses, such as loss of self-esteem and loss of trust
4. Assimilating the event into the person's sense of self

Unresolved Sexual Trauma

Unresolved sexual trauma occurs when the victim does not deal with the feelings or reactions to the experience, neither assimilating nor adapting to the sexual assault. Typically, unresolved sexual trauma occurs more often in women who have little or no intervention to support them during the acute phase of rape trauma or who experience subsequent victimization. Women who at the time of the attack face chronic life stressors, lack social support, suffer poor self-esteem, or have been victims before are also more likely to experience unresolved sexual trauma.[6,5,19] Another risk factor in unresolved sexual trauma is the woman's place in the life cycle; young women and those for whom the sexual assault was their first sexual experience may have delayed recovery from rape trauma. The nurse may suspect unresolved sexual trauma when the following conditions are present:

1. The person develops persistent phobic symptoms, such as fear of being alone or going out.
2. The person retreats from sexual themes and has lowered self-esteem and guilt feelings.
3. A relatively minor event triggers the symptoms of the rape trauma.
4. The anniversary date of the sexual assault brings on symptoms of the rape trauma.
5. The person totally avoids contact with members of the opposite sex.
6. Relationships with family and friends shift in negative ways toward withdrawal, unusual anger, or silence; negativity may represent displacement of feelings toward the assailant.

A type of unresolved sexual trauma is seen in a silent reaction to rape, wherein the rape victim has never discussed the sexual assault with anyone.

RECOVERY FROM RAPE TRAUMA

A community intervention program can help the victim recover from rape trauma. This program is a coordinated effort to bring together all bureaucratic systems—medical, legal, police, and judicial—and support systems of the victim and family toward the common goal of helping her resolve the crisis and reorganize her life. Public education and community awareness are other essential components of a comprehensive community intervention program. Aims of community intervention include the following:

1. The police are knowledgeable and concerned about the crime and effective in apprehending the assailant.
2. Medical treatment is administered with care, and good evidence is collected.
3. The district attorney's office works closely with the police, medical, and forensic science departments to ensure apprehension and conviction of the assailant.

4. The public is educated and assured of the effectiveness of responses from the various systems involved with the victim of rape or sexual assault.

When these aims have been met, victims are more willing to report the assault and more likely to work through the events surrounding the attack successfully. The victim must have careful, caring interactions with each system she encounters after the assault. Trained counselors available through victim support programs also can assist the victim and her family and friends by providing crisis counseling during the immediate trauma and through resolution and reorganization. When a crisis center or victim support program is not available, hospital and emergency room nurses can use crisis intervention techniques to offer supportive counseling to the woman experiencing rape trauma syndrome.

Application of the Nursing Process to Victims of Rape and Sexual Assault

ASSESSMENT

Assessing a victim of rape or sexual assault begins at the initial encounter. This may take place in an emergency room, hospital, physician's office, or a counseling center.[2,8,38,40]

Assessing the victim's physical status is necessary to determine the extent of external and internal injuries and to begin planning appropriate medical interventions. The victim's appearance and the condition of her body must not be altered, because physical evidence is essential to the apprehension and prosecution of the assailant. First aid may be administered to the victim, but further medical attention should be conducted in conjunction with the medical team responsible for the collection of evidence in sexual assault cases.

When assessing the victim's emotional state, the nurse first attends to her primary concerns, offering information and reassurance in these areas before addressing other issues. Some women focus on concerns for physical safety. Others have anxiety about significant others; for example, a woman may ask, "What will I tell my husband?" Accepting these concerns and providing supportive care can calm the victim and can begin establishing a therapeutic alliance. Emotional assessment also includes determining the victim's perception of the event, her coping behaviors, and her situational and social supports (Box 40-2).

Of particular importance in assessment is the role of self-blame,[48] especially the distinction between maladaptive and adaptive uses of self-blame. The nurse must continually assess the victim's use of self-blame. *Behavioral self-blame* represents adaptive, control-oriented responses. Attribution is made to a controllable, modifiable source ("I should not have walked home so late at night. I won't do that again"). The victim can believe that she can avoid similar experiences in the future and thereby have a sense of regaining control and decreased helplessness. *Characterological self-blame* is maladaptive and associated with depression and helplessness. Attribution is made to character—an internal, relatively nonmodifiable source.

Behavioral self-blame can serve three needs in positive adaptation: the needs for perceived control over one's life, to preserve belief in a just world, and to find meaning for negative life experiences. Anxiety is reduced by providing a reason for the rape through self-blame. When self-blame is helpful to the victim, it may be inaccurately viewed by others, who may try to dissuade the victim from the self-blame beliefs. Awareness that expression of negative affect and behavioral self-blame may be helpful can assist the nurse in carrying out the nursing process. Further, the nurse must have realistic expectations about the length of recovery time.[11]

NURSING DIAGNOSIS

When analyzing the assessment data provided by the rape victim and her significant other, the nurse may arrive at many possible nursing diagnoses. Some of the accepted nursing diagnoses that are appropriate in guiding nursing intervention for the rape victim include the following:

1. Physical needs
   a. Risk for Infection
   b. Risk for Trauma
   c. Altered Nutrition: Less than body requirements
   d. Pain, acute
   e. Sleep Pattern Disturbance
   f. Sexual Dysfunction
2. Emotional needs
   a. Anxiety
   b. Rape-Trauma Syndrome
   c. Spiritual Distress
   d. Impaired Social Interaction
   e. Powerlessness
   f. Fear
   g. Body Image Disturbance, Self Esteem Disturbance, Altered Role Performance, Personal Identity Disturbance
   h. Ineffective Individual Coping
   i. Ineffective Family Coping: Compromised, Disabling

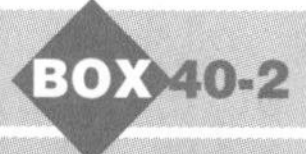

Therapeutic Dialogue: Making Contact With a Rape Victim

Ann B, a 20-year-old college student, called the crisis line of a metropolitan hospital. She was referred to the obstetrics-gynecology clinic of the hospital and spoke with a staff nurse in the clinic.

Client: I'm calling for some information.

Nurse: Yes, I'm Ms Smith; how may I help you?

Client: I've been staying with a friend for the afternoon. We were going to watch the game on television. He went out to get some things at the grocery. The doorbell rang and a man wanted to use the phone to get his car started. He came in and then, and then, well I don't know what to do. I'm alright; he didn't hurt me, but I don't know what to do. He left. I'm okay. Johnny came back and, and what should I do?

Nurse: I think you are telling me that you've been attacked. I'd like to help; could you tell me your name? Your first name is fine if that's all you want to share now.

Client: Ann.

Nurse: Ann, I am a nurse here in the clinic. When a woman has been attacked, she can come here. We can help you and see that you have medical attention. A rape crisis counselor is available to stay with you while you see the doctor and talk with the police.

Client: Oh, do I have to talk to the police? I'm really all right. He didn't hurt me. I don't have any cuts or anything, but I don't know what to do. It was so dumb of me to let him come in. I don't know how I could have been so dumb!

Nurse: Ann, you weren't dumb. You did what many people would do when they want to be helpful. Lots of women have done the same thing. You may not have been hurt, but you may need medical attention. The best thing you can do now is come in. You don't have to talk to the police if you don't want to. The crisis counselor can talk with you and explain what the police can do and then you can decide. But it would be good to see a doctor. John can come with you, and he can be with you. You don't have to come by yourself. We don't have to tell anyone about this, but you do need to see a doctor.

In this initial contact, the nurse is establishing a climate of supportiveness for Ann by providing her with information and being directive in regard to the immediate steps that she must take to meet her health care needs.

Nurse: Ann, I'm going to be here when you come in. I'll look for you and introduce you to the counselor. The doctor will want to examine you. You need to have some medicine so you won't get an infection. Would you like John to bring you?

Client: Yes, I guess so. He can bring me.

Nurse: That will be good. It will be better if you come now. Don't take a bath or shower, but just come now as you are. Can I give John directions? (The nurse then talked with John and gave him directions to the hospital and the clinic.)

Nurse: John, I know this must be upsetting for you.

John: That crazy s.o.b. I'd like to find him and string him up. I don't know how this could have happened. If I'd just stayed home. . . .

Nurse: John, I know you are angry. Right now, though, Ann needs you to be calm. She is blaming herself for what's happened. She may think your anger is at her for doing something she thinks is stupid, letting the man in the house. Ann needs medical attention now, and while you're here, you can talk with the rape crisis counselor to decide what to do next.

DISCUSSION

During an initial contact with a rape victim, it is essential to address the state of disequilibrium that the victim experiences after the attack by providing her with information and specific actions that she can take. These directions offer her structure and a sense of control to counteract her feelings of help-

continued

BOX 40-2 (Continued)

lessness and of being overwhelmed. The information should be given in a warm, supportive, personal manner. This form of interaction opens an avenue through which the victim can begin to develop a trusting relationship with the nurse or other health care provider.

In this situation, the nurse assessed John's immediate reactions to the rape and his ability to support Ann during the initial phase of the crisis. After allowing John to express his anger and acknowledging his feelings, the nurse focused on providing directives to him on how he could help Ann at this time. In this way, the nurse assisted John in gaining a sense of control and purposefulness for his feelings.

Note that in this initial contact, the nurse did not probe for information about the attack. The primary goal of the interaction was to begin the process of trust building and provide information about the specific steps that the woman needed to take. The nurse did not initiate discussion of issues that are common to rape victims but addressed only those issues brought up by Ann, that is, her feelings of shame and guilt.

After trust has been established and the immediate need for medical attention has been met, Ann and John will be counseled individually to assess their perceptions of the event, their situational supports, and their coping mechanisms. Planning for therapeutic interventions will be based on these assessments. Ann and John will also be counseled together to facilitate their understanding and sharing their feelings. Separately and together, Ann and John will be involved in anticipatory planning for the events and feelings to come.

j. Altered Family Process
k. Altered Growth and Development
l. Impaired Verbal Communication
m. Knowledge Deficit concerning physical and emotional responses and health care needs

PLANNING

Setting goals for the victim of rape or sexual assault includes plans to aid the woman during the immediate, interim, and long-term phases of rape trauma syndrome. Immediate concerns are the promotion of the victim's physical well-being and the collection of evidence to be used in legal proceedings. Planning during the first hours after an assault should include the following:

1. Medical attention to the victim
2. Notification of significant people in the victim's life
3. Plans for the victim to leave the medical facility
4. Plans for the victim's immediate safety
5. Plans for follow-up contact with a crisis counselor during the interim period

During the interim period, the first few days after an assault, plans must be made to recontact the victim, refer her to a victim support center, or continue supportive counseling. Long-term plans should include providing support at certain times of stress, such as police investigations, court proceedings, and the anniversary of the attack.

INTERVENTION

Building Rapport and Trust

The primary goal of nursing intervention is establishing a therapeutic alliance with the victim. Important to this goal is nonjudgmental acceptance of the victim. It is not unusual for the woman to feel dirty, guilty, or in other ways unacceptable. She must feel that the revulsion society expresses about sexual assault in general is not directed at her in particular. The nurse should respond to the woman's verbal and nonverbal expressions of need. Because the victim may misinterpret any questions or comments not directly related to her immediate situation as blaming or rejecting, the nurse should delay probing questions until the therapeutic alliance is established. The woman's recent experience of objectification intensifies her self-consciousness. She is much more sensitive to others' reactions yet less able to interpret others' behavior rationally.

> My memories of going to the emergency room are blurred. What stands out is how repulsive I felt when I went into the OB-GYN waiting room. Who else would be in an OB-GYN waiting room in the middle of the night but pregnant women? I had to find a small corridor to be in where no one could see me, where I couldn't upset a woman about to give birth or be confronted with the horrible travesty of sexual intercourse I had just experienced. Later, I could view the irony of the situation—at the time I just felt so exposed and repulsive.

Preparing the Victim for Medical Events

After establishing rapport with the victim, the nurse should begin to prepare her for the events she will encounter in the emergency room and during interactions with hospital, police, and other personnel. Preparation for these events is essential, because most women will not have any knowledge or experience to guide them in the immediate crisis.[16,23] The nurse should give the woman brief, concrete explanations of what is going to happen to her and why. This information provides the victim with a needed sense of control and boundaries. Preparation for the physical examination helps the victim view the examination as essential to her well-being, rather than as further physical intrusion. Her calmness and cooperation assist in the collection of evidence for the apprehension and prosecution of the rapist. In this immediate rape crisis, the nurse determines the victim's emotional needs. Does she want a support counselor to stay with her? Does she want family or friends called? Does she need assistance from the social services department of the hospital?

Encouraging Ventilation About the Assault

Once physical needs have been addressed, the victim can use the therapeutic relationship to begin her necessary ventilation about the assault. She should be encouraged to talk about the event and about her feelings. Early and full ventilation helps the woman regain a sense of control; by experiencing acceptance in the face of the degrading details of the rape, she is assisted to regain self-worth. When the assault is reported to the police, the victim will be questioned by many people, all of whom will be strangers to her. Few of these people will have sufficient time to develop a strong therapeutic alliance with her. Talking out the experience with a nurse or other mental health professional will prepare the victim for the investigations to follow.

Exploring Physical Safety Concerns

During the immediate contact with the victim, the nurse explores the woman's concerns for her own physical safety. Where will she go after leaving this initial contact? With whom will she leave? How can the nurse intervene to increase the woman's feeling of physical safety at this time?

> I had to feel safe again. The first things I did were to make physical changes for safety. A locksmith changed and added new locks; a carpenter changed the windows and doors. I was lucky I could afford to do these things, because they helped. I could be alone in my house. But still, the vulnerable feeling stayed with me a long, long time. Even now, 2 years after, I sometimes feel edgy at night and get up to check the locks several times at night. It helps to have a "safe room." The police recommend this—have one room, preferably your bedroom with a phone in it. Add deadbolt locks to any door leading into the room. Any suspicious sound or activity, you can lock yourself in the room and call the police.

Providing Anticipatory Guidance for Significant Others

The rape victim likely will express concern for her family and friends. The nurse offers anticipatory guidance to significant others by talking with them and guiding them in their responses to the victim. Helping family and friends explore their feelings, particularly feelings of anger, can free them from the intensity of these feelings and enable them to be more sensitive to and supportive of the victim.[17,52] Significant others may engage in a "conspiracy of silence" because they believe the less said, the better. This silent approach only intensifies the victim's feelings of guilt, shame, and unworthiness of love.

Making Follow-up Plans

The victim and nurse must agree on an intermediate follow-up plan. The nurse may refer the victim to a counseling center or decide to continue working with her through telephone counseling. The nurse must note several phone numbers where the woman may be reached. The woman may not return home, particularly if the assault occurred in her home, and may choose to stay with family or friends for several days. The victim should not be called at work, unless she agrees to this in advance.

Preparing the Victim for the Interim Phase

The victim should be instructed about the medical follow-up she will need during the interim phase. Although she may appear calm and in control at this time, the nurse should not assume that she will be able to recall any verbal information given to her. She always should receive written instructions for medication and doctors' appointments, reinforced with verbal instructions. The written information can be reassuring at the moment and in the future.

> I know they told me why I had a shot of penicillin. I know I knew it, but when I called my doctor for a follow-up appointment, they scheduled me for blood work. I asked what for. It was as though my mind couldn't deal with the possibility of VD and had rejected that information completely when I was in the emergency room. It made me nervous about what else I had forgotten . . . was I taking the antipregnancy medication the right way, so it would work?

Promoting Reorganization

The victim should feel she can recontact the nurse in the days following the assault to ask questions, talk, and share feelings. The nurse can assist the woman by giving her specific, written instructions about how to reach her and the best times to call.

During reorganization, the nurse intervenes by counseling on the telephone or through face-to-face

Nursing Care Plan 40-1

The Client Who is a Victim of Rape or Sexual Assault

Ms. M, a thirty-five year old woman, was admitted to the emergency department of the local hospital at 2 AM. She drove herself to the hospital after being raped by a man on their second date. While resisting, she received several bruises; at present, she has slight vaginal bleeding. She is distressed and crying, afraid she is pregnant or has contracted an STD. "I can't stay at home," she says, "I can't go back there. What will I do? He knows where I live."

Nursing Diagnosis

Risk for Injury: trauma related to violent physical and sexual assault

Outcome

Client will show no signs of untreated injuries or follow-up medical appointments.

Intervention	Rationale
Provide physical care to treat injuries (lacerations, bruises), prevent pregnancy, and treat infection.	Physical care of the client promotes recovery from traumatic injuries.
Ensure accurate evidence collection to promote apprehension and conviction of the assailant.	Careful collection of evidence is an essential part of bringing the assailant to justice.

Evaluation

Client recovers from physical injuries of rape or sexual assault.

Nursing Diagnosis

Risk for Infection related to sexual assault

Outcome

Client will show no signs of infection on follow-up medical appointments.

Intervention	Rationale
Give clear, concise explanations to the victim about procedures and their rationale.	Assessment and prompt intervention reduce the course of the infection.
Give specific, written directions regarding follow-up medical appointments and medication administration.	During the crisis of the rape aftermath the victim is likely to not hear or to misinterpret directions.

Evaluation

Client develops no infections.

Nursing Diagnosis

Rape trauma syndrome related to aftermath of rape crisis.

Outcome

The client will name and discuss her feelings about the event within one week.

continued

Nursing Care Plan 40-1 *(Continued)*

Intervention	Rationale
Communicate nonjudgmental acceptance through nonverbal means (tone of voice, facial expression, touch); approach in consistent and nonthreatening manner.	A nonjudgmental, nonthreatening approach allows the development of trust and decreases victim's anxiety and fear.
Delay probing questions about the details of the attack until after trust has been established.	Establishing a trusting relationship with the nurse helps the client express feelings about the rape in a supportive environment.

Evaluation

Client works through her feelings associated with the rape and recovers from the experience.

Nursing Diagnosis

Risk for Ineffective Individual Coping related to anxiety about rape experience.

Outcome

Client will identify effective coping skills and positive coping outcomes within 2 weeks after the rape.

Intervention	Rationale
Provide opportunities for the victim to talk freely about the event, the feelings aroused, and the meaning of the event to her.	Measures to reduce or manage anxiety associated with rape include verbalization of feelings, positive self-talk, and support of significant others.
Encourage the victim's family and friends to ventilate their feelings and to demonstrate acceptance and understanding of her.	Support of significant others is an important factor in the victim's recovery.
Provide anticipatory guidance for police investigations, medical questioning, and court proceedings.	Anticipatory guidance helps the victim prepare for future, potentially traumatic events.

Evaluation

Client uses effective coping skills and functions in an adaptive mode.

contact or by monitoring the woman's coping and adaptive behaviors. Anticipatory guidance is extremely helpful during the weeks and months following the attack (Nursing Care Plan 40-1).

If the rapist is apprehended, the victim should be given information about the court process. It may be helpful for her to rehearse her testimony to prepare her for the painful retelling in front of strangers. She also may benefit from exploring how she will feel relating the events in front of strangers. Often, apprehension and court proceedings occur after the woman has begun reorganizing her life. She may have moved past the acute phase of rape trauma syndrome and may have begun to adapt and live her life once again. The prospect of the trial will renew her feelings of vulnerability and fear. This stress point in her life can be navigated with the support of a nurse-counselor. The woman needs to be prepared for the potential outcome of the trial, explore her feelings about it, and consider how she will cope with the actuality. Not every case is prosecuted; not every rapist is convicted.

> I think I was the craziest during the trial. I kept telling myself it was nothing compared to the real thing, but I was even more consumed with thoughts about it all than I had been in the first weeks after the rape. I guess my denial system was not as strong then as it had been right after the rape. It never occurred to me that there might not be a resolution, one way or the other. I had thought about the possibility of the guy getting off, I had thought about how I would feel when I saw him again. But it never occurred to me that there could be a hung jury! No resolution, and the thought of doing it all again was almost more than I

thought I could cope with. I was so ready to have it done and over with, finally. Not to have that finality was crushing.

Considering the Nurse's Feelings and Attitudes

Just as society has stereotypical views about rape and sexual assault, so does each person. Nurses must face their own fears about rape, their anger, and their feelings of helplessness. Understanding and acknowledging these feelings allows nurses to attend to the feelings of victims. There may be times and circumstances for which a nurse has not prepared, however. Some events may be so gruesome that nurses find them intolerable. A supportive network is as valuable for nurses as it is for victims. Nurses need someone with whom they can share feelings about the events they encounter. It is beneficial for nurses and other health care professionals to take active roles concerning the theme of sexual assault; for example, organizing a rape prevention seminar for colleagues or friends or contacting police to evaluate home for physical safety. Nurses can reassure themselves and counteract feelings of helplessness and fears of victimization by taking active steps to ensure their own safety.[6,11]

EVALUATION

Few women are prepared for rape or sexual assault. The feelings that result are overwhelming. Although recovery from rape trauma may follow a generalized pattern of behaviors, each woman brings to the experience a unique array of personal coping skills, personality characteristics, history with stress, and social networks. The nurse must evaluate each encounter with the victim to monitor the progress of coping and the effectiveness of interventions. Through this evaluative process, the nurse may determine that another mode of therapy would be more beneficial. For some women, the assault will precipitate a major breakdown in coping skills, or adequate coping skills will not be available. Individual therapy with a clinical nurse specialist, psychologist, psychiatrist, or social worker may be the referral of choice.[37,43]

◆ Chapter Summary

This chapter has discussed the theoretical perspectives of sexual assault, the findings of recent research about rape and its victims, and therapeutic interventions by nurses and other mental health care providers. Chapter highlights include the following:

1. Theoretical perspectives of rape and sexual assault include historical references, legal definitions, psychological reactions, and sociological views as means of examining types of assaults and characteristics of assailants.
2. Rape trauma syndrome is the process of adaptation experienced by the victim of rape as she strives to overcome her feelings of vulnerability, fear, and helplessness and as she tries to regain her sense of equilibrium. It can be viewed as a post-traumatic stress disorder.
3. Unresolved sexual trauma and silent reaction to rape delay or inhibit a woman's recovery from the rape crisis.
4. Community intervention programs encompass the medical, legal, police, and judicial institutions with which the victim of rape or sexual assault must interact.
5. Nursing assessment of the victim of rape or sexual assault focuses on the woman's physical and emotional state, concerns for physical safety, anxiety about significant others, perception of the event, coping skills, and availability of support people.
6. Planning for the victim who has just been assaulted includes medical attention and physical safety. Intermediate and long-term planning consist of continued contact with the victim, supportive counseling, and help with reorganizing life.
7. The aim of nursing intervention for the victim of rape or sexual assault is to develop a therapeutic alliance that will help her begin to ventilate her feelings and explore what life changes she wants to make.
8. Preparation for medical events, police investigations, and court proceedings helps demystify these procedures for the woman.
9. Anticipatory guidance is necessary for the family and friends of the rape victim to help them explore their own feelings and identify ways to become more supportive of her.
10. Follow-up plans for medical appointments and supportive counseling help the victim reintegrate and reorganize her life.
11. To enhance their therapeutic potential, nurses must recognize and face their own fears and stereotypical views of rape and sexual assault.

Review Questions

1. Which of the following statements about rape and sexual assault is false?
   A. Rape involves force or threat of force.
   B. Rape is a crime of sex motivated by sexual desire.
   C. Rape and sexual assault are crimes of violence and force.
   D. Sexual assault refers to forcible sexual acts against the victim's will.

2. Sexual assault that occurs when a woman consents to be with a man, but does not consent to sex with him is called
   A. confidence rape.
   B. accessory-to-assault.
   C. date rape.
   D. sex-stress rape.
3. Treatment of sex offenders is best undertaken through all of the following EXCEPT
   A. behavioral techniques.
   B. confrontational techniques.
   C. aversive conditioning.
   D. psychoanalytical approaches.
4. Ms. Cindy L is brought to the emergency room by the police following a rape in her apartment laundry room. She sits quietly and answers the nurse's questions carefully. You believe that Cindy
   A. must not have been threatened with violence.
   B. is suffering anxiety and fear but has a controlled reaction to the crisis.
   C. will have a rapid resolution of her crisis.
   D. should remember all of the nurse's health teaching.

◆ References

1. Braen GR, Martin CA, Warfield MC, Engelberg J: Rape and the Rape Trauma Syndrome. South Med J 78 (October): 1230–1235, 1985
2. Brownmiller S: Against Our Will. New York, Simon & Schuster, 1975
3. Burgess AW: Rape Trauma Syndrome: A Nursing Diagnosis. Occup Health Nurs 33 (August): 405–406, 1985
4. Burgess AW, Holmstrom LL: Rape Trauma Syndrome and Post Traumatic Stress Response. In Burgess AW (ed): Rape and Sexual Assault: A Research Handbook, pp 46–60. New York, Garland, 1985
5. Burgess AW, Holmstrom LL: Recovery From Rape and Prior Life Stress. Res Nurs Health 1: 165–174, 1978
6. Burgess AW, Holmstrom LL: Rape: Crisis and Recovery. West Newton, MA, Awab, 1985
7. Burkhart BR, Stanton AL: Sexual Aggression in Acquaintance Relationships. In Russell G (ed): Violence in Intimate Relationships. Old Tappan, NJ, Spectrum Press, 1985
8. Burt MR: Cultural Myths and Supports for Rape. J Pers Soc Psychol 38 (February): 217–230, 1980
9. Calhoun L, Selby J, Warring L: Social Perceptions of the Victim's Causal Role in Rape: An Exploratory Examination of Four Factors. Human Relations 29: 517–526, 1976
10. Damrosch SP: Nursing Students' Assessments of Behaviorally Self-Blaming Rape Victims. Nurs Res 34 (July–August): 221–224, 1985
11. Damrosch SP: How Perceived Carelessness and Time of Attack Affect Nursing Students' Attributions About Rape Victims. Psychol Rep 56 (April): 531–536, 1985
12. Ellis E: A Review of Empirical Rape Research: Victim Reactions and Response to Treatment. Clin Psychol Rev 3: 473–490, 1983
13. Ellis GM: Acquaintance Rape. Perspectives in Psychiatric Care 30 (1): 11–16, 1994
14. Field HS: Attitudes toward Rape: A Comparative Analysis of Police, Rapists, Crisis Counselors, and Citizens. J Pers Soc Psychol 36: 156–179, 1978
15. Feldman-Summers S: Conceptual and Empirical Issues Associated with Rape. In Walker MJ, Brodsky SL (eds): Sexual Assault: The Victim and the Rapist. Lexington, MA, DC Health, 1976
16. Flynn L: Interview: Women and Rape. Medical Aspects of Human Sexuality 8 (May): 183–197, 1974
17. Foley T: Family Response to Rape and Sexual Assault. In Burgess AW (ed): Rape and Sexual Assault. New York, Garland, 1985
18. Frazier P, Borgida E: Rape Trauma Syndrome Evidence in Court. Am Psychol 40 (September): 984–993, 1985
19. George LK, Winfield-Laird J: Sexual Assault: Prevalence and Mental Health Consequences. Final Report Submitted to National Institute of Mental Health, 1986
20. Greer JG, Suart IR (eds): The Sexual Agressor: Current Perspectives on Treatment. New York, Van Nostrand Reinhold, 1983
21. Groth NA: Men Who Rape: The Psychology of the Offender. New York, Plenum Press, 1979
22. Groth NA, Burgess AW, Holmstrom LL: Rape: Power, Anger, and Sexuality. Am J Psychiatry 134: 1239–1243, 1977
23. Heinrich LB: Care of the Female Rape Victim. Am J Primary Health Care 12 (11): 9–16, 1987
24. Kanin EJ: Date Rapists: Differential Sexual Socialization and Relative Deprivation. Arch Sex Behav 14 (June): 219–231, 1985
25. Kilpatrick DG, Saunders BE, Amick-McMullan A, Best CL, Veronen LJ, Resnick HS: Victim and Crime Factors Associated With the Development of Crime-related Post-Traumatic Stress Disorder. Behav Ther 20: 199–214, 1989
26. Kilpatrick DG, Veronen LJ, Saunders BE, Best CL, Amick-McMullan A, Paduhovich J: The Psychological Impact of Crime: A Study of Randomly Surveyed Crime Victims. National Institute of Justice, Grant No. 84-IJ-CX-0039, Final Report, 1987
27. Koss MP: The Scope of Rape: Implications for the Clinical Treatment of Victims. Clin Psychol 36 (4): 88–91, 1983
28. Ledray LE: The Sexual Assault Nurse Clinician: A Fifteen-year Experience in Minneapolis. J Emergency Nurs 18 (3): 217–222, 1992
29. Lindemann E: Symptomotology and Management of Acute Grief. Am J Orthopsychiatry 45: 813–824, 1944
30. McCarthy BW: A Cognitive-Behavioral Approach to Understanding and Treating Sexual Trauma. J Sex Marital Ther 12 (Winter): 322–329, 1986
31. MacDonald J: Rape: Offenders and Their Victims. Springfield, IL, Charles C. Thomas, 1971
32. Mayer RA, Boggio NT: The Adolescent Rape Victim. Emergency Medicine 24 (3): 98–100, 1992
33. Marinelli RD: Acquaintance Rape: A Case Study Approach. J Health Education 25 (2): 106–107, 1994
34. Masters WH: Sexual Dysfunction as an Aftermath of Sex-

ual Assault of Men by Women. J Sex Marital Ther 12 (Spring): 35–45, 1986
35. Moore HA, Zusman J, Root GC: Noninstitutional Treatment for Sex Offenders in Florida. Am J Psychiatry 142 (August): 964–967, 1985
36. Moynihan BA, Duggan KC: The Rape Crisis Team: Consultation to Critical Care. Dimen Crit Care Nurs 1 (6): 354–359, 1982
37. Ochberg FM (ed): Post-Traumatic Therapy and Victims of Violence. New York, Brunner/Masel, 1988
38. Oliver M, Van Der Voort M: Caring for the Rape Victim...In Many Cases, Emergency Medical Personnel Are the First Face-to-Face Contact. Emergency 15 (3): 30–31, 1983
39. Popiel DA, Susskind EC: The Impact of Rape: Social Support as a Moderator of Stress. Am J Community Psychol 13 (December): 645–676, 1985
40. Resick PA, Jackson TL: Attitudes toward Rape Among Mental Health Professionals. Am J Community Psychol 9: 481–490, 1981
41. Riesenberg D: Motivations Studied and Treatments Devised in Attempt to Change Rapists' Behavior. JAMA 257 (February): 899–900, 1987
42. Riesenberg D: Treating a Societal Malignancy-Rape. JAMA 257 (February): 726–727, 1987
43. Rose DS: Worse Than Death: Psychodynamics of Rape Victims and the Need for Psychotherapy. Am J Psychiatry 143 (July): 817–824, 1986
44. Ruckman LM: Rape: How To Begin the Healing. Am J Nurs 92 (9): 48–51, 1992
45. Sampselle CM: The Role of Nursing in Preventing Violence Against Women. J Obstet, Gynecol, Neonatal Nurs 20 (6): 41–47, 1991
46. Santiago JM, McCall-Perez F, Gorcey M, Beigel A: Long-Term Psychological Effects of Rape in 35 Rape Victims. Am J Psychiatry 142 (November): 1338–1340, 1985
47. Seigel JM, Burnam MA, Stein JA, Golding JM, Sorenson SB: Sexual Assault and Psychiatric Disorders: A Preliminary Investigation. Final Report for National Institute of Mental Health Grant, 1986
48. Steketee G, Foa EB: Rape Victims: Post-traumatic Stress Responses and Their Treatment: A Review of the Literature. Clin Psychol Rev 3: 417–433, 1983
49. Tyra PA: Older Women: Victims of Rape. J Gerontological Nurs 19 (5): 7–12, 1993
50. Von JM, Kilpatrick DG, Burgess AW, Hartman CR: Rape and Sexual Assault. In Rosenberg ML, Fenley MA (eds): Violence in America: A Public Health Approach. New York, Oxford University Press, 1991
51. Walker MJ, Brodsky SL (eds): Sexual Assault: The Victim and the Rapist. Lexington, MA, DC Health, 1976
52. Wilcox BL: Social Support, Life Stress, and Psychological Adjustment: A Test of the Buffering Hypothesis. Am J Community Psychol 9: 371–387, 1981
53. Wyer RS, Bodenhausen G, Gorman TF: Cognitive Mediators of Reactions to Rape. J Pers Soc Psychol 48 (February): 324–338, 1985

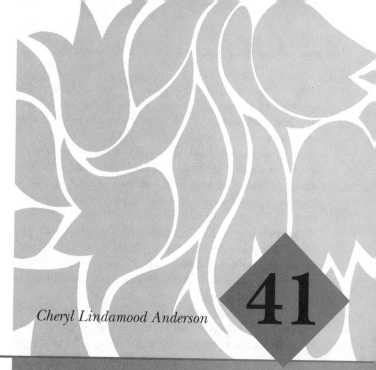

Violence Within the Family

Cheryl Lindamood Anderson

41

Peter, Peter pumpkin eater
Had a wife and couldn't keep her.
He put her in a pumpkin shell
And there he kept her very well.
There was an old woman who lived in a shoe.
She had so many children she didn't know what to do.
She gave them some broth without any bread.
She whipped them all soundly and put them to bed.

Physical, emotional, or verbal abuse can appear in any relationship. Outbreaks of violence in the family are usually quickly denied and concealed to maintain the family's ideal image as nurturing, protecting, and guiding its members. Violence in the parent–child relationship, however, has been recognized and researched for more than 3 decades. More recently, studies of violent child–parent and male–female partner relationships have emerged. Nonetheless, society still does not understand a great deal about violent families.

Violence among family members is a complex issue intertwined with many factors, such as alcohol, poverty, stress, and an ongoing cycle of violence. These factors are not necessarily the causes of violence within the family, but they may influence the development of family violence.

This overview of violence in the family focuses primarily on the violence directed at abused children, women, and elders. Brief attention is given to the violence among adolescents and young adults as victims and perpetrators within family and courtship situations. The chapter describes physical, sexual, and emotional abuse and their consequences. To describe the assaulted individual, the term victim, rather than survivor, is used to indicate the magnitude of harm suffered by the incident(s). It must be recognized, however, that many individuals assaulted as children or adults are clearly survivors. The incidence, traditional and current theoretical applications, and dynamics of family violence are discussed. A major emphasis is the nursing process—assessment, nursing diagnosis, planning, intervention, and evaluation—as applied to the abused client and family.

Learning Objectives

On completion of this chapter, you should be able to accomplish the following:

1. *Discuss types of child abuse, and identify short- and long-term consequences to victims.*
2. *Define six types of child abuse.*
3. *Discuss the difficulty in documenting abuse.*
4. *Identify some predictors of potential child abuse.*
5. *Identify some predictors of parents who are at high risk of abusing their children.*
6. *Contrast the characteristics of the battering mate and the battered spouse.*
7. *Compare the roles of victim and batterer in dating and courtship violence.*
8. *Contrast the characteristics of the adult batterer and the battered elder.*
9. *Describe the strengths, limitations, and usefulness of the legal system in dealing with child, spouse, and elder abuse.*
10. *Apply the nursing process to the care of the abused and abusing individual and family.*
11. *Discuss the relevance and application of past and current theories to the problem of family violence.*
12. *Recognize and discuss the nurse's feelings, experiences, and behaviors that may affect therapeutic effectiveness or lead to personal burnout.*

◆ Child Abuse

Child abuse is difficult to define precisely, and incorporates many realms. Parents Anonymous recognizes six types of child abuse:

1. Physical abuse: acts of commission, such as burning or beating a child
2. Physical neglect: acts of omission or inadequate parenting abilities, such as improper feeding or clothing
3. Emotional abuse: attitudes directed toward the child that may be harmful to emotional development
4. Emotional neglect: lack of parent–child interaction
5. Sexual abuse: involvement of the child with a parent or adult family member in activities ranging from sex play to actual intercourse
6. Verbal abuse: assaults on the child that are verbally degrading, such as constant ridicule

Documenting any type of abuse except obvious physical abuse is difficult; therefore, health care providers must be aware of specific clues that indicate potential or suspected abuse. All violent families are not alike. They differ in their specific situations, in the circumstances surrounding the abuse, and even in the degree or nature of abuse directed at the child. Table 41-1 gives physical and behavioral indicators of four types of child abuse and neglect.

The Model Child Protective Services Act defines an abused or neglected child as a person younger than 18 years whose physical or mental health or welfare is harmed or threatened with harm by acts of omission on the part of the responsible caregiver.[52] Physical abuse may include injuries resulting from excessive corporal punishment.

When considering the various forms of child abuse, less than 5% of these maltreatments occur in isolation.[82] Verbal or sexual abuse seldom occurs without some other component of maltreatment. Earlier onset of verbal abuse and emotional neglect is associated with greater severity and frequency of maltreatment.[82]

PHYSICAL ABUSE

Researchers agree that physically abusing parenting behaviors are a consequence of many factors, with some of the most potent being stress, family resources, social isolation, or a combination of all.[20] Definitions of discipline and punishment vary. Having experienced a particular form of punishment as a child is a significant

Table 41-1

Physical and Behavioral Indicators of Child Abuse and Neglect

Type of Child Abuse and Neglect	Physical Indicators	Behavioral Indicators
PHYSICAL ABUSE	Unexplained bruises and welts: On face, lips, mouth On torso, back, buttocks, thighs In various stages of healing Clustered, forming regular patterns Reflecting shape of article used to inflict (electric cord, belt buckle) On several different surface areas Regularly appear after absence, weekend, or vacation	Wary of adult contacts Apprehensive when other children cry Behavioral extremes: Aggressiveness Withdrawal
	Unexplained burns: Cigar, cigarette burns, especially on soles, palms, back, or buttocks Immersion burns (sock-like, glove-like, doughnut-shaped on buttocks or genitalia) Patterned like electric burner, iron, and so forth Rope burns on arms, legs, neck, or torso Unexplained fractures: To skull, nose, facial structure In various stages of healing Multiple or spiral fractures Unexplained lacerations or abrasions: To mouth, lips, gums, eyes To external genitalia	Frightened of parents Afraid to go home Reports injury by parents
PHYSICAL NEGLECT	Consistent hunger, poor hygiene, inappropriate dress Consistent lack of supervision, especially in dangerous activities for long periods Unattended physical problems or medical needs Abandonment	Begging, stealing food Extended stays at school (early arrival and late departure) Constant fatigue, listlessness, or falling asleep in class Alcohol or drug abuse Delinquency (eg, thefts) States there is no caretaker
SEXUAL ABUSE	Difficulty in walking or sitting Torn, stained, or bloody underclothing Pain or itching in genital area Bruises or bleeding in external genitalia, vaginal, or anal areas Venereal disease, especially in preteens Pregnancy	Unwilling to change for gym or participate in physical education class Withdrawal, fantasy, or infantile behavior Bizarre, sophisticated, or unusual sexual behavior or knowledge Poor peer relationships Delinquent or runaway behavior Reports sexual assault by caretaker
EMOTIONAL MALTREATMENT	Speech disorders Lags in physical development Failure to thrive	Habit disorders (eg, sucking, biting, rocking) Conduct disorders (eg, antisocial, destructive) Neurotic traits (sleep disorders, inhibition of play) Psychoneurotic reactions (hysteria, obsession, compulsion, phobias, hypochondria) Behavior extremes: Compliant, passive Aggressive, demanding Overly adaptive behavior: Inappropriately adult Inappropriately infant Developmental lags (mental, emotional) Attempted suicide

(From Heindl C, Krall C, Salus M, Broadhurst D: The Nurse's Role in the Prevention and Treatment of Child Abuse and Neglect. Washington, DC, HEW publication #[OHDS] 79-30202, 1979.)

risk factor for parents currently approving of that type of punishment for their children.[18]

Incidence of Physical Abuse

Physical abuse may be defined along a continuum of behaviors and consequences from slaps, punches, and pushing to beatings and from no visible marks to major body damage and death. Inclusion of all forms of abuse are not considered in all cases because they are not reported. An estimated 6.9 million children have been assaulted by their parents at a rate of 110 incidents per 1,000 children. Mortality and morbidity of physical child maltreatment are approximately 10% to 15%.[67]

False allegations of abuse are also common due to lack of information, spite, or vengeance. Another form of abuse, Munchausen syndrome by proxy, occurs when a parent, generally a mother, fabricates an illness in her child[63] (Case Study 41-1). Lifetime psychiatric histories of these mothers have revealed personality disorders, alcohol abuse, and history of self-harm.[15]

41-1 Case Study

Munchausen Syndrome by Proxy

A 23-month-old was admitted to a children's hospital with a history from the mother of apnea, perioral cyanosis, shaking spells, and periods of unresponsiveness occurring multiple times during the 24 hours prior to admission. Some episodes reportedly required mouth-to-mouth resuscitation. The client had two previous hospitalizations elsewhere and was maintained at home on an apnea monitor. A complete medical evaluation was normal. Information from other sources revealed gross inaccuracies in the social history and that two previous workups for apnea had been normal. During psychiatric evaluation of the mother, she admitted fabricating the child's history. She did not keep subsequent psychiatric appointments, reporting time constraints of a fictitious job. When legal proceedings were begun to remove the child from the home, she robbed the person with whom she was staying and left the state. The social service agency in another state was contacted, and the child and mother were found with relatives. The child was placed in foster care, and the mother committed herself to a psychiatric hospital.

Questions for Discussion

1. How are the medical treatments abusive to the child?
2. What signs indicate that the mother may need treatment rather than the child?

SEXUAL ABUSE

A common definition of sexual abuse is forced, tricked, or coerced sexual behavior between a young person and an older person.[43] Older definitions of sexual abuse include an age difference of at least 5 years between victim and perpetrator.

Sexual abuse of children can include pornographic photographs, rape, molestation, child prostitution, and incest; however, other sexual activities, such as exhibitionism, fondling, French kissing, ejaculation, masturbation, oral sex, and anal sex, may be more common. Rape and actual intercourse may represent only 10.5% of reported cases of sexual abuse in children.[37] Sexual abuse may interfere with a child's normal, healthy development by producing a situation with which the child is unable to cope physically, emotionally, or intellectually. Often a sexually abused child suffers anxiety, shame, or guilt. Research has revealed that professionals, nonprofessionals, and psychiatric clients' opinions regarding the severity of child sexual abuse are consistent and coincide with clinical observations and empirical evidence.[29]

Incidence of Sexual Abuse

The actual incidence of sexual abuse is unknown because no precise national statistics exist; however, it may be higher than the incidence of physical abuse.[119] More than 133,000 children are known to be sexually assaulted; many others remain undetected or are inaccurately determined not to have been abused.[25] Estimates of the prevalence of sexual abuse range from 6% to 62% of the population for female victims and 3% to 31% of the population for male victims.[87] The wide variation may be explained in part by methodological factors, such as different definitions of sexual abuse.

Victims often know their assailants; as many as 80% of sexual abuse victims are abused by people known to them. Young children have a significantly increased risk of being assaulted by a known assailant in a familiar environment, such as the home.[37]

Characteristics of Sexually Abusing Adults and Their Victims

Two general characteristics may describe those who sexually abuse their children: lack of impulse control, sometimes as a result of transient stress or as a characteristic of the abuser, and a confusion of roles, wherein the child is regarded not as a child but as the object of the adult's needs. These characteristics of the parent-surrogate may be seen in all types of child abuse.[119]

Research has failed to identify characteristics that consistently discriminate between sexual offenders and nonoffenders. The offender may be passive, introverted, sociopathic, alcoholic, socially isolated, or inadequate.

The offender has low self-esteem, emotional immaturity, and difficulty relating to age-appropriate peers, and often has a chaotic and dysfunctional family of origin.[50,101] The likelihood of molestation is increased within a dysfunctional family.[102] Various types of personality disorganization and sexual identity confusion, younger age, and past or present involvement with the criminal justice system may interact with situational factors, such as alcohol or drug abuse, marital discord, and accessibility to young girls leading to sexual abuse.

Both parents may be distant and inaccessible, stimulate a sexual climate in the home, or keep family secrets, such as an extramarital affair.[103] Nonoffending mothers may suffer severe emotional problems due to the disclosure of abuse, attempt suicide, and actually be victims of abuse by the partner. Other mothers may be a major support and resource for the sexually abused child. The majority of nonoffending mothers believe their children's allegations and often file formal complaints.[30]

It is unclear what factors increase a child's risk for sexual abuse.[34] Girls are victimized more often, although boys are also victims. An underreporting of male victimization occurs because many male victims are abused by adolescent boys, and the narrow age difference leads to a label of "inappropriate sex play" rather than abuse.[96] Although both male and female victims are at equal risk for physical trauma, boys are more likely threatened with physical sexual trauma. As with girls, the majority of boys are abused by male offenders.

Victims of incestuous sexual abuse are frequently characterized as being the oldest daughter of a family, approximately 8 years old when the incestuous relationship begins, and involved in the relationship for an average of 5 years. Behavioral responses of these children toward the abuser and the abusive incident can be described as passive. The children expect other adults to perceive what is happening and protect them. When this does not happen, the child's level of trust diminishes.[37] Later, if a female victim enters therapy, she is typically 20 to 25 years old, married, and presenting to the therapist with marital problems.[119] All victims of sexual abuse do not enter therapy or counseling. They may feel they have no signs and symptoms of dsyfunction. Others who choose to present for treatment early, rather than later, usually are individuals who reported their abuse to law enforcement, were older when abuse began, had an abuse of long duration, and experienced more sexual acts.[66]

Short- and Long-Term Victim Consequences of Sexual Abuse

There is no typical symptom profile of a child who has experienced sexual abuse.[74] Many victims of childhood sexual abuse experience depression, low self-esteem, guilt, and interpersonal difficulties.[74] Not all children display significant symptoms. Sexually abused children may exhibit nightmares, anger and hostility, withdrawal from activities, academic problems, daydreaming, aggressive behavior, and overcompliance or anxiousness to please. Other behavioral problems seen in older abused children include alcohol and drug abuse, promiscuity, prostitution, suicide attempts, and entrance into cults.

A more recently recognized occurrence in children exposed to repeated sexual or physical abuse is a dissociative disorder or post-traumatic stress disorder (PTSD).[43] The psychological impact of sexual abuse on adolescents is noted in reported confusion about sexual identity and sexual norms or equation of sex with love and caring.[33]

Health care concerns for sexually abused children and adolescents include the possibility of pregnancy; eating disorders, such as anorexia or bulimia; and sexually transmitted diseases (STDs).

As high as 10% of children assessed for sexual abuse have STDs.[4] Health care professionals knowledgeable about sexual abuse and STDs and trained to do a sexual assault examination need to be present when a child is admitted. Children tend to regard the medical examination for sexual assault with more fear than an ordinary doctor's visit, but the child's fear and pain can be minimized.[70] See Case Study 41-2 and Box 41-1 for information about the evaluation of prepubertal children with STDs. Total care of these children includes care of injuries, evaluation of risk for pregnancy, evaluation of risk for STDs, and crisis intervention.[71]

Adults with a history of childhood sexual abuse report rageful behavior, disrupted marriages, dissatisfaction with marital relationships, and a tendency to be religious nonpractitioners.[35]

Also noted among adult women sexually abused during childhood is an increased risk of adult alcohol abuse, marriage to an alcohol abuser, or becoming a victim of date or marital rape.[38] More recently recognized in adults with a history of abuse or trauma is the diagnosis of dissociative identity disorder (DID), which includes a continuum of symptoms from PTSD to multiple personality.[109] As many as 80% to 90% of individuals diagnosed with multiple personalities report a childhood history of abuse[28] (see Chapter 32, Dissociative Disorders). Further research may address whether

41-2 Case Study

The Prepubertal Child With A Sexually Transmitted Disease

Cindy was 10 years old when she entered the labor and delivery area in active labor. A female companion was at her side. She was seen once in a prenatal clinic several months before, and her prenatal history was sketchy.

Present information noted that the father of the baby was an 18-year-old next door neighbor. Cindy lived with her mother and eight siblings in a poor area of town. Prenatal history also noted the appearance of condylomas extending from the rectal area up for approximately 5 in. Cindy stated that the clinic doctor had indicated that "after delivery, the situation would be taken care of." Progress notes referred to future laser surgery after delivery.

Questions for Discussion

1. How would you ensure that Cindy received client education and follow-up care?
2. Is there evidence that Cindy has been sexually abused?
3. How would you prepare for reporting and providing legal intervention in this case if necessary?

the effects noted in the victims are specific to sexual abuse and trauma or to emotional abuse in general.

EMOTIONAL ABUSE

Emotional abuse and neglect and verbal abuse may be considered together as emotional maltreatment because of their similar predictors and consequences. The emotionally maltreated child may or may not also be physically or sexually abused, but physically abused children are always emotionally maltreated. For a parent–child relationship to be emotionally abusive, there must be an action or series of actions or omissions by the parents that have caused emotional injury or harm to the child. It is unfortunate that often the true extent of injuries inflicted by emotional abuse cannot be seen until later in life; even then, the disordered behaviors of the adult may not be connected to the emotional abuse received as a child.

An emotionally maltreated child and an emotionally disturbed child may display similar behavior, but the parents' actions may help to differentiate the cause of the problem. Parents of an emotionally disturbed child generally recognize that there is a problem and seek help, whereas the parents of an emotionally maltreated child may blame the child for the problem and refuse or delay offers of help. The parents of the emotionally maltreated child may at times appear unconcerned about their child's welfare.[52]

◆ Spouse Abuse

Increased evidence indicates that domestic violence is often associated with the use of alcohol and drugs, unemployment and underemployment, and child or parent abuse. As many as 90% of female batterers were victims of abuse as children. Furthermore, it has been estimated that one in three abused women abuse their children as well.[99]

Domestic violence may refer to an abused man. Abuse toward the man in a relationship is not uncommon, especially emotional or verbal abuse, although many dismiss or ignore it. It is likely that more than 1 million husbands are abused by their wives annually.[104] The problem is largely ignored because of men's embarrassment in reporting abusive incidents. The abused man may fit the macho stereotype but be very cautious of his use of power, or he may be ill, feeble, old, passive, dependent on the woman, and self-blaming. These men stay in violent marriages for many of the same reasons

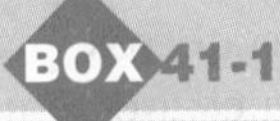

BOX 41-1

Suggestions for Evaluation of Prepubertal Children With Sexually Transmitted Diseases

Report to a local child protection agency.
Report to a local health department.
Elicit a history of sexually transmitted disease from all contacts: caretakers, relatives, playmates, family members.
Examine child for evidence of child abuse.
Prepare saline wet mount from the vagina.
Perform a VDRL.
Perform gonorrhea cultures from vagina, urethra, rectum, and pharnyx.
Perform herpes and *Chlamydia* cultures as necessary.

(Adapted from Neinstein L, Goldenring J, Carpenter S: Nonsexual Transmission of Sexually Transmitted Diseases. Pediatrics 74:69–75, 1984)

battered women do, including emotional dependence, economic dependence, or custody of children.

◆ Dating or Courtship Violence

Abuse occurs between live-in lovers, common law couples, homosexual couples, and dating or courtship partners. Half of all dating relationships entail some violence or sexual exploitation.[75] Nearly 3% of college students report severe forms of aggression toward one another, such as punchings or beatings.[94]

Although violence or other clues may be warnings to the couple, marriage may be attempted anyway, perhaps owing to society's romantic view of courtship. Such courtship behaviors, however, set the stage for marital problems, including escalated violence and marital rape.[75] The belief may persist that with a loving and supportive relationship, the abuse will vanish. Often partners equate violence in the relationship with love.[24] Both beliefs are myths.

Reasons for violence within courtship and dating relationships vary. Jealousy and disagreements about sex or drinking are commonly reported reasons for aggression.[95]

Effective intervention into the problems of marital or courtship violence works on three levels: primary (preventing negative courtship interaction), secondary (targeting high-risk couples), and tertiary (remediation with people involved in violent or exploitative relationships).[75] The best way to address marital or courtship violence is before it occurs.

Primary intervention for marital or courtship violence emphasizes education and developing problem-solving skills. Education of couples involves conflict management, dealing with issues of jealousy and rejection, using drug and alcohol, communicating, and understanding sexual signals. Additional educational emphasis enhances empathy and understanding between partners, decreases adversarial attitudes, provides partners with information on courtship violence, and identifies the strength of a support group of peers in preventing violence and exploitation. Partners responding to marital or courtship violence or distress by asking advice from friends or family or seeking sympathy from others often feel better about the stressful situation and avoid dating violence.[14]

Secondary intervention provides education and problem-solving techniques to partners previously in violent relationships or home situations. Partners struggling with conflict issues in relationships also may be targeted. Learning to negotiate and compromise is essential.[94]

Tertiary intervention emphasizes the identification of the group needing services. Counseling may help people work through the issues of past violence. Box 41-2 discusses adolescents as victims and perpetrators of abuse.[75]

◆ Elder Abuse

As the elderly population increases, more adult children will be caring for their elderly parents because of the shortage of home care and long-term facilities. The frustration and stress encountered in caring for someone elderly, possible financial stress, medical problems, and potential marital strain of keeping an elder parent in the home are some of the factors leading to elder abuse.

Early work on elder abuse noted a similarity in definition and consequences between battered children and battered elders that prevented complete assessments and effective treatments for the elderly. The elderly individual is not a child but an autonomous adult and therefore can be an aggressor or exposed to types of maltreatment absent in child abuse.[111] In many ways, elder victims of abuse are similar to other adult victims of abuse. The use of alcohol by adult caregivers of the elderly equates with the use of alcohol found in other domestic violence cases.[6]

Elder abuse does not always involve physical abuse. The following are four definitions of abuse:

1. Physical abuse: willful and direct infliction of pain and injury
2. Neglect: lack of attention, abandonment, or confinement by family members or society
3. Psychosocial abuse: withholding decision-making power and affection or social isolation
4. Exploitation: dishonest or inappropriate use of the elder's money, property, or other resources[91]

Elderly people are not always the victims of a frustrated son or daughter; the majority are abused by their partners. In a 1988 study of 2,020 community dwelling elders in Boston, 58% were abused by their spouses, and only 24% by their children.[90] Elderly men are at greater risk than elderly women, because elderly men are more likely to be part of a marital pair than are elderly women. Abuse among an elderly pair, in many instances, may have been ongoing for many years without recognition.

Assaults of older victims typically are underreported, especially elder sexual assault. Elders reporting assault generally present with genital injuries and state location of assault at home by an unknown assailant.[80]

◆ Incidence and Significance

Statistics on the number of children, women, and elders abused each year within families vary widely. Problems in documenting and reporting lead to an estimation of

BOX 41-2

Adolescents as Victims and as Perpetrators of Abuse

AS VICTIMS

The dynamics of the family in which adolescent abuse occurs appear to be different from those of the family in which abuse of younger children occurs. Much of the stress related to an occurrence of adolescent abuse may result from the parent's experience of stress at the same time the adolescent is facing the stresses of identity, independence, and autonomy. Parents of adolescents appear to be facing their own developmental crisis—that of midlife—when the children are teenagers. The increased strain from the two concurrent developmental crises can place the adolescent at risk for maltreatment.

It has been suggested that there are three distinguishing patterns of adolescent maltreatment:

1. Parents are disorganized and overwhelmed with life and see their teenager as disrespectful and unresponsive.
2. More violent means of control are sought as the adolescent becomes stronger and bigger.
3. Families are described as child oriented; therefore, the abuse begins when the child tries to separate from the family.

Individual personalities and inherited traits, developmental stages of the individuals involved, reactions to these developmental stages, and social, cultural, and situational factors structure and limit the ways in which a person may respond to stress (eg, by becoming abusive).

Adolescent maltreatment is not a commonly recognized form of abuse because a bigger, stronger adolescent victim of abuse evokes less sympathy than a smaller child victim. It is assumed the teenager can take care of himself or leave the situation—as many do, becoming teenage runaways.

Some differences have been noted between maltreated teenagers and maltreated younger children. In the case of adolescent maltreatment, the perpetrator is often male and the victim is female, the opposite to abuse of younger children. Adolescent abuse is often self-reported rather than reported by other individuals. Many adolescents who are abused come from families with histories of alcohol or drug abuse by parents and of spousal abuse, rather than childhood abuse to the teenager. Education and income levels may be higher in the family of adolescent abuse than in families abusing the younger child. Because the adolescent is a victim of abuse from a family with different dynamics and, as a teenager, requires different services for different needs, the adolescent victim cannot be overlooked.

(Adapted from Doueck H, Ishisaka A, Sweany S, Gilchrist L: Adolescent Maltreatment. Journal of Interpersonal Violence 2 [June]: 139–154, 1987)

AS PERPETRATORS

Estimates suggest that about 20% of perpetrators are adolescents; however, some surveys suggest that up to 50% of all child sexual abuse is committed by offenders who are younger than 18 years. Preadolescents make up an additional 5% to 10% of perpetrators. Abusive incidents may vary from genital viewing and fondling to actual intercourse. Some incidents are typical of date rape or acquaintance rape in which peer pressure forces the issue of sexual activities.

Many adolescent perpetrators are socially isolated and lonely, seeking out younger children for repetitive acts of sexual activity. If disclosure is not brought about and appropriate interventions instituted, abuse will continue to other children. It is common for the siblings of the adolescent perpetrator to be victims of this type of abuse, but the young children in the extended family of such an adolescent can also be frequently abused.

(Adapted from DeJong AR, Finkel MA: Sexual Abuse of Children. Curr Probl Pediatr 20 [9]:489–567, 1990)

abuse among children and women. The First National Family Violence survey estimated in 1975 that 1.5 million children between 3 and 17 years old and living with two parents were abused. A replication of that study in 1985 showed a 47% decline in abuse, indicating that 705,000 fewer children were the victims of violence in 1985.[44] This optimistic report was not fully credited in the scientific community; however, it may illustrate the efforts of society to deal with the major problem of child abuse.

More than 92% of young adults, however, report physical punishment during childhood and 50.7% report punishment during adolescence.[67] Nevertheless, each year 2,000 children die in circumstances suggestive of abuse or neglect.

Estimates of the number of women who are abused each year range from 1 million to 28 million.[55,69,73] Severe and repeated battering occurs in 10% to 50% of heterosexual couples. Approximately 1 in 10 women who are in intimate heterosexual relationships, encountered in any health care setting, are victims of abuse by a male partner.[21]

Statistics place the range of elder abuse between 500,000 and 1.5 million cases annually.[98] Because reporting is sparse, various studies offer other estimates of elder abuse. The victim's or the abuser's shame or guilt may also contribute to a failure to report. Such violent acts as being beaten or attacked with a weapon often are too painful to report. Many incidents of abuse are not reported because of fear of retaliation or lack of opportunities to change the abusing situation. Many battered women and elders and battering parents describe the abuse as an accident.

Unfortunately, health care providers may unintentionally discourage the reporting of abuse by their actions or comments. A parent may know he or she is exceedingly harsh with the child's discipline and seek help, only to face ridicule and debasement from the health care professional. If this happens, the family may turn to one hospital after another for care, or they may stop seeking medical intervention altogether.

Every state has a mandatory law for reporting child abuse, with the underlying intention that not reporting suspected child abuse is a misdemeanor. In addition, no state requires that the reporter of abuse have actual proof of abuse or neglect before reporting. The law may specify that a person must report "suspected" incidents or include the phrase "reason to believe" in the report.[16] The report of suspected child abuse states that a child *may* be abused, not that the parents are abusers. Responsibility for the abusive actions should be determined by a qualified professional.

Along with increased reporting of suspected abuse have come increased false allegations of abuse. More than half of reported incidences of child abuse are found to be unsubstantiated.[118] The nurse can help avoid misdiagnosing child abuse by taking these steps:

1. Be aware that false allegations are common and can have tragic consequences for the family.
2. Become aware of cases in which misdiagnosis is common, such as cultural practices and diseases that may mimic injury or sexual abuse charges.
3. Be aware of child abuse laws in your state, and work to better the system.
4. Remember that no tool is 100% accurate in diagnosing abuse of children.
5. Give parents every chance to present their side of the situation.
6. Document all information obtained in interviews with the child, family, and significant others.

Laws for reporting abuse of partners are less clear than laws for reporting child or elder abuse. Although it is generally accepted that a woman should not be abused by her partner, each state handles the situation of partner abuse differently, with inconsistent legal interventions (Box 41-3, Table 41-2). Several states now require, however, that health care professionals suspecting partner violence must provide referrals and resources to women before discharge.

◆ Theories of Violence and Aggression as They Relate to Family Violence

IMPULSE AND MALADAPTATION

Various disciplines have developed theories that explain violence in general or a particular aspect of family violence. Early works on violence discuss a death instinct that directs a destructive drive[40] or an inherited maladapted behavior toward self or others.[76] Other theories suggest that aggression and violence are learned behaviors,[10] a result of acute social disorganization,[100] or consequent to the situation that confronts them (symbolic interactionism).[8]

THEORETICAL AND CONCEPTUAL FRAMEWORKS OF FAMILY VIOLENCE

Theories relevant to the violence experienced between family members suggest a cycle of violence, a learned helplessness framework, and a social exchange and conflict framework.[19,105] Systems theory as applied to family functioning and relationships offers a suggestion that violence between family members is the product of a system rather than chance aberration or the product of inadequate socialization or disturbed personalities.[107] Restak suggests an association between poor mother–infant interaction and potential child abuse as a basis for a psychobiological theory of the origin of violence.[93]

The best known model of child abuse may be that promulgated by Helfer and Kempe. In its most simplistic form, this model suggests the possibility of abuse any time a child, a parent, and stress are present within a family.[53]

Years of continued research on child abuse have illustrated that most theoretical or conceptual frameworks are limited in scope and characterize only a small number of abusive families.[22] Not all abused children have mentally incompetent or psychotic parents, and not all stressful families abuse their children.

The inability of previous theories to describe all abusive families and the knowledge that several factors appear to occur together to cause abuse have led to the development of the *human ecological* theory of child abuse. This theory comes from the separate ideas and work of Garbarino and Belsky, who draw heavily on Bronfenbrenner's model of the ecology of human de-

BOX 41-3

Legal Issues in Family Violence

CHILD ABUSE

Less than 20 years ago, only 11 states had laws requiring the reporting of child abuse. Professionals often hesitated in reporting abuse because of not knowing what to report or to whom to report it.

Today, there is a mandatory reporting law for child abuse in all states. Failure to report is a misdemeanor. Reports can be made to the Child Welfare Service, a county attorney, or a law officer. Problems still exist in reporting cases of abuse because all states have different reporting statutes in regard to the following areas:

1. Types of instances that must be reported
2. People who must report
3. Time limits for reporting
4. Manner of reporting (written, oral, or both)
5. Agencies to which reports must be made
6. Degree of immunity conferred on reports[120]

The major purposes of mandatory reporting laws are to protect the victim of abuse from repeated attacks, provide social services to families, and improve the methods of identification and investigation of suspected abuse cases. Investigation into the reported child abuse is the second step of involvement in the situation and is a direct consequence of a filed report. An investigation has three purposes:

1. To determine if abuse or neglect is occurring
2. To determine if the child is at risk within the home
3. To determine if that risk is serious enough to warrant intervention guaranteeing the child's safety[120]

BATTERED WOMEN

Legal protection for the battered woman is less well developed. At times the legal system may encourage the wife to return home rather than to file a legal complaint against the batterer.

Different states have various civil remedies for battered women, such as protective orders, temporary restraining orders or vacate orders that generally include time limits.

Protective orders helping to protect the woman and her children at day care facilities can be crim inally enforceable.

Other civil remedies can be issued only if the wife is filing for, or has been granted, a divorce. Shelter services may be minimal to nonexistent in some states. Special police training to handle domestic abuse is increasing. Some police, however, will still not issue a warrant for arrest unless violent acts are observed by legal authorities.

As many as 33% of police officers may not know they can make a warrantless arrest without making an observation of the violence.[32] Often if an arrest is made, the woman, out of fear of retaliation, may later drop the charges. Several states and/or counties now have a "no drop" policy when abuse is suspected and charges have been filed. Marital rape is also a legal issue. As of 1989, 14 states still provide the wife with no choice in whenever or however her husband decides to have sex.[32] Spousal abuse is listed as a misdemeanor, a felony, or assault and battery according to the state; however, an attitude continues to prevail viewing spousal abuse as a private matter to be worked out by the couple.

ELDER ABUSE

When it comes to protecting elderly individuals and determining nurses' legal responsibilities, each state has its own legislation. There is no federal policy.

Forty-two states now have mandatory elder abuse or neglect reporting laws[77]; other state laws cover the elderly and disabled adult (over 18) together. Nurses must report abuse; however, each state designates to whom they must report. The time between reporting and investigating the abuse differs from state to state. In most states, the definition of abuse covers physical abuse, neglect, and exploitation of the elderly; however, many specifics are identified by each state's law.[110]

Although some progress has been made concerning the legal issues in family violence, much more is necessary. Children, women, and the elderly still are not safe from abuse within their own families; society appears at times to condone the violence. This "private matter" of family violence must be turned into a public matter. Only an increased awareness of violence and its consequences will lead to changes in our legal system.

Table 41-2

New Legal Considerations for Domestic Violence in the State of Texas

Item	Status
PROTECTIVE ORDERS	
Dropping fee for protective order	Awaiting governor's signature (Texas)
Disallowing court to automatically drop a protective order because a divorce is pending	
Denying protective order respondents the ability to purchase firearms	
Ordering of a temporary protective order (good for 30 days) until full protective order in place (good for 1 year)	Signed into law (Texas)
STALKING	
Removing requirement of 2 reports before legal actions can be taken	Signed into law (Texas)
Requiring immediate notification to victim of release of batterer from jail, holding facility, prison	
Cooperation with Child and Adult Protective and Regulatory Services	
Requiring Department of Protective and Regulatory Services document abuse of battered women while investigating elder and child abuse	Awaiting governor's signature (Texas)
MEDICAL REPORTING	
Requiring medical professionals suspecting victims of domestic violence to provide referrals for shelter and safety assistance and document in medical records	Signed into law (Texas), September 1, 1995
RESOLUTIONS	
Requesting Higher Education Board to evaluate and encourage domestic training in all higher education institutions	Awaiting governor's signature (Texas)

velopment.[12,17,41] Their focus on the relationship between humans and their environment allows for a much clearer understanding of child abuse; this focus considers its multiple causes, such as individual personality and environmental stressors. Separate work by Garbarino and Belsky has led to a theoretical framework consisting of four levels of analysis that subsume almost all explanations of child abuse to date:

1. Ontogenic development, which considers the history of abuse in abusing parents and parental expectations of children
2. The microsystem, which considers infant and child characteristics and marital stress or conflicts
3. The exosystem, which considers the world of work and the neighborhood (eg, social isolation)
4. The macrosystem, which considers the attitude of society about violence in general

Anderson is continuing work on this theory.[2,3] Continued research and the development of conceptual and theoretical frameworks will expand the knowledge of family dynamics that contribute to family violence.

◆ Characteristics of Abusive Family Members

ABUSIVE PARENTS

Unquestionably, parents are the most common batterers in cases of child abuse, but distinction between biological, adoptive, or step-parents is often not made. Other individuals, such as foster parents, friends, and lovers of the parent(s), may also be involved.

Parents may have minimal parenting skills, poor family functioning, history of child abuse and neglect, unrealistic expectations for the children, low child acceptance or child centeredness, high levels of verbal aggression between mother and child, and high levels of stress.[67] Heightened abuse potential has been associated with single parent or nonparent custody.[67]

Violent families commonly illustrate poor communication patterns between members and lack of parental emotional support.[79] Other parental abusive characteristics reported in the literature have been categorized into four major areas: socialization factors, biological factors, cognitive and affective factors, and behavioral factors[79] (Box 41-4).

Abusing parents often identify their children as provoking the violence, rating their children as having emotional and behavioral problems.[67] Parents at high risk for potential abuse have described their children as aggressive, antisocial, and prone to injuries.[67] Other children prone to abuse may be noted as physically or mentally challenged.

Family violence is highly influenced by parental or child characteristics and a number of sociocultural variables. Clearly an assessment of parent, child, and family

BOX 41-4

Perpetrator Variables Associated With Physical Child Abuse

Socialization factors
- Demographics
- Childhood history of abuse

Biological factors
- Neurological and neuropsychological characteristics
- Physiological reactivity
- Physical health problems

Cognitive and affective factors
- Self-esteem and ego strength
- Locus of control
- Perceptions, attributions, and evaluations of child behavior
- Expectations of child behavior
- Life stress or distress
- Depression
- Other personality factors

Behavioral factors
- Alcohol and drug use
- Social isolation
- Parent–child interactions
- Parental discipline strategies

Note: Many of these categories overlap.
(Milner J, Chilamkurti C: Physical Child Abuse Perpetrator Characteristics. Journal of Interpersonal Violence 6:345–366, 1991.)

characteristics is essential in understanding potential contributors to abusive behaviors.

Behavioral indicators of abusing parents may include some of the following traits:

1. Lack of concern about the child
2. Attempt to conceal the child's injury or protect the identity of the abuser
3. Routine use of harsh, unreasonable, and age-inappropriate punishment of a child
4. High demands from the abuser's own parents
5. Inability to provide emotionally for self as an adult
6. Expectations that children will fill an emotional void
7. View of the child as a small adult capable of meeting the abuser's needs[52]

ABUSIVE SPOUSES AND PARTNERS

Men who batter are often characterized by having a need to control, an inability to recognize anger, low self-esteem, dependency conflicts, a fear of intimacy, and violent family backgrounds.[92] Abusers in treatment have reported feelings of powerlessness and an intolerance to being controlled.[88] Control of the partner may be gained by physical or psychological means.

A dominant influence on the male abuser is societal expectations of men, resulting in rigid sex role expectations. When boys deviate from the male sex role stereotype, they are punished with shaming remarks. The male bravado results from men being denied their own emotional experience and feeling ashamed of their longings and feelings. Shame leads to powerlessness, which is unacceptable to men. With the male bravado, violence and abuse often ensue. Abusive behaviors maintains the control.[88]

ELDER ABUSERS

Research on elder abuse indicates an abuser profile of the caregiver that is useful to health professionals' assessments. It includes the following elements:

1. Middle aged or older
2. Often a spouse but may be daughter or son
3. Experiencing stress, such as financial problems, medical problems, marital conflict, or unemployment
4. Increased demands of caretaking role depleting family resources
5. Resentful of role reversal with parent
6. Low self-esteem
7. Impaired impulse control
8. Possible abuse as a child[91]
9. Substance abuse[77]

Also, the caregiver may exhibit the following behaviors during contacts with the elderly victim:

1. Acts excessively concerned or unconcerned
2. Treats elder like a child or nonperson
3. Shows minimal eye contact or verbal contact with the elder[91]

As the health care professional interacts with the caregiver, other behaviors may be noticed, such as refusal to permit hospitalization of the elder, failure to visit the elder if admitted to a hospital, blame of the elder for the injury, or refusal to allow the elder to be interviewed alone.[91]

An elderly person's dependence on a spouse or child seems to be a strong indicator for abuse due to the stress that such a burden of care presents. Health care providers need to consider that some elderly people may support dependent abusers and stay in abusive situations because they perceive that their spouses or children still need them.[89]

◆ Effect of Violence on Victim and Family

EFFECT ON THE CHILD

The most obvious and life-threatening consequence of abuse is the physical damage to the victim. Medical damage to the children reflects varying degrees of medical risk. Severe health complications can occur well after the injury was sustained. Physically abused children may indicate early developmental delays, neurological soft signs, serious physical injuries, or skin marking and scars.[67] "Shaken baby syndrome," a less recognized form of physical abuse, may lead to whiplash-induced intracranial and intraocular bleeding and no external signs of head trauma.[27] Sexually abused children may report nightmares, enuresis, gastrointestinal problems, red and swollen labia, insomnia,[21] vaginal tears, bruising, or STDs.

Abuse within the home affects the child immediately or later. The abused child may be characterized by any of the following behaviors:

1. Appears wary of physical contact with adults
2. Seems frightened by parents
3. Stares in a vacant or frozen manner
4. Seeks affection from everyone
5. Manipulates adults to get attention
6. May not cry when approached by an examiner or react in a frightened manner during painful procedures[52]

School-age children may exhibit loss of school days, deficit in reading skills and expressive language, poor grades and academic performance, evidence of low self-esteem, aggression, and social and peer difficulties.[67] Psychologically, children exposed to long-standing, repeated exposure to extreme events (physical or sexual trauma) may exhibit such reactions as massive denial, repression, dissociation, identification with the aggressor, absence of feelings, rage, and unremitting sadness or depression.[67] Unrecognized and unresolved rage and sadness can lead the child victim of abuse to either sue the parents[64] or, more tragically, kill the parents.[51]

As many as 90% of children may be affected by violence indirectly, including those seeing the violence or its after-effects.[60] Simply witnessing abuse in the home influences the child's later adult behavior; boys who witness abuse show more abusive behavior as husbands than those who do not.[56,97,116] Girls raised in an environment of approved violence may be more likely to marry violence-prone men.

Children who are not directly abused themselves but are caught in the middle of parental marital discord also may demonstrate behavior problems, such as anxiety disorders, truancy, or aggression. The learning of a cycle of abuse may be demonstrated in these people's abusive dating relationships, marriages, parenting behaviors, or elderly caretaking.

EFFECT ON THE WOMAN

The physical effects of abuse on the woman are generally recognized through injuries of the head, neck, or shoulders, with black eyes being the most common lesion. Other injuries may result from being pushed against walls or down stairs.

Characteristic behaviors of battered women include fearfulness, jumpiness, and distance seeking. Emotional and financial dependency, a rigid adherence to patriarchal sex roles, low self-esteem, and a socially learned pattern of violence are also noted.

Psychological symptoms associated with the trauma of being battered can include anxiety, fears, recurrent nightmares, sleep and eating disorders, numbed affect flashbacks, hypervigilance, and increased startle responses.[59] A history of physical or sexual abuse among female inpatients is associated with dissociative symptoms in adulthood.[109] Battered women experience a number of symptoms of psychological trauma.

Battered women often feel powerless, defeated, and fearful in a battering relationship. In an effort to cope, the use of drugs and alcohol is common. The presence of one or more addictions appears to be more common among women indicating partner or childhood abuse than among women reporting no history or current violence.[1] More severe consequences of battering may be suicide, suicide attempts, or homicide (Case Study 41-3).

Spousal killings are fairly gender equal; for every 100 men who kill their wives, 75 women kill their husbands.[114] While the numbers of killings may be nearly equal, this does not imply symmetry in husbands' and wives' actions and motives. Unlike women, men often hunt down and kill spouses who leave them, kill wives as a part of a planned murder-suicide, kill in response to infidelity, kill after a lengthy period of coercive abuse and assault, and kill the woman and children together. Women often kill after years of abuse, when resources are depleted, and in self-defense.[114]

According to the woman's perception of the abuse, her reactions may vary. Women may seek shelter protection, legal intervention, or temporary or permanent severance of the relationship, or they may appear to do nothing at all. Staying in a shelter not only provides protection to the woman and child, but also may change patterns of violence among the family after leaving the shelter. A 6-month follow-up of families from a shelter indicated less child abuse than in the year preceding the stay at the shelter.[45] Many of the women, however, were not living with the battering spouse. Postshelter

41-3 **Case Study**

Maria, a Battered Wife

Maria and James lived together for several years in a common-law relationship. They rented a small but adequate apartment in a poorer section of Los Angeles. Although the first few years together had been good, lately James had begun to drink more heavily and hit Maria. One night, Maria was hurt badly by his physical abuse and required a 3-day stay in the hospital. Maria realized then that her situation was not going to improve and made plans to file charges against James and move from their apartment.

Pursuing the issue to court was hampered by several legal obstacles, but Maria persisted. In court, the judge asked James to leave Maria alone, and James promised that he would comply.

Three months later, Maria had found a new apartment and a job; however, James discovered where Maria lived, barged in on her, and hit her, which led to another hospitalization for Maria. Again in court, the judge asked James to leave Maria alone, and, once again, James promised that he would.

Several months later, James returned. Maria tried to fight, but in the struggle, Maria's eye was "put out" with a broom handle. After her hospitalization Maria again returned to court and heard the same exchange between the judge and James. She was terrified and moved to another location, but James found her again and beat her severely. After that hospitalization, Maria told the court she had done everything possible to prevent James from finding her and described her multiple hospitalizations. Still, the judge only asked James to stay away from Maria. When Maria returned to her apartment that night, she took out the small gun she had bought for protection. Unable to use it on another human being, she shot herself. She died before reaching the hospital.[50]

Questions for Discussion

1. What are some of the common characteristics of abusive families illustrated by this violent family?
2. Discuss the legal ramifications and failures involved in this case history. What should have been done?
3. When Maria was in contact with health care professionals, what could have been done to prevent future abuse?
4. Outline a nursing assessment of Maria and James and parallel interventions for them.

(From Langley R, Levy R: Wife Beating: The Silent Crisis, pp 71–84. New York, Simon and Schuster, 1977)

advocacy services for the first 10 weeks indicated increased social support for the battered women, increased quality of life, less depression, less emotional attachment to assailants, increased personal sense of power, and decreased physical abuse over time.[108]

Why women return to a violent relationship has been explored with a number of women (Box 41-5). A woman will make the decision to leave when she has had enough, and the positives are outweighed by the negatives. This time of separation, however, is one of the most dangerous times for the woman. Many women will return home again and again before making a permanent separation.

The legal system does not always protect the battered woman. In some states, unless the abuse is witnessed by the police, no arrest of the abuser may be made, despite bruises or other injuries. Once the police leave the home, the man may retaliate with another beating because the wife called the police. Obviously, women seeking legal intervention may find that the legal system does not necessarily work in their favor (see Case Study 41-3). Often, a woman who reports abuse and files a complaint against the batterer later drops the complaint. A woman may drop charges because of fear of retaliation, fear of cutting off the breadwinner from the family system, love for the batterer, or pressures from those in the legal system who have been through this process and "wasted paperwork" many times before. Because dropped complaints occur, however, some states have waived the option of dropping a complaint once it has been filed.

For women who follow through with the legal system, suggestions to help ensure safety include running away and hiding from the batterer, arresting the batterer, and applying for restraining or protective orders. Arresting the batterer can lead to family stressors, such as imposed unemployment and income reduction, anger, resentment, and later additional abuse toward the victim. Nevertheless, arresting the batterer is the preferred response to domestic violence for several rea-

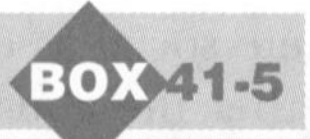

Why Women Stay

SITUATIONAL FACTORS

- Economic dependence
- Fear of greater physical danger to themselves and their children if they attempt to leave
- Fear of emotional damage to children
- Fear of losing custody of children
- Lack of alternative housing
- Lack of job skills
- Social isolation resulting in lack of support from family or friends and lack of information regarding alternatives
- Fear of involvement in court processes
- Cultural and religious constraints
- Fear of retaliation

EMOTIONAL FACTORS

- Fear of loneliness
- Insecurity about potential independence and lack of emotional support
- Guilt about failure of marriage
- Fear that husband is not able to survive alone
- Belief that husband will change
- Ambivalence and fear about making formidable life changes

(From Barnett ER, Pittman CB, Ragan CK, Salus MK: Family Violence: Intervention Strategies, p. 16. Washington, DC, U.S. Department of Health and Human Services, 1980)

sons. Arrest conveys the message to the batterer, the victim, and society that domestic abuse is a crime, and the batterer is responsible for the behavior. It also appears to deter future violence.[32]

Protective orders provide protection of the victim and children by barring the batterer from the victim's residence. Further abuse and harassment are also deterred. A protective order is criminally enforceable, and police can make an arrest with probable cause if the order is broken.

Increased training and education for policemen and judges help the problem of domestic violence enormously. Many police departments provide special training to officers for intervening in situations of domestic violence, but many departments do not. By 1983, 28 states had laws allowing police to make warrantless arrests (arresting the batterer on probable cause with no actual witnessing of the abuse).[32]

The decision to arrest is based on several factors, including the policeman's knowledge that a warrantless arrest is an option. Arrest occurs most often when the policeman's safety is threatened, a felony is committed, a weapon is used, the victim is seriously injured, future violence is likely, there is a history of frequent calls from the household, the batterer is under the influence of drugs or alcohol, the victim has been previously injured, there has been prior legal action (such as restraining order), or the victim insists on arrest.[32]

Battered women turn to shelters and emergency facilities when abuse is severe. Nurses have ample opportunity to intervene, even though the outcome may be the woman's return to the same situation. The nurse can use the time to support or care for the woman and educate her about her alternatives and options for safety, rather than ignoring the woman, treating her rudely, and provide nothing but emergency medical care. Some battered women arrive in the emergency department high on drugs or alcohol, combative, and angry. A woman may appear evasive, uninterested in working on her problems, irresponsible for caring for herself, and generally troublesome.[68] Caring for these victims is not an easy task, and a nurse's negative attitude prevents addressing the battering issues and leads to incomplete assessment and intervention.

EFFECT ON THE ELDERLY

Physical consequences of elder abuse may be noted as unexplained alopecia, bruises, abrasions, fractures, falls, welts, hematomas, grip marks, or bleeding. Signs of neglect may include dehydration, malnutrition, poor skin condition, unkempt appearance, muscle contractures, oversedation, or lack of needed hearing aid or glasses. Indicators of psychosocial abuse may be low self-esteem, invalid guilt, passive or withdrawn behaviors, or hopelessness. Exploitation of the elderly may be noted in the hospital or the community in paternalism by health care professionals, lack of understanding or unnecessary custodialism, victimization by con artists, and illegal use of the elder's money or property by family members or others.[91]

Embarrassment may prevent an elderly person from reporting abuse. In some situations, the elder may accept the abuse as deserved because he or she once abused the now-abusive adult when the adult was a child. The elder also may fear retaliation by the abuser and lack alternatives for care.

Sadly, society's response to elder abuse has been long in coming. The broken body of a small child always stirs the emotions, but the broken body of an elder may not. Many elderly and infirmed are not treated with respect, but are warehoused in boarding homes where they are stored like furniture rather than being regarded as humans.[36] No wonder the reality of elderly abuse has only recently been recognized.

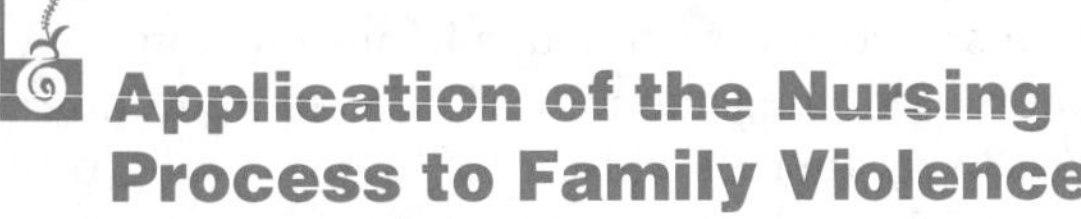

Application of the Nursing Process to Family Violence

ASSESSMENT

Assessing and Diagnosing the Battered Child

A child with a history of being battered or who is at risk for abuse may be under a nurse's care in any clinical setting with any injury. The nurse is in a unique position to detect potential and probable abuse, saving a child's life.

Screening Families for Possible Child Abuse. Assessment of predictors for high-risk children of abuse involves an investigation of many factors, such as child, parent (caregiver), environment (home), and community. Parenting styles and attitudes and values regarding discipline and punishment also need to be known. The nine categories of indicators of abusive families require assessment:

1. Generational abuse (history of childhood or partner abuse, attitude about violence)
2. Prenatal characteristics (lack of prenatal care, denial of pregnancy)
3. Intrapartum characteristics (labor and delivery concerns, postpartum separation of mother and newborn immediately after delivery)
4. Postpartum characteristics (no interest in infant, does not hold, no chosen name, poor eye contact)
5. Infant and child characteristics (multiple births, physically challenged, low birth weight, premature)
6. Parental characteristics (drug or alcohol use or history)
7. Family characteristics (unemployment, financial concerns)
8. Stress and life crisis
9. Social isolation (residence location, unlisted phone)

Research by the author has led to the development of a tool based on these most significant indicators for identifying potential parenting problems and subsequent child abuse (Box 41-6).[2,3] Additional efforts aimed at more effective identification of mothers who are at risk for problems in parenting have been made by others. Any of these predictors alone or in combination may not indicate abuse; however, they are signals to health professionals of needed interventions for optimal parenting and healthy families.

Investigating Child Abuse. Once a report of suspected abuse or neglect is made, an investigation of the family commences. The first item in a complete social assessment of the family is determining whether the abused child is safe in his or her present surroundings by examining the following issues:

1. Are weapons available to the abuser?
2. Have weapons been used, or may a weapon possibly be used, in the present abusive situation?
3. Is there use of alcohol or a history of abuse of alcohol?
4. Is there talk of murder or suicide?

Following the assessment of the danger to the child, the remainder of the social assessment, including family strengths and weaknesses, is completed.

Evaluating the Child's Physical Health. During assessment, the nurse assists with medical evaluation of the child, including making proper referrals for physical examination, radiographs, and laboratory studies. Nurses and medical personnel also cooperate with child protective services personnel and share information that will contribute to a thorough social assessment.

The multidisciplinary approach to diagnosing, evaluating, and planning the treatment of victims of child abuse and neglect has been widely advocated and adopted by hospitals and community-based services.[58] The multidisciplinary team, commonly composed of a physician, nurse, social worker, psychologist (and possibly a chaplain and lawyer), has been most effective in fulfilling a central role in acquiring extended and nonduplicated services needed to reduce the suffering of child abuse victims.

Traditionally, the nurse is responsible for obtaining specific health data, such as the parent's explanation of the child's injury, whether the explanation correlates with the type of injury, and the child's history of trauma or health problems. The child who is accident prone or has frequent health problems should be further assessed.

Physical assessment focusing on the condition of the skin questions if the child has bruises, scars, or lacerations. Preventive health practices are determined by questioning whether the child's immunizations are current and whether the child is examined by a physician on a regular basis. The child's nutritional status is assessed through dietary history and the age-appropriateness and adequacy of the diet.

Assessing the health of the sexually assaulted child includes an assessment of vaginal tears and lacerations, perineal bruising, or discharge. Proof of recent sexual contact may include the presence of motile or nonmotile sperm in the vagina, anus, or mouth or on the skin.[71] When collecting evidence for a sexual assault examination, three types of evidence are useful to prove an assault has occurred:

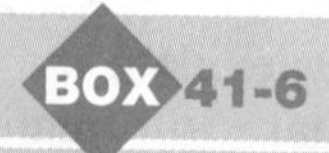

Assessing Parenting Behaviors and Subsequent Child Abuse

PARENTING PROFILE ASSESSMENT*

Assessment of Client (Through Mother)	Yes	No	Unsure
Moderate to severe discipline as a child (5)	___	___	___
Past or present spousal abuse (3)	___	___	___
Perception of stress (4.5)	___	___	___
Moderate to severe life change unit score (4.5)†	___	___	___
High-school education or less (3)	___	___	___
Rare involvements out of home (1.25)	___	___	___
Little or no prenatal care (2.5)	___	___	___
Does not feel good about herself (3.5)	___	___	___
Feels like running away (3)	___	___	___
Age at first birth under 20 (2)	___	___	___
Assessment of Family (Through Mother)			
Unlisted or no phone (1)	___	___	___
Difficulty communicating with family members (3.5)	___	___	___
History of unemployment over a 2-month period (of usual provider) (2)	___	___	___
Currently underemployed or unemployed (usual provider) (2)	___	___	___
Family involvements with police (2)	___	___	___
Less than $20,000 a year income (2.5)	___	___	___
Assessment of Discipline Methods (Through Mother)‡			
Curses at child(ren) when disciplining (3.5)	___	___	___
Child(ren) show(s) evidence of punishment after disciplining (cuts, bruises, missed school) (3)	___	___	___
Perceives discipline of child(ren) as harsh (3)	___	___	___
Calls child(ren) names when disciplining (3.5)	___	___	___

SCORING OF RISK ASSESSMENT

Scores for each variable are located in parentheses beside the variable. The scores match the scoring value on the original data collection instrument.

For each "yes" answer, add in the appropriate score. Unsure statements are not scored. More than three "unsures" compromises the validity of the risk assessment score.

After totaling the score, review the assessment for the *presence of all five following variables:*

Income under $20,000 a year
High-school education or less
Family involvements with police
Perceives discipline of child(ren) as harsh
Moderate or severe life change unit score

ALERT FOR ABUSE

Check Appropriate Box

Possible parenting problems and risk for child abuse: over 21 points or the presence of all five variables (these families require a follow-up home visit) ☐

Minimal parenting problems and low risk for child abuse: 21 points and under and absence of one to five variables (follow-up for families is optional) ☐

Uncertain risk: no additional children at home for immediate assessment of discipline methods by mother or three or more "unsures" checked (follow-up required for additional information) ☐

Follow-up
Scheduled for ______________________
____

* *Timing of a repeat home assessment is indicated by the at-risk status of the mother. A reassessment of variables may be required to determine additional areas of risk and necessary interventions.*

† *Tool to assess life change unit score must accompany this tool.*

‡ *If assessment is made in hospital between mother and first newborn, observations of this area will need to be deferred until home follow-up.*

(Copyright 1986, Anderson C. Reprinted with permission from Anderson C: Assessing Parenting Potential: Alerting Nursing Professionals of Risk for Child Abuse. Pediatr Nurs [September/October]: 323–329, 1987)

1. Evidence of force or coercion against victim's will
2. Evidence indicating the identity of the assailant
3. Evidence indicating that sexual assault occurred within the specific time frame[71]

Although the sexual assault examination needs to be thorough and comprehensive, most children do not perceive the examination any more negatively than a regular physical examination. The fear and pain from the examination can be minimized and effectively managed for most children.[70]

Evaluating the Child's Psychosocial Status. Information about the child's social history, family supports, composition of the household, and economic status is gathered by the nurse and by medical and child protective personnel. The nurse asks about the child's typical daily activities, the parent's description of the child, the child's school performance, extracurricular activities, and developmental level of functioning. Specifically, the nurse notes whether the parents describe positive or negative aspects of the child's character and whether the parents see the child as doing well in school and at home.

The nurse must pay particular attention to the quality of the parent–child interaction, the degree of parental cooperation with or resistance to medical treatment, the degree of parental concern about the situation, and the adequacy of the parents' coping abilities. Do the parents see a need for change in their home situation? Are they aware of their own involvement in the abuse or neglect? Do they want to keep the family intact and work together to solve their problems? Descriptive assessments of the affectional ties within the family and the available supports for the parents provide essential information.[52] Are there, for example, any other adults or older children at home who can assume some family responsibilities?

A child brought into the emergency room as a suspected victim of abuse should be admitted to the hospital. Hospital admission allows time for thorough evaluation and protects the child from an immediate abusive situation. Parents may permit the admission of their child and may feel relieved that the child is removed from the home. If the parents do not want to leave the child at the hospital and health care workers require additional time to complete the evaluation of the suspected abuse, the hospital can request a court order to retain the child for a specific length of time.

Diagnosing Abuse. The nurse and other health care providers should consider numerous factors when formulating a diagnosis of child abuse. Do the parents present a contradictory history? Is the cause of injury projected onto another person? Did the parents wait an unduly long time before seeking care for the child? Is there poor maternal or paternal attachment? Is a history provided that does not adequately explain the injury? Are the parents reluctant to share information with medical personnel? Have the parents gone from one hospital to another? Are the parents difficult to locate after the child's admission to the hospital?[53] Is the hospital far from the family's home?[46]

Certain factors to consider when diagnosing abuse specifically concern the child at risk. Does the child have an unexplained injury? Does the child show evidence of poor care, malnutrition, repeated injuries, fractures, burn marks, bite marks, or skin injuries, particularly bruises?[46] Table 41-3 describes bruises at various stages of healing. Does the child appear to take care of the parent?

A diagnosis of sexual abuse may be by disclosure from the child. A first-time disclosure may be made to other family members or during a formal investigation for suspected abuse. Disclosure during investigation is contingent on many issues, including the nature of the investigative interview, use of "nonleading questions" and nonjudgmental style, age of the child, and previous disclosure to others.[65]

Legally, it is mandatory for professionals, such as nurses, who suspect child abuse to report their suspicions to the appropriate authorities (police or child protective services). If the responsible health care provider fails to report suspicions of child abuse, it is the nurse's responsibility to do so within hospital protocol.

Assessing and Diagnosing the Battered Wife

An identification of child abuse may be tied to the abuse of a partner (man or woman) as well. Some women abused by their partner in turn abuse their children, and some men abuse both partner and children. Women abused by mates are twice as likely to abuse their children than are women not abused by their mates.[45] An alert nurse may identify abused women in almost any health care facility, such as an outpatient

Table 41-3

Stages of Healing of Bruises

Color	Age
Red to red-blue	Less than 24 h
Purple to dark blue	1–4 d
Green to yellow-green	5–7 d
Yellow to brown	7–10 d
Disappearance	1–3 wk

(From Gill F: Caring for Abused Children in the ED. Holistic Nurs Pract 4 [November]: 37–43, 1989)

clinic, emergency room, prenatal clinic, or even at home during a visit by a public health nurse.

Identifying the Battered Woman. The acutely battered woman in the emergency room is likely to come to the hospital without her partner, state that she has no private physician, and present with the complaint of an altercation or a fall. These characteristics, along with a high incidence of skull and facial contusions, assist the nurse in identifying a victim of battering. The nurse may also note a delay between injury and seeking medical treatment, hesitancy in providing information regarding the injury, or minimization of the injury. Sometimes a battered woman may enter the emergency room with a battered child or present with drug overdose or alcohol intoxication, which contributes to the difficulty of accurately assessing the underlying problem. A history of repeated injuries, particularly around the head, neck, or breasts, or an injury that is not adequately explained should alert the nurse's suspicions and encourage a closer investigation of the woman's situation.[21]

In screening high-risk women for potential or current abuse, knowledge of family background and interaction patterns is helpful. The nurse should consider the history of abuse in the partner's family of origin, partner abuse in previous marriages or relationships, child abuse of either partner or children of the couple, history of alcohol or drug abuse,[72] or previous suicide attempts.[23] Additional clues include unequal power positions in family, helplessness, possessiveness of mate, depression, and low self-esteem.

Between the acute battering incidents, the woman may visit her family doctor and complain of insomnia, abdominal pain, headaches, or nervousness. These physical manifestations of the woman's anxiety frequently are precipitated by her knowledge that the battering is cyclical and that the next episode is approaching. Unfortunately, many clinicians fail to investigate these complaints and their relationship to the battering, and prescribe sedatives and tranquilizers.

Diagnosing Abuse. The history of the battered woman is likely to reveal serious bleeding injuries; broken bones of the vertebrae, pelvis, jaw, or extremities; and burns from scalding water, cigarettes, or hot appliances.[99] The history must be taken with sensitivity to the woman's embarrassment, hesitancy, evasiveness, fears, excuses for the "accident," and cultural or ethnic identity. The nurse must be aware of the cultural issues important to the battered woman that may affect her response to treatment.[21] Nurses must view the battered woman's behaviors from a cultural perspective, including consideration of the woman's family structure, gender roles, marriage patterns, sexual behaviors, contraceptive practices, childrearing practices, diet, dress, religion, migrant status, occupation, self-treatment strategies, and lay healers.[21]

The battered victim may offer subtle clues about her situation; therefore, the health care professional should remain alert to their appearance. The abused woman may hint or state directly that she wants to speak privately with the health care provider. Most women are hoping the health care provider may ask about the abuse. If abuse is suspected but clues are indecisive, the woman must be asked direct questions. To gain the most accurate information, use direct questioning. Ask how the partner generally resolves conflict when angry. Questions such as "How often does your mate hit (slap, punch, push) you?"provide more information than closed-ended questions such as "Does your partner hit you?"

Other behaviors characterizing many battered women appear to fit the pervasive pattern of a self-defeating behavior disorder. The person may avoid pleasurable experiences, be drawn to situations in which there is suffering, or prevent others from helping her.[39] Because of this observation, psychiatrists and feminists battled the inclusion of the self-defeating personality disorder in the fourth edition of the Diagnostic and Statistical Manual of Mental Disorders (see Box 41-7 for DSM-IV categories for abuse and neglect). A decade of research has shown that all eight criteria describing the self-defeating personality appear in female victims of violence.[39] Feminists fear that labeling the battered woman as self-defeating would strip her of custody of her children by labeling her mentally ill—a step backward in recognizing and intervening in the social problem of battered women.

Assessing and Diagnosing the Battered Elder

Several clues, many of which are applicable to any victim of violence, may suggest abuse or neglect of the elderly client:

1. Client brought to health care facility by a person other than the caregiver
2. Frequent repeat visits to health care facility for various injuries
3. History of going from doctor to doctor
4. Delay between time of injury and seeking help
5. Inconsistency between explanation of injury and clinical findings[98]
6. Any of the previously mentioned behaviors by victim or caregiver
7. Any of the previously mentioned signs of injury or abuse

Particular high-risk situations may place the elderly at greater risk for abuse:

BOX 41-7

DSM-IV Categories for Problems Related to Abuse or Neglect

PHYSICAL ABUSE OF CHILD

This category should be used when the focus of clinical attention is physical abuse of a child.

SEXUAL ABUSE OF CHILD

This category should be used when the focus of clinical attention is sexual abuse of a child.

NEGLECT OF CHILD

This category should be used when the focus of clinical attention is child neglect.

PHYSICAL ABUSE OF ADULT

This category should be used when the focus of clinical attention is physical abuse of an adult (eg, spouse beating, abuse of elderly parent).

SEXUAL ABUSE OF ADULT

This category should be used when the focus of clinical attention is sexual abuse of an adult (eg, sexual coercion, rape).

1. Care needs exceed or soon will exceed caretaker's abilities.
2. Caregiver is experiencing frustration in giving care.
3. Caregiver is demonstrating signs of stress.
4. Living situation includes substance abuse by caregiver.[6]
5. Family has a history of abuse.[98]

Some of these assessment clues may be more applicable to the battered elder who is alone, physically or mentally debilitated, and residing with children (or other caregiver, excluding mate). Most elderly people are abused by their mates, not their children. A situation involving elder abuse may be an ongoing relationship of violence for an entire family. In these situations, assessment applicable to partner violence is more appropriate. In many cases, however, the caregiver is elderly, and the abuse may be far from deliberate. These families need understanding and help regarding alternatives for care and other necessary resources. The characteristics of the elderly victim or caregiver in isolation do not necessarily lead to maltreatment of the elderly, but in association with a crisis, they can.[57]

NURSING DIAGNOSIS

With increasing awareness of family violence and its implication to the field of nursing, the potential for violence was introduced in the taxonomy of nursing diagnoses in 1980. Most leading researchers in the field of family violence agree that primary attention should be focused on the prevention of violence within families rather than on curing the existing dysfunctional family. As discussed previously, several predictors have been identified that may influence a family to become violent. Each of these predictors may be an etiology for various nursing diagnoses regarding the potential for violence.

The following examples of nursing diagnoses may guide care in and out of the hospital setting:

1. Risk for Family Violence (specifically, child abuse) related to lack of family support and medical care during pregnancy; identification of unliked traits in the child that are seen in one or both parents
2. Risk for Family Violence (specifically, child or partner abuse) related to increased daily use of alcohol and drugs; inability to communicate effectively among all family members; lack of social involvements with family and friends; increase in perceived or actual stress currently or continuing for long periods of time; history of child abuse to one or both parents
3. Risk for Elder Abuse related to adult caregiver's history of abuse as a child by elderly; increased caregiver stress due to increased dependency of elder

The use of nursing diagnoses will enable nurses to understand, assess, and intervene better with the violent or potentially violent family (Nursing Care Plan 41-1).

PLANNING

The nurse planning interventions for abusing and abused clients must be aware of personal feelings concerning battering incidents and display a nonjudgmental attitude toward the family. Previous knowledge of and experience with abusing families will help the nurse create an accepting atmosphere. A judgmental remark uttered irresponsibly will only intensify the family members' shame and guilt. Acceptance and willingness to work openly with the family, on the other hand, will promote the attainment of long-term goals to prevent further abuse.

One major goal in working with violent families is to promote trust between the nurse, the abused victim, and the abusing family member. This goal may or may not be reached, depending on the kinds of experiences the family has already had with health care professionals. Trust is encouraged and accomplished only with time.

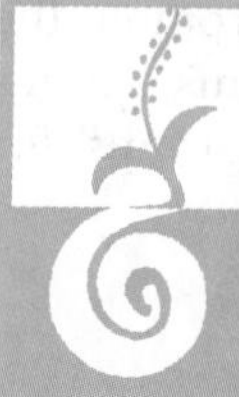

Nursing Care Plan 41-1

Parents in a Violent Relationship

Maria D is seen regularly at the emergency room with bruises, bleeding, and intense psychological distress. At times she is intoxicated. She admits that her husband, Don, has hit her after they argue about money or infidelity. The family has been referred for counseling and they have attended on a sporadic basis. They recently moved to the city so that Don could work at an engineering job. Their main recreation is spending time at a neighborhood bar. They have three young children, ages 2, $3^1/_2$, and 6 years. Maria says that Don is "not mean" to the children, but that they become frightened when the parents fight. She says that sometimes she yells at the six year old, "At least he's old enough to understand what I tell him to do." She also complains that the $3^1/_2$ year old still wets his bed at night "to get me mad."

Nursing Diagnosis

Risk for Altered Parenting, related to violent pattern of parental interactions and unrealistic expectations of children

Outcome

Parents will acknowledge cycle of abuse and learn and use new parenting skills.

Intervention	Rationale
Encourage parents to return to family counseling.	Family counseling focuses on resolving communication and relationship issues.
Encourage parents to attend Parents Anonymous groups; provide other community resources to strengthen parenting skills.	Support from other parents and information about normal child development decrease sense of isolation.
Praise parent's use of new parenting skills.	Support and praise enhances repetition of healthier parenting behavior.

Evaluation

Parents demonstrate new, healthier parenting behaviors to break cycle of abuse.

Nursing Diagnosis

Ineffective Individual Coping related to use of alcohol as method to handle stress

Outcome

Clients will identify and use alternative measures to cope with stress.

Intervention	Rationale
Encourage client to acknowledge the negative effects of alcohol use.	Denial is a common defense mechanism used by alcohol-dependent individuals. Recognition and admission of alcohol as problem is first step in changing behavior.
Refer to Alcoholics Anonymous.	Participation in A.A. effectively assists individuals to maintain sobriety.
Teach alternative stress reduction measures such as: use of support persons; use of problem-solving techniques; engaging in relaxing activities.	Use of measures to handle stress will provide alternative to reliance on alcohol.

Evaluation

Client reports use of methods other than alcohol use to reduce stress.

Discussion and planning with the violent family should be conducted in a private, quiet, nonthreatening environment. The nurse should encourage the family to verbalize some of their goals. The family's active participation in the planning process reminds them that the role of the health care provider is *not* to make the family's decisions or tell them what to do. Family members should be asked what changes they want to occur within the family and how they see these changes taking place. Comprehensive planning always incorporates the family's own goals.

The nurse should provide the family with information on available alternatives. This may be especially important for the battered woman, who may not view her immediate departure from the family as a viable alternative. When a battered woman chooses to remain with her abusing mate, plans must be made to maintain her safety within the home. Sometimes a woman will delay her decision to leave the battering environment until she is financially prepared or has developed greater confidence in her abilities.

Counseling a battered woman or elder may best be done without the family at first. Cojoint therapy (with both partners present) has worked well for some battering couples but not for others. A victim of abuse may not be able to provide accurate or complete information to the nurse in the presence of the abuser.

The nurse should provide a battered woman with information on nearby shelters, support groups, and counseling options. Within the safety of a shelter, the woman may learn how to become more independent through the development of skills that will prepare her financially if she decides to leave the family unit. Some shelters have emergency funds to help the battered victims with essential, immediate expenses. Child care alternatives also should be discussed.

The nurse may even help the woman locate a new place to stay. Because of the increased demand for shelters and their scarceness in some communities, most shelters impose a time limit on the woman's stay; therefore, the woman must make some decisions about her future. It is unfortunate that there are relatively few intermediate shelters where a woman can stay as she continues to work out her plans for the future. An intermediate (stage two) shelter allows the woman to continue to develop her job skills and care for her children within a protected environment. A new concept in shelter care is being explored, in which arrangements are made for battered women to live in the community with nonabusive families. The influence of these nonabusive families as role models is being researched for expected outcomes. Society's heightened awareness of the battering phenomenon should lead to greater community involvement and the development of more shelters for the acute and intermediate stages of abuse and recovery. This awareness also should promote the activities of support groups, such as Parents Anonymous, for abusive parents and support groups for abused elders.

INTERVENTION

The Nurse's Feelings

The nurse can intervene effectively only after establishing trust and rapport with the abusing family. While involved with the family, the nurse is exposed to information about the abuse that is often painful to acknowledge and accept. Admittedly, the nurse may feel a certain amount of anger or disgust when intervening with an abusing family.

Dealing with violent families can be stressful for the nurse. The nurse is expected to provide unending support and understanding, but who cares for the caregiver? Box 41-8 lists strategies that can help the nurse dealing with violent families to avoid burnout.

Working with helpless infants and children who have been sexually assaulted or beaten stirs up a wide spectrum of feelings in any person concerned with the health and well-being of others. Nurses should be actively involved in a support group in which they can ventilate and work through their own personal feelings of anger or possible experiences of abuse.

Recognizing and reporting child abuse by nurses appear to be affected by the type of abuse identified. Higher priorities are set for victims of sexual abuse than physical abuse and emotional abuse.[85] When the victim is an adult, nurses and medical students often blame the victim for an assault or for staying in the abusive situation.[5,13]

Intervening With the Abused Child

Nursing interventions for the abused child begin with required medical and surgical care; however, in the midst of physical treatment, the child's emotional needs must not be forgotten. To initiate a trusting relationship with the abused child, the nurse should explain all tests and procedures in terms the child can understand before they are done. The nurse should talk, sing, and play with the child to establish rapport, keeping in mind that the child may not welcome the nurse's touch. The nurse should ascertain that the child will permit touch before approaching.

Planning the Child's Care. After the immediate danger to the child has passed, the nurse begins to formulate goals relating to future safety and psychosocial development. Major goals include improving the child's self-esteem; developing more positive interpersonal relationships between the child and family; helping the child communicate feelings verbally or through art,

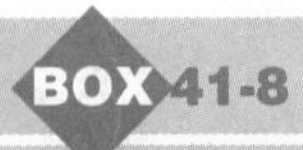

Strategies for Avoiding Burnout

PROFESSIONAL ARENA

1. Value professional convictions.
2. Foster open communication with the family and care team.
3. Promote research efforts addressing family protection issues.
4. Use available professional resources (social workers, chaplains, psychiatric clinical nurse specialists).
5. Continue to learn new information.

PERSONAL ARENA

1. Validate self-worth to maintain self-esteem.
2. Eat a balanced diet.
3. Obtain sufficient rest.
4. Understand and monitor self-behaviors.
5. Be alert for signs of exhaustion and burnout.
6. Set up "contract" with understanding coworker to verbalize feelings confidentially in uncensored framework.
7. Spend times with friends where "shop talk" is prohibited.
8. Spend time away from workplace; take mental health days when really needed.
9. Assume responsibility for seeking professional help when needed.
10. Recognize when it is best to move on to another type of work without guilt feelings.

(Adapted from Gill F: Caring for Abused Children in the ED. Holistic Nurs Pract 4 [November]: 37–43, 1989)

books, or play; helping the child channel aggression constructively; and promoting a sense of security and predictability.

Accepting the child, recognizing and commenting on abilities, and providing activities in which the child excels will promote positive self-esteem (Nursing Care Plan 41-2).

One novel approach to helping abused children is *bibliotherapy,* or treatment through books.[86] Through bibliotherapy, children can gain insight into the problem of abuse, use books as a medium through which to discuss their problem, be helped to focus attention outside of self, and be helped to discuss objectively a situation in a story similar to their own.

If the parents are unable to change their behaviors, the only safe place for the child may be a foster home or a temporary shelter. Consistency and follow-up care are essential.

Intervening with the abused child once the danger period is over requires comprehensive planning and working toward a series of long-term goals. Repairing the child's physical and emotional damage takes time, as does unlearning the cycle of violence (Nursing Care Plan 41-3, p. 847).

Intervening With the Abusive Parents

Accepting the Parents. Intervening with abusing parents immediately after an abusive incident may severely test the nurse's ability to remain nonjudgmental and accepting of clients. Parents who feel they can honestly relate their feelings to a trusting, nonjudgmental professional generally provide some information during the admission interview. The nurse must allow the parents to ventilate their feelings. If the nurse is not able to allow this, another health care professional should be found who is capable of working with the family.

Health care professionals need to communicate honestly with parents regarding the report filed and the possible outcomes. A feeling of faith that the parents can learn to parent is important to express. Praise and attention to the parents can help promote parental self-esteem and confidence. Intervention with the family must involve confidentiality, the establishment of realistic goals within a specific time frame, measurable and observable short-term goals, and specific plans for each involved agency to prevent duplication of services and consistency of care.

Community resources, such as Parents Anonymous, parenting guidance centers, planned parenthood, and individual and group therapy, may also benefit the parents. Emphasis in Parents Anonymous is on teaching the parent to identify needs that are not being met, to establish a support system within the group, to increase interpersonal skills, and to take action toward meeting needs for affiliation, nurturance, and self-esteem.[61] Many changes in abusive mothers have been reported, especially after 18 months or more of continuous involvement in the group. Mothers state that they have become more assertive and self-confident and better able to handle stress. They demonstrate better parenting skills, appear less impulsive, and take more responsibility for their own behaviors (Box 41-9, p. 848).[61]

The court may require some parents to undergo psychiatric consultations or therapy before the abused child is returned to the home. Such referrals can help the battering parents communicate their feelings and frustrations more appropriately, develop a more positive self-concept, arrange time for themselves, learn appropriate developmental expectations

Nursing Care Plan 41-2

The Physically Abused Child

Nine year old Tommy is sent to the nurse's office by a concerned gym teacher. Tommy has welts and bruises on his back and legs, which appear to be from being beaten by a belt. When asked, Tommy said that he got the marks roughhousing with his friends. The nurse points out that those sorts of marks would be different, and explains that she is there to help. Tommy admits, "My Dad hits me when I'm bad," and says that his father is not pleased with his poor academic performance. He rationalizes that his father is "old fashioned" and that he doesn't want anyone to know that he is stupid and has such poor grades.

Nursing Diagnosis

Self-esteem Disturbance related to internalizing parental view that child is "stupid"

Outcome

Client will express positive attributes about self.

Intervention	Rationale
Communicate acceptance through verbal and nonverbal means; praise the child's good work or efforts; reassure that he is not to blame for the abuse	Acceptance of the child and demonstration of positive regard reinforces that he is a worthwhile person and not to blame for the abuse.
Help child identify positive aspects of self	Child with negative self view may need assistance in identifying positive attributes.

Evaluation

Child reports positive feelings about himself.

Nursing Diagnosis

Fear, related to physical abuse by parent

Outcome

Child will remain safe, ie, free from violence or abuse, and express trust in adult care provider.

Intervention	Rationale
Report child abuse to state protective services.	All 50 states have laws mandating the reporting of child abuse.
Intervene in the abusive situation as a caring, supportive adult.	This gives the child the message that adults can be trusted.
Provide a consistent environment and be available to listen to the child.	Consistency and availability help the child develop trust.
Support child for not tolerating abuse and for reporting abuse.	Support facilitates movement from role of victim to role of survivor.

Evaluation

Child reports positive feelings about self and interacts openly with care provider.

Nursing Care Plan 41-3

The Sexually Abused Child

The C family shared a summer beach house with another family, friends of the parents. After the end of summer, the C family's eight year old daughter, Mara C, told her mother that the 17 year old son of the other family had forced her to perform sexual acts with him. Mara is vague about the nature of the activity. He had intimidated her by saying that if she told anyone, he'd say that she had a crush on him and was lying.

Nursing Diagnosis

Anxiety, related to sexual abuse

Outcome

Child will express feelings and participate in therapy; parents will agree on a plan to demonstrate support to child.

Intervention	Rationale
Assure child that she is not to blame.	Reassurance decreases child's guilt, anxiety, and fear.
Interview the child alone; encourage child to recount experience either verbally or through pictures or drawings, role-playing, or therapeutic play; record and clarify meanings of child's particular words.	Providing a safe environment allows the child to explain the events of the abuse and express feelings openly.
Help parents show continuing love and support to the child, and work through their own guilt and anger.	Parental support is critical in determining a positive outcome for child; parents need help in working through their feelings about the abuse.
In cooperation with parents, praise child's courage in speaking up, and reinforce child's self esteem.	This reinforces that child should not feel "guilty" for being coerced, and provides basis for rebuilding self-image.

Evaluation

Child expresses feelings and thoughts about sexual abuse and receives love and support from parents.

for their child, and recognize that their problem is not unique.

Approaching the Entire Family. Nursing intervention must be directed at the entire family, not at one individual. The true abuser of a child within the family would not necessarily have to be identified for effective interventions to be implemented with the abusive family.

When intervening with the family, the nurse must maintain confidentiality, establish realistic goals within a time frame, formulate short-term objectives that are measurable and observable, define specific plans for each involved agency to prevent duplication of services, and promote consistency of care through the involvement of as few people as possible.[52]

Intervening With the Abused Partner

In the immediate phase of intervention, the battered woman's injuries must be treated medically or surgically as required. If her injuries are not severe enough to warrant hospitalization, the nurse must consider letting the woman go home.[99]

Choosing to go home is a common decision and an alternative the nurse must accept. Walking through the safety issues with the woman who has chosen to return home is essential. Follow-up with the woman would be the ideal intervention.

A follow-up of women who choose to enter a shelter and are provided postshelter advocacy services reveals increased social support for women, increased quality of life, less depression, less emotional attachment to assailants, and an increased sense of personal power.

BOX 41-9

An Open Letter From a Member of Parents Anonymous

Dear Friends,
I feel that to get my point across, I must reach out and touch each of you with some of my innermost feelings. I'll call myself Sally, because Parents Anonymous (P.A.), the author, and editor have respected the philosophy of P.A. which allows me to remain unknown. It has taken me 28 years of searching to find out who I am and like her! I am a P.A. parent.

When I heard P.A. deals with child abuse, I couldn't believe *I* abused my children! I've never left a cut or bruise on my kids; they have no scars—or do they?

In society today, we see child abuse mentioned in the paper when Jane Doe burns her child in hot bath water, or Fred Smith beats his girlfriend's child to death, or Mary Jones, 16 years old and only a child herself, leaves her baby in the care of a stranger, who then disappears with the child. Abuse and neglect can muster feelings like, "Hang 'em from the nearest tree," or "What kind of awful person would do such a thing?" It's true, these things happen every day, everywhere in the world. My questions to you are these: What brings a person to the point of hurting someone they love? Since when is whipping with belts, paddles, hairbrushes, and shoes a "normal" form of discipline? When is leaving children alone 2 to 6 hours a day to avoid babysitting costs, calling them derogatory names, or forcing a child to eat every bit of food an adult puts on the plate "normal" childrearing?

Physical and sexual abuse turn our children into abusive adults. Abuse is a cycle and is passed on, in one form or another, from generation to generation. Child abuse "hunters" can only intensify the problem by putting parents in jail, removing children from their homes, and so on.

Parents Anonymous is a self-help support group, which simply means the group supports you in your efforts to become better parents. Parents Anonymous is a support system with no guarantee that if you attend six meetings, your abusive traits will go away. What P.A. does is emotionally support you as you cope with the tasks of being a parent while struggling to live in a tough world.

When I attended my first meeting of P.A. I thought that no one could ever understand what I was feeling. I heard some of the problems of members of the chapter and realized that not only did we have a lot in common, I left feeling like things weren't nearly as bad for me as they were for others!

Not everyone can attend group meetings such as M.A.D.D., A.A., or P.A. This should be understood, and parents should not be pressured into a group atmosphere. The key word is support, and this support can be sought from clergy, therapists, counselors, good friends, or close relatives. It is important to know that somebody cares. Any of us becomes very defensive when confronted with our own family's problems. Being nonjudgmental of the parents and what they've done is an important part of beginning a trusting relationship with the parents. If a child has never "driven you crazy," it will be very hard for you to understand what a parent goes through before and after an abusive episode.

Child abuse has no economic class—as a matter of fact, it can't be pinpointed to any race, creed, or color. There are, however, many common denominators, such as stress, employment, and finances, but one significant factor is the generational cycle. If you were abused as a child, chances are you will have a tendency to abuse your children. We were raised hearing "tapes." "Don't do as I do, do as I say!" "A good spanking never hurt you." As parents, we "replay" those tapes. By seeking help and learning to admit to ourselves that we can never be "perfect" parents, we start to grow as better people and better parents.

I have three children. They are now, 10, 6, and 2 years old. My problems are not larger or smaller than when I joined P.A. (my children were 5 and 2 then). They are just *different* now. I've come to grips with the fact that my problems will never go away; they will just keep changing. What I have learned is a new way of coping with them so the stress in my life doesn't affect my children as much. Learning this takes each person his or her own time, and some people never learn it at all. I have learned this with support and guidance from P.A. chapters.

Parents Anonymous builds self-esteem. If you've heard all your life that you're worthless, you begin to feel that way about yourself. If you don't like yourself, even a little, then nothing much else makes you happy. Parents Anonymous helps you find the "good guy" and the "ugly green monster" in yourself. To recognize and separate these, to learn what triggers your anger, and why your kids "push buttons" are all a part of P.A. Through a chapter meeting we can take one or several problems to the group each week and get many ideas on what to do the next time it occurs. Options! Support! Hope!

Many parents come with the same frustrations, and just knowing "I am not alone" helps. It takes time and patience to work through years of feeling the anger, hurt, despair, and frustration that has led to abuse problems. Parents Anonymous helps work through those times to break the cycle of child abuse in the family.

continued

BOX 41-9 (Continued)

I started out as a parent in P.A. with great needs, and in the chapter in Springfield, Illinois, I discovered the self-worth and strength to get through some really tough times. Now I want to help special families learn to deal with their tough times. With every meeting, training session, seminar, or workshop, I learn more about the ifs and whys of family violence. I have so many caring friends at P.A. that these groups have become families in themselves. Now, I am a chapter sponsor with great hopes of helping families the way mine was, and still is, by being involved in P.A.

My advice to you as nurses who may come in contact with family violence is to remain open. It takes a great deal for a parent to arrive at the point of abuse. Be willing to listen without judgment while remaining honest about your feelings and open to growth. I also warn you to be sufficiently aware of your own feelings so that you might "pass," if the case or situation warrants it.

I've talked about hope, support, encouragement, openness, honesty, caring, trust, and love. I've told you from my heart how I feel about P.A.

I wish each of you success in your nursing education and career and, most of all, in your parenting experiences, which are, however stressful, the most rewarding of all.

Sincerely,
Sally

Abuse, however, may continue.[108] Thorough assessment and accurate record-keeping in cases of suspected abuse are extremely important.

Treating the Battered Woman. When a battered woman is identified, the nurse must create a situation in which the woman can be comfortable, supported, and free to discuss her feelings confidentially. The nurse must know and provide the available referrals for the battered woman, such as women's shelters and legal aid agencies.

The nurse may recommend marital counseling for the couple if both partners see the abusing problem as one needing intervention. More often, the woman seeks counseling or group therapy alone and then later drops out. Battered women have a high drop-out rate from psychotherapy for the following reasons:

1. The woman is afraid of the partner's retaliation.
2. The woman wants to avoid the stigma of being in therapy and being a battered woman.
3. Therapy is seen as another promise of help that will ultimately fail.
4. Some women are seriously locked in their abusive situations and do not want to scrutinize their problem further.
5. The offer of help is premature.

Battered spouses appear to pass through an abuse cycle that may influence the battered woman's use of referrals.[112] The *tension build-up stage,* is characterized by increased verbal abuse and minor physical abuse, decreased meaningful communication, and increased anxiety or anxious depression. The battered woman may seek help because of complaints of psychosomatic problems, such as headaches and insomnia; she may appear, at this time, more amenable to using resources and accepting information about domestic violence and future safety.

The following stage, the *acute episode,* begins when the tension exceeds the couple's ability to cope. Battering may be initiated by the man or woman. During this stage, the woman may enter the emergency room if injuries warrant or a woman's shelter for protection if injuries are not life-threatening. In the emergency room, the degree of injury, denial, humiliation, or the use of substances may prevent an accurate diagnosis of abuse, but once made, the woman may be amenable to assistance.

The last stage, *reconciliation,* is entered when the couple temporarily resolves the state of increased tension. The reconciliation stage is generally shorter than the previous stage, and the battering couple can reenter it repeatedly. As the couple reconciles more frequently, this stage becomes shorter.[112] Follow-up by the woman on resources or referrals made at this time is generally lacking.

Treating the Battered Pregnant Woman. Frequently, battering begins or becomes worse during pregnancy.[21] The question of potential battering must be addressed each time the woman enters into the health care facility for prenatal care or delivery because battering may not occur until the last trimester. Battering must be ruled out any time a woman presents with trauma or injury. Trauma to the abdomen may cause antepartal hemorrhage or premature labor or fetal consequences.[75] Violence during pregnancy may be the partner's attempt to terminate the pregnancy and therefore eliminate the stress of an additional child in the family.[99] Battered women have three times the number of abortions and two times the number of miscarriages as nonbattered women.[121] Commonly overlooked, battering during pregnancy may be present in nearly half of all women assessed.[56] Surveys of women in shelters have found 44% to 100% of these women report battering during pregnancy.[54]

The pregnant woman who leaves her husband enters a complex prenatal period. The progress of the mother and fetus must be safeguarded through close prenatal supervision.[99] The battered pregnant woman may need to visit the health professional more frequently and may need to be seen without appointments during the more disorganized periods of her life.[99] Intrapartally, caregivers must be made aware of the abusive situation and must focus their care on raising the battered woman's self-esteem and providing understanding and support.

Treating the Battered New Mother. After the battered woman gives birth, pediatric caregivers need to offer additional support. The arrival of a first infant into the home is one of the most common events precipitating the occurrence of abuse.[112] If the abused woman elects to return home with the newborn, the nurse must be committed to including the mate in the plan of care. The nurse may have no alternative except to prepare the woman for possible abuse with plans for her own safety and that of the infant. Before the new mother returns to her home, the nurse should encourage her to know the location of the nearest shelter, to obtain extra keys to the car, to keep a few necessities packed and hidden away until needed, and to keep handy the name of someone to call for support and assistance.

Unplanned or unwanted pregnancies have also been identified as significant precipitating factors in partner abuse. Birth control information and Planned Parenthood agencies are helpful resources for the battered woman to help her select an appropriate method of child spacing.[99]

Treating the Batterer. Working with the man who batters can be challenging. As when dealing with abusive parents, the nurse must be nonjudgmental and open without condoning the situation. Nearly 150 men's programs have emerged in the last 5 years.[47] These programs are aimed at improving control of impulses and anger and offsetting the imposing social and institutional supports that predispose men to commit violence against women.[47] Agencies that do exist suggest group sessions; however, it is difficult to get men to attend group sessions because of intimidation and guarded thoughts and feelings. Problems occurring in group therapy include denial, victim blaming, feelings of loneliness, and attrition when attendance is not mandated by law.[47] Other interventions for male batterers are to keep a diary or "anger journal," record physical signs of anger, and learn to take time outs.[83] If the batterer can become involved in a therapy or self-help group and get in touch with his feelings and emotions regarding the abuse, the violence can be stopped.

Perpetrators of sexual abuse may not be physically abusive to the victim and require different interventions and resources. Many professionals believe that while perpetrators are in counseling, they should be separated from the family. Recontact with the family, if advised, should proceed slowly and in stages.[84]

Honest communication and rapport are essential for an effective interview with the perpetrator. Interviewers vary according to their manner of collecting data from the perpetrator; however, several strategies, as follows, may be considered useful:

1. Be familiar with the research on sex offenders.
2. Remain in control during the interview.
3. Do not "tip your hand" (allow offender to assume you know a great deal of his history, not just a part).
4. Interview all family or collaterals separately.
5. Use multiple data sources (psychological tests, medical records).
6. Emphasize what happened and not why it happened.
7. Use behavioral descriptors (molester or rapist mean different things to different people).
8. Ask direct questions.
9. Develop a "yes" set of questions (helps with agreement and cooperation with offender).
10. Ignore answers believed to be untruthful. (Points will require confirmation later and evaluator will be free to rephase question in nonconfrontive manner.)
11. Repeat questions.
12. Avoid multiple questions.
13. Ask questions quickly (prevents premeditation on part of offender).
14. Alternate support and confrontation.
15. Frame disclosure as positive action.[78]

Intervening With the Battered Elder

Subjective and objective data are assessed by the nurse in a respectful and nonjudgmental manner. Elder abuse is a complex problem with dynamic and variable origins; knowledge of the facts of abuse alone is insufficient for total care. Nurses must be aware of community resources for the elderly victim and caregiver. These resources can help the elderly lead active and fulfilling lives. Specific resources for the elderly include legal aid, medical assistance, visiting nursing, nutrition services, physical and occupational therapy, adult day care, counseling and educational services, and shelters. Informal support systems and self-help groups are important to the elderly victim and caretaker. Day care centers for abused elderly and abused children to attend together are available in some communities.

Interventions for the abused elderly have often been less than effective by professionals due to the attitudes of professionals toward the elderly.[122] While elderly

Americans are abused only slightly less commonly than children, less cases of elder abuse than child abuse are reported. Additionally, while states spend an average of $22 per child for protective services, only $2.90 is spent for each elderly person[122] (Nursing Care Plan 41-4).

Providing Community Education

What can nurses do to help battered victims and families? Participation in public workshops and forums on family violence will help to raise community consciousness and prompt the establishment of task forces on battered women, support groups for elders, and additional shelters. Nurses frequently answer "hot lines" for battered women and organize self-help support groups. Community education can help by making victims aware of shelters, emergency funds, and community mental health centers. The experience, knowledge, and research of nurses can help educate other professionals regarding the dynamics of family violence.

EVALUATION

The effectiveness of treatment for abusing and abused people depends strongly on society and its awareness of battering within the family. The community's involvement with the problem of abuse will influence how readily it provides needed shelters and education. Changes in the legal system and special task forces in police departments that deal with the family will determine the effectiveness of treatment for the violent family.

The nurse's evaluation of therapeutic interventions must first address the issue of the client's safety: Is the person who has been a victim of abuse safe from the likelihood of future abuse? The family's participation in the

Nursing Care Plan 41-4

The Battered Elder

Mrs. A is a seventy-year-old woman reporting to the emergency room with a sprained wrist and facial bruises. Her demeanor is shy and withdrawn; she seems reluctant to talk to the nurse about how she received her injuries, while implying that she does not wish to return home. Before being discharged, when asked directly, she admits that her husband inflicted the injuries on her, and that she has never told anyone before.

Nursing Diagnosis

Fear, related to being physically abused by a family member

Outcome

Client will devise a plan to maintain safety or to leave abusive situation, if desired, identifying supportive persons to assist her.

Intervention	Rationale
Approach client in a nonjudgmental manner; interview them privately and confidentially regarding the abuse.	Client who has suffered abuse is likely to feel shame; respectful treatment reinforces sense of worth.
Be available as a listener and source of support regarding client's experiences, feelings, and fears.	Encouraging client to describe experiences and express fears is the first step to changing secretive patterns.
Assist the client in identifying her own strengths; help her reach an awareness that resources and alternatives exist.	Identification of strengths and available resources offer the client hope.
Provide client with information about community resources and services; women's shelters, legal aid, assertiveness training workshops, job skill development programs.	Information and skills training provide client with ability to make plans to improve living situation.

Evaluation

Client reports reduced fear, improved self-worth, and plans to improve living situation.

planning and implementation of treatment will increase the acceptance and therefore the value of the treatment.

An effective network or support group is needed to help rehabilitate abused and abusive family members. The evaluation process should be continuous. Follow-up with violent families must be continued until the learned pattern of violent behavior is extinguished.

◆ Chapter Summary

This chapter has summarized some of the literature of the past 2 decades in the area of child, elder, and woman abuse. Abuse and neglect can occur among any family member; further discussion of others does not imply a problem of lesser significance or importance. The chapter has presented the following major points:

1. Six specific types of abuse recognized by Parents Anonymous are physical abuse, physical neglect, emotional abuse, emotional neglect, sexual abuse, and verbal abuse.
2. Physical abuse is more empirically observable than emotional abuse and therefore predominates in the available literature on family violence; however, physical abuse may be the least common form of abuse within the family.
3. Emotional maltreatment and sexual abuse are probably more common than major physical trauma to children.
4. The incidence, significance, and impact of all forms of family violence are tremendous.
5. Family violence can be directed at any family member, including man, woman, fetus, child, young or old.
6. Half of all dating relationships entail violence or sexual exploitation.
7. Although early research on the causes of family abuse emphasized the personality deficits of abusers, more recent studies have focused on financial stress, drug dependency, marital discord, and other factors.
8. The nurse must recognize the characteristics of abusing families and the effect of abuse on the entire family, rather than limiting attention to the individual victim.
9. Nursing assessment of the battered child includes the identification of the predictors of abuse and vulnerable infants, physical and psychosocial information about the child, and specific data about the injury.
10. Assessment of the battered woman often reveals a history of repeated injuries, psychosomatic complaints, and drug and alcohol abuse.
11. Elder abuse is less frequently recognized and may be considered less important because of the limited respect that society gives to the elderly.
12. It is difficult but important for the health care professional to document all types of abuse within families.
13. The goals and principles of intervening with the abused victim and family focus on an accepting, objective, and nonjudgmental approach to the family.
14. Health care providers must be familiar with the available community resources and their usefulness to the client and family.
15. Because abuse of women, children, and elders often occur together in a family, the nurse or other health care professional may need to intervene on behalf of more than one family member.
16. Nurses must become aware of and face their own feelings about working with the violent family.
17. Nurses need to become involved in the area of social change through consciousness raising, community education, and the legal process.

Critical Thinking Questions

1. *Identify five common descriptors of the abusing family.*
2. *List at least five signs or symptoms indicating potential or probable abuse in an adult woman.*
3. *Discuss four strategies that can be used when interviewing a sexual abuse perpetrator.*
4. *Consider the following situation, and decide whether or not you think there has been sexual abuse:*

   Subjective Data

   Becky, 3 years old, was brought to your office by her mother. Yesterday Becky complained to her mother that her "private parts itch." When her mother looked at her bottom, she noticed that the skin surrounding her vulva and anus was thin and white, had some red streaks, and had an area that was excoriated and ulcerated. Becky's mother normally works evenings and depends on a babysitter to help Becky bathe and get ready for bed. Occasionally the sitter's boyfriend comes over in the evening to study with her. Becky's father works for the government and is currently completing a 3-month assignment in Alaska. Becky's only other caregiver is her maternal grandmother. Becky's mother wonders whether Becky has an infection or if the boyfriend may be sexually abusing her. She wants you to check Becky before she talks to the babysitter.

(continued)

Objective Data

Becky is bright, happy, alert, and very articulate for a child of 3 years. When you ask her why she came to see you today, she states, "Because my privates itch." When asked who touches her private parts, she states, "Susan (the babysitter) touches me on my privates after my bath to help me dry." When asked who else touches her on her private parts, she states, "My mother and sometimes my grandmother, and that's all." She denies that anyone has hurt her there. There are no bruises, tears, scars, or any other lesions visible.

1. *On the basis of the history and physical examination, what are your differential diagnoses?*
2. *Which diagnosis do you select and why?*
3. *What is your treatment plan?*
4. *What follow-up is necessary?*

(Used with permission from: Jonides L, Walsh S, Rudy C: Is This Sexual Abuse? Journal of Pediatric Health Care 8: 87, 1994)

Review Questions

1. Munchausen syndrome by proxy is characterized by the following:
   - **A.** A true medical illness
   - **B.** An undiagnosed psychological illness
   - **C.** A report of abuse due to spite or vengeance
   - **D.** A fabricated medical illness
2. A sexually abusive perpetrator is often characterized by the following traits:
   - **A.** Psychotic or undiagnosed mental illness
   - **B.** Difficulty relating to age-appropriate peers
   - **C.** Reports dysfunctional family of origin
   - **D.** Nonuser of drugs or alcohol
   - **E.** B and C
3. Consequences of child sexual abuse may include the following:
   - **A.** Pregnancy
   - **B.** STDs
   - **C.** Dissociative identity disorder
   - **D.** Addictions
   - **E.** All of the above
4. All of the following comments are true of elder abuse except:
   - **A.** The abused victim may be dependent on the caregiver for needs.
   - **B.** The caregiver may be old, with limited resources.
   - **C.** Abuse, if by partner, probably is a long-lasting pattern.
   - **D.** Consequences of elder abuse are minimal and infrequent.
5. Marital rape is theoretically still accepted in how many states?
   - **A.** 35
   - **B.** None
   - **C.** 14
   - **D.** 47

◆ References

1. Anderson C: Addictive Patterns Among Battered Women: A Pilot Study. Addictions Nursing network 4: 94–100, 1994
2. Anderson C: A Preliminary Profile of Abusive and Non-Abusive Mothers. Unpublished PhD dissertation, Texas Woman's University, 1985
3. Anderson C: Assessing Parenting Potential: Alerting Nursing Professionals of Risk for Child Abuse. Pediatr Nurs (September/October): 323–329, 1987
4. Anderson C: Childhood Sexually Transmitted Diseases: One Consequence of Sexual Abuse. Public Health Nurs 12: 58–63, 1995
5. Anderson C: Health Care Professionals' Reactions to Battered Women Who Kill Their Mates. (unpublished research) Presented at Southwestern Sociological Association, San Antonio, 1991
6. Anetzberger G, Korbin J, Austin C: Alcoholism and Elder Abuse. Journal of Interpersonal Violence 9: 184–194, 1994
7. Appleton W: The Battered Woman Syndrome. Ann Emerg Med 9 (February): 84–92, 1980
8. Athens L: Violent Crime: A Symbolic Interactionist Study. Symbolic Interaction 2 (Spring): 56–69, 1978
9. Avison W, Turner J, Noh S: Screening for Problem Parenting: Preliminary Evidence on a Promising Instrument. Child Abuse Negl 10: 157–170, 1986
10. Bandura A: Aggression: A Social Learning Analysis. Englewood Cliffs, NJ, Prentice-Hall, 1973
11. Bauer W, Twentyman C: Abusing, Neglectful and Comparison Mothers' Responses to Child-Related and Non-Child-Related Stressors. J Consult Clin Psychol 53: 335–343, 1985
12. Belsky J: Child Maltreatment: An Ecological Integration. Am Psychol 35 (April): 320–333, 1980
13. Best C, Dansky B, Kilpatrick D: Medical Students' Attitudes about Female Rape Victims. Journal of Interpersonal Violence 7: 175–188, 1992
14. Bird G, Stith S, Schladale J: Psychological Resources, Coping Strategies and Negotiation Styles as Discriminating Violence in Dating Relationships. Family Relations 40 (January): 45–50, 1991
15. Bools C, Neale B, Meadow R: Munchausen Syndrome by Proxy: A Study of Psychopathology. Child Abuse Negl 18: 773–788, 1994

16. Broadhurst D: The Educator's Role in the Prevention and Treatment of Child Abuse and Neglect. Washington, DC, Department of Health, Education and Welfare (Pub. No. OHDS79-30172), 1979
17. Bronfenbrenner U: The Ecology of Human Development. Cambridge, Harvard University Press, 1977
18. Buntain-Ricklefs J, Kemper K, Bell M, Babonis T: Punishments: What Predicts Adult Approval. Child Abuse Negl 18: 945–955, 1994
19. Burr W, Hill R, Nye F, Reiss I (eds): Contemporary Theories About the Family, vol 2. New York, Free Press, 1979
20. Burrell B, Thompson B, Sexton D: Predicting Child Abuse Potential Across Family Types. Child Abuse Negl 18: 1039–1049, 1994
21. Campbell J, Humphreys J: Nursing Care of Survivors of Family Violence. St. Louis, CV Mosby, 1993
22. Campbell J, Humpreys J: Nursing Care of Victims of Family Violence. Reston, VA, Reston Publishing Company, 1984
23. Candib L: Naming the Contradiction: Family Medicine Failure to Face Violence Against Women. Family and Community Health 13 (November): 47–57, 1990
24. Cate RM, Henton JM, Koval JE, Christopher TS, Lloyd SA: Premarital Abuse: A Social psychological Perspective. J Fam Issues 3: 79–90, 1982
25. Chaffin M: Assessment and Treatment of Child Sexual Abusers. Journal of Interpersonal Violence 9: 224–238, 1994
26. Conte J, Schuerman J: The Effects of Sexual Abuse on Children: A Multidimensional View. Journal of Interpersonal Violence 2 (December): 380–391, 1987
27. Coody D, Brown M, Montgomery D, Flynn A, Yetman R: Shaken Baby Syndrome: Identification and Prevention for Nurse Practitioners. Journal of Pediatric Health Care 8 (March/April): 50–55, 1994
28. Curtain S: Recognizing Multiple Personality Disorder. J Psychosoc Nurs 31: 29–33, 1993
29. Davenport C, Browne K, Palmer R: Options on the Traumatizing Effects of Child Sexual Abuse: Evidence for Consensus. Child Abuse Negl 18: 725–738, 1994
30. Deblinger E, Hathawat C, Lippmann J, Steer R: Psychosocial Characteristics and Correlates of Symptom Distress in Nonoffending Mothers of Sexually Abused Children. Journal of Interpersonal Violence 8: 155–169, 1993
31. Dunford FW, Huizinga D, Elliot D: The Omaha Domestic Violence Police Experiment: Final Report to the National Institute of Justice and the City of Omaha. Boulder, CO, 1989
32. Eigenberg H, Moriarty L: Domestic Violence and Local Law Enforcement in Texas: Examining Police Officers' Awareness of State Legislation. Journal of Interpersonal Violence 6 (March): 94–102, 1991
33. Finkelhor D: The Trauma of Child Sexual Abuse: Two Models. Journal of Interpersonal Violence 2 (December): 348–367, 1987
34. Finkelhor D, Baron L: High Risk Children. In David Finkelhor (ed): A Sourcebook on Child Sexual Abuse. Beverly Hills, CA, Sage, 1986
35. Finkelhor G, Hotaling G, Lewis IA, Smith C: Sexual Abuse and its Relationship to Later Sexual Satisfaction, Marital Status, Religion and Attitudes. Journal of Interpersonal Violence 4 (December): 379–400, 1989
36. Fitch J: Stopping Elderly Abuse. Journal of Emergency Medical Services (April): 50–53, 1986
37. Flynn E: Preventing and Diagnosing Sexual Abuse in Children. Nurse Pract 12 (February): 47–54, 1987
38. Fox K, Gilbert B: The Interpersonal and Psychological Functioning of Women who Experienced Childhood Physical Abuse, Incest, and Parental Alcoholism. Child Abuse Negl 18: 849–858, 1994
39. Franklin D: The Politics of Masochism. Psychology Today (January): 53–57, 1987
40. Freud S: The Ego and the Id. Riviere J (trans). Strachey J (ed). New York, WW Norton, 1962
41. Garbarino J: The Human Ecology of Child Maltreatment: A Conceptual Model for Research. J Marriage Fam 39: 721–732, 1977
42. Gaylord J: Wife Battering: A Preliminary Survey of 100 Cases. Br Med J 1 (January): 194–197, 1975
43. Gelles R, Conte J: Domestic Violence and Sexual Abuse of Children: A Review of Research in the Eighties. J Marriage Fam 52 (November): 1045–1058, 1990
44. Gelles R, Strauss U: Is Violence Towards Children Increasing? Journal of Interpersonal Violence 2 (June): 212–223, 1987
45. Giles-Sims J: A Longitudinal Study of Battered Children of Battered Women. Family Relations 34 (April): 205–210, 1985.
46. Gill F: Caring for Abused Children in the ED. Holistic Nurs Pract 4 (November): 37–43, 1989
47. Gondolf E: Men who Batter: An Integrated Approach to Stopping Wife Abuse. Holmes Beach, FL, Learning Publications, 1990
48. Graziano A, Lindquist C, Kunce L, Munjal K: Physical Punishment in Childhood and Current Attitudes. Journal of Interpersonal Violence 7: 147–155, 1992
49. Gruber A, Heck E, Mintzner E: Children Who Set Fires. Am J Orthopsychiatry 51 (July): 484–487, 1981
50. Hanson R, Lipovsky J, Saunders B: Characteristics of Fathers in Incest Families. Journal of Interpersonal Violence 9: 155–170, 1994
51. Heide, K: Parents Who Get Killed and the Children Who Kill Them. Journal of Interpersonal Violence 8: 531–545, 1993
52. Heindl C, Krall C, Salus M, Broadhurst D: The Nurse's Role in the Prevention and Treatment of Child Abuse and Neglect. Washington, DC, Department of Health, Education and Welfare (Pub. No. OHDS79-30202), 1979
53. Helfer R, Kempe CH: Helping the Battered Child and His Family. Philadelphia, JB Lippincott, 1972
54. Helton A, McFarland J: Battered and Pregnant: A Prevalence Study. Am J Public Health 77: 1337–1339, 1987
55. Hendrix MJ, LaGodna G, Bohen C: The Battered Wife. Am J Nurs 78 (April): 650–653, 1978
56. Hilton N: Battered Women's Concerns About Their Children Witnessing Wife Assault. Journal of Interpersonal Violence 7: 77–87, 1992
57. Hirst S: The Abused Elderly. J Psychosoc Nurs Mental Health Care 24 (October): 37–45, 1986
58. Hochstadt N, Harwicke N: How Effective is the Multidis-

ciplinary Approach? A Follow-Up Study. Child Abuse Negl 9: 365–371, 1995

59. Houskamp B, Foy D: The Assessment of Posttraumatic Stress Disorder in Battered Women. Journal of Interpersonal Violence 6: 367–375, 1991
60. Hughes H: Impact of Spouse Abuse on Children of Battered Women. Violence Update August: 1, 9, 1992
61. Hunka C, O'Toole A, O'Toole R: Self-Help Therapy in Parents Anonymous. J Psychosoc Nurs Ment Health Care 23: 24–31, 1985
62. Johnson R: Aggression in Man and Animals. Philadelphia, WB Saunders, 1972
63. Jones J, Butler H, Hamilton B, Perdue J, Stern P, Woody R: Munchausen Syndrome by Proxy. Child Abuse Negl 10: 33–40, 1986
64. Kaslow F: Children who Sue Parents: A New Form of Family Homicide? Journal of Marital and Family Therapy 16: 151–163, 1990
65. Keary K, Fitzpatrick C: Children's Disclosure of Sexual Abuse During Formal Investigation. Child Abuse Negl 7: 543–548, 1994
66. Kendall-Tackett K: Characteristics of Abuse That Influence When Adults Molested as Children Seek Treatment. Journal of Interpersonal Violence 6: 486–494, 1991
67. Kolko D: Characteristics of Child Victims of Physical Violence. Journal of Interpersonal Violence 7: 244–276, 1992
68. Kurz D: Emergency Department Responses to Battered Women: Resistance to Medicalization. Social Problems 34: 69–81, 1987
69. Langley R, Levy R: Wife Beating: The Silent Crisis. New York, Simon and Schuster, 1977
70. Lazebnik R, Zimet G, Ebert J, Anglin T, Williams P, Bunch D, Krowchuk D: How Children Perceive the Medical Evaluation for Suspected Sexual Abuse. Child Abuse Negl 18: 739–745, 1994
71. Ledray L: The Sexual Assault Examination: Overview and Lessions Learned in One Program. Journal of Emergency Nursing 18: 223–232, 1992
72. Lichtenstein V: The Battered Woman: Guideline for Effective Intervention. Issues in Mental Health Nursing 3 (July–September): 237–251, 1981
73. Limandri B: The Therapeutic Relationship with Abused Women. J Psychosoc Nurs 25 (February): 9–16, 1987
74. Lipovsky J, Saunders B, Murphy S: Depression, Anxiety, and Behavior Problems Among Victims of Father-Child Sexual Assault and Nonabuse Siblings. Journal of Interpersonal Violence 4 (December): 452–469, 1989
75. Lloyd S: The Darkside of Courtship: Violence and Sexual Exploitation. Family Relations 40 (January): 14–20, 1991
76. Lorenz K: On Aggression. New York, Harcourt, Brace, 1966
77. Matlaw J, Spence, D: The Hospital Elder Assessment Team: A Protocol for Suspected Cases of Elder Abuse and Neglect. Journal of Elder Abuse and Neglect 6: 23–37, 1994
78. McGrath R: Assessment of Sexual Aggressors: Practical Clinical Interviewing Strategies. Journal of Interpersonal Violence 5: 507–520, 1990
79. Milner J, Chilamkurti C: Physical Child Abuse Perpetrator Characteristics. Journal of Interpersonal Violence 6: 345–366, 1991
80. Muram D, Miller K, Cutler A: Sexual Assault of the Elderly Victim. Journal of Interpersonal Violence 7: 70–77, 1992
81. Neinstein L, Goldenring J, Carpenter S: Nonsexual Transmission of Sexually Transmitted Diseases. Pediatrics 74: 69–75, 1984
82. Ney P, Fung T, Wickett A: The Worst Combinations of Child Abuse and Neglect. Child Abuse Negl 18: 705–714, 1994
83. Nikstaitis G: Treatment for Men Who Batter. J Psychosoc Nurs Ment Health Care 27: 33–36, 1985
84. O'Connell M: Reuniting Incest Offenders With Their Families. Journal of Interpersonal Violence 1: 374–387, 1986
85. O'Toole A, O'Toole R, Webster S, Lucal, B: Nurses' Responses to Child Abusers. Journal of Interpersonal Violence 9: 194–207, 1994
86. Pardeck J: Bibliotherapy with Abused Children. Fam Society 71 (April): 229–235, 1990
87. Peters S, Wyatt G, Finkelhor D: Prevalence. In David Finkelhor (ed): A Sourcebook on Child Sexual Abuse. Beverly Hills, CA, Sage, 1986
88. Petrik N, Petrik-Olsen R, Subotnik L: Powerlessness and the Need to Control. Journal of Interpersonal Violence 9: 278–284, 1994
89. Pillemer K: The Dangers of Dependency: New Findings on Domestic Violence Against the Elderly. Social Problems 33 (December): 146–158, 1985
90. Pillemer K, Finkelhor D: The Prevalence of Elder Abuse: A Random Sample Survey. Gerontologist 28: 51–57, 1988
91. Podnieks E: Elder Abuse: It's Time We Did Something About It. Can Nurs (December): 36–39, 1985
92. Potter S: Men in Violent Relationships. Dallas, TX, Family Violence Miniseries, 1989
93. Restak R: The Brain: The Last Frontier. New York, Doubleday, 1979
94. Riggs D: Relationship Problems and Dating Aggression. Journal of Interpersonal Violence 8: 18–36, 1993
95. Riggs D, O'Leary KD, Breslin FC: Multiple Correlates of Physical Aggression in Dating Couples. Journal of Interpersonal Violence 5 (March): 61–74, 1990
96. Roane T: Male Victims of Sexual Abuse: A Case Review Within a Child Protective Team. Child Welfare LXXI (May/June): 231–239, 1992
97. Rosenbaum A, O'Leary K: Children: The Unintended Victims of Violence. Am J Orthopsychiatry 51 (October): 692–699, 1981
98. Ross M, Ross PL, Ross-Carson M: Elderly Abuse. Can Nurs (February): 37–39, 1985
99. Sammons L: Battered and Pregnant. MCN 6 (July/August): 246–251, 1981
100. Scott J: In Endleman S (ed): Violence in the Streets. Chicago, Quadrangle Books, 1968
101. Simkins L: Characteristics of Sexually Repressed Child Molesters. Journal of Interpersonal Violence 8: 3–18, 1993
102. Simon L, Sales B, Kaszniak A, Kahn M: Characteristics of Child Molesters. Journal of Interpersonal Violence 7: 211–226, 1992

103. Smith H, Isreal E: Sibling Incest: A Study of the Dynamics of 25 Cases. Child Abuse Negl 11: 101–108, 1987
104. Steinmetz S: The Battered Husband Syndrome. Victimology Int J 2 (March): 499–509, 1978
105. Steimetz S: The Cycle of Violence: Assertive, Aggressive, and Abusive Family Interaction. New York, Praegle Publication, 1977
106. Stevens-Simon C, McAnarney E: Childhood Victimization: Relationship to Adolescent Pregnancy Outcome. Child Abuse Negl 18: 569–575, 1994
107. Straus M: A General Systems Theory Approach to a Theory of Violence Between Family Members. Soc Sci Inform 12 (June): 105–125, 1973
108. Sullivan C, Campbell R, Angelique H, Elby K, Davidson, W: An Advocacy Intervention Program for Women With Abusive Partners: Six Month Follow-Up. American Journal of Community Psychol 22: 101–121, 1994
109. Swett C, Halpert M: Reported History of Physical and Sexual Abuse in Relation to Dissociation and Other Symptomatology in Women Psychiatric Inpatients. Journal of Interpersonal Violence 8: 545–556, 1993
110. Thosaben M, Anderson L: Reporting Elder Abuse. Am J Nurs 85 (April): 371–374, 1985
111. Utech M, Garrett R: Elder and Child Abuse. Journal of Interpersonal Violence 7: 418–428, 1992
112. Walker L: The Battered Woman. New York, Harper-Colophon Books, 1979
113. White J, Humphrey J: Women's Aggression in Heterosexual Conflicts. Aggressive Behavior 20: 195–202, 1994
114. Wilson M, Daly M: Who Kills Whom in Spouse Killings? On the Exceptional Sex Ratio of Spousal Homicides in the United States. Criminology 30: 189–209, 1992
115. Wolfe D: Child-Abusive Parents: An Empirical Review and Analysis. Psychol Bull 97: 462–482, 1985
116. Wolfe D, Jaffe P, Wilson S, Zak L: Children of Battered Women: The Relationship of Child Behavior to Family Violence and Maternal Stress. J Consult Clin Psychol 53: 657–665, 1985
117. Wolff J: Bite Marks: Recognizing Child Abuse and Identifying Abusers. Fam Society 71 (October): 496–498, 1990
118. Wong D: False Allegations of Child Abuse: The Other Side of the Tragedy. Pediatr Nurs 13 (September/October): 329–335, 1987
119. Sexual Abuse of Children: Selected Readings. Washington, DC, Department of Health and Human Services (Pub. No. OHDS78-30161), 1980
120. The Police Perspective in Child Abuse and Neglect. Gaithersburg, MD, International Association of Chiefs of Police, 1977
121. Anon: Trouble and Strife. Nurs Times (Aug): 32–33, 1986
122. Anonymous: Elder Abuse and Neglect. Council Report JAMA 257: 966–971, 1987

Suicide

Bruce Payne Mericle

42

I am now the most miserable man living. If what I feel were equally distributed to the whole human family, there would not be one cheerful face on earth.

Abraham Lincoln

Abraham Lincoln is believed to have suffered through several periods of severe depression. His previously noted comment is not unusual for someone suffering with a diagnosable major depressive disorder. The presence of a mental disorder, including schizophrenia, substance abuse, borderline personality, and the mood disorders, is a primary risk factor to consider when assessing for suicidal ideation.[9,18,36]

Many mental disorders, including depression, result in psychic pain that becomes unbearable and may result in death.[9,50] *Schneidman*[45,46] *wrote that "unendurable psychological pain" is a universal characteristic of people who attempt or commit suicide (p 124).*

In addition to the presence of psychopathology, substance abuse and stressful life situations also play important roles in suicide. For example, the rock star Kurt Cobain, who committed suicide in 1995, was severely depressed and had a history of heroin abuse.[16]

Demographic variables, including age, gender, ethnicity, and degree of physical wellness, influence risk for suicide. Understanding the characteristics of suicidal ideation and behavior is important, because suicide is the eighth leading cause of death in the United States today. It accounts for 1.4% of all American deaths.[37]

As an isolated act, suicide often is perplexing. While it certainly is the individual's last desperate message to the world, nurses and other health care providers must know that most individuals do not want to end their life when they attempt suicide. Rather, they are seeking relief from the unbearable emotional or physical pain described by Schneidman.

The purpose of this chapter is to help the reader understand the nature of suicidal behaviors and identify factors that place some at risk. By studying the research literature and the professional experiences of clinicians, nurses are better able to understand how health care professionals can assist suicidal people to find healthier ways of coping with stress.

Throughout this chapter, the reader is introduced to a variety of theories about suicidal behavior, its incidence, and at-risk populations. The assessment phase of the nursing process is used as a method for identifying those at risk and as a means for planning, implementing, and evaluating care. Prevention of suicide and care of suicide survivors are also discussed. Following a brief description of legal responsibilities, ethical issues, including the possibility of professional involvement in assisted suicide, are discussed.

Learning Objectives

On completion of this chapter you should be able to accomplish the following:

1. *Understand suicide as a form of self-destructive behavior.*
2. *Discuss factors related to the incidence of suicide and populations affected.*
3. *Discuss sociological, psychological, and biological theories of the development and dynamics of suicide.*
4. *Apply the nursing process to the care of clients exhibiting suicidal behavior.*
5. *Recognize and discuss your own feelings and behaviors that may affect the suicidal client, his or her significant others, and survivors of suicide.*
6. *Discuss legal and ethical issues, including much publicized issues of assisted suicide and the responsibilities of health care professionals.*
7. *Correctly answer the 10-item suicide fact or myth quiz (Box 42-1).*

◆ Incidence and Populations Affected

In 1994, the National Center for Health Statistics[37] published the most recently available data (1991) concerning demographic variables for suicides in the United States. Suicide continues as the eighth leading cause of death among all age groups. It is the third leading cause among 15- to 24-year-olds, following unintentional death and homicide.[36] White people are twice as likely to die by suicide as nonwhite people. The ratio of male to female suicides in the United States is increasing, and as of 1991, for every woman who commits suicide, four men will die at their own hands. More than 70% of all U.S. suicides are committed by white men.[36,37]

The most recent statistics indicate an alarming increase in the number of elderly who take their lives.[10,11] The suicide rate among very old men (85 years and older) is 75.1 suicides per 100,000 population compared with an 11.8 per 100,000 overall suicide rate. The population of elderly American men is now the group at highest risk.[36]

United States ethnic groups demonstrating the highest suicide rates are the Native Americans and Alaska natives.[20,21,36] Rates, however, vary considerably from tribe to tribe. Situational stress, including availability of adequate housing and access to health care, are two important factors that contribute to tribal variances.[21]

Geographically, rates are highest in the western mountain region and lowest along the Northeast seaboard. This latter fact may be related to easier access to health care along the Atlantic coast.

◆ Etiological Theories

Why people commit suicide is a question that continues to interest researchers and clinicians. People attempt to end their lives for many reasons. For some, it is an escape from poor physical health, often accompanied by chronic pain; for others, it resolves social alienation or unbearable intrapsychic pain. For others, it is an escape

BOX 42-1

Suicide Quiz: Statement of Fact or Myth

The 10 statements below are designed to test preconceived notions you may hold about people who attempt or commit suicide. Place an F if you believe the statement is a fact or an M if it is a myth. Each statement is addressed as part of the chapter discussion. You may compare your beliefs as you read or check them against the answers that appear in Box 42-3 at the end of the chapter.

____ 1. Only depressed people commit suicide.
____ 2. Alcohol is implicated in more than 50% of all completed suicides.
____ 3. Suicide is the third leading cause of death among teenagers.
____ 4. A 60-year-old man is more likely to commit suicide than an 85-year-old man.
____ 5. Most women who commit suicide do so with a drug overdose.
____ 6. Most people who kill themselves leave a suicide note.
____ 7. African American men have a higher suicide rate than white American men.
____ 8. Of all human feelings, guilt feelings are the best predictor of suicide risk.
____ 9. Asking a person if he or she feels suicidal will increase his or her risk of suicide.
____ 10. Psychiatric mental health professionals generally are more cautious than the average citizen about admitting that they are feeling suicidal.

from years of suffering with mental illness. For example, the suicide rate among the chronic schizophrenic population is much higher than the national average. Further, one research study of Vietnam veterans suffering with posttraumatic stress disorder demonstrated that exposure to significant stress coupled with poor physical health and social isolation are believed to contribute to increased risk for suicide.[6]

Age and gender are important factors that contribute to who will attempt versus who will commit suicide. Age and gender also influence the reasons for suicide and the methods chosen. These factors are discussed in greater depth later in this chapter.

Most people who attempt suicide have recently experienced a period of increased stress. Suicide among the young is often associated with interpersonal discord, rejection by a friend when peer approval is critical, or job loss or financial problems.

Among the elderly, losses are often clustered. Significant factors may include deteriorating health, loss of lifelong friends, or loss of financial independence.[10,11]

SOCIOLOGICAL THEORIES

Durkheim, considered by many to be the founder of modern suicidology, based his early observations of suicidal behavior on social statistics available in Europe during the late 19th century. He postulated that individuals committed suicide because they lacked purpose in life (egoistic suicide), sensed social normlessness (anomic suicide), or gave up living for a greater good (altruistic suicide).[14]

Edwin Schneidman, a contemporary expert on suicide, began his work in the early 1950s. He conceptualizes suicidal behavior within a sociological *crisis* framework.[28,45] Several of his concepts are important for nurses caring for suicidal individuals. They include the following notions about the person:

- Is exclusively focused on unbearable pain
- Communicates some form of trauma (poor health, rejection)
- Communicates the idea of cessation (eternal sleep, death)
- Is in a state of great disturbance (crisis)
- Communicates ambivalence (seeing death as the only way to be rid of the pain but yet *not* wanting to die)

Recently, a counter social force has been identified as important for protecting individuals from depression and therefore possibly from suicide. That force is the presence of a social support system of family or friends. These social systems seem to be of greater importance for the mental health of the young, while involvement in religious and community groups is more significant for preventing depression in the older adult.[17]

PSYCHOLOGICAL THEORIES

Psychoanalytic View

At about the time Durkheim studied suicide from a sociological perspective, Sigmund Freud was studying it from a psychoanalytic point of view. Freud defined two drives basic to all people: eros, the drive toward life, and thanatos, the drive toward death. Based on his psychological theory, Freud proposed that suicidal behavior emerged when the "death drive" took precedence over the "life drive." This shift in the intrapsychic forces of an individual, he believed, occurred in response to the real or imagined loss of a significant object.

The image of the loved one, with all its concomitant feelings, was internalized. The individual who felt abandoned by the lost love object experienced anger, and this anger, lacking an outlet, was turned toward the self. The ultimate act of self-destruction (suicide) resulted as an overwhelming depressive response to the loss.[31]

Contemporary assessment for risk of suicide requires evaluation of the extent of recent losses as part of the systematic development of a data base.

Interpersonal View

Later psychological theories, although not completely rejecting Freudian thought, viewed suicide as the result of an interpersonal and intrapsychic crisis. The individual experiences interpersonal discord, which leads to conflict and ambivalence about continuing to live. Suicide becomes the means for resolving interpersonal conflict.[46]

Today, a standard of care for suicidal people includes appealing to healthy ambivalence by suggesting that it is possible to resolve conflict in ways other than dying.

BIOLOGICAL THEORIES

Recently, biological explanations for self-destructive behavior have been investigated, although the search has yet to identify a strong link between biological processes and suicidal behaviors. Serotonin provides inhibitory control over aggression in many animals.[56,58] When insufficient serotonin is available in the brain, the result may be excessive aggressive behavior, including self-directed aggression.

Mann and colleagues studied the autopsied brains of 21 victims of violent suicides (gunshot wounds, hanging, and jumps from heights) and found statistically significant increases in the postsynaptic frontal cortices' binding sites when compared with matched controls.[32] Increased binding decreases the availability of serotonin for regulation of aggressive behavior.

5-HIAA (5-Hydroxyindoleacetic acid) is a metabolite of serotonin and is normally found in spinal fluid. Nordstrom and coworkers studied 92 men and women who had attempted suicide to determine if low concentrations of cerebrospinal fluid 5-HIAA would predict risk for suicide. The clients were followed for 1 year. Within this year, 11 (12%) of the research subjects committed suicide. The authors concluded that low cerebrospinal fluid 5-HIAA predicts short-range suicide risk and supports the serotonin hypothesis of suicide risk.[38]

A recent study concluded that low serum cholesterol is positively correlated with attempted suicide.[19] Cholesterol is believed to be a biological marker of serotonin. Thus, low serum cholesterol would suggest low serotonin availability and reduced inhibition of aggression.

Much more research is necessary before we fully understand the relationships of biological alterations to suicidal behavior; nonetheless, it is an area that promises to provide some answers in the future.

◆ Dynamics of Suicide

A person contemplating suicide generally perceives himself or herself as isolated. This isolation is manifested often as actual physical distancing or as a sense of aloneness. The person may experience feelings of guilt, hopelessness, helplessness, and worthlessness. Of these feelings, hopelessness and worthlessness are strong predictors of suicide.[43] Many suicide notes written by people who have committed suicide express such feelings.[28] Because the suicidal person's feelings are overwhelming, he or she is unable to initiate or respond to social interactions.

As a result of discussions with suicidal clients and from examination of suicide notes, theorists have gleaned an understanding of the emotional components of suicide. The emotional state of the suicidal person is characterized by depression and anger. The suicidal person's desire to be free of pain or to be dead is often coupled with a simultaneous desire to be saved. Ultimately, however, the suicidal gesture has unique meaning for the individual and must be explored to be understood.

These dynamics, the interplay between the suicidal person and his or her environment, form the basis for intervention.

Application of the Nursing Process

ASSESSMENT

Estimation of Risk

Accurate assessment of the estimation of risk is the key to developing a nursing care plan for the suicidal client. Through development of a knowledge base, observation, and thoughtful listening, the nurse examines the client's current life situation, behaviors, and verbalizations for clues of suicidal intent. During the assessment process, issues to be explored include the client's request for help, the presence and nature of a suicide plan, the client's mental status, the client's lifestyle, and the availability of support systems. Thus, theoretical knowledge and clinical judgment guide the nurse in estimating the extent of risk amid a complex set of behaviors and thoughts.

Risk Factors

The identification of risk factors is considered a major part of suicide prevention.[49] The following discussion focuses on six identified risk factors.

Age. Children younger than 14 years rarely (less than 1% of all suicides) commit suicide. Therefore, they are not usually considered a population at risk (Fig. 42-1).

Between the ages of 18 and 30 years, the rate rises dramatically. The rate of suicide for this group has more than doubled since 1950.[24,39] Many of the people in this age group are also those found in the military, colleges, or prison. All three systems produce a significant number of suicides.[30]

There has been much public debate about the possible effect of the "heavy metal" subculture on this age group, because the lyrics of some heavy metal music address suicide. At least one study, conducted by Stack and others, concluded that the heavy metal subculture tended to draw those who are already at high risk for suicide (eg, white men) and therefore did not directly increase the risk for suicide among this population.[52]

The elderly, those 65 years or older, also account for a significant number of suicides. In elderly American men, the older the man, the greater the risk for suicide. Men older than 85 years are the population at highest risk today.[37]

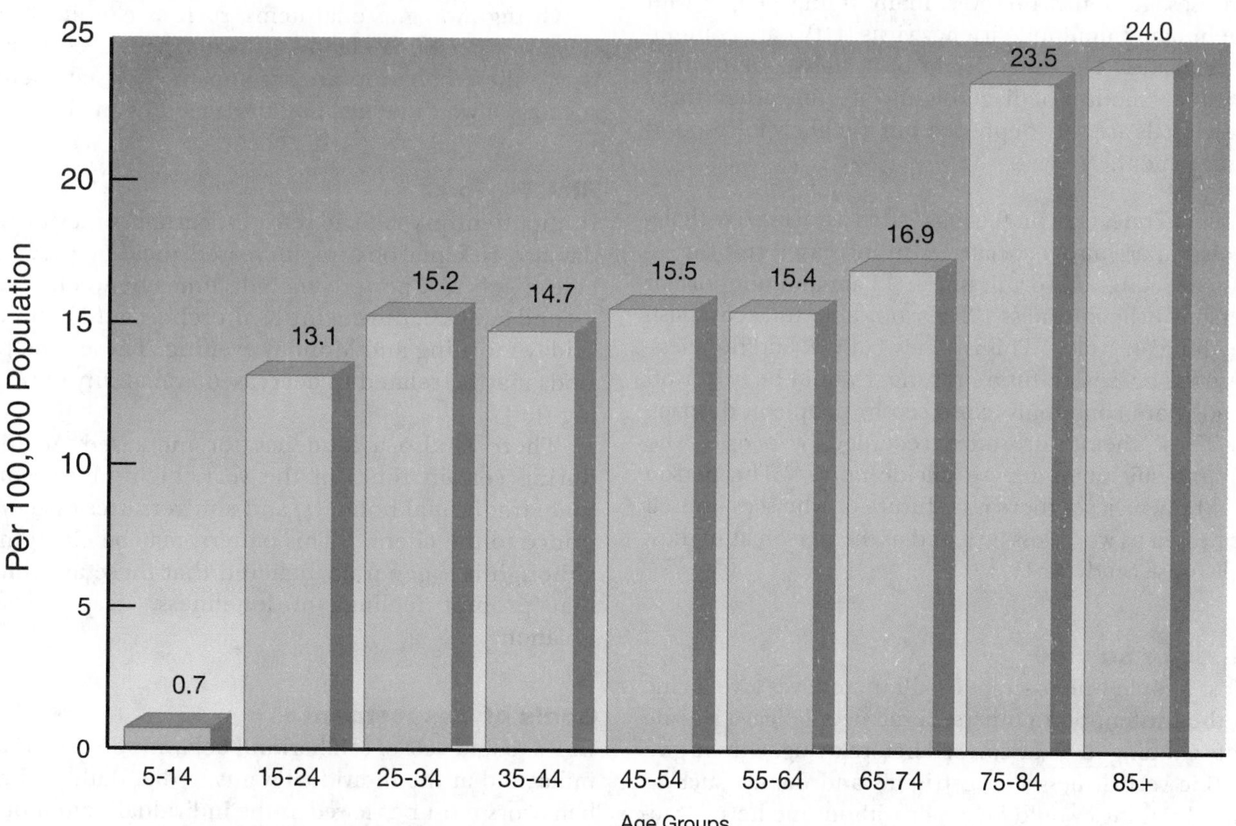

Figure 42-1. Suicide based on age per 100,000 population. (Adapted from National Center for Health Statistics: Vital and Health Statistics Mortality Surveillance System: Models from the Second Year. Series 20 (22): Hyattsville, MD, October, 1994)

Gender. As noted previously, four times as many men commit suicide as women. This is particularly true for white men. However, the majority of people who attempt suicide are women.[36]

Ethnicity. Native Americans and Natives of Alaska continue to be over-represented in the population of those who commit suicide. Stressful lifestyles and endemic alcoholism in some tribes contribute to this high rate among Native Americans.[21,30]

Mental Disorders. Nearly 20% of men and women diagnosed with depression or bipolar disorder will die by their own hands. Ten to fifteen percent of people with schizophrenia die by suicide, 10 to 15 times the national rate.[30] Those with borderline personality, a disorder characterized by impulsive behavior, also have a 10% rate of suicide.[29]

Finally, substance abuse is frequently associated with suicide. Autopsies suggest that as many as 50% of all suicide victims have alcohol or some other drug in their blood at the time of death.[36]

Medical Illness. Until recently, deteriorating health was a problem of the very old. Most suicides were completed by the elderly suffering with cancer or other terminal illnesses. Recently, however, many young people with the human immunodeficiency virus (HIV) are committing suicide.[4] The latter deaths occur most often within the first 9 months of diagnosis and at a time when these individuals are very depressed but are likely to respond to treatment.[3,4]

Feeling Tone. Certain feelings, often associated with depression, are also associated with increased risk for suicide. Feelings of worthlessness ("I am an unimportant person"), helplessness ("I am not able to accomplish anything"), guilt ("This is all my fault"), and hopelessness ("There is no future for me; I would be better off dead") are commonly expressed by people in despair.

These themes are often recorded by people who commit suicide and leave suicide notes.[28] The person who fully believes there is no future or who sees himself or herself as worthless is viewed as the person at highest risk (Case Study 42-1).

Clues to Suicide

Most people who attempt to kill themselves give a clue of their intention to others. Some people leave suicide notes hoping to be discovered before dying. Others give cryptic verbal messages to friends and family, such as "Maybe things would be easier without me here." Suicidal intent may also be communicated behaviorally, either directly or indirectly. Table 42-1 lists examples of some behavioral clues.

Behavioral Changes

Depressed and suicidal people frequently lack the energy to act on their thoughts until the vegetative symptoms, including fatigue, loss of appetite, and psychomotor retardation, lift.

However, a sudden sense of calm in a previously distraught client may signal a decision to attempt suicide. As clients who begin antidepressant therapy begin to feel more energetic, they may be at greater risk because they now have the energy to carry out a plan. It is important, therefore, to keep in mind that antidepressant therapy, which has an effect in 2 to 4 weeks, may briefly increase the risk for suicide.

Subtle changes in expected patterns of behavior are perhaps the most important indicators of increasing suicide risk, although they may be difficult to interpret. The turmoil of a person considering suicide may be manifested as increased anxiety, insomnia, poor concentration, anorexia, or somaticism. The person may also express anger or despair.

People close to the suicidal person are often best able to monitor these subtle changes in behavior. Therefore, nursing staff and family must be cognizant of any change that may suggest that the client is more vulnerable. This is especially true during known periods of increased risk.

Giving away personal items, such as clothing, may suggest a person is planning suicide. This is especially true if these behaviors are accompanied by statements, such as "I won't be needing these clothes any longer."

Risk Periods

In inpatient psychiatric settings, certain times of the day are risk periods for increased incidence of suicide. High risk periods include times between 10:30 PM and 5:30 AM, during intrashift report, and between Friday morning and Monday evening. These time periods may be related to decreased availability of nursing staff.[57]

There is also a tendency for increased suicides during certain times of the year, including springtime, traditional holidays, and anniversaries of significance to the client.[40] This pattern may be changing, although it is generally believed that these are times that prompt feelings of loneliness, despair, and isolation.

Goals of Assessment

Clues to and acts of self-harmful behavior do not always indicate that the individual wants to die. Rather, these behaviors must be viewed as the individual's attempt to communicate a dramatic message; that is, the behaviors are a cry for help. The goals of assessment include the following:

42-1 Case Study

The Client Contemplating Suicide

Tim Williams sat in his apartment alone, wating for the police to arrive. He had just finished talking with a member of a local suicide hotline and after a 30-minute discussion, agreed to be evaluated for possible admission to a psychiatric facility.

Tim grew up in a small, rural community along the New Jersey coast. For as long as he could remember, he wanted to be a police officer. He, like his parents, had a strong sense of right and wrong. It was in part his value system that prompted him to apply to the local police academy shortly after graduation from high school. He hoped that in some way he could make a difference and make the small community in which he lived a better place.

Two years after joining the force, Tim rekindled a relationship with a woman he had dated several times. One year later, they were married. The marriage seemed to go well for about the first year. After that, Tim's wife noticed that Tim began stopping at a local tavern after finishing work on the 3 PM to 11 PM shift. Initially he would stop for one beer, but over time, he stayed until the bar closed.

When Janet, his wife, confronted him about his drinking, he accused her of not understanding the pressures of being a cop. She found it difficult to talk with him because he often said that he was capable of handling his own problems. Finally, the couple agreed to separate, and ultimately the marriage ended in divorce.

Shortly after divorcing Janet, Tim applied for a position in the police department of a large metropolitan police force. He was offered the job based on his record of performance and the recommendation of his former chief of police. Tim was known by his colleagues as an excellent officer.

Tim called the suicide hotline on New Year's Eve. He was scheduled off duty and had no plans to party. To the contrary, it was the first major holiday he had spent away from his family and the first since his divorce. Earlier in the day, he decided he would "celebrate" alone, and had purchased a bottle of champagne. He began drinking early in the evening and by 10 PM, he was feeling very depressed. He thought about his failed marriage and his sense of aloneness. It was at that point that Tim removed his service revolver from its holster and stared down the barrel.

By the time the police arrived, Tim had placed his revolver back in its holster. He was taken to the admission area of the nearest psychiatric hospital.

The psychiatric nurse on duty in the admission suite greeted Tim and suggested that they talk briefly. She noted that Tim indeed appeared very depressed. He spoke in a low tone of voice as he related that he had been feeling sad for at least the past year. He had, in fact, contemplated suicide on several occasions, but this was the first time in which he actually removed his gun from its holster.

He was admitted to a closed unit for further evaluation and for treatment. The admitting psychiatrist placed Mr. Williams on one-to-one observation to decrease the risk of suicide. The results of a physical examination and routine laboratory studies suggested a physically healthy 27-year-old man.

Mr. Williams' treatment included the use of an SSRI (selective serotonin reuptake inhibitor) antidepressant, an anger management group, and referral to a substance abuse counselor for further evaluation of his drinking patterns.

Initially, during anger management group sessions, Tim was reluctant to talk. It was important to him that as a police officer that he "keep his problems to himself." After several sessions in which he saw others seeming to benefit from talking, Tim began to talk about his sense of isolation and aloneness.

Three days after admission, the one-to-one observation was changed to every hour checks. This was based on Tim's ability to make a clear verbal agreement not to harm himself.

At the end of 2 weeks, Mr. Williams was discharged with a referral to outpatient treatment and was to continue taking the SSRI as prescribed.

Questions for Discussion

1. What circumstances in Mr. Williams' life place him at greater risk for suicide than the general population?
2. What are the advantages of interventions, such as anger management, for clients such as Mr. Williams?
3. What are the advantages and disadvantages when deciding to change observation from one to one to a less restrictive intervention when a person is at risk for suicide?
4. What factors are likely to decrease the risk of suicide once a client has been discharged to the community?

Table 42-1

Clues to Suicide

Verbal	Nonverbal
DIRECT "I can't stand it—I'm going to kill myself." "I could die without pain by taking all my pills."	Actions such as taking pills, cutting wrists, making a noose
INDIRECT "My family would be better off without me." "Pray for me." "I won't be here when you get back."	Risk-taking lifestyles Giving away possessions Purchasing a cemetery plot Sudden sense of calmness

- Establishing the probability that the individual will act to harm himself or herself
- Determining the meaning of the wish to self-harm
- Providing data for initiating a therapeutic relationship
- Determining the extent of protective nursing care that will be necessary

Data are obtained through direct interview of the client and discussions with significant others. Your personal values will influence your interpretation of data and therefore must be considered.

Interviewing Strategies

Client assessment is an interpersonal process. During the initial interaction, it is important to establish a warm atmosphere that communicates concern and interest. Calling the client by name demonstrates an attitude of respect and offsets feelings of worthlessness. Verbally acknowledging the client's perception of the situation, including fears and sense of desperation, helps to convey a willingness to understand the situation. Touch may be used judiciously to establish a bond of reassurance and support. Questions should be in response to content provided by the client and should be clearly and directly stated. Avoid euphemisms, such as "doing yourself in." Instead, ask directly, "Are you feeling suicidal?" Use of the word suicide actually conveys to the client, "I understand how desperate you feel." Box 42-2 provides an example of one initial assessment focused on determining suicidal risk.

Interviewing the Family

Family and friends should be included in discussions about the risk of suicide. They may provide insights concerning usual coping strategies and previously undetected suicidal risks. This is particularly true if the client is unable to provide information, for example, following ingestion of pills.

Data gathered may aid the nurse in identifying precipitants to the suicidal act. Health care workers, including emergency room nurses, may be able to provide valuable information. Questions directed to others must be phrased in a manner that protects client confidentiality.

Values and Attitudes

Because suicide assessment is a dyadic process, the nurse's own values, moral beliefs, and attitudes toward self-destructive behavior have great influence on responses to the client. Therefore, caregivers must be cognizant of personal feelings and attitudes about people who attempt to take their own lives. The following questions address some of the issues that must be considered by clinicians because they have ethical and moral implications:

- Do you believe that suicide is ever justifiable?
- Do you believe that people who attempt suicide are trying to gain attention?
- Do you think that suicide is not really preventable?

Answering these questions and discussing the responses with peers will help you identify your feelings and reactions to the suicidal person. This self-awareness will then aid in responding to the client with greater objectivity and empathy.

Societal attitudes also influence how we treat suicidal individuals. Although suicide is rarely considered a criminal act, many societies and cultural groups consider suicide an immoral act. Some religious groups believe that suicide is a sin and promulgate rules against self-destructive behavior. However, during social crises, such as war, proscriptions against suicide may give way to the value of giving one's life for a greater good. While social sanctions against suicide may dissuade potential victims, they also contribute to the stigma attached to suicidal people and their families.

BOX 42-2

Therapeutic Dialogue: Assessing Suicidal Risk

Nurse: (During admission interview.) Mike, I'd like to know more about why you came to the hospital.

Client: Well, after I lost my job, I just stayed around the house. The kids, you know (looking at the floor), after they go to school, I'm pretty much alone. And my wife, well it's awful, but she's got to work. We really need the money.

Nurse: Uh, huh. (Trying to reestablish eye contact with client.) You're alone most of the day, and your wife and children are busy with work and school. Sounds like you've felt lonely and a bit worthless.

Client: You don't know what it's like. (Meeting nurse's eye contact.) There's just no other choice. They're all caught up in their own things. They don't need me; I'm just a burden. (Mournful facial expression.)

Nurse: Mike, you're telling me that you feel like a burden and that you have no other choice. What is the choice?

Client: Well, I thought it would be better for them, and anyway, what's left for me? I'm not a man anymore.

Nurse: You seem quite desperate. I wonder if you've thought of killing yourself?

Client: Uh, no, uh, well, there's the insurance, but she wouldn't hear of it. She's the one that called the doctor. I just don't know. (Twisting wedding ring on his finger.)

Nurse: (Slowly and softly.) Sometimes when a person's life seems worthless and hopeless, he sees sucide as a reasonable choice.

Client: Yeah—I know (hesitates). I had those pills from my wife's operation, and the kids were at school. I would've been alone, and I could've slept.

Nurse: Let me make sure I understand you—you've been thinking about killing yourself and had a plan. Is that right?

Client: Well, yeah, but she came home for her purse and saw the pills out and started yelling. I wasn't really sure—I still don't know. Then she made me come here.

Nurse: How are you feeling now that you're here?

Client: I guess it's okay. She really is right.

Nurse: Do you still have thoughts of killing yourself?

Client: I don't know. Sometimes. I don't know.

Nurse: I'm sure the past few weeks have been rough for you. For now, I want to work with you to keep you from killing yourself and to help you figure out what you want to do to make things different.

DISCUSSION

The client in this interview displays a moderate risk of suicide. He experiences suicidal thoughts and has a specific plan of moderate lethality but low accessibility to the means or method. The client demonstrates a depressed affect with feelings of hopelessness and worthlessness. His risk of suicide is also judged as a moderate risk based on the significant factors of job loss, role change, and loss of status. The client expresses ambivalence about dying and appears to have a supportive family structure. The fact that the client agreed to be hospitalized for psychiatric treatment suggests that he has some degree of motivation.

The nurse uses therapeutic communication techniques to establish rapport with the client and gather assessment data. She responds to the feelings and the content expressed by the client. The nurse directly inquires about the client's suicidal thoughts and involves him in establishing a treatment plan that will promote autonomy and provide support.

Content of the Assessment

Assessment of the client must explore the following six areas:

- How the client entered the health system
- The client's intent when he or she used self-destructive behavior
- Presence of a suicide plan
- Current mental status
- Availability of support systems
- The client's predominant lifestyle

Entry into the Health Care System. Assessment of the client at risk for suicide includes an examination of how the person initially sought help. Did the person call a suicide hotline? Did he or she call the physician? Did he or she ask a friend to take him or her to the hospital? The greater the individual's volition in seeking help, the greater the chance that early intervention will prevent a death by suicide.[15,53]

The Client's Intent. Determining the meaning of the self-destructive thoughts or acts for the individual is an ongoing process. Initially, questions should be directed toward determining the nature of the immediate crisis and the effect the person desires from the self-harm act. It is important to listen for clues to the client's intent—does the client want to die, or is he or she seeking relief from unbearable stress? By examining the desired client goal, assessment and intervention can be geared toward providing safety and meeting the expressed needs of the client.

Because clients at high risk for killing themselves display severe anxiety and poor concentration, exploration of the meaning of suicide is limited initially to overt, conscious motives. In-depth exploration of the factors leading to the suicide attempt is delayed until after the crisis has passed and the person is no longer at risk of acting on impulses.

All people think about suicide. However, to certain individuals, suicidal ideation is not an intellectual tour through the options of life and death but an actual plan to end life. In the assessment process, the nurse distinguishes between clients who use self-destructive behavior to end their lives and those who are attempting to reach another goal. Through systematic assessment, the examination of content surrounding suicidal ideation can determine the how, where, when, and what of self-destruction.

The Suicide Plan. When assessing a potentially suicidal individual, ask directly, "Are you planning to kill yourself?" The directness of the question lets the client know you take him or her very seriously and understand the level of his or her distress.

If the client admits to a plan, further assess for the intended method. Generally, the more lethal the method (use of a firearm, hanging, self-immolation, or jumping from a height), the greater the risk. Once the intended method has been determined, assess whether or not the resource is available. A person who intends to shoot himself or herself and who has a firearm and ammunition at home is in more immediate danger than a person without a gun.

The intended location for the suicide is also an important consideration. A person who plans to go to a remote wooded area is generally believed to be at greater risk than one who attempts suicide where he or she is likely to be rescued.

Although the rule of thumb is the more specific the plan, the greater the risk of suicide, all suicidal ideation must be taken seriously. Compare, for example, the plan of a young man who states that he will hang himself with a bed sheet in his room as soon as the staff member leaves with that of a another man who wants to "take a few pills to end the pain." While the former is more serious, both men should be considered at risk because the intensity of risk varies over time.

In summary, three critical factors, outlined by Schneidman[46] determine in large part whether or not a person is successful in committing suicide:

- The lethality of the plan ("I will shoot myself")
- Availability of resources ("I have a gun in my possession")
- Likelihood of being rescued ("I will do it in the woods")

Mental Status Examination. After determining whether or not a client has a plan for ending his or her life, evaluation of the mental status is in order. It should include estimation of the client's level of anxiety, mood, and thought organization. Clients with a moderate to severe level of anxiety are at greater risk for deliberately acting on their suicidal thoughts. In a panic state, the person may make an impulsive, haphazard attempt at suicide; low levels of anxiety rarely result in suicide.[23] However, immediately prior to a suicide gesture, the anxiety of the client may drop because he or she now has a plan that will eliminate the pain. Generally by then, the mood of the person is depressed and hopeless. Disorganized thought and impaired judgment leave the person more vulnerable to an accidental suicide.[44]

Availability of Support Systems. The nurse must evaluate the client's available support systems. Although the presence of family and friends tends to lower the risk of suicide, problems in any of these relationships with significant others may have precipitated the suicidal gesture.[1]

Realistic assessment of availability of support systems is important because the client, from a sense of isolation and alienation, may be unable to know and make therapeutic use of available family and friends.

The Client's Lifestyle. Examination of the client's current and usual lifestyle is also important. What type of coping mechanisms does the client use? Is the client defense oriented or task oriented? Has there been a change in the client's appetite, interest in sex, sleep patterns, or interpersonal relationships? A marked change in any of these behaviors may signal changing suicidal intent. Stability of lifestyle is also important. Is the suicide ideation the result of a sudden, significant change, or has the person been dysfunctional for an extended time? A history of a stable lifestyle, including good job and social functioning, reduces the risk of suicide.

Estimation of the Risk for Suicide

Once the initial assessment of suicidal risk has been completed, the health care team must interpret the data to determine the suicidal risk. The extent of risk is not an absolute; rather, the use of clinical judgment allows the nurse to infer level of risk based on an understanding of the available clinical data. It is better to assume a greater risk than a lesser risk until staff members have a better understanding of the client's potential for committing suicide.[8] Table 42-2 provides some guidance for estimating a client's potential for suicide.

Careful, accurate documentation of the six factors—suicide clues, means by which client sought help, suicidal plan, mental status, available support systems, and lifestyle—provides for continuity of care and meets the nurse's legal responsibilities. Documentation includes making notations in the client's chart and in the written nursing care plan.

Formulating a Nursing Care Plan

As with any clinical problem, the nursing care plan provides a structure for determining client needs, establishing priorities, generating interventions, and evaluating the benefits of care given. Nursing Care Plan 42-1 provides a sample Nursing Care Plan for a suicidal client.

NURSING DIAGNOSIS

The formulation of nursing diagnoses is an essential component of the nursing process. The client's potential for self-harm, level of coping skills, degree of hopelessness, and use of support systems can be addressed in nursing diagnoses. In turn, the diagnoses guide or prescribe nursing interventions. Some examples of nursing diagnoses for the suicidal client include the following:

- Hopelessness related to rejection by spouse
- Ineffective Individual Coping related to impulsivity, characterized by multiple suicide attempts
- Risk for Injury related to high risk for suicide

PLANNING

Planning involves bringing together the nurse's assessment and judgment with the client's perceptions to formulate an appropriate approach to treatment. This includes an assessment of risk and discussion among team members and with the client about what is most important for meeting the client's needs. The focus during the planning phase includes the measures needed to protect the client while maximizing his or her autonomy.

Table 42-2

Assessing the Degree of Suicide Risk

	Intensity of Risk		
Behavior or Symptom	*Low*	*Moderate*	*High*
Anxiety	Mild	Moderate	High, or panic state
Depression	Mild	Moderate	Severe
Isolation, withdrawal	Some feelings of isolation, no withdrawal	Some feelings of helplessness, hopelessness, and withdrawal	Hopeless, helpless, withdrawn, and self-deprecating
Daily functioning	Fairly good in most activities	Moderately good in some activities	Not good in any activities
Resources	Several	Some	Few or none
Coping strategies, devices being used	Generally constructive	Some that are constructive	Predominantly destructive
Significant others	Several who are available	Few or only one available	Only one or none available
Psychiatric help in past	None, or positive attitude toward	Yes, and moderately satisfied	Negative view of help received
Lifestyle	Stable	Moderately stable	Unstable
Alcohol or drug use	Infrequently to excess	Frequently to excess	Continual abuse
Previous suicide attempts	None, or of low lethality	One or more, of moderate lethality	Multiple attempts of high lethality
Disorientation, disorganization	None	Some	Marked
Hostility	Little or none	Some	Marked
Suicide plan	Vague, fleeting thoughts but no plan	Frequent thoughts, occasional ideas about a plan	Frequent or constant thought with a specific plan

(From Hatton CL, McBride S: Suicide: Assessment and Intervention. Norwalk, CT, Appleton-Century-Crofts, 1984.)

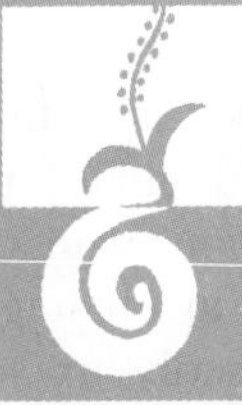

Nursing Care Plan 42-1

Suicidal Client: Moderate Risk

Mrs. J, a 60-year-old woman, was admitted to the inpatient psychiatric unit following an overdose of oxycodone/acetaminophen (Percocet). She has been living alone in her house for the past year since her husband of 40 years died of lung cancer. She had provided care for him in her home with the assistance of a home health hospice program. The hospice staff have followed her for grief counseling on a monthly basis since her husband's death. Mrs. J has two children who live out of the area and have been able to visit on a sporadic basis. She has had one previous episode of major depression, which occurred following her mother's death 5 years ago.

The hospice nurse initiated the referral for treatment when she found Mrs. J in her home with the open bottle of Percocet. She had taken approximately five tablets when the nurse arrived. Upon admission, the psychiatric nurse notes that Mrs. J has continued to verbalize the desire to die, saying, "My life is over; there is no use going on. I'm useless and deserve to die." She is unkempt and has not showered in several days. The staff nurse assigned to Mrs. J develops the initial nursing care plan, establishing two priority nursing diagnoses.

Nursing Diagnosis

Ineffective Individual Coping related to feelings of worthlessness and hopelessness as evidenced by expression of suicidal ideation

Outcome

Client will not act on suicidal ideation.

Intervention	Rationale
Provide suicide assessment as needed.	Degree of risk of suicide changes with time. Ongoing suicide assessment permits the nurse to determine suicide level and adjust frequency of observation.
Document level of risk and appropriate plan on client's chart.	Documentation allows for ongoing evaluation of fluctuations in risk of suicide and aids in future planning.
Establish a contract with client that she will not hurt herself and will report to nursing staff if she begins to feel suicidal.	Suicide contracts give the client some responsibility for controlling actions and encourage her to come to staff for support when feeling more suicidal.
If suicide risk increases, implement a higher risk plan and inform the client and all involved caregivers.	By implementing a higher risk plan, you communicate your concern to the client. Staff involved in care must know that the client is more at risk for suicide.

Evaluation

Client remains safe from self-harm.

continued

There is always concern that a professional misjudgment will result in the death of the client receiving care. However, risk is inherent when attempts are made to provide client autonomy.

Additionally, repeated contacts with chronically suicidal clients may lead to feelings of frustration and anger. The sense of futility that health care providers experience while caring for the person with repeated nonlethal suicide attempts may lead them to underestimate the client's need for safety.

Treatment Settings

When planning care, consideration is given to the immediate treatment environment and the usual living situation of the client. In the inpatient setting, the nurse uses the resources of nursing and non-nursing team mem-

Nursing Care Plan 42-1 (Continued)

Nursing Diagnosis

Alteration in activities of daily living related to feeling hopelessness and worthless as evidenced by inattention to personal hygiene

Outcome

Client will maintain activities of daily living.

Intervention	Rationale
Approach the client and encourage her to meet her daily hygiene needs.	Seeking out the client demonstrates concern for well-being.
If the client is unable to perform an activity of daily living, offer to assist her.	Offering assistance promotes completion of an activity yet continues to expect some independent behavior from the client.
When giving directions, keep instructions concise. Offer information just before it is needed.	Clients who are depressed often have a decreased ability to concentrate and lose short-term memory.
If necessary, write down activities you expect a client to complete.	Written instructions provide a reference for the client who is forgetful and avoid embarrassment by eliminating the need for the client to ask for repeated instructions.

Evaluation

Client performs activities of daily living such as independent grooming/bathing.

bers to formulate and implement the treatment plan. Community care of the suicidal client demands that the nurse and client together discuss the supports to which the client will have access once discharged. Family members, friends, and a suicide hotline are important resources. A more detailed discussion of hospital- and community-based care of the suicidal client follows.

Short-Term Goals

Nursing care plans for the client with suicidal thoughts or behaviors are directed toward providing safety and interpersonal support. Short-term goals include the following:

- The client will not act on a suicidal plan.
- The client will talk with staff about suicidal thoughts.
- The client will take steps to resolve relationship issues and lifestyles that increase the risk of suicide.

Long-Term Goals

Long-term goals focus on helping the client resolve the issues that precipitated the suicide crisis and develop less destructive coping mechanisms. Long-term goals include the following:

- The client will be free of suicidal ideation.
- The client will use task-oriented reactions to stress.
- The client will resolve issues related to problematic relationships and lifestyles that increase the risk of suicide.

INTERVENTION

Suicidal clients are encountered in their homes, in community hospitals, in emergency rooms, on psychiatric units, and through telephone calls to crisis intervention hotlines. The number of suicidal people encountered in the general hospital is increasing as those with chronic illnesses, including acquired immunodeficiency syndrome, seek medical care.[13]

Although the settings in which nursing care is provided vary, nursing actions focus on the following three concerns:

- Reducing the risk of suicide
- Exploring with the client the lifestyles or stressors that precipitated the suicidal crisis
- Assisting the client to develop new ways of coping

All three actions are important; the emphasis placed on each varies depending on the client situation. The following description of interventions may be used by nurses in any setting but for discussion purposes, are grouped according to several types of treatment settings.

Community Intervention

With the advent of managed care, it is not unusual for clients in acute crisis to be treated in the community. When the potential for suicide is an issue, the community health nurse must be cognizant of the nature of crisis, know how to help, and recommend hospitalization when the risk of suicide is high.

Understanding the Meaning of the Crisis. The nature of a crisis is such that it is time limited and demands change. Thus, during a suicide crisis, the client may be receptive to additional assistance and the opportunity to try new coping mechanisms.[1,26]

Mobilizing Coping Skills. To respond effectively, the nurse must clarify the meaning of the suicide crisis to the client and to those around him or her. By exploring precipitating stressors and responding to the client's words and feelings, the person is helped to identify the meaning of this life event. The practitioner can then, in conjunction with the client and significant others, decide if adequate support systems are available and decide if the client is able to cope adequately outside the hospital. This is accomplished by asking the client what type of assistance he or she believes is needed. Questions such as, "What can I do for you?" and "What would be helpful to you?" indicate interest and decrease any sense of despair and hopelessness.

The use of joint problem solving helps to establish a plan of assistance and may include contacting identified supports, contacting a suicide hotline if necessary, and arranging for another form of treatment if the crisis is unresolved.

Whatever the circumstances, initial contact with a suicidal client should not be terminated until he or she can state a specific plan of action for preventing self-destructive behavior. The client must identify effective coping behaviors and be able to use them.

The Need for Hospitalization. A person at high risk for suicide in the community should be encouraged to enter a psychiatric inpatient unit of a hospital or other treatment facility. The assistance of family or friends may be elicited to convince the client of the need for hospitalization. If the client refuses hospitalization, the nurse must determine with whom the client can remain until the crisis has passed. Never indicate that the client can be magically protected from his or her impulses. If the client agrees to be hospitalized, several interventions are likely.

Hospital or Treatment Center Intervention

Providing Environmental Support. The hospitalized suicidal client may already have made one suicide attempt but remains at risk to make another or may have entered the hospital as a means to resist acting on suicidal impulses. In addition to interpersonal support provided in the community, the nurse now uses the hospital setting to provide safe environmental support for the client.[41] Hospitalization should be viewed as a continuation of treatment in the community, not a result of treatment failure in the community.

People at high risk for suicide are placed in a protective environment, such as a closed unit. These units provide for safety by restricting access to potentially hazardous objects, such as scissors, razors, light bulbs, and knives. To preserve client dignity, as many personal items as possible should remain in the client's possession. However, items such as belts often are temporarily removed for the person's safety.

The nurse administering medication to the client at risk must ensure that all medications are swallowed. The client may sequester medications for later use in an in-hospital suicide attempt or while on a home visit.

Demonstrating Concern and Offering Help. Therapeutic interpersonal contacts are used to decrease the client's sense of isolation. Verbal contact every 1 to 2 hours reinforces the nurse's interest and concern. Realistic reassurance may be given, such as informing the client that staff are immediately available until the suicidal crisis passes and will work with the client to help him or her resist the suicidal urge.

Conversations should address the client's healthy, functional living. This may include focusing on activities of daily living, such as hygiene, eating, and dressing. Extensive discussion and exploration of the reasons for the suicidal behavior should be avoided until the risk of suicide has decreased.

The severe social isolation of the high-risk suicidal client can be combated by regular, frequent contact with consistent personnel. Because the client is not likely to approach the staff, staff must seek out the client. The number of staff working with the client should be limited, and the client should know that staff are available. The client should know who is available, how often someone will make contact, and how to notify a nurse if the client does want to make contact.

The highly impulsive client may require very close observation (one staff member to one client), even while in a protected environment. An alternative intervention for a client at somewhat less risk is to have nursing personnel keep the individual within eyesight.

As the client becomes less suicidal and the nurse wants to give the person more autonomy, the client may be asked to check in with staff every 30 to 60 minutes.

At these times, it is customary to ensure that the client is not currently suicidal and willing to come to staff if he or she begins feeling suicidal before the next check-in period.

Impulsive behavior may also be controlled through use of quiet rooms that provide a safe and less stimulating environment. The client should understand that the use of a quiet room is to provide support by decreasing environmental stimuli and is never used as a punitive measure. Statements such as, "This time out is to help you regain control" acknowledge that you believe the client can control his or her own behavior.

Establishing a "No Suicide" Contract. Once the initial crisis is resolved, the individual may no longer be at high risk for suicide and may be allowed more freedom. It is imperative at this time that the nurse establish a "no suicide" contract with the client who is now at moderate to low risk. In this contract, the client must repeat verbatim to the nurse that he or she will not accidentally or intentionally kill himself or herself. The no suicide contract specifies the length of time for which the contract is valid and is renewed before it expires. Accurate documentation of the specifics of the contract must be noted in the client's chart.

If a client is unable to make a no suicide contract, the ambivalence may manifest itself as an attempt to alter the wording of the contract. For example, the client might say, "I will try not to kill myself" or "I might be able to keep the agreement." Insistence on the exact wording of the contract promotes honesty and reinforces to the client his or her responsibility for controlling impulses. If a client is unable to make a no suicide contract, environmental supports, such as those noted previously, should be used.

Promoting Decision Making and Autonomy. Simple decisions required to carry out activities of daily living are often difficult for suicidal clients because they are preoccupied with their suicidal thoughts. Therefore, it is important to encourage clients to make decisions concerning when they will bathe and what they will wear. Aiding the client in decision making decreases isolation by providing contact with a helping professional; it also maintains a sense of dignity through self-direction and tends to decrease feelings of helplessness.

Exploring Client Strengths. The suicide crisis should be viewed as a dramatic but ineffective means of communication. It is an attempt to send others an important message: "I am hurting." Although it is important to acknowledge the person's pain, it is also important to assist the client to focus on strengths. One way to do this is to help the person to identify stressors that contributed to the development of suicidal ideation. From there, the client may begin to look at other more healthy coping mechanisms to resolve the situation.

Often clients who threaten or make suicidal gestures have established poor coping patterns. Nursing intervention should be directed toward strengthening healthy coping patterns or developing new patterns. Discussing alternatives with clients assists them in identifying other ways of dealing with stressors. Continued use of methods that have been useful in the past can be reinforced.

Protecting the Thought-Disordered Client. Clients who have thought disorders, including those with schizophrenia, may be at additional risk for making impulsive, self-destructive gestures. For example, schizophrenic individuals may use self-harmful behaviors as a means of reality testing (cutting their wrists to see if blood will flow) or in response to auditory command hallucinations.[44] It is not uncommon for "the voices" to tell a person, "You are no good; you should kill yourself." Providing a safe environment in which the client is closely observed and assessed for hallucinatory experiences limits the potential for impulsive, self-destructive behavior based on poor reality testing.

Postsuicide Intervention

Prevention of suicide is the primary goal of treatment. The interventions previously described are intended to prevent suicide in people already in the health care system. However, many contact a suicide hotline as a method for seeking assistance. Conversely, postvention services are designed to assist survivors of suicide adjust to the loss and should be available to anyone close to the deceased person, including professional caregivers.[12,51,54,55]

Suicide Prevention Services. Suicide centers were developed in the 1950s to provide access into the health care system for individuals considering suicide but who were not yet in treatment.[45,46,47] The pioneering work of the Los Angeles Suicide Prevention Center illustrates the effectiveness of crisis intervention service in helping potentially suicidal individuals postpone the decision to kill themselves.[46] Since the late 1950s, volunteer groups and professional clinics have established crisis services nationwide to deal with the suicidal person. These services provide anonymous telephone hotlines and limited face-to-face counseling to people at risk. Crisis intervention services use crisis theory to help people resist deciding to commit suicide and obtain needed therapy.

Community workers, other than those professionally trained, may also encounter and work with suicidal individuals. The clergy, public health personnel, and the police all may provide support to a suicidal individual.

In England, The Samaritans have offered support and counsel to suicidal people since the early 1900s.[47] Their efforts began after noticing that suicidal people benefited from the availability of a compassionate listener. The willingness of a volunteer to listen may communicate to a suicidal person that he or she has worth and that life is not hopeless.

Unfortunately, despite the availability of effective hotlines and inpatient psychiatric care, some people do kill themselves. The act of suicide is an interpersonal act and therefore affects everyone significant to the person. Nursing care does not end with a completed act; nurses must continue to work with the survivors of suicide to resolve their reactions.

Survivors of Suicide. The term survivor-victim is used to describe the dual role of the survivor of suicide.[47] Those left behind experience anger, frustration, guilt, and ambivalence in addition to the grief associated directly with the death.[14] Many family members describe a sense of shame and embarrassment following a suicide. Estrangement by well-meaning relatives is a common phenomenon because often they do not know how to respond. Out of uncertainty and fear, friends and relatives may decide it is better "not to rock the boat."

Resynthesis of Survivor-Victims. Using Resnick's model of resynthesis, survivor-victims may be guided through the stages of resuscitation, rehabilitation, and renewal.[42] During the resuscitation stage, normally the first 24 hours following notification of the suicide, the nurse offers assistance related to dealing with the shock of the death.

Emphasis is placed on funeral and burial arrangements and with helping the survivor-victims to acknowledge the finality of the death. During rehabilitation, survivor-victims are encouraged to mourn the death of the person and express any unique reactions to the suicide. This may be accomplished either by meeting with a person individually or by including him or her as a member of a therapeutic group. The renewal phase, characterized by acceptance, is a time for helping the survivor-victims integrate the suicide experience into their own lives.

Health Care Survivor-Victims. A professional who has been involved in the suicide of an individual needs the same opportunities to grieve as do others.[7,12,34]

Professional caregivers also have a responsibility to review and analyze circumstances surrounding the suicide of a client under their care. The process by which this is accomplished is called a psychological autopsy.

When a client commits suicide, nursing and other care staff also experience feelings of anger and guilt. Frequently, a suicide elicits a sense of failure among personnel. During a psychological autopsy, staff gather to review the client's behaviors and actual death act.[7,47] The purpose of the autopsy is to examine the clues to determine if any were missed and to learn from the evaluation of this situation. The psychological autopsy does not attach blame to any member of the health care team.

Following the death of one client by overdose, the staff of one unit met on three occasions to discuss the death and their reactions to it. Staff members verbalized feelings of frustration at their lack of power to keep the client from killing himself. They also expressed anger toward the client for "doing it to them." Examination of the clues revealed that the client, a chronically depressed young man, had not established a therapeutic alliance with any of the staff. No changes in eating and sleeping patterns were noted. Based on the evaluation of this client's suicide, the staff modified the existing assessment protocol on the unit to include a verbatim report of an interaction with every potentially suicidal client during every shift.

EVALUATION

Evaluation of the care of the suicidal individual includes examining all phases of the nursing process. The first goal is identification; that is, did the nurse correctly identify the individual as being at risk for suicide? Expertise in assessing for suicide potential comes not only from following a systematic process, but also from performing suicide risk assessments and receiving verification from colleagues. Evaluation of the assessment phase should reveal that the nurse accurately assessed the suicide risk of all people receiving care.

Evaluation of the planning and implementation of care provided is an ongoing process. The information gathered in the daily evaluation of a nursing care plan forms the basis for determining if the client continues to be at risk. Reassessment should include reevaluation of the goals of therapy, the effectiveness of interventions, and the progress the client is making. Intrashift reports, team conferences, and peer supervision sessions are particularly good times to reassess care.

◆ Professional Practice Issues

LEGAL ISSUES

State mental health laws and administrative orders govern the manner in which clients at risk for self-harm are to receive care. Some suicidal clients who have refused treatment may be hospitalized under state commitment procedures. It is the responsibility of professional nurses to know the laws that govern nursing practice regarding suicidal clients.

Hospital inpatient units will have written policies and procedures that guide nursing practice. You would be expected to know the institution's policies and procedures. Policies usually define the frequency for as-

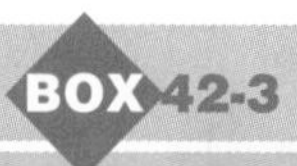

Answers to Suicide Quiz

1. Myth: Although major depression is frequently a factor, not all people who commit suicide meet the DSM-IV criteria for this diagnostic category.
2. Fact: Most people who commit suicide have a history of substance abuse; often that drug is alcohol.
3. Fact: Unintentional death (accidents) is the leading cause of death for this age group; suicide ranks third.
4. Myth: The very old (85 years and older) now have the highest rate of suicide in the United States.
5. Myth: Firearms are the method of choice for women and men.
6. Myth: Although statistics vary, only about 15% leave a suicide note.
7. Myth: White men have the highest rate of suicide when compared with African American men and to African American and white women.
8. Myth: Research suggests that feelings of hopelessness ("there is no future for me") are a more reliable predictor of risk for suicide than other feelings.
9. Myth: To the contrary, asking a person if he or she feels suicidal usually conveys the notion, "I am concerned about you" and therefore tends to decrease suicidality.
10. Fact: People in the role of mental health professional often believe they must appear as the epitome of mental health.

sessment of suicide risk and the extent to which a client is protected. For example, clients who have been assessed as being at low risk may be asked to contact a staff member every hour, whereas a person at high risk may require continual eye contact by assigned nursing staff.

Documentation of assessments and of nursing care provided are essential to provide a written record of the client's status and of nursing interventions used to assist the client.

ETHICAL ISSUES: ASSISTED SUICIDE

The professional nurse is ethically bound to protect clients who are at risk for self-harm. The ethical codes established by the American Nurses Association[2] provide a base from which nurses practice. Additionally, it is assumed that nurses will do nothing to harm or shorten the lives of clients in their care.

The publication of Humphry's book, *Final Exit,*[27,33] in 1991 focused attention on health care providers and others who assist individuals who are unable to kill themselves to commit suicide. Other factors, including increasing numbers of elderly American citizens with chronic illnesses[22,35] and the number of people infected with HIV, have added to this interest in assisted suicide.[3] For example, in 1993 in San Francisco, the Hemlock Society held a "suicide workshop" attended by more than 130 HIV-infected gay men. The purpose of the workshop was to educate people on how to commit suicide.[5]

There are important research findings to keep in mind regarding suicidal ideation among the chronically and terminally ill. Ninety-five percent of all suicidal clients have a diagnosable psychiatric disorder.[25] Treatment for many of these individuals often results in elimination of suicidal ideation and a greater desire to live, despite serious illness.

Beyond the improvement gained with treatment, nurses need to practice within the law. Assisting a person to commit suicide is clearly outside the realm of nursing practice for ethical and legal reasons.[48]

◆ Chapter Summary

All forms of self-destructive behavior are potentially life-threatening. This chapter has focused on use of the nursing process for caring for the client at risk for suicide. Major points of this chapter include the following:

1. Suicide occurs as a response to life situations within an intrapersonal and interpersonal context.
2. Although we tend to view suicidal behavior from intrapsychic and interpersonal theoretical models, there is growing evidence that biological factors may be involved in prompting self-harm.

3. The suicidal person feels anger, isolation, desperation, hopelessness, and ambivalence.
4. The suicide act is intended to communicate a dramatic message and has many meanings. It is viewed as a cry for help.
5. Nursing assessment is used to estimate risk, discover the meaning for the client of the suicidal ideation, and provide a basis for planning protective care.
6. Six factors that guide assessment are the presence of clues to suicide, the means by which the person sought help, the suicide plan, and the person's mental status, support systems, and lifestyle.
7. Nursing care is planned in collaboration with the client, significant others, and the psychiatric staff.
8. Nursing interventions focus on providing safety and establishing a therapeutic alliance.
9. One goal of nursing is to assist the client to express the meaning of the suicide attempt.
10. Therapeutic intervention also focuses on assisting the client to establish more constructive coping skills.
11. Nursing intervention continues after a completed suicide through postvention activities with survivor-victims.
12. Evaluation of nursing care is based on two questions: Were the clues identified early enough to permit intervention? Was the intervention appropriate and effective?
13. Psychological autopsies are a valuable tool by which professionals can express their feelings of anger and frustration at the behaviors of clients who commit suicide. Autopsies also provide an opportunity to evaluate care that was given to improve nursing practice for future clients at risk for suicide.

Critical Thinking Questions

1. *Discuss several considerations that must be taken into account when planning protective care of a person at risk for suicide.*
2. *Discuss legal and ethical implications of a nurse asked to assist a client to commit suicide.*

Review Questions

1. Which of the following people is statistically at greatest risk for suicide?
   - **A.** A 10-year-old boy
   - **B.** A 16-year-old girl
   - **C.** A 40-year-old woman
   - **D.** A 65-year-old man
2. The most common method of suicide among women is by
   - **A.** firearms.
   - **B.** hanging.
   - **C.** overdosing with drugs.
   - **D.** poisoning.
3. The majority of people who commit suicide leave a suicide note.
   - **A.** True
   - **B.** False
4. Which of the following feelings is most predictive of suicide risk?
   - **A.** Aloneness
   - **B.** Guilt
   - **C.** Helplessness
   - **D.** Hopelessness

◆ References

1. Aguilera D, Messick J: Crisis Intervention, 5th ed. St. Louis, CV Mosby, 1986
2. American Nurses' Association: Code for Nurses With Interpretative Statements. Kansas City, MO, American Nurses' Association, 1985
3. Aro A, et al: Fear of Acquired Immunodeficiency Syndrome and Fear of Other Illness in Suicide. Acta Psychiatr Scand 90: 65–69, 1994
4. Beckett A, Shenson D: Suicide Risk in Patients With Immunodeficiency Virus Infection and Acquired Immunodeficiency Syndrome. Harvard Review of Psychiatry 1: 27–35, 1993
5. Brinkley S: Workshop of Deliverance: Teaching the Methods of Death. Philadelphia Gay News July 16–22: 1, 1993
6. Bullman T, Kang H: Posttraumatic Stress Disorder and the Risk of Traumatic Deaths Among Vietnam Veterans. J Nerv Ment Dis 182 (11): 604–609, 1994
7. Bultema J: Healing Process for the Multidisciplinary Team: Recovering Post-Inpatient Suicide. J Psychosoc Nurs 32 (2): 19–24, 1994
8. Campbell L: Depression: Acute Care in the Hospital. Am J Nurs 288–291, 1986
9. Chew K, McCleary R: A Life Course Theory of Suicide Risk. Suicide and Life Threatening Behavior. 24 (3): 234–244, 1994
10. Conwell Y: Suicide in the Elderly. Consensus Development Conference on the Diagnosis and Treatment of Depression in Late Life. Washington, DC, National Institute of Mental Health, November 4–6, 1991
11. Conwell Y, Rotenburg M, Caine E: Completed Suicide Age 50 and Over. J Am Geriatr Soc 38: 640–644, 1990
12. Cooper C: Patient Suicide and Assault: Their Impact on Psychiatric Hospital Staff. J Psychosoc Ment Health Nurs Serv 33 (6): 26–29, 1995
13. Cooper-Patrick L: Identifying Suicidal Ideation in General Medical Patients. JAMA 272 (22): 1757–1762, 1994
14. Durkheim E: Suicide (Spaulding J, Simpson G, Trans). Glencoe, Il, Free Press, (Originally published 1897), 1951

15. Earle K, et al: Characteristics of Outpatient Suicides. Hosp Community Psychiatry 45 (2): 123–126, 1994
16. Gelman D: The Mystery of Suicide. Newsweek April 18: 44–53, 1994
17. George L: Social Factors and Depression in Late Life. Consensus Development Conference on the Diagnosis and Treatment of Depression in Late Life. Washington, DC, National Institute of Mental Health, November 4–6, 1991
18. Godfrey A: Mortality Surveillance System: Models From the Second Year. Hyattsville, MD, National Center for Health Statistics Series 20 (22): 38, DHHS Publication #95-1859, 1994
19. Golier J, et al: Low Serum Cholesterol Level and Attempted Suicide. Am J Psychiatry 152 (3): 419–423, 1995
20. Gregory R: Grief and Loss Among Eskimos Attempting Suicide in Western Alaska. Am J Psychiatry 151 (12): 1815–1816, 1994
21. Group for the Advancement of Psychiatry: Suicide and Ethnicity in the United States, Report #128. New York, Brunner/Mazel Publishers, 1989
22. Ham R, Meyers B: Late Life Depression and Suicide Potential. Washington, DC, American Association of Retired Persons (Pamphlet), 1993
23. Hatton C, Valente S: Suicide: Assessment and Intervention, 2d ed. Norwalk, CT, Appleton-Century-Crofts, 1984
24. Hazell P: Adolescent Suicide Clusters: Evidence, Mechanisms and Prevention. Aust N Z J Psychiatry 27: 653–665, 1993
25. Hendin H, Klerman G: Physician-Assisted Suicide: The Dangers of Legalization. Am J Psychiatry 150: 1, 143–145, 1993
26. Hradek E: Crisis Intervention and Suicide. J Psychosoc Nurs 26 (5): 24–27, 1988
27. Humphrey D: Final Exit: The Practicalities of Self-Destructive and Assisted Suicide for the Dying. Eugene, OR, The Hemlock Society, 1991
28. Leenaars A: Suicide Notes: Predictive Clues and Patterns. New York, Human Sciences Press, 1988
29. Linehan M, et al: Interpersonal Outcome of Cognitive Behavioral Treatment for Chronically Suicidal Borderline Patients. Am J Psychiatry 151 (12): 1771–1776, 1994
30. Lipschitz A: Suicide Prevention in Young Adults: AGE 18-30. Suicide and Life-Threatening Behavior 25 (1): 155–169, 1995
31. Litman R: Sigmund Freud on Suicide. Bulletin of Suicidology July: 112–113, 1968
32. Mann JJ, et al: Increased Serotonin 2 and B-adrenergic Receptor Binding in the Frontal Cortices of Suicide Victims. Arch Gen Psychiatry 43 (October): 954–959, 1986
33. Marzuk P, et al: Increase in Fatal Suicidal Poisonings and Suffocations in the Year Final Exit Was Published: A National Study. Am J Psychiatry 151 (12): 1813–1814, 1994
34. Mericle B: When A Colleague Commits Suicide. J Psychosoc Nurs 31 (9): 11–13, 1993
35. Moore S: Rational Suicide Among Older Adults: A Cause for Concern. Arch Psychiatric Nursing VII (2): 106–110, 1993
36. Moscicki E: Epidemiology of Suicidal Behavior. Suicide and Life Threatening Behavior 25 (1): 22–35, 1995
37. National Center for Health Statistics: Advance Report of Final Mortality Statistics, 1991. NCHS Monthly Vital Statistics Report 42 (2 Supplement): Hyattsville, MD, Public Health Service, 1994
38. Nordstrom P, et al: CSF 5-HIAA Predicts Suicide Risk After Attempted Suicide. Suicide and Life Threatening Behavior 24 (1): 1–14, 1994
39. Pearce C, Martin G: Predicting Suicide Attempts Among Adolescents. Acta Psychiatr Scand 90: 324–328, 1994
40. Phillips D, Lio J: The Frequency of Suicides Around Major Public Holidays: Some Surprising Findings. Suicide and Life Threatening Behavior 10 (Spring): 41–50, 1980
41. Reid W, Long A: The Role of the Nurse Providing Therapeutic Care for the Suicidal Patient. J Adv Nurs 18: 1369–1376, 1993
42. Resnick HP: Emergency Psychiatric Care (NIMH). Bowie, MD, Charles Press Publishers
43. Rickelman B, Houfek J: Toward An Interactional Model of Suicidal Behaviors: Cognitive Rigidity, Attributional Style, Stress, Hopelessness and Depression. Archives of Psychiatric Nursing IX (3): 158–168, 1995
44. Robins E: Psychosis and Suicide. Biol Psychiatry 21 (7): 665–672, 1986
45. Schneidman E, Farberow N, Litman R: The Psychology of Suicide: A Clinical Guide to Evaluation and Treatment, revised ed. Northdale, NJ, Jason Aronson, 1994
46. Schneidman E: Definition of Suicide. New York, John Wiley & Sons, 1985
47. Schneidman E: An Overview: Personality, Motivation and Behavior. In Hankoff L, Einsidler B (eds): Suicide Theory and Clinical Aspects. Littleton, MA, P.S.G. Publications, 1979
48. Schwarz J, Kowalski S: Rhetoric and Reasoning on Assisted Suicide: An Exchange of Views. Nursing and Health Care 15 (1): 46–49, 1994
49. Silverman M, Maris R: The Prevention of Suicidal Behaviors: An Overview. Suicide and Life Threatening Behavior 25 (1): 10–21, 1995
50. Slaby A, Garfinkel L: No One Saw My Pain: Why Teens Kill Themselves. New York, WW Norton & Company, 1994
51. Smith B, et al: Exploring Widows' Experiences After the Suicide of Their Spouse. J Psychosoc Nurs 33 (5): 10–15, 1995
52. Stack S, et al: The Heavy Metal Subculture and Suicide. Suicide and Life Threatening Behavior 24 (1): 15–23, 1994
53. Stenager E, Jensen K: Attempted Suicide and Contact With the Primary Health Authorities. Acta Psychiatr Scand 90: 109–113, 1994
54. Sterner A, Howell C: Hiding and Healing: Resolving the Suicide of a Parent or Sibling. Archives of Psychiatric Nursing V (6): 350–356, 1991
55. Van Dongen C: Agonizing Questioning: Experiences of Survivors of Suicide Victims. Nurs Res 39 (4): 224–229, 1990
56. Volavaka J: Neurobiology of Violence. Washington, DC, American Psychiatric Press, 1995
57. Vollen K: Suicide in Relation to Time of Day and Day of Week. Am J Nurs 75 (March): 263, 1975
58. Yehuda R, et al.: Neuroendocrine Aspects of Suicidal Behavior. Neurologic Clinics 6 (1): 83–101, 1988

Community-Based Care

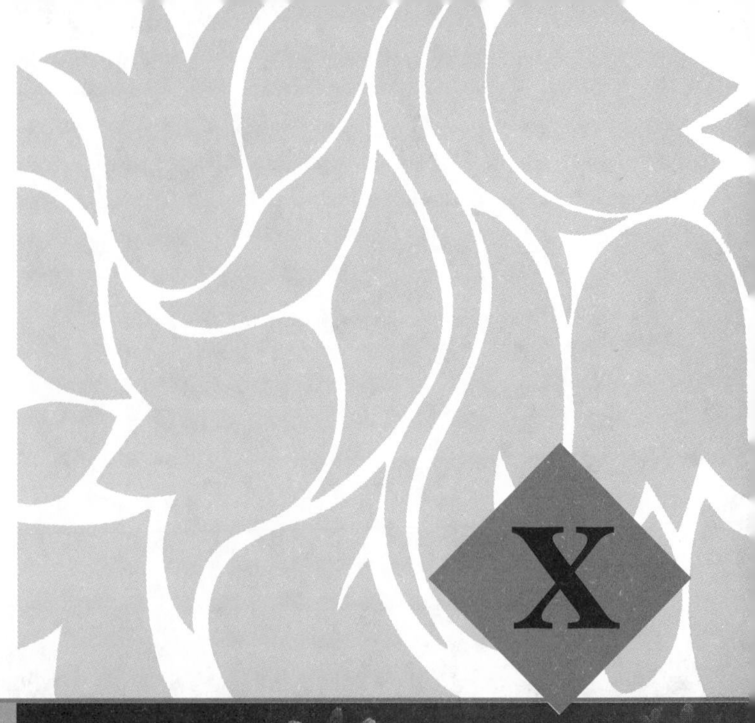

X

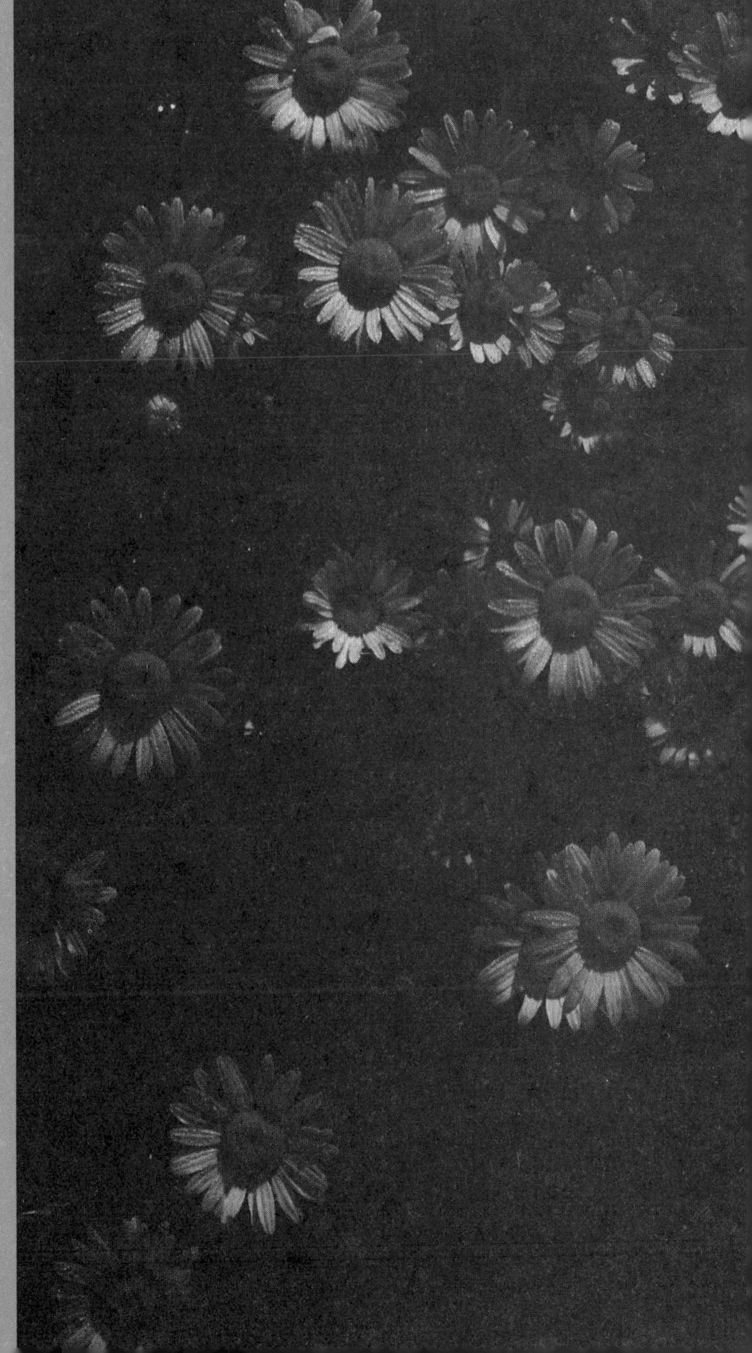

Community Mental Health

Mary Huggins
Marilyn Jaffe-Ruiz

43

A good part of the struggles of mankind center around the task of finding an expedient accommodation—one, that is, that will bring happiness—between this claim of the individual and the cultural claims of the group: and one of the problems that touches the fate of humanity is whether such an accommodation can be reached by means of some particular form of civilization or whether the conflict is irreconcilable.

Sigmund Freud, Civilization and its Discontents

Community mental health is an idea, a philosophy, and an enactment that came to fruition in 1963 with the late President John F. Kennedy's "bold new approach."[24] *Interest in the care of people with mental illness in the community has waxed and waned, depending on the political, social, and economic climate. Through the 1960s and 1970s, the community mental health movement enjoyed momentum and prosperity, but this interest subsided in the late 1970s and 1980s. The early 1990s saw a new concern for homeless individuals or those who are homeless and mentally ill. Although the enthusiasm and the financial and political support for community mental health services have diminished, many of the important principles of care that evolved can still be applied to psychiatric-mental health treatment in which nurses continue to play an important role.*

This chapter presents a brief history of community mental health and a look at existing trends. The role of the nurse has become increasingly important in this evolution in providing comprehensive mental health services.

Learning Objectives

On completion of this chapter, you should be able to accomplish the following:

1. *Define the term community mental health.*
2. *Describe the philosophy on which community mental health is based.*
3. *Identify five essential services of the community mental health care delivery system.*
4. *Differentiate among primary, secondary, and tertiary prevention in community mental health nursing.*
5. *Analyze various factors that influence trends in community mental health.*
6. *Describe the role of the nurse in community mental health.*

◆ Defining Community Mental Health

Community mental health is best defined operationally and philosophically. The phrase *community mental health* describes a change in focus of psychiatric-mental health care from the individual to the individual's interaction with the environment. It also describes a place where comprehensive care is delivered: outside of hospitals, in the least restrictive setting, and hopefully at home or as close as possible to the client's place of residence. Community mental health includes "all activities undertaken in the community in the name of mental health."[8]

Additionally, community mental health focuses on an assessment of the community—its populations, stressors, and strengths. Mental health problems are seen not only as residing within a person whom it would be advantageous to treat in a noninstitutional setting, but also as residing within specified groups. To accomplish treatment for these groups, the Community Mental Health Centers Act of 1963 identified five components of service, which have become almost synonymous with community mental health:

1. Inpatient services
2. Outpatient services
3. Partial hospitalization
4. Emergency services
5. Consultation and education

Although not in law and not used consistently, the public health precepts of health promotion and prevention (or primary prevention), early case finding and prompt intervention (or secondary prevention), rehabilitation (or tertiary prevention), and mechanisms for continuity of care have provided community mental health with a useful conceptual basis. Recently, prevention has been de-emphasized; however, these concepts remain a basic orientation for the community mental health movement.

PRIMARY, SECONDARY, AND TERTIARY PREVENTION

On a community level, prevention is geared toward individuals and specialized populations. Early childhood and parent education programs, infant stimulation programs, and early socialization play groups attempt to effect *primary prevention* of mental disorders. Although these programs are valuable for most families, they are especially so in families with more apparent risk factors (eg, those with crack-addicted pregnant teenagers and homeless families).

Secondary prevention is provided by crisis intervention services, including hot lines, walk-in services, brief psychotherapy, and hospitalization when necessary. Consumer education groups and self-help groups also play a role in providing support to individuals and families during periods of increased stress or exacerbation of symptoms. Psychoactive medication also is a therapeutic measure of secondary prevention.

Rehabilitation, or *tertiary prevention,* and continuity of care need to be available to all socioeconomic groups in the way of family supports, home services, residential placements, and halfway houses. Liaison workers, reliable friends, family members, or sponsors need to be helped to negotiate complex systems of care and to advocate for the client.[11]

PHILOSOPHICAL BASES

There is an important philosophical premise of community mental health: a shift from the belief that all mental illness is intrapsychic and amenable to psychoanalytic treatment to a belief that the whole population may need psychiatric treatment. The interaction of people and their environment, acknowledging early psychological struggles, is seen as the cause of emotional disorders; societal stressors are seen as contributing to a person's ills.

Another philosophical premise of community mental health is the belief that mental health services should be available to all who need them regardless of personal characteristics, such as age, ability to pay, or place of residence. Individual freedom, long-term relationships in small groups, and community organization are valued activities and qualities that have been incorporated into community mental health care.[25] There has been a recent change from the biological or medical model to a biopsychosocial model, encompassing services from all health and social service disciplines.[30]

Service delivery to clients has been modified to eliminate long-term custodial care and explore new avenues for treatment (ie, free-standing community mental health and nurse-managed centers, treatment units of community hospitals, and the streets, where teams of mental health workers deliver treatment to people who are homeless and in need).[17] Most recently, continuous treatment wrap-around services have been developed to provide the level and intensity of treatment intervention needed to keep people in their homes as an alternative to institutions.[37] Wrap-around services are a continuum of benefits organized around an individual enrollee's treatment needs. The trend has been toward decreasing costs and increasing use of medications to ensure treatment participation and cooperation. Nurses and other mental health professionals have become increasingly involved in the assessment and treatment of social ills. Mental health workers have become involved in tenant advocacy, legal issues, and school problems, along with traditional psychological issues.

Research into the outcomes of community psychiatric care as provided by nurses and others must be expanded.[28,9] The role of the nurse as an important and cost-effective clinician in community psychiatric care needs to be better established.

HISTORY AND INFLUENCES

The community mental health movement has been hailed as a revolution in psychiatry, with the shift of care from people in institutions to populations in the community—a precursor to the development of community support systems (see Chapter 45, Community-Based Care and Rehabilitation). This change in the focus of care, or movement, has the same magnitude of impact as that of Phillippe Pinel removing the chains from mental patients and Sigmund Freud introducing psychodynamic concepts.[32]

Advances in psychopharmacology have played a large, but often unstated, role in community-based mental health treatment. With the advent of major tranquilizers in the early 1950s, people could be treated in less restrictive environments and were psychologically amenable to other treatment modalities, such as the verbal therapies of individual, group, and family therapy.

Before 1963, responsibility for care and treatment of people with mental illness fell to state and local governments. The Community Mental Health Centers Act of 1963 was the first piece of federal legislation providing large-scale funding for the building and staffing of treatment centers for mental illness.[7] However, the federal government began to return this responsibility to state and community governments with its Omnibus Reconciliation Act of 1981.

This historical overview documents increasing federal responsibility for funding of mental health services through the 1970s, culminating in the Public Law 97-35, which began the trend in the federal government's passing of the funding responsibility back to the states. Mandated by the Community Mental Health Centers Act of 1963, the focus of mental health care shifted from people in institutions to communities organized into catchment areas that consist of 270,000 and 420,000 people.[34] Community mental health centers were built and staffed to provide comprehensive and continuous care with an emphasis on prevention. Minorities, children, and elderly people were identified as groups whose needs were incorporated into the legislation of the 1970s. Direct service joined with indirect services to provide consultation and education to schools, religious organizations, courts, nonpsychiatric health professionals, and families as caregivers. Shifts in funding continued throughout the 1980s and early 1990s. Use of Medicaid and Medicare dollars expanded to cover a variety of mental health professionals and services in community settings. Concomitant with this expansion of public dollars was the influence of health care reform and the increasing development of health maintenance organizations. Most recently, the Medicaid reform process has provided a major challenge to the funding of community mental health services. The relationship between the public and private sectors, although complex, is being invited to form new partnerships to address this changing environment. New challenges are erupting daily as Medicaid reform and the managed care evolution continue. Community mental health services must seek ways to continue to remain viable financially and still remain true to their basic core values (Table 43-1).

Table 43-1

Historical Review of Community Mental Health

Date	Event	Impact
1946	Congress passes the National Mental Health Centers Act	National Institute of Mental Health created
1955	Mental Health Study Act	Joint Commission on Mental Illness and Mental Health established
1960	Report of Joint Commission of Mental Illness and Mental Health	Action for Mental Health published
1963	Report on Mental Illness and Mental Retardation from the President to Congress	Community Mental Health Centers Act passes
1975	Congress extends Community Mental Health Centers Act 29	Continued federal funding for building and staffing of Centers
1977	General Accounting Report	Provides impetus for establishment of Community Support Program
1978	President's Commission on Mental Health 31	Reports to President on status of Mental Health services
1981	Omnibus Reconciliation Act (Public Law 97–35)	Shifts responsibility back to states
1990s	Expanded use of Medicaid and Medicare dollars Health Care Reform	Increased service variety in community settings Development of health maintenance organizations expanded
1992	Congress established the Center for Mental Health Services (Public Law 102–321)	Provides assistance to states in improving and increasing the range of services
	Public Health Service report "Healthy People 2000: National Health Promotion and Disease Prevention Objectives"	Sets national priorities for the promotion of health and the prevention of disease

Application of the Nursing Process to Community Mental Health

The community mental health nurse has the opportunity to work with the person and the social system. Stressors that impinge on people in the human–environment interaction are often social in nature. At the same time, this provides the health professional with an opportunity to supply additional interactions to improve a person's coping ability. Services and programs do not substitute for real relationships with people who are not paid to like an individual. These real connections are the primary supports that sustain each of us.[15] Nurses complement their usual role through directing individuals to maximize contact and providing support.[12]

Historically, nurses have played a key role in providing mental health services in the community by combining public health and psychiatric nursing knowledge. One study identified 22 roles nurses play in community mental health; the most frequently identified roles included therapist, cotherapist, collaborator on the interdisciplinary team, consultant, liaison, case finder, and crisis intervention worker.[32]

ASSESSMENT AND NURSING DIAGNOSIS

The community mental health nurse assesses the person and the available relevant community resources, living arrangements (including housing and significant others), health, job and economic status, cultural background, and religious affiliation. Stress in any one or more of these areas may interact with a vulnerable person to produce psychiatric-mental health problems.

The nurse's assessment of the client in the community considers several factors, including economic conditions that contribute to the rate of mental illness. The following questions are pertinent to this assessment: What is the current economic, social, and political climate? How are these likely to affect the client's system? What additional services might need to be provided during times of financial need?

Sociocultural status often affects a client's economic conditions. Many minority groups in this country are disproportionately represented among the underemployed and unemployed members of society. Additionally, many people use health care providers who are indigenous to their cultural group. In some communities, medicine men and women, herbalists, and spiritualists may be front-line primary care providers. The nurse needs to be sensitive to how the health care system is viewed by the client and vice versa. Often, because of economic, cultural, or language barriers, obtaining health care has been a frustrating or discouraging experience for the client.

A client with a strong *support system* is better able to solve problems effectively. Who are the important people to the client? What are their relative states of health or illness? How involved are they able or willing to be? What role(s) does the client serve for them? Many people who are mentally ill, especially if they are chronically ill, live in isolation. What service, religious, and self-help groups are available?

Transportation to a health care agency is often a problem. How accessible is the agency to the client? Are outreach services provided? Are alternative means of transportation available? Is reimbursement provided? Transportation is of particular concern for the elderly and for the individual with serious mental illness who formerly might have received treatment in a state institution.[20]

Some clients are representative of populations with special needs; some communities have organized services around such people. Examples of special populations are people with mental illness who are elderly, have acquired immunodeficiency syndrome, are young, are substance abusers, are homeless, or are developmentally disabled.[41] Does the client or the family fit into a special needs category? If so, what resources are available for referral to special needs services in the community?

The type of living facilities certainly reflects how a person receives care or performs self-care. In what type of dwelling does the client live? Is it safe?[35,23] Is there adequate plumbing, heating, refrigeration, and air circulation? Can the client live without supervision? Are halfway houses, group homes, or adult homes with supervision available if necessary? How receptive is the community to people with mental illness?[22,26,29] Services for homeless mentally ill people must include finding homes and the proper supports to assist the client in the community.

The community mental health nurse, as case manager, assesses the client's needs and the services available. For example, the nurse might think a client could manage at home by attending a day treatment program, but if no day treatment program is available, acute care hospitalization may be necessary.

The nurse analyzes the data gathered about the client's life situation and about the community and determines the level of need. This analysis leads the nurse to identify diagnoses prompting the plan and the nursing interventions.

PLANNING

The nurse and other members of the treatment team carefully evaluate the client's needs and the community resources before beginning the planning process. Planning takes into consideration the goals that the client, family, and significant others want to achieve. Realistic, attainable, short-term goals are imperative to reduce frustration and facilitate successful treatment outcomes. For example, including information regarding the individual's preferences (eg, job, interests) within the assessment process enhances predictability for positive outcomes.[10]

INTERVENTION

A useful framework for planning a community mental health intervention is the public health model of health promotion and primary, secondary, and tertiary prevention. The nurse may be a primary care provider by working with clients (as individuals, families, or groups) to identify their needs and facilitate treatment through collaboration and referral.

Primary Prevention

Primary prevention aims to prevent illness or disorder before it occurs. To accomplish this goal, the nurse must anticipate the needs of special populations and provide counseling and other needed services, for example, to those undergoing a developmental or situational crisis. Brief, short-term, supportive services to families undergoing bereavement or experiencing other losses are considered primary prevention. Nurses provide these services in public health and mental health settings by identifying and strengthening coping abilities; for instance, the nurse might foster a client's use of intellectualization to mobilize energy to find resources during a family crisis. Another nursing intervention is the development of appropriate community mental health services, such as senior citizens' hot-lunch and drop-in programs to reduce the isolation of elderly people while meeting their nutritional needs. Children of homeless families need a tremendous amount of intervention to prevent psychological, physical, social, and cultural disturbances.

Another example is that of a middle-age man who is depressed after losing a job. The man may require individual therapy to intervene in the depression, while his family may need help adjusting to the modification of roles resulting from this loss. On a community scale, food subsidies, housing programs, and stimulation of employment may be needed to promote mental health (Case Study 43-1 and Nursing Care Plan 43-1).

Secondary Prevention

Secondary prevention reduces prevalence through early case finding and prompt intervention. Rapid, available, and accessible treatment and referrals to appropriate services are essential. Short-term hospitalization, inten-

(text continues on page 886)

Nursing Care Plan 43-1

Intervening in a Family's Crisis

Mr. Alan is a 45-year-old engineer in the aircraft industry. He lives with his 42-year-old wife and two daughters, Mary, age 14, and Jane, age 18.

The aircraft plant in their community has recently been shut down because of a slowdown of growth in that industry. Mr. Alan has lost his $35,000-a-year position, as have most of his neighbors.

Mrs. Alan is a homemaker. She has not worked outside the home since her oldest daughter was born. Before that time, she worked as an executive secretary. Periodically during their marriage, Mrs. Alan suffered from periods of depression, specifically after the loss of her parents and when the family moved from an urban to a more suburban environment. Each episode of depression was treated by brief psychotherapy and antidepressant medication.

This year, Jane has begun college in a neighboring state and Mary is a freshman in high school. Mary has had increasing difficulty with school. She has been truant, and her grades have fallen from her usual A's to barely passing marks. In the classroom, she seems lethargic and demonstrates a poor attention span. Because of these problems, the homeroom teacher referred Mary to a school nurse.

The school nurse took a complete health history and performed a physical assessment of Mary. In the course of the interview, Mary told the nurse that she is upset and worried about her parents. She said that they have been fighting constantly since her father lost his job 1 month ago, and she's worried that her mother will get "sick" again. Mary also told the nurse that she has been frightened and unable to sleep.

During their conversation, the nurse observed that Mary's speech was slurred and her reaction time slowed. The nurse asked Mary if she was using any drugs. Mary stated that since she has been unable to sleep, she had been smoking marijuana and sometimes takes "downs" a friend gave her.

The nurse realized that to help Mary, she would have to meet with the whole family. She told Mary that she was going to call her parents in to meet with them and Mary's teacher together.

The next day, the meeting took place. Mr. and Mrs. Alan were very concerned about the teacher's report of Mary's behavior. They too were upset about their home situation and were therefore not paying as much attention as usual to Mary, although they noticed and were worried about the changes in her behavior. Mrs. Alan admitted to feeling depressed and worried that she might not be able to function in a job outside her home. Mr. Alan expressed that he felt numbed by his job loss. Their financial problems are further compounded by the expenses of Jane's tuition and room and board. Also, because Mr. Alan's job is terminated, so are his health insurance benefits.

The school nurse helped the family recognize their need for help and suggested that she refer them to the community mental health center. The family seemed relieved by the suggestion and cautiously accepted the referral.

The Alan family (including Jane) visited the community mental health center 2 days later. The community mental health center nurse gathered the initial intake and assessment information. She identified the family to be in crisis precipitated by Mr. Alan's recent job loss. This loss of job has meant a loss of family income, alteration in roles with resultant marital discord, and drug abuse by the younger daughter. The older daughter, Jane, felt guilty about being away, worried, and angry about the possibility of being made to return home from college.

After the assessment and during the planning of strategies for intervention, the nurse realized that even though the Alan family is unique, these same issues were confronting many other families in the area. The family as a whole and each individual member needed assistance.

The nurse analyzed her data and shared with the Alan family her assessment, validating their concerns and desires. She elicited their thoughts and ideas about the interventions, which she then presented to the Mental Health Center's treatment team.

Her suggestions are incorporated in the following Nursing Care Plan.

continued

Nursing Care Plan 43-1 *(Continued)*

Nursing Diagnosis

Ineffective Grieving/Crisis Resolution: Compromised related to father's job loss, youngest daughter's involvement in drugs secondary to father's job loss, mother's depression, and increased financial concerns

Outcome

Family members will use support services to assist in current crisis.

Intervention	Rationale
Encourage open communication among family members.	Lack of open communication during times of stress promotes misperceptions about problems and increases family members' sense of isolation.
Assist members to identify their own concerns during current crisis.	Identification of individual concerns promotes each member's sense of self.
Explain and coordinate support options for community assistance for family, including the following: 1. Individual brief psychotherapy and family therapy 2. Support group for individuals who have lost a job 3. Financial assistance; health insurance provisions; food subsidy program; family therapy 4. Drug treatment for adolescents 5. School work-study programs or part-time job to help defray college expenses	Community mental health intervention includes services that promote primary and secondary prevention. Identification of relevant community resources is an essential part of intervention. The nurse addresses each family member's individual problem and the problems impacting on the family as a whole.
Communicate openly with representatives from community agencies with which family becomes involved to increase members' use of services.	Promoting continuity of care is an important part of the role of the community mental health nurse.

Evaluation

Family members will demonstrate effective coping skills while dealing with current family crisis.

Continuation of Case Study and Follow-up Community Involvement

The community mental health nurse recognizes that other families similar to the Alans may be experiencing increased stress and possibly crisis related to the shutdown of a major community industry. The nurse discusses with the mental health team these concerns. The team identifies a goal of promotion of primary and secondary prevention for families affected by the industry closing. Planning for intervention includes contacting the local unemployment Center and the local Department of Welfare to discuss areas in which services could be coordinated in the current community crisis. The local high school nurse who initiated referral for the Alan family will also be contacted to collaborate on ways in which students at risk can be identified to provide early intervention.

Questions for Discussion

1. *Which of the five essential components of community mental health did the nurse use to intervene with the Alan family?*
2. *What other alternatives, based on the principles of community mental health, might the school nurse have suggested if a community mental health center were not available in the community?*
3. *Which of the interventions planned for the Alan family are examples of primary prevention? Which are examples of secondary prevention?*
4. *What are the various biopsychological stressors that contributed to the Alan family's problems?*
5. *How is the role of the community mental health nurse similar to and different from other nursing roles?*
6. *How do you compare the principles and philosophy of community mental health with other treatment approaches?*

sive outpatient treatment, medication, and partial hospitalization are some of the approaches through which secondary prevention is accomplished. Nurses frequently provide this care in emergency rooms to the suicidal client, in inpatient units, and in psychiatric and other health care clinics. The nurse intervenes by fostering a therapeutic relationship, restructuring the environment, bringing in services, providing respite or halfway house care, and using psychopharmacological agents to strengthen the client's coping mechanisms. For the person who is homeless, a livable and safe shelter is an imperative intervention.

Tertiary Prevention

Tertiary prevention aims to reduce long-term disability through rehabilitation, aftercare, and resocialization. The nurse assesses clients' stress levels and coping behaviors and encourages new patterns of adaptive behavior and new coping skills. One client goal, for example, may be to learn to talk out problems rather than to attack someone.

Deinstitutionalization of large numbers of psychiatric clients during the late 1960s and 1970s (and continuing to the present) made the tertiary prevention level of care the focus of much attention by communities, politicians, and health care workers. Many communities with insufficient resources were not equipped to absorb large numbers of psychiatric clients into their neighborhoods. Additionally, the stigma attached to psychiatric illness and the possible occurrence of deviant social behavior resulting from mental disturbance make this type of disorder not acceptable to the majority of people.

The overall goal of community mental health nursing is to provide the optimal level of mental health care for a community and its members. It is not sufficient to treat an individual's ills without treating the larger societal issues. It is counterproductive for a person who has been deinstitutionalized to come to a mental health clinic and receive medication, supportive psychotherapy, supplemental security income, and food stamps if there is inadequate or no housing and no meaningful work.

The community mental health nurse assists clients by identifying needs, problems, strengths, and resources; making referrals and linkages; offering therapeutic support; and encouraging effective problem solving. In addition, the nurse needs to work actively as an advocate promoting legislation for innovative approaches to preventing problems and caring for people with mental illness in communities.[5]

EVALUATION

Legislative pressures are moving the mental health system from process to outcome evaluations. Although complete agreement regarding the tools to be used in measuring outcomes has not been achieved, there is some agreement regarding the outcomes to measure. The center for Mental Health Services has developed a "Mental Health Report Card," which focuses on recovery, self-management, and personhood. Overall access to treatment, treatment methodologies, treatment outcomes, and consumer satisfaction are some of the areas being measured. The following outcomes are specifically addressed:

- Reduced symptomatology
- Extent of adverse effects from treatment
- Change in substance abuse patterns
- Functioning and productivity
- Psychiatric inpatient readmissions
- Positive change as defined by consumers
- Social integration
- Living in housing of choice
- Involvement in the criminal justice system
- Report of increased respect and dignity

One scale in practical use is the Goal Attainment Scale, which measures individual functioning levels; other scales emphasize the burden or impact on the community and specifically stress areas such as use of jails and crisis services. New information regarding the assessment of individual and community functioning is being developed. Resources for these tools would be the Center for Mental Health Services, the National Institute for Mental Health, or the International Association of Psychosocial Rehabilitation Services (IAPSRS). Tools developed by the IAPSRS Research Committee show promise in outcome measurement on the individual and community level. Funding, policy setting, and critical issues depend on the clarity of outcome studies. To say a client is or is not better or that a community has mental health services adequate for its population is difficult in the absence of clear-cut criteria.[38] Identified areas for study include:

1. Program quality that conforms to standards
2. Values of specific treatment
3. Safety and efficacy, rather than usual and customary practice
4. Administrative structure
5. Program designs
6. Target populations of clients
7. Outcome indices, such as reduction of symptoms and vocational and social rehabilitation

Unfortunately, little research in the social sciences shows direct cause-and-effect findings. Instead, results are likely to be descriptive and inconclusive. The ambiguities of the social systems model, though frustrating, offer the mental health practitioner, especially nurses, an opportunity for diverse and creative practice. A shift from a single-causality to a multicausality mode of explanation of emotional disorders, which includes biological, environmental, psychosocial, sociological, and spiritual stressors, is essential for providing holistic care.

◆ Trends Affecting Community Mental Health Care Delivery

The hopes, enthusiasm, and plentiful deferral funding that characterized 1963 have diminished in the 1990s. The state of the economy, unemployment, homelessness, high crime rates, and a conservative political climate all diminish the prospects of community mental health making a significant impact on mental illness. Nevertheless, these times may spawn some new ideals for effective community-based mental health services in which nurses may play an important therapeutic role. Much research is needed to demonstrate beneficial outcomes with cost-effective service. Preventive treatment, identification of potential at-risk populations, and diverse treatment modalities using various practitioners need to be examined.

Some gains of the community mental health movement include a reduction of population and an unlocking of doors of state hospitals, literally and figuratively, to operationalize the notion of treatment in the least restrictive setting; a decreased emphasis on expensive analytical therapies as a major form of psychiatric treatment; and a de-emphasis on psychiatrists as the only legitimate care providers to enable other professionals (eg, registered nurses, social workers, psychologists, and paraprofessionals) to play a more active role in care. Mental health care providers have broadened the scope of services available to a wider range of the population.

The plight of homeless people with mental illness has prompted a reexamination of the issues surrounding asylum for those who have the need and the right to treatment yet may not be in a position to seek it voluntarily. Forced intervention raises the complementary question regarding the right of the individual to refuse treatment.

Community mental health must provide for comprehensive and continuous care that is available and accessible to all members of the population. It must involve the orderly uninterrupted movement of clients among the diverse elements of the service delivery system. Strong linkages and communication networks need to be established without a duplication of efforts or negation of important components.[4]

The need remains to develop primary prevention and mental health promotion systematically, from prenatal care to care for people as they age. Secondary prevention, acute care, and early case finding should be available through community hospitals. People with emotional disorders require services to alleviate stressors and to strengthen coping skills; these services (or tertiary care) include financial, housing, educational, food, recreational, and social services in a homelike setting with backup services as needed.[18,19,26]

Greater emphasis and appreciation should be given to self-help groups and transitional and respite facilities. Families of people with mental illness are better equipped to provide supportive care on a continual basis if they, too, have support services, education regarding the illness, and opportunities for separation from the disturbed family member.

The need for mental health services will not diminish in the future. At any time, approximately 22% of the American population suffers from a clearly diagnosable mental illness. This is between 35 and 50 million individuals.[42] Of these individuals, millions do not receive any care. At the same time, unfortunately, funding for mental health services is disappearing. With the shift of funding from the federal level to the state and community level, mental health services are being reduced. According to the National Community Mental Healthcare Council, "The dreams of the 1960s are in stark contrast to the emerging realities of the 1990s."[33] The "bold new approach" of the 1960s must be evaluated and redesigned to preserve the humanistic intent of community mental health as we approach the 21st century.

◆ Chapter Summary

This chapter has traced the development of the community mental health movement in the United States and the current challenges facing American communities. Other chapter highlights include the following:

1. Community mental health services are designed to provide comprehensive, continuous care to populations who need them.
2. The aims of community mental health are health promotion, prevention of illness or disorder (primary prevention), limitation of disability (secondary prevention), and rehabilitation (tertiary care).
3. Mental health workers, professionals and paraprofessionals, are used in addition to psychiatrists to provide mental health care to individuals, families, and communities.
4. The shift in funding from federal to state and local levels has reduced mental health services and endangered the viability of community mental health.
5. The community mental health nurse applies the nursing process to provide comprehensive services to clients.

Critical Thinking Questions

1. *Describe ways that a professional nurse can participate in primary prevention to influence the state of a client's mental health.*
2. *Discuss ways that advances in psychopharmacology have changed psychiatric nursing and influenced the role of the psychiatric nurse in community-based mental health care.*
3. *Describe ways that the philosophy of nursing and the philosophy of Community Mental Health are similar and provide an explanation regarding these similarities.*
4. *Discuss key roles that nurses frequently play in providing community-based mental health care and explain why nurses often are filling in these key roles.*

Review Questions

1. The term community mental health describes which of the following?
   - **A.** Change in focus from the individual to the individual and environment
   - **B.** A place where care is delivered
   - **C.** An assessment of the environment
   - **D.** Services delivered in the community
   - **E.** All of the above
   - **F.** A, B, and C only
2. Tertiary prevention is synonymous with which of the following services?
   - **A.** Crisis intervention
   - **B.** Educational groups
   - **C.** Community assessment
   - **D.** None of the above
   - **E.** All of the above
3. The philosophical premise of community mental health is limited to the following groups of people:
   - **A.** All who need them, regardless of payment mechanisms
   - **B.** Individuals with managed care providers and government entitlement
   - **C.** Individuals needing services from a community psychiatrist only
   - **D.** All of the above
4. The nurse in a community mental health center evaluates which of the following areas?
   - **A.** The individual and his or her mental health stressors
   - **B.** The individual within a social system
   - **C.** Transportation
   - **D.** Housing
   - **E.** Services available to meet the needs of the individual
   - **F.** A and E only
   - **G.** All of the above

◆ References

1. Aiken L: Unmet Needs of the Chronically Mentally Ill: Will Nursing Respond? Image 19 (Fall): 121–125, 1987
2. Albee G: The Fourth Mental Health Revolution. J Prevention 1: 67–70, 1980
3. Antai-Otong D: Concerns of the Hospitalized and Community Psychiatric Client. Nurs Clin North Am 24 (September): 665–673, 1989
4. Bachrach L: Community Care for Chronic Mental Patients: A Conceptual Analysis. Am J Psychiatry 138 (November): 1449–1451, 1981
5. Bazelon Center for Mental Health Law: What Does Fair Housing Mean to People With Disabilities? The Housing Center May: 1994
6. Bellak A, Mueser K: A Comprehensive Treatment Program for Schizophrenia and Chronic Mental Illness. Community Ment Health J 22 (Fall): 186, 1986
7. Biegel A, Levinson A: The Community Mental Health Center: Strategies and Programs. New York, Basic Books, 1972
8. Bloom B: Community Mental Health: A General Introduction. Monterey, Brooks/Cole, 1977
9. Bond GR, McDonel EC: Vocational Rehabilitation Outcomes for Persons With Psychiatric Disabilities: An Update. Journal of Vocational Rehabilitation 1 (3):9–20, 1991
10. Bond GR, Deitzen L: Predictive Validity and Vocational Assessment: Reframing the Question. In Gluekauf RL, Sechrest LB, Bond GR, McDonel EC (eds): Improving Assessment in Rehabilitation and Health. Newbury, CA, Sage, 1992
11. Brooker C: The Health Education Needs of Families Caring For A Schizophrenic Relative and the Potential Role for Community Psychiatric Nurses. J Adv Nurs 15: 1092–1098, 1990
12. Carling P: Promoting Social Integration. In Carling P (ed): Coming Home: Integrating People With our Communities. New York, Guilford Press, 1994
13. Collins-Colon T: Do It Yourself. J Psychosoc Nurs 28 (6): 25–29, 1990
14. Connolly P: Services for the Undeserved. J Psychosoc Nurs 29 (1): 15–20, 1991
15. Curtis L: Social Integration: Inviting, Including, in Community. Community, Center for Community Change Through Housing and Housing Support 4 (1):1–3, 1994
16. Fagin C: Psychiatric Nursing at the Crossroads: Quo Vadis. Perspect Psyciatr Care 19 (34): 79–106, 1981
17. Flaskerud J: The Effects of Culture-Compatible Intervention on the Utilization of Mental Health Services by Minority Clients. Community Ment Health J 22 (2): 127–140, 1986
18. Forker J: The Community as the Site for Psychiatric-

Mental Health Nursing Clinical Practicum. J Professional Nursing 4 (November-December): 447–452, 1988

19. Fredo L: Learning Diversity: Accommodations in Colleges and Universities for Students With Mental Illness. Boston, Community Support Network News, Center for Psychosocial Rehabilitation, 1994
20. Hagebak J, Hagebak B: Serving the Mental Health Needs of the Elderly: The Case for Removing Barriers. Community Ment Health J 16 (4): 263–275, 1980
21. Hicks M: The Community Sojourn From the Perspective of One Who Relapsed. Issues in Mental Health Nursing 10: 137–147, 1989
22. Johnson P, Beditz J: Community Support Systems: Scaling Community Acceptance. Community Ment Health J 17 (Summer): 153–160, 1981
23. Jonikas J, Cook J: Safe, Secure and Street Smart: Empowering Women With Mental Illness to Achieve Greater Independence in the Community. Chicago, Thresholds National Research and Training Center, 1993
24. Kennedy JF: Message From the President of the United States Relative to Mental Illness and Mental Retardation. House of Representatives, Document No. 58, 88th Congress, 1st Session. Reprinted in Bloom B: Community Mental Health: A General Introduction. Monterey, CA, Brooks/Cole, 1977
25. Lamb HR, Zusman J: A New Look at Primary Prevention. Hosp Community Psychiatry 32 (December): 843–848, 1981
26. Mancuso L: Case Studies on Reasonable Accommodations for Workers With Psychiatric Disabilities. Center for Mental Health Services, The California Department of Mental Health and California Department of Rehabilitation, Sacramento, CA, 1993
27. McCausland M: Deinstitutionalization of the Mentally Ill: Oversimplification of the Issues of the Mentally Ill. Adv Nurs Sci 9: 24–33, 1987
28. Mindnich D, Hart B: Linking Hospital and Community. J Psychosoc Nurs 33 (1):25–28, 1995
29. Ozarin L: Community Alternatives to Institutional Care. Am J Psychiatr 133 (January): 69–72, 1976
30. Palmer-Erbs V, Anthony W: Incorporating Psychiatric Rehabilitation Principles into Mental Health Nursing. J Psychosoc Nurs 3 (3):36–44, 1995
31. President's Commission on Mental Health: Report to the President From the President's Commission on Mental Health, vols 1 and 2. Washington, DC, Government Printing Office, 1978
32. Ramshorn MT: Mental Health Services. In Haber J, et al (eds): Comprehensive Psychiatric Nursing, pp 10–17. New York, McGraw-Hill, 1978
33. Ray CA, Finley JK: Did CMHCs Fail or Succeed? Analysis of the Expectations and Outcomes of the Community Mental Health Movement. Administration and Policy in Mental Health. 21 (4):283–293, 1994
34. Reiger DA, Boyd JH, Burke JD, Rae DS, Myers JK, Kramer M, Robins LN, George LK, Karno M, Locke BZ: One-Month Prevalence of Mental Disorders in the United States. Arch Gen Psychiatry 45 (November): 997–986, 1988
35. Reidy D: Shattering Illusions of Difference. Resources 4 (2):3–6, 1992
36. Report of the Task Force on Community Mental Health Programs. Am J Psychiatry 139 (May): 705–708, 1982
37. Schaftt G, Randolf F: Innovative Community Based Services for Older Persons With Mental Illness. U.S. Department of Health and Human Services, Center for Mental Health Services CSP, Rockville, MD, 1994
38. Schulberg H: Outcome Evaluations for the Mental Health Field. Community Ment Health J 17 (Summer): 132–142, 1981
39. Simpson K: Community Psychiatric Nursing—A Research Based Profession? Adv Nurs 14: 274–280, 1980
40. U.S. Department of Health and Human Services: Caring for People With Severe Mental Disorders: A National Plan of Research to Improve Services. Washington, DC, National Institute of Mental Health, National Advisory Mental Health Council, 1991
41. U.S. Department of Health and Human Services: CMHS Mission From a Bulletin of the Center for Mental Health Services, Rockville, MD, May, 1994
42. Welch M, Boyd MA, Bell D: Education In Primary Prevention. In Psychiatric Mental Health Nursing for the Baccalaureate Student. Int Nurs Rev 34 (5): 126–130, 1987

Psychosocial Home Care

Nina A. Klebanoff

44

Heidegger sees that home means more than a house and the merely casual possession of domestic things. Hestia makes a house a home by endowing it with soul. It is her gift to reveal how my dwelling serves as an outward expression of my inward self and how the image of the inmost center of a dwelling, its hearth, serves as the most adequate, the most inevitable, image of the essence of self.

Martin Heidegger,
Remembrance of the Poet

Home health care is an aspect of home care. Home health care nurses provide skilled nursing on a visiting basis to clients in need of care. Psychosocial home care *nursing practice is an approach complementary to but distinct from the medical, or disease, model of mental health and mental illness. The prefix* psycho- *(from the Greek* psyche*) signifies the human mental, behavioral, and emotional structure—mind, soul, consciousness, or spirit. The term* social *signifies the individual client, family, and community in which they reside and their relationship to and interaction with humanity or society. This chapter discusses the historical, philosophical, and theoretical foundations of psychosocial home health care nursing, the role of the nurse in the provision of psychosocial home health care, and central issues and trends in the field.*

Learning Objectives

On completion of this chapter, you should be able to accomplish the following:

1. *Define home health care nursing, and identify the need for psychosocial home health care nursing.*
2. *Describe the historical, philosophical, and theoretical foundations on which psychosocial home health care nursing practice is based.*
3. *Identify the essential components of psychosocial home health care nursing practice.*
4. *Discuss the appropriate candidates for referral to psychosocial home health care nursing service.*
5. *Differentiate among the role aspects and functions of the psychosocial home health care nurse.*
6. *Apply the nursing process to the care of a client and family in their home.*
7. *Analyze various factors that influence trends in psychosocial home health care.*
8. *Explore the relationships among psychosocial home health care nursing, community or public health, and community mental health.*

◆ Defining Psychosocial Home Care

Home care, including psychosocial home care, is one part of a comprehensive health and mental health care system. It aims to provide an array of health-related services to clients and families in their places of residence. These residences include residential care facilities, group homes, and private homes of clients or their family members. Home health care is an aspect of community health nursing[58] *not* an alternative to institutional care. It is one of the most rapidly growing and changing fields in health care today, even though it is one of the oldest forms of ambulatory health care.

SERVING CLIENT AND FAMILY NEEDS

Because nurses are the major providers of home care, they can coordinate and manage home health care effectively. Other suitable service components for home care, singly or in a multitude of combinations and sequences, include but are not limited to the following:

1. Medical services
2. Social work services
3. Psychological services
4. Physical therapy
5. Occupational therapy
6. Vocational therapy
7. Speech therapy
8. Recreational therapy
9. Respiratory therapy
10. Dental services
11. Pharmacy services
12. Intravenous and parenteral therapy
13. Enterostomal or wound therapy
14. Nutritional services
15. Homemaker, home health aide or assistant, and companion services
16. Transportation services
17. Laboratory services
18. Use of durable and disposable medical supplies and equipment

The individual needs of the client and family determine which services are to be arranged and coordinated in the home. In home care, the word *family* means anyone in the client's life who is able and willing to take some responsibility for helping the identified home care client.

PROVIDING HOME HEALTH CARE

In general, home health care services are provided by the following:

1. Official or public agencies operated by state or local governments
2. Private and voluntary nonprofit agencies operated by boards of directors
3. Combinations of official and voluntary nonprofit agencies operated by both sources or a new board
4. Hospital-based agencies administered by the hospital's board of directors
5. Proprietary (for profit) agencies administered by the owner
6. Individual or group partnerships of nurses or other health professionals providing home care services on a private or charitable basis

Box 44-1 outlines the ways in which these types of services are reimbursed. Box 44-2 identifies various

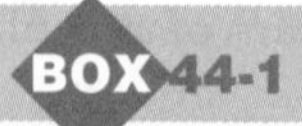

Sources of Reimbursement for Home Health Care Services

Psychosocial home care services may be paid for in the following five ways:

1. Medicare, the program of the federal government, will pay for psychosocial home care services if the client has a primary psychiatric diagnosis, has been evaluated by a psychiatrist (and reevaluated every 60 days by one), and is homebound. Homebound status, in general, means that a client is unable to leave home either due to illness or injury (eg, physical reasons, such as unsteady gait, shortness of breath after 10 ft, or a fracture); or because psychiatric illness, to some degree, makes it unsafe to leave home unsupervised; or because of a refusal to leave the place of residence. Medicare provides cost-based reimbursement under Part A coverage. Payment is based on the lesser of aggregate allowable cost or customary charges. There are region-specific fee screens for skilled nursing and other disciplines.
2. Medicaid, a federally and state-funded program, is a state-administered program of reimbursement for home care services, among other functions. Each state has its own criteria for eligibility and reimbursement for psychosocial home care services. Some states do not cover psychosocial home care at all, while others cover it if there is a primary medical diagnosis. Managed Medicaid coverage varies locally within a state, if at all.
3. Many third-party payers (private health insurance companies, managed care organizations, and health maintenance organizations) follow the guidelines set forth by Medicare. Others, however, adhere to their own rules and regulations, which may or may not cover psychosocial home care nursing services. With the presence, increase, and benefit of home care services, some health insurance companies are paying for home care services on a case-by-case basis. Coverage for home health care is usually at 80% of reasonable and customary charges from home health organizations. However, to date there are no industry standards regarding reimbursement of this type of services.
4. Some clients pay directly for psychosocial home care services, mainly because they do not meet the criteria for Medicare, Medicaid, or private health insurance coverage or do not have private health insurance. Some agencies or providers charge a flat rate, while others have a sliding fee scale (based on the client's ability to pay). A client also may choose to pay directly for psychosocial home care services to continue desired services in the home beyond the period authorized by an insurance company or the government programs.
5. Some agencies and people have funds to pay for home care on a charity basis for those in need of psychosocial home care services but for whom no funding sources exist.

home health care referral sources. Every home care situation has more or less psychosocial aspects. Home care services are customized for each client, depending on needs or problems and the needs of the home health care provider and the reimburser. Because of the psychosocial and wellness orientation of community health nursing, a psychiatric nurse working in this setting is more aptly titled a psychosocial nurse rather than a psychiatric nurse.

GOALS OF PSYCHOSOCIAL HOME HEALTH CARE

The two goals of home health care are to gain, regain, maintain, or restore the client's optimal state of health and independence and to minimize and rehabilitate the effects of illness and disability before or after institutionalization. Specific goals of psychosocial home care nursing are to prevent hospitalization and provide

BOX 44-2

Referral Sources for the Psychosocial Home Health Care Nurse

Hospital discharge planners
Nurses, physicians, social workers
Clients and former clients
Family members and caregivers
Landlords, neighbors, bank personnel
Health departments
Police and fire departments, postal service
Community agencies and clergy
Interdisciplinary staffings
Managed care organization representatives

the least restrictive alternative for treatment. For example, a client might be able to go to his or her own home following discharge from a psychiatric hospitalization, rather than to a nursing home or the home of a family member, because of the availability of psychosocial home care services. The need and demand for psychosocial home care nursing services are likely to continue to increase because of the following factors:

1. Most people prefer to remain in their homes and to be as independent as possible.
2. Psychiatric inpatients have been deinstitutionalized to an increasing degree.
3. Home care cases are increasingly complex.
4. Consumers increasingly expect holistic care, which includes the psychological, social, spiritual, and environmental or ecological realms, in addition to the physical factors of health care.
5. Home care in general, and psychosocial home care in particular, is cost-effective.

THE PSYCHOSOCIAL CLINICAL NURSE SPECIALIST

Figure 44-1 illustrates the components of the three roles of psychosocial nurses in home care. A *psychosocial clinical nurse specialist* is defined as follows: a master's-prepared nurse with psychiatric and mental health assessment and intervention skills who is eligible for, or has already received, the American Nurses Association (ANA) certification as a specialist in adult psychiatric and mental health nursing.[59]

As minimal preparation, a nurse should possess a baccalaureate degree in nursing to function as a generalist nurse in community health or home health care. Pyschosocial home health nurses must have within the last 5 years at least 2 years of recent acute psychiatric inpatient experience. They must also have recent medical-surgical or related experience because often psychosocial home care clients are physically compromised.[31] A specialist is prepared to provide advanced practitioner skills as a clinician, administrator, teacher, or researcher. It is recommended that psychosocial home care services be provided by a master's-prepared and certified nurse.[41]

◆ History of Psychosocial Home Care

Conceptually, home health care takes into account cultural, historical, professional, economic, political, philosophical, social, pharmacological, technological, and ecological factors. Home care has been delivered in the United States since the 1950s.[70] Approaches were patterned after the service delivered in Amsterdam, Holland.[49] In the late 1960s and early 1970s, during the height of the community mental health movement, efforts were directed toward providing home care for the mentally ill, especially the elderly mentally ill.[70] The 1983 report of the Joint Commission of Mental Illness and Health sped the process of supporting mental clients in society through the deinstitutionalization of mental inpatients and a focus on community care instead of hospital-based care.

PRINCIPLES OF PSYCHOSOCIAL HOME CARE

Most home care agencies share the following basic principles and philosophy:[60]

1. As long as it is medically, socially, and economically possible, adults want to remain in their own homes and communities and should be permitted to do so.
2. Clients who need long-term care often present many overlapping challenges and problems.
3. The whole individual must be considered.
4. Services must be coordinated and integrated.
5. Cost-effective care requires direct payment at the level of program delivery.
6. High quality long-term care should be affordable.

Additionally, the following premises guide the clinical approach of the psychosocial home care nurse and a psychosocial specialty team or service:

1. Client care is maximized when integrated into a comprehensive care plan that takes into account the client and family and their environment, self-concept, functioning level, coping mechanisms, stressors, and sociocultural perspective.

Clinician

Teacher

Consultant

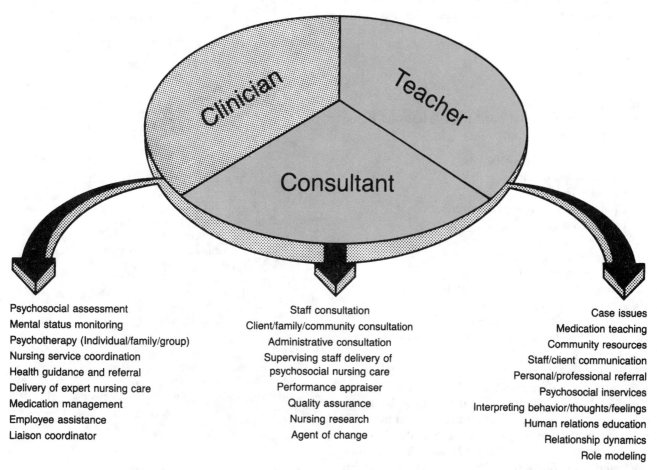

Psychosocial assessment
Mental status monitoring
Psychotherapy (Individual/family/group)
Nursing service coordination
Health guidance and referral
Delivery of expert nursing care
Medication management
Employee assistance
Liaison coordinator

Staff consultation
Client/family/community consultation
Administrative consultation
Supervising staff delivery of psychosocial nursing care
Performance appraiser
Quality assurance
Nursing research
Agent of change

Case issues
Medication teaching
Community resources
Staff/client communication
Personal/professional referral
Psychosocial inservices
Interpreting behavior/thoughts/feelings
Human relations education
Relationship dynamics
Role modeling

Figure 44-1. Role aspects of the psychosocial clinical nurse specialist in home care. (Klebanoff NA, Casler CB: The Psychosocial Clinical Nurse Specialist: An Untapped Resource for Home Care. Home Healthcare Nurse 4: 37, 1986; reprinted with permission from Hospital Publications, Inc.)

2. A client's or family's reaction to an alteration in mental health status, mental disability, or mental illness is often influenced by whether the condition is permanent, temporary, degenerative, or unknown.
3. Care of a client is based on the idea of therapeutic use of self, the setting and attaining of goals for health status enhancement, and the development of the client's ability to develop personal resources within a realistic level of functioning.

ECLECTIC NATURE OF PSYCHOSOCIAL HOME CARE

The biopsychosocial model interacts with theories from adaptation, behaviorism, systems, cognitive therapy, community mental health, communications, crisis intervention, family therapy, developmental perspectives, self-care, interpersonal, social learning, and nursing models and from other theoretical models discussed elsewhere in this textbook; these provide fertile ground for an individualized approach to psychosocial home care. Usually, the psychosocial home care nurse will use a blended or eclectic approach to meet the needs of a home care client. However, theories of crisis intervention, Orem's self-care nursing theory, and behavioral therapy can guide psychosocial home care.

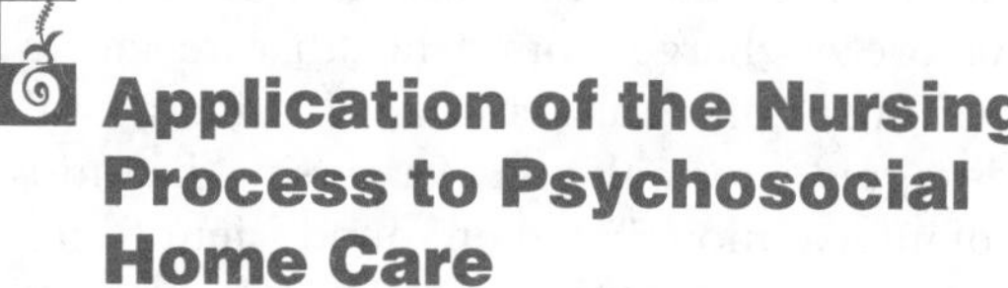

Application of the Nursing Process to Psychosocial Home Care

The psychosocial home care nurse has the unique privilege of working with the client and family on their own turf, because psychosocial home care nursing services are delivered in the place of residence. The nurse must remember that the home is part of a larger community and social system and that the provision of home care services involves many different disciplines and services. Cultural influences also play a large part in the planning and delivery of psychosocial home care nursing services. Some cultural differences pertinent to home care are identified in Box 44-3.

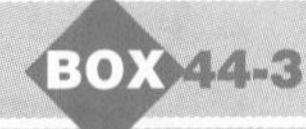

Cultural Factors Influencing Psychosocial Home Health Care Nursing Practice

The following cultural factors should be assessed in each psychosocial home health care situation:

1. Family structure
2. Race and ethnic origin
3. Countries of residence
4. Dietary habits and nutritional variables
5. Religious and spiritual practices
6. Ways of communicating, use of language
7. Use of appreciation of art, music, drama, and so on in the home
8. Dress and clothing habits
9. Health and mental health behavior, beliefs, patterns
10. Illness and mental illness behavior, beliefs, patterns
11. Healing health beliefs and practices
12. Influence of external beliefs
13. Perceptions of health care providers
14. Other family beliefs, values, customs, rituals, and habits

ASSESSMENT

Indications for Care

Critical indicators of the need for psychosocial home care include the following:

1. Mental health status changes
2. Health status changes
3. Changes in material welfare
4. Changes in the home environment
5. Family changes
6. Changes in social support network
7. Changes in psychosocial functioning
8. Changes in motivation
9. Need for health or medication teaching
10. Need for anticipatory guidance
11. Psychiatric crisis or emergency
12. Changes in leisure time or diversionary activities

Standards of Care

In accordance with the ANA Standards of Home Health Nursing Practice (Box 44-4), the psychosocial home care nurse assesses the client and family and available personal and community resources. (See also the ANA Statement on Psychiatric-Mental Health Clinical Nursing Practice and Standards of Psychiatric-Mental Health Clinical Nursing Practice.)[1] The legal necessity of documenting all nursing activities in the home supports the use of the nursing process as guided by the Standards of Home Health Nursing Practice. Most states have enacted legislation that details the rights of populations receiving care at home, especially the elderly. National associations have printed materials outlining the rights of people receiving care in their homes (Box 44-5). In accordance with Standard III, Data Collection, the nurse continuously collects and records data that are comprehensive, accurate, and systematic. Information assessed before discharge from a health care facility, during the initial home care visit, and during all subsequent visits guides formulation of a nursing diagnosis, planning of interventions based on sound scientific and theoretical foundations (Standard II, Theory), and evaluation of nursing care. Data collection for assessment purposes includes the following in conjunction with Standard III:

1. Physical, emotional, intellectual, psychological, social, cultural, religious, spiritual, community, and environmental history; support systems; lifestyle factors; and stressors
2. Client's and family's growth and development, dynamics, perceptions, vulnerabilities, risk factors, and current and past coping strengths or mechanisms
3. Sleep, rest, and activity patterns; appetite and nutritional-metabolic patterns; elimination patterns; other patterns and habits affecting health, knowledge, and motivation
4. Self and role-relationship enactments and patterns, including sexuality-reproductive patterns
5. Mental and emotional status, including thought processes, perceptual patterns, and cognitive functioning
6. Understanding of and receptivity to home care and expectations of the psychosocial home care program

The psychosocial nurse collects objective and subjective data in a standardized, succinct, and systematic manner regarding the psychosocial indicators for home care, resources, and parameters for assessment. Many sources are available from which to collect these data, including community health nursing texts.

Data Gathering Methods

A client and family members or other significant people (eg, neighbors or a rabbi) are the primary sources for assessment data through history taking, interviewing,

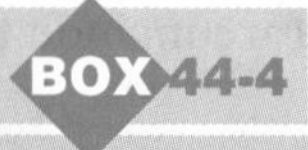

ANA Standards of Home Health Nursing Practice

Standard I. Organization of Home Health Services

All home health services are planned, organized, and directed by a master's- prepared professional nurse with experience in community health and administration.

Standard II. Theory

The nurse applies theoretical concepts as a basis for decisions in practice.

Standard III. Data Collection

The nurse continuously collects and records data that are comprehensive, accurate, and systematic.

Standard IV. Diagnosis

The nurse uses health assessment data to determine nursing diagnoses.

Standard V. Planning

The nurse develops care plans that establish goals. The care plan is based on nursing diagnoses and incorporates therapeutic, preventive, and rehabilitative nursing actions.

Standard VI. Intervention

The nurse, guided by the care plan, intervenes to provide comfort, to restore, improve, and promote health, to prevent complications and sequelae of illness, and to effect rehabilitation.

Standard VII. Evaluation

The nurse continually evaluates the client and family's responses to interventions in order to determine progress toward goal attainment and to revise the data base, nursing diagnoses, and plan of care.

Standard VIII. Continuity of Care

The nurse is responsible for the client's appropriate and uninterrupted care along the health care continuum, and therefore uses discharge planning, case management, and coordination of community resources.

Standard IX. Interdisciplinary Collaboration

The nurse initiates and maintains a liaison relationship with all appropriate health care providers to ensure that all efforts effectively complement one another.

Standard X. Professional Development

The nurse assumes responsibility for professional development and contributes to the professional growth of others.

Standard XI. Research

The nurse participates in research activities that contribute to the profession's continuing development of knowledge of home health care.

Standard XII. Ethics

The nurse uses the code for nurses established by the American Nurses Association as a guide for ethical decision making in practice.

physical assessment, mental status examination, and reporting that various diagnostic and psychological tests were performed. The nurse will need objective, independent verification of information gathered in the client's home. The home environment itself provides valuable assessment information (Box 44-6, p. 899). Various flow sheets and forms of nursing progress notes are available for use in data collection in home health care and psychosocial home health care nursing. Usually the agency offering the home health care services provides these forms for the nurse's use. As data are collected and organized, nursing diagnoses relative to the mutually identified problems are formulated. The nurse includes the client and family in the nursing process, because they are integral to planning, implementation, and evaluation of home care services. Also during the assessment phase, once the necessity for and acceptance of home care have been established, the nurse determines the resources, equipment, and disciplines that will be needed in the home and initiates referrals for them.

NURSING DIAGNOSIS

Data collection during the psychosociocultural assessment—subjective verbal data, objective nonverbal data, symptoms, signs, etiology, risk factors, and critical indicators—ends the assessment phase of the nursing process and begins the decision-making process: formulating a nursing diagnosis. Standard IV, Diagnosis, of the Standards for Home Health Nursing Practice addresses this phase. Nursing diagnosis starts with identifying actual health problems or needs requiring immediate attention. The nurse also notes potential problems that can be prevented or dealt with quickly if they become actual problems (Box 44-7). Because of the added complexity of home care, clients likely will have more than one nursing diagnosis. The most com-

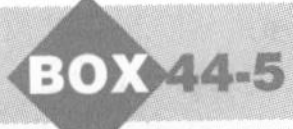

National Associations and Organizations Concerned With Home Health Care

American Hospital Association Division of Ambulatory and Home Care Services
840 North Lake Shore Drive
Chicago, IL 60611
312-280-6000

American Association for Continuing Care
1101 Connecticut Avenue, N.W.
Washington, DC 20036
202-857-1194

American Federation of Home Health Agencies
1320 Fenwick Lane, Suite 500
Silver Spring, MD 20910
301-588-1454

American Nurses Association
1101 14th Street, N.W., Suite 200
Washington, DC 20005
202-789-1800

Council of Community Health Services
National League for Nursing
10 Columbus Circle
New York, NY 10019
212-582-1022

The Association of Ambulatory Behavioral Healthcare
901 N. Washington St.
Suite 600
Alexandria, VA 22314
703-836-2274

National Association of Home Care
205 C Street, N.E.
Washington, DC 20002
202-547-7424

National Homecaring Council
67 Irving Place
New York, NY 10003
212-674-4990

mon psychiatric diagnoses seen in psychosocial home care are found in Boxes 44-8 and 44-9 (p.901).

PLANNING

Goal Setting

Nursing diagnoses give the psychosocial home health care nurse needed information to formulate short- and long-term goals with the client and family. Examples of short-term goals in psychosocial home care include the following:

1. The client and family will participate in the home physical therapy program three times for at least 10 minutes in each 24-hour period.
2. The client will not attempt to harm herself or himself in any way until the psychosocial home care nurse returns within 24 hours.
3. The client and family will identify in writing at least five factors that lead to anxious feelings within 48 hours of the client's admission to home care services.

Short-term goals usually are immediate, realistic steps that are to be taken for long-term goals to be met. The time perspective in home care is longer than that in an acute care psychiatric hospital. For example, at the onset of home care services, the nurse may visit daily, which would facilitate setting 24-hour goals, whereas if home visits are made weekly, biweekly, or monthly, the client and family and the nurse will couch goal statements in longer time frames. Because home care services are provided on an episodic, intermittent basis, very long-term or enduring goals usually will not be met for months or years after discharge from psychosocial home care services. A few examples of long-term goals appropriate for the psychosocial home care setting are as follows:

1. The client will perform relaxation exercises for at least 15 minutes daily for the next 6 months.
2. The client and family will attend monthly Alliance for the Mentally Ill support group meetings.
3. The client will reestablish and maintain sexual activity at the level specified before the onset of depression.

A sample home health clinical pathway is shown in Table 44-1 (p. 902).

Client and Family Outcomes

Some general outcomes are expected in psychosocial home care nursing:

1. Maximizing the client's level of independence through health promotion, maintenance, and restoration
2. Preventing complications in the home through health teaching, education about psychoactive medication, and sharing information about community resources
3. Averting or minimizing a psychiatric crisis through anticipation and planning
4. Delaying admission to a nursing home or other long-term care facility

Other long-term outcomes that can result from psychosocial home care services are the client's ability to

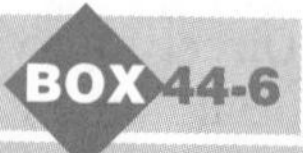

Psychosocial Home Health Safety Assessment

On the first psychosocial home health visit, complete this checklist to determine objectively the level of safety in the home. Administer other appropriate assessments as indicated (eg, suicide assessment, falls risk assessment). Make corrective actions as necessary.

	YES	NO
Are there dangerous objects (eg, guns, knives, scissors) or items (ie, tools) in the home? (If so, list:)	____	____
Is the client or family willing to remove the dangerous objects or items from the home care setting?	____	____
Does the client have suicidal or homicidal ideation?	____	____
Has the client ever attempted suicide in the past?	____	____
Do any of the prescribed medications pose a risk for overdosage?	____	____
Is there a telephone within easy reach of the client?	____	____
Are emergency numbers easily available to the client and the caregivers?	____	____
Is oxygen being used in the home?	____	____
Are functional fire alarms present?	____	____
Are any electrical devices damaged?	____	____
Are there any hazardous materials, substances, or waste in the home environment?	____	____
Is there proper lighting, ventilation, heating, and cooling?	____	____
Does the client need assistance to ambulate?	____	____
Does the client have a history of falls, cardiovascular disorder(s), neurological dysfunction(s), musculoskeletal disorder(s), vision impairment or hearing loss, urinary urgency or incontinence?	____	____
Does the client have any other condition or take any medications that would affect balance, blood pressure, or level of consciousness?	____	____
Is the client confused, agitated, or in denial regarding the need for assistance?	____	____
Any other risks in the psychosocial home care environment? (If so, list:)	____	____

________________ ________________ ________________

Client Name/# RN Name/Signature Date

maintain ties with the family network and community and to maintain a greater sense of control by helping to determine health, mental health, or mental illness care needs. Home and community assessment contributes to effective, efficient, and appropriate discharge planning. Psychosocial home care nursing contributes invaluable insight to the client, the family, and other team members; this insight influences the overall plan of care, support, and follow-up. Two client populations are appropriate for referral for psychosocial home care nursing services:

1. Clients and families who demonstrate actual or potential nursing diagnoses and client or family conditions suitable for psychosocial home care, including psychoactive medication management for clients who are newly diagnosed with, or have exacerbations of, psychiatric (medical) disorders
2. Clients with new or exacerbated nursing or medical diagnoses (not of a psychosocial, psychiatric, or mental illness or health nature) complicated by the presence of factors described in item 1

The most common specific population groups to be served include the elderly, people with problems in living, people with psychosocial responses to their health conditions (especially after accidents or with long-term physical problems such as chronic obstructive pulmonary disease and cancers), and people with long-term or enduring mental illness. The nursing care plan written for use in psychosocial home care nursing practice outlines the specific actions that will be taken by the nurse, client,

BOX 44-7

The Most Common North American Nursing Diagnosis Association (NANDA) Diagnoses in Psychosocial Home Health Care

1.1.2.2 Altered Nutrition: Less than body requirements
1.3.1.1 Constipation
2.1.1.1 Impaired Verbal Communication
3.1.1 Impaired Social Interaction
3.1.2 Social Isolation
4.1.1 Spiritual Distress (distress of the human spirit)
5.1.1.1.1 Impaired Adjustment
5.2.1 Ineffective Management of Therapeutic Regimen (individual)
5.1.2.1.1 Ineffective Family Coping: Disabling
6.2.1 Sleep Pattern Disturbance
6.4.1.1 Impaired Home Maintenance Management
6.5.2 Bathing/Hygiene Self Care Deficit
6.5.3 Dressing/Grooming Self Care Deficit
7.1.2 Self Esteem Disturbance
7.2 Sensory/Perceptual Alterations (Specify) (Visual, auditory, kinesthetic, gustatory, tactile, olfactory)
7.3.2 Powerlessness
8.1.1 Knowledge Deficit (Specify)
8.3 Altered Thought Processes
9.1.1 Pain
9.1.1.1 Chronic Pain
9.2.1.1 Dysfunctional Grieving
9.2.2 Risk for Violence: Self-directed or directed at others
9.2.2.1 Risk for Self-Mutilation
9.2.3 Post-Trauma Response
9.3.1 Anxiety
9.3.2 Fear

and family unit to achieve the mutually agreed-on goals and outcomes to the identified needs or problems. Nursing Care Plans 44-1 and 44-2 (pp. 903–905) provide examples from each of the two main client populations and selected aspects of their psychosocial nursing care plans.

INTERVENTION

The psychosocial home care client's specific goals and outcomes lead to individual interventions in the home. Interpersonal, intellectual, and technical skills are used during this phase of the nursing process, which is addressed by Standard V, Intervention. Direct interventions used in the home by the psychosocial home care nurse include the following:

1. Comprehensive in-home assessment
2. Crisis intervention
3. Medication administration, monitoring, and teaching about responses, indications, actions, and interactions
4. Individual, couple, family, and group counseling and psychotherapy
5. Verbal or written contracts with the client
6. Health guidance and referral
7. Client advocacy
8. Case management activities
9. Mental, emotional, physical, and spiritual observation, interpretation, and evaluation
10. Health care team coordination
11. Liaison activities
12. Reporting to physician about client response to home environment, medication responses, medical follow-up, new signs and symptoms relative to the client's status
13. Supervision of team members (eg, home health assistant)
14. Role modeling or social skills education
15. Teaching (see Table 44-2, p.906)
    a. Diet, special diet
    b. Disease, illness, wellness
    c. Management of illness
    d. Stress reduction
    e. Risk factors
    f. Safety measures, accident prevention
    g. Management of activities of daily living
    h. Emergency measures
    i. Positive coping behaviors
    j. Administration of treatments, medications
    k. Rehabilitative exercises, when indicated
    l. Community resources to help attain state of optimal functioning, client well-being, and psychosocial rehabilitation

The psychosocial nurse also may intervene to correct actual or potential safety hazards:

1. Structural integrity of the residence
2. Heating, cooling, ventilation
3. Stairways and ramps
4. Storage of dangerous objects and fluids
5. Storage of medications
6. Mats and throw rugs
7. Gas and electrical appliances
8. Number of people per square footage
9. Cooking and bathing facilities
10. Nature of neighborhood
11. Sanitation

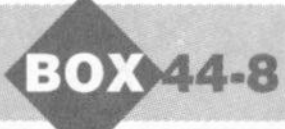

BOX 44-8

The Most Common Psychiatric Diagnoses in the DSM-IV in Psychosocial Home Health Care

Schizophrenia, Disorganized Type
Schizophrenia, Paranoid Type
Schizoaffective Disorder
Delusional Disorder
Brief Psychotic Disorder
Psychotic Disorder Due to [General Medical Condition] With Delusions
Major Depressive Disorder, Single Episode Severe Without Psychotic Features
Major Depressive Disorder, Single Episode Severe With Mood Incongruent Psychotic Features
Bipolar Disorder, Single Manic Episode Severe Without Psychotic Features
Bipolar Disorder, Single Manic Episode Severe With Mood Incongruent Psychotic Features

The nurse who works in the home care setting also intervenes in indirect ways. Indirect home care includes the nurse's actions that affect the home care situation but do not involve personal contact with the client or family. The psychosocial home care nurse may need to provide an in-service for the home care agency staff or a community group and to participate in agency orientations, team conferences, discharge planning meetings, and recertification sessions.

EVALUATION

According to Standard VII, Evaluation, the nurse continually evaluates the client's and family's responses to interventions to determine progress toward goal attainment and to determine the needed revision to the data base, nursing diagnoses, and plan of care.[3] Plans for discharge from home care services are made early in the course of home care, ideally during the initial visit. This helps the client reach measurable, customized goals. The nurse, client, and family determine whether the goals for home care have been met. In home care, changing client needs and status necessitates a dynamic and continual revision of, and addition to, the data base and nursing care plan. Chart audits, reviews by regulatory agencies, peer reviews, and the various home health agency certification processes also evaluate the quality and effectiveness of home care services. All involved in the home care case—client, family, nurse, other home health care team members, physician, and others—evaluate the client's progress toward and attainment of goals. As the client and family become increasingly able to care for the client, the nurse and other home health team members decrease the intensity and frequency of their visits. Discharge from home care services includes making provisions for aftercare, if indicated, and other types of case management and coordination of community resources (see Standard VIII, Continuity of Care).

OTHER CONSIDERATIONS

Two related practices in home nursing care overlap psychosocial home health care. They are hospice care and care of the person living with acquired immunodeficiency syndrome (AIDS). Many excellent texts and articles discuss hospice care. Chapter 48, The Client on the HIV Spectrum, discusses hospice care and mental health interventions for clients with AIDS and their families.

NURSES' ATTITUDES AND FEELINGS

According to Burgess, certain characteristics or traits are helpful to psychosocial home care nursing:

1. "Self-starter" approach to work
2. Good physical assessment skills
3. Superb clinical judgment
4. The ability to communicate effectively with clients, family members, other health team members, and others in the community

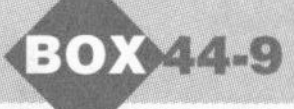

BOX 44-9

The Most Common International Classification of Diseases, Ninth Revision (ICD-9) Diagnoses in Psychosocial Home Health Care

Schizoaffective Type
Schizophrenia
Depressive Psychoses, Single Episode
Bipolar Affective Disorder
Affective Psychosis
Paranoia
Psychosis, NOS
Panic Disorder
Conversion Disorder
Neurotic Depression
Acute Stress Reaction
Depressive Disorder

Table 44-1 Home Health Clinical Pathway—Psychiatric Focus

Patient Name: ______________ Sex: ____ Age: ____

Clinician: __________ Physician: __________

Diagnosis: ______________ DSM IV: __________ CPT: __________ Medicare #: __________

Payor Source: ______________ Current Medications: ______________

Chief Complaint in Patient's Words: ______________

TREATMENT GOALS: 1) Increased level of functioning
2) Monitoring of medication regimen via patient education
3) Identification and activation of familial or community resources

Assessment	Planning	Interventions	Evaluation
1) Risk potential: —suicidal —homicidal —potential detox —acute psychosis	1) Do not enter a home if a patient is threatening or has a weapon.	1) Notify M.D., consider inpatient care	1) Support System: —medication compliance —viable suicide plan
2) Homebound status: Excessive social isolation	2) Number of planned visits weekly	2) Document contributing symptoms to homebound status.	2) Reevaluate homebound status at each visit.
3) Appearance, mood, affect, speech, mental status, presence of audio/visual hallucinations	3) Arrange a visit where primary caregiver is present.	3) —Consider referral to social worker. —Encourage dialogue.	3) —Verbal and non-verbal communication —Home environment
4) —Medication compliance —Medication teaching needs	4) Plan and rehearse med administration with patient and/or caregiver; encourage self-reliance	4) —Stress importance of med compliance. —Signs & symptoms of adverse drug reaction —Dietary considerations	4) Document compliance or absence of and notify M.D. if necessary.
5) Socioeconomic needs	5) Identify community resources available to the client.	5) Refer to social worker for unmet socioeconomic needs.	

CRITERIA LISTED ABOVE IS ONLY A GUIDELINE AND IS NOT INTENDED TO BE A STANDARD OF CARE

Strategic Clinical Systems, Inc., 3715 Mission Ct., Granbury, Tx 76049, (817) 326-4239. PsychPaths™

Darla Belt, RN & Vickie Pflueger, RNC—Authors

5. Efficient organizational skills
6. Well-honed time management techniques
7. The ability to prioritize work
8. The ability to function independently with minimal supervision
9. A good and growing working knowledge of community, state, and national resources and referral sources[10]

Additionally, it is helpful if the psychosocial home care nurse is comfortable in various settings with diverse home and family arrangements. A high comfort level for differences helps a nurse respond to the intrinsic dignity, worth, and value of clients and their significant others. A nurse working in this arena must be able to explain health care benefits to clients and their families, feel comfortable discussing financial arrangements with responsible parties, and market the service to others. Discussing financial arrangements, and in some instances collecting fees, can lead to anxious feelings in a nurse who is not accustomed to these matters.

Unfortunately, home health care nurses are isolated from one another, from other health care professionals, from their supervisors, and from a shared work setting. Also, safety considerations in the community and home setting necessitate common sense and extra precautions, such as carrying a cellular telephone. For these reasons, the home health care nurse is susceptible to frustration, resentment, sadness, and fear. Additionally, home health care nursing requires an unusually large amount of paperwork and necessary documentation that must be completed within stringent time spans for reimbursement purposes; this adds to the potential for burnout. Two other main features of home care can be viewed as disadvantages. The first is the considerable overlapping of professional and personal boundaries in this realm. The second is the fact that the psychosocial home care nurse may not have as much privacy and

Nursing Care Plan 44-1

Psychosocial Home Care of a Client With Delusions

Mrs. RB is a widowed 76-year-old female with no children who has worked as a homemaker all of her life. After 52 years of marriage, her husband suffered a massive and fatal heart attack in their home one month ago. She believes, however, that her husband is not at home because he has "taken ill" and that she can cure him. She is convinced that he is having an affair with a neighbor and that if she repeats a certain chant in the crawl-space of their home, he will "get well and come home" and that "I'll be better, too."

Mrs. RB is conversant but vigilant. Her social network includes 2 neighbors and a nephew, whom she sees "as often as I want to." Currently she refuses to leave her home. Formerly she attended the Baptist Church but no longer does; she states that she does "not feel in control of my soul."

She has no previous history of psychiatric difficulties. Other than her own parents, who died many years ago, she had no prior experience with significant losses. She denies that her husband is dead when her nephew points it out to her. She says she doesn't know why her nephew is making such a fuss and that she doesn't need any help. By her report she has been sleeping fewer than 3 hours per night ("because I have to keep up the chanting") and eats only one small meal a day ("I just don't feel like eating"). She has lost 18 lbs in the past month.

Severe problem with primary support group. Global Assessment of Functioning is 50. Score on the Geriatric Depression Scale is 10. Philadelphia Geriatric Center Morale Scale is 12.

No known physical health problems currently or in the past, according to her nephew and husband's physician; however, she has not been to a doctor "in years." Physical exam findings within normal limits. Cranial nerves intact.

Neatly dressed in a house dress with appropriate grooming. Eye gaze downcast. Predominant affect of fear, anxiety, and apprehension. Comprehension and speech adequate. Magical thinking and delusions regarding whereabouts of spouse; no suicidal or homicidal ideation; oriented to self, date, place, and situation; recent and remote memory and recall intact; follows a three-stage command correctly. Judgment intact except about spouse; major defense is denial. Moderately unmotivated to deal with this problem.

Not currently taking any medication. No history of drug/alcohol abuse. Does not and has never smoked cigarettes.

Home clean and neat, and in good repair, with adequate access and parking. In a generally quiet, safe neighborhood; client states that she feels safe in her own home. No gross safety hazards noted.

Able to perform activities of daily living. Can use the telephone without help; prepares own meals and does own housework. Relies on nephew to get to places out of walking distance; nephew also helps manage her money.

Nursing Diagnosis

Altered Thought Process related to feelings of anxiety and depression secondary to recent loss, nutritional deficits, altered sleep patterns, and possible organic factors

Outcome

Client will express decreased delusions and identify feelings and stressors underlying delusional beliefs.

Intervention	Rationale
Establish a therapeutic alliance with client in a one-to-one client-nurse relationship.	Clients who form a positive alliance with their caregivers are more likely to have better outcomes.
Involve client and nephew in structured psychosocial home visits to actively listen to her and promote thought processing and clear communication of thoughts.	Effective communication helps client solve problems; a nonjudgmental attitude improves sense of self-worth and self-identity.

continued

Nursing Care Plan 44-1 (Continued)

Intervention	Rationale
Avoid arguing, reasoning with or challenging her delusions; provide comfort, support, and feedback to client.	Attempts to correct delusional beliefs increase anxiety, which reinforce the client's need to rigidly adhere to the false beliefs. Emotional comfort and support enhance self-esteem.
Explore with client the events that trigger delusions; discuss anxiety and other feelings underlying her delusions.	Exploring delusional topics helps to understand the dynamics of the delusions; delusions will become less necessary as client learns to cope with her feelings of loss.
Teach the client alternatives and ways to control her thoughts with recreation, distraction, and positive coping/relaxation techniques (e.g., watching TV, reading, listening to soothing music, deep breathing, and recalling pleasant times, places, and people).	These alternative measures reduce fear, anxiety, and other uncomfortable feelings.
Monitor, teach, and promote sleep, hygiene, hydration, elimination, nutrition, and orientation measures.	Less physical and psychological stress, and fewer mental status alterations, occur when the client has adequate sleep and hydration, regular elimination, and sufficient nutrition.
Encourage the client to engage in here-and-now conversations with neighbors and nephew; establish and post a daily schedule that sparks interest in the here-and-now world.	Reality-based interactions reinforce her contact with reality; social skills are best fostered in a safe, familiar context.
Teach client and nephew to monitor and report signs of impaired thought processes and set criteria to determine when to seek further professional help.	Monitoring of judgment, distractibility, hygiene, and so on, permits earlier and more successful intervention.

Evaluation

Client reports no delusional thoughts and demonstrates improved self-care and social skills.

control over the environment in the home as is found in an institutional setting. Many families who receive home care have multiple problems, and the psychosocial home care nurse may experience a sense of helplessness, sadness, or anger in attempting to provide comprehensive care in a limited time with less than ideal resources.

On the other hand, home health care nurses enjoy a high level of responsibility, autonomy, and decision making; direct access to clients and families; the satisfaction of working collaboratively with other health team members; the opportunity to work as a client advocate; and some measure of control over their schedules, which allows them to complete work at home. The psychosocial home care nurse is able to observe and work with people on their own turf, where clients are perhaps more likely to share information with the nurse and the nurse can see the obvious and subtle details that influence a client's optimal functioning. Another advantage of home care is that it is often more economical and cost-effective than institutional care. This appeals to the many psychosocial nurses who want to work with clients and their families, as opposed to "doing to" them.

Finally, in keeping with the notion of giving care in the least restrictive setting possible, home is often the first choice if the appropriate supports are in place. An awareness and processing of personal emotional and physical feelings are of utmost importance for any nurse practicing in this area. Psychosocial home health care nurses need support. Meetings with multidisciplinary team members provide a time for all to share their thoughts and feelings and to gain support from each other. Conferences with peers or supervisors can also serve this purpose. To continue to meet the challenge of this aspect of the complex American health care system, the psychosocial nurse must rest, rejuvenate, and reflect on the positive aspects of providing psychosocial home health care.

Nursing Care Plan 44-2

Psychosocial Home Care of a Client With Bipolar Disorder

Mr. J, age 34, has a history of bipolar disorder, which has been treated in the past with lithium carbonate and intermittent hospitalizations, approximately every 2 years. Recently his spouse filed for divorce and he became suicidal. They have been married 7 years and have no children.

Mr. J was hospitalized following an automobile accident in which he sustained multiple internal injuries and a broken left leg. He had stopped taking the lithium before his accident; during the hospital stay he was given phenothiazines. Shortly before his discharge, he was again started on lithium carbonate. His spouse moved out of their condominium while he was in the hospital, but she agreed to assist with his care at home until he was more independent. A hospital-based social worker made the referral to a home care agency that sent a psychosocial clinical nurse specialist into the home to visit. The nurse monitored his physical status, his risk of self-harm, and his adherence and response to lithium therapy including monitoring with the Young Mania Scale. The nurse also provided supportive psychotherapy, referral to community resources, and instruction and support to him and his wife regarding his care at home.

The psychosocial home care nurse arranged for physical therapy and monitoring of serum lithium levels. Mr. J's spouse began to attend support group meetings held by the local chapter of the Depressive and Manic Depressive Association.

Nursing Diagnosis

Risk for Violence: Self-directed or directed at others

Outcome

Client will sign no-suicide contract and call the crisis and suicide telephone hotline as needed.

Intervention	Rationale
Continually assess risk for harm to self and others; monitor with suicide lethality scale.	Assessment of risk factors allows for prompt and effective intervention.
Assess home environment for dangerous objects and weapons and have them removed from the home, at least temporarily; limit the amount of medication prescribed at any one time.	Removal or restriction of weapons, dangerous objects, and medications reduces the possible means of self-harm.
Contract a no-suicide agreement verbally and in written form.	A no-suicide agreement reduces the client's risk of self-harm.
Instruct client, spouse, and other family members to notify nurse and/or physician of suicidal ideation and intent; formulate an emergency or crisis plan which includes hospitalization as needed.	Client and family will be prepared to deal with suicidal thoughts or actions following instruction and planning with nurse.
Make appropriate referrals to mental health professionals in the community, including telephone numbers to call.	Referral to mental health professionals provides sufficient resources for client.
Help client mobilize his coping skills and resources.	Mobilization of his coping skills and resources increases his competency and efficacy.

Evaluation

Client does not harm himself and reports no further suicidal intent.

Table 44-2

Client and Family Teaching

Content	Teaching Activity	Evaluation
Provide an explanation of possible causes of the delusional thoughts and client's bizarre behavior.	Enumerate and describe the precipitating stressors and predisposing factors that might trigger the delusional thoughts and maladaptive behavior. Obtain and give printed reference materials and other resources.	The family correctly identifies the possible etiologies (ie, recent death of spouse, feelings of anxiety, nutritional deficits, sleep disturbance, and possible organic cause) of the client's thoughts and behavior.
Define and describe signs and symptoms of impaired thought process.	Define the spheres of unimpaired thought process.	The family identifies signs of cognitive impairment (eg, changes in thought and speech, bizarre behaviors, ambivalence in decision making, impaired impulse control and behavior, distractibility, changes in self-care, hygiene and grooming) and reports them to the psychosocial home health nurse or other health care provider.
Refer to community resources.	Provide a thorough list of community referrals and resources. Discuss the needs and resources as required by the client's needs, condition, and interests. Meet with staff members of selected community programs and services. Visit meetings and programs of selected resources and self-help programs.	Caregiver, family members, and client describe various programs that will give relevant services according to the client's and family's needs. Caregiver and client contact suitable programs and self-help groups when indicated.

◆ Trends in Psychosocial Home Health Care Nursing

The future of psychosocial home health care nursing practice in the United States will be affected by the incidence of mental illness, demographics, and legislative and political trend. The 1990s will be a time of new service dimensions, innovation, and quality improvement. Preferred provider arrangements and proprietary joint ventures to provide durable medical equipment are two examples of this changing business climate. National trends, referrer needs, and the preferences of individual communities and consumers will greatly affect the successful delivery of psychosocial home health care nursing services.

Approximately 2 to 5 million people with long-term or enduring mental illness live in the United States, and most of them live in their communities. The elderly population is growing at a dramatic rate. Alzheimer's disease affects 5% to 10% of the population older than 65 years and increases proportionally in people older than 85 years. Maintaining a person affected by a cognitive brain disorder in the home or facilitating transfer to a temporary or permanent facility is often a function of the psychosocial home health care nurse. Long-term service or intensive care management is needed to support this population in the home. However, most home care services are reimbursed on a short-term or intermittent basis. Legislation to authorize long-term home care services has been proposed but remains to be enacted. Bills permitting directly reimbursable community nursing services, including home health care, are in the demonstration phase. Managed care arrangements with capitated reimbursement are being incorporated into the home health arena.

Other needs include respite care for family members of clients who live at home to prevent hospitalization, institutionalization, caretaker burnout, client abuse, and overload. Also, women and elderly people from minority groups are especially susceptible to mental health and mental illness problems as a result of discrimination and will increasingly need attention in terms of psychosocial home health care. Improving coping methods and strengthening family care bonds will help to meet this burgeoning demand.

The ANA identifies societal and political forces that influence and shape the delivery of home health care nursing services. The societal forces include the following:

1. The rate of living older Americans is increasing disproportionately to the total population.
2. Traditionally, women have provided health care for youth and aging parents; more than half of all adult women now must work or choose to work outside the home and are therefore not available to care for family members.
3. The traditional support system of the extended family has been almost eliminated by the increasing mobility of society and the ever-increasing rate of single-parent family units and female heads of households.

Governmental responses to societal demands, changes, and spending trends have changed health care financing patterns. Political forces identified by the ANA that influence the provision of home health care services include the following:

1. Increased private third-party payment and government-financed health care programs, beginning in the 1960s, have promoted an increase in the demand for and use of health care services.
2. Shorter hospital stays with earlier discharges of more acutely ill clients from institutions have called attention to the need for home health care services; these shorter hospital stays have been prompted by prospective, diagnosis-related, and managed health care plans.[3]

◆ Chapter Summary

This chapter has discussed home health care in general and psychosocial home health care nursing in particular. Chapter highlights include the following:

1. Home health care nursing and psychosocial home health care nursing are aspects of community health nursing and the community health movement.
2. Psychosocial home health care nursing is *not* an alternative to institutional care; the reverse is the case.
3. The goals of psychosocial home health care are to assist the client and family to gain, regain, maintain, or restore the optimal state of health and independence; to minimize and rehabilitate the effects of illness and disability before or after institutionalization; and to prevent institutionalization altogether when possible.
4. The nursing process is used by the psychosocial home health care nurse to provide comprehensive services to clients in their places of residence.
5. Various social, legislative, and political forces make it likely that the need and demand for psychosocial home health care services will continue to increase.
6. The business climate of the 1990s will increase the demand for precise accounting of services and a greater tolerance for ever-increasing paperwork.

Critical Thinking Questions

1. *Briefly describe some of the components of an in-home mental wellness program.*
2. *Name two of the benefits of psychosocial home health care nursing to clients, caregivers and family members, and physicians.*
3. *What steps can the psychosocial home care nurse take to ensure personal safety?*
4. *Discuss the place of psychosocial home care on the continuum of mental health services.*

Review Questions

1. All of the following are true regarding psychosocial home interventions except which of the following?
   A. Psychosocial home care is less threatening and restrictive than hospitalization.
   B. Psychosocial home care is more comfortable than hospitalization.
   C. Psychosocial home care is more expensive than inpatient hospitalization.
   D. Psychosocial home care can be a part of a discharge plan.
2. Which of the following client conditions meets a criterion for homebound status?
   A. There are frequent absences from the home for shopping.
   B. The client refuses to leave home because of severe depression or paranoia.
   C. The client attends a day treatment program for socialization purposes.
   D. The client drives a car.
3. Which of the following groups are potential referral sources for psychosocial home health care?
   A. Former psychosocial home care clients
   B. Members of the clergy

C. Hospital-based psychiatric nurses
D. All of the above

◆ References

1. American Nurses' Association: Standards of Community Health Nursing Practice. Kansas City, MO, American Nurses' Association, 1973
2. American Nurses' Association: Standards of Psychiatric and Mental Health Nursing Practice. Kansas City, MO, American Nurses' Association, 1982
3. American Nurses' Association: Standards of Home Health Nursing Practice. Kansas City, MO, American Nurses' Association, 1986
4. Bernstein LH: The Role of the Physician in Home Care. Public Health Nursing 4 (1): 2–4, 1987
5. Brince J: The Psychiatric Patient: Hospital Care—Home Care. Caring 7: 12–16, 1986
6. Brooker B: Community Families: A Seven-Year Perspective. J Community Psychol 8: 147–151, 1980
7. Brooker B: A New Role for the Community Psychiatric Nurse in Working With Families Caring for a Relative With Schizophrenia. Int J Soc Psychiatry 36 (3): 216–224, 1990
8. Burgess A, Lazare A: Psychiatric Nursing in the Hospital and the Community. Engelwood Cliffs, NJ, Prentice-Hall, 1990
9. Burgess W, Ragland EC: Community Health Nursing Philosophy, Process, Practice. Norwalk, CT, Appleton-Century-Crofts, 1983
10. Carson VB: Bay Area Health Care Psychiatric Home Care Model. Home Healthcare Nurse 13 (4): 26–35, 1995
11. Chenoweth B, Spencer B: Dementia: The Experience of Family Caregivers. Gerontologist 26 (3): 260–266, 1986
12. Davies J, Janosik E: Mental Health and Psychiatric Nursing: A Caring Approach. Boston, Jones and Bartlett, 1991
13. Dean C, Gadd EM: Home Treatment for Acute Psychiatric Illness. British Journal of Medicine 301: 1021–1023, 1990
14. Duffy J, Miller MP, Parlocha P: Psychiatric Home Care. Home Healthcare Nurse 11 (2): 22–28, 1993
15. Ellenbecker CH, Shea K: Documentation in Home Health Care Practice. Nurs Clin North Am 29 (3): 495–506, 1994
16. Falvo DR: Multicultural Issues in Patient Education and Patient Compliance: A Special Report, Excerpted from Effective Patient Education: A Guide to Increased Compliance, 2d ed. Gaithersburg, MD, Aspen Publishers, 1995
17. Frank A, Gunderson J: The Role of the Therapeutic Alliance in the Treatment of Schizophrenia. Arch Gen Psychiatry 47: 228–236, 1990
18. Frisch N: Home Care Nursing and the Psychosocial-Emotional Needs of Clients. Home Healthcare Nurse 11: 64–65, 70, 1993
19. Gillis LS, Koch A, Joyi M: The Value and Cost-Effectiveness of a Home Visiting Program for Psychiatric Patients. S Afr Med J 77: 309–310; 312, 1990
20. Halloran T, Huggins M: A Five-year Directional Statement and Plan for Mental Health Services for the Adult Chronically and Seriously Ill. Hennepin County, MN, Mental Health Division, Department of Community Services, 1980
21. Harper MS: Providing Mental Health Services in the Homes of the Elderly. Caring 8 (6): 4–53, 1989
22. Harris M, Solomon K: A Study of Client Acceptance of Various Professionals in Psychiatric Home Visits. Hosp Community Psychiatry 28 (9): 661, 1977
23. Harris MD: Psychiatric Evaluation and Therapy. Home Healthcare Nurse 11: 66–67, 1993
24. Hatch C, Schut L: Description of a Crisis-Oriented Psychiatric Home Visiting Service. J Psychiatr Nurs 18 (4): 31–35, 1980
25. Health Care Financing Administration Home Health and Hospice Manual Regulations (HIM—11). Baltimore, MD, Sections 204 & 205, 1989
26. Hellwig K: Psychiatric Home Care Nursing: Managing Patients in the Community Setting. J Psychosoc Nurs 31 (12): 21–24, 1993
27. Helton M, Gordon S, Nunnery S: The Correlation Between Sleep Deprivation and the Intensive Care Unit Syndrome. Heart Lung 9: 31–35, 1980
28. Hildebrandt DE, Davis JM: Home Visits: A Method of Reducing the Pre-Intake Dropout Rate. J Psychiatr Nurs Ment Health Serv 13 (5): 43–44, 1975
29. Holland L: Mental Health Supportive Home Care Aides. Caring 12: 44–48, 1993
30. Home Health Care Team: Randomized Trial of a New Team Approach to Home Care. National Center for Health Services Research, Grant #HS03030, 1982
31. Planning and Program Development for Psychiatric Home Care. Journal of Nursing Administration 23 (11): 23–28, 1993
32. Kelley JH, Lehman L: Assessment of Anxiety, Depression, and Suspiciousness in the Home Care Setting. Home Healthcare Nurse 11: 16–20, 1993
33. Kemmerer B: Psychiatric Home Health Care Reduces Costs and Improves Patient Satisfaction. Psychiatry and Substance Abuse Issue Tracking, April. Washington, DC, Health Care Advisory Board, 1994
34. Krauss JB, Slavinsky AT: The Chronically Ill Psychiatric Patient and the Community. Boston, Blackwell Scientific, 1982
35. Kruse EA, Jones G: Development of a Comprehensive Suicide Protocol in a Home Health Care and Social Service Agency. Journal of Home Health Care Practice 3 (2): 47–56, 1990
36. Kruse EA, Wood M: (1989). Delivering Mental Health Services in the Home. Caring 6: 28–34; 59, 1989
37. Laben JK, McLean CP: Legal Issues and Guidelines for Nurses Who Care for the Mentally Ill. Thorofare, NJ, Slack, 1984
38. Lehman L, Kelley JH: Nursing Interventions for Anxiety, Depression, and Suspiciousness in the Home Care Setting. Journal of Home Healthcare Nursing 11: 35–40, 1993
39. Lipsman R, Fader D, Harmon J: Developing Home-Based Mental Health Services for Maine's Older Adults. Pride

Institute Journal of Long Term Home Health Care 2 (1): 29–38, 1992
40. Marvan-Hyam J: Occupational Stress of the Home Health Nurse. Home Healthcare Nurs 4 (3): 18–21, 1986
41. Mellon SK: Mental Health Clinical Nurse Specialist in Home Care for the 90s. Issues in Mental Health Nursing 15: 229–237, 1994
42. Menenberg SR: Somatopsychology and AIDS Victims. J Psychosoc Nurs Ment Health Serv 25 (5): 18–22, 1987
43. Menosky J: Occupational Therapy Services for the Homebound Psychiatric Patient. Journal of Home Health Care Practice 2 (3): 57–67, 1990
44. Muijen M, Marks I, Connolly J, et al: Home Based Care and Standard Hospital Care for Patients With Severe Mental Illness; A Randomized Control Trial. British Journal of Medicine 304: 749–753, 1992
45. Omdahl DJ: Preventing Home Care Denials. Am J Nurs 8 (August): 1031–1033, 1987
46. Pai S, Nagarajaiah: Treatment of Schizophrenic Patients in Their Homes Through a Visiting Nurse—Some Issues in the Nurse's Training. Int J Nurs Stud 19: 167–172, 1982
47. Phillips L, Rempusheski V: Caring for the Frail Elderly at Home: Toward a Theoretical Explanation of the Dynamics of Poor Quality Family Caregiving. Advances in Nursing Science 8 (4): 62–84, 1986
48. Pigot HE, Trott L: Translating Research into Practice: The Implementation of an In-Home Crisis Intervention Triage and Treatment Service in the Private Sector. American Journal of Medical Quality 8 (3): 138–144, 1993
49. Querida A: The Shaping of Community Mental Health Care. In Breslau LD, Haug MR (eds): Depression and Aging Causes, Care, and Consequences, p 201. New York, Springer, 1983
50. Quinlan J, Ohlund G: Psychiatric Home Care: An Introduction. Home Healthcare Nurse, 13 (4): 20–24, 1993
51. Rice R: Suicidal Thoughts and Ideation. Home Healthcare Nurse 11: 67, 1993
52. Richie F, Lusky K: Psychiatric Home Health Nursing: A New Role in Community Mental Health. J Community Ment Health 23 (3): 229–235, 1987
53. Schipske G: Documenting Care for the Patient at Home. The Coordinator 3 (4): 19–21, 1984
54. Sharpe D: Community Nursing—Psychiatry in the Home. Nursing Mirror 150 (2): 34–36, 1980
55. Solomon K, Harris MR: A Study of Client Acceptance of Various Professionals in Psychiatric Home Visits. Hosp Community Psychiatry 28 (9): 661–665, 1977
56. Soreff SM: Indications for Home Treatment. Psychiatr Clin North Am 8 (3): 563–575, 1985
57. Soreff SM: Psychiatric Home Care Revisited: Its Scope and Advantages. Continuum, Spring 1 (1): 71–78, 1994
58. Stanhope M, Lancaster J: Community Health Nursing: Process and Practice for Promoting Health. St. Louis, CV Mosby, 1984
59. Stanton L, Heymans G: A Pilot Study to Evaluate Visiting Nurses' Services to Chronic Psychiatric Patients. Hosp Community Psychiatry 28 (2): 97–101, 1977
60. Steffl BM, Eide I: Long-Term Care: Discharge Planning, Home Care, and Alternatives. In Steffl BM (ed): Handbook of Gerontological Nursing, pp 498–512. New York, Van Nostrand Reinhold, 1984
61. Thoaben M: Depression in the Medically Ill Homebound Patient. Journal of Home Health Care Practice 2 (3): 33–38, 1990
62. Thobaben M: Developing a Psychiatric Nursing Home Health Service. Caring 6: 10–14, 1989
63. Thobaben M, Kozlak J: Home Health Care's Unique Role in Serving the Elderly Mentally Ill. Home Healthcare Nurse 2(3): 16–20, 1990
64. Todd J: Community Nurse: CPN–A Life Line Keeping Psychiatric Patients at Home. Nurs Mirror 147 (15): 46–48, 1978
65. Townsend M: Drug Guide for Psychiatric Nursing. Philadelphia, FA Davis, 1990
66. Trimath M, Brestensky J: The Role of the Mental Health Nurse in Home Health Care. Home Health Care Practice d2 (3): 1–8, 1990
67. Van Dongen CJ, Jambunathan J: Pilot Study Results: The Psychiatric RN Case Manager. J Psychosoc Nurs 30: 11–14, 1992
68. Wagner BD: Innovations in the Geriatric Continuum of Care. Continuum 1 (1): 51–60, 1994
72. Wasson W, Ripeckyj A, Lazarus LW, Kupferer S, Barry S, Force F: Home Evaluation of Psychiatrically Impaired Elderly: Process and Outcome. Gerontologist 24: 238–242, 1984
70. Weiner LW, Becker A, Friedman TT: Home Treatment: Spearhead of Community Psychiatry. In Breslau LD, Haug MR (eds): Depression and Aging Causes, Care, and Consequences, pp 201–202. New York, Springer, 1983
71. Weinstein S: Specialty Teams in Home Care. Am J Nurs 84 (3): 342–345, 1984
72. West DA, Litwok E, Oberlander K, Martin DA: Emergency Psychiatric Home Visiting: Report of Four Years' Experience. J Clin Psychiatry 41 (4): 113–118, 1980

Community-Based Care and Rehabilitation

Mary Huggins

45

There are bridges in geography
. . .from Manhattan to Brooklyn
There are bridges in music
There are bridges in life. . .
. . .birth
. . .marriage
. . .death
There are bridges
. . .between genders
. . .between cultures
. . .between philosophies of healing

Bobette Perrone, H. Henrietta Stoeckel, and Victoria Kruger, "Bridges" in Medicine Woman; Curanderas and Women Doctors, *1990*

A community support system is defined as a "network of caring and responsible people committed to assisting a vulnerable population to meet their needs and develop their potentials without being unnecessarily isolated or excluded from the community."[29] *This definition encompasses the basic philosophy of care meant to address humanely the needs of adults with severe and persistent (severe) mental illnesses that seriously limit their ability to function in the primary areas of daily living. Before the Community Support Program (CSP), a federal initiative, these people had been labeled deinstitutionalized. In the 1970s, a General Accounting Office report publicly recognized that the social policies surrounding deinstitutionalization were not effectively addressing the basic needs of people with severe mental illness.*

In an attempt to address these issues, the Community Support Service Branch was established in the National Institute of Mental Health (NIMH). This program was transferred to the newly formed Center for Mental Health Services in 1992. The purpose of the Branch was to promote community support systems in all areas of the country. Since its establishment, this movement has made an amazing impact on the delivery system of broad-ranged services and support needed for this special population to live in the least restrictive environment. The movement also recognizes the need for quality of life. Much has been learned. Much is left undone. This chapter presents a historical and philosophical context for the development of community support systems, explores the effects of the community support movement on delivery systems, and projects trends that will affect continued delivery of community-based care.

Learning Objectives

On completion of this chapter, you should be able to accomplish the following:

1. *Define the term community support system.*
2. *Describe the philosophical context of the community support initiative.*
3. *Identify the essential components of a community support system.*
4. *Explain the relationship of case management and service coordination to the effectiveness of a community support system.*
5. *Compare at least five models for the delivery of community support services.*
6. *Describe the impact of community support systems on clients and their families.*
7. *Identify the trends that affect social policy regarding the care of people with severe mental illnesses.*
8. *Describe the role of the nurse in a community support system.*

◆ Definition of Community Support System

Like community mental health (see Chapter 43, Community Mental Health), a community support system must be defined philosophically and operationally. The changing focus and locale described in the definition of community mental health is built on and refined in the definition of community support systems. Not only does an effective community support system require all the components of community mental health, it also requires elements of systems theory. It is "more than a list of necessary service components. . .the range of service components must be organized into an integrated system."[2]

A community support system can be seen as a systems model that delivers community-based care for a specific population formerly requiring admission to hospitals for significant portions of their lives. This system includes a range of life supports (health, mental health, and rehabilitation services), social networks, housing arrangements, and educational and employment opportunities. It not only delivers these specific services, but also can be exemplified by several program models. Conceptually, a community support system operates on the system level through the linkage of a network of agencies dedicated to providing services to support people with severe mental illnesses in the least restrictive environment; on the program level, community support systems operate through various program models.

The network is coordinated by a single agency responsible for organization and coordination of the system and for negotiation among the various agencies forming the network of services. This agency is responsible for articulating the philosophical and operational basis for the network and allows active participation of all people with an investment in the system (ie, the consumer, family member, government official, and provider). The community support system is not a single model but embraces and incorporates many models to provide comprehensive services to meet the diverse needs of the population. To achieve the comprehensiveness needed to address the needs of people with severe mental illness, a community support system maintains flexibility, allowing for incorporation of the positive elements of several generic models, such as the medical, rehabilitation, and social support models, while promoting a seamless system of service delivery.

Essential components of a community support system are as follows:[26]

1. Identification of and assertive outreach to the population at risk to inform the individual of available services and to ensure access to needed services, which may include arranging for needed transportation
2. Provision of adequate mental health care, including diagnostic evaluations, prescribed medications, periodic reviews, management of psychotropic medication therapy, and community-based psychi-

atric or psychological services, counseling, and treatment that may be specialized (eg, substance abuse treatment)
3. Development of linkages to provide access to medical and dental services, including help in applying for medical assistance benefits, and provision of health services in vivo and transportation to appointments
4. Provision of 24-hour quick-response assistance to enable the family and individual to cope more effectively with crises while maintaining the individual's status as a functioning community member; requires the availability of crisis options on a 24-hour basis provided by trained professionals at various sites when necessary, including at home, in the criminal justice system, or on the job
5. Provision of psychosocial and vocational services through various rehabilitative options for an indefinite duration, focusing primarily on improving the individual's ability to function in normal social roles (eg, training in daily living and community living skills, development of social skills, interests, and leisure activities) and assistance in finding and making use of appropriate employment and vocational services
6. Provision of a range of rehabilitative and supportive housing options based on choice and offering the necessary degree of support, incentives, and encouragement for the individual to accept increasing responsibility for his or her own life
7. Provision of backup support, assistance, consultation, and education to families, friends, landlords, employers, and community agencies and referrals to family self-help or advocacy programs (eg, the National Alliance for the Mentally Ill, Reach) to maximize the benefits of individuals living in the community and minimize problems associated with their presence
8. Recognition and involvement of concerned community members and endorsement of the natural support system, including consumer and family self-help groups, churches, community organizations, commerce, and industry in the development and implementation of community support systems on the systems level
9. Assistance in the application for entitlements (eg, financial, medical, and housing and other benefits) crucial to meeting basic human needs, including assistance in obtaining food, clothing, shelter, general medical and dental care and assistance in ensuring that personal safety has been taken into account
10. Protection of the individual's rights, provision of information regarding basic civil rights and available resources, and access to advocacy and grievance procedures to ensure that appropriate mechanisms are in place to protect these rights
11. Availability of case management (a single person or team) responsible for helping the individual make informed choices, ensuring timely access to needed assistance, providing opportunities and encouragement for self-help, and coordinating all services to meet the needs of the individual
12. Provision of these components through an integrated system that is responsive to the individual's needs, including special needs (eg, elderly people, young adults, people who are homeless and mentally ill, people in the criminal justice system, people who are developmentally disabled or hearing impaired)

An overriding element of these components is respect for each person's dignity and individual needs and empowerment rather than dependency. The goal is to enable people with a severe mental illness to remain in the community and function at optimal levels of independence. People who constitute this population are diverse and have unique concerns, abilities, motivations, and problems. Therefore, the guiding principles of a community support system are based on services that provide for the following:

1. self-determination
2. individuation
3. normalization of settings and offerings
4. least restrictive appropriate settings
5. maximization of mutual assistance and self-help[15]

In addition, the system needs to be culturally competent (guided by the provision of coordinated, flexible, racially and culturally appropriate services that focus on the individual's strengths) and held accountable to the consumers of the services.

The CSP has been an effective model to focus attention at all levels of government on people with severe mental illness. Effective CSPs "have positive sanction for their activities and service function from the highest level of local and state administration."[15] This includes visibility and continuing support from all levels of government—city, county, and state—to affect services at the systems level (eg, police, housing authorities, and local planning boards). This attention has helped to publicize the conditions under which this vulnerable population must exist and to identify the needs of people with severe mental illness as a priority.

◆ Background Information

When the Community Mental Health Centers Act established community mental health centers (CMHC) throughout the nation, a series of pharmacological breakthroughs led to the development of several new drugs. This combination promised a new era in the treatment of long-term mental illness—deinstitutionalization. By 1974, residents in public mental institutions had declined to 216,000 compared to 559,000 in 1955.[32] This placement in the community occurred without the needed supports to maintain basic community living. Most CMHCs and other programs were ill-equipped and unprepared to assume responsibility for needed support services. Deinstitutionalization resulted in a depopulation of public mental institutions without the concomitant establishment of needed supports or adequate funding for community alternatives.

Deinstitutionalization is not the sole cause of the system's problems. Long-term neglect of people in need has been at least equally responsible. As the era of depopulation progressed, former clients of the state hospitals began the revolving door syndrome. With the lack of community alternatives and the tightening of admissions to the state hospital, recidivism was imminent. As numbers grew, attention turned to the living conditions under which deinstitutionalized people must live. Conditions in many communities were as bad as those in institutions, with isolation, neglect, nontreatment, and sometimes physical abuse added to the mental illness.[27]

In addition, a number of younger people experiencing mental illness began to be extruded from their home communities. In past years, this younger group would have been hospitalized, but closing of the public hospitals and tightening of admission criteria precluded their admission. Thus, added to the increasing population of people who were deinstitutionalized were these young people who had never been in an institution. Combined with these individuals were the ever-increasing number of homeless people with mental illness.

In this environment, CSP was conceived. Several studies (eg, a report from the General Accounting Office) and newspaper, magazine, and television accounts focused on deinstitutionalization. Attention was brought to bear on the lack of services to promote growth and autonomy and provide support to people with mental illness in the community. As a result, in 1974, NIMH formed an ad hoc committee that culminated in a task force recommendation to establish community alternatives encompassing the essential components needed for people with mental illness to live in the community. With unexpended federal funds from Hospital Improvement Program grants, the CSP initiative was launched on a shoestring in 1977. Since 1977, all 50 states, the District of Columbia and several U.S. territories have developed CSPs. This initiative prioritized the problem, thereby giving it the attention needed to develop models of care, including other areas of human services (eg, housing and employment) and coordinating the system.[30]

In 1992, Congress established the Center for Mental Health Services under Public Law 102-321 to assist states to improve and increase the range of qualitative service offerings in response to the expanding numbers of individuals with mental illness, their families, and their communities. The CSP was incorporated into this Center under the Public Health Service. The Public Health Service developed a report "Healthy People 2000: National Health Promotion and Disease Prevention Objectives," which includes the setting of national priority areas for the promotion of health and the prevention of diseases. This report includes several objectives relating to mental health and mental disorders. The CSP remains integral to the implementation of these objectives as they relate to severe mental illness.

◆ Philosophical Basis of Community Support Systems

Community support systems encompass a philosophy based on values that act on three levels: the individual, the agency, and the network. These values are centered on the individual, allowing the consumer to be central to the system. As such, the individual maintains involvement in decisions that affect the needed services. The central theme of community support is empowerment, recognizing the following three tenets:

1. All people are valuable and should be afforded dignity, respect, and the opportunity to take full advantage of their human, legal, and social rights.
2. Every human being is capable of growth, development, and learning.
3. Services should be provided in a normative and socially valued way.

PRINCIPLES OF PSYCHIATRIC REHABILITATION

These values can be embodied in various settings. However, certain principles have been identified as basic to psychiatric rehabilitation settings:[3]

1. The primary focus is on the improvement of the capabilities and the competence of the person with psychiatric problems, even the most disabled. The alleviation of symptoms is secondary.
2. Insight is not a primary goal; rather, the focus is on the person's ability to function.
3. The provision of services is eclectic and uses a variety of therapeutic constructs.
4. Improvement of vocational outcomes is a central focus.

5. Emphasis on positive expectations and hope is essential to the process.
6. A deliberate increase in dependency, as in sheltered settings, may be a first step in the process.
7. Active participation and involvement of the individual in rehabilitation, the operation of programs, and the delivery of services is sought to provide rehabilitation with, rather than to, the individual.
8. Development of individual skills and environmental resources is fundamental in the rehabilitation process.

Thus, the comprehensive network of services recognizes and emphasizes continuity of care, in many cases for an indefinite time.

◆ Access

An effective community support system embraces a comprehensive spectrum of services for people with severe mental illness and their relatives. These services are not related to the specific content of a particular program model but are part of the programs's philosophy, operating style, and leadership.[15] Several models providing access to the community support system have been identified. These models may be developed singly or in combination.[27] Each must contain the essential components of an effective community support system, either within the program or by means of linkages to the provider system. Although all program models share similarities, they differ in comprehensiveness and in the degree to which services are provided or brokered. Additionally, these models are based on individually tailored program plans with realistic goals based on an assessment of the individual's strengths and weaknesses.

PROGRAM MODELS

The services in these program models are delivered for the most part in real-life communities (in vivo), as opposed to hospital settings, to promote the transfer of learning through modeling and immediate reinforcement. These sites include, but are not limited to, home, school, and work. Five examples are briefly described.

Psychosocial Rehabilitation Model

The psychosocial rehabilitation model evolved from Fountain House, which was founded by a group of clients in New York City in 1948. This model is generally organized as a clubhouse with members who are full participants in the program operation. Services usually are divided into four major areas:

1. social or recreational
2. vocational
3. residential
4. educational

Members are provided the opportunity to participate in a wide variety of activities relating to the management of the program (eg, meal preparation, newsletter publication, janitorial services) and decision making regarding program operation. Evaluation indicates that this model is effective in reducing hospitalizations and improving community functioning, particularly in the area of vocation and independent living for long-term members.[6]

Fairweather Lodge Model

The Fairweather Lodge model was begun in 1960. It uses the hospital as a training center for clients who subsequently move into the community to live in a lodge and operate a small business. Group norms and peer support form the foundation of this model. All members of the lodge participate fully in the lodge and the workplace, using appropriate work roles and habits. Evaluation indicates a reduction in recidivism and an increase in community employment activities.[11]

Training in Community Living Model

This model (also known as the program of assertive community treatment) was begun in the 1970s in Madison, Wisconsin. It involves in vivo teaching of basic coping skills in the client's environment. It is an extremely directive approach, taking treatment to the individual through role modeling and support and treating the individual as a responsible citizen. The hospital is used only in extreme cases. This model emphasizes the importance of clinical management, including appropriate medications and medication monitoring. It teaches the individual about symptoms, the relationship of the symptom to stress, and how to control the symptom.

Research indicates that this model is effective in helping the individual to maintain stability in the community. Stability is exhibited by increased work productivity, decreased symptomatology, decreased hospitalization, decreased unemployment, and increased satisfaction with life.[34]

Consumer-Run Alternative Models

The consumer-run alternative models endorse that the planning, administering, delivery, and evaluation of services is done for consumers by consumers. Philosophically, this is a self-help model. Its core is voluntary participation, consumer control, and empowerment. Several such alternatives have been developed. Social, recreational, and educational services frequently are added to the core drop-in center, which may also include community and public education and advocacy at the individual and public policy levels. Consumer alternatives have also been started in the areas of residential, crisis, and vocational services.

Several states have developed offices devoted to consumer programming and advocacy within the state office of mental health. The Michigan Department of Mental Health has collected data that indicate a highly successful experience overall based on high attendance and high levels of reported satisfaction. Additional research has been recommended to assess the negative effects on consumers who staff these alternatives.[19] In addition to the establishment of an office in the Ohio State Department of Mental Health specific for consumer issues, Ohio has made an evaluator available to assist consumer-run programs in the development of a sound and consumer-acceptable evaluation.

Community Worker Models

The community worker models rely on ordinary citizens to provide a range of community support services. These services are generally provided on a part-time paid or volunteer basis. Services include friendship, emotional support, teaching of community living skills, and assistance in accessing appropriate services. The community worker complements professional mental health services by modeling appropriate behaviors and monitoring the individual's level of functioning. Two primary variations of this model exist.

The community supportive care variation (Rhinelander model), originating in rural Wisconsin, pays lay citizens to function as community support workers. It emphasizes one-to-one relationships.

The Compeer variation uses volunteers to provide caring, supportive relationships. It originated in Rochester, New York, as an adjunct to therapy, filling in for a lack of natural supports.

Evaluation of these variations suggests a reduction in rehospitalization rates and days and positive changes in the individuals's ability to socialize and cope in the community.[7,9]

◆ Public Policy and Trends

The CSP is a system change initiative. Therefore, public policy issues needing attention become the focus or are identified by the development of an effective community support system. Certain areas of concern have become obstacles at worst, and challenges at best, to the delivery of community-based care for people with severe mental illness. The following is a list of major issues providing significant challenges:[31]

1. In the United States, 22% of adults experience severe mental illness, creating diseases with a debilitation potential similar to chronic heart disease; 12% of all children are affected by mental and emotional disturbances.
2. Approximately one-third of the 600,000 people who are homeless on a given night have a serious mental illness; more than half also have a substance abuse problem.
3. Recent estimates indicate that nearly 7% (54,000) of all inmates have a serious mental illness and that 12.5% (95,000) inmates require some psychiatric attention.
4. Of the more than 40 million adults with a mental illness requiring treatment, only one in four receive the needed treatment.
5. Many of the more than 1.5 million individuals suffering from human immunodeficiency virus or acquired immunodeficiency syndrome also experience severe psychological distress.
6. Culturally relevant services are not available as a matter of course for people of color (eg, Native Americans, African Americans) and thousands of refugees and detainees (including former political prisoners from Vietnam and their families, Pentecostal refugees from the former Soviet Union, Mariel Cubans).

◆ Effects of Chronicity in Severe Mental Illness

A growing body of knowledge identifies mental illness as a disease of the brain. Severe mental illness must be recognized as a chronic condition, much like multiple sclerosis, chronic heart disease, and other chronic, debilitating diseases. This recognition would counter the myth of a quick cure. It also would diminish the belief that people with a severe mental illness can live without supportive treatment, such as medication, and varying degrees of treatment intensity and length as the need arises. Additionally, gross confusion between the disease and the symptoms occurs, perpetuating the myth that severe mental illness precludes opportunities for rehabilitation. According to Pepper, "in failing to specify the differences between chronic mental disorder and long-term social disability, we perpetuate the myth that they are synonymous. In fact, the social disability is separate and its development is neither inevitable or incurable. Such confusion victimizes patients with a chronic disorder by denying them the opportunity for rehabilitation of their social disorder."[21]

RESOURCES

Conflicting federal, state, and local mandates have precluded the targeting of resources (funds and staff) to the community. This can be best documented simply by looking at the dramatic shift of funding responsibility in the last 30 years.

In the late 1960s, most costs for this population rested with state governments (primarily in state hospitals). More recently, responsibility for the provision of community-based care has rested at the local government level, with federal payments and reimbursements to support the individual. However, responsibility for overall planning and policy making has remained at the state level. Funding bases that were not intended to support people with mental illness have become the core for community-based treatment (Medicaid and Supplemental Security Income). At present, Medicaid funding, although limited in noninstitutional settings, is the major source of health care funding for poor people, including most people with severe mental illness. This has resulted in inappropriate admissions to nursing facilities and other institutions simply to receive appropriate care. In some states, commitment laws have been promulgated in an attempt to stem inappropriate admissions to state hospitals. Families of people with severe mental illness are becoming active in attempts to loosen these laws. This activity is due both to the difficulty in admitting their loved ones and to their sense that hospitalization is necessary to address appropriately the individual's needs.

Reliance on Supplemental Security Income as the major source of financial support for people with severe mental illness allows little opportunity for choices. Many of these people live in unlicensed facilities with little or no follow-up care. The average monthly stipend is such that little is left after paying the rent. Opportunities are limited or nonexistent due to the lack of funds for recreation, clothing, and transportation. Additionally, these limited stipends can buy only a level of housing most generally found in the poorer areas of the inner city; thus, the so-called social services ghetto is established.[13]

Further, a person who gets a job generally remains in low-paying and entry level positions and risks losing the limited benefits that have been made available (eg, access to health care).[33] This situation is further complicated by the mental illness, which in many cases is exacerbated by stress. A person who is rehospitalized or is unable to work on a long-term basis loses benefits and medical insurance. Some legislative efforts have been developed in recognition of the person's ability to work on a sporadic or part-time basis. However, efforts made in this area may be moot as Congress moves toward the elimination of federal programs that support the housing, vocational, and basic health benefits for disabled individuals. Unless safety net services remain intact, serious problems resulting in reinstitutionalization may occur.

REINSTITUTIONALIZATION

Due to the fundamental lack of public policy to date and the potential dissolving of the current infrastructure, serious problems are surfacing associated with reinstitutionalization of people with severe mental illness. This is occurring in hospitals and jails. As responsibility for people with severe mental illness remains in limbo, local government is being overwhelmed by the large numbers of inadequately housed or homeless people. This increases the number of people coming to the attention of the local authorities—taken to jails or committed to a hospital.

SAFETY NET SERVICES

Regulation and legislation must emphasize the establishment of community support services as an essential safety net, including case management and interagency cooperation in all local areas. Data have underscored the effectiveness of case management and community supports on the increased quality of life for people involved in these programs. Historically, these services have not been eligible for Medicaid and other sources of funding. Payment for case management, day treatment, psychosocial programs, housing supports, and other community supports and parity for outpatient and other health care coverage are essential to any funding of community treatment alternatives.

Mainstream resources at the local and state level are equally important in the development of effective community-based alternatives to meet the needs of individuals being discharged from state hospital and nursing facilities (as required under the Nursing Home Reform Act of 1987).[10,25] The passage of the Americans With Disabilities Act and the Fair Housing Act provides for protection of individual rights; this is a springboard for the development of a comprehensive community support system.[4,16,14]

STIGMA

General ignorance regarding mental illness is perpetuated by the media. Sometimes this ignorance is exhibited as frustration about the person's inability to be cured; other times it is exhibited as fear of the person's perceived differentness. Whatever the basis, the outcome is stigma and discrimination. Stigma may take place at the job location, resulting in not being hired or hired for only entry-level, low-expectation positions. Stigma in housing can take the form of refusing to rent to a person with mental illness or raising the rent just above the fair market rate, thus precluding the use of a subsidy. Stigma may take the form of developing restrictive zoning that regulates where the person can live.

Stigma may take place on the street, when passersby avert their eyes and avoid interaction. Although it is clearly discriminatory to refuse jobs and housing based on a person's diagnosis, fear regarding personal safety and community welfare has allowed these practices to continue. Further, the frustration of seeing a person with "an obvious illness" not receiving cared has escalated the stigma, hindering community acceptance.

At the forefront of the antistigma campaigns are consumer and family movements. These groups demand to be involved in the development of treatment alternatives. They provide advocacy and knowledge regarding the disease—including realistic expectations—to other consumers, family members, and the general public. In many parts of the county, consumers and families are involved in antistigma media watches and public education and advocacy.

Consumers and family members are increasingly involved at the decision-making levels of government, helping to shape future policies and practices. In many states, legislation requires consumer or family member participation at the decision-making level (eg, the Minnesota Comprehensive Mental Health Systems Act).

In adapting the Principles of Psychiatric Rehabilitation, Anthony has provided a challenge of hope as an "essential ingredient"—hope for recovery and as a guiding vision of the future.[1]

REFORMS

Social and health care reforms must be assessed to ascertain their effectiveness as proposed public policy. Although total agreement on needed reforms has not been reached, the following reforms are being viewed with some unanimity:

1. The development of a comprehensive policy for people with severe mental illness in the least restrictive alternative should range from prevention to hospitalization (noting that in some instances, hospitalization is the least restrictive alterative) and should include accommodation for acute episodes. This policy should recognize the need for supportive housing and other community support services, including recreation, jobs, and medical, dental, and mental health services.[8,21,24,5]
2. Government policy and funding must be directed toward the development of a comprehensive, unified, seamless network of community support services in each community. According to Pepper, "state governments, being the repositories of constitutional responsibility for the mentally ill, [must] take the initiative in developing policies" addressing the following areas: entitlement of citizens to intensive interventions funded by private insurance when available and by public funding when it is not; comprehensive, integrated outpatient alternatives and community support services when needed; and integrated services for people with dual disabilities.[21]
3. Active initiatives are needed from the federal government in the development of federal policy regarding financial resources and regulations so that quality community-based alternatives can become a reality.[21]
4. Antistigma efforts should focus on the general population to promote an understanding of mental illness, incorporating research about the illness as a chronic disease.
5. Active initiatives for health care reform should include parity for mental health services, recognizing that although people with severe mental illness typically do not do well in mainstream health maintenance organizations, new systems designed to address the high-risk consumer may have potential.[18]

Although many other needs in the area of public policy are evident, initiatives begun by the federal CSP must continue so that safety net services are in place and trends resulting in untoward outcomes, such as reinsitutionalization in hospitals and jails, can be averted. Community support services have been acknowledged nationally in the role of working with existing resources to develop community alternatives.[24] The emphasis on social integration providing bridging for people with psychiatric disabilities to "participate in all aspects of community life" (housing, employment, school, recreation) is the basis of social integration.[22,28]

◆ The Nurse's Role

As in community mental health, the nurse is in a unique position to assess individual and community supports. Further, the nurse has the ability to focus on a particular situation while retaining a holistic approach. Such an approach blends physical, mental, and social needs with community environmental norms.

Nurses are unique in their ability to bridge the gap between the hospital and community, the psychiatrist and community caregiver, and the public and other health care providers.[20] Nursing education emphasizes teamwork and sharing of responsibility with others to an extent rarely found in other professions. Nurses understand the needs and responsibilities of 24-hour programming. When included on community teams, nurses enhance the teams' understanding of treatment alternatives, medications and side effects, and the importance of client education and teaching to reduce stress and alleviate episodes.[12] This unique background is underscored as clients in the community are treated with drugs (eg, clozapine [Clozaril]) that require assertive outreach and monitoring to encourage compliance. Nurses understand the importance of physical movement to decrease muscle atrophy and other long-term effects resulting from lack of full range-of-motion exercise frequently associated with mental illness.

The combination of inpatient, public health, and psychiatric nursing knowledge based on good physical assessment skills is imperative in community-based programs. Understanding the role of stress offers the nurse the ability to provide the integrative link among community resources, housing, vocation, social relationships, and psychiatric episodes; the nurse helps to separate the disease from the social disability.[21] Nurses educate the consumer, professional, and public regarding the disability, medication effects or side effects, interventions to diminish harm, and effects of stress on mental disorders.

Nurses have traditionally worked with natural support systems to develop care plans. In many parts of the country, nurses have initiated contact with tribal healers, curanderas, midwives, or other healers in the implementation of this plan. Integration of the nursing care process into the community support system is therefore a logical extension of the nurse's role.

◆ Chapter Summary

Research indicates that community support is crucial to quality of life for people with severe mental illness in the community. This chapter has presented an overview of the development of community support systems and the essential issues and trends in community-based care. The following points are among those discussed:

1. The goal of community support systems is to enable people with severe mental illness to remain in the community and function at optimal levels of independence.
2. A community support system encourages participation of all people in the system—consumers, family members, government officials, and providers—to deliver a full range of life-supportive care. The Community Support Service Branch, now part of the Center for Mental Health Services, promotes community support systems in all areas of the country.
3. Services are based on guiding principles that promote self-determination and individuation. Important goals are to achieve normalization of setting in the least restrictive environment, and to provide supportive, neutral assistance in a culturally competent way.
4. Essential components of a community support system include: active outreach efforts; help in ensuring access to services; psychosocial and vocational development programs; rehabilitative and supportive housing options; crisis intervention services; family and community education programs.
5. Several effective program models have been identified. In the psychosocial rehabilitation and Fairweather Lodge models, community members participate in activities that relate to program management and operation. The PACT model emphasizes clinical management of symptoms and development of coping skills. Consumer-run alternative models are self-help programs based on voluntary participation and personal empowerment. Community worker models rely on ordinary citizens to supplement and enhance professional mental health services.
6. Consumer and family movements have been increasingly active in promoting the destigmatization of mental illness, developing treatment alternatives, and helping to shape policy at all levels of government.
7. Nurses can serve as an important link between hospital and community, and can bring essential knowledge and skills to a community-based treatment team.

Critical Thinking Questions

1. *In what ways can nurses affect the outcome of mentally ill clients in the community?*
2. *What skills do nurses have that enable them to be "bridges" in community-based care?*
3. *What mental health needs does a client in the community have that differ from those of an institutionalized client?*
4. *Why are there such a variety of community support systems models that are currently used to deliver community-based care?*
5. *What are the underlying needs of the mentally ill that support the need for social and health care reforms?*

Review Questions

1. When defining an effective community support system, what factors need to be considered?
   A. The needs and functioning level of people with serious mental illness

B. A basic philosophy of care based on values and guiding principles
C. A specific model program
D. All of the above
E. A and B only

2. A community support system delivers community-based care through linkage to a network of agencies. This network provides the following services:
   A. Mental health services
   B. Rehabilitation services
   C. Medical service
   D. Social support services
   E. All of the above
3. The primary focus of a community support system is to
   A. Eliminate symptoms.
   B. Focus on functioning.
   C. Bring rehabilitation to the individual.
   D. Develop skills and improve outcomes.
   E. All of the above
   F. B and D only
4. The nurse provides for which of the following services in a community support system?
   A. Medication monitoring
   B. Group therapy
   C. System advocate
   D. All of the above
   E. A and B only

◆ References

1. Anthony W: Recovery From Mental Illness: The Guiding Vision of the Mental Health Service System in the 1990s. Psychosoc Rehab J 16: 11–24, 1993
2. Anthony W, Blanch A: Research on Community Support Services What We Have Learned. Psychosoc Rehab J 12 (3): 55–81, 1989
3. Anthony W, Cohen M, Cohen B: Psychiatric Rehabilitation. In Talbot J (ed): The Chronic Mental Patient: Five Years Later. New York, Grune & Stratton, 1984
4. Bazelon Center for Mental Health Law: What Does Fair Housing Mean to People With Disabilities? The Housing Center: 1–27, May, 1994
5. Bond G: Applying Psychiatric Rehabilitation Principles To Employment: Recent Findings from Schizophrenia. In Ancill RJ, Holiday J, Higgenbottom J (eds): Exploring the Spectrum of Psychosis. Chichester, NY, John Wiley and Sons, 1994
6. Bond G, Dincin J, Setze P, Witheridge T: The Effectiveness of Psychiatric Rehabilitation: A Summary of Research at Thresholds. Psychosoc Rehab J 7 (4): 6–22, 1984
7. Cannady D: Chronics and Cleaning Ladies. Psychosoc Rehab J 5 (1): 13–16, 1982
8. Carling PJ, Ridgway P: A Psychiatric Rehabilitation Approach To Housing. In Anthony W, Farka M(eds): Psychiatric Rehabilitation: Program and Practices. Baltimore, Johns Hopkins University Press, 1989
9. Compeer Program: Annual Report 1984–1985. Rochester, NY, Compeer, 1985
10. Cook J, Jonikas J, Soloman M: Models of Vocational Rehabilitation for Youth and Adults With Severe Mental Illness: Implications for America 2000 and the ADA. American Rehab 18 (3): 6–11, 1992
11. Fairweather G: The Prototype Lodge Society: Instituting Group Process Principles, New Directions for Mental Health Services-The Fairweather Lodge: A Twenty-Five Year Retrospective. San Francisco, Jossey-Bass, 1980
12. Huggins M: A Model Case Management System in a Local CSS: Community Support Network News, Vol 4, No 4. Boston University Center For Psychiatric Rehabilitation, December, 1985
13. Jonikas J, Cook J: Safe, Secure and Street Smart: Empowering Women with Mental Illness to Achieve Greater Independence in the Community. Chicago, Thresholds National Research and Training Center, 1993
14. Kincaid J: The ADA and Section 504: Legal Mechanisms for Achieving Effective Supported Education: Community Support Network News, Vol 10, No 2. Boston University Center for Psychiatric Rehabilitation, 1994
15. Libermann R, Kuehnel T, Phipps C, Cardin V: Resource Book for Psychiatric Rehabilitation: Elements of Services for the Mentally Ill. Camarillo, CA, Center fir Rehabilitation Research and Training in Mental Illness, UCLA School of Medicine, 1984
16. Mancuso L: Case Studies on Reasonable Accommodations for Workers With Psychiatric Disabilities. Center for Mental Health Services, The California Department of Mental Health and California Department of Rehabilitation, Sacramento, CA, 1993
17. Manderscheid RW: CSP Research Accomplishments: Community Support Network News, Vol 4. No 2. Boston University Center For Psychiatric Rehabilitation, October, 1987
18. Mechanic D, Aiken L: Improving the Care of Patients With Chronic Mental Illness. N Engl J Med 317 (26): 1634–1638, 1987
19. Mowbry C, Chamberlain P, Jenning M: Final Report: Consumer Run Alternative Services: Demonstration and Evaluation Projects 1982–1984. Lansing, MI, Research and Evaluation Division, Michigan Department of Mental Health, 1984
20. Palmer-Erbs V, Anthony W: Incorporating Psychiatric Rehabilitation Principles Into Mental Health Nursing. J Psychosoc Nurs 3 (3): 36–44, 1995
21. Pepper B: A Public Policy for the Long-Term Mentally Ill: A Positive Alternative to Reinstitutionalization. Am J Orthopsychiatry 57 (3): 452–457, 1987
22. Reidy D: Shattering Illusions of Difference. Resources 4: 2, 3–6, 1992
23. Rubenstein L, Koyanagi C, Manes J: Mental Health Funding. Hosp Community Psychiatry 38 (4): 410–412, 1987
24. Searight HR, Handal PJ: Psychiatric Deinstitutionalization: The Possibilities and the Reality. Psychiatr Q 58 (3): 153–166, 1987
25. Schaftt G, Randolf F: Innovative Community Based Ser-

vices for Older Persons With Mental Illness. U.S. Department of Health and Human Services, Center for Mental Health Services CSP, Rockville, MD, 1994

26. Stroul B: Introduction to the Special Issue: The Community Support System Concept. Psychosoc Rehab J 11 (2): 5–8, 1987
27. Stroul B: Models of Community Support Services: Approaches to Helping Persons With Long-Term Mental Illness. National Institute of Mental Health, Community Support Program, Rockville, MD, 1986
28. Sullivan A: Supported Education, Past, Present and Future. Community Support Network News, Vol 10, No 2. Boston University Center for Psychiatric Rehabilitation, 1994
29. Turner J: Comprehensive Community Support Systems for Severely Mentally Disabled Adults: Definitions, Components and Guiding Principles, rev ed. National Institute of Mental Health, Rockville, MD, 1986
30. U.S. Department of Health and Human Services: Caring for People With Severe Mental Disorders: A National Plan of Research to Improve Services. National Institute of Mental Health, National Advisory Mental Health Council, Washington, DC, 1991
31. U.S. Department of Health and Human Services: CMHS Mission, from a Bulletin of the Center for Mental Health Services. Rockville, MD, Center for Mental Health Services, 1994
32. U.S. Department of Health and Human Services: Toward a National Plan for the Chronically Mentally Ill: Report to the Secretary by the Department of Health and Human Services Steering Committee on the Chronically Mentally Ill. Washington, DC, DHHS, 1980
33. Viccora E, Perry J, Mancuso L: Exemplary Practices In Employment Services For People With Psychiatric Disabilities. Alexandria, VA, National Association of State Mental Health Program Directors, 1993
34. Weisbrod BA, Test MA, Stein LI: Alternatives to Mental Hospital Treatment II: Economic Benefit-Cost Analysis. Arch Gen Psychiatry 37 (April): 400–408, 1980

Mental Health Intervention With the Medical Client

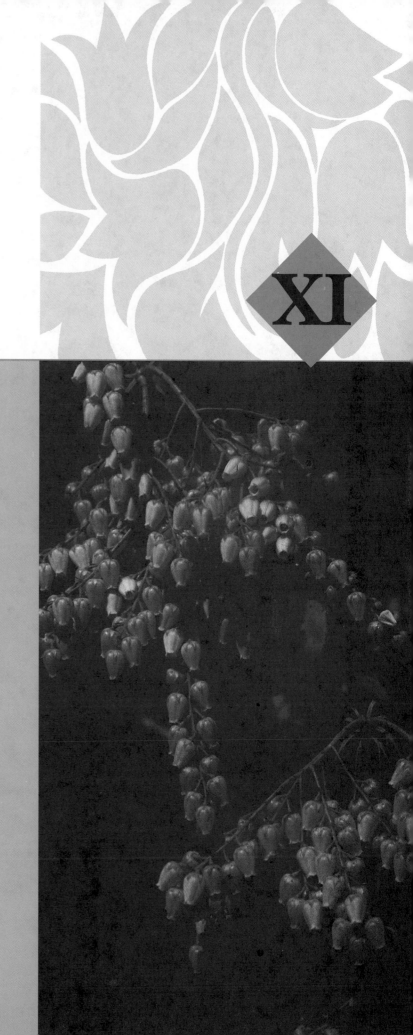

XI

Psychosocial Impact of Acute Illness

Sherill Nones Cronin
Cynthia Ann Pastorino

46

Surgical Ward

They are and suffer: that is all they do.
A bandage hides the place where each is living.
His knowledge of the world restricted to
The treatment that the instruments are giving.
And lie apart like epochs from each other
—Truth in their sense is how much they can bear;
It is not talk like ours, but groans they smother—
And are remote as plants; we lie elsewhere.
For who when healthy can become a foot?
Even a scratch we can't recall when cured.
But are boist'rous in a moment and believe
In the common world of the uninjured, and cannot
Imagine isolation. Only happiness is shared,
And anger, and the idea of love.

W.H. Auden, Collected Poems

Acute illness and hospitalization produce a number of physiological and psychological stressors for clients and their families. Acute illness also influences their ability to cope with stress. The concepts of uncertainty, hardiness, and social support help to explain how people cope with trauma, surgery, or acute illness and guide nursing interventions to facilitate positive psychosocial response. These concepts also help us understand the effects that nurses experience when working with acutely ill people.

Learning Objectives

On completion of this chapter, you should be able to accomplish the following:

1. *Identify stressors associated with hospitalization and acute illness.*
2. *Describe the process and functions of coping.*
3. *Explain the role that uncertainty and hardiness play in the coping process.*
4. *Identify individual and disease-related characteristics that influence coping.*
5. *Discuss the family's role during acute illness.*
6. *Identify nursing diagnoses that may be associated with the psychosocial impact of acute illness and hospitalization.*
7. *Describe interventions that nurses can use to reduce uncertainty and enhance coping efforts of the client and family.*
8. *Identify strategies to promote well-being in nurses who care for acutely ill clients.*

◆ Stress and Coping

Hospitalized clients experience stress from various sources, including physiological dysfunction, circadian rhythm disturbances, and limited access to family, familiar objects, and surroundings. Uncertainty regarding the illness, its consequences, and the effects it may have on significant others adds to the stress of the illness experience. Because of the complex nature of the mind–body interaction, we have only a beginning understanding of the multiple effects that stress can have on individuals.

Stress can be defined as "a relationship between the person and the environment that is appraised by the person as taxing or exceeding his or her resources and as endangering well-being" (p 572).[4] How the person reacts to stress depends on two processes: cognitive appraisal and coping.

Cognitive appraisal is a two-phase process through which the individual evaluates the stressor and its potential effect on well-being. In the first phase, primary appraisal, the person evaluates what is at stake in the event. For example, is the person's life, or that of a loved one, in jeopardy? Is there a potential threat to occupational or family roles? Is there a risk of chronic health problems or disabilities? A range of personality characteristics, including values, beliefs, and hardiness (see following discussion), helps the individual define those stakes that are relevant. In the second phase, secondary appraisal, the person evaluates what, if anything, can be done to overcome the stressor or to modify its harmful effects. That is, to what extent will a particular action relieve the danger? In this phase, various coping options are evaluated.

Coping refers to the person's cognitive and behavioral efforts to manage, reduce, master, or tolerate the stressor and its effects. Coping has two major functions: dealing with the problem that is causing distress (problem-focused coping) and dealing with the emotions that arise from the problem (emotion-focused coping). People use both forms of coping in most stressful situations. The specific ways, or strategies, that are used depend largely on the resources that are available and the constraints that may inhibit their use in a specific situation.[11]

Problem-focused coping strategies are aimed at changing or managing the situation. They include such behaviors as planful problem-solving, seeking information, and aggressive efforts to alter the situation. Problem-focused strategies tend to be used more when dealing with aspects of a situation that are appraised as changeable.

Emotion-focused coping strategies are aimed at changing or managing the individual's reaction to the situation. They include such behaviors as wishful thinking, escape or avoidance behaviors (eg, drinking, using drugs, exercising), rationalization, accepting responsibility, using humor, and developing a positive outlook. Emotion-focused strategies are used more when the individual sees few, if any, options for affecting the outcomes.

Individuals usually have a repertoire of coping strategies that they have used successfully in the past. When faced with a stressful encounter, they may "try out" a number of these strategies to find the best approach for the situation. Flexibility in coping strategies is advantageous; it allows individuals a variety of responses and thus the ability to come to terms with the experience and use it to further growth and adaptation. However, it is important to remember that the hospital environment may limit people's coping skills. After discharge to a more familiar environment, individuals may feel more free to use coping methods that help them relieve stress.

SOCIAL SUPPORT

A factor that may affect the client's appraisal and response to stress is social support. *Social support* is defined as an exchange of resources between individuals that is perceived by the provider or recipient as enhancing the well-being of the recipient. Several types of support may be provided: *instrumental support,* the provision of direct help, such as financial support or assistance with household chores; *informational support,* the giving of needed information, such as help with problem-solving; *emotional support,* the communication of love, caring, trust, or concern; and *spiritual support,* augmentation of an individual's faith or relationship with God or facilitation of ties to a clergyman.[5]

Social support may serve as a buffering mechanism to reduce the negative effects of stress. It may do this by altering appraisal of the stressful event or by intervening between the experience of stress and the onset of negative outcomes by assisting with reappraisal of the situation, inhibiting maladaptive responses, or facilitating adaptive responses. As a result, effective coping can occur, and positive coping outcomes will result. The simple presence of family members, however, does not necessarily indicate that a client has adequate social support.

UNCERTAINTY

A factor that may interfere with an individual's coping efforts is uncertainty. *Uncertainty* is a cognitive state created when an event occurs that cannot be adequately defined or categorized due to lack of information.[8] The degree of uncertainty produced is influenced by the complexity of the event, the amount of ambiguity surrounding the event, and other situational factors, such as previous experiences.

The client hospitalized for an acute illness or trauma is in a situation filled with uncertainty, often unable to recognize unfamiliar sights and sounds, interpret medical jargon, identify expectations of the staff, or predict a daily routine. The illness may also have made bodily functions or symptoms unpredictable. Unfamiliar procedures and treatments may further increase the client's sense of uncertainty and loss of self-mastery.[15] Uncertainty may continue after hospital discharge if the client is not clear about what he or she can (or cannot) do after leaving the hospital; the symptoms the client may experience and the expected progress may also be unpredictable.

The experience of uncertainty can range from a vague sense of feeling unsettled to being completely overwhelmed and unable to cope with the situation. How a person appraises an uncertain event influences his or her response. A person who is unsure about a diagnosis or the severity of the illness may focus on the possibility that things will work out alright. Thus, the uncertainty may facilitate hope.[1] However, uncertainty is usually threatening because there is no clear perception of what will happen next. Effects of this uncertainty may include a limited sense of control over the event and an increased sense of helplessness. As a result, the individual may experience fear, excessive worrying, rumination, and anxiety. Coping processes may be immobilized because the person may not know what to do to help or change the situation and therefore may do nothing.

HARDINESS

Hardiness helps to explain individual differences in coping with acute illness; it encompasses personality characteristics that enable a person to remain healthy in the face of stressful life events.[13] Hardiness may help a client adapt to the stressors of chronic and acute illness by influencing the individual's perception of the stressors, the coping strategies chosen, or the social resources used.[12]

Personal hardiness has three dimensions: control, commitment, and challenge. *Control* involves the belief that personal resources can be used to appraise, interpret, and influence health-related stressors. In a client with acute illness, actual control may be limited. However, the perception of control motivates the individual to seek explanations as to why something is happening and to be actively involved in making decisions regarding care. *Commitment* refers to having a sense of purpose and involvement in health-related activities appropriate for the client's specific situation, for example, participation in deep-breathing exercises when very ill. *Challenge* refers to the reappraisal of a stressor as an opportunity for personal growth, rather than as a threat to security.[9] Individuals who welcome challenge are able to use available resources to cope with the stressors they experience.

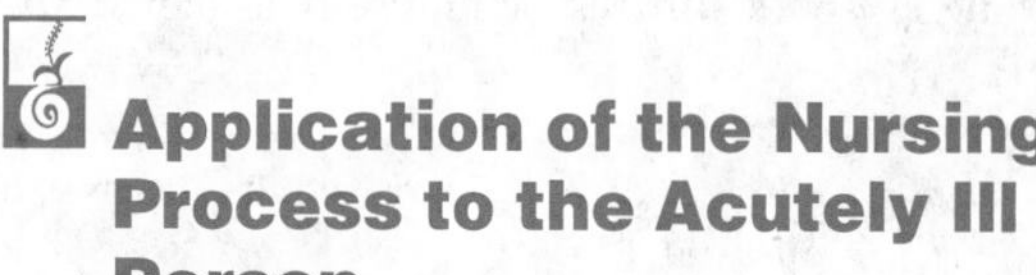

Application of the Nursing Process to the Acutely Ill Person

ASSESSMENT

Psychosocial assessment of the acutely ill client should include a determination of the impact and meaning of the acute illness experience. This includes individual perceptions and characteristics, such as new and ongoing stressors in the client's life, the meaning of the stressors to the client, and personal resources that affect the client's ability to cope with them. Disease characteristics, such as the degree of uncertainty involved, and environmental factors, such as level of social support available, should also be assessed.

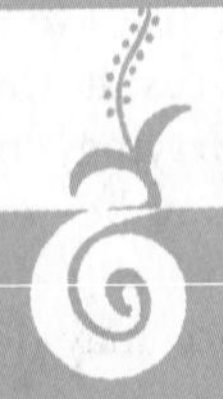

Nursing Care Plan 46-1

Family Stress During Critical Illness

Mr. S, 55 years old, was admitted to the critical care unit for treatment following an acute myocardial infarction (MI). He had been shoveling snow and developed severe chest pain and shortness of breath. Initial electrocardiogram testing revealed changes consistent with an acute MI.

The nurse who admitted Mr. S to the coronary care unit noted that he had a strained facial expression and asked many questions about the monitoring equipment being used. His wife expressed concern and told the nurse, "He should have waited until our son came home to shovel that driveway." Mr. S's 22-year-old son arrived in the unit and loudly complained about the lack of information he received about his father's condition.

In carrying out the prescribed treatment measures for Mr. S's acute MI, the nurse also recognizes that the family is responding to stress. The partial nursing care plan that follows addresses the psychosocial needs of the family.

Nursing Diagnosis

Anxiety related to situational crisis and/or loss of control

Outcome

Client will verbalize decreased anxiety.

Intervention	Rationale
Encourage client to verbalize specific concerns and actively listen.	Verbalization helps client recognize existence of anxiety. Active listening and acceptance validate client's worth and communicate that help is available.
Provide simple, clear explanations of tests, treatments, symptoms, and client's progress.	Adequate information helps client distinguish between realistic concerns and exaggerated fears; reducing possible sources of uncertainty decreases anxiety.
Reduce environmental stimuli such as excessive noise level and bright lighting.	Excessive sensory stimuli, such as that found in critical care units, disrupt normal circadian rhythms and sustain anxiety.
Teach client simple relaxation strategies (eg, slow, deep breathing exercises; progressive muscle relaxation).	Relaxation strategies reduce muscle tension, provide distraction, and counteract escalating anxiety.

Evaluation

Client's anxiety is decreased; he discusses his concerns, practices relaxation techniques, and appears restful.

continued

Individual Perceptions and Characteristics

The assessment of new and ongoing stressors may be difficult in the crisis atmosphere of acute illness, when the nurse and client are preoccupied with the situation at hand. However, knowing how the client and family perceive the current situation, how they have approached other stressors in the past, what additional stressors they are experiencing, and how they deal with uncertainty assists the nurse in developing an effective plan of action.

The experience of acute stress, on top of existing physical, emotional, or spiritual stressors, can be overwhelming and can leave the client and family exhausted and unable to meet their basic physiological and emotional needs. How previous crises have been handled may suggest coping style preferences (eg, information seeking, distraction, humor, denial). This information can be used to guide intervention planning for this episode. However, although the client and family may have coped effectively in the past, this acute episode

Nursing Care Plan 46-1 *(Continued)*

Nursing Diagnosis

Ineffective Family Coping related to presence of multiple stressors and lack of support systems

Outcome

Family members will verbalize feelings and seek information and support from the nurse, other health care providers, and/or other support systems.

Intervention	Rationale
Establish a calm and trusting atmosphere that conveys mutual respect, collaboration, and assurance.	A trusting and empathetic relationship between the nurse and family members helps the family keep or redefine hope about client's outcome, manage discouraging news, and develop confidence in the health care team.
Keep open, honest lines of communication with family members; identify a consistent contact person in the family.	Frequent communication in jargon-free and comprehensible language helps the family develop a realistic view of the situation. Having a consistent contact person reduces the chance of misinterpretation of incomplete information.
Facilitate family comfort and the satisfaction of basic needs.	To provide support for the client and each other, family members must receive adequate rest, nutrition, and hygiene.
Develop mechanisms for additional support to family members (eg, support groups).	Support groups provide a forum for sharing information and coping strategies with others.
Allow family members frequent access to client.	Family proximity has comforting effects on both the client and family members. The more serious the client's condition, the more intense is the family's need to remain close.

Evaluation

The family manages the stress of the client's illness, supports him in the hospital, communicates openly, and engages in self-care.

may represent an overwhelming challenge and may necessitate the introduction of new coping strategies.

It is important to ascertain the meaning of the illness event to the client and family. Each illness or traumatic event carries unique individual and cultural meanings. Some are associated with social stigma, for example, acquired immunodeficiency syndrome. Some may have varying cultural connotations; for example, a gunshot wound carries different meanings depending on how the injury occurred. Some may be accompanied by feelings of guilt if the individual or family assigns blame for the illness, for example, an acute cardiac event in a client who has continued to smoke despite health warnings.

Personal characteristics and abilities may also influence how a client copes with the crisis of physical illness. These include intellectual abilities, communication skills, experience with the health care delivery system, personal insight, and emotional, financial, and social resources. Thus, each person brings unique skills to a coping situation. Assessment of these individual attributes helps the nurse select or adapt interventions to enhance coping efforts.

Characteristics of the Disease

The nurse should consider the following characteristics of the disease when assessing the impact of acute illness on the client and family:

1. timing of the disruption, including duration and amount of preparation or time to plan (ie, was this illness expected or unexpected? Is the illness a result of an acute or chronic process?)
2. severity of the illness

3. degree of physiological stress, such as the degree of pain, disability, or loss of function
4. predictability of the illness and symptoms (Clearly defined situations offer known behavioral options.)
5. factors involved in the disease or treatment process that may influence the client's response, such as circadian rhythm disruption, lack of privacy, noise (sensory overload or deprivation of meaningful sounds and events), loss of control, loss of contact with loved ones and familiar objects, and loss of routine

Severe illnesses will vary in their predictability and consequences. For example, a head injury is often accompanied by overwhelming uncertainty regarding ultimate client outcome. Effects may be transient or permanent, with mild to profound intellectual, functional, and other sequelae. Treatment choices may have tremendous implications for the future functioning of the client and family. However, immediately following notification regarding the injury, the family is expected to make treatment and legal decisions affecting the injured person, often based on very little information and at a time of severe stress. The family's response to such a situation is, understandably, often one of extreme stress and anxiety.

Family Assessment

Family assessment is guided by knowledge of the most common stressors that families experience during an episode of acute illness. These include concern about an uncertain prognosis; fear that the client will experience intense pain, disability, or death; lack of privacy; unfamiliarity of environments; separation from loved ones; disruption of support systems; and changes in family roles. These stressors evoke anxiety in the family and lead to an overriding perception of threat. Family members may respond to this threat with feelings of panic, anger, denial, frustration, impatience, or hopelessness.

The strategies that families use to cope with acute illness or trauma are as varied as individuals' coping strategies. Additionally, families may use a variety of strategies to deal with the multiple stressors involved. For example, for a family coping with cancer and the effects of chemotherapy, these strategies may include allowing the family to become a buffer between the ill person and others and cognitive actions, such as providing information, softening the blow, being present, resisting disruption of family and individual routines, and preserving the client's sense of self. Again, knowing what coping behaviors have been effective in the past can help the nurse in selecting interventions to ease the impact of the illness event.[5]

The level of stress in the family may also persist after the event, even when the physiological problem is resolving. For example, family members may exhibit a delayed reaction to a trauma once the loved one is out of danger and they realize the full impact of the experience. Caregiver stress—especially at the time of discharge from the hospital—is common. This stress may be demonstrated as hostility toward the nurses or the hospital as caregiving is turned over to the family, and formerly denied uncertainties and insecurities surface. Because anxiety and predictability influence coping effort, the better prepared the family is and the more predictable the care or outcome, the easier it is for the family to cope with their new role.

NURSING DIAGNOSIS

The nature of the acute illness will determine which physiological nursing diagnoses may apply. Possible psychosocial nursing diagnoses may include the following:

1. Anxiety related to situational crisis, lack of knowledge, or loss of control
2. Ineffective Family Coping related to presence of multiple stressors and lack of support systems
3. Altered Role Performance related to impaired physical functioning
4. Altered Body Image related to perception of disfigurement and dysfunction
5. Self Esteem Disturbance related to changes in ability to perform basic self-care skills
6. Impaired Verbal Communication related to presence of artificial airways

PLANNING

The overall goal of nursing interventions is to support effective coping strategies used by the client and family. This support enables the client and family to gain a sense of self-control by focusing energy on the task at hand, managing the uncertainty associated with the experience, reducing the negative effects of stress, and fostering hope. During a time of crisis, long-term goals are not of immediate concern; short-term, realistic goals are needed to help the client and family reestablish equilibrium (Nursing Care Plan 46-1, pp. 928–929).

The presence of a consistent, informed contact person is an invaluable asset to the family. A clinical nurse specialist (CNS) may assume the role of contact person and interpreter of events for the client and family. The CNS can also assist the staff in the development of an individualized plan of care.

The family's need for support and information is great during serious illnesses. The CNS may help to establish methods to address these informational needs. One such method is the formation of support groups for the families of the critically ill.[2] In a support group, family members can unburden their concerns and fears to others in similar circumstances.[6] Members can also help each other by offering examples of coping strategies that they have found useful. Critical care support groups tend to have short-term membership, because the need for this type of acute intervention resolves as the client's condition changes.

Attention to the family's physical and emotional needs enables them to cope more effectively with the crisis and in turn, more effectively support the ill family member.[10] Furthermore, just as family members need access to the ill member, so does the client require closeness to loved ones.[3] Research has demonstrated that family proximity results in positive client outcomes, such as improved orientation, decreased anxiety, and increased sleep.[14] In the last decade, most intensive care units have recognized the positive effects of flexible, less restrictive visiting times than those permitted in the past. This flexibility balances the need for physical closeness with the requirements of physical care and encourages communication and collaborative relationships between family and staff (Case Study 46-1).

46-1 Case Study

Helping A Family Through A Crisis of Trauma

Mr. C, a 70-year-old businessman, was critically injured in an automobile accident. The accident occurred 60 miles away from the nearest trauma center, so Mr. C was flown to the center by helicopter. On arrival, the extent of his injuries was noted: multiple fractures, including both legs, ribs, and right arm; and a closed head injury with loss of consciousness. Mr. C was quickly moved to the intensive care unit for treatment. He was intubated, placed on a ventilator, and given vasopressors to maintain his blood pressure.

Meanwhile, his 64-year-old wife was notified of the accident by the county sheriff. She was unable to contact her sons and drove to the hospital by herself. On arrival, she was directed to the ICU where she saw her husband of 40 years intubated, unconscious, and attached to multiple monitors and IV lines.

Questions for Discussion

1. Discuss the possible stressors that Mrs. C might be experiencing.
2. What immediate needs of Mrs. C should the nurse assess?
3. What actions could friends and family take to help Mrs. C during the initial crisis?
4. Discuss interventions the nurse could initiate to facilitate Mrs. C's adaptation.

INTERVENTION

The nurse promotes a positive psychosocial response by sharing information, offering emotional support and positive coping strategies, and promoting health and hardiness.

Sharing information is as significant as any other type of care provided. The client's perceptions, feelings, decisions, and actions are shaped by the information received. The need for information begins at the moment of admission. Decisions made in those initial hours of the physical crisis may influence treatments, finances, and ethical and legal matters. When under stress, the client and family may be unable to grasp the meaning of papers they are signing or information they are receiving. Thus, information must be concrete and understandable.

A client's anxiety or distress from frightening procedures is decreased by explaining expected sensory experiences associated with the procedures. Sensory information describes in concrete terms what will be felt, tasted, seen, or smelled during a procedure; how the environment will look; and the duration and sequence of events. This information may help allay anxiety by decreasing the discrepancy between what is expected and what is experienced. For example, knowing the specific sensations associated with suctioning may assist the client to interpret those felt sensations as normal and therefore less frightening and uncertain.

Sensory information may also be used to assist the client to predict or interpret the symptoms associated with an illness or its treatment. If symptoms are perceived as unpredictable or uncontrollable, the client is left with a sense of panic or helplessness and futility. Knowing what symptoms to expect and what the symptoms mean provides the client with a sense of mastery and self-confidence. The nurse validates the interpretation of symptoms so that nuances of change can be recognized and managed (Box 46-1).

Family informational needs can be met in a variety of ways. Information booklets and videos can help meet the need for concrete information. Telephone contact is an efficient way to keep families updated on the client's condition. Additionally, pagers allow families to leave the hospital to attend to work or family responsibilities, knowing they can be contacted immediately if an emergency arises.[7] Family meetings or rounds can facilitate information dissemination and prevent sending confusing or "mixed" messages.

Emotional support assists the client to maintain self-confidence, self-worth, and feelings of hope. Although

BOX 46-1

Coping With the Uncertainty of Critical Illness

Mr. F is admitted to the emergency department with complaints of chest tightness, numbness and tingling in the left arm, and some shortness of breath. He has a history of coronary artery disease and myocardial infarction and underwent coronary angioplasty 2 months ago. He delayed coming to the hospital when this episode began because "this didn't feel exactly like the same kind of pain that I had before. I didn't think it was anything to get excited about." He also states, "I just had that balloon procedure done. How could I be having more problems with my heart? Are they going to do that treatment again? I don't think that's necessary, do you?"

1. What is generating the uncertainty that Mr. F is experiencing? Think about all the possible sources of uncertainty in this situation.
2. What should the nurse do? In thinking about your answer, consider first what the nurse should assess. Remember that not all of Mr. F's uncertainty is related to his prognosis. Second, think about the possible misunderstandings or misinterpretations that seem to be present. What information or clarification should the nurse provide? Third, think about what the nurse could do to assist Mr. F's use of more facilitative coping strategies. How can the nurse help Mr. F sort out the various aspects of the stress he is experiencing and indentify ways to cope with them?

finding the cause of an illness usually is not a priority in the initial phase of the experience, the process of assembling the story of the event becomes important as time passes. The individual needs to tell and retell the story in order to define and come to terms with the illness and its impact. The nurse assists in this process by encouraging the telling of the story, defining the situation and interpreting the events, and reframing the event as the client and family progress through the crisis. These cognitive restructuring strategies allow the client and family to come to terms with the experience and then to focus energy on problem solving.

At times, the client and family may blame themselves or others for the illness. The nurse may hear comments from family members such as "I told him he should stop smoking" and self-blaming comments from the client. There may be an element of truth in these statements, but at the time of acute illness it is counterproductive to focus on feelings of inadequacy. The client and family must be able to forgive themselves and move on.

The nurse promotes hardiness and adaptation by suggesting specific stress-reducing activities. In an attempt to make the environment more normal, for example, the nurse may attend to the noise level on the unit. Meeting the client's and family's basic needs helps reduce the perception of stress. Other stress-reduction activities include providing physical exercise; maintaining a normal sleep-rest-activity cycle; providing music therapy; offering relaxation techniques, such as massage; and encouraging reduced consumption of caffeine and nicotine. Obviously, a time of crisis is not the time for making major lifestyle changes. However, the nurse can build on the client's readiness and interest in health to initiate a healthier lifestyle.

EVALUATION

The nurse evaluates the effectiveness of interventions through behavioral indicators of reduced stress and reengagement in usual activities. A high level of stress may persist for several weeks after an acute episode and is influenced by the expectations and outcomes of the illness and how needs were met during the time of crisis. Follow-up assessments and ongoing interventions may be necessary to help the client and family resume their usual activities and quality of life.

◆ Effects on the Nurse

The stresses of nursing are many—hard physical work, an endless stream of information, rapidly changing work environments, emotionally draining client situations, and a degree of uncertainty regarding client circumstances and future directions. The ever-expanding knowledge base in health care may leave the nurse feeling inadequate and frustrated as new procedures and protocols supplant the familiar. The nurse may feel ambivalent as to whether treatment plans truly reflect the client's needs and values as compared with those of the hospital or other involved parties. Often the nurse must mediate among client, physician, and health care institution to provide appropriate, quality nursing care.

The concept of hardiness may play an important role in preventing caregiver burnout. Nurses can assess their own hardiness and determine ways to increase it. To establish a sense of control and minimize the effects of uncertainty, the nurse needs adequate educational preparation and continued mentoring in any nursing situation. Orientation programs that facilitate the development of mentoring relationships are the most advantageous. The importance of a relationship between the novice nurse and a more experienced nurse cannot be overemphasized. This relationship builds personal hardiness through the nurturance of competent clinical practice. The verbal and nonverbal support of a mentor can reduce the uncertainty of a situation and increase the novice nurse's sense of mastery.

Just as nurses intervene with clients and families in crises to promote health, they must also intervene with other nurses to promote occupational and personal well-being. Many strategies suggested for clients are also appropriate for nurses. These include attending support group meetings; reframing critical clinical events; using exercise, distraction, relaxation, and massage; and reducing intake of caffeine and other stimulants.

◆ Chapter Summary

This chapter examines the psychosocial stresses of, and responses to, acute illness, with emphasis on the following points:

1. The concepts of social support, uncertainty, and hardiness are a useful framework for examining stress and coping in acutely ill clients, their families, and the nurses who care for them.
2. Nurses must assess the impact of physiological crises on the client and family and their ability to cope with the impact.
3. Realistic goals and plans are based on prioritized nursing diagnoses.
4. The nurse intervenes to promote health, hardiness, and adaptation and reduce negative effects of stress.

Review Questions

1. What are the two major functions of coping?
2. What are the four types of social support that family members may provide?
3. Which situation would be more difficult for a client and family to cope with: the terminal phase of a prolonged bout with cancer or a sudden, massive myocardial infarction with no previous symptoms?
4. What are the three components of hardiness, and how do they enhance a person's adaptation to stress?
5. The rationale for providing sensory information to acutely ill clients is to
   - A. Promote feelings of control.
   - B. Decrease parasympathetic sensations.
   - C. Decrease sensitivity to pain.
   - D. Avoid sensory deprivation.
6. Which would *not* be considered one of the primary needs of families of acutely ill clients?
   - A. Access to the client
   - B. Knowledge that competent and caring nursing care is being provided
   - C. Assurances about the future
   - D. Information regarding the client's care
7. All of the following may help to reduce the effects of stress associated with the nursing role *except*
   - A. Discussion with coworkers.
   - B. Reassessment of negative clinical incidents.
   - C. Serving as unit resource person.
   - D. Watching television.

◆ References

1. Bailey JM, Nielsen BI: Uncertainty and Appraisal of Uncertainty in Women With Rheumatoid Arthritis. Orthopaedic Nursing 12: 63–67, 1993
2. Byrd JA: Critical Waiting: Families in Crisis—How Nurses Can Help the Other Victims of Critical Illness. Ultrastat: Essential Issues for Advanced Critical-Care Nursing 1 (3): 1–6, 1994
3. Dracup K: Challenges in Critical Care Nursing: Helping Patients and Families Cope. Critical Care Nurse (August Supplement): 3–9, 1993
4. Folkman S, Lazarus RS, Gruen RJ, DeLongis A: Appraisal, Coping, Health Status, and Psychological Symptoms. J Pers Soc Psychol 50: 571–579, 1986
5. Halm MA: Support and Reassurance Needs: Strategies for Practice. Critical Care Nursing Clinics of North America 4: 633–643, 1992
6. Harvey C, Dixon M, Padberg N: Support Group for Families of Trauma Patients: A Unique Approach. Critical Care Nurse 15 (4): 59–63, 1995
7. Henneman EA, Cardin S: Need for Information: Interventions for Practice. Critical Care Nursing Clinics of North America 4: 615–621, 1992
8. Hilton BA: Perceptions of Uncertainty: Its Relevance to Life-Threatening and Chronic Illness. Critical Care Nurse 12 (2): 70–73, 1992
9. Jennings BM, Staggers N: A Critical Analysis of Hardiness. Nurs Res 43: 274–281, 1994
10. Leske JS: Needs of Adult Family Members After Critical Illness: Prescriptions for Interventions. Critical Care Nursing Clinics of North America 4: 587–596, 1992
11. McHaffie HE: Coping: An Essential Element of Nursing. J Adv Nurs 17: 933–940, 1992
12. Narsavage GL, Weaver TE: Physiologic Status, Coping, and Hardiness as Predictors of Outcomes in Chronic Obstructive Pulmonary Disease. Nurs Res 43: 90–94, 1994
13. Tartasky DS: Hardiness: Conceptual and Methodological Issues. Image 25: 225–229, 1993
14. Titler MG, Walsh SM: Visiting Critically Ill Adults: Strategies for Practice. Critical Care Nursing Clinics of North America 4: 623–632, 1992
15. White RE, Frasure-Smith N: Uncertainty and Psychologic Stress After Coronary Angioplasty and Coronary Bypass Surgery. Heart Lung 24: 19–27, 1995

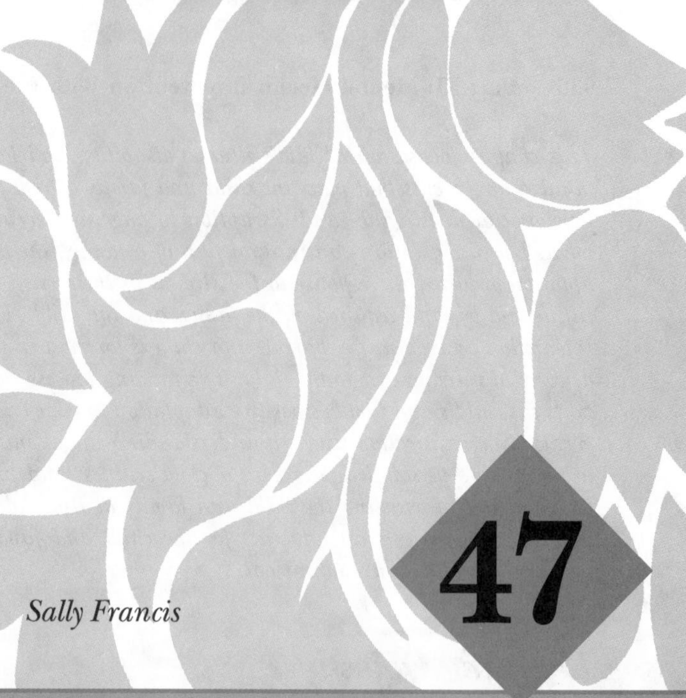

The Child at Risk: Illness, Disability, and Hospitalization

Sally Francis

47

Whenever I approach a child, his presence inspires two feelings in me. Affection for what he is now, and respect for what he may one day become.

Louis Pasteur

This chapter focuses on a child's illness, disability, and hospitalization, events that place the child and family at risk for psychosocial disturbance and disruption to ongoing development. Because a child is an integral part of a family, the adaptation required in response to the stresses of these crises is influenced by, and required of, the family and the child. The interaction between nurse, parent, and child is foremost in the delivery of nursing care to the child. The nursing process supports the child's and family's positive adaptation to these crisis events. Communication and self-understanding are essential to the nurse's personal coping with a child's illness and professional role of assisting the child and family at risk. Additionally, the nurse is an advocate for the child and family within the health care environment.

Learning Objectives

On completion of this chapter, you should be able to accomplish the following:

1. *Discuss the overlay of illness, disability, and hospitalization on the developmental needs of children.*
2. *Describe the influences of hospitalization, parent–child attachment, and communication on the child's and family's positive adaptation.*
3. *Apply the nursing process to the care of ill, disabled, or hospitalized children.*
4. *Describe the nurse's role of advocacy for children in health care and for their families.*
5. *Discuss the nurse's use of personal coping measures and collegial support in the provision of psychosocial care to children at risk due to illness, disability, or hospitalization.*

◆ Development and the Overlay of Illness, Disability, and Hospitalization

All people arrive at adulthood having developed from the dependency of an infant who must rely on the external world for survival. Successful passage through the phases of development leads to a sense of the self as separate from the external environment and capable of using the external world to provide for survival. The person becomes self-reliant and interdependent with others in the environment. This is accomplished in childhood by acquiring skills and resolving developmental crises. The crises of illness, disability, and hospitalization are frequently added to the normal, although monumental, developmental vicissitudes. These events may place the child at risk for decreased opportunity for physical survival and for unsuccessfully managing the developmental tasks that lead to satisfying, productive adulthood. On the other hand, these crises also provide opportunities for the child and family to acquire skills for coping with, mastering, and adapting to stress.[35]

A developing child is an integral part of a family unit; the stresses of illness, disability, and hospitalization are disruptions for the family and for the child.[33] For example, the family's daily routines are altered by trips to the health care setting. The parents' relationship is altered by sleeping arrangements and family responsibilities divided between home and hospital. Siblings experience disruptions as they become secondary to the ill child and are cared for by neighbors or relatives.[14] Hospital bills, medication costs, and time off work result in financial strains. As one child takes on the client role, other family members shift in their roles and functions within the family. These disruptions in the family's daily living, routines, and roles require adaptation by all family members.[11,14,20,50]

Adaptation becomes more complex when the illness is a chronic condition or disability. The family unit must make ongoing adjustments with each phase of the illness.[37] Consider the family with a child with leukemia. At the time of diagnosis, there is an acute phase of stress and disequilibrium. With the onset of remission, the family begins adjusting. As the remission extends over time, the family adapts; however, disruption occurs again when the child relapses, necessitating adjustment that may be followed by another remission. Stress, disequilibrium, adjustment, and adaptation may recur several times as the disease process and treatments continue.[83]

When the chronic illness or disability lasts for months and years, the child and family must make new adjustments and adaptations with each developmental phase through which the child passes.[23] For example, the child with congenital abnormalities must cope with disruptions in daily living resulting from staged surgical corrections, while the evolving processes of body image, sexual identification, self-esteem, and mastery take on different emphases with each stage of psychosexual development. This overlay of illness on developmental behaviors is also seen when the usual storm and stress of adolescence is compounded in the child with diabetes who uses noncompliance with treatment as a vehicle for expressing typical adolescent rebellion.

The parents' feelings of grief and guilt for what the child is, or could have been, further complicate the family's adaptation. The family may mourn the loss of the fantasized child. The family's feelings about their actual child's disability and their perceptions of the stresses caused by the disability influence their adjustment to the stressors. The support available to the family and the understanding and acceptance of their feelings also influence adaptation. *Adaptation* is the end state of adjusting to the changes brought about by the illness, disability, or hospitalization. How the child and family perceive the stress influences how they cope. The nurse affects the child's and family's perceptions of, understanding of, and responses to stress and subsequently, their adaptation. By providing support and assistance in mastering stress, the nurse mediates the family's adaptive responses. To do so, the nurse must understand the effects of hospitalization, parent–child attachment, and communication as factors influencing the child at risk.

HOSPITALIZATION

Whether as a mental health consultant or as a pediatric clinician, the nurse often becomes involved with a child and family on admission into the hospital. Admissions take three general forms:

1. Emergency admissions for which there is little time for advance preparation
2. Planned admissions for elective events, such as diagnostic workups and surgery
3. Episodic admissions, that is, one of multiple hospitalizations for a chronic condition

Entry into the health care system is a time of stress for the child and family. The amount of stress experienced by the child and family and the opportunities for mediation of the stress vary with the type of admission.[2,3] The nurse has a greater opportunity to initiate planned interventions with planned or episodic admissions than with emergency admissions. Admission to the hospital carries the potential for psychological upset, which will have a disruptive effect on the child's development (Box 47-1). This disruption occurs in about 25% of all pediatric hospitalizations. Children with multiple admissions during the first 4 years of life are the most vulnerable to the effects of psychological upset. On the other hand, another 25%

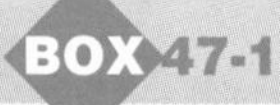

47-1

Psychosocial Needs of Children in Hospitals

A HISTORICAL PERSPECTIVE

Reports of hospital conditions during the first part of the 20th century described stringent aseptic conditions that were enforced to counteract the threat of untreatable cross-infections. In these hospitals, children were isolated from one another, contact with staff was restricted, and parents were permitted very limited visiting.

The studies of maternal–child separations in the 1940s by Rene Spitz and Anna Freud brought the term *maternal deprivation* into focus. James Robertson, a colleague of Anna Freud, applied the study of mother–child separations to hospitalized children. His findings, published in 1958, documented adverse effects of hospitalization on children and brought about reforms in pediatric care in English hospitals.

In the United States, interest in the emotional care of hospitalized children developed throughout the 1950s. Impetus came from the first major U.S. study to document the psychological effects of hospitalization on children. Conducted by Dane Prugh in Boston, the study found that adverse psychological disturbance resulting from a child's hospitalization could be mediated by unlimited parental visiting, provision of play, preparation programs for children, and support of staff and parents.

Research and clinical concern continued in the 1960s and led to the formation of a multidisciplinary organization focused on the psychosocial needs of children in health care—the Association for the Care of Children in Hospitals. In 1980, the name of this organization was changed to the Association for the Care of Children's Health to reflect changing patterns of health care, such as the expanded role of outpatient care in chronic illness.

The thrust of research from the mid-1960s through the 1970s focused on the use of preparation to decrease children's anxiety in health care. Clinical settings also developed or expanded therapeutic play programs to provide emotional support to children. The development of the clinical nurse specialist role and primary nursing in pediatrics further strengthened the provision of care based on the developmental needs of children. Research studies by Douglas, reported in 1975, and a supporting study by Quinton and Rutter documented the prolonged trauma experienced by some children as a result of hospitalization and identified children at psychiatric risk.

In the last decade, increased recognition of children at risk and awareness of the growing population of chronically ill and handicapped children has led to a new focus on *family-centered care*. Legislative, educational, and health care systems have begun to recognize the family as the constant in a child's life and to understand the need to include the family in planning and carrying out services for the child. Hospital and ambulatory care increasingly view health care as a partnership between professional staff and families, a partnership that supports physical and psychosocial care.

of children admitted appear to benefit psychologically from hospitalization. The remaining 50% of children admitted into hospitals are neither unusually negatively affected nor do they benefit psychologically by hospitalization.[44,59]

The previous statistics affirm an imperative of pediatric health care: to examine a child's experiences in hospitalization. The goal of this examination is to minimize the potential negative psychological effects and maximize the opportunities for psychological benefit from prolonged hospitalization (Box 47-2). Benefits can occur when the child and family view hospitalization as a stressful event that can result in positive adaptation, an event that can lead to growth in self-confidence, self-esteem, and mastery. As hospitalization supports the child's physical well-being, it can support—and may in fact enhance—the child's emotional well-being. Hospitalization at the time of initial diagnosis of a chronic illness or disability begins the process of adjustment for the family. Whether diagnosis is made at birth or later, the family experiences initial feelings of shock and disbelief. Disruption occurs and adjustment begins.

The Ontario Child Health Study compared large numbers of children with and without chronic illness.[9-11] The findings suggest that chronic illness does not guarantee resulting psychopathology in children, siblings, or families. However, a greater risk for psychological disturbance was substantiated. Protective factors have been found in a wide range of studies; these include family functioning with harmony, self-esteem, mastery behaviors, and available social support systems. Families with higher adaptation have been identified as having more family cohesion and greater moral or religious emphasis. The latter characteristic gives positive attribution (meaning) to the chronic illness and provides a belief system that gives support and makes sense out of what has happened to the family.[26,62]

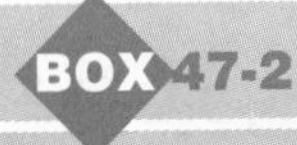

47-2

Prolonged Hospitalization and Immobilization

Special needs arise when infants, children, or adolescents experience prolonged hospitalization. At greatest risk are infants. Organizing the environment to facilitate the development of trust and cognitive processes is essential.[61] The challenge to the nurse is to collaborate creatively with the family and other health care disciplines to "normalize" the environment, that is, to incorporate essential life experiences into the hospital setting. Included can be such activities as developing a schedule for the baby's day, which promotes predictability and decreases disruptions and unnecessary people; using adaptive toys (homemade or commercial products) that enhance stimulation and organization of sensory modes; and providing support programs for *all* family members, such as respite time for the parents and sibling involvement with the infant in the hospital.

Equally challenging to the nurse's creativity is the immobilized child. Whether immobilization results from treatment and equipment or from surgical intervention, the child's experience of powerlessness can be a risk to positive coping and eventual adaptation. Again, environmental manipulation can counteract the necessary restrictions. Most important is the recognition that mobility is the child's primary way of exerting control, expressing tension and anxiety, and exploring the environment. The nurse must recognize the child's attempts to compensate for the loss of mobility and facilitate adaptive behaviors that give the child feelings of control and mastery.

A common response of children to immobilization in an intensive care unit is to withdraw from the environment by refusing to make eye contact. Another common behavior is seen when a child in traction uses the nurse call button incessantly. Providing realistic choices is a first step in assisting the child to regain feelings of control. Providing outlets for tension and anxiety, through verbalization and adaptive activity, further assists the child in compensating for the loss of mobility. Support and structure also are provided by increasing peer contacts and continuing normal routines, such as schoolwork.

Peer contact was maintained for a child who was in traction and in isolation through daily bingo games held in the play room; the child participated by telephone. Audiotapes made by the child and sent home to siblings, who sent their own tape-recorded messages back, provided an outlet for the child's energy and a readily available comforting device. Daily sessions with fantasy, such as reading stories involving action, allowed the child to identify with and vicariously become an action hero, mastering challenges. Through assessment and planning, the nurse can help the child regain feelings of control to counteract the powerlessness of immobility.

PARENT–CHILD ATTACHMENT

Evidence clearly indicates the importance of the child's primary emotional support figure being present during the hospitalization.[8,69,83] The child's anxiety aroused by unfamiliar surroundings and people and by painful events is secondary to the anxiety aroused by separation from his or her primary object relation. Although this is evident for young children, it also applies to older children for whom regression is a normal response to the physical and emotional demands of illness and hospitalization.[22] Providing emotional support to the child must begin with efforts to continue the support provided by the child's primary attachment. Usually this primary attachment is to the parents, particularly the mother. On the child's entry into health care, the nurse plays an important role in continuing the parent–child attachment. The nurse explains to the parents the need for *rooming-in,* that is, allowing the parents unlimited stay in the child's room. The nurse refers the parents to the social work department to acquire financial assistance or to other services, such as child care, that will make the parents' rooming-in possible.

After ensuring continuing parent–child attachment, the nurse next directs efforts toward decreasing the parents' anxiety. Young children mirror their parents' anxiety. Interventions to reduce the parents' distress typically also reduce the child's anxiety.[81] The nursing process is based on the child's needs and the parents' ability to meet these needs. This is not always as easy as it may seem. The nurse continually examines personal feelings toward the parents. For example, it may be easier to provide comfort and support to a 2-year-old child who has ingested cleaning fluid than to be supportive of negligent parents. However, the parents' perceptions of health care, formulated during this initial hospitalization, will influence the family's positive adaptation to future admissions, surgical procedures, and clinic visits. The acceptance and support offered to the parents by the nurse help them clarify their own feelings of guilt. This may lead to greater receptiveness to the nurse's instructions for home care and to role modeling and education promoting more effective parenting, limit setting, and discipline for their child. The nurse who does not acknowledge his or her own feelings of blame toward the parents may unconsciously exclude them from participation in the child's physical and emotional care. As the parents become increasingly uncomfortable in the climate provided by the nurse, they may withdraw from the nurse's efforts at instruction and perhaps withdraw from their child. By ignoring or discounting feelings evoked by the parents, nurses unwittingly sabotage their own efforts to implement the nursing process and promote the child's adaptation.

COMMUNICATION

The nurse conveys attitudes and feelings that influence the behavior of clients. Communication is a key element when caring for children at risk from illness, disability, and hospitalization. Verbal communication conveys warmth, acceptance, empathy, and caring; however, communicating these attitudes through nonverbal means is more important.[8,24,30]

The nurse has many functions and duties to perform in pediatrics, including the administration of drugs, therapies, treatments, and other tasks relating to machines and equipment. How the nurse performs these functions communicates a level of caring that influences the child's and family's coping. For instance, the necessary physical restraint of a child during a lumbar puncture can convey caring and support of the child's efforts, however limited, for self-control, or can indicate punitive retaliation against the child's actions, which are judged as willfully immature and hostile. The difference is observed in the nurse's physical handling of the child, tone of voice, and facial expressions. Through these communications, the nurse can convey a supportive, humanistic concern for the child as a person or can convey a mechanical, task-oriented outlook, in which the child is perceived as an object to be controlled. The former attitude is health inducing, because it promotes the child's coping with stress; the latter attitude, in its dehumanization of the child, adds to the child's psychological stress and places the child at further risk.

Successful communication with a child and family is built on an understanding of their problems, needs, and strengths obtained from the nursing assessment and on the recognition and acceptance of personal feelings and attitudes.[28,30]

Application of the Nursing Process to the Child at Risk

Each child and family is unique, as is each course of hospitalization of a child. The degree of physical disability and psychological distress resulting from illness varies from child to child.

The complexity of facts and possibilities and the feelings they arouse may seem overwhelming; however, by keeping the goal—minimizing psychosocial distress—in focus, the nurse maintains the commitment to children at risk. The nurse assists the child's and family's positive adaptation by performing tasks within the perspective of providing emotional support. The nursing process provides a framework within which information is organized and nursing intervention planned.

The nurse has an opportunity to assist the child and

family in defining the stressors as opportunities for growth rather than as events that are overwhelming, beyond personal control, and causing disorganization and disturbance. The nurse best supports the child's positive adaptation through the nursing process, beginning with the first step—assessment.

ASSESSMENT

The goal of assessment is to gather and organize information to aid the nurse in caring for the child at risk. The assessment incorporates information about the child, family, and resources available in the health care setting.

Developmental Level

Assessment of the child begins with exploring the child's developmental level. With what psychosocial issues is the child dealing? How does the child process events and information? What fears, general and specific to health care, are typical of children at a particular age? Box 47-3 outlines common fears and anxieties of children. Chronological age, combined with an understanding of theories of psychosexual, ego, and cognitive development, provide guidelines for nursing assessment.[5,25,32]

Environmental Influences

Environmental influences affecting the child's response to the stresses of illness, disability, and hospitalization are assessed by gathering information about the child's specific illness or disability, previous life experiences, and family.[61]

Nature of the Illness or Disability. Research has not substantiated a causal relationship between a specific illness or disability and a psychological disorder in a child. Nevertheless, knowledge about specific diagnoses does provide the nurse with information about the typical kind of hospitalization required, treatments prescribed, and medical events that the child will encounter; pain and physical discomfort anticipated; type and number of intrusive procedures expected; any outward physical signs of the disease or disability; and required treatments to which the child and family must adjust. This and other

BOX 47-3

Common Fears and Anxieties of Children in Health Care

DEVELOPMENTAL PHASE	FEARS AND ANXIETIES
Infancy	Separation anxiety
Toddlerhood	Separation anxiety Fear of the unknown Fear of strangers
Preschool age	Separation anxiety Anxiety about body intrusions, intense need for body intactness Anxieties aroused by egocentric thought, fantasies, magical thinking Fear of punishment aroused by guilt, as child feels he or she is the cause of the illness or disability Fear of body mutilation
School age	Fear of body injury Fear of pain Fear of loss of respect, love, and emerging self-esteem Anxiety related to guilt Fear of anesthesia
Adolescence	Fear of loss of identity and control Anxiety about body image and changes in physical appearance Fear of loss of status in peer group Anxiety related to long-term implications of illness or disability

information related to a specific illness or disability have implications for the nurse in planning and carrying out interventions to support the child's adaptation.

Previous Life Experiences. The child's response to the stress of illness and hospitalization is influenced by previous experiences, particularly those perceived as stressful. Hospitalization may be the first stressful experience encountered by the child and family. If so, the child's repertoire of responses and skills will be limited because of little experience in responding to stress.

Other children have had many opportunities to develop coping skills in response to stress. The child whose family moved a great distance 2 months before the child's hospitalization or whose mother began full-time work after giving birth to the family's second child certainly will have had practice with coping. Such recent changes in the child's life may intensify feelings of vulnerability and insecurity.

Previous stressful life experiences may influence the child's perception of the immediate stress. What, for example, is the meaning of hospitalization to a 10-year-old girl whose maternal aunt died with cancer in a hospital 3 months earlier? Knowing about the child's previous life experiences that the child and family perceive as stressful helps the nurse understand the child's responses to the immediate stress and affects planing and interventions.

Family. The greatest environmental influence on a child is the family. The family constellation, ability to organize daily activities, socioeconomic level, cultural-ethnic makeup, and previous life experiences have implications for nursing care of the child.[45,47] Several factors relate to the child's vulnerability to psychological disturbance resulting from hospitalization. For example, children from chaotic, disorganized families experiencing chronic family distress—called *families with high psychosocial disadvantage*—have the greatest risk for psychiatric disturbance resulting from hospitalization.[52]

Assessment of the family's cultural-ethnic orientation has obvious implications for nursing care.[4,35,66] What language does the family speak? What language can they read? Can they understand the language that the nurse speaks? Perhaps less obvious are the cultural implications for behavioral responses to health care. For example, in Hispanic families, it may be more difficult for a mother to remain with her child in the hospital and to make decisions if she is not accompanied by her husband.

The family's religious beliefs and practices influence their perceptions and coping with stresses of illness. For example, the refusal of blood transfusions by Jehovah's Witnesses may complicate medical care and increase the anxiety of staff, which in turn, compounds the stress on the family. The family's previous life experiences alert the nurse to changes to which they may still be adjusting and that may have depleted their resources for dealing with the stress of the child's illness. Of particular concern is information about loss and grief. Is the family mourning the illness or death of a significant person at the time of the child's hospitalization? How emotionally available are the parents and family members to the child as the child experiences the stresses of illness, disability, and hospitalization?

The mother of an 18-month-old child was observed sleeping throughout the remainder of the day of the child's admission to the hospital and the following day. The mother seldom roused when the child cried or fretted. When talking with the mother, the nurse explored possible reasons for the extended sleep. Suspecting a depressive reaction, the nurse questioned the mother about recent events in the family's life. Although there had not been other illness in the family, the mother's aunt—a close emotional support to her—had died in a car accident 2 days earlier. This information not only assisted the nurse's assessment and plans for care of the child, it also facilitated the nurse's interaction with and personal reactions to the family. The information enabled the nurse to extend empathy and acceptance to the mother, rather than to judge her a "bad" mother because she was unresponsive to her child.

Idiosyncratic (Personal) Attributes of the Child

Assessment of the child's developmental level and of environmental influences on the child must be augmented with an understanding of the child as an individual. What is the child's temperament and personality?[81] Does the child typically move toward new experiences, or is the child shy? What is the child's pain tolerance?[53] What coping mechanisms does the child use to defend against stress?[3,5,25,37] What words does the child use to refer to body parts and functions? Is there a transitional object that provides comfort, such as a blanket or doll? What are the child's preferences—dietary, play activities, nap and bedtime routines? By what name does the child prefer to be called? What was the child like before the illness; that is, what was the child's premorbid personality? Gathering and analyzing information about the child specific to personality and temperament increase the nurse's understanding of the child's responses to the stressors in illness, disability, and hospitalization. It also allows the nurse to implement nursing actions in ways that minimize the strangeness of the health care setting and convey to the child and family the nurse's deep commitment to the child as a person, not an object, in health care.[46]

The nurse analyzes the assessment data to determine the health problems of child and family and to formulate nursing diagnoses. Analysis also helps the nurse understand and clarify personal feelings toward a child and family. For example, understanding that a child's physical expression of anger is a typical response of 2-year-olds, that a child's refusal to find comfort in the nurse's arms is usual in separation anxiety, and that this particular child is described as "a difficult baby" by the mother can help the nurse remain supportive of the child. Through understanding based on assessment of the child, the nurse remains supportive rather than withdrawing because he or she has personalized the child's rejection of nursing efforts.

Assessment of the Health Care Setting

A final aspect of assessment that influences the implementation of the nursing process is the health care setting's ability to meet the psychosocial needs of the child and family. What resources are provided by the physical environment? What departmental or program resources are available? Finally, what is the affective environment of the health care setting? The assessment of the child and family is combined with an assessment of the health care setting's ability to provide for the needs of the child; this total assessment affects the planning and interventions.

The Physical Environment. No hospital or health care setting is ideal; all have assets and limitations that affect the delivery of care to clients. One setting may be particularly supportive of the needs of young children but meet few of the typical needs of adolescents. For example, the pediatric unit may have a large playroom but no space that offers privacy or peer interaction for the teenagers.[16] If there are limited provisions for rooming-in, what will the nurse have to do to make the parent comfortably available to the child? If the pediatric unit does not have a playroom, what can the nurse improvise as space for children to be actively engaged in constructive play?

Department and Program Resources. Departments within the health care setting offer resources the nurse uses in planning care. For example, the dietary department assists in meal planning to meet individual preferences, enhancing the child's nutritional intake and providing more familiar, comfortable mealtimes. The social work department provides financial referrals for families and support and counseling for parents. The child life and child development department (sometimes known as play therapy or children's activities department) provides developmental assessments, supervised play and activities based on assessments, and support for children's understanding and mastery of the health care experience.[1] The volunteer department may provide "parent surrogates" for children whose parents must return to work. Foster grandparent programs are used in this capacity in many children's hospitals in the United States.

The Affective Environment. Does the formal philosophy of the health care setting and nursing department emphasize the psychosocial needs of children and families and family-centered care? Does the informal group attitude welcome parents or feel they are a nuisance? How much support will the nurse receive from the other staff and departments in meeting the psychosocial needs of families?[2] The answers to these questions help the nurse integrate psychosocial care into the physical care of children.

NURSING DIAGNOSIS

The nurse caring for a child who is physically ill or disabled and the child's family uses the assessment data to formulate nursing diagnoses that guide intervention. Appropriate diagnoses could include the following:

1. Altered Growth and Development related to prolonged or repeated hospitalizations, chronic illness, physical disability
2. Fear of invasive or painful procedures related to inadequate comprehension of the medical event, lack of opportunity to use medical play to work through the procedure or event, parental anxiety
3. Ineffective Individual Coping related to overwhelming stimuli of medical environment, lack of comprehension of the medical experience
4. Ineffective Family Coping: Compromised related to serious illness of child, separation of siblings during child's hospitalization, absence of parent from home while staying with hospitalized child
5. Diversional Activity Deficit related to separation from home and usual activities, separation from siblings and peer group, restrictions of illness or disability and treatment

PLANNING

Treatment plans are drawn from the information provided in the assessment of the child and family and the health care setting. Planning includes goal setting, resource use, and discharge planning.

Development of Trust, Understanding, and Mastery

Three concepts are paramount to planning for the child at risk—trust, understanding, and mastery. If the nurse uses these concepts in planning interventions, the psychosocial needs of the child and family will be integrated into nursing care. The nurse must ask such questions as, "How can I assist in the child's and family's development of trust?" "How can I assist in their understanding?'' ''How can I assist in their development of mastery of the stresses they encounter in health care?'' ''What goals can I establish around these concepts?'' ''How can I plan to use the resources available to assist in their trust, understanding, and mastery?'' ''What discharge plans are necessary to continue their mastery?''

Goal Setting

Without goals, the nurse has limited knowledge and limited ability to direct the nursing process. Although treatment plans for physical care of pediatric diagnoses may be standardized in some settings, plans for psychosocial care cannot be standardized. The health care setting necessitates individualization of treatment plans. The nurse plans the performance of required physical care in an emotionally supportive manner.[46]

Treatment plans should be individualized but share some common goals. The primary goal should be to minimize the potential for psychosocial disturbance in the child as the state of physical health is restored or supported. A second goal should be to maximize the opportunities for psychosocial benefit as the child's physical well-being is restored or supported. A third should be to help the child develop trust, understanding, and mastery of the stressful experiences in health care.

Goals specific to an individual child and family, which may lead to positive adaptation, should also be made in the planning process. These goals should include the use of resources available in the health care setting.

A 5-year-old child is admitted for intravenous antibiotic therapy to treat cystic fibrosis. The admission is one of many that the child has experienced, and the hospital and treatment are familiar to the child; however, the child has great difficulty with intrusive procedures. As the nurse plans care, a specific goal for this child will be to develop positive coping with intrusive procedures. Resources available in this particular setting that the nurse plans to use are consistent nursing assignments and the child life and child development program.

Consistent nursing facilitates the child's development of trust. The formation of a therapeutic alliance with the nurse assists the child in perceiving intrusive procedures as necessary steps to feeling better rather than as retaliation or punishment. The child life and child development program provides unhurried opportunities for the child to play out feelings and anxieties aroused by medical procedures. This play, often called medical play, facilitates the child's mastery of aggressive, angry feelings. The presence of the child life specialist during medical play provides support and boundaries for the child's expression of feelings.[63]

Discharge Planning

Discharge planning begins with the assessment of the child and continues throughout hospitalization. For example, instructing parents in home care is most successful when a therapeutic alliance has been formed with the family, a process that begins on admission. The child's specific illness or disability may dictate any particular referrals needed. Discharge planning also includes preparing the family for changes in the child's behavior, either specific to the diagnosis or as common reactions to hospitalization.[57] Discharge plans also should include follow-up contact to assess the child's adjustment and any concerns of the parents.

Finally, discharge planning should include the concept of closure, that is, the ending of an experience marked by a sense of resolution, which can include feelings expressed by the individuals toward one another. This is particularly important for a child who has experienced lengthy hospitalization. Closure of the hospital experience gives the child permission to move on in the process of adaptation—to move back into the family and home and other relationships, while retaining the esteem of the people left behind in the health care setting.

A simple closure device is saying to the child, ''John, you have done it! You have been here with people you didn't know, and you had things done to you that hurt, but you did it! You made new friends in the playroom, you painted your Mom some pictures, and you took your medicine, which helped you feel better. Now you get to go home. You did it! You helped me and the doctor help your kidney. Thank you!''

This small speech, accompanied by a congratulatory handshake, conveys a strong message of mastery to a 7-year-old and takes very little time from the nurse's busy routines.

INTERVENTION

Nursing interventions to support a child at risk due to illness, disability, or hospitalization are directed toward the following:

1. External or environmental factors that influence the child's and family's experience of the stressors
2. Influencing the child's and family's perceptions of the stressful experience
3. Support for family-centered care (Box 47-4)

The concepts of trust, understanding, and mastery are applied to internal and external factors. For example, providing rooming-in for the parent of a 4-year-old is an environmental intervention that enhances the child's ability to trust. Preparing the child for surgery enhances the child's understanding and mastery by in-

BOX 47-4

Family-Centered Care

Advances in medical technology, economic trends in health care and rising hospital costs, and development of home health care services, the consumer movement, and federal initiatives in health care (and in education) for the handicapped provided momentum in the 1980s and early 1990s for emphasis on family-centered care.

As described by the Association for the Care of Children's Health, the elements of family-centered care are as follows.[27,55]

1. Recognition that the family is the constant in the child's life, while service systems and personnel within the systems fluctuate
2. Facilitation of parent–professional collaboration in all levels of health care (care of the individual child, program development, implementation and evaluation, and policy formation)
3. Sharing of unbiased and complete information with parents about their child's care in appropriate, supportive ways on an ongoing basis
4. Implementation of policies and programs and provision of emotional and financial support to meet the needs of families
5. Recognition of family strengths and respect for different methods of coping
6. Understanding and incorporating developmental needs of children and their families into health care delivery systems
7. Encouragement and facilitation of parent-to-parent support
8. Design of health care delivery systems that are flexible, accessible, and responsive to families

By incorporating these elements in the organization and delivery of care, the nurse provides support to children that increases the psychosocial support to families and decreases risk to children in health care.

fluencing the way the child feels about the surgical procedure.[38,58]

Setting Priorities

Nurses set priorities based on assessment data, goals, and plans for individual clients. This provides the nurse with a guide for allocating the resources of time and energy. Priorities should reflect the child's degree of vulnerability for psychosocial disturbance in illness, disability, and hospitalization. Children most vulnerable to psychiatric disturbances are those in the first 4 years of life who have had multiple hospital admissions and who are from psychosocially disadvantaged families. These children should receive the greatest allocation of the nurse's time and energy that can be devoted to psychosocial care. These priorities must coincide with the priorities for required physical care. Other priorities are children of any age assessed as being vulnerable to stress in illness, disability, and hospitalization. Vulnerability is seen in the following children who:

1. have recently have experienced severe stress, such as a death in the family, parents' divorce, or parental illness.
2. have experienced a recent series of stressful events.
3. Were in mild to moderate psychological distress before the hospital admission.
4. cannot understand communication as it is usually performed in the health care setting, communicate in another language, or have severe hearing or visual deficits.
5. have limited life experiences and limited repertoires of behaviors with which to respond to stress.
6. have experienced recent illness or hospitalization that may or may not be related to the present condition.
7. have defects from birth, such as blindness or deafness.[52]

Finally, the nurse considers as priorities interventions that will be growth producing for all clients.[34,87] The child's psychosocial growth is enhanced as he or she adjusts positively to the stresses of illness, disability, and hospitalization. Not all nursing interventions can be planned in advance; some are of an acute crisis nature. As nurses gain experience working with children at risk, they gain greater flexibility in intervening in acute emergency situations.

> A 6-year-old with esophageal varices begins hemorrhaging. The child is alert as the "stat" call is made; the room fills with staff and a cardiac monitor is rushed in. The child looks at the monitor, which has not yet been activated, and cries out in extreme fear, "I'm dying! I'm dead! The line is straight. The line is straight!"
>
> Those participating in this acute emergency will certainly be sensitive to the need for simple explanations in future emergencies when the child is alert and aware of the activities.

In a global sense, and in each specific instance, the nurse must ask, "How can I promote this child's development of trust, understanding, and mastery?"

These three concepts are used to organize nursing interventions.

Interventions to Support and Develop Trust

Interventions to support and develop trust involve external factors, such as changes in the physical environment, in conjunction with interpersonal behaviors, such as communication. The nature and flavor of the interventions vary. Developing trust with a 15-month-old focuses on the presence of the parenting figure; with a 15-year-old, it depends on verbal communication and its congruence with nonverbal messages. Interventions in the physical environment may include the following:

1. Maintaining the child's tie with primary emotional support figures (rooming-in)
2. Ensuring continuity of care in nursing assignments
3. Maintaining the child's tie with family (sibling visiting)
4. Maintaining the child's tie with peer group, for older children and adolescents
5. Structuring delivery of care so that intrusive procedures are not done in the child's bed or room
6. Structuring delivery of care so that routines and rituals associated with activities of daily living (eg, meals, naps, bathing, bedtime) can be continued during hospitalization

Nursing interventions to support trust, which are based on interpersonal behaviors, may include the following:

1. Spending nonstructured, non–task-oriented time with the child and parents
2. Postponing intrusive procedures, whenever possible, until the child and parents recognize the nurse as a trusted individual
3. Communicating openness and trustworthiness through nonverbal signals and congruence of verbal and nonverbal messages
4. Using communication skills of active listening, inviting requests, attending, showing warmth, self-disclosure, and feedback

Interventions to Support and Develop Understanding

Developing and supporting the child's and family's understanding directly affect their stress levels as the nurse mediates their perceptions of the stressors. Observation of young children in health care shows that their fantasies of what will happen often are more frightening than the real events. Through preparation, the child learns about the reality—what he or she will see, hear, feel, and be expected to do. Sensory preparation, which imparts information about what the child will see, hear, and feel, has been successful in decreasing children's anxiety during health care procedures.[35]

The nurse reduces the child's anxiety by relating to the child's concrete feelings rather than by explaining the medical details. For example, an explanation of what happens during the surgery is not appropriate, because the child will not feel during this time. Explaining that a mist that feels cool and soft will be blowing in his or her face when awakening after surgery is important, however. Experiencing the feeling of the mist during presurgery preparation enhances sensory preparation for the child.

Extensive research and clinical literature have shown that understanding can be developed through preparation and client education.[13,29,38,59] Interventions to promote understanding include the following:

1. Preadmission preparation
2. Stress point preparation, immediately before each potentially stressful experience, such as injections, venipunctures, or going to a new location in the hospital
3. Preparation for diagnostic procedures
4. Preparation for surgical procedures
5. Client education to teach child and parents about inpatient and home care, for example, teaching a child newly diagnosed with diabetes to self-administer insulin

The nurse integrates the concept of developing understanding through preparation into all nursing tasks. At each point of potential stress, the nurse gives the child some advance knowledge of what to expect, particularly what he or she will feel.[43] How the nurse presents the information depends on the child's cognitive development, what the child can expect sensorially, and a brief explanation of why.

Answering the question of "why" is important to develop understanding for the child and for parents and other family members.[43] Children's concepts of illness and causality follow developmental trends aligned with cognitive development as described by Piaget.[36,40,64,65] Young children functioning at the concrete operational level need brief, specific, unambiguous, object-related explanations of why things are being done to them.

Older children who can grasp cause-and-effect relationships benefit from simple analogies. Adolescents who have begun abstract thinking may require more detailed information with explanations of the implications for treatment. Giving suitable explanations for health care events lets the child understand that there is a plan for care, that he or she is not being subjected to disturbing events at the whim of more powerful individuals, and that boundaries and limits are known and shared. The impact of regression in health care also must be considered in the child's understanding. A child may regress to a lower level of cognition during stress.

A further aspect of interventions to support understanding relates to the structuring of events. As much as possible, the nurse should structure routines of care to follow a course that can be known to the child. It is desirable, wherever possible, to follow routines the child experiences at home. For school-age children, simple charts of the daily activities and calenders to mark the days and special events will help them understand the process and reinforce the ending of the hospitalization.

By developing a child's understanding of what is to happen, when, and why, the nurse intervenes in the child's perception of the stress. Fantasies become anchored in reality; overwhelming fear of the unknown becomes a manageable known. Parents' perceptions take on more realistic concerns, thereby decreasing the anxiety they project to the child. Numerous movies, filmstrips, coloring books, and children's books have been developed for pediatric preparation and client and parent education. Materials that most closely approximate the reality and provide behavioral modeling for the child most effectively decrease children's anxiety.[59]

Interventions to Support and Develop Mastery

A final group of interventions uses the development of trust and understanding to activate the child's coping with stressors. *Mastery* describes positive coping with stress, which encourages adaptation. Illness, disability, and hospitalization present as life crises that disrupt reality as experienced by the child and family. These life events involve changes to which the child must react. Coping is the process through which the child comes to terms with the changes in reality. Coping devices are the choices in ways of using resources, new structures, and integrations developed by the child to respond to the changes in the environment. Defense mechanisms also are part of the overall coping effort.[17,29] Changes and stressors in the environment demand coping. Adaptation, a return to equilibrium, results from coping. Mastery is positive adaptation, the successful use of coping devices to come to terms with the environment. It is the child's ability to respond to and use the environment constructively.

Resilience, the ability to bounce back from adversity, depends on family cohesion, external support systems that reinforce a child's coping efforts, and self-esteem. Personal relationships and task accomplishment greatly influence self-esteem.[21] Task accomplishment involves positive achievements in school, work, social relationships, and nonschool activities. It can include coping skills, stress inoculation techniques, and social problem-solving skills.[43, 52] Self-esteem also is enhanced by past successful coping and by positive appraisal by others.[56]

In one study of chronic illness in children, the following four adaptive patterns were identified in those who did not develop debilitating psychological symptoms during the course of their diseases:

1. Intellectualization
2. Identification with medical staff
3. Denial in the service of hope
4. Idiosyncratic rituals[22]

Interventions to support these adaptive patterns from the onset of the illness or disability lead to mastery. *Intellectualization* contributes a sense of organization to the ego's assimilation of anxiety (Box 47-5). *Identification with medical staff,* when combined with intellectualization, fosters a strong desire to care for one's own body.

> Identification is seen when a child develops a trusting bond with a particular nurse. The child likes the nurse and knows from pleasurable interchanges between them that the nurse likes her. Because this nurse believes a particular treatment will be helpful, the child also adopts this belief and wants to do what is necessary to help herself.

Denial in the service of hope alleviates the painful external reality of sickness and allows courage and hope to assist the endurance of unreasonable suffering. *Idiosyncratic rituals* are patterns of behavior developed to cope with, or get through, particular aspects of illness or treatments. The rituals bind staff and client together in a shared, nonpathological routine. Unless the ritual interferes with the client's care, staff should not disrupt it, because it offers a playful yet formalized sequence that provides boundaries for the child's anxiety. The ritual enhances the child's feeling of belonging and personal distinctiveness.

> A 6-year-old boy having difficulty with intravenous injections begins chanting, "I think I can; I think I can; I think I can," when he sits down in the treatment room and continues this chant throughout the procedure. This chant is taken from the children's book, *The Little Engine That Could.* At the conclusion of procedures, the child and nurse exclaim together, "I knew I could!" This ritual is repeated whenever the child has intravenous infusions. It brings shared mastery to the child and nurse and recognition and praise for the child's attempts to hold his arm immobile and cooperate as a team member in his care.

These adaptive patterns of behavior that allow the child to manage and master the changes in the environment relate to the internal and external perceptions. Interventions may support mastery through mediating the child's internal or external, physical

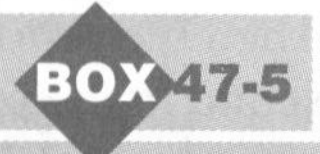

Supporting Children's Use of Intellectualization

A common misconception among young children is that they have somehow caused their illness.[36,64] Telling the child many times in different ways that he or she did not cause the illness develops appropriate intellectualization, which reduces guilt and anxiety.

A 3-year-old girl playing with a doll picked it up, gave it a big swat on the bottom and said, "You've been bad! You have to go to the hospital!" An observing health care provider said to the child and her mother, "Lots of children think they have been bad and that's why they come to the hospital. But you know, you haven't been bad; those other kids haven't been bad. You came to the hospital so your hurt in your stomach would be helped to go away. Your mother knows you weren't bad. She brought you to the hospital so we can help you feel better and help the hurt go away." The mother then picked up the child and gave her a big hug, echoing these statements and adding, "Mommy and Daddy love you." Later, the child was playing with the doll and imitated the words and actions of the mother. This child was using intellectualization, that is, thinking about her experience in ways appropriate to her developmental level, as a coping mechanism.

Intellectualization in an older child was graphically illustrated when an 11-year-old boy requested that pictures be taken of him while he underwent a lumbar puncture. Previously, he had great difficulty with the procedure, was uncooperative, and could not maintain positioning. He could not mentally visualize what was being done to him. The pictures helped him see what was being done, think about what was happening, and understand why positioning and cooperation were important. The pictures were also important as concrete means to help the child think about the experience after it was over and develop mastery. For several days after the procedure, the boy would say to adults entering his room, "Say, do you want to see what I did?" He would then display the pictures with pride at his accomplishment.

environment. Play is a most useful means for supporting mastery.

Play. What is play? It is not the equivalent of adult recreation. Erikson states the following:

> The playing adult steps sideward into another reality; the playing child advances forward to new stages of mastery. I propose the theory that the child's play is the infantile form of the human ability to deal with experience by creating model situations and to master reality by experiment and planning.[15]

Play, he further states, is "an indispensable harbor" used for "overhauling of shattered emotions after periods of rough going in the social seas." It is a device for mastering anxiety-producing aspects of hospitalization and illness or disability. Piaget views play as a means of assimilation. New experiences, such as the stressful events of illness, are assimilated and accommodated into the child's structure.[41] One study looked specifically at the use of play in hospitals by children 3 to 8 years old. The youngest children first established a trusting relationship with the adult in the play setting and then moved to the manipulation of toy objects. Older children used toys rather than the adult to orient, establish familiarity, and then achieve pleasure in the mastery of function. Once familiarity was established, they moved into supportive peer play.[60]

The play environment and the child's use of play can be used to assess and support trust and understanding.[63] Play interventions support mastery by affording the child the opportunity to be actively involved in structuring, controlling, and recreating the stresses of the hospital and illness events. This is most dramatically seen in *medical play,* dramatic play using props of real medical equipment in which the child plays being a client and a caregiver. When this play is nondirective (ie, not designed toward a specific learning objective), the process of mastery is facilitated.

Expression of Feelings. Other interventions that support mastery encourage the child to express feelings through art, story telling, books, and peer-group discussions. Efforts that facilitate communication between parents and child help overcome the "conspiracy of silence" and lead to shared mastery of feelings.

Stress Immunization

Many nursing interventions are protective mechanisms or *stress immunization.* As with all interventions to increase the child's understanding, preparation and play activities afford an opportunity to anticipate the stress event. The child can mentally rehearse the event, become desensitized, and practice coping strategies. Early preparation for a future stress event immunizes the child to the negative effects of the stress experience. Successful management becomes protective as the child's cognitive appraisal is altered from a negative to a sense of accomplishment. For example, one intervention to decrease a child's fear of needles combined reading a story about the event, drawing pictures, discussing fears and fantasies, reading a poem, and playing with medical instruments. This intervention successfully decreased anxiety and fear and increased cooperation during injections. Two additional techniques for children 5 years and older require few materials and little time: thought stopping and relaxation training. Parents can carry out these techniques with their child, activating the child's and the parents' coping skills.

Thought stopping involves substituting reassuring information each time the child begins to think about an upcoming stress event. The child, with the parent and nurse, generates the reassuring information and memorizes short phrases that convey the meaning. For example, a child with daily venipunctures used these positive statements: "It doesn't take too long; I get a prize when it is over; it will help the doctors help me." Her reassuring facts were: "My mother can stay with me; I can go to the playroom when it's over." Using thought stopping gradually weakens fear responses. In addition, the child develops a resource that decreases feelings of helplessness and increases mastery.

Relaxation training teaches the child to focus attention on his or her body, tighten and relax different muscles, and breathe deeply. The same progression should be used each time so that the process becomes familiar. The training should take place many times in a nonstressful setting. When the child has learned the process of relaxation, the parent can coach the child in the process during a stressful event.[43]

Positive Feedback to Child and Family. The nurse further supports mastery through interventions that mediate the child's self-esteem. The Roy Adaptation Nursing Model discusses this as interventions in the self-concept mode.[48] Self-concept is determined through interaction with others.[48] The nurse intervenes by providing positive feedback to the child and family about their successes, however small (Box 47-6).

School Activities. Providing school activities for the child who is hospitalized or homebound builds the child's self-esteem as new academic skills and information are learned successfully. This intervention in the physical environment enhances the child's internal perceptions.[52]

EVALUATION

The final component of the nursing process, evaluation actually is an ongoing process that begins with the child's entry into the health care system. Evaluation is a feedback loop for the nursing process. At any point in the process, evaluation determines the success or appropriateness of other aspects of the process. Evaluation is based on observation and analysis. Observing a child's behavior, analyzing it, and thinking about its

BOX 47-6

Reinforcing Self-Esteem

"Amy, I know it hurts you to have your injections. When you held your leg still, counted to three, squeezed your mom's hand, and said, 'Ouchie!' you helped me! Thank You!"

It is not uncommon to observe children's anger expressed in play. Children will say to a doll, "I'm the nurse, and I'm going to give you a shot. Don't you cry or I'll give you another one!" The nurse who observes such expressed anger may feel dismay to realize the careful support of the child has seemingly gone unrecognized by the child.

However, what is really happening is ventilation of natural anger and retaliation in an acceptable way. Children do have anger and should be allowed to express it. Anger need not represent a personal rejection of the nurse's efforts. If one finds it difficult to accept the display of children's anger, the nurse might need to question his or her personal support system and look for ways to feel good that are not dependent on a child's total acceptance.

In one setting where psychosocial care is a priority, the nurses try to have some pleasant physical interaction with young children after an invasive procedure. The nurse will say something like, "Judy, I know the needle I gave you hurt. I wish I didn't have to hurt you, but that is the only way to give this medicine. Now that the hurt is over, can I give you a hug? I want to help you feel good, too." Most children eagerly and positively respond to this request. Parents also seem to appreciate this extra display of caring for their child.

Occasionally, a child will refuse. If the nurse takes this refusal as a personal rejection, further distress is placed on the child. when the nurse accepts the child's refusal and says, "That's okay, Judy. Some other time maybe we can do something nice together—when you want to," the nurse conveys a deep acceptance of the child as an individual and a belief in the child's basic worth and hope for better things to come.

meaning and probable causes confirm or modify the analysis of assessment data and subsequent plans. Evaluating the child's response to interventions may lead to developing other interventions, continuing present interventions, or developing a new plan of care.

Self-Reflection

Evaluation also offers the nurse an opportunity for self-reflection: "How am I doing?" "How do I feel?" "How am I coping?" "What stresses am I experiencing in working with this child and family?" Therapeutic use of self when working with the child at risk is a primary organizing factor in the nursing process. Conveying an openness, acceptance, and warmth actualizes the development of trust. Understanding, developed through preparation, enables clear, appropriate communication between the nurse and child and family. Ego strength in the nurse is necessary to allow and accept the child's negative feelings.[28] At times, the nurse's defense mechanisms may aid in coping. At other times, they may interfere with personal coping and with assisting the child and family in positive coping. An example of this interference is the nurse's denial of pain when, in truth, bearing the child's pain is difficult for him or her. For example, a nurse may say to a child, "There, that was just a little stick. It didn't really hurt so bad. Don't cry." The nurse is actually saying that she hates to hurt children and does not want the child to cry because he or she will have to face the fact that he or she did hurt the child. The nurse must continually evaluate the effectiveness of defense or coping mechanisms and processes. Working with ill or disabled children in a hospital or health care setting can be emotionally painful and draining. There are times of helplessness: The child's physical pain continues, the disability cannot be reversed, disease progress cannot be arrested, or death is an approaching reality. Anger is a natural expression of helplessness. How and where the nurse directs anger is important. Evaluating professional and personal effectiveness is enhanced by awareness of other defense or coping mechanisms, such as denial, repression, projection, intellectualization, and overidentification.

Need for Personal and Professional Supports

Working with children can stir up the "child" in each of us. Unresolved issues in our developmental past may be brought into preconscious awareness and may evoke unpleasant feelings. Acknowledging and accepting these feelings, understanding oneself, and developing personal support systems and professional support systems within the work setting all aid in caring for children at risk.[4]

◆ The Nurse's Role as an Advocate

While knowledge of the psychosocial needs of children in health care has progressed, the application of such knowledge has lagged Decisions about the allocation of funds and resources often are made by people far removed from the literature and research findings. The medical model, built on concrete observations and manipulation of observable data, is frequently resistant to the "soft" sciences. Changing routines of care to meet psychosocial needs of children acknowledges that providing health care can be detrimental to children's development; those caring for children are reluctant to admit that while helping, they also inflict pain. Regardless of these and other explanations, the need to provide for the psychosocial requirements of children and families exists. As an advocate, the nurse educates about, facilitates, and models more effective care of children.

Advocacy occurs when the nurse shares with other health care providers information that helps them understand the child and family. This may be done through verbal communication, as when giving a change-of-shift report, or written communication in the nursing progress notes. Advocacy may also take the form of volunteering to present nursing inservice education programs organized around psychosocial issues. Frequently, advocacy for individual children takes the form of sharing information that makes caring for the child easier for other staff. For example, the nurse may share tricks of the trade with a laboratory technician who must collect blood samples from a child. Advocacy also takes place when the nurse shares information with the parents. It is not uncommon to see parents placing unrealistic demands for behavior on their child. The parents might say to their child, "You're a big boy now—don't cry!" By explaining pain and the usefulness of expressing pain for the child's emotional and physical well-being, the nurse promotes quality care for the child.

At times, advocacy is best accomplished by helping others identify, intellectually and emotionally, with the child and family.

> One child used a ritual of stalling and gaining control before he could participate in intrusive procedures. He seemed to need more time than other children. This need for time was interpreted by one staff member simply as stalling that served no useful purpose other than taking up time. Another nurse observed, "Did you ever dive off the high-dive board when you were little? I can remember climbing the ladder, getting to the top, walking out to the end of the board, and I just couldn't make myself jump. I wanted to. I would back up a little, take forward steps, and then stand again. I just couldn't do it at first. I'd take an-

other try, and finally I would be able to. I think this is what Jeff does. He's just getting himself ready for the big plunge." The first nurse, with a strong remembrance, exclaimed, "I used to do that when I was doing backward dives off the high dive. Was I ever scared!" With an analogy she could appreciate, this nurse was able to understand the child's need for "just a little more time" to get ready for frightening events.

Advocacy also occurs during staff meetings when health care providers discuss ideas and reach decisions about routines of care for children and their families. Speaking up on ways to provide health care that meet the institution's needs and the psychosocial needs of children and families demonstrates for others the importance and possibility of combining and meeting both needs. Reading journals, talking with people from other health care settings, and attending educational conferences impart information about how best to care for children and families in pediatric settings.

Accepting the role of advocate involves realizing that advocacy can minimize the potential for psychosocial disturbance and maximize the opportunities for benefit to children by facilitating physical care. By reducing the emotional stress component of the client's illness, the child is left with more metabolic resources in reserve to deal with the disease.[29]

◆ Chapter Summary

This chapter has discussed the child in health care from the perspective of the stress-adaptation theory. Illness, disability, and hospitalization are life crises for a child and family; the impact of these events can affect the child's developmental progress. Major points of the chapter include the following:

1. Children with chronic conditions have increased risk for difficulties in psychological development.
2. Children with multiple admissions to the hospital in the first 4 years of life are the most vulnerable to psychological disturbance.
3. The nurse recognizes and analyzes the influences of hospitalization, parent–child attachment, and communication when applying the nursing process.
4. Assessment of the child at risk for psychosocial disturbance in health care includes gathering information about the child's developmental level, the environmental influences on the child (such as the nature of the specific illness or disability, the child's previous life experiences, and the child's family), and personal attributes of the child.
5. Planning and interventions for the child who is ill, disabled, or hospitalized are evaluated for effectiveness in supporting the child's and family's development of trust, understanding, and mastery of the stresses involved in health care.
6. Preparation for experiences encountered in health care and the use of play are common yet crucial psychosocial interventions.
7. Mastery allows children to be active on their own behalf, to turn from being passive victims to assuming participatory roles.
8. Interventions to support mastery allow the child active exploration of feelings, as in nondirective play and expressive arts; enhance the child's and family's self-concept and self-esteem; and promote family-centered care.
9. Evaluating the effectiveness of nursing intervention is based on observation and analysis of the child's and family's behavior and self-reflection.
10. The nurse's acceptance of the advocate role, coupled with the responsibility to minimize potential psychological disturbances and maximize growth potentials, affords the challenges and rewards of nursing for children.

Review Questions

1. The effects of the overlay of chronic illness and disability on development may be seen when
   - **A.** a toddler refuses to eat the food being fed him.
   - **B.** an adolescent with diabetes refuses to comply with the medical regimen.
   - **C.** an infant has recurrent ear infections requiring surgery.
   - **D.** a parent stays in the hospital room of a latency-age child with a physical disability.
2. Which group of children are most vulnerable to psychological distress resulting from hospitalization?
   - **A.** Adolescents with chronic illness
   - **B.** Preadolescents who have life-long disabilities
   - **C.** School-age children who have never been hospitalized
   - **D.** Children under 4 years with multiple admissions to the hospital
3. What is the *most* important intervention to decrease emotional upset in a child who is in a hospital or health care setting?
   - **A.** Presence of her/his primary emotional support person
   - **B.** Preparation for medical events
   - **C.** Age-appropriate and clear communication
   - **D.** Availability of play materials
4. Which of the following would not help the child at risk develop trust, understanding, and mastery?
   - **A.** Consistent nursing care
   - **B.** Therapeutic alliance with caregivers
   - **C.** Discouragement of expression of feelings
   - **D.** Medical play

5. Common fears and anxieties of school-age children in health care are
   A. separation anxiety and fear of strangers.
   B. anxiety about body image and fear of loss of status among peers.
   C. fear of bodily injury and fear of loss of love and respect.
   D. anxiety about bodily intrusions and fear of bodily mutilation.

◆ References

1. Amercian Academy of Pediatrics, Committee on Hospitalized Care: Child Life Programs. Pediatrics 91 (3): 671–673, 1993
2. Amico J, Davihizar R: Supporting Families of Critically Ill Children. Journal of Clinical Nursing: 3 (4): 213–218, 1994
3. Austin JK: Assessment of Coping Mechanisms Used by Parents and Children With Chronic Illness. MCN 15 (2): 98–102, 1990
4. Beardslee WR, DeMaso DR: Staff Groups in a Pediatric Hospital: Content and Coping. Am J Orthopsychiatry 52 (October): 712–718, 1982
5. Bossert E: Factors Influencing the Coping of Hospitalized School-Age Children. Journal of Pediatric Nursing: Nursing Care of Children and Families 9 (5): 299–306, 1994
6. Bowlby J: Separation: Anxiety and Anger. New York, Basic Books, 1973
7. Brookins GK: Culture, Ethnicity, and Bicultural Competence: Implications for Children With Chronic Illness and Disability. Pediatrics 91 (5): 1056–1062, 1993
8. Burke SO, Kauffman E, Costello EA, Dillon MC: Hazardous Secrets and Reluctantly Taking Charge: Parenting a Child With Repeated Hospitalizations. Image—Journal of Nursing Scholarship 23 (1): 39–45, 1991
9. Cadman D, Boyle M, Offord DR: The Ontario Child Health Study: Social Adjustment and Mental Health of Siblings of Children With Chronic Health Problems. Dev Behav Pediatr 9: 117–121, 1988
10. Cadman D, Boyle M, Szatmari P, American DR: Chronic Illness, Disability and Mental and Social Well-being: Findings of the Ontario Child Health Study. Pediatrics 79: 805–813, 1987
11. Canam C: Common Adaptive Tasks Facing Parents of Children with Chronic Conditions. J Adv Nurs 18 (1): 4–53, 1993
12. Douglas JB: Early Hospital Admissions and Later Disturbances of Behavior and Learning. Dev Med Child Neurol 17 (August): 456–480, 1975
13. Droske S, Francis S: Pediatric Diagnostic Procedures. New York, John Wiley & Sons, 1981
14. Drotar D, Crawford P: Psychological Adaptations of Siblings of Chronically Ill Children: Research and Practice Implications. Dev Behav Pediatr 6: 355–262, 1986
15. Erikson E: Childhood and Society. New York, WW Norton, 1950
16. Francis S, Myers-Gordon K, Pyper C: Design of an Adolescent Activity Room. Children's Health Care 16 (4): 268–273, 1988
17. Freud A: The Ego and Mechanisms of Defense. New York, International Universities Press, 1966
18. Freud A: The Role of Bodily Illness in the Mental Life of Children. In Eissler RS, Freud A, Kris M, Solnit A (eds): Physical Illness and Handicap in Childhood, pp 1–12. New Haven, Yale University Press, 1977
19. Friedman MM: Transcultural Family Nursing: Application to Latin and Black Families. J Pediatr Nurs 5 (3): 214–222, 1990
20. Gallo AM, Breitmayer BJ, Knafl KA, Zoeller L: Stigma in Childhood Chronic Illness: A Well Sibling Perspective. Pediatric Nursing 17: 21–25, 1991
21. Garmezy N: Resilience in Children's Adaptation to Negative Life Events and Stressed Environments. Pediatr Ann 20 (9): 459–466, 1991
22. Geist RA: Onset of Chronic Illness in Children and Adolescents: Psychotherapeutic and Consultative Intervention. Am J Orthopsychiatry 49 (January): 4–23, 1979
23. Gudas LJ, Koocher GP, Wypij D: Perceptions of Medical Compliance in Children and Adolescents with Cystic Fibrosis. Dev Behav Pediatr 12 (4): 236–242, 1991
24. Hass DL, Gray HB, McConnell B: Parent/Professional Partnerships in Caring for Children With Special Health Care Needs. Issues in Compehensive Pediatric Nursing 15 (1): 39–42, 1992
25. Hauck MR: Cognitive Abilities of Preschool Children: Implications for Nurses Working With Young Children. J Pediatr Nurs 6 (4): 230–235, 1991
26. Hinds PS, Martin J: Hopefulness and the Self-Sustaining Process in Adolescents With Cancer. Nurs Res 37 (6): 336–340, 1988
27. Hostler SL: Family-centered Care. Pediatr Clin North Am 38 (6): 1545–1560, 1991
28. Lauterbach SS, Becker PH: Caring for Self: Becoming a Self-reflective Nurse. Holistic Nursing Practice 10 (2): 57–68, 1996
29. Lazarus R, Folkman S: Stress, Appraisal, and Coping. New York, Springer Publishing, 1984
30. MacPhee M: The Family Systems Approach and Pediatric Nursing Care. Pediatric Nursing 21 (5): 417–423, 1994
31. McLeod SM, McClowry SG: Using Temperament Theory to Individualize the Psychosocial Care of Hospitalized Children. Child Health Care 19 (2): 79–85, 1990
32. Mulhern RK, Wasserman AL, Friedman AG, Fairclough D: Social Competence and Behavioral Adjustment of Children Who Are Long Term Survivors of Cancer. Pediatrics 83 (1): 18–25, 1989
33. Patterson JM: Family Resilience to the Challenge of a Child's Disability. Pediatr Ann 20 (9): 491–499, 1991
34. Patterson JM, Gaber G: Preventing Mental Health Problems in Children With Chronic Illness or Disability. Child Health Care 20 (3): 150–161, 1991
35. Pellegrini DS: Psychosocial Risk and Protective Factors in Childhood. Dev Behav Pediatr 11 (4): 201–209, 1990
36. Perrin EC, Sayer AG, Willett JB: Sticks and Stones May Break My Bones...Reasoning About Illness Causality and

Body Functioning in Children Who Have a Chronic Illness. Pediatrics 88 (3): 608–619, 1991

37. Perrin JM, MacLean WE: Children with Chronic Illness: The Prevention of Dysfunction. Pediatr Clin North Am 35 (6): 1325–1335, 1988
38. Peterson L: Coping by Children Undergoing Stressful Medical Procedures: Some Conceptual, Methodological, and Therapeutic Issues. J Consult Clin Psychol 57: 380–388, 1989
39. Phillips M: Support Groups for Parents of Chronically Ill Children. Pediatric Nursing 16 (4): 404–406, 1990
40. Piaget J: The Language and Thought of the Child. New York, Meridian Books, 1953
41. Piaget J: Play, Dreams and Imitation in Childhood. New York, WW Norton, 1962
42. Pless IB, Power C, Peckham CS: Long-term Psychosocial Sequelae of Chronic Physical Disorders in Childhood. Pediatrics 91 (6): 1131–1136, 1993
43. Poster EC: Stress Immunization: Techniques to Help Children Cope with Hospitalization. Matern Child Nurs J 12 (Summer): 119–134, 1983
44. Quinton D, Rutter M: Early Hospital Admissions and Later Disturbances of Behavior: An Attempted Replication of Douglas' Findings. Dev Med Child Neurol 18 (August): 447–459, 1976
45. Randall-David E: Strategies for Working With Culturally Diverse Minorities and Clients. Washington, DC, Association for the Care of Children's Health, 1989
46. Radwin LE: Knowing the Patient: A Process Model for Individualized Interventions. Nurs Res 44 (6): 364–370, 1995.
47. Rawlins PS, Rawlins TD, Horner M: Development of the Family Needs Assessment Tool. West J Nurs Res 12 (2): 201–214, 1990
48. Riehl J, Roy Sr C: Conceptual Models for Nursing Practice. New York, Appleton-Century-Crofts, 1974
49. Robertson J: Young Children in Hospitals. New York, Basic Books, 1958
50. Ross-Alaolmolki K, Heinzer MM, Howard R, Marszal S: Impact of Childhood Cancer on Siblings and Family: Family Strategies for Primary Health Care. Holistic Nursing Practice 9 (4): 66–75, 1995
51. Rutter M: Prevention of Children's Psychosocial Disorders: Myth and Substance. Pediatrics 70 (December): 883–894, 1982
52. Rutter M: Psychological Resilience and Protective Mechanisms, Am J Orthopsychiatry 57 (3): 316–360, 1987
53. Savedra MC, Tesler MD, Holzemer WL, Brokaw P: A Strategy to Assess the Temporal Dimension of Pain in Children and Adolescents. Nurs Res 44 (5): 272–276, 1995
54. Seideman RY, Kleine, PF: A Theory of Transformed Parenting: Parenting a Child With Developmental Delay/Mental Retardation. Nurs Res 44 (1): 38–44, 1995
55. Shelton TL, Jeppson ES, Johnson BH: Family-centered Care for Children With Special Health Care Needs. Washington, DC, Association for the Care of Children's Health, 1987
56. Sieving RE, Zirbel-Donish ST: Development and Enhancement of Self-Esteem in Children. J Pediatr Health Care 4 (6): 290–296, 1990
57. Snowdon AW, Kane DJ: Parental Needs Following the Discharge of a Hospitalized Child. Pediatric Nursing 21 (5): 425–428, 1995
58. Thompson ML: Information-Seeking Coping and Anxiety in School-Age Children Anticipating Surgery. Children's Health Care 23 (2): 87–98, 1994
59. Thompson RH: Psychosocial Research on Pediatric Hospitalization and Health Care. Springfield, IL, Charles C. Thomas, 1985
60. Tisza V, Hurwitz I, Angoff K: The Use of a Play Program for Hospitalized Children. J Am Acad Child Psychiatry 9 (July): 515–531, 1970
61. Turner-Henson A: Mothers of Chronically Ill Children and Perceptions of Environmental Variables. Issues in Comprehensive Pediatric Nursing 16 (2): 63–76, 1993
62. Varni JW, Rubenfeld LA, Talbot D, Setoguchi Y: Family Functioning, Temperament, and Psychologic Adaptation in Children With Congenital or Acquired Limb Deficiencies. Pediatrics 84: 323–330, 1989
63. Wolfer J, Gaynard L, Goldberger J, Laidley LN, Thompson R: An Experimental Evaluation of a Model Child Life Program. Children's Health Care 16 (4): 244–254, 1988
64. Yoos HL: Children's Illness Concepts: Old and New Paradigms. Pediatr Nurs 20 (2): 134–140, 1994
65. Youngblut JM: Children's Understanding of Illness: Developmental Aspects. AACN Clinical Issues in Critical Care Nursing 5 (1): 42–48, 1994

The Client on the Human Immunodeficiency Virus Spectrum

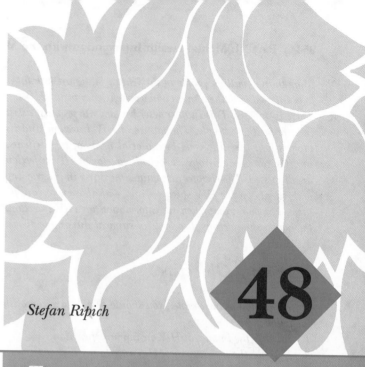

Stefan Ripich

The first time I heard about it I was standing in my kitchen. I was about to go out shopping for my youngest's birthday party. The phone rang. It was this doctor calling me about my son Bernard. He used all these words I can't pronounce. And then he said, "Do you understand what I've told you?" I said yes. Right before he hung up he said, "So you know he has AIDS." That's the first time I heard the word. I turned white.

William M. Hoffman,
As Is

More than 1 million people in the United States are estimated to be infected with the human immunodeficiency virus (HIV).[12] *There is no cure. This chapter describes how nurses must assist in care for these people. The nature of HIV infection and its progression, the numerous psychosocial needs of these clients, and the complex neuropsychological sequelae of HIV infection are discussed. The chapter also guides the nurse in intervening with clients on the HIV spectrum and with those who care for them. For more comprehensive information on HIV infection, the reader should consult a medical-surgical nursing textbook.*

Learning Objectives

On completion of the chapter, you should be able to accomplish the following:

1. *Identify the impact of HIV on immune function.*
2. *Describe the progression of HIV infection.*
3. *Evaluate your own feelings about caring for a client on the HIV spectrum.*
4. *Identify the potential psychosocial problems and neuropsychological complications associated with HIV infection.*
5. *Apply the nursing process to caring for a client on the HIV spectrum.*

◆ Overview of HIV Infection

Viruses are minute fragments of protected genetic material. They enter cells, usurp cellular function, and direct the cells to abandon all normal activities and only create new viruses. A virus can be thought of as a loaded gun—not as a living creature, but as something with potentially disastrous effects given the right sequence of events.

Viruses are remarkably specific considering their simple nature. They commonly have a lipoprotein coat (also manufactured by their host cell), which helps them to find exactly which cells they can infect to support their own replication. Because viruses use the biological machinery of their host cells, there are very few differences between viruses and hosts. This makes it nearly impossible to intervene to destroy the virus without also harming the host. Although information about viruses and HIV in particular is rapidly changing, one fact remains: According to today's thinking, acquired immunodeficiency syndrome (AIDS) is incurable.

ETIOLOGY AND INCIDENCE

Similar to other viruses, HIV affects only specific cells. Its particular host cell is the human CD4 cell, an important part of the human immune system. CD4 cells (formerly called T cells) defend against very primitive invaders such as fungi, yeasts, and other viruses; HIV invades CD4 cells and takes over their functions. Soon, the CD4 cells are too busy replicating more HIV to perform their own immune function.

Once the host has been infected with HIV, other immune system components form antibodies to fight the HIV. Detection of these antibodies in several laboratory tests is, in most cases, positive proof that the person was exposed to HIV. Such a person is said to be *HIV-positive.* It takes about 3 months after exposure for today's antibody tests to shift into a positive range.

Ironically, even though the host's immune system may be devastated by HIV, other immune functions can remain intact. When immune system depletion results in several specific infections (called *opportunistic infections* because the infectious agents use the opportunity of a compromised immune system to infect a host), the person is diagnosed as having AIDS. Knowing that HIV invades cells that defend against primitive organisms helps to explain why people living with AIDS commonly suffer from such opportunistic infectious agents as *Candida albicans* (thrush), herpes zoster, and *Pneumocystis carinii* pneumonia, and such cancers as Kaposi's sarcoma and various lymphomas.

This chapter deals with all people infected with HIV, regardless of their wellness status. Because physical symptoms of HIV infection can range from remaining absent for many years to causing death from an AIDS-related opportunistic infection, HIV-positive people are referred to as being on the HIV *spectrum.* Problems requiring psychiatric nursing intervention can affect people at all points on the HIV spectrum. About 600,000 people in the United States have been diagnosed with AIDS.[12] For each person diagnosed with AIDS, as many as 10 people may be HIV-positive. Spread of HIV occurs through exchange of body fluids that contain the virus; it cannot be spread through casual contact. It must have a portal of entry, such as a tear in a mucous membrane (as might occur through sexual contact) or access to the bloodstream (as might occur in transfusions or injections with contaminated needles). Another possible transmission route is from a mother to her fetus. These specific modes of transmission place certain groups of people at greater risk for HIV infection than others; in general, gay men, intravenous drug users, and sexual partners of intravenous drug users have been hit the hardest in the AIDS epidemic. However, HIV is spreading into the heterosexual population. All nurses, regardless of their area of practice, have had or soon will have contact with HIV-positive people.

Progression of HIV Infection

Soon after exposure to HIV, the body mounts a response to the virus, commonly causing severe mononucleosis-like symptoms characterized by fatigue and swollen glands. This response, termed a *conversion reac-*

tion, usually occurs 4 to 6 weeks after initial infection. During this time, a person does not have sufficient antibodies to shift the HIV screening test into the positive range and would appear to be HIV negative. After 8 to 12 weeks, the person usually has sufficient antibodies to shift the test into the positive range.

The next phase of HIV infection is characterized by several years of latency, during which no physical signs of illness are apparent. The person may be psychologically aware that he or she has a life-threatening illness, but no health problems exist yet. He or she may view HIV infection as a punishment for some form of behavior; a gay man may experience a resurgence of previously resolved internalized homophobia. Some people describe a sense of worry or impending doom during this phase, while others describe a sense of grief related to a loss of options for the future, given the uncertainty about the amount of time they have left to live. Some may feel compelled to remain in jobs they dislike to avoid interrupting health insurance coverage. Others may be interested in forming a primary relationship or starting a family but wonder how they can find a partner who will love them if they are HIV-positive. Many are well enough and at the appropriate developmental stage to focus on career and relationships but feel their HIV status thwarts their dreams and aspirations.

Eventually, the immune system weakens as more CD4 cell blood counts correlate with increasing health problems. In this compromised state, the person may suffer from such generalized problems as fatigue, swollen lymph nodes, periodic fever, or other annoying but non–life-threatening health problems. During this phase and in the asymptomatic phase that precedes it, the person commonly becomes obsessed with his or her CD4 count. Laboratory values are seen as indicators of health status, and falling CD4 counts often precipitate feelings of depression, anger, and helplessness.

Inevitably, whatever denial may have served as an effective coping mechanism is defeated as CD4 cells drop or the first opportunistic infection appears. What was once known and understood only on an intellectual level becomes a physical reality to be dealt with at every turn—every 4 hours when a pill is taken or with every swallow of a throat made sore by an oral yeast infection. These clients need medical intervention and psychosocial support to help resolve this crisis.

Several years into the progression of the HIV, a person usually faces periodic health problems that may require hospitalization. Most often, however, the HIV-positive person is at home with illnesses of varying severity. The person may be too sick to work and may face financial stresses. Such issues as finding suitable and affordable housing; providing for dependent family members, such as children or parents; and perhaps even having a partner also dying of AIDS cause increased stress. For a person too sick to leave the home or from a stigmatized risk group with limited social support (such as gay men and drug abusers), social isolation becomes increasingly problematic. Also, self-image may be dramatically altered secondary to weight loss or disfiguring Kaposi's sarcoma lesions. The correlation between increased isolation and increased prevalence of illness is significant; as isolation increases, the symptoms of physical illness develop faster.[6]

Finally, in most cases, about 1 decade after initial infection, the person progresses to an AIDS diagnosis and is in the final stages of his or her life. Resolution of grief, life review, and approaching death are important issues.

◆ Attitudes About HIV and AIDS

Although every nursing student is admonished to pay attention to his or her feelings to avoid bringing personal issues into the nurse–client relationship, the client on the HIV spectrum requires one further step. Beyond examining personal feelings, the nurse also should examine the role of cultural myths that attempt to answer the terrible question, "Why is AIDS happening?"

MYTHS ABOUT AIDS

As stories or belief systems found in every culture, myths serve several important purposes. Myths bind generations together by transmitting cultural beliefs from one generation to the next. They help explain catastrophic events to decrease anxiety for a whole culture. Myths also hurt and alienate people, explain events inaccurately, and increase anxiety among individuals.

Several myths seek to explain AIDS.[8] For instance, some people believe that AIDS is a punishment for wrongdoing or immorality. Although many religions have done away with the notion of an angry, vengeful god who smites the wicked, this myth remains pervasive in American culture (think of the expression "hit by a bolt of lightning" or "may God strike me dead"). Somewhere in the nurse's consciousness—and in the consciousness of the HIV-positive person—may be the myth that AIDS results from bad behavior. The last thing a person living with AIDS needs is a caregiver who believes, however well intentioned, that the HIV-positive individual is waging a hopeless and predestined battle with an angry God. We know that AIDS is caused by a virus and not anything supernatural. A behavior can be done repeatedly, but if the virus is not present, the infection cannot occur.

Another myth is that AIDS is a new age messenger sent to teach us new ways of getting along. According to this myth, only when we collectively learn to reach out in love and acceptance will the world be rid of AIDS.

A similar myth is that AIDS is the result of a sick earth. Some point to world events as evidence that things are out of control. According to those who believe this myth, phenomena like feline leukemia (a disease similar to AIDS in cats) and reports of AIDS in species as different from each other as cows and dolphins suggest that the environment has become so contaminated that illness and disease are bound to follow.

Myths of mysterious, top-secret covert activities by the federal government or big business take many different forms. One is that AIDS is the result of a government germ warfare experiment that went wrong. Another, supposedly supported by the fact that Africa has been so hard-hit by AIDS, is that AIDS started when the government shipped a large cargo of inferior-quality hepatitis vaccine there. Still another myth is that AIDS is not caused by HIV, but HIV is an elaborate ruse devised to allow pharmaceutical companies and the health care system to reap big profits from expensive drugs and treatments.

THE NURSE'S ATTITUDES

The nurse may have feelings that are unrelated to transmission of HIV but are tied to caring for any chronically ill or dying client. When dealing with a client in the early stages of HIV infection, the nurse struggles to maintain the client's health and quality of life. Simultaneously, the nurse must struggle with the responsibility of helping the client and his or her loved ones understand the reality of HIV infection and the client's uncertain future. This dichotomy between optimism and reality is often frustrating and disheartening. Although the nurse supports life and joins in the therapeutic relationship, he or she is also forced to realize that this relationship may ultimately end in the client's death.

As the disease progresses, the nurse must face the future honestly with the client. The nature of HIV infection often requires an intense, collaborative nurse–client relationship. The nurse must assist the client understand the future, prepare for potential problems, and hopefully cope with these problems with dignity. The nurse becomes a primary person in rallying resources to sustain the client's quality of life. This is perhaps the most difficult time for the client and the nurse, because the client's coping skills are increasingly challenged.

Eventually, the nurse, the client, and the client's loved ones must prepare for the client's death. The nurse may feel a deep sense of frustration as every attempt to prevent disease progression fails. Nurses also must deal with feelings of grief while preparing emotionally for the death of a client for whom they have provided so much care and support. Nurses may need to seek support to help resolve these feelings.

◆ Psychosocial Aspects of HIV Infection

People on the HIV spectrum have varied psychosocial needs that change with time. This section identifies people at risk for special psychosocial needs and reviews these needs as they change with disease progression.

IDENTIFYING RISKS

Many people who are anxious about their HIV status are hesitant to discuss the matter with health professionals because they are embarrassed or fear recrimination. Clients may offer subtle cues as to the nature of their fears but will not always bring these fears into the open. The nurse should address issues regarding HIV and AIDS with *every* client, not just those in known risk groups. As people are exposed to more AIDS information (and misinformation), adequate education needs to be a part of every interaction with clients. The nurse's open, nonjudgmental attitude will encourage a concerned client to verbalize his or her fears, as will the presence of literature, posters, or other information in the care setting, which conveys the message that AIDS is an acceptable topic of discussion.

Anxiety about being tested for HIV status is common, and in many areas, pretest and post-test counseling is required by law. During this counseling, the nurse explores several key areas. First, what does the client understand about the meaning of a positive or negative test result? A client may perceive a positive result as a death sentence. Second, how will the client deal with a positive test result? A particularly troubled client may have inadequate coping mechanisms to deal with a positive result and may increase drug or alcohol use to blunt fear, sadness, or anger. In contrast, another client may be inspired by a positive result to regain control of his or her life and be motivated to engage in health-promoting behaviors. The nurse can identify clients with inadequate coping mechanisms and make the appropriate referrals for ongoing psychotherapy or support. Third, will a positive test result increase a client's risk of suicide? The nurse may be hesitant to ask this question but should raise it with every client who comes for HIV testing. The suicide rate for men with AIDS is 66 times higher than in the general population;[9] thus, the nurse needs to assess for suicide potential in every client considering HIV testing. When a client expresses thoughts of hopelessness or self-harm, the nurse should explore these thoughts in more depth. Often such thoughts are based on misinformation, which the nurse can dispel. When the client persists in these thoughts after further discussion, referral for further evaluation is indicated (see Chapter 42, Suicide).

Whatever concerns the nurse might have regarding these three issues—the meaning of the HIV test result, coping mechanisms, and suicide risk—should not deter the nurse from advising testing for a client who fears he or she may be HIV-positive. Early detection and prompt intervention can only enhance the duration and quality of life for the client on the HIV spectrum.

Another important group at risk for psychosocial difficulties is those who love and care for the client on the HIV spectrum (some of whom may be HIV-positive themselves). These caregivers are often subject to tremendous physical and psychological burdens in caring for a chronically ill loved one. Because they may be part of an alternative family structure, such as a gay union, an extended family structure found among gay and lesbian people, or two unmarried heterosexual people, they may lack the social supports afforded the traditional family.

Nursing traditionally has valued a holistic approach to care and has viewed environmental considerations as essential in planning nursing intervention. The person living with AIDS, like everyone, exists within an environmental context. Caregivers also exist in this context. Nursing support for the person living with AIDS frequently may mean nursing support for the caregiver and the client. Because these caregivers often are outside readily identifiable family structures, the nurse needs to be vigilant for their presence and provide extra attention to their needs.

IDENTIFYING PSYCHOSOCIAL NEEDS

One of the greatest cruelties of AIDS is its unpredictability.[11] The client on the HIV spectrum must live with the uncertainty of life on a daily basis. The ways in which the nurse assists this client in adjusting to this uncertainty have long-range effects.

Early Stage

A client invariably reacts to a positive HIV test result with anxiety (Case Study 48-1). Obviously, this anxiety is legitimate and is intensified by a fear of dying. For example, a client may report increased anxiety associated with loss of a primary relationship or employment because of his or her HIV status. This client may fear disclosing his or her HIV status to loved ones or employers.

The client may experience other emotions as well. Early on, the client learns the meaning of his or her diagnosis in terms of consequences on life plans. Many clients on the HIV spectrum are at a developmental stage where career and family are important tasks. People in American society are encultured at an early age that a person's value is based on what he or she produces, whether that is monetarily or emotionally. As a result, self-esteem issues are often tied to external events. The client at an early stage on the HIV spectrum is faced with many difficult decisions. Although the client may have a realistic desire to accomplish life goals, he or she may need to face the fact that lofty goals may not be attainable and that just living day to day is an adequate achievement. For the younger client, dreams about a career may no longer be available, whereas the middle-aged client may have to relinquish dreams about a comfortable retirement. The client is forced to make important trade-offs, frequently resulting in grief due to loss of dreams and diminished self-esteem due to inability to achieve life goals.

Another factor associated with decreased self-esteem is a sense of shame associated with being on the HIV spectrum. This shame may take several forms. First, HIV-positive people are still stigmatized by society and made to feel like pariahs. Signs of this stigmatization are everywhere, and the message is easily internalized; people with HIV are diseased and unclean. The nurse assists the client in confronting these feelings by casting doubt on their validity.

Second, the client may feel a profound sense of shame associated with how he or she was infected. This feeling may be particularly strong in a homosexual client. A gay man or lesbian commonly grows up receiving powerful messages that his or her sexual orientation is immoral and shameful. Many internalize these messages and are able to attain a sense of self-acceptance only after years of struggle. This self-acceptance may be eroded on receiving a positive HIV test result. The person may feel that homosexuality caused the infection and may feel shame and regret. The nurse can assist the client in coping with these feelings by helping him or her see that HIV caused the infection, not the client. Often, this may be a client's first experience with this kind of unconditional positive regard, and the nurse may need to role model this kind of acceptance.

Third, the client may feel shame in interpersonal relationships. The client may feel unlovable because of the HIV-positive status and may feel profound shame associated with the ability to transmit the virus. The client may describe feelings of being a lethal weapon, capable of infecting anyone through intimacy. Every nurse should know how HIV is transmitted and be able to counsel clients in ways to reduce the risk of transmission. Assisting the client in feeling lovable is an important way of decreasing this shame.

Despite the many psychosocial implications, it is a reasonable goal to assist the HIV-positive client in re-

Case Study

A Client at the Beginning of the HIV Spectrum: Tim

The following was related by Tim, a 26-year-old man who recently learned he tested positive for HIV:

> I found out about my HIV status about 3 months ago. It was pretty rough because my dad died just after that. I had this awful flu about a year ago that wouldn't go away, and I kept trying to get an appointment with this HMO I belong to. Anyway, it went on for about a month, and I still couldn't get in. Finally I went in and they thought that something was really the matter with me but they didn't know what. So they just let me go. Anyway, sometime later a bunch of us from church decided to go in to get tested at the free clinic. I had been practicing safe sex for a long time, so I thought I was in the clear. I only agreed to go to support my friend who was really scared to death. Well, we went in together to get tested. We had our blood drawn together after we got counseled. Two weeks later, we go in to get our results, and it turns out that I'm positive and he's negative! I was shocked, and I kept saying "Wait! This isn't supposed to be happening!" Then my dad died. I felt really sad, and when we had dinner after the funeral and there was this empty chair there, all I could keep thinking was "Am I next?" I finally told my family, and I'm pretty lucky I guess. My mom says she's sure that I'll lick this thing because I'm so hard headed. She may be right. Anyway, I don't like to say I'm HIV positive. I say to people I'm HIV challenged. Or if I do say I'm HIV positive, I mean it like HIV *positive,* you know? Like this somehow has to be a positive experience.

Questions for Discussion

1. Coping with stress is complicated when several stressors are operating at once. Tim described two major stressors: learning that he is HIV positive and his father's death. Based on the other things Tim said, is he subject to any other stressors that you might want to assess? What might you want to explore in terms of Tim's support systems?
2. What about the natural history of HIV infection might explain Tim's difficulty with his HMO?
3. Although Tim seems upbeat, do any clues in his statement alert you that something is bothering him? What do you know about grief reactions that might apply? What defense mechanisms can you identify?

solving these issues and finding contentment. Denial may be an important and appropriate coping mechanism for the client during this time. When a client's reaction to early-stage HIV infection is maladaptive or interferes with any area of the client's life, it requires prompt and effective intervention. The nurse should never downplay psychosocial issues as unimportant or simply a part of the disease. Assisting the client to deal with these issues can help enhance quality of life.

Middle Stage

This stage, in which the client first begins to experience symptoms, commonly is the most challenging time for the client and nurse.[9] It can be a heartbreaking time for the client's loved ones also. As the client begins to experience a decline in health, coping mechanisms are tested more severely (Nursing Care Plan 48-1). The denial that is so common in many illnesses no longer adequately prevents the client's distress. Second, central nervous system (CNS) involvement may make the client respond differently to internal or external stressors.

Until now, the client may have been able to use denial and other coping strategies to subdue worries. In the middle stage, however, the onset of symptoms strips away denial, and the client may experience increased anxiety and a sense of doom. Uncertainty about the future often becomes painful as the client attempts to regain control over his or her health but cannot.

These first symptoms may be as subtle as a change in energy level or as devastating as a neuropathy that

Nursing Care Plan 48-1

A Client in the Middle of the HIV Spectrum: Sandra

The following was related by Sandra, a 37-year-old woman who has known of her HIV-positive status for 5 years:

> Well, I got it from my husband. He uses drugs. Well, I should say he *used* them, since he's in jail now. I hear he's coming out soon. My kids don't know anything yet and I don't want them to, you understand? It's just like I don't want them to have to deal with it at school. But they won't be for long because we're gonna be moving soon. I don't want him coming out of jail and coming around here bothering me. I just got my life back together after this last trip I went through in the hospital. That was terrible. My mother came over to stay with the kids, and she can't handle them. Sometimes I feel like I can't either. But they're all I've got now. I'm gonna move though, to a secret place where nobody will find me. I just keep on doing the best I can, but I worry a lot too. I mean, what's going to happen to these kids? Lots of times I'm too sick to keep on them about homework and stuff. They always want to go out and play, but it's not safe around here for that. And I worry about me too. Seems like every little cough I get, or every little cold I think "Oh please Lord don't let me die" . . . but then it goes away. Only thing is once it's gone I just don't feel better . . . I just keep wondering if not now, then when?

Questions for Discussion

1. *Sandra did move to another place, and then another. What are some of the environmental factors that you should consider when planning Sandra's care? What resources might be helpful to Sandra?*
2. *How do you feel about Sandra's worries that something could happen to her children? How might that affect the care provided for Sandra? Do you feel differently about Sandra than you do about someone who contracted HIV from homosexual sex or an injection of illicit drugs with a contaminated needle?*
3. *Existential philosophers believe that confronting our own mortality is the most important task we can undertake. Sandra clearly is pondering the uncertainty of her life. Would you be inclined to offer hope to Sandra? Would you be comfortable assisting her to explore these issues? What if she verbalized an understanding that her diagnosis is terminal?*

Nursing Diagnosis

Powerlessness related to difficulty dealing with feelings associated with unmanageable events

Outcome

Client will initiate realistic plans for care of self and children.

Intervention	Rationale
Encourage client's expression of feelings of anxiety and fear regarding her health status and the future of her children.	Expressing feelings allows client to clarify issues and mobilize resources.
Help client identify and use support systems, such as resources to help with finances, health care, and child care.	Supportive people and agencies provide the assistance client needs to cope with her multiple stressors; a range of community resources allows the client to receive needed services at present and in the future.

Evaluation

Client makes and follows through on plans for children's and her own care.

leads to paralysis. Regardless of severity, this initial loss, and fear of future losses, can be extremely distressing. The nurse should assist the HIV-positive client to express feelings and identify the positive aspects of life and health that he or she still has. At this stage, the client on the HIV spectrum must realistically accept his or her health status.

Self-esteem and body image may be affected by HIV-related illnesses when the client experiences alterations in appearance or loss of independence when he or she requires increasing help with self-care. The nurse can assist the client by exploring these issues and offering support. The nurse may act as an important bridge between the client and family or between the client and other caregivers during this stage.

The client may express a profound sense of loss of the illusion that he or she would be the "lucky one" who never got sick. The client may be forced to face the loss of the myth that he or she had unlimited time to live. This can be an agonizing time for the client and a time when a positive outlook may be most important in sustaining health-promoting behaviors.

The client's family, too, has important psychosocial needs during this period. The nurse provides them with information about the client's illness and more importantly, may be the only person to whom family members can express their grief, sense of burden, fears, and anger. Often, a family that once was fragmented by rejection of the client's lifestyle is drawn unwillingly into the caregiving role, or the client who once rejected his or her family may have to call on them for assistance. Sometimes family members that had been absent from the client's life suddenly reappear and attempt to usurp the client's autonomy or the authority of the client's primary caregiver in deciding important issues about care. The nurse often must be a mediator in these situations. Working with clients and families requires that the nurse fulfill the role of client advocate, with the client's wishes as the primary concern.

During this phase, it is appropriate for the client, family, and health care team to open a dialogue about loss and death. The nurse often plays a key role in these dialogues, which should occur before life-threatening complications are likely. Death may be a frightening topic for all involved, including the nurse, but one of the most important messages that the nurse can convey is that death, no matter how tragic or premature, is an inevitable and natural part of life and can be faced with peace and dignity.

The nurse recognizes that clients and their families can approach death with peace when they have been encouraged to verbalize their feelings and have been allowed to make their own decisions about those things within their control. Often a client expresses fear of pain as death approaches; the nurse should provide reassurance that any pain that occurs can be controlled. A client may have a specific preference about where he or she wants to die. The nurse cannot make any guarantees but can assist the client and family in making all possible preparations to fulfill this desire.

Although all clients face unforeseen events that may leave them unable to express their wishes, while they are well, they may want to express exactly which measures they want taken to sustain their lives. The nurse serves an important role in encouraging the client to verbalize these feelings and providing further explanation of specific life-sustaining interventions, such as emergency intubation, cardiopulmonary resuscitation, and indefinite mechanical ventilation. In most states, these wishes can be translated into living wills, and the nurse should encourage the client to make such a declaration.

A client also may have specific wishes about what is done after death. The nurse should encourage expression of wishes about funeral services or disposal of property. A parent may worry who will care for his or her children; in most cases, a legal will drawn up by an attorney is required. The nurse can assist the client in dealing with his or her feelings of sadness related to this heartbreaking issue.

Late Stage

By the late stage of AIDS, the client ideally has reached a realistic level of acceptance regarding his or her health status and uncertain future (Case Study 48-2). The client may have the capacity to enjoy life on a day-to-day basis but has several tasks left to accomplish. The client may be faced with physical or cognitive difficulties that hinder daily function and may need support in verbalizing a continued sense of loss as health declines or as memory or cognition decreases. Also, the client may rely on the nurse for continued acceptance despite increasing physical dependence or alterations in appearance. Such environmental factors as money, housing, relationships, and health care may impinge as stressors on the client's psyche. The nurse must assist the client in dealing with this stress and maintaining a positive outlook.

Life review—looking at one's life and making peace with it—becomes an important task in the late stages of HIV infection as the client makes final preparations for death. The goal of life review is to achieve a sense of completion regarding one's life. The nurse can assist the client in identifying what has been accomplished, what is yet to be accomplished, and what never will be accomplished. The client may express joy about certain aspects of life and grief about those things left undone. The client's family also must do a life review as they recall past events and make peace with what has occurred. The nurse should assist the family in understanding and experiencing their own grief and then in reconsolidating without the physical presence of the client.

48-2 **Case Study**

A Client at the End of the HIV Spectrum: Ken

The following was related by Ken, a 42-year-old man with AIDS:

> Well, I guess I've been through it all by now. I have so few T cells left I've got each one of them named! I've had crypto, and toxo, and KS, and thrush . . . but I just keep plugging along. I don't know how I do it. I try to keep a positive attitude, and I just want to be able to say that if I died tomorrow I would have lived a full life today. Sometimes I get so tired, though, you know? I mean, I had these Kaposi's lesions on the veins inside my legs and my legs were swollen. So I went through all this radiation and it went away. Next thing it comes right back on the end of my penis and I have to go get my penis irradiated. They were wonderful and all, and very respectful, but it just gets to me. And then, you know, I'll be sitting there waiting an hour to get my treatment and I'll think to myself, "OK, this isn't worth it anymore," but then right away I stop myself and say, "Wait, Ken! Stop! Don't do that to yourself! Life is worth living. Life is *good*," and you know something? From where I'm sitting right now, and I know this sounds strange when you look at me, I believe life *is* good and even if I am going to die I don't want to miss a single minute of what I have left.

Questions for Discussion

1. Ken identified two important CNS complications of HIV infection that he has experienced. Suppose that he reports a persistent, gradually worsening headache and winces when he turns his head to look at you. What might you suspect?
2. How would you react if one day Ken told you that he feels that life is not worth living anymore and that he wants to stop treatment? What would you assess? How would you feel and what would you do if he told you that he wanted to end his suffering?
3. Ken is a warm and open person who often speaks in public about his illness and experience. If you could ask him anything at all, what would it be? If you could tell him anything, what would you want him to know?

◆ Neurophysiological Aspects of HIV Infection

When caring for any client on the HIV spectrum, the nurse must consider CNS involvement as an overlay for understanding the client's description of what is happening to him or her. About 10% of all clients with AIDS report neurological complaints as the first symptoms; another 40% develop serious neurological problems.[5] As many as 80% to 90% of these clients exhibit some CNS damage on autopsy.[5]

A client may report subtle problems that may appear related to depression but require further evaluation. These subtle changes may appear as irritability, a change in handwriting, forgetfulness, or numerous other symptoms that first may seem trivial. Such early changes may indicate the progression of CNS involvement that can damage the client's personality, ability to think, and ultimately, ability to perform self-care. As CNS functions deteriorate, the client becomes unable to act or interact in the ways he or she once did. The client may struggle to compensate for these subtle changes or may rationalize the new deficits as being related to mood or fatigue or as temporary. Often, the client slowly withdraws from family and friends and may appear to be depressed. Early symptoms of CNS involvement are difficult to distinguish from clinical depression.[5]

Family and friends may find themselves puzzled and disappointed by the client's response. As the client becomes less able to interact, he or she may be less able to reciprocate intimacy. Decreased intimacy between the client and caregivers can lead to an increased sense of burden on the part of the caregivers. The nurse can support caregivers in this crucial time by offering support and encouraging them to attend to their own needs and the needs of the client.

There are four main causes of CNS involvement in the client on the HIV spectrum, each with its own devastating effects: direct HIV infection of the brain, spinal cord, and peripheral nerves; opportunistic infections; lymphomas; and toxic effects of treatments.

DIRECT INFECTION BY HIV

Clients with CNS involvement often have a complicated array of problems known as *AIDS dementia complex* (ADC). Most evidence points to direct infection from HIV as the cause; ADC also is the most common cause of neurological problems in clients on the HIV spectrum.

The physical manifestations of HIV infection of the CNS involve cerebral atrophy, white matter pallor, ventricular enlargement, and sometimes cavities in the brain or spinal cord called *vacuoles.* Neuropsychological assessment reveals a general slowing of cognitive and sensorimotor functions. These findings are consistent with a progressive, subcortical dementia (similar to Huntington's and Parkinson's diseases), involving clumsiness with or without weakness in the arms and legs, social withdrawal, apathy, and personality changes.[5]

Early symptoms of ADC may present as difficulty in concentrating, especially when the task requires extended effort. The client may describe forgetfulness or an inability to do familiar tasks. The client may notice this forgetfulness in subtle ways but as the disease progresses, may be forced to compensate in elaborate ways. The client may become depressed and withdrawn, especially as walking becomes difficult. Changes in handwriting or speech are often experienced at this stage, and the nurse may notice an absence of spontaneous verbal or motor responses.

Fortunately, the drug AZT also crosses the blood–brain barrier and seems to reverse cognitive and motor symptoms. Research that promotes early use of AZT does not address neurological outcomes, but because HIV invades the CNS early, treatment with AZT actually may prevent ADC. However, AZT has side effects that sometimes mimic ADC or other opportunistic infections.

OPPORTUNISTIC INFECTIONS

Toxoplasmosis

Of the three major diseases associated with opportunistic infection of the CNS, by far the most common cause of cerebral mass lesions is *toxoplasmosis.*[1] Toxoplasmosis is caused by a protozoan that enters the body through the gastrointestinal tract, moves into the bloodstream, and infiltrates the brain. In nonimmunocompromised people, the protozoan causes a vascular inflammation that results in a thrombosis, then coagulation necrosis, and ultimately a cyst in the brain. In immunocompromised people, the acute phase continues with multiple abscesses deep in the brain.

Symptoms of toxoplasmosis include lethargy, weakness, and seizures. Depending on the location of the abscess in the brain, it can produce many paralytic symptoms, including hemiparesis, dysphasia, and sensory deficits. The main difference between toxoplasmosis and other opportunistic infections is that toxoplasmosis presents with specific, unilateral, focal neurological findings versus the others that present with generalized symptoms.

Herpesvirus

Three types of *herpesviruses* can attack the CNS: cytomegalovirus (CMV), herpes simplex (types I and II), and herpes varicella zoster. The herpesviruses can diffuse CNS inflammation with such symptoms as stiff neck, headache, confusion, and lethargy and may even progress to coma or death. Of the three types of herpesviruses, CMV has a particular effect on the retina, producing retinal detachment that causes progressive blindness. The course of the herpes infection depends on how well the client's immune system is functioning but is complicated when several viruses are active simultaneously.

Cryptococcal Meningitis

As many as 10% of all people living with AIDS will contract *cryptococcal meningitis.* The causative organism is a common fungus found in soil, which enters the body through the respiratory system. This infection can begin with minor symptoms, such as headache or stiff neck, but it can produce lethargy and focal problems if intracranial pressure is increased due to hydrocephalus. Mainly, however, the client will describe a severe frontal headache over the eyes that is not relieved with any pain reliever and that is present all the time even when awakening.

LYMPHOMAS

Lymphomas once accounted for only about 2% of all primary brain tumors in the United States. Today, lymphomas occur in clients on the HIV spectrum nearly as often as meningiomas (the most common type of noncancerous brain tumor) occur in the general population. Lymphomas typically grow deep within the brain's structures in the thalamus, corpus callosum, or ventricles or between the two cerebral hemispheres. Multiple lesions are common.

Because of their location, lymphomas are like toxoplasmosis; they produce symptoms associated with localized functions. For example, the client may experience one-sided weakness, visual loss, memory loss, confusion, or loss of specific function associated with the area affected. About one-third of clients with these lesions experience seizures.

TOXIC EFFECTS OF TREATMENTS

Any drug that crosses the blood–brain barrier can produce neurological symptoms. A client's new neurological problems may be related to the frequently changing medications used to treat other problems. The client may have added an over-the-counter drug (including dietary supplements or plant or animal extracts) that interacts with other medications. In clients with HIV infection of the CNS, common drugs may have stronger or different effects than usually anticipated.

AZT is commonly used to fight HIV infection and can have side effects that mimic early ADC or other opportunistic infections. Clients sometimes report headaches, nausea, malaise, or depression. Amphotericin B (used to treat cryptococcal meningitis), pyrimethamine (used to treat toxoplasmosis), and many chemotherapeutic agents can cause seizures. Flucytosine (used to treat cryptococcal meningitis) and ganciclovir (used to treat CMV) have been known to cause confusion, drowsiness, and hallucinations. Certain drugs in combination might cause symptoms that mimic CNS involvement; these symptoms would probably not occur if each drug were used alone. AZT has been known to interact with sedatives to produce a profound slowing of mental and physical activities that resembles the effects of Parkinson's disease.

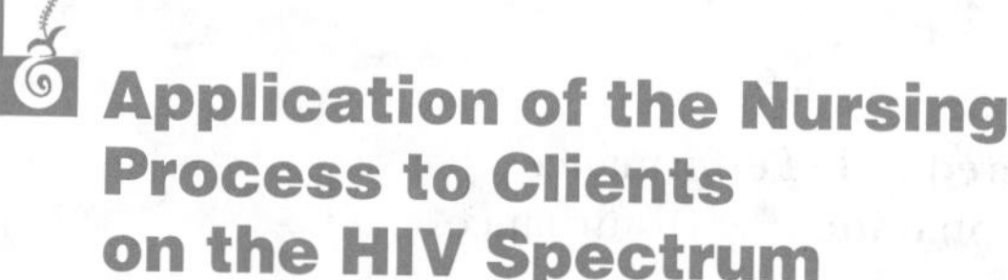

Application of the Nursing Process to Clients on the HIV Spectrum

Holistic nursing care involves the body, mind, and spirit of the client and nurse. Besides providing routine physical care, the nurse must apply the nursing process to assess and intervene for the client's psychosocial and neuropsychological problems.

ASSESSMENT

The client on the HIV spectrum requires constant and consistent scrutiny.[5] In some cases, timely and accurate nursing assessment can mean the difference between temporary and permanent damage, independence and physical debilitation, or even life and death. However, the therapeutic relationship between the client and nurse can be complicated by factors beyond the client's or nurse's control. For example, an extremely agitated or irritable client may drive a wedge into the relationship and insist that it is the nurse's fault. The client may be increasingly forgetful or apathetic and be identified as noncompliant when he or she misses appointments or inconsistently complies with treatment regimens that require regularity. The client may have driven off friends and family by being despondent; these symptoms can progress long before anyone realizes that this behavior is part of the illness.

Most nurses are familiar with global tools for assessing neurological status, such as the Mini-Mental Status Examination, in which clients offer information about their orientation or perform simple tasks. These measures are well suited to the general population but fall short in detecting the subtle neurological changes in the client on the HIV spectrum.

The first and most important way of detecting subtle changes may be the therapeutic relationship and intuitive understandings of baseline function of the client. Just by talking with the client, the nurse often can discern that something is amiss in the client's behavior. The nurse should always follow through on any intuitive suspicions with more definitive assessment.

The nurse can incorporate more structured assessments into regular assessments or even into the daily care routine. These assessments can be informative. For example, most people can recall a series of about seven numbers. If the client cannot remember more than four numbers, then the nurse would suspect memory deficit. Often, when provided with the appropriate questions, the client can identify subtle changes that he or she previously may not have noticed or dismissed as unimportant (Table 48-1). Sensory function might be assessed by asking the client to identify sharp, dull, or soft objects touched to the extremities or fingertips while the eyes are closed.

The nurse can assess motor function by asking the client to perform such activities as touching his or her nose with a finger with eyes closed or by alternately promoting and supinating the hands on the thighs. Difficulty or clumsiness might suggest CNS involvement. Assessing the client's gait or the quantity and quality of spontaneous movements also provides important assessment data. The nurse can also assess higher levels of functioning, such as abstract thinking or problem solving. A client's response to a proverb, such as "a stitch in time saves nine" might indicate concrete thinking, which impairs the ability to learn new behaviors or to apply past learning to new situations. How a client responds to a hypothetical situation might provide information about the client's ability to make important decisions. For example, if clients cannot identify what they might do if they found a sealed letter with a stamp

Table 48-1

Assessing Early Changes in Mental Status

Cognitive Functioning Questionnaire

We want to know if you have any recent concerns about your thinking or mental functioning. We are not trying to find out about life-long problems. Circle Yes only if the problem described has developed or become worse recently (within the last few months to a year). Otherwise, circle No. Please be sure to circle either Yes or No for every item, even if you are uncertain.

Are you more forgetful than usual?	Yes	No
Do you forget new things, like the names or phone numbers of people you've just met?	Yes	No
Do you have more trouble than usual thinking of the names of people you meet unexpectedly?	Yes	No
Do you have trouble finding the right word, even though you know what you want to say?	Yes	No
Do you have trouble organizing your thoughts when you're talking to people?	Yes	No
In conversations do you "miss" things or forget almost immediately what people say to you?	Yes	No
Do you find that even though you know the things you have to do, you forget to do them at the right time?	Yes	No
Do you have trouble concentrating when there's a lot of activity going on around you?	Yes	No
Is it hard to keep your mind on something, like reading or watching television, even when you are in quiet surroundings?	Yes	No
Do you find you have to stop and think about tasks that you used to be able to do automatically or with very little thought?	Yes	No
Do you have trouble planning, organizing, or carrying out complex tasks (for example, working out your time schedule, balancing your checkbook, planning and preparing a meal for several people, following complex directions)?	Yes	No
Do you seem to have trouble getting started with things, even though you have the desire and the ability to do them?	Yes	No
Do you find or do people tell that you have made mistakes in carrying out tasks, even though you were not aware of any problems at the time?	Yes	No
Does your thinking seem slower than usual?	Yes	No
Have you found that you seem less in control of your behavior or feelings than usual (for example, talking more, acting more impulsively, getting irritated or sad more easily)?	Yes	No
Have people said that your personality or behavior seems different from usual?	Yes	No
Has your interest in your job, hobbies, sports, and so forth dropped?	Yes	No
Are you avoiding social contacts, family, friends, and so forth?	Yes	No
Are you having any trouble with your motor coordination, for example, stumbling, being clumsy, dropping things, having sloppier than usual handwriting?	Yes	No

(From Griggens CC, Mack JL: 1990, unpublished material. Used with permission.)

on it, how can they identify what life-support measures they want performed on their behalf?

NURSING DIAGNOSIS

Formulating nursing diagnoses for the client on the HIV spectrum involves considering all relevant psychosocial and neurological factors. The nurse should keep in mind that pertinent diagnoses will fluctuate as the client alternates between inpatient and outpatient care and progresses further along the HIV spectrum. Important nursing diagnoses for the client on the HIV spectrum include the following:

1. Sensory/Perceptual Alterations
2. Self Esteem Disturbance
3. Body Image Disturbance
4. Social Isolation
5. Dysfunctional Grieving
6. Self-Care Deficit
7. Altered Role Performance
8. Personal Identity Disturbance
9. Spiritual Distress
10. Hopelessness
11. Altered Family Processes
12. Anxiety
13. Risk for Infection
14. Risk for Injury

PLANNING AND INTERVENTION

Nursing intervention for the client on the HIV spectrum is directed at supporting the client in remaining as autonomous as possible during varying health states. The nurse must use counseling skills to assist the client through alternating cycles of independence and dependence.

When a relatively healthy person is confronted by

HIV infection, the nurse uses crisis intervention and traditional counseling skills to assist the client in coping on intellectual, emotional, and spiritual levels. For a client with deeply ingrained dysfunctional behavior patterns, the nurse must carefully cull from a mass of assessment data those dysfunctional behaviors that were part of the client's baseline evaluation from those that result from inadequate coping in times of stress. The nurse pays careful attention to boundaries and addresses issues that are amenable to counseling. Long-term psychotherapy may be of great benefit to the client on the HIV spectrum; however, it may require that the nurse have additional education and experience.

The client also may benefit from attending support group meetings. A support group can help enhance the client's sense of control and reduce the isolation associated with chronic illness. Listening as others relate their experiences and fears can normalize and diminish the client's own fears. Support groups also can play an important educational role as clients discuss their treatments and ways of solving day-to-day problems.

Often the nurse assumes an important teaching role when the client is first diagnosed, followed in some sense by a learner role once the client takes charge of the illness and develops a voracious appetite for information. During both of these phases, the nurse must remain aware of the intellectual and contextual factors operating within each client's experience and use appropriate interactive styles. The nurse also must convey an open attitude that encourages the client to express essential assessment data, fears and concerns, self-care strategies, use of alternative therapies, and so forth.

There are three main areas for consideration when intervening with CNS deficits in the HIV-positive client: intellectual and cognitive function, sensorimotor function, and personality or behavioral disturbances. These areas are interrelated in varying ways for each client, requiring individualized planning and intervention.

When intellectual function is impaired, the nurse must make adjustments in the way care is provided, the nature of interactions with the client, expectations of the client, and the environment in which the client operates. The nurse must adjust the way care is provided by relying on written or visual cues for the client rather than verbal directions. Verbal directions must be phrased in a way that the client can remember and understand, for example, breaking lengthy directions into short, simple steps.

The nurse may need to make adjustments in the nature of interactions with the client, for example, calling the client to remind him or her of upcoming appointments. Information from the client may need to be verified with significant others. The nurse may need to interact in ways that are consistent with the client's familiar ways of interacting. Abrupt changes in the client's routine need to be minimized. The client may need extra support for socialization, and isolation must be avoided.

The nurse may need to adjust expectations of the client in the presence of HIV infection. Teaching must be confined to simple ideas or tasks. Written material should supplement teaching, and caregivers may need to be included in teaching to a greater degree than usual. Decision-making options should be provided only to the client's tolerance level. For a client who has impaired abstract thinking or problem-solving ability, the nurse may need to provide extensive support in translating learning into new situations.

The nurse may need to adjust the environment for the client with CNS involvement. Stimuli should be controlled for the client who has difficulty concentrating, especially if teaching is to occur. The nurse may need to provide external supports to help the client, such as appointment books or phone directories. The nurse may need to structure the day for the client, and in an inpatient setting, the nurse may need to make frequent checks on the confused client. The client's room and bathroom should be labeled. The nurse may need to make sure that there are no abrupt changes in the client's living space.

When sensorimotor function is impaired, the client requires special safety measures and support. Before the client bathes, the water temperature should be checked. Attention to problems associated with immobility (such as skin breakdown and deep vein thrombosis) is essential, and the nurse may need to assist with ambulation. Problems with bowel and bladder incontinence may require the nurse to assess for other problems, such as urinary tract infection, burning on urination, or skin breakdown. A client with sensorimotor difficulties may need to be encouraged to speak slowly or point to what he or she wants.

For a client with personality or behavioral disturbances, the nurse must intervene in a manner that preserves self-esteem. A client's behavior is more easily redirected than controlled. The environment becomes a focus for nursing intervention as the nurse removes agitating stimuli while providing safety. The nurse may need to teach stress management techniques or limit contact with anxious family members or friends. Most of all, the nurse may need to pay careful attention to his or her own feelings about this type of client when the client is demanding or hostile. Maintaining a therapeutic nurse–client relationship may be the most important intervention of all. First and foremost, the nurse must retain the unconditional positive regard so commonly discussed in psychiatric settings.

EVALUATION

The nurse and the client on the HIV spectrum face unique concerns in developing their relationship related to the presence of a third person: the physician. Perhaps unlike in any other nurse–client–physician triad, the client on the HIV spectrum often perceives the nurse as the facilitator of life-sustaining care from the physician. When difficulty arises in the relationship, the client may be reticent to express his or her concerns for fear that the nurse might become an obstruction to his or her ability to access the physician. Indeed, in today's health care setting, in which many nurses work in advanced practice, it may be a reasonable (although erroneous) assumption that the nurse intervenes for the physician. Thus, evaluation of nursing intervention is valid only to the extent that clients openly air their grievances regarding their care.

Traditional evaluation strategies are effective with the client on the HIV spectrum but are enhanced when goal setting stays close to the prognostic realities of the client's health status. Although no health care provider can predict the exact duration of anyone's life, denial of the client's status by the nurse can lead to goals that are unrealistic and unattainable. When faced with yet another failure, the client is set up for frustration. Thus, goals should reflect the uncertainty of the client's life.

◆ Chapter Summary

This chapter describes the psychiatric nursing considerations for the person on the HIV spectrum. It reviews the natural history of the illness, the psychosocial needs of the client, and the neuropsychological implications of HIV infection. The major points outlined in this chapter are as follows:

1. In HIV, the virus invades the host and diminishes the host's ability to fight off primitive organisms. The host is then prey to numerous life-threatening opportunistic infections.
2. The time between initial infection and death is very long, so HIV-positive clients are conceptualized as being located somewhere along a continuum. Each place on the continuum has psychosocial and neuropsychological sequelae.
3. Early in the spectrum, the client may express fear, grief, or anxiety related to his or her HIV status. Many life goals must be reconsidered. Denial is a common coping mechanism at this time.
4. As the client progresses on the HIV spectrum, denial is no longer adequate as a coping mechanism. The client must deal with uncertainty about the future, especially related to his or her health. This middle phase of the illness is often described as the most difficult phase.
5. In the final stages of illness, the client must make peace with his or her life and with impending death. Life review is an important task.
6. The client's family has a complex set of needs related to their sense of anger or loss. They require nursing support for their role as caregivers.
7. The nurse's attitudes are frequently affected by myths that explain the reason for AIDS. Also, the nurse faces specific emotional issues related to care of the client on the HIV spectrum.
8. There are four main mechanisms behind CNS involvement of HIV infection: direct action of HIV, opportunistic infection, lymphomas, and side effects of treatments.
9. Three main opportunistic infections are associated with HIV infection: toxoplasmosis, herpes, and cryptococcal meningitis. One particular type of herpesvirus is CMV, which attacks the retina.
10. Ongoing assessment is essential to the care of the client on the HIV spectrum. It may mean the difference between temporary or permanent damage, independence of physical debility, or even life or death.
11. Assessment strategies can be incorporated into other nursing activities to promote better understanding of neuropsychological function. Appropriate interventions are based on the client's ability to function.
12. The nurse must consider three aspects of CNS involvement when planning care: intellectual or cognitive deficits, sensorimotor deficits, and personality or behavioral changes.
13. The nurse may need to make several adjustments when providing care for the client on the HIV spectrum. These adjustments occur in the kind of care provided, the nature of the interactions, expectations of the client, and the client's environment.

Review Questions

1. Explain how the presence of the HIV in the human host results in depletion of immune function.
2. Explain why the current epidemiological figures that report the number of AIDS cases may underrepresent the seriousness of the AIDS epidemic.
3. Detail the relationship between the conversion reaction and seroconversion.
4. What are the typical coping mechanisms found in HIV-positive individuals during the various stages of their illness?
5. Explain how the myth that AIDS is a punishment for bad behavior is destructive when it is believed

by the client. Explain how it is destructive when it is believed by the nurse.

6. How would you convey that HIV is an acceptable topic of conversation between your clients and you?
7. What are the three specific considerations when interacting with a client receiving the results of his or her HIV test?
8. How are anxiety and decreased self-esteem associated with the client in the early stages of HIV infection?
9. Why is the middle stage of HIV infection often described as the most challenging for the client and for the nurse?
10. Describe the four major causes of CNS problems in the HIV-infected individual.
11. Identify the three main areas for consideration when intervening with the HIV-positive client, and describe how they interrelate to require highly individualized planning and intervention.
12. Describe the process by which the nurse differentiates inadequate coping from deeply ingrained dysfunctional behaviors.

◆ References

1. Burgess AP, et al: A Longitudinal Study of the Neuropsychiatric Consequences of HIV-1 Infection in Gay Men. Psychol Med 24 (4): 897–904, 1994
2. Ciricillo SF, Rosenblum ML: AIDS and the Neurosurgeon: An Update. Adv Tech Stand Neurosurg 21: 155–182, 1994
3. Griggens CC, Mack JL: Personal Communication. December 1: 1991
4. Kaplan RM, et al: Validity of the Quality of Well Being Scale for Persons With Human Immunodeficiency Virus Infection. Psychosom Med 57 (2): 138–147, 1995
5. Lin N, Dean A, Ensel W (eds): Social Support, Life Events, and Depression. Orlando, FL, Academic Press, 1986
6. Lipton SA: Neuronal Injury Associated With HIV-1 and Potential Treatment With Calcium Channel and NMDA Agonists. Dev Neurosci 16 (3–4): 145–151, 1994
7. Lovette J: Five Myths About AIDS. White Crane 11, 1991
8. Marzuk PM, et al: Increased Risk of Suicide in People With AIDS. JAMA 259: 1333–1337, 1988
9. Ripich S: Psychosocial Issues Faced by Persons With AIDS. J Psychosoc Nurs 32 (11): 49–51, 1994
10. Soloway B, Hecht FM: Preparing for Disease and Disability. AIDS Clin Care 2: 76–77, 1991
11. Santa Clara County (CA) Board of Health: Surveillance Report. March: 1995
12. Williams K, Ulvestad E, Antel J: Immune Regulatory and Effector Properties of Human Adult Microglia Studies in Vitro and in Situ. Advancements in Neuroimmunology 4 (3): 273–281, 1994
13. Wyness MA: AIDS Dementia Complex: Guidelines for Nursing Care. Axone 16 (2): 37–46, 1994

Professional Issues in Psychiatric-Mental Health Nursing

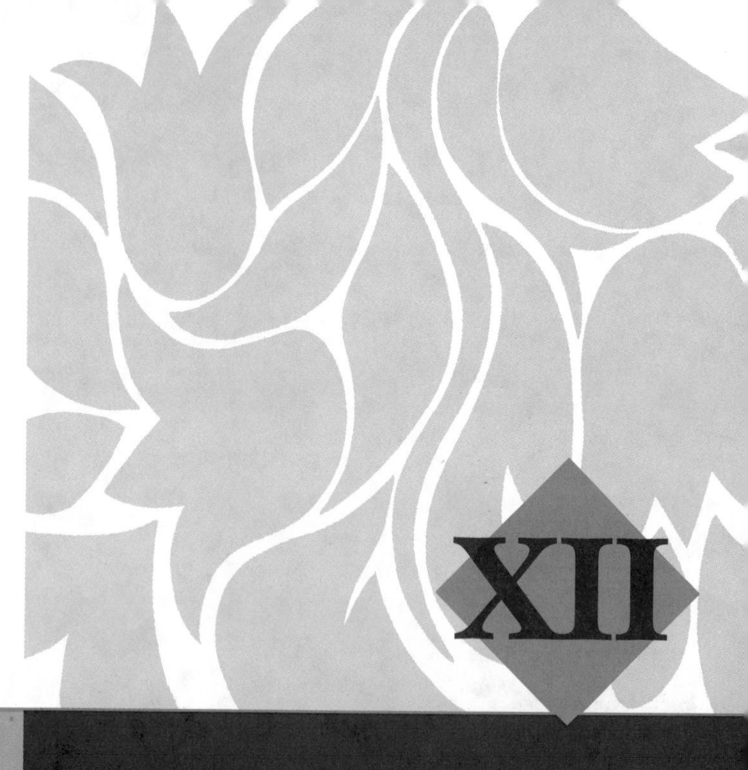

XII

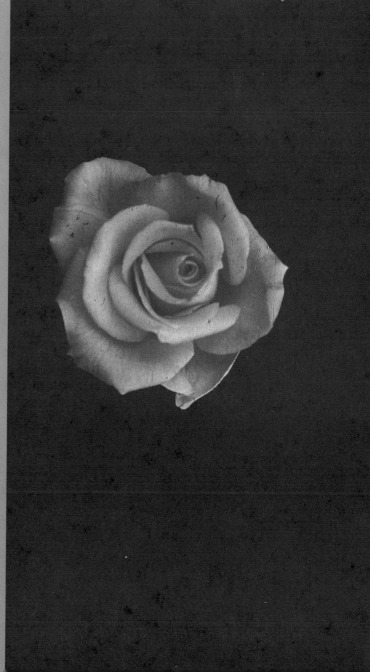

Legal Implications of Psychiatric-Mental Health Nursing

Virginia Trotter Betts
Robin S. Diamond

49

Like the five blind men, each grasping a different part of the fabled elephant and each describing a different beast, so the perceivers of the therapeutic state have seen in it diverse realities. Some have viewed it as a humanistic boon. Others have portrayed it as the first rational endeavor for the scientific control of deviant behavior. Still others have compared it to the infamous Star Chamber proceeding–the royal Tudor court that dispensed arbitrary punishments without proper regard for the safeguards that the law usually provided for the liberty of the subject.

Nicholas Kittrie, **Informed Consent: A Guide for Health Care Remedies,** *1981*

Probably no other specialty area of nursing demands as great a need for knowledge of the law and its effect on nursing practice as psychiatric-mental health nursing. Health care consumers are becoming increasingly knowledgeable about legal issues, rights, and remedies and have improved access to legal counsel through legal clinics, the American Civil Liberties Union, and other protective rights conscious groups. Box 49-1 provides a historical perspective on legal trends in mental health care. Psychiatric-mental health nurses and other health care professionals must be aware not only that their practice must meet their own professional standards, but also that those professional standards must adhere closely to legal standards as developed through case or statutory law.

Psychiatric nurses are responsible for the services that they perform and for those that they do not perform. They are responsible for accurate assessment, careful planning, competent implementation, and purposeful evaluation. If psychiatric nurses are not aware of the national expectations for clinical practice, the impact on clinical practice of new laws arising from cases decided in the court system, and proposed and past legislation affecting mental health care, it seems unlikely that they can provide the quality of care that would safeguard clients' rights, protect clients' safety,

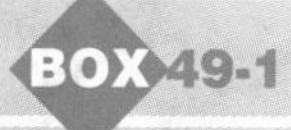

Past and Present Legal Trends in Mental Health

For the last few hundred years, society has dealt with its mentally disturbed members in a variety of ways. Until recently, the principal method was to segregate them from the general population.
This isolation from society is reported in K. Jones's *Lunacy, Law & Conscience:*

16th century: Deranged were expelled, shipped off, executed.
17th century: Insane were locked up in jails and houses of correction.
18th century: Madmen were confined in madhouses.
19th century: Lunatics were sent to asylums.
20th century: Mentally ill are committed to hospitals.
1980's–1990's: Social and economic initiatives attempt to maintain the mentally ill outside of hospitals. Crisis teams that go to the client's home are being used by community mental health centers. Home health behavioral services are springing up in most areas of the country.

Present laws regarding the treatment of the mentally ill evolved from the Common Law of England. During the 11th century, the King of England was responsible for the care of the insane if there were no kinsmen. By the beginning of the 14th century, the church and the lord of the manor were responsible for the mentally ill. Then, in the early 14th century, Edward II proclaimed the King's responsibility toward the mentally ill. The national law of guardianships extended to this class of people, and they were again made the duty of the crown. The term *parens patriae* was used by W. Blackstone to refer to the power and the responsibility of the state to care for the disabled members of society.

At first, the mentally disabled who came to the new world were dealt with informally by the colonists. Families locked up their mentally ill relatives in back rooms or outhouses. Other who had nowhere to go wandered from place to place or were confined in jails with criminals, drunkards, and other social outcasts. The *parens patriae* power of the King then was officially assumed by the states.

In 1752, Philadelphia Hospital was opened. The nation's first general hospital, it also provided treatment to the mentally ill. During this period, Pinel's and Luke's work in France and London regarding the "moral treatment" of the mentally ill implied a mental condition that was curable in an appropriate psychological and social environment.

By the middle of the 19th century, it was obvious that the corporate hospitals were unable to meet the needs of the mentally disabled. This caused social crusaders, such as Dorothea Dix, to assist with funding, building, and enlarging public mental hospitals. Despite their humanistic purposes, these hospitals actually allowed for an era of custodial treatment by the unwarranted commitment of thousands of homeless people in overcrowded hospitals with little regard for any legal protective processes.

To combat these increasingly unacceptable conditions, the clients' rights movement developed; the movement supported the concept of deinstitutionalization of the mentally ill. During the last decade, the deinstitutionalization concept and its implementation have been at the forefront of mental health care delivery. Community mental health centers have opened their doors to provide necessary psychiatric treatment to people who do not require inpatient hospitalization. As a result of this community approach, inpatient psychiatric numbers have decreased dramatically since the early 1950s, and within the last 10 years, the criteria for judicial commitment have been narrowed considerably.

continued

BOX 49-1 (Continued)

Deinstitutionalization had mandated the development of more than 2,000 public mental health centers to provide care for the mentally ill for whom inpatient care is not necessary, leaving hospital facilities to care for those who are not functioning safely in society due to mental illness. The integration of the mentally ill into the general population has engendered a great deal of political and social controversy and conflict. This conflict is not likely to be resolved until the stigma attached to mental illness is replaced by an increased understanding of mental health and illness by society or until the health delivery system develops community support services, such as housing, employment, and accessible aftercare that facilitate social integration of the formerly hospitalized mental health client population.

Legal rights and remedies for the mentally ill are still evolving. One of the most frequently litigated issues is the right to refuse psychotropic medication. New statutes resulting from judicial decisions have had a major impact on the care and treatment of the mentally ill. The passage of the Americans with Disabilities Act provides broad civil rights protection for people with mental illnesses in the workplace, housing, and education. Dramatic changes in health care financing following the failure of passage of health care reform are complicating the availability and the accessibility of mental health services. Managed care companies are revolutionizing the way individuals gain access to and providers deliver behavioral health care services. In managed care's initial stages, costs, not quality, appear to be dominating delivery system changes.

(Source: Jones, K: Lunacy, Law, and Conscience. London, Routledge and Kegan Paul, 1955; Kaimowitz v Michigan Department of Mental Hygiene, *2 Prison Law Reporter: 433;* Parham, Commissioner, Department of Human Resources of Georgia et al v J.L., et al, *422 US Reports 584, 1979)*

or further nurses' influence or power on the interdisciplinary mental health team.

This chapter first identifies the legal authority of professional nursing practice and acknowledges the evolving expansion of nursing's scope of practice. It then defines a standard of quality care as set by professional nurses and demonstrates the impact on this standard by current case law. The chapter also clarifies some differences in important legal concepts that may seem somewhat similar to the novice. Some of these differences include the following:

1. *Competency to stand trial versus competency to handle affairs*
2. *The tort actions of malpractice and assault and battery*
3. *Criminal or civil status of clients in inpatient institutions and the difference in voluntary and involuntary civil status rights*

It is imperative that nurses learn to value, respect, and seek out knowledge about laws, legislation, and the legal processes that regulate, impede, and facilitate professional nursing practice. The major goal of this chapter is to prepare nurses to include legal principles in their psychiatric-mental health nursing practice to benefit and protect the nurse and to enhance the quality of client care.

Learning Objectives

On completion of the chapter, you should be able to accomplish the following:

1. *Identify and discuss some legal issues basic to accountable nursing practice: nursing practice and malpractice, informed consent, confidentiality, and record keeping.*
2. *Identify the basic rights of mentally ill people.*
3. *Differentiate between voluntary and involuntary civil commitment.*
4. *Differentiate between criminal and civil commitment.*
5. *Discuss the differences between the competency to stand trial and general legal competency.*
6. *Differentiate between the rights of voluntary and involuntary clients.*
7. *Identify nursing implications for the right to refuse treatment and other important client rights.*
8. *Plan actions for ensuring accountability for psychiatric-mental health nursing practice, including using the American Nurses Association (ANA) Standards of Clinical Nursing Practice, integrating quality improvement into practice, seeking appropriate legal consultation, and participating in political activity for public policy change.*

◆ Legal Issues Basic to Accountable Psychiatric-Mental Health Nursing Practice

NURSING PRACTICE AND MALPRACTICE

Nursing Practice Acts

Nursing as a profession is given effect in each state by the promulgation of the nurse practice act by each state legislature. Each state nurse practice act defines nursing, describes the scope of nursing, and identifies limits on nursing practice within that state. Although the nurse practice act may differ in each state, the recently amended (1990) definition of nursing in the Tennessee Nurse Practice Act is similar to many of the evolving acts in the nation. The act immediately highlights some recognized independent and dependent areas of nursing practice (Box 49-2). Reviewing the specific activities mandated in the Tennessee Nurse Practice Act reveals that only "the administration of medications and treatment as is prescribed by —" is a service that could be considered dependent for the nurse; that is, it is dependent on the acts (orders) of someone else.[34] The rest of the mandated activities are acts that nurses can, should, and must do on their own initiative because clients need and should reasonably expect these nursing actions. Nurses are responsible and accountable for these nursing acts and are responsible for performing them in a manner that is safe for the client.

Barriers to the practice of psychiatric-mental health clinical nurse specialties remain. In addition to complex reimbursement practices, other barriers include lack of recognition of the clinical nurse specialist as an advanced practice nurse, limitation of diagnostic and prescriptive authority to nurse practitioners, difficulties in obtaining hospital privileges, and limited entry to managed care panels.

However, nursing is expanding its scope and roles as a result of increasing nursing education, health access needs in communities, and the strong political activities of nursing organizations, especially the ANA and state nurses associations. With this broadened scope comes new challenges, responsibilities, and opportunities. As of the summer of 1995, advanced nurse practitioners have prescriptive authority in 48 states and receive third-party reimbursement from private insurers in 43 states and Medicaid reimbursement in 48 states.[3] As nurses overcome barriers to practice across the nation, they are increasing access to the quality, cost-effective care consumers need.

Nursing Malpractice

Malpractice is a particular kind of tort action brought by a consumer plaintiff against a defendant professional from whom the consumer plaintiff feels that he or she has received injury during the course of the professional–consumer relationship. Malpractice is professional negligence.

For a plaintiff consumer to receive money damages by successfully suing a professional nurse for malpractice, the consumer plaintiff must prove the following five elements of nursing negligence:

1. The nurse professional had a duty to use due care toward the plaintiff.
2. The nurse professional's performance fell below the standard of care and was therefore a breach of that duty.

BOX 49-2

Professional Nursing Defined (TCA 63-7-103)

(a) The practice of professional nursing means the performance for compensation of any act requiring substantial specialized judgment and skill based on knowledge of the natural, behavioral, and nursing sciences, and the humanities as the basis for application of the nursing process in wellness and illness care.
Professional nursing includes:
(1) Responsible supervision of a patient requiring skill and observation of symptoms and reactions and accurate recording of the facts;
(2) Promotion, restoration and maintenance of health or prevention of illness of others;
(3) Counseling, managing, supervising and teaching of others;
(4) Administration of medications and treatments as prescribed by a licensed physician, dentist, podiatrist, or nurse authorized to prescribe pursuant to Section 63-7-123;
(5) Application of such nursing procedures as involve understanding of cause and effect;
(6) Nursing management of illness, injury or infirmity including identification of patient problems.

(b) Notwithstanding the provisions of subsection (a), the practice of professional nursing shall not include acts of medical diagnosis or the development of a medical plan of care and therapeutics for a patient, except to the extent such acts may be authorized by Tennessee Code Annotated Sections 63-7-123, 63-7-207 and 68-1-602.

3. As a result of the failure to meet the standard of care, the plaintiff consumer was injured, and the nurse's action was the proximate cause of the injury.
4. The act in which the nurse engaged could foreseeably have caused an injury.
5. The plaintiff consumer must prove his or her injuries.

In a malpractice action against the nurse, the proof of the standard of care becomes an essential and important ingredient. Expert witness testimony is usually presented by both sides to give the jury the perspectives of experts on professional practices and standards. The appropriate expert witness for psychiatric nursing practice is another psychiatric nurse who would have knowledge about what the standard of care in the particular case should have been.

Such expert testimony is presented in the case and is submitted with all other testimony and evidence to the jury for a decision. The jury is asked by the court to apply the reasonable person test to the facts in the case at hand. The *reasonable person test*, as applied to the nurse defendant, is what the reasonably prudent nurse would have done under similar circumstances if that nurse came from the same or a similar community (Box 49-3). To decrease liability for malpractice, psychiatric nurses must keep their professional practice within the bounds that their nurse peers would consider reasonable and appropriate. The law of negligence seeks a peer standard for reasonableness of action—not a quality performance standard of excellence.

In the history of malpractice litigation, nurses have been protected from direct suits by clients due to the perception that they are either dependent on the physician for orders or are employees of an institution. Attorneys, using the "deep pocket" theory of recovery, tended to sue as direct defendants either the well-insured physician or the employer-hospital rather than the nurse. With the advent of consumerism, the recognition of professional nursing as an independent discipline, and the awareness that most nurses are self-insured against malpractice liability, there is an increasing trend to sue the individual nurse as a codefendant along with the physician and the facility.[22]

This trend has many implications for nursing practice and for the profession. As nurses are being held increasingly responsible and monetarily liable for nursing practice and malpractice, nursing must and will take control of nursing practice issues, such as staffing, educational qualifications and competencies, and role definition on the health care team.

When nurses are found liable for less-than-adequate nursing care, employers are usually found liable to the plaintiff under the legal theory of respondeat superior. *Respondeat superior* states that the acts of employees are attributable to the employer for the purpose of being responsible for damages to injured third parties.[27] Good-quality client care provided by nurses greatly decreases malpractice litigation and successful recovery against professional and corporate defendants. Good-quality client care can only be legally proved by clear, concise, accurate, complete, and outcome-oriented documentation. The medical record is the best source of legal protection in a malpractice suit.[15]

INFORMED CONSENT—A BASIC RIGHT

All clients have a right to informed consent before health care interventions are undertaken. The performance of health care treatments or procedures without the client's informed consent can result in legal action against the primary provider and the health care agency. A client will prevail in a lawsuit alleging battery (the unpermitted touching of another) if it can be proved that the client did not consent to the procedure.[27]

Consent is an absolute defense to battery, and informed consent is required in health care situations. *Informed consent* can be defined as that given in an interaction or series of interactions between the treating provider and the client that allows the client to consider fully information about the treatment that is being proposed (eg, the way it will be administered, its prognoses, its side effects, its risks, the possible consequences of refusing the treatment, and other treatment alternatives).[30]

In the case of Canterbury v. Spence (1972), the court said that the client could truly be informed only if the primary provider shared with the client all things that "the patient would find significant" in making a decision on whether to permit or to participate in a particular treatment regimen.[11] Elements of informed consent include the following:

1. Adequate and accurate knowledge and information
2. An individual with legal capacity to consent
3. Voluntarily given consent[18]

As a broad mandate for informed consent, the U.S. Congress in Omnibus Budget Reconciliation Act (1990)[24] passed the Patient Self-Determination Act (PSDA),[24] which went into effect on December 1, 1991. The PSDA requires that health facilities provide clear information in writing to every client concerning the client's legal rights to make decisions about his or her health care, including the right to accept or refuse treatment.

Special Consent Considerations in Psychiatric Settings

A major problem with consent arises with psychiatric clients because the validity of their competence to agree to a procedure is usually questioned. Many mental health

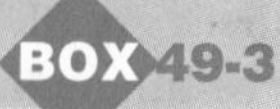

Practice or Malpractice?

A 23-year-old, married graduate student, Mr. T became severely depressed over a 3-week period. He was increasingly despondent, was unable to study, and discussed suicide with his family and friends on frequent occasions during the 3-week period. He finally became so immobilized that he requested voluntary admission to the psychiatric unit of the local general hospital.

The unit was a 32-bed, open-ward therapeutic community treatment center and the nursing model was primary nursing. Mr. T's primary nurse, Ms. D, met him on admission and completed a nursing history in a hurried manner. She did not include the client's wife in the history-taking process, nor did she directly inquire about suicidal thoughts, gestures, or plans despite his obvious depression.

Ms. D's nursing history and her participation in the interdisciplinary team conference to develop the treatment plan for the client included information about his health status, drug allergies, the stressors of graduate school, and his deteriorated eating and sleeping habits. Information from and about the client's family was omitted, as well as the client's and his wife's perceptions of the severity of the problem and their goals for hospitalization.

After 10 days on the unit, Mr. T evidenced an improved mood and energy level. He approached the nurse, Ms. D, with a request for a weekend pass. Ms. D championed his request in the team meeting noting his increased energy, his compliance and "good" behavior, and his voluntary admission status.

The team, relying on Ms. D's judgment, agreed that she could facilitate his pass. Without further assessment or activity, Ms. D provided him with the weekend pass. The client left the unit at 2:00 P.M., went to his home, and took an overdose of medication, part of which was provided for him for his pass and part of which he had acquired on his own before admission. He died before he was discovered by his wife when she returned home from work; she had not been informed that a pass was to be granted to her husband.

The wife sued the primary nurse, the hospital, and the attending physician for negligence and wrongful death.

If you were called as an expert witness to evaluate Ms. D's standard of care and her possible liability, both personally and jointly, what would you consider?

1. Inadequate history taking and initial assessment, especially lack of family participation in the process
2. Limited scope of assessment
3. Poor understanding of dynamics of depression indicated in client assessment
4. Lack of understanding of the meaning of voluntary status
5. No planning with the family for goals for treatment or continuity of care
6. Limited evidence of use of the ANA Standards of Practice

It is doubtful that this primary nurse and her treatment team colleagues met the "reasonable person" test in the case of Mr. T. As his caretakers, they had a duty to do so. They breached their duty and his harm was foreseeable. Their inappropriate actions toward him were legally significant factors in his death, and death, is a monetarily compensable injury.

Therefore, it is likely that, by providing each element of negligence, the client's wife will be able to recover money damages from the defendants. Malpractice does occur in psychiatric settings due to acts of both commission and omission.

clients certainly are capable of giving informed consent. They are aware of their surroundings, they understand what is being said, they are making their decisions based on what they think is best for them, and they are doing it without coercion.

Nevertheless, some clients are not able to give informed consent. It may be questionable whether clients already determined by the court to be incompetent for the purposes of handling civil and business affairs possess the ability to make treatment decisions. Likewise, some clients who have not been so adjudicated are so clearly impaired by their psychiatric illness that a true understanding of what is being said is not possible, and they are therefore unable to give valid consent. Because of this unreliability, major nursing considerations for informed consent in psychiatric-mental health practice are the constant monitoring and observing of clients for the following:

1. A state of legal capacity or competence when they are asked to give informed consent
2. Continuing understanding of the information that they have been given
3. Power and opportunities to revoke consent at any time during a course of treatment[30]

Substituted Consent. When a client is unable to give informed consent, health care providers should obtain substituted consent for the necessary treatment or procedure. *Substituted consent* is authorization given by another person on behalf of one who is in need of a procedure or treatment. Substituted consent can come from a court-appointed guardian or in some instances, from the client's next of kin. If the client has not previously been adjudicated incompetent to handle personal affairs and if the law so permits and no next of kin are available to give substituted consent, the health care agency may initiate a court proceeding to appoint a guardian so that the procedure or treatment can be carried out.[30]

Nurses and other health care providers need to know the statutory requirements for obtaining substituted consent. The nurse functioning in the role of client advocate also needs to know whether a client has been adjudicated incompetent and whether consent from a next of kin or a guardian is a legally acceptable substitution for the client's consent. Ensuring legally adequate informed consent before treatment is an important part of the psychiatric nursing care plan. If an emergency exists, the client can be given medication without consent to prevent harm to self or others.[13]

The Nurse's Role

Regarding informed consent, the nurse is the client's advocate, the physician's colleague, and the facility's excellent employee by continuing evaluation of a client's ability to give informed consent and his or her willingness to participate and continue in a treatment modality. Unless serving as the primary provider, it is not the nurse's responsibility to obtain informed consent; that is an activity between the client and the primary provider. It is the nurse's prerogative to pursue actively the observations as outlined previously to protect the client's rights during treatment. Every agency should clearly define the nurse's role in obtaining a client's signature on a consent form. A joint signing between the primary provider and client at the time of the decision is a preferred method of documenting consent; many agency policies and consent forms reflect this preference.

CONFIDENTIALITY

In nursing practice, it is acknowledged that the data generated through interpersonal relationships and indirect sources with and about clients are confidential. It is a professional and an ethical duty to use knowledge gained about clients only for the enhancement of their care and not for other purposes, such as gossip, personal gain, or curiosity. The confidentiality of verbal and written information must be maintained. This is especially true in the care of mentally ill clients.

Despite some advances, there continues to be a tremendous stigma attached to anyone labeled with a diagnosis of mental illness. Any breach of confidentiality of data about clients, their diagnoses, their symptoms, their behaviors, and the outcomes of treatment can certainly affect the rest of their lives in terms of employment, promotions, marriage, insurance benefits, and so forth. However, a delicate balance must be maintained by the practitioner. With managed care companies being the payers for behavioral health services, providers (hospitals, nurses, social workers, physicians) have to provide clinical information to the managed care company case manager to justify admission and continued treatment of clients. "Fiscal informed consent" should be obtained from the client or family.[13] It is the provider's responsibility to know the legal requirements regarding clinical confidentiality and the requirements of the managed care company to be informed of the clinical condition of the client for reimbursement. Thus, psychiatric nurses cannot be too careful with records, reports, and care plans.

Responsible Record Keeping

According to the Bill of Rights of the American Hospital Association, each client has a right to a written record that enhances care.[2] Records are legal documents that can be used in court; therefore, all nursing notes and progress records should reflect descriptive, nonjudgmental, and objective statements. Examples of significant data include here-and-now observations of the client through the use of the nurse's senses, an accurate report of what is said and done for the client, and a description of the client outcomes of the care provided.[19]

Verbal communication and data sharing are important, especially on treatment teams and units that use interdisciplinary approaches to client care. The verbal sharing should be straightforward, forthright, descriptive, and unopinionated and should be shared only with those involved in the client's care and treatment. It is wise in a psychiatric institution to have an established methodology of reminding staff about their professional and legal responsibilities for confidentiality, such as an annual signing of a form that promises the maintenance of client confidentiality.

Privileged Communication

Privileged communication is provided by statute in each state. The statute delineates which categories of professionals are given the legal privilege not to be required to reveal conversations and communications with a citizen. Although statutes differ from state to state, the statutes customarily provide privilege to physicians, attorneys, clergymen, and in some states, psychologists, nurses, and other health care providers. Psychiatric nurses should be aware of statutory privileged communication, and if the nursing privilege is limited or nonexistent, they should know what typical boundaries to set in therapeutic interviews. In the absence of statutory privileges for nurses, communications between the nurse and client may be required to be repeated in court through the subpoena process. Therefore, sharing sensitive or incriminating data should not be encouraged.

Some cases have involved the issue of the appropriate circumstances that warrant breach of the confidential relationship with a client. A leading case in this area is Tarasoff v. Board of Regents of University of California (1974), which held that therapists may have a duty to protect a person who is threatened by a client.[32] Subsequent decisions discuss the issues of foreseeable violence and the amount of control that the therapist could reasonably use to prevent the harm.[10] In these types of cases, courts have said that the mandate on therapists to hold clients' verbalizations in confidence is cut off when those confidences include threats on the lives of other people.

Courts have held that although the duty of confidentiality between client and therapist should be recognized, a higher duty to protect the public safety intervenes and subsumes the duty of confidentiality. There are no nursing cases per se on this point, but it is important to know that threats to other people cannot be ignored or unattended, especially when there is some reasonable opportunity for the client to follow through on these threats.

Other types of situation in which a breach of confidentiality may be required by law include child abuse allegations and allegations of sexual misconduct made against a therapist.

◆ Providing Legally Acceptable Nursing Care: Rights Issues

BASIC RIGHTS OF PSYCHIATRIC CLIENTS

An important issue in psychiatric-mental health nursing care is the recognition of the basic rights of clients. This is particularly true because the treatment of mentally ill clients tends to be more coercive, less voluntary, and less open to public awareness and scrutiny than are the treatment and hospitalization of other types of clients.

When psychiatric clients enter a hospital, they lose their freedom to come and go, to schedule their time, and to choose and control activities of daily living. If also adjudicated incompetent, they lose the freedom to manage financial and legal affairs and make many important decisions.[14]

Because of the loss of these important freedoms, the courts and advocates of psychiatric clients closely guard and value the rights that the psychiatric client retains. Some of these rights include the right to communicate with an attorney, the right to send and receive mail without censorship, the right to visitors, the right to the basic necessities of life, and the right to safety from harm while hospitalized.

Certainly, treatment issues sometimes arise that call for a limitation on visitors. Clients may be included in a behavior modification treatment program that requires the earning of tokens to secure certain privileges or articles. However, clients have a right to challenge such restrictions, and the treatment facility may have to prove the value or necessity of such rights abridgements.[14]

Use of restraints and seclusion as treatment approaches is considered suspect, because such approaches reflect a flavor of possible punishment; therefore, the when, where, why, and how long of restraints and seclusion need to be addressed by policy in every psychiatric facility. Many states have developed statutes to define the use of restraints and seclusion within psychiatric units. The Joint Commission for the Accreditation of Healthcare Organizations is currently refining the standards for the use of restraints and seclusion.

Clients have limited rights to be paid for work within institutions. Forced or even voluntary labor by clients without payment violates the principles of law in our society. The amount of payment considered adequate for client labor is still not clearly defined in each state.[14]

Clients have the right not to be subjected to experimental treatments nor to be subjects in research projects without their informed consent. Because of the complexity of informed consent issues with psychiatric clients, as discussed previously, institutions with programs involving research or experimental treatment approaches must have institutional review boards to evaluate such projects and programs and to approve or disapprove them based on strict client-protection criteria. Humane research approaches that entail no undue risks to clients but have strong expectations of benefit and that allow clients to withdraw from the project at any time are usually viewed favorably by these human subjects committees if clients give voluntary consent to participate.[14]

Nursing Implications for Provision of Rights

Nursing has long espoused that one of its important roles in the health care system is to act as a client advocate. Nowhere is the advocacy role more important than in the psychiatric care system as an assessor of and spokesman for the protection of client rights.

Discussing rights within treatment teams, including these rights in the nursing care plan, and ensuring that methodologies for rights protection are included in facility and unit policies and procedures are nursing activities that fulfill the client advocate role (Table 49-1). One important resource that nursing should request is

Table 49-1

Nursing Care Guidelines to Maintain Legal Rights of Clients

Outcome 1: Client feedback will reflect satisfaction with nursing care.

Intervention	Rationale
Provide minimum of "reasonable person" standard of care in use of nursing process to deliver client care.	Breach of guidelines for safe practice and standards of care, such as the ANA Standards of Psychiatric-Mental Health Nursing Practice, can provide basis for negligence and malpractice suits.
Attend periodic inservice workshops that review legal and ethical issues.	Responsibility to update knowledge base continually is essential to the practice of safe nursing care.

Outcome 2: Clients' right to informed consent will be maintained.

Intervention	Rationale
Apply elements of informed consent, including the following: 1. Person must be competent. 2. Person must have ability to refuse consent. 3. Person must have adequate information for consent, including information regarding alternatives to treatment. 4. Consent must be legal.	A basic client right is the right to have control over their own bodies. Physician has the legal obligation to ensure that clients are giving informed consent, with the nurse's observation and assessment of client being considered.
Observe and document client behavior that indicates that consent is valid.	Client record reflects specific nursing assessment of current behaviors, and appropriate nursing action needs to be taken if consent is questioned or invalidated.
Record and report any discrepancies in consent or behavior, revocation of consent, or other issues to client's physician.	Nurse acts as client advocate and has interdependent role of assessment of consent, compliance, and consent revocation with the physician.

Outcome 3: Clients' right to confidentiality of health data will be protected.

Intervention	Rationale
Protect client record and chart, and share data only with client authorization.	Client's written authorization is necessary before information in records or charts can be shared.
Maintain communication about client and client care between treatment team members.	Information about client care can be shared among treatment team members to provide continuity.
Use policy and procedures that reflect nurse's duty to protect in cases of threats to harm other people.	Nurse has responsibility to breach confidentiality to protect others from harm.

Outcome 4: Clients' rights will be protected.

Intervention	Rationale
Review policies and procedures of unit to ensure that they are in accordance with client rights.	Policies and procedures need to be in place that comply with protection of clients' rights.
Attend inservice training on legal issues, such as voluntary or involuntary commitment and treatment consequences.	As a member of psychiatric treatment team, the nurse has a responsibility to ensure that client care is in compliance with legislation and statutory laws dealing with commitment and treatment issues.
Suggest that legal consultation be obtained for new decision, update, review of policy and procedures, and case consultation.	A legal consultant should be available to staff.
Use the ANA Quality Assurance Model to provide the basis for a quality assurance program.	Nurse must develop or participate in quality assurance programming. Ongoing audits should be performed on each diagnostic category of frequent client population.

ongoing legal advice and consultation in the area of client rights.

CLIENT STATUS AND SPECIFIC LEGAL ISSUES

When psychiatric clients are hospitalized, the type of admission is vitally important. Various admission statutes reflect differing client rights and staff treatment responsibilities. Civil commitment admissions include the following:

1. Voluntary admissions
2. Emergency admissions
3. Involuntary commitments (indefinite duration)

Each state has specific statutory regulations pertaining to each admission status that mandate procedures for admission, discharge, and commitment for treatment.

Voluntary Admissions

Clients who present themselves at psychiatric facilities and request hospitalization are considered *voluntary admission* clients. Likewise, clients evaluated as being of danger to themselves or to others or being so seriously mentally ill that they cannot adequately meet their own needs in the community but who are willing to submit to treatment and are competent to do so have voluntary admission status.

Voluntary clients have certain rights that differ from the rights of other hospitalized clients. Specifically, voluntary clients are considered competent unless otherwise adjudicated and therefore have the absolute right to refuse treatment, including psychotropic medications, unless they are dangerous to themselves or others, as in a violent destructive episode within the treatment unit.[28]

Voluntary clients do not have an absolute right to discharge at any time but may be required to request discharge. This time delay gives the health care team an opportunity to initiate a procedure to change a client's admission status to involuntary if the client meets the necessary statutory requirements. Many clearly mentally ill people can be voluntarily treated but cannot be required by the state to be treated in any setting if the client refuses. Therefore, numerous mentally ill people whose behavior causes family, community, and social problems do not and cannot receive psychiatric care if they are unwilling to be voluntary clients.

Involuntary Admissions

Clients are considered to have *emergency involuntary admission* status when they act in a manner that indicates that they are mentally ill and due to the illness, likely to harm themselves or others; they are taken into custody and detained in a psychiatric facility.[33] The exact procedure for the initial evaluation is defined by state statute, as is the possible length of detainment and attendant treatment available.

All emergency admission clients are admitted to facilities for the purposes of diagnosis, evaluation, and emergency treatment. At the end of the statutorily limited admission period, the client must be discharged, changed to voluntary status, or attend a civil hearing to determine the need for continuing treatment on an involuntary basis.

During the time of the emergency admission, the client's right to come and go is restricted, but the right to consult with an attorney to prepare for a hearing must be protected. Clients may be forced to take psychotropic medications, especially if they continue to be dangerous to self or others, but more invasive procedures, such as electroconvulsive therapy (ECT) or psychosurgery, are not permitted. No treatment should impair the client's ability to consult with an attorney at the time of a hearing.[33]

A person who refuses psychiatric hospitalization or treatment but poses a danger to self or others, who is mentally ill, and for whom less drastic treatment means are unsuitable may be adjudicated to *indefinite involuntary admission* status in a psychiatric hospital for an indefinite period.[33] The exact legal procedure may differ in each state, but the standards for commitment are similar (Case Study 49-1).

To deprive a person of liberty to the extent of involuntary commitment is a serious matter, and the legal protections are strict. Addington v. Texas (1979), requires that in a civil hearing before involuntary commitment, the standard of proof of "mentally ill and dangerous to self or others" must be beyond that of a "preponderance of the evidence" (the prior civil commitment standard) and must be instead "clear and convincing evidence" (a much higher standard).[1] This Supreme Court standard of the protection of the right to liberty must be reflected in the statutes of each state concerning commitment procedures.

It is for clients who are indefinitely involuntarily committed that many of the issues of psychiatric client rights have been pursued. Other evolving rights are discussed in a later section of this chapter.

LEGAL ISSUES OF SPECIAL CLIENT POPULATIONS

Forensic Psychiatric Clients

Mental health professionals become involved with clients who are charged with criminal acts in two major circumstances: for the evaluation of a defendant's competency to stand trial and concomitant pretrial treatment if needed and for the evaluation of a defendant's

Case Study

Committable and not Committable

A Case of Mental Distress—not Committable

Mrs. A, a 65-year-old widow, had lived alone for 25 years. Her neighbors frequently expressed concern among themselves and to the local authorities about Mrs. A's unusual lifestyle and eccentric behavior. Their complaints were generally based on tales told to them by neighborhood children. The observations of the neighborhood children included reports that Mrs. A slept during the day but stayed up all night, ate strange foods such as raw meat and 10 pounds of sugar every 2 weeks, and talked to herself aloud. The only public place in which Mrs. A was ever seen was in the church on Sunday mornings.

Finally, a neighbor called the police who picked up Mrs. A while she was in her yard placing tree branches in strange patterns. She was then admitted as an emergency admission to the local state mental hospital. The various psychiatric team members' assessments and psychological diagnostic testing results were presented at the hearing, along with testimony from other experts and testimony from the neighbors. The descriptive nursing observations of Mrs. A's behavior for the 5 days prior to the hearing were a most important part of the expert evidence and testimony.

The mental health assessment indicated that Mrs. A's rather odd behavior was the result of her suffering from primary degenerative dementia. The court found that, even though Mrs. A exhibited rather bizarre behaviors at times, her mental condition, as indicated by the testimony, did not generate a tendency for her to harm either herself or others. Likewise, the testimony did not indicate that her condition would prevent her from using community resources in a manner adequate for continued self-care.

Therefore, the court determined that Mrs. A was not judicially committable to an inpatient psychiatric unit. Nevertheless, the court did find the need for follow-up care by a visiting nurse from the local mental health center to monitor Mrs. A's nutrition, self-care, and any further progression of her mental illness that might eventually require hospitalization.

A Case for Involuntary Civil Commitment

Jim, a 20-year-old single white man, lived at home with his parents while attending college classes at the community college. For the past 2 months, Jim's behavior had become increasingly bizarre. Finally, he did not sleep, did not eat, and did not attend class. He left his parents' house at all times of the day and night, which caused a great deal of disturbance. When his father attempted to reason with him, he became increasingly agitated and stormed out of the house.

The parents were not aware of any drug use; however, they are aware of the fact that Jim had been drinking large amounts of beer. Jim lost a lot of weight and failed to care for his personal hygiene.

Although Jim had become very agitated, he had never made any threats toward anyone nor had he exhibited any assaultive behavior. He became increasingly preoccupied with the Bible; when his parents questioned his strange behavior, he responded that he was an apostle and that he was only doing what God told him to do. About 1 month ago, Jim's parents persuaded him to visit the local mental health center, but when the therapist suggested inpatient treatment at a psychiatric hospital, Jim stormed out of his office.

One night, with Jim standing on the patio "preaching the gospel," and disturbing the whole neighborhood, his parents, feeling completely helpless and frightened, called the local police department. The police transported Jim to the state psychiatric facility where he stayed for 5 days on an emergency admission status, after which time he attended his hearing.

During the hearing, Jim was still hyperactive to the point that he could not sit still. Based on the testimony of both the physician and the nurse regarding Jim's mental condition and behavior, the court found that Jim met the standards for civil judicial commitment on two grounds. First, his hyperactivity secondary to his mental illness was resulting in loss of appetite, loss of weight, and insomnia to the extent that his physical health was compromised. Second, his increasing agitation and preoccupation with religion, also secondary to his mental illness, was potentially an antecedent to a situation in which he could lose control and harm others. Therefore, Jim was returned to the psychiatric hospital for continued treatment on a nonvoluntary, civilly committed basis with no judicial pronouncements about his competency status.

mental condition at the time of an alleged crime and concomitant treatment if the defendant pleads and is acquitted on an insanity defense. This specialized area of mental health care is called *forensic psychiatry.*

Competency to stand trial refers to a defendant's mental condition at the time of the trial. Mental health professionals determine whether the defendant is competent by assessing the following in the defendant:

1. Ability to assist attorney with defense
2. Understanding of the nature and consequences of the charge against him or her
3. Understanding of courtroom procedures

If the defendant is incompetent to stand trial, treatment begins with the defendant being judicially committed to a psychiatric hospital with a forensic unit. Treatment of incompetent defendants includes, but is not limited to, medication, individual and group psychotherapy, and education about courtroom proceedings and the current legal predicament. A defendant can exhibit signs and symptoms of mental illness but still be competent to stand trial.

A decision handed down by the U.S. Supreme Court in Jackson v. Indiana (1972) resulted in state statutes designed to protect the rights of criminal defendants who continue to be incompetent to stand trial by virtue of their mental illness.[16] These defendants can no longer be detained for an indefinite time without the benefit of the same type of commitment hearing to which all civilly committed clients have a right. In other words, these pretrial defendants should be returned to court as soon as they are competent to stand trial, and this should be the primary goal of pretrial treatment.

If the defendant chooses to plead an insanity defense, mental health professionals are involved in evaluating the defendant's mental condition at the time of the alleged crime. Four different standards or tests determine whether an insanity plea is a valid defense.

The earliest standard that achieved wide acceptance in the United States was the M'Naughten rule, established in England in 1843. This is the *right-wrong test,* which states that if at the time of his or her criminal act, the defendant suffered from a disease of the mind that so affected reason that he or she was unaware of the nature and quality of the act or that the act was wrong, then he or she is to be found not guilty by reason of insanity.

The second test, the *irresistible impulse rule,* broadened the M'Naughten rule. This test retained the language of the M'Naughten rule but also provided that a person acting in response to an irresistible impulse also lacked criminal responsibility, even though he or she knew the wrongfulness of the act.

The third test, the *Durham rule,* provided that a person lacked criminal responsibility if his or her acts were the product of a mental disease or defect. This rule was not widely used.

The fourth test was adopted by the American Law Institute and is the most widely used today. It provides that a person is not responsible for a criminal act if he or she was suffering from a mental illness at the time of the act, was unable to appreciate the wrongfulness of the act, and was unable to conform his or her conduct to the requirements of the law.

If a defendant is found not guilty by reason of insanity, the legal implication is that because of a mental condition, the defendant could not form the deliberate intent necessary to constitute mens rea. *Mens rea* is the mental element necessary for a defendant to be convicted of a crime; it involves a notion of deliberate criminal intent and foresight of the consequences.

A person found not guilty by reason of insanity is involuntarily admitted to a psychiatric facility for a statutorily defined evaluation period. During this time, mental health professionals evaluate the need for hospitalization and any other appropriate disposition. On completion of the evaluation, the court is notified of the recommendations, at which time a hearing may be scheduled to determine the court's order for release or for continuation of mandatory commitment for treatment. As soon as clients are considered not committable, they must be released into the community, possibly with some mandatory requirements for aftercare.

There is a great deal of controversy involving the verdict of not guilty by reason of insanity, particularly after the John Hinckley acquittal in the assassination attempt against President Ronald Reagan in 1981. As a result of this controversy, some states have passed a "guilty but mentally ill" plea, meant to mandate psychiatric treatment of mentally ill criminals in correctional facilities. This plea has not yet passed constitutionality scrutiny; although it is popular in principle, it may not be the final answer to a difficult balancing problem between the rights of victims and the rights of mentally ill offenders.

Ideally, the mental health team responsible for providing forensic evaluations and services is composed of a psychiatrist, a clinical psychologist, a social worker, a psychiatric-mental health nurse clinical specialist, and other nursing personnel who are active in the client's evaluation and treatment. Nurse clinical specialists can be valuable members of the mental health team. They are specially trained to perform mental status examinations and to function as individual and group therapists. In some states, they are qualified to be trained in competency evaluations and to testify in court as expert forensic witnesses.

Registered nurses are likewise valuable in the evaluation and treatment of these clients. Their nursing assessments, nursing observations, nursing interventions, knowledge of medications, and accurate documentation contribute to the formulation and implementation of a treatment plan to ensure that these clients with special needs are given the highest quality of care possible.

Juvenile Psychiatric Clients

A special population of psychiatric clients is minors or juveniles. Until recently, parents or guardians have had almost an absolute privilege to admit their minor children younger than 18 years for mental health treatment. This absolute right has been eroded somewhat by state recognition of some rights of more mature children (12–18 years old) to protest such treatment.[14]

In 1979, the U.S. Supreme Court, in Parham v. J. L. et al, gave a more definite standard for juvenile admissions to which state statutes and hospital policy should conform.[25] The Supreme Court held that juveniles can be authorized for admission by their parents but that accompanying the admission, some *neutral fact finder* should determine whether statutory requirements for admission are satisfied. Further, an adversarial hearing for admission is not required, nor does due process require that the fact finder be legally trained or be a hearing officer.[25] By ruling in this way, the Court balanced competing interests of the rights of parents and guardians to control the lives of their children with the right of children to due process prior to limitation on their liberty.

Psychiatric-mental health nurses need to be mindful of these procedural protections for the benefit of their juvenile clients. Limiting hospitalization to statutory requirements is an important advocacy activity for juvenile psychiatric clients.

MAJOR EVOLVING LEGAL RIGHTS

Right to Treatment

The idea that psychiatric clients have a legally actionable right to psychiatric treatment began to develop in the late 1960s and culminated in the early 1970s in the Circuit Court case of Wyatt v. Stickney (1971).[36] The case provided innovative statements about the rights of civilly committed mentally ill clients in state hospitals. The court stated that such clients do have certain treatment rights, which include the following:

1. Treatment must give some realistic opportunity to improve or be cured.
2. Custodial care is insufficient to meet treatment requirements.
3. A lack of funding does not excuse a state from treatment responsibilities.
4. Commitment without treatment violates the due process rights of clients.[36]

Perhaps the most important pronouncement in this case concerns the three determinants for the adequacy of treatment, which are a humane environment, a qualified staff in adequate numbers, and individualized treatment plans.[36] This case gave the nation guidance about treatment rights; however, because it was not reviewed by the Supreme Court, it is not totally generalizable.

The Supreme Court decision on O'Connor v. Donaldson (1975)is commonly thought to be the leading case for the right to treatment.[23] However, the decision states that no state can confine a nondangerous mentally ill person in a state hospital who is capable of surviving safely in the community alone or with the help of willing, responsible family or friends.[23] There is still no clear national standard on the right to treatment of involuntarily civilly committed clients or on the right of the state to commit involuntarily mentally ill people for treatment. Future cases will decide these issues.

Treatment in the Least Restrictive Environment

Over time, through dicta and decisions, courts have given guidance to the mental health system on many matters, including standards about the settings in which treatment should occur. As early as 1969, in Covington v. Harris, the court held that a person treated involuntarily should receive such treatment in a setting that is least restrictive to liberty but will still meet treatment needs.[12] Least restrictive environments can be community resources instead of hospitalization, open wards instead of locked wards, or outpatient care instead of inpatient care.[14] Because of this client right, nurses need to assess constantly a client's condition and status so that more or less restrictive treatment alternatives can be applied based on the client's evolving needs.

Right to Refuse Treatment

The doctrine of informed consent implies that clients have a right to choose or refuse medical and health treatment. Certainly, health care providers, through interpersonal relationships and client education, may try to convince clients about the need for certain treatments, but only in rare or life-threatening instances do courts intervene in clients' negative treatment decisions.

Voluntary Clients. Following this principle of judicial noninterference, voluntary clients who have not been adjudicated incompetent have an absolute right to refuse treatment and to choose between treatment alternatives. They cannot be forced to take medications, be research subjects, or be involved in invasive treatments, such as ECT or psychosurgery. Only in rare cases of severe behavioral acting out that threatens self or others can a voluntary client be forced to take psychotropic medications.

Involuntary Clients. The rights of involuntarily committed clients to refuse treatment are less clearly defined than are the rights of voluntary clients. Rennie v. Klein (1981) and Rogers v. Okin (1979) are the leading cases to give guidance on this unsettled issue.[28,29] The courts have been prone to state that involuntary clients cannot refuse tried and true treatments that promote recovery, such as psychotropic medication; however, protections must be applied for more risky procedures with more extreme side effects or consequences, such as ECT, insulin shock, or psychosurgery. In Mills v. Rogers (1982, on appeal of Rogers v. Okin), the Supreme Court seemed to favor a standard that would confer no absolute right of involuntary clients to refuse treatment but that treatment decisions would be left to the judgment of professionals who would consider client rights in their treatment decisions.[29]

There is much controversy and litigation about the rights of involuntary clients to refuse treatment; therefore, the psychiatric nurse must be aware of the most recent case law about this issue. Unit and facility policies need to remain current and should clearly reflect that as treatment becomes more invasive, has increased risk, or demonstrates questionable results, it is more important that the client's right to refuse be honored.

Right to Aftercare

Care in the community following psychiatric hospitalization is needed to prevent readmission and to ensure the rehabilitation of former inpatients. There is no absolute legal right at this time to aftercare programs unless such a right is provided by state statutes. It is not inconceivable that case laws may evolve to mandate aftercare services as a right of mental health clients.

In conjunction with other members of the interdisciplinary team, nurses plan for aftercare treatment. As knowledgeable and responsible citizens, nurses voice their concern at all levels of the political system to see that psychiatric clients have access to adequate aftercare services, such as outpatient counseling, medication follow-up, vocational placement, and sheltered living environments.

◆ Strategies for Ensuring Quality and Accountability in Nursing Practice

STANDARDS OF PRACTICE OF THE AMERICAN NURSES ASSOCIATION

The ANA has developed clinical standards of practice for generic and specialty areas of practice. The generic standards apply to all professional nursing practice and are guidelines or norms for practice. A review of the generic standards indicates that nurses must use the nursing process in therapeutic relationships with clients. In other words, nurses will assess, diagnose, document, report, plan, implement, and evaluate client care with the client, family, and significant others.[4] The focus of nursing practice is on the client's attainment or restoration of physical and mental health. Nurses are uniquely able to view clients holistically and to engage in a process with clients that has as its aim care and growth. Using the ANA Standards of Clinical Nursing Practice as a base for performance evaluation will ensure such practice. In psychiatric settings, nurses should use ANA specialty standards for psychiatric mental health nursing in addition to the generic ones because both reflect professional and legal expectations.[6]

QUALITY IMPROVEMENT PROGRAMMING

Another major strategy for improving quality and accountability in nursing is the *nursing quality improvement program.* The ANA has developed a national program emphasizing that nurses should implement the standards of nursing practice through development of and participation in systematic quality improvement endeavors.[4]

The ANA has developed a conceptual model for quality improvement (Fig. 49-1). Using this model as the conceptual basis for quality improvement facilitates nurses' and other health care practitioners' understanding of quality improvement and demonstrates that quality care is ensured to consumers and is not merely an exercise used for accreditation or reimbursement verification.

Numerous nursing activities fit into the ANA quality model, including client care audit, peer review, client classification and acuity rating, the nursing clinical ladder, medical care evaluation, and nursing care planning. A psychiatric audit is a procedure through which client care in psychiatric settings can be measured for its effectiveness in providing care to population categories in psychiatric settings. The ANA Model for Quality Improvement can be used in a psychiatric audit as a way of conceptualizing the audit activity as a dynamic process. The process includes values classification, criteria development, client care measurements, identification of care successes and failures, development of alternative care approaches, and introduction of change into the psychiatric setting.[4] The dynamic audit process is never complete until a complete reaudit is accomplished to evaluate the effectiveness of change.

Audit criteria should include the measurement of

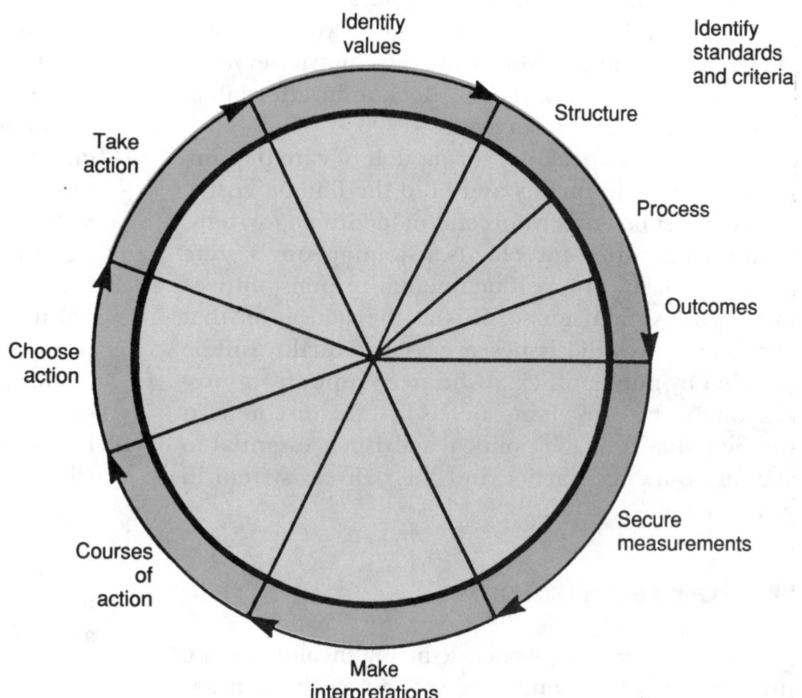

Figure 49-1. Quality assurance model.

the health team's awareness of the legal rights and remedies available to clients. Criteria that address the client's legal needs are important, especially in the psychiatric setting. Nurses should voluntarily and enthusiastically join in quality improvement programs for the purpose of systematically evaluating client care to improve care for all consumers.

LEGAL CONSULTATION

Psychiatric health professionals also need to know how and when to obtain appropriate legal consultation on an ongoing basis. First, the attorney consulted must be aware of the issues in mental health law to assess the institution's policies and procedures and to provide a review for the staff in a problem-solving, rather than policing, manner. Second, some arrangements should be made to have such an attorney offer continuing education programs on a regular basis to review with the staff updates on court decisions and recent legislation that would affect care in the psychiatric unit. Also, having legal consultation readily available on a case (client) consultation basis when the staff is endeavoring to ensure legal accountability is extremely valuable. Most institutions should provide this kind of legal consultation, if requested, for the benefit of their clients and to protect the institution from potential liability.

POLITICAL ACTIVISM AND CLIENT CARE

In September 1994, the 103rd Congress of the United States ended its debate on comprehensive health care reform—a proposal strongly backed by nurses of America. The plan before the nation would have guaranteed universal access to quality and affordable care, and the basic benefits included parity for mental health services. In the aftermath of the debate, massive health industry restructuring is occurring due to alternated financing mechanisms with an overwhelming emphasis on decreasing costs of health care services.

In the rush to decrease costs, concerns about quality and access seem to have faded. The 104th Congress has an ambitious agenda to slow the growth of Medicare and Medicaid, and the financing and delivery modes favored appear to be managed care, block grants without federal mandates, and promotion of self-responsibility.

As health care professionals, nurses have developed a variety of public policy plans for the nation's health and have used political action, such as lobbying, endorsing "health-friendly" candidates and working in their campaigns, fund raising, and voting to make these plans a near reality.[20] The failure of reform and the potential negative fallout for client care make future policy and political activism even more important. When less money and investment are provided for health care, the most disadvantaged, vulnerable, and stigmatized services receive less. Therefore, unless there is a concerted voice by providers, clients, and advocates of psychiatric services, there is likely to be a serious decline in affordable, quality mental health services.

Nurses must speak out for models of care that improve access and quality and hold the line on costs.[8] Nurses must be equally forceful in identifying systems that do not work for clients.[21] Joining one's state nurses association is a fundamental responsibility of every professional nurse. It is at the state level that care, costs, provider issues, access, and quality will be decided by public officials who need input from professionals who put clients' needs first. Involvement in public policy through political activism is essential to shaping nursing practice and the delivery system in years to come.

◆ Chapter Summary

The legal impact on psychiatric-mental health nursing practice is immense and subtle. The psychiatric nurse who evaluates practice in an attempt to improve the nursing profession and the health of clients does so not from legal demands, but from professional standards. Nevertheless, nursing practice must meet certain legal standards and must adjust its course as new legal standards evolve. Capable and challenged nurses have legal knowledge about client care; it is to them that many clients will turn for information, advocacy, and protective justice.

Chapter highlights include the following:

1. Nurses have independent and dependent areas of nursing practice and are liable for maintenance of a responsible standard of care to clients in both of these areas of practice.
2. A failure to meet the standard of care that results in an injury to a client or consumer makes the nurse liable for nursing negligence or malpractice.
3. Nurses have a duty to participate in the issues of informed consent, which are basic rights of clients; failure to obtain informed consent from a client prior to a procedure can result in a civil action against the physician and the health care agency on the theories of assault and battery or malpractice.
4. Clients also have a right to rely on the appropriateness and confidentiality of their medical records and data.
5. Confidentiality is an ethical, professional, and legal responsibility and is in many instances mandated by statute.
6. Privileged communication is determined by statute for certain professional groups and their clients.
7. Some cases indicate that confidentiality must be breached when the public safety is in jeopardy, as when clients threaten to harm other people.
8. To provide legally acceptable nursing care in psychiatric-mental health settings, nurses must be informed about a variety of issues, including recognized client rights, and they must take responsibility with other health team members to see that client rights are protected.
9. Client rights may differ due to the civil or criminal nature of commitment proceedings, the voluntariness of a civil commitment, the purpose of the criminal commitment, and the age of the client.
10. Psychiatric-mental health caregivers must identify client status and client rights and secure adequate consultation as client rights evolve.
11. Strategies for enhancing the quality of psychiatric-mental health nursing care, thereby ensuring quality care and accountability by nursing to consumers, are as follows:
    - Nurses must practice with the ANA Standards of Clinical Nursing Practice as their normative base.
    - Nurses must develop and participate in quality improvement programming, including psychiatric audits.
    - Nurses must request and secure ongoing continuing education and consultation with attorneys knowledgeable in mental health law.
    - Nurses must participate in public policy and political action to improve health and mental health care.

Critical Thinking Questions

1. *Under what legal doctrine are employers named in a legal action against their employers (ie, when the employer-hospital is sued along with the nurse)?*
2. *Name the elements of "informed consent."*
3. *What is the nurse's responsibility in obtaining informed consent?*
4. *How has managed care altered the responsibility of health care providers to release information?*
5. *How long can psychotropic medication be administered during a psychiatric emergency?*
6. *List four basic rights of psychiatric clients.*
7. *Does a civilly committed adolescent have the same rights as a civilly committed adult?*
8. *What does the least restrictive doctrine mandate with regard to where a client can obtain treatment?*

Review Questions

1. List the five elements of nursing negligence.
2. What is the "reasonable person" test?
3. When is informed consent not required when administering psychotropic medications?
4. What is the significance of the Tarasoff decision?
5. Define forensic psychiatry.
6. What is the significance of the Parham decision?
7. How do ANA Standards of Clinical Nursing Practice define the focus of nursing practice?

◆ References

1. *Addington v Texas,* 99 Supreme Court Reporter 1813, 441 US Reports 418 (1979)
2. American Hospital Association: A Patient's Bill of Rights. Chicago, American Hospital Association, 1994
3. American Nurses Association: Analysis and Comparison of Advanced Practice Recognition with Medicaid Reimbursement and Insurance Reimbursement Laws. Washington, DC, American Nurses Association, 1995
4. American Nurses Association: Quality Assurance Workbook. Kansas City, MO, American Nurses Association, 1976
5. American Nurses Association: Standards of Clinical Nursing Practice. Washington, DC, American Nurses Association, 1994
6. American Nurses Association: Statement on the Scope and Standards of Psychiatric Mental Health Clinical Nursing Practice. Washington, DC, American Nurses Publishing, 1994
7. American Nurses Association: Nursing's Agenda for Health Care Reform. Kansas City, MO, American Nurses Association, 1991
8. Baradell J: Cost Effectiveness and Quality of Care Provided by Clinical Nurse Specialists. Journal of Psychological Nursing 32 (3): 21–24, 1994
9. Barback F (ed): Mental Health Law News. Ohio, Interwood Publications
10. Beck JC: The Psychotherapist's Duty to Protect Third Parties from Harm. Mental and Physical Disability Law Reporter 2 (March-April), 1987
11. *Cantebury v Spence,* 464 Federal Second Reporter 772 (1972)
12. *Covington v Harris,* 419 Federal Second Reporter 617 (1969)
13. Dasco S, Dasco C: Managed Care Answer Book. New York, Panel Publishers, 1995
14. Ennis B, Emery R: The Rights of Mental Patients. New York, Avon Books, 1978
15. Feutz SA: Preventive Legal Maintenance. J Nurs Adm 17 (January): 8–10, 1987
16. *Jackson v Indiana,* 46 US Reports 715 (1072)
17. Jones K: Lunacy, Law, and Conscience. London, Routledge and Kegam Paul, 1955
18. *Kaimowitz v Michigan Department of Mental Hygiene,* 2 Prison Law Reporter 433
19. Kerr AH: Nurses Notes—That's Where the Goodies Are. Nursing 75 (February): 34–41, 1975
20. Krauss J: Health Care Reform: Essential Mental Health Services. Washington, DC, American Nurses Publishing, 1993
21. Krauss J: How Well Will We Manage Care. Archives of Psychiatric Nursing 8 (6): 339, 1994
22. Menzes: The Negligent Nurse: Rx for the Medical Malpractice Victim. Tulsa Law Review 12: 104, 1976
23. *O'Connor v Donaldson,* 422 US Reports 563 (1975)
24. OBRA, Public Law 101–508
25. *Parham, Commissioner, Department of Human Resources of Georgia et al v J.L., et al* 422 US Reports 584 (1979)
26. OBRA, Patient Self-Determination Act, 199 4206 and 4571
27. Prosser W: Law of Torts. St. Paul, MN, West Publishing, 1971
28. *Rennie v Klein,* 653 Federal Second Reporter 836 (1981)
29. *Rogers v Okin,* 478 Federal Supplement Reporter 1342 (D. Mass. 1979); aff'd in part, rev'd in part, *Rogers v Okin,* 634 Federal Second Reporter 650 (1st Cir 1980); vacated and remanded; sub nomine *Mills v Rogers,* 457 US 291 (1982); on remand, *Rogers v Okin,* 738 Federal Second Report 1 (1st Cir 1984)
30. Rossoff AJ: Informed Consent: A Guide for Health Care Remedies. Rockville, MD, Aspen Systems, 1981
31. Smith JW: Hospital Liability. New York, Law Journal Seminars Press, 1995
32. *Tarasoff v Board of Regents of University of California,* 592 Pacific Second Reporter 553 (1974)
33. Tennessee Code Annotated, Section 33-6-103
34. Tennessee Code Annotated, Section 63-7-101 et seq.
35. Weiner B, Wettstein R: Leagal Issues in Mental Health Care. NY and London, Plenum Press, 1993
36. *Wyatt v Stickney,* 325 Federal Supplement Reporter 781 (1971)

Research in Psychiatric-Mental Health Nursing

James McColgan, Jr.
Mary Ann Sweeney

50

RULE 1. We are to admit no more causes of natural things than such as are both true and sufficient to explain their appearances.

Isaac Newton,
Rules of Reasoning in Philosophy

This chapter presents an overview of the research process in nursing. Special emphasis is placed on two key areas that integrate research skills with a well-rounded nursing practice base. The first area is use of published research reports. Nurses need to identify reports that may be relevant to nursing practice and after evaluating these reports, incorporate important findings into their routine nursing practice. The second area of emphasis is involvement in the steps of the research process. Because learning is enhanced by participation, practical suggestions are included with the beginning researcher in mind.

Learning Objectives

On completion of this chapter, you should be able to accomplish the following:

1. *Define nursing research, and recognize broad distinctions among the main types of research.*
2. *Discuss the varied ways that the research process can be incorporated into the role of the nurse.*
3. *Locate published nursing research reports and other sources of research-related information.*
4. *Read, evaluate, and use information from research studies.*
5. *Develop a strategy for active participation in activities related to nursing research.*

◆ Understanding Nursing Research

DEFINITION AND PURPOSE OF RESEARCH

One way of gathering and processing information related to nursing is through the research process. Unfortunately, the mention of the word research often triggers immediate, unfavorable reactions in many professionals. Whether or not they realize it, nurses have been doing research for quite some time.

Research is one way to gather and process information. It is used routinely by all types of professional groups. The research process is a series of formalized steps that can be followed by nurses, psychologists, biologists, or any professionals to obtain objective data or information. *Nursing research* has "application to the study of all nursing problems with the goal of expanding the theoretical basis of nursing through the discovery of new knowledge."[7]

THE RESEARCH PROCESS

The steps of the research process provide a structured and consistent approach to information gathering. Flexibility at each step of the research process allows a study to be specifically tailored to each new and unique situation. Information gained in a study must be as accurate as possible. It should also be useful and above all, unbiased by the investigator's point of view. Many safeguards have been devised to help researchers collect "good" or "clean" information and to help them sort out its true meaning.

Scientific Method Applied to Nursing

The *scientific method* is a set of deliberate steps to be followed when approaching any question. Broadly defined, these steps are identification of the question, collection of relevant facts concerning the question, analysis of these facts, development of an approach to investigate the question, investigation and collection of data, analysis of findings, and interpretation and application of the investigation's results. These same steps are used in the nursing process. When faced with the question of how best to care for a client, the nurse assesses the client, identifies a nursing diagnosis, develops a plan of nursing care, implements it, evaluates its effect, and revises it as necessary. The steps of the nursing process are the scientific method applied to development of a nursing care plan. Table 50-1 compares the steps of the scientific method with those of the nursing process.

The scientific method is the most effective way of determining relationships between variables, thereby enabling a scientist to understand, predict, and to a degree, control their behavior.[6] It can be applied by practitioners of any professional discipline to obtain objective information.

The nursing role is expanding to include the use of scientific research methods at many different levels of expertise. Nursing students, faculty members, and clinical nurse practitioners in all types of settings are becoming increasingly involved in nursing research

Table 50-1

Comparison of Scientific Method and Nursing Process Steps

Scientific Method	Nursing Process
Collection of relevant facts	Assessment
Analysis of facts	Nursing diagnosis
Development of approach to investigation	Planning
Investigation and collection of data	Implementation
Analysis of findings	Evaluation
Interpretation and application of findings	Revision

throughout the course of their normal work routine (Box 50-1).

Nurses are fortunate that their work entails a variety of interesting experiences and situations. The selection of research topics can be as varied as the types of roles that nurses perform.

The best introduction to the realm of research is to read it. Find examples in the literature of studies that cover issues or questions that interest or are important to you. You can locate reading material in books, journals, indexes, and abstracts. Your objective should be to locate, read, and assess the results of a research project; if applicable, use your new knowledge in nursing activities.

There are many ways to implement the research process, depending on the objectives of the individual conducting the study. Table 50-2 summarizes the main points of the six most common types of research approaches. After reading your first few research reports, select a report, and compare it with the characteristics presented in Table 50-2.

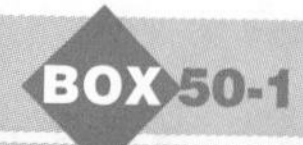

BOX 50-1

Examples of Recent Psychiatric Nursing Research Studies

A Theory of Transformed Parenting: Parenting a Child with Developmental Delay/Mental Retardation, *Nursing Research,* 44 (1), 1995. Authors: Ruth Young Siedeman and Paul F. Kleine.

Child Bereavement After Paternal Suicides, *Journal of Child and Adolescent Psychiatric Nursing,* 8 (2, April–June), 1995. Authors: Janet Grossman, David C. Clark, Deborah Gross, Lois Halstead, and James Pennington.

Chronic Sorrow: The Lived Experience of Parents of Chronically Mentally Ill Individuals. *Archives of Psychiatric Nursing,* IX (2, April), 1995. Author: Georgene G. Eakes.

Exploring Widows' Experiences After the Suicide of Their Spouse. *Journal of Psychosocial Nursing,* 33 (5), 1995. Authors: Barbara J. Smith, Ann M. Mitchell, Audrie A. Bruno, and Rose E. Constantino.

Hardiness and Death Attitudes: Predictors of Depression in the Institutionalized Elderly. *Archives of Psychiatric Nursing,* VIII, (5, October), 1994. Author: Janine K. Cataldo.

Living with Depression: Family Members' Experiences and Treatment Needs. *Journal of Psychosocial Nursing,* 34 (1), 1996. Author: Terry A. Badger.

Maintenance of Self-Esteem by Obese Children. *Journal of Child and Adolescent Psychiatric Nursing,* 8 (1, January–March), 1995.

Psychological Correlates of Adolescent Depression. *Journal of Child and Adolescent Psychiatric Nursing,* 8 (4, October–December), 1995. Authors: Diane Brage, Christie Campbell-Grossman, and Jennifer Dunkel.

Severity of Depression, Cognitions, and Functioning Among Depressed Inpatients With and Without Coexisting Substance Abuse. *Journal of the American Psychiatric Nurses Association,* 1 (2, April), 1995. Author: Jaclene A. Zauszniewski.

The Development of the Self-Care Ability to Detect Early Signs of Relapse Among Individuals Who Have Schizophrenia. *Archives of Psychiatric Nursing,* IX (5, October), 1995. Author: Cynthia Baker.

◆ Using Published Research

THE RESEARCH REPORT

The first step in using research findings in nursing practice is learning how to read and understand published reports. When you are comfortable reviewing the purpose and content of research reports, you can begin to evaluate their results and apply the findings appropriately to nursing theory and practice.

The four major sections of a research report are the introduction, methodology, results, and discussion. Each area contains essential information for your comprehension of the research study and its possible applications to nursing practice.

Introduction

The introduction of the research report describes the problem that was investigated and provides related background information. The description of the problem, usually found in the first paragraph, is typically a declarative statement describing the overall purpose of the study. An example is "The purpose of this study is to investigate the relationship between blood pressure and levels of psychological stress." An interrogative statement of the research problem may be used to question the nature of the relationship between the variables being studied. An example of this type of problem statement is "What is the relationship between blood pressure and levels of psychological stress?"

A simple definition of the study is particularly important at the outset of a research report. The focus of the

Table 50-2

Characteristics of Various Research Approaches

Philosophical	Historical	Case Study	Methodological	Survey	Experimental
TIME FRAME					
Present, past	Past	Present, past	Present	Present	Present, future
RESEARCH OBJECTIVES					
Trace development or present status of abstract ideas.	Discover existing facts and combine to draw conclusions.	Provide indepth analysis of subject that usually includes historical aspects.	Develop instruments to measure variables; test statistical procedures for appropriateness.	Discover new facts about subjects; make conclusions and interpretations.	Predict events; discover cause-and-effect relationships under controlled conditions.
DATA COLLECTION SOURCE					
Documents	Personal and public documents, records, artifacts; interviews in limited circumstances	Combination of data from subjects, documents, and artifacts	Subjects for pretesting, reliability, and validation of instruments	Subjects	Subjects
TYPE OF RESEARCH REPORT					
Narrative only	Narrative, sometimes objects or artifacts	Narrative with occasional numerical data; can include objects or artifacts	Numerical with accompanying narrative statements	Narrative that usually includes numerical data	Narrative with great emphasis on numerical data

study will be one or more variables. Variables may be defined as characteristics or traits. In the hypothetical example given previously, the variables in the problem statement are "blood pressure" and "psychological stress." The variables being investigated are identified and defined in general terms in the introduction but are definitely refined in the methodology section of the study.

The introduction should help you understand what is being investigated and why this is an important topic for scrutiny. The background of the problem is presented through a review of related literature. The literature review should be exhaustive and demonstrate the author's comprehensive grasp of the topic. It should cite key studies that have been conducted about the problem, describe the findings of previous studies, and identify questions concerning the problem that have yet to be answered. Although the literature review is not intended to provide an expert level of knowledge or understanding concerning the problem area, it should give you an appreciation for where the problem under investigation fits into the realm of nursing theory and practice.

Methodology

The methodology section of the research report describes the mechanics by which the study was conducted. It includes a description of the population and sample, research instrument, data collection methods, and data analysis procedures. The detailed information in this portion of the report is needed to provide a clear understanding of the procedures used so they can be evaluated or replicated by you and other researchers.

Population and Sample. The *study population* is the entire group of subjects possessing the qualities desired by the researcher. As a hypothetical example, a researcher may want to investigate the relationship between blood pressure and psychological stress in American men older than 40 years who live in urban settings. In this example, the study population would include all men older than 40 years living in American cities.

The *sample* is a subset of the study population—the group of people selected from the population to participate in the research study. The sample of the population described in the previous example could be men older than 40 years living in Dallas, New York, San Francisco, or any other American city.

The research report should describe in as much detail as possible the population and criteria used to select the sample. This description should include how many individuals were selected, how they were chosen, and the procedures used to obtain consent from the individuals for participation in the study.

Research Instrument. The description of the research instrument includes its format, validity, and reliability. The instrument itself might be a questionnaire, an interview schedule, or machinery or equipment (eg, a sphygmomanometer). For the first two types of instruments, the number, type, and some examples of the items should be included in the research report. For the latter, the description should include the device's brand name and model and how it collects data. The great number and variety of instruments available to researchers makes knowledge of a particular instrument's format crucial to understanding this aspect of data collection.

Validity refers to an instrument's ability to measure the variable(s) under investigation in the research study. *Face validity* is the degree to which the instrument appears related to what is being studied. The determination that a research instrument has face validity need not be made by someone familiar with the area under study. The focus of face validity is on the apparent ability of the instrument to measure what the researcher intends to measure.

Content validity refers to the degree to which the instrument collects representative data related to the variable being measured. To establish content validity, the researcher asks subject matter experts from the area under investigation to assess the degree to which items in the instrument will measure the variable(s) under study. Content validity is the degree of agreement between experts that in their judgment, the instrument will measure or collect the desired data.[8]

Construct validity is more difficult to establish. Constructs are concepts that are not directly observable, such as human reasoning, intelligence, or stress. One means to establish construct validity is to collect data with the instrument and compare it with data collected by an alternative means of measuring the variable. For example, the instrument could be administered to a group that is also observed by judges for the construct. The amount of agreement between the data collected by the instrument and the observations of the judges is the level of construct validity. Another means of establishing construct validity is to administer the instrument to a group known to possess the construct that the researcher wants to measure.

In the hypothetical research study, we might use a questionnaire to measure anxiety, because constructs are intangible, and anxiety is a manifestation of the construct stress. To establish construct validity, we would administer our questionnaire to a group that we know demonstrates characteristics of anxiety. Such a group might be clients with a clinical diagnosis of anxiety disorder who display high levels of anxiety. This would be our *known group*. A research instrument that has construct validity will collect data corresponding to the characteristics of the known group. If our questionnaire has construct validity, the responses of the known group would indicate that they have high levels of stress. Still another means of establishing construct validity is to compare the instrument with one already known to measure the construct. In this method, both instruments are administered to the sample, and the data collected are compared for agreement. The amount of agreement between the two instruments is the level of construct validity.

Criterion-related validity is used to predict future performance. This validity is established by *post facto* identification of characteristics related to successful performance of a task. The characteristics are formulated into an instrument that should then identify individuals who will successfully perform the tasks desired. When establishing the criterion-related validity of an instrument, the researcher focuses not on the collection of data itself, but rather on how well the data collected predict future events and outcomes. Instruments with criterion-related validity are often used in business and industry to identify potential employees who are able to behave in desired manners or perform desired tasks. The varied types of validity are important when assessing the value of the instrument used to obtain data from subjects.

Reliability of a research instrument refers to its consistency, its ability to collect the same kind of data in repeated administrations and in a variety of situations. One of the more common ways of determining reliability is termed *test-retest reliability*. To establish this reliability, the researcher administers the instrument to a sample group and after a specified period (from 2 weeks to several months), readministers the same instrument to the same sample group. An instrument with a high degree of test-retest reliability will collect similar data on both occasions. When reading a research report, you need to know that the instrument collects data consistently before believing its findings.

Data Collection. After describing the instrument, the research report should describe the data collection methodology—how the sample was selected from the study population and how the data were collected. In this portion of the report, you should find sufficient details to replicate the research report.

The description of how the sample was selected should explain its source and the criteria used to select or exclude individuals from it. Continuing with our hypothetical research study, we might state that our sample will be selected from male pedestrians at the intersection of Main and Lamar Streets in downtown Dallas who answer yes to the questions "Are you older than 40 years?" and "Do you live in Dallas?" To select our sample, we would stand at the designated intersection and address these questions to male passersby. Those answering yes to both questions would be included in the sample; those answering no to either one would not be included.

The description of the data collection method may be general or complex, depending on the instrument format used. The methodology of using mechanical instruments or paper and pencil measures with established reliability and validity may be described in general terms if the instrument's specific administration procedures have been followed by the researcher. More complex descriptions of the methodology are required when researchers adapt an instrument or its administration procedure to meet their particular needs. In the former case, you may be referred to the original instrument; in the latter case, the researcher should report the methodology in sufficient detail to enable you to replicate it. In our hypothetical research study, the description of the data collection method should include how the questionnaire was completed by the study participant and how his blood pressure was measured.

Data Analysis. The final area in the methodology, the data analysis plan, describes processing of the raw data and the procedures, usually statistical, that will be used to tabulate the data. Processing may range from hand scoring items on a test or questionnaire to coding data for computer analysis. Statistical procedures used by researchers are classified as descriptive or inferential.

Descriptive statistics are used to summarize the characteristics of the data collected. The most commonly used descriptive statistics are frequencies and mean (or average) scores. The descriptive statistics that might be included in a research report about our hypothetical study are highest, lowest, and average stress levels measured by our questionnaire; highest, lowest, and average systolic and diastolic blood pressures measured with our sample; and the age of the oldest and youngest participants and the average age of the study sample.

Inferential statistics are used to test hypotheses and develop conclusions about the population from the results of the sample. Unlike most descriptive statistics, inferential statistics require the application of complex mathematical formulas. For this reason, a computer is often used for this type of data analysis. The type of data collected (nominal, interval, ratio, or ordinal) determines which inferential statistical test can be used for analysis. Each reports a numerical value for its specific statistic that is compared with a table of values for that test. If the numerical value of the statistic falls at or above the table's designated value for the level of significance desired, the relationship between the variables is supported. The level of significance is important because it describes the extent to which researchers are willing to be wrong about their conclusions. The standard level of significance used in research is 0.05. This means that the researcher wants to be correct 95% of the time when stating that there is a relationship between variables and wrong only 5% of the time. When describing the data analysis plan, the researcher should name the statistical test that will be used and specify the acceptable level of significance.

Results. This section of the research report describes the implementation of the data analysis plan. The discussion should focus first on the overall characteristics of the data by using descriptive statistics. The discussion should highlight important characteristics rather than reporting each item singly. Most of the data may be presented in a table. When using this format, though, the researcher must focus on the clarity of the table itself. A table that is confusing or complicated makes the data it contains worthless. Not every piece of data collected should be discussed individually, but the highlights of the data should be discussed thoroughly.

Data analysis and interpretation should follow a logical sequence. One way is to follow the sequence established by the order of the hypotheses or research questions. The analysis of the data should report the statistical values obtained and their levels of significance. The researcher should also state whether or not a hypothesis was supported or in the case of research questions, whether a relationship was implied.

Research in which hypotheses or relationships are not supported also has value. The absence of a relationship or lack of significant findings in a research study has important implications.

Discussion

The discussion portion of the research report describes the conclusions the researcher has drawn from the study and suggests implications of this information in regard to nursing practice. The discussion should review, in broad terms, the various aspects of the study: the hypotheses or research questions, sample, research instrument, and major results. Often the researcher will compare the obtained results with other similar studies. The conclusions must be specific and clearly based on the study results. The results direct and limit the conclusions that the researcher may make. The conclusions describe what has been learned from the study, summarizing what was and was not found, what was answered, and what remains unanswered.

The implications of the findings described by the researcher suggest practical uses for the information learned. As an example, returning to our hypothetical research study, our conclusions might be that there is a direct relationship between stress levels reported by our sample and their measured systolic and diastolic blood pressures. The implication of our research results might then be that our study population may reduce systolic and diastolic blood pressure by reducing stress level. Implications also include predictions of the impact that the results may have on the theory or practice of nursing. In our hypothetical research study, we might suggest the need for primary preventive nursing interventions.

The research report usually concludes with suggestions concerning the future directions of research in this area. Often the researcher will suggest a larger sample or different population. Sometimes, based on the results, the researcher may suggest a different approach for a new study.

The discussion portion of a research report is considered by many to be its substance, but the discussion must be considered within its overall context. The conclusions and implications of a research report must be viewed in relation to specific information about such factors as the size of the sample, the soundness of the instrument and methodology, and the data analysis plan. Weakness in any of these areas reduces the value and applicability of the study's conclusions and implications. Box 50-2 provides guidelines for extracting, summarizing, and evaluating information from research reports.

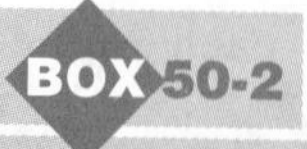

Research Reading Guidelines

Use the following guide to extract and summarize in your own words research studies that you read:

1. Reference (in bibliography format)
2. Introduction
   a. Research problem
   b. Purpose of the study
   c. Summary of relevant points in the literature review
3. Methodology
   a. Variables
   b. Instrument(s)
   c. Sample
   d. Data collection plan
   e. Data analysis plan
4. Results
   a. Summary of main results
   b. Interesting additional findings
5. Discussion
   a. Conclusions
   b. Implications
6. Evaluation
   a. Your comprehension level of the report (easy, difficult, complicated)
   b. Overall value of the study (very worthwhile, average, questionable)

◆ Protection of Subjects' Rights

The ethics surrounding the conduct of research studies must be considered. The nurse conducting a research study has the dual roles of researcher and nurse. As a researcher, the nurse must implement the study's methodology and collect the desired data. As a nurse, the researcher continues to have the nursing responsibility of promoting the health needs of the person. The issues with which the nurse-researcher should be concerned include the person's right not to participate, informed consent, confidentiality, and anonymity.

RIGHT TO REFUSE TO PARTICIPATE

A person has the right to refuse to participate in any research study for any reason. No other person or institution may deny or override this right. Furthermore, a person may not be coerced into agreeing to participate in a research study. Nurses should be aware of a client's involvement in a research study and the circumstances surrounding this involvement, even when they are not directly involved in the research themselves.

RIGHT TO INFORMED CONSENT

Informed consent means that the person has the right to be fully informed about what participation in the research study involves, how it might affect him or her, the time commitment required, and any possible risks involved. To obtain informed consent, the nurseresearcher must explain these aspects of the study to the person in nontechnical language. The nurseresearcher must be careful not to affect or bias the information that will be forthcoming from the person, while answering all questions about the study as fully and honestly as possible. Obtaining informed consent from potential research subjects can be time consuming for the researcher, but it will pay dividends by increasing the level of each subject's participation.

RIGHT TO CONFIDENTIALITY AND ANONYMITY

Confidentiality and anonymity are often considered synonymous by researchers; however, they are not the same thing. *Confidentiality* is the person's right to privacy concerning the data provided to the researcher. Researchers may ensure confidentiality of data by various methods, such as replacing names with code numbers. *Anonymity* is each person's right to privacy as a participant in the research study. The most common manner in which well-meaning researchers violate a subject's anonymity is by specifically identifying the source of the study's sample in the research report. For example, a researcher who identifies the sample as "the senior class of nursing students at Plain State College" has not provided anonymity to the research subjects. Although the research report must contain specific information concerning the criteria for selection of the sample and its characteristics, the specific source need not be revealed.

The nurse researcher must be cognizant of the rights of subjects involved in research studies. As a professional, the nurse must balance the requirements of these rights and the research process itself. Above all, as a nurse, the researcher must support and protect subjects' rights.

◆ Participating in Nursing Research

DEVELOPING NECESSARY SKILLS

Three steps help develop the skills necessary to participate in nursing research. The amount of participation increases from step to step. The steps should be approached in order.

Step 1: Read as Many Studies as Possible

You can gain greater understanding, depth of knowledge, and confidence in identifying the steps of the research process by reading and critiquing examples in the professional literature. Journals, indexes, and abstracts will provide you with a starting point for locating nursing-related research articles. Box 50-2 will help you to analyze and evaluate research reports.

Step 2: Practice Individual Steps of the Research Process

You need not undertake a complete study to gain experience in research-related activities. Start with one step of the research process that involves a skill you can develop to do your job better—for example, summarizing and analyzing data. Look over the data analysis sections of other research reports and try to summarize your own client-related data in a similar way. In other words, construct a table that presents the key points, and then make several summary statements about the information in your table.

Perhaps you need to present a summary of the current literature regarding a procedure at a team conference. Study the introductory sections of published research studies to see how various articles are summarized, condensed, and combined. Note how the authors give credit to the original sources and how they present reports with conflicting results.

Step 3: Replicate a Published Study

The best way to acquire an understanding of the research process is to become actively involved in it. A good way for you to begin is to use a previously conducted study as an example. Use it as a step-by-step pattern, just as a tailor would when making a garment. For instance, check the literature to see if any related articles have been published since the date of the research report. Use the same instrument, if possible, or a close facsimile. Your tables will already be laid out, but the data will be new. You'll learn a lot about the practical steps of conducting a project while having your own set of backup instructions.

Nurses just starting out in research often think that they must reinvent the wheel. This can be frustrating, whereas replication of a previously conducted study is not only less frustrating, but also more instructional. Replication of previously conducted studies is a necessary step in the process of building sound theoretical knowledge. Also, replications of studies are appearing more frequently in the nursing literature.

TIPS ON CONDUCTING SMALL RESEARCH PROJECTS

The following 10 steps will help you get started toward becoming a professional who uses research meaningfully in any area of nursing practice:

1. Define a topic about which you want to find out more. Your interest level will help spur you on to explore the topic further. Note two things—the types of articles you tend to read when you look through professional journals and the aspects of nursing about which you think a lot. The first step is to summarize your idea or interest in a few words, such as "communicating with confused patients" or "exploring nurses' reactions to dying patients."

The idea does not need to be crystal clear, just a start in a direction that is interesting to you.

2. Find several studies that have been published on this general topic or that are closely related to it. You may find a related study that has been done by researchers in another discipline, such as psychologists or social workers. Use these studies to begin to build a research folder. Your research folder will be your collection of ideas and information about your topic. Summarize the main points of the research report, or make a copy that you can put in your folder for later reference. Find several articles about your topic that may not be formal research studies, and add them to your folder. The more you know about a particular topic, the better. Note the articles that authors mention often in their bibliographies. Read and gather those as well.
3. Pick out one aspect of one of the studies in your folder, and develop a plan to replicate it in a limited fashion. Use a study or parts of several studies as a pattern to follow. For instance, suppose a study on communicating with confused clients contrasts two different types of nursing intervention. Use the two approaches as part of your nursing care, and observe the results. Add some notes about your findings to your folder. Talk with other experienced nurses to find out their views and experiences on the subject. With your previous reading and thinking about the topic, you will quickly be able to spot and explore new ideas. Add all this to your growing research folder.
4. Talk to colleagues about your interest and the material you have gathered. See if you can find someone who would like to work with you on this type of study. It is often more stimulating to work with another researcher or even a small group. That way, you can share the work and have a built-in audience for discussing various aspects of your study. If you want to pursue it by yourself, try to locate someone with some research experience with whom you can consult and discuss ideas.
5. Write out a simple study plan. Define what you intend to study, and outline the steps you plan to take to complete your project. Keep it simple and straightforward. You can do another project later if you want to investigate some other aspect of the topic.
6. Polish your proposal outline with advice from expert sources, such as a basic textbook or someone who has previously conducted a research project. Do not be afraid to investigate your resources; many health care institutions provide assistance to employees who want to carry out small-scale studies. Try to project the time it will take you to complete the tasks on this polished version of the outline. Then double each time frame to give yourself leeway. Periodic checks of your project calender will help keep you on schedule. You will need a tentative budget, but you can keep the costs of important work to a minimum, as other researchers have demonstrated.[3]
7. Identify the steps you need to follow to gain permission to conduct your study. Usually, you will need to submit a written request to an institutional review committee. Use your outline as a basis for the proposal to this group.
8. Attend workshops, continuing education classes, or university courses in research-related topics. You may even find someone with whom to consult or a research partner there.
9. Keep a record of all your study activities. You may want to write about the study at a later time.
10. Offer to give a small inservice program about your study. You can communicate your procedures and findings and hopefully stimulate more interest and discussion about your study.

◆ Chapter Summary

This chapter has explained the research process as an effective way to gather and process information; it has examined some of the components of nursing research. Chapter highlights include the following:

1. The research process can be applied by any professional interested in obtaining data or information.
2. Safeguards in the steps of the research process provide structure and consistency to information gathering.
3. Research reports contain four components:
    - a. Introduction, the problem investigated and related background information
    - b. Methodology, the population and sample, research instrument(s), and procedures for data collection and analysis
    - c. Results, the analysis and interpretation of the data
    - d. Discussion, the conclusions drawn from the study, the implications of the findings in relation to nursing practice, and suggestions for possible uses of the information
4. Each person has the right to refuse to participate in research studies, the right to informed consent, and the right to confidentiality and anonymity.
5. The expanding role of nurses includes participation in nursing research and the use of nursing research to improve psychiatric-mental health nursing practice.

Review Questions

1. Which of the following statements best describes nursing research?
   - A. Nursing research is a step in the nursing process.
   - B. Nursing research is a scientific process that requires advanced training and education to implement effectively.
   - C. Nursing research is the application of the scientific method to the study of questions and problems related to nursing theory and practice.
   - D. Nursing research is the process by which nurses can help keep their clinical practice up to date.
2. What information will the introduction of a research report give to you?
   - A. A description of the problem that was investigated
   - B. An overview of the method(s) used to collect the data
   - C. Preliminary analysis of the data that were collected
   - D. A description of the implications that the study results have for nursing theory and practice
3. What is the first step in developing your skills as a nurse researcher?
   - A. Replicate a published research study.
   - B. Join a research support group.
   - C. Enroll in an introductory statistics course at your local college.
   - D. Read all the research studies you can.
4. The ethical conduct of nursing research is important. Imagine yourself in the role of nurse-researcher. With which of the following statements would you agree?
   - A. As a nurse conducting a research study, my priority is the implementation of my data collection methodology.
   - B. A person has the right to refuse to participate in my research study for any reason, and when faced with this situation, I should not try to persuade or coerce participation.
   - C. As a researcher, I must be able to separate my nursing responsibility toward the person from my responsibility to conduct my study.
   - D. I can use technical nursing terms and jargon to answer a potential subject's questions and obtain informed consent.

◆ References

1. Cronenwett LR: Effective Methods for Disseminating Research Findings to Nurses in Practice. Nurs Clin North Am 30 (September): 429–438, 1995
2. Downs FS: A Source Book of Nursing Research, 3d ed. Philadelphia, FA Davis, 1984
3. Holstrom L, Burgess A: Low-Cost Research: A Project on a Shoestring. Nurs Res 31 (March–April): 123–125, 1982
4. Kirchhoff KT: Issues and Challenges in Clinical Nursing Research. Nurs Clin North Am 28 (June): 271–278, 1993
5. Munhall P: Nursing Philosophy and Nursing Research: In Apposition or Opposition? Nurs Res 31 (May–June): 176–177, 1982
6. Polit DF, Hungler BP: Nursing Research: Principles and Methods, 4th ed. Philadelphia, JB Lippincott, 1991
7. Sweeney MA, Olivieri P: An Introduction to Nursing Research: Research, Measurement, and Computers in Nursing. Philadelphia, JB Lippincott, 1981
8. Waltz CF, Bausell RB: Nursing Research. Design, Statistics, and Computer Analysis. Philadelphia, FA Davis, 1981

Career Profiles in Psychiatric-Mental Health Nursing

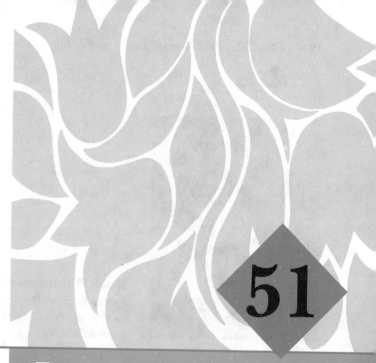

The progressive world is necessarily divided into two classes—those who take the best of what there is and enjoy it—those who wish for something better and try to create it.

Florence Nightingale,
Cassandra, *1851*

Work is love made visible.

Kahlil Gibran,
The Prophet, *1923*

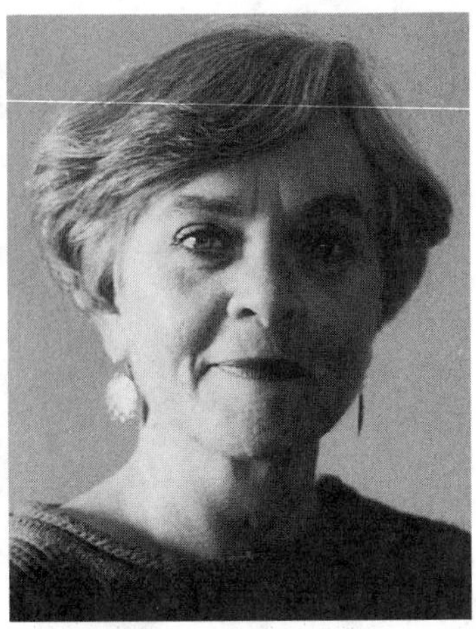

Beth Bonham, MSN, RN, CS
Family Support Services Program Director
Indiana Juvenile Task Force, Inc.
Indianapolis, Indiana

I am so very fortunate to be a nurse! What other single educational preparation could offer such diverse career opportunities as critical care, public health, college professor, elementary school counselor, and child or adolescent psychiatric nursing? What other profession offers such diverse clinical settings as a client's kitchen table, a college classroom, a dying client's bedside, or a juvenile court?

My road to psychiatric mental health nursing has been circuitous, but in reflecting on 26 (I can't possibly be that old!) years of practice, the paths, byways, and resting places have all interfaced. I was a critical care nurse who stood at an intubated client's bedside, holding his hand and having a conversation with him, and he couldn't speak. I implemented behavior modification plans for long-term ventilator clients for whom everyone else was tired of caring—and before I knew what the term meant! I sat, frustrated, in a client's living room *knowing* there was something else to say but not having the knowledge or skills to practice family therapy. I sat in a room full of educators who wanted to start an elementary school counseling program and told them why they needed a psychiatric-mental health nurse to initiate it. I developed a psychiatric-mental health curriculum for a baccalaureate nursing program because I am committed to teaching those coming up behind me. I did these things because I didn't know they couldn't be done, and I knew they needed to be done. I listened to people, observed people, and trusted my knowledge. I once had a supervisor who called me arrogant. I think she used the wrong "a" word—I think she really meant "audacious." The things I did had scientific rationale and always were in the best interest of the client.

Wanting to stay in nursing and remain marketable, I researched which nursing specialty would allow continued professional and personal growth. I discovered psychiatric-mental health nursing, and then I discovered (I believe it was revealed to me) child psychiatric nursing. I had come home (and I went full circle, I might add—my highest state board scores as a new graduate were in psychiatric nursing).

I chose psychiatric-mental health nursing because it channeled my critical thinking, problem solving, verbal, written, and risk-taking skills. It offered a foundation for behavior—mine and clients'. It offered a host of like-minded spirits who were independent thinkers and who were supportive. It offered career challenges in a variety of community settings. It offered a vehicle to grow professionally and truly learn what being an accountable, committed, and responsible person means. It offered new skills and positions of which I had never dreamed. It offered a specialty of stimulation and "can do" rather than "you can't." These offerings are why I chose psychiatric-mental health nursing and certainly why I remain. The challenge and hope that is psychiatric nursing are visited daily.

I am currently employed by the Indiana Juvenile Justice Task Force, Inc. as the Program Director of the Family Support Services Program. I developed the program on a nursing process model of assessment, intervention, implementation, and evaluation. Our clients are juvenile delinquents and their families. The program is psychotherapeutic—individual, family, and group therapies are offered weekly. Families are asked to identify their strengths, and together we develop mutual goals. Most parents are concerned with learning how to communicate, discipline, and parent their adolescent children. Most youth are concerned with peer relationships, staying out of trouble, and getting a job or completing high school. The program is intensive and home based. The family specialist interacts with the youth daily, and counseling occurs in the home; staff do not have an office. Family counselors serve as liaisons between all systems that affect the youth and family—education, employment, health care access, probation, court, and other agencies. All of the youth have had some kind of psychiatric treatment before becoming adjudicated. Many have a roller coaster history of psychopharmacological treatment with little or no follow-up. Many have past or current histories of substance abuse, sexual abuse, single parenting, and early school failure. Many 16-year-old teenagers have only one high school credit. A mutual treatment plan is developed with measurable goals identified. With intentional small caseloads—urban family specialists have six youths, rural specialists have seven—daily interaction, and swift consequences of behavior, we see changes within 4 to 6 months. Family specialists wear many hats—counselor, advocate, policeman, role model, coach, and liaison to the community. Many youths attain verbal, social, study, and relationship skills they never before possessed. We believe in positive reinforcement and use that with youths and adults. Termination from the program is celebrated, and the youth tells the juvenile judge in court why he or she is ready to be discharged successfully.

As the Program Director, I incorporated individual and group clinical supervision. The staff need support too. Relationship building with community stakeholders is critical. I meet with the various systems' representatives to assess how we're doing and what can be done differently. Research and evaluation are key components, and we use several different tools to evaluate program effectiveness and integrity and youth and adult behavioral changes. My role has become more administrative as the program has enlarged, but clinical supervision keeps me close to the issues.

This role in psychiatric-mental health nursing has numerous interesting, joyful, and challenging aspects. It is interesting to learn a new discipline and the language of juvenile law. It is joyful to see an adolescent gain insight into his or her behavior, watch a parent hug a child for whom he or she had lost hope, and see the interdisciplinary model in practice as community stakeholders problem solve. It is challenging to watch a program grow and be able to change directions as needed. It is challenging to accept that a youth needs a more restrictive environment and equally challenging to assist in finding one that the youth needs, not one that needs the youth. It is also challenging to recognize my own professional and personal development. I struggle with the *clinician versus administrative* role and constantly seek a balance of the head and the heart.

I offer advice to novice nurses thinking of entering psychiatric-mental health nursing. Find a mentor wherever you go. Another's wisdom can lighten your load. Be creative. Develop "unorthodox" interventions. Seek out and work at interdisciplinary dialogue and collegiality. There is much to be learned from and shared with others. There *is* enough work for everyone. Volunteer for committees in your agency. It's a wonderful way to learn, take risks, and be recognized. Become a member of one professional nursing organization. The support and information are vital for your development. As a brand new child and adolescent psychiatric nurse graduate, I became a member of the Association of Child and Adolescent Psychiatric Nurses (ACAPN). In that group I not only found and received support and information, but my leadership skills were tapped and developed. After holding a variety of offices for the local and state ACAPN over a period of ten years, I eventually became national President of the ACAPN. Look beyond the obvious. What is already is—how can *you* make a difference?

I see psychiatric-mental health nursing on the brink of opportunity. We need well-educated, articulate, and compassionate nurses. We need to see this as an economic and a mental health care issue. We need to define clearly who we are, what outcomes people can expect, and how they can get there. I see mental health care positioned in a variety of community settings—some of which aren't known yet. You will discover that—those of you who are becoming educated problem solvers, critical thinkers, and risk takers.

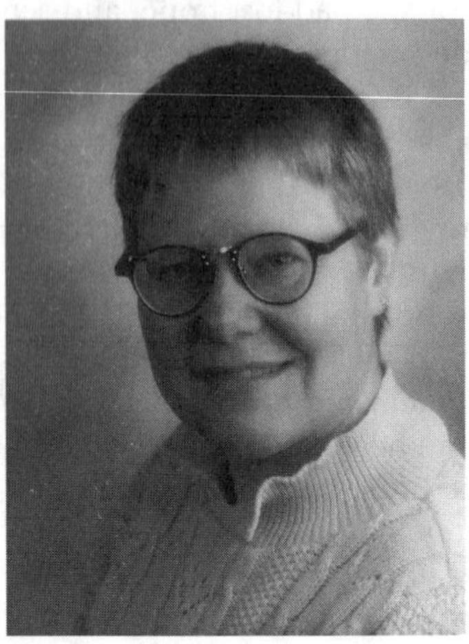

Sharon E. Byers, RN, MSN, CS
Clinical Nurse Specialist
Children and Family Services Department
Minneapolis, Minnesota

I am working on a grant-funded project to provide mental health outreach to homeless children, primarily children of homeless families but also unaccompanied homeless youth. I wrote this grant in response to what I saw as a tragedy of unmet needs among children in temporary situations; they are not yet hooked up to medical benefits and are experiencing a lot of trauma in the experience of homelessness and the family stresses that led to the homelessness.

Homelessness is a way of life for a frighteningly increasing number of people, about one-third of whom are younger than 18 years. My focus is to make contact with these children and adolescents and their families when possible; offer my services of assessment, crisis intervention, and short-term therapy; and refer them for longer term services in the community. To do this, I also have to educate the community service providers—providers of general services to the homeless and providers of general mental health services—about the special mental health risk factors, needs, and sensitivities of homeless youth. Part of my job consists of providing and arranging for this type of "cross-training." I also must become a part of several teams in numerous agencies where I can make contact with these children and young people. I am fortunate to have good relationships with shelters and other agencies staffed with experienced and dedicated people who send me referrals from school programs, healthcare-for-the-homeless clinics, and drop-in and multiservice centers for the homeless. Because the family and children are in crisis in many aspects of their lives, I do not attempt to address deeper issues; instead, I focus on immediate symptoms in response to losses and stress, such as low self-esteem, inability to focus, regression, anger, and fear. I do this work through play therapy and developmentally appropriate interview styles. I also consult with parents and refer them for any needed mental health services. In addition to services provided in agencies where children are found, I do street outreach as part of a collaboration of agencies providing services to homeless youth in the Minneapolis-St. Paul area. I make contacts with young people on the street, in coffee houses, and in drop-in sites for homeless youth.

I am also administrating a grant I wrote 1 year ago to provide specialized case management services to gay, lesbian, bisexual, and transgender (GLBT) homeless youth. Many of these are homeless because of their sexual orientation; many have been forced into prostitution and with that, the lifestyle of a chronic drug abuser. The ability to trust adults is fragile or nonexistent among these young people. Many are in constant crisis and prefer to depend for their support on "street families," who themselves are without resources and lack many necessary coping skills. Relationships have to be developed slowly with this population; the case manager tries to provide support and encouragement to allow the development of internal motivation to take a risk and try to work it out with the world, accept housing and employment, and return to school. Home is usually not a viable option for these youths, but independent living and some sort of peace with family are reasonable goals. As part of this project, I help facilitate a support group for homeless GLBT youth, provide counseling and crisis intervention, and encourage acceptance of referrals to gay-friendly counseling services in the community. The case manager focuses on day-to-day problem solving and skill development for making change and becoming independent. He helps build bridges between these youth and youth-serving agencies in the community. I help him measure changes seen and evaluate our effectiveness for our funding agency and for future projects of this type.

All of this work takes place in the context of my membership on a mental health crisis team for children and youth, a part of Family and Children's Mental Health of Hennepin County in Minneapolis, Minnesota. Before my involvement with the grant projects, I served on the crisis team, responding to calls from schools, parents, group homes, foster homes, and temporary shelters for children and youth. Our primary goal was to ensure safety for children in mental health crisis. To this end, we assessed for and arranged hospitalizations for children in life-threatening situations, such as seriously self-destructive, suicidal, and homicidal states. We provided special support to the seriously emotionally disturbed children on the case loads of the children's mental health case managers. We arranged respite care when possible and needed, provided problem-solving negotiations with families and other caregivers to support a good placement, and consulted with shelter and group home staff to ensure appropriate treatment planning for the child. Another aspect of this position on the crisis team was the assessment of 16- and 17-year-olds for mental health commitment. This involved in-depth assessment of the youths and all available records and interviews with families, hospital staff, and other professionals involved in providing mental health and social work services to these children. The team examines all the information gathered and decides whether or not to support the commitment and then passes this information on to the county attorney for further consideration.

I consider myself to have had a very rich work life in my 21 years as a nurse. I have worked medical-surgical nursing on a special care unit and psychiatric staff nursing on mental health units of hospitals. I have provided individual, group, couple, and family psychotherapy to young adults, middle adults, older adults, children, and adolescents. I have provided case management to chronically mentally ill adults in transition from long-term state hospital stays and mobile outreach to mentally ill homeless adults and children. I have taken on many of these roles within the same agency in which I now work and in a variety of other agencies in other cities and parts of the country. I have enjoyed consultation and inspiration from other nurses and many professionals in the mental health field.

The thing I like most about nursing is that we are trained to look at the whole person, adapt to a variety of settings and work teams, and provide the specific service appropriate to the client at that time. This training and study have allowed me to develop many skills in working with people with a range of mental health concerns and to adapt to many job settings and responsibilities. My advice to new graduates is to explore your interests and talents and keep alive the creative spirits with which you were born. The world is changing so fast that only skill and creativity can make the difference in meeting the needs of client populations.

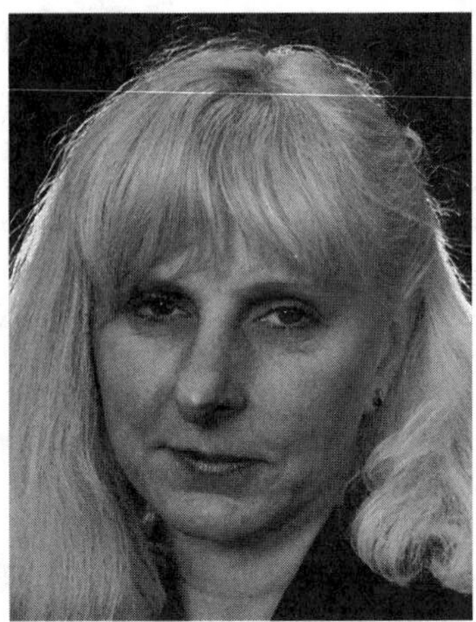

Susan E. Caverly, ARNP, MA, CS
Research/Clinical Instructor,
Department of Psychosocial and Community Health Nursing,
University of Washington, Seattle, Washington;
Psychiatric Nurse Practitioner

My role as a psychiatric nurse is best described as a work in progress. My first interests in the specialty arose from desire to work with terminally ill people and their significant others to help them resolve and cope with grief issues. I later practiced in the emergency setting providing crisis intervention services to people with mental illness and those faced with tremendous situational stress. I am currently engaged in clinical practice as a Psychiatric Nurse Practitioner with prescriptive authority and have a research practice as university faculty. The research project with which I am involved is an evaluation of public mental health service outcome change in response to regulatory waivers.

In Washington state, the nurse practice act recognizes psychiatric-mental health clinical specialists as Advanced Registered Nurse Practitioners (ARNPs). Psychiatric Nurse Practitioners are also eligible to request prescriptive authority for legend drugs within our scope of practice. (Legend drugs are medications that are not restricted by pharmacy schedule as controlled substances.) This environment has shaped the alternatives for practice that have been open to me. In some instances, my practice has been limited because the demand for professionals with my qualifications has been primarily in the area of psychiatric diagnosis and clinical management, including medication prescription. However, the ability to work as an autonomous practitioner, receive third-party reimbursement, and prescribe psychiatric medications has opened more practice opportunities than it has closed.

The practice I have chosen allows and requires me to integrate the biopsychosocial components related to the evaluation and treatment of mental illness. I interpret this to include the health status of the individual, the psychosocial and cultural factors that contribute to health status and use of mental health services, and the environmental context of the community in which the individual must function. This understanding of my role permits me to intervene within my scope of practice in a wide array of situations using a broad range of psychiatric nursing skills. On any clinic day, I may rule out thyroid disorder as the cause of psychiatric symptoms by ordering laboratory tests or requesting a physical examination; assess whether sleep difficulties and anxiety are associated with substance dependence; provide psychotherapy and family education and prescribe medication to treat symptoms of depressed mood and panic experienced by a person with post-traumatic stress disorder; and medicate or hospitalize an acutely psychotic person with a diagnosis of bipolar disorder. The challenges of my practice coupled with the need to provide care in an efficient yet safe and individually tailored manner are stimulating, at times taxing, and always humbling.

In my private practice, I have the luxury to be more flexible with regard to the amount of time that I spend with individual consumers. I have tried to develop a sliding fee scale that is responsive to the person's ability to pay for psychiatric care. The people with whom I work in private practice are frequently situationally stressed as opposed to suffering major mental illness. Often the goal of therapy is to improve capacity to work effectively or to develop coping and self-management skills. I prescribe psychoactive medications to treat anxiety and depression, but the assessment and intervention occur before symptoms reach the severe and disabling level that is commonly the case in public sector practice.

The research component of my practice is important to me. The mental health care delivery systems we develop as a community or country must provide accessible, high-quality care, and they must be affordable. Collaborative projects between mental health authorities and university researchers provide mental health administrators, professionals, and researchers the opportunity to pool economic and skill resources to generate knowledge while informing and perhaps reforming the system of care. It is exciting to be a part of this process.

As I think about the path that led me to become a Psychiatric Nurse Practitioner, the key factor was the frustration I felt as I attempted to intervene in psychosocial problems that presented in my general or oncology nursing practice. There was never adequate time to attend to these problems; the pressing needs of the physical illnesses precluded prioritization of the mental health needs. As I came to realize my preference to care for the most severely ill, I was also able to see that people with mental illness are among those who are the most severely ill. Finally, the feeling of having a special capacity and skill to intervene in situations from which other nurses turned helped me to recognize the significant contributions made by psychiatric nursing.

In my role as a psychiatric nurse practitioner, I am forced to consider the differences and similarities between what I do and what a psychiatrist might do. Accounting for individual differences, I find that the skills I have as a psychiatric nurse prepare me for a broader practice than that of most psychiatrists. I am more able to acknowledge that not everyone I treat will get well and that my role may be palliative and supportive. I am comfortable learning from consumers when my academically learned interventions don't work or don't fit. The pragmatism and advocacy of nursing create the possibility for a healing psychosocial dynamic between the psychiatric nurse and the consumer. The relationship is grounded in a mutual respect and collaboration not necessarily common to all disciplines.

Although I value the nurse–consumer relationship, I find biological and pharmacological interventions to be useful and at times amazing. When a person responds to a psychotropic agent that has been appropriately prescribed, it can be dramatic and profound. I am very biologically biased. Prescriptive practice has been a professional journey crossing traditional boundaries between nursing and medicine. It is clear to me that medicine and nursing overlap in terms of activities but that this shared practice does not detract from the professional identities of either discipline. In my practice, I think, act, and view myself as an advanced practice psychiatric nurse who assumes a substitutive role for that of a psychiatrist. I do not seek recognition as a "parapsychiatrist."

Perhaps the most frustrating aspect of my work as a Psychiatric Nurse Practitioner is the need to spend a significant part of my time pushing at practice barriers. The other issue I find draining is the difficulty nursing has in remaining a solid coalition rather than engaging in subspecialty political splintering. If I were to have a magic wand, I would obliterate the barriers to practice for all competent health care practitioners (not only nurses). I would also coalesce nursing into a group with collective professional identity, a minimal desire to limit the practice of other disciplines, and a strong sense of political and community responsibility to the people for whom we care.

I believe that the future for psychiatric nursing holds great promise. However, there will undoubtedly be some quivering of the ground, and psychiatric nurses will need to sell our value to those who purchase health care. Managed mental health care will challenge psychiatric nurses at all levels of practice to find efficient models of care and to document the contribution of psychiatric nursing to mental health and physical health outcomes. We must become not only good nurses and responsible employees, but contractors and business people who understand the cost of providing specialty services and the cost offset of failing to provide access to these services. Our consumer advocacy role will be stretched as we find our place in this competitive yet flexible and elastic new environment.

My advice to novice psychiatric-mental health nurses is to become accomplished in general psychiatric and specialty psychiatric nursing. Approach the unstable health care environment as a gift; breathe deeply, and find the capacity for flexibility in terms of role characteristics, community practice site, and means of remuneration. Psychosocial skills will be invaluable as health care reform efforts unfold, and psychiatric nurses will assume new, as yet undeveloped, roles. We must be alert for windows of opportunity created by forces to reform the health care system; we cannot afford to expend energy guarding a potentially anachronistic domain.

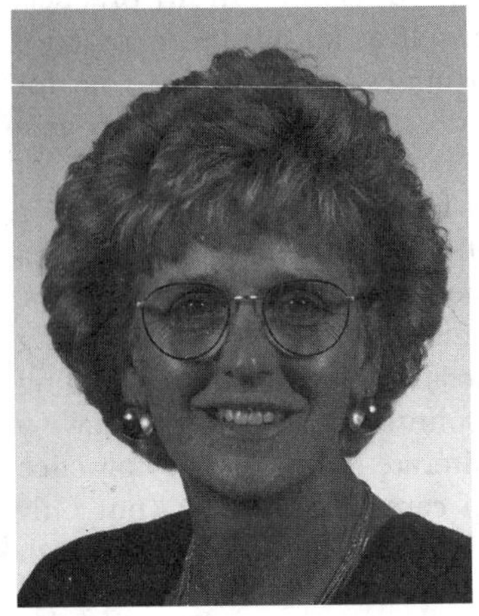

Phyllis M. Connolly, PhD, RN, CS
San Jose State University
School of Nursing
San Jose, California

My role in psychiatric-mental health nursing includes a full-time position as Professor in the School of Nursing at San Jose State University, and my primary assignment is the undergraduate baccalaureate program. I teach through a faculty practice model in the School of Nursing's Nurse-Managed Center. The population on which I focus my research, practice, and teaching are people with serious mental illness living in the community.

I also coordinate the Transdisciplinary Collaboration Project, which involves extensive collaboration with local mental health system service providers, consumers, families, consumer advocacy groups, faculty from the College of Social Work, Department of Occupational Therapy, Communications Disorders, and the Therapeutic Recreation Program.

I'm certified as a clinical specialist in adult psychiatric-mental health nursing by the American Nurses Association and a trained facilitator in the Moller-Wer Simultaneous Consumer/Family Education Model. Thus, in my private practice, which currently focuses on the simultaneous consumer-family education program, I integrate students' course objectives in the advanced undergraduate and graduate program into my practice and their learning.

I didn't choose psychiatric-mental health nursing until I started my graduate program in psychiatric-mental health nursing. I had been practicing in acute medical-surgical hospital nursing for 15 years and was considering graduate education but was unsure of which area of speciality I should pursue.

During that mulling time, I observed what I believed to be a large proportion of stress-related illnesses in the hospital, requiring a large amount of preoperative teaching, diabetic teaching, medication education, and cardiac rehabilitation. I had also started working in a new all registered nursing primary care acute care facility and began to see what nursing should really be—a collaboration with the client in meeting their goals and needs. As I began to see the need for prevention in chronic illness, the area of stress management became more interesting to me. I decided the area of nursing that would give me the most skills and competencies, particularly in the area of stress management, would be psychiatric nursing. That was and is the most meaningful area of nursing for me.

I remain in the field because I believe I can make a difference in the lives of people in the areas of prevention, restoration, and rehabilitation. I am also able to make a difference in the way my students view and treat people with mental illness.

My advice to novice nurses thinking of entering psychiatric-mental health nursing is to find a mentor. I would suggest finding an expert master's prepared clinical specialist and ask that person to mentor you. I would also be sure that your physical and psychosocial assessment skills are honed.

The future of psychiatric-mental health nursing is exciting and full of challenges and opportunities. Much more care will be delivered in the home and the community. Teaching families and consumers will take on an even greater significance in accessing care and managing symptoms. More technology will be used for distance supervision, continuing education, health promotion, self-help, and health evaluation. Managed care will drive more efficient and effective systems of care. Psychiatric-mental health nurses will be needed as providers of direct services, researchers and developers of new knowledge and techniques, case managers, and executives.

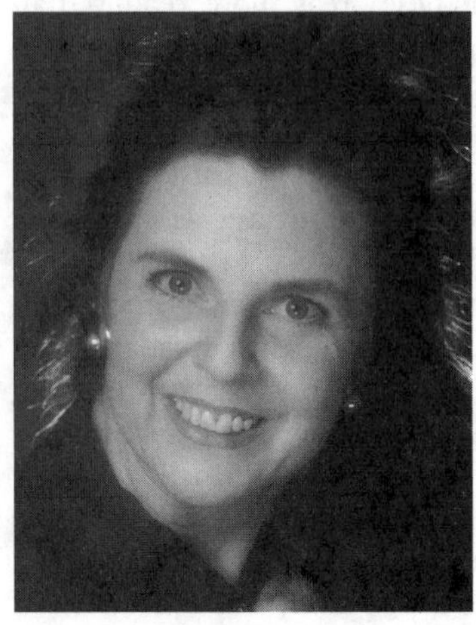

Karen K. Dewey, RN, CS, MS
Assistant Professor
School of Nursing
Weber State University
Ogden, Utah

My role in psychiatric-mental health nursing is that of Assistant Professor teaching psychiatric nursing for the Associate Degree Nursing Program. I have also worked as a staff nurse on the behavioral health units (acute, adolescent, adult, and drug and alcohol units) and as a psychiatric home care nurse for McKay-Dee Hospital (Ogden). While working on my graduate degree, I did the quality assurance piece for the Behavioral Health Department. My internship was spent doing individual and group psychotherapy at the YCC (Ogden Women's Crisis Center) and at Weber County Mental Health Department. In December 1995, I received my certification as a Clinical Specialist in adult psychiatric and mental health nursing and hope to develop a private practice in combination with my teaching responsibilities.

It is my belief that I did not choose psychiatric-mental health nursing. Rather, it chose me. It was the easiest rotation for me as a nursing student at Weber State College. Listening to clients relate their concerns and fears was the most rewarding part of the job. In fact, I couldn't wait to get done with the routine chores of nursing so that I would have time to sit with clients and hear their concerns. I found that this also seemed to reduce clients' anxiety significantly.

When I came to the end of my Associate Degree program and started thinking about where I would work, I received a call from McKay-Dee Hospital asking me to come in for an interview. Ruth Brown, the psychiatric nursing instructor, had given my name as a student who had done well in the psychiatric nursing rotation. By the end of the interview, I had a job. I started working on the acute psychiatric unit and loved it. The clients seemed to trust me and feel relaxed. Many times, when a client was agitated, he or she did not need restraints if I sat with him or her. It was very rewarding and a boost to my ego.

In retrospect, as so many people in the health care field, I'm sure personal issues entered into my career choice. Two of our four children suffered from chronic illnesses, and both have died from complications of their illnesses. Our oldest daughter, Tracy, was born with a rare brain disease (hypsarrhythmia) and was profoundly retarded. She lived at home with us for 22 years. Our second oldest daughter, Julie, died in May 1995 from complications of diabetes. I believe that our entire family has learned great lessons from these two extraordinary people. My husband, Bill, is a very sensitive, caring individual, and our other two children, Kristy and Greg, are also wonderful, caring people.

As a teacher, I try to encourage my students to look at life and view their clients in a different way. I emphasize being nonjudgmental ("love the person; hate the behavior"), caring about the individual while maintaining proper boundaries, and really listening to what the client is saying. Students are also encouraged to look at their own issues to be able to care for others in a nonjudgmental way. These things are very important to me because of my personal experiences with health care systems in the role of a parent. I have met some very caring individuals and some individuals who were quite unprofessional. From a quality assurance point of view, clients who are treated in a caring manner will tolerate genuine mistakes much more readily from health care professionals. People who feel that they have had their concerns taken seriously are much more satisfied, even if their concerns cannot be remedied.

Psychiatric nursing is a very exciting field. It is, in

my opinion, the basis for all other fields of nursing. As for the future, it seems that there will be a great need for more psychiatric home care programs and for more psychiatric nurses to practice in community settings. I believe that nursing clinics would fill a great community need and that Clinical Specialists in psychiatric and mental health nursing are the people who could provide effective and efficient mental health care to communities. Psychiatric nurses have the expertise to provide mental health education in a variety of settings (ie, schools, hospitals, clinics, and the county mental health systems).

Clients coming into the system with mental health problems seem to be younger and younger. Perhaps we, as psychiatric nurses, need to be focusing on educating the children in grade school regarding stress reduction and ways to promote good mental health. Teenagers need to have information on good parenting skills and childhood developmental issues *before* they need them. Young teenage fathers need to have interventions to help them deal with the responsibilities and stress of their new roles, as do the mothers. Nurses have the expertise and can intervene in these areas more readily than some other professionals because of their medical knowledge and assessment skills. Nurses also are trusted and accepted by the public because of our reputation for caring.

The thing I would like to instill in my students is that caring *about* their clients is as important as caring *for* them. This can make a big difference in the outcome of a client. Many times we do make a difference, and we don't even know it. Last summer, my husband and I took our grandson out to a fast food restaurant. The girl who waited on us said, "Is your name Karen? You took care of me at the Behavioral Health Institute a few years ago. I wanted you to know that since then, I finished high school, and I'm working here this summer to earn money for college. I start in the fall. I just wanted to thank you." As I said, we *do* make a difference. We just don't always know it.

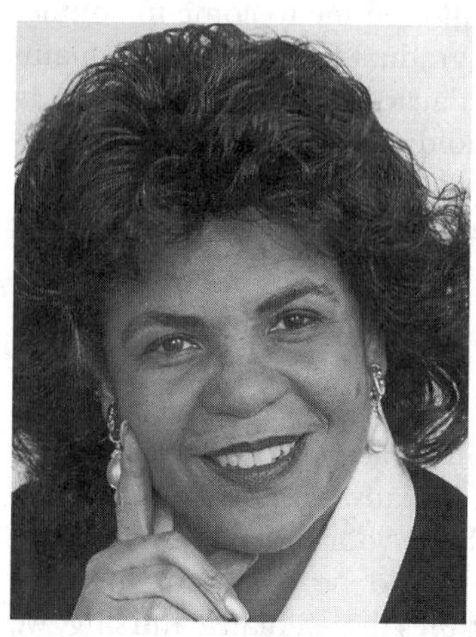

Patricia Nottingham Dzandu, MS, RN, CS, CNAA
Nursing Manager, Psychiatry Services
Veterans Administration Medical Center
Hampton, Virginia

The foundation for my nursing career began at Hampton Institute (Hampton University) where I received a BSN degree. After graduation, I moved to New Haven, Connecticut to work as a staff nurse on a 15-bed inpatient psychiatric unit at Yale New Haven Hospital. This was an exciting time for me because I was an active participant in research protocols for lithium carbonate, cerebrospinal fluid, and depression. I practiced next to the top psychiatrists in the world, and these experiences have stayed with me more than many others. Why? It afforded me the opportunity to witness the positive effects of medication for our client population and have a "bird's eye" view of the research.

During my 8 years at Yale New Haven Hospital, I attended the University of New Haven and received a master's degree in community psychology. My interest blossomed into acute psychiatric nursing and primary prevention related to reducing the despair of mental illness through early intervention and detection in community-based programs. This period in my career allowed me to begin my research on children of mentally ill parents from a community-based model.

Several years later, I returned to Virginia to assume a psychiatric nurse case manager role for an outpatient mental health clinic. My community psychology background paid off in that I became a medication nurse and group therapist for a 75-client case load. The realities of mental illness will continue to play an important part in my view and concern for clients.

Finally, after considerable thought, I entered the nursing administration world with my first position as Director of Nursing for the Psychiatric Institute of Richmond, a campus-like setting offering inpatient and residential care for children and adolescents. My career then consisted of nursing director positions for Peninsula Psychiatric Hospital in Hampton, Virginia; Richland Hospital in Fort Worth, Texas; and Harris-Methodist Hospital in Bedford, Texas. Nursing administration became my niche, which was completely opposite from how I got started. However, I had a desire to participate as a change initiator after witnessing during my formative practicing years the need for nurses to be engineers and designers of client care systems. My appreciation for the negative effects of mental illness as seen in my earlier research participation at Yale and the public outpatient mental clinic continue to resurface in my current roles in psychiatric nursing.

The changes in the psychiatric industry forced me to alter my academic preparation. My master's degree in psychology was not the correct match for my career path in nursing administration. Therefore, I returned to school after 12 years to pursue a master's degree in psychiatric nursing-nursing administration from Texas Woman's University. This prepared me for other opportunities as the psychiatric industry continued to change.

My current role is that of Nursing Manager for a 70-bed psychiatric service at Veteran's Administration. My role is a combination of clinical nurse specialist and manager. My emphasis is to supervise a nursing staff of all levels and to assist in the movement of our service to increase alternatives to inpatient care. I also participate in establishing and maintaining staffing patterns, group supervision, milieu program design, and performance reviews; I participate with other allied health providers on joint committees and projects. I am an active member in the Nursing Services Administrative Council, research committees, and quality improvement initiatives.

The challenge of this role has been to maintain an efficient department or units amidst a cost-driven environment. Each day for the last 20 years I have had to keep a pulse on resources and be able to provide effective client care. What has benefited me the most is to see the gold mine of resources available on our Veteran's Administration campus on which our clients can piggyback. My challenge is to be able to coordinate the flow of services campus-wide to benefit our psychiatric clients.

The Texas experience during the psychiatric hospital investigations was the most challenging time because of the scrutiny and criticism placed on the industry. This sparked my efforts to start the Psychiatric-Mental Health Conference/Practice Group for Texas Nurses Association-District III, Fort Worth, Texas. It is my belief that during hard times, nurses need to support one another, ascertain correct facts, and use effective coping mechanisms to make it through the day to day scrutiny. As a result, we captured positive nursing care projects that had been implemented in our district. They were bound and distributed to our membership. In fact, the message was "Job well done, nurses of Tarrant County." The greatest benefit was the networking and support that counteracted despair and isolation. This project opened up the opportunity for me to coordinate the same model for the Virginia Nurses Association-District 10, Hampton, Virginia. I am Chairperson for the Clinical Nursing Practice Group, which encompasses all specialty areas. The format is the same as used in Texas, whereby nurses present a nursing care project and research. At the end of the year, a bound collection of abstracts is developed for distribution. Many nurses have never presented, and this is one way to disseminate our worth and teach all levels of nurses the art of capturing the good through documentation.

In addition to my primary and secondary roles as described, I am Adjunct Faculty at Hampton University School of Nursing Graduate Department. I teach nursing administration, group dynamics, and community mental health. This has allowed me to come in contact with undergraduate and graduate students while maintaining my primary psychiatric-mental health roles. My advice to nurses is threefold:

1. Keep up with trends, and match your educational qualifications to fit the change. Take risks and be a change initiator, instead of waiting for the change to happen without your input, regardless of how small it is.
2. Get involved in nursing groups to facilitate networking and document your practice. Take advantage of quality improvement initiatives as one vehicle to assess, record, and evaluate your outcomes.
3. Take care of yourself, and be conscious of stress management. Many times in psychiatric nursing, we focus on others before ourselves.

I also encourage students or novice nurses to think about leadership and management in our field. Much emphasis has gone to the nurse practitioner tract, which is appropriate, but I am concerned about future leadership in nursing. It's workable, dynamic, and creative.

The future of psychiatric nursing is promising. I tell students that psychiatric nursing transcends all of the nursing specialties. You cannot isolate or deny the benefits of the professional nurse–client relationship. The market is changing, however, and we may not see traditional positions in psychiatric nursing anymore. The inpatient setting is declining, but opportunities in home health care clinics, outpatient clinics, and schools are developing. There will still be inpatient beds, but the rapid turnover will be greater. I encourage nurses to seek certification in psychiatric nursing because this may be a deciding factor for employment requirements as the industry changes. Regardless, I am proud to be a part of the profession of psychiatric nursing.

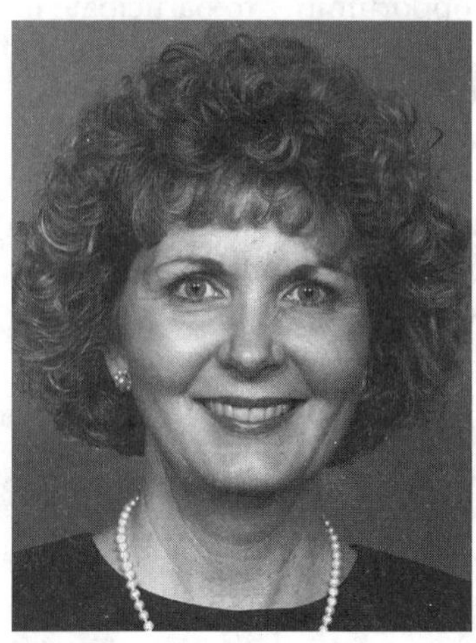

Diane L. Faucher, MSN, RN, CS
Superintendent
Austin State Hospital
Austin, Texas

Although I am serving as CEO of a 352-bed Joint Commission for the Accreditation of Healthcare Organizations (JCAHO)-accredited state hospital, I consider myself to be a practicing psychiatric-mental health nurse. It is frustrating when people, especially nurses, ask me when in my career I left nursing. I am equally dismayed when I hear nurses in mental health service settings who have nontraditional roles talk about "when they used to be" nurses.

When I became a nurse, and later when I became attracted to psychiatric-mental health nursing, I never dreamed that my career path would lead me to management. I started my nursing career as a licensed vocational nurse and entered professional nursing through a career ladder approach that included associate, baccalaureate, and master's degree programs. Although this was at a time when little was available in the way of advanced placement opportunity and I had to cover some learning content more than once, I have always been grateful that fate led me through a ladder approach to education. This experience has given me a view of the health care system from a variety of perspectives, and I've had the opportunity to become socialized in a variety of roles.

My early nursing career was in an acute care medical-surgical setting. I will always be glad for this time in my career, not only because of the richness of experiences, but also for the foundation of knowledge that I accumulated. I first became interested in psychiatric-mental health nursing as a baccalaureate student when I spent a day following a hospital psychiatric nursing supervisor through a routine day, which included a luncheon meeting at the local mental health association. This was exciting stuff! Seeing the linkage between hospital-based acute care and community-based services was a new experience for me.

This experience became the first step in my career as a psychiatric-mental health nurse. I went on to a master's degree program at the University of Texas at Austin. It was 1977, and times were good. The National Institute of Mental Health was still awarding psychiatric nursing stipends, and the university had a wonderful psychiatric program. I was assigned to Austin State Hospital for my individual and group therapy experiences. Working at a private psychiatric hospital part time and taking graduate courses with labs in a state hospital were enlightening experiences. I found public sector nursing more rewarding. Except for a 2-year period in which I taught community mental health nursing at the baccalaureate level, I have worked in either public community-based or hospital-based services ever since.

I have held a number of positions since beginning a career in mental health services, including serving as a clinical nurse specialist, a coordinator of licensure for private mental hospitals in Texas, a quality assurance consultant, and a special assistant to the Commissioner of the Texas Department of Mental Health-Mental Retardation, an organization employing more than 30,000 people. There are two primary reasons that I love my field of practice and genuinely enjoy coming to work every day: 1) the challenge and joy of serving people with the greatest needs and 2) the ongoing opportunities for growth and job diversity that I have experienced in public mental health services.

One of the most interesting and challenging features of being a nurse is that nurses are actually prepared by education and experience to do just about anything in the field of health care planning, deployment, and administration. However, we are not socialized to know it! Our colleagues do not always believe it. I see this as a major opportunity for nurse educators and practicing nurses.

Why is no one surprised when a psychiatrist, psychologist, or psychiatric social worker becomes an administrator, but it is almost always a surprise for a nurse to do so? To begin with, I never had a single teacher, supervisor, or mentor suggest to me that a nurse could be anything more influential in an organization than nursing director. We have never been taught to envision a career as a CEO, and if we do so, we are seen as abandoning the profession.

This perception of abandonment is not just a belief held by my nursing colleagues; it is often a perception of other professionals and the general public. A couple of years ago, a nurse and a physician both received presidential appointments at the same time. The news coverage noted that the new Surgeon General was a physician and that the new head of the Social Security Administration had once been a nurse. I rest my case.

The world of psychiatric-mental health services is changing at a pace previously not experienced or envisioned. Not only is the entire system of service delivery changing, its effects are being felt by consumers and providers, especially nurses. I just saw a hospital publication with a cover story entitled, "Faded Glory-Is this Nursing's Last Stand?" Does it have to be this way? Is it inevitable? Not at all!

The psychiatric-mental health services of yesterday are quickly becoming the behavioral health managed care system of today. I would extend two challenges to new graduates interested in this field of practice and to currently practicing psychiatric nurses. First, develop an understanding of the changes that are inevitable, and within them, find new opportunities for nursing practice. With the increased emphasis on measurable outputs, outcomes, and efficiencies, be willing to develop new approaches to the delivery of nursing care. As hospital units and many hospitals are closing down, develop more requisite variety, that is, the ability to expand nursing practice in new settings and with new approaches. If we do not do this, others will do it for us at the expense of the nursing profession.

In Texas, the public mental health service system is glued together by one of the strongest case management systems in the nation. There are thousands of case managers serving Texans with serious mental illness, yet hardly any are nurses. This is because the nursing profession did not seize any opportunities to participate in the planning of the case management system in the beginning, and subsequently nurses have been unwilling to take on a nontraditional role. This is in a state where the first case managers were public health nurses on horseback! In the few places where nurses are case managers, they are doing a terrific job and making a real difference. To be successful, they have identified a case management role that is unique from other case management roles, including serving consumers who have complex psychiatric problems, are medically fragile, and are on medications requiring special monitoring. Professional nurses are finding success in serving ACT Teams, a primary care model that delivers assertive community treatment. Nurses must be willing to think outside traditional roles and treatment models to be successful.

The second challenge I would extend relates to nurses' role in management. I would ask new graduates to consider a career goal that includes being a manager or a CEO, even if it is "outside" of nursing. What better way to have a positive influence on the practice of nursing. For those already well into a career, it's not too late. If you wait to make a job advancement move until you feel completely ready, you have probably waited too long. Even if you don't have such aspirations, support nurses who do, and support new graduates to not limit aspirations within a glass ceiling.

Nurses belong in leadership roles and understand many aspects of health care that others do not. Nurses have many power skills and may not even be in touch with some of them! A few years ago, I was taking a total quality management course with other non-nurse managers, and most of the content focused on the application of a systemic problem-solving process in management and decision making. This was a new concept for most; for me, it appeared to be nothing more than the nursing process. Nurses are good managers because of their ability to use this scientific process and because of other strengths, including advocacy skills, communication skills, negotiation skills, and the comfort we feel with the team approach. If we want psychiatric-mental health nursing to not "fade away," we must be part of the design team for the behavioral health systems within the managed care environment of tomorrow.

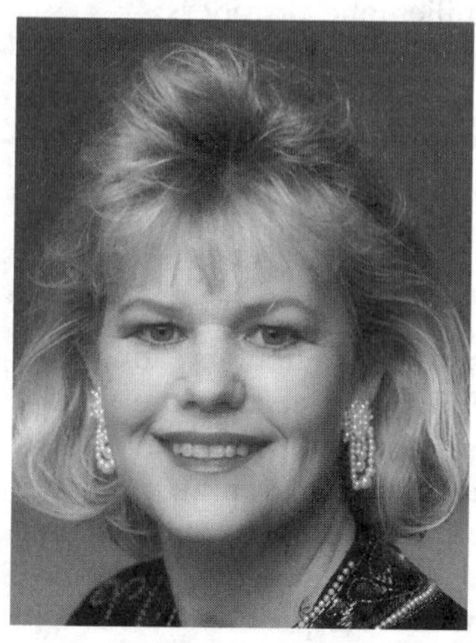

Kimberly Littrell, APRN, CS, CGP
President and CEO
Promedica, Inc.
Tucker, Georgia

I began my career in psychiatric-mental health nursing at the age of 19. Our first clinical rotation at nursing school was in psychiatry. As students, we were thrust on the floor of an acute treatment unit at the university teaching hospital in our second week of classes. Without our uniforms, hats, or stethoscopes to protect us, we were immersed in a world unknown to us as neophyte clinicians. I will never forget how all the students huddled together in a group in the day room as if we would be devoured should we separate; I remember the frustration of our instructor as we were told to "go out and contract" with a client for our training experience. The other students rushed on to the unit and contracted with all the "good" clients: borderlines, depressed women, and bipolars. One young woman with schizophrenia was the only client who had not been approached by a student. This 22-year-old woman was 8 months pregnant and had been transferred from the state hospital to deliver her baby. In the 1970s, it was customary to discontinue antipsychotic medication when a woman became pregnant, so this client had been off medication for several months. Our sessions consisted of her pacing up and down the hallways, barking and growling at me, hiding under the bed, and attempting to spit at me. Not knowing how to make contact with her, I paced with her, read her the newspaper while she hid under the bed, and shared my candy. Although I was never sure how much of my presence and "chatter" she absorbed, something amazing occurred in those first few weeks of my training. I began to feel comfortable on the unit, and as I sat on the floor with my client, I became a respectful observer of the "life" on a psychiatric unit. I appreciated the genuine suffering that the clients were experiencing, their individual stories, and their struggles toward recovery. They were not the "crazy" people whom as a child I had been taught to fear and avoid, but unique individuals whose illness was just as serious as anyone in the intensive care unit. My client began to tolerate my presence and even sat beside me for short periods. As the days became weeks, she finally delivered a healthy baby boy. She was placed on trifluoperazine (Stelazine) and was stabilized enough to return to the state hospital. On the day of her discharge, she told me, "Although I acted like an animal, you were the only person who didn't treat me like an animal." Those were very powerful words for someone 19 years old to hear! I became hooked on psychiatric nursing and focused my entire senior year on refining my assessment and intervention skills. I worked every other weekend as an assistant on the unit and was the only student who chose psychiatry for my practicum experience.

After graduation, I went to work at a state hospital in Georgia and requested to be on the "chronic" unit. I was constantly challenged to find ways into the psychotic world of the clients—how to communicate with them in spite of their delusions, understand their neologisms, and teach them about their illness and medications in ways they could understand. After 2 years, I returned to graduate school and focused my thesis on personal space and territoriality in schizophrenia. I continued to work on the weekends and was fortunate to have exposure to group therapy in my new work site. The mode of treatment appealed to me, particularly for working with adults with schizophrenia. I received additional training and supervision and have since obtained my certification in group therapy. After I was awarded my Master's degree, I was selected as a research nurse on a National Institute of Mental Health grant, *Treatment Strategies in Schizophrenia.* This 5-year, multicenter study analyzed treatment interventions of depot medication and psychoeducation. I was afforded the opportunity to train with leaders in the field of schizophrenia; people whose work I had read and referenced were now my mentors and teachers.

My experience and training at the National Institute of Mental Health ignited a fire inside me—how to effectively implement the *theories* of treatment into actual clinical practice. I began designing the "ideal" program for people with schizophrenia. It would include a multidisciplinary treatment team, comprehensive services, residential services, state-of-the-art antipsychotic medications, and research.

In 1986, I opened the first totally comprehensive treatment center for adults with schizophrenia in the United States. Schizophrenia Treatment and Rehabilitation, Inc. (STAR) had gone from an idea to reality. At STAR, we conducted investigational drug studies on the new antipsychotic medications and analyzed their effects on reintegration. During the next 7 years, the program received multiple commendations, awards, and recognitions for work in the field of schizophrenia and mental health. In 1993, I went to Los Angeles to work as the technical advisor on a movie about my work at STAR. The ABC made-for-television movie *Out of Darkness* starring Diana Ross aired in January 1994 and was truly a magical experience for me. In that same year, I was given the Mental Health Professional of the Year award by the Alliance for the Mentally Ill. Charter Medical Corporation offered to buy my program to expand their continuum of care and incorporate specialized outpatient treatment in their services. Through our alliance, I was able to open two more programs, one in Indianapolis and one in Orlando. In 1995, I received the Award for Excellence in Clinical Practice from the American Psychiatric Nurses Association. I have now started my second company, Promedica Research Center. We are conducting investigational studies in the areas of pharmacology, group therapy, and reintegration strategies. We also develop psychoeducational materials for consumers, families, and providers.

I chose to enter psychiatric nursing because I found it stimulating, interesting, challenging, and rich with opportunity. Throughout my 20 years in the field, I have always felt there was more to learn and experience. I believe that we, in psychiatric nursing, have the opportunity to change and improve the health care delivery system through our own efforts if we are willing to take the chance! I have been an entrepreneur, creating business based on my perception of needs in the field. I believe nursing is the best equipped profession to treat mental illness by the nature of our training. Our understanding of the physical, emotional, and spiritual components of individuals gives us a unique perspective on the human condition; this perspective is lacking in other disciplines.

I am excited about the potential for psychiatric nursing and would strongly recommend this area as a career path. I see the trend in health care to recognize psychiatric nursing as a speciality area. Advanced practice nurses are receiving prescriptive authority, privileged communication, and the ability to involuntarily commit clients. Psychiatric nurses have opened clinics, home health agencies, and private practices and are thriving in the dual role of nurse and business person. With the reconfiguration of health care occurring at a mind-boggling rate, I believe privatization of mental health will continue well into the next millennium. This will give nurses the opportunity to be as independent in their practice as they choose to be. I believe that our training provides nurses with superior methods of healing and furnishes the self-confidence, motivation, and pleasure to work in this challenging field that can, at times, be analogous to a labyrinth. We are in a unique time that enables us to move beyond traditional roles and limitations in our practice. As Lamb once said, "The measure of choosing well, is whether a man likes what he has chosen." I like what I have chosen.

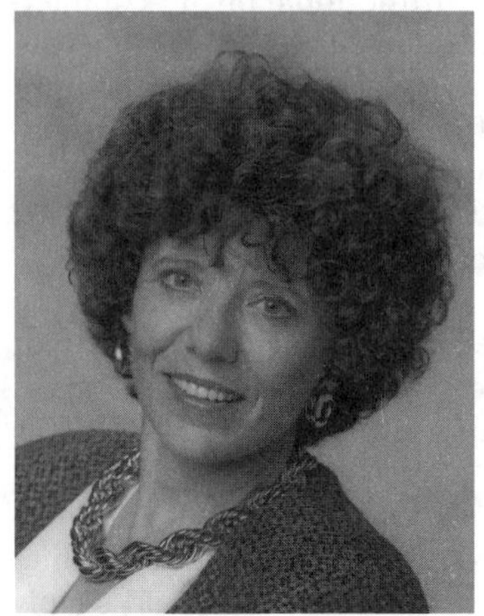

Wanda Krystyna Mohr, PhD, RNC
Program Director
Psychiatric Mental Health Division
School of Nursing
University of Pennsylvania
Philadelphia, Pennsylvania

My roles in nursing throughout my lifetime have been varied. I did not begin as a psychiatric-mental health nurse. I fell into the specialty serendipitously. I received my diploma from a 3-year school of nursing in New Jersey in 1966. I was not the world's best student at the time, and I was constantly in trouble for my oppositional nature and my tendency for pushing the boundaries of what I saw as a highly arbitrary and rigid discipline. Part of that opposition was a penchant for taking on difficult causes and siding with the underdog point of view—the theme of my life and career, although I didn't know it at the time.

I began my nursing career as a medical-surgical nurse at the Presbyterian Hospital of the Columbia-Presbyterian Medical Center in New York City in the late 1960s. It was an invaluable experience in which I became thoroughly grounded in the basic practice of nursing. It afforded me the opportunity to work among superb practitioners in a world class medical center. I continued in medical-surgical nursing, working in a variety of roles in outpatient and inpatient settings until I moved to Texas in the late 1970s. I decided to return to school. Because there were no advanced nursing programs in the area, I "made do" and received a bachelor's degree in literature and psychology. I followed this with a master's degree in psychology with a focus on adolescent problems. Part of the advanced degree was a requirement that we conduct a research project. This was my first taste of research and writing, and I was hooked. Shortly after my graduation in 1984, I entered into a private practice multidisciplinary clinic with the dean of my behavioral sciences program, and I specialized in adolescent problems. However, I was neither happy with the role as a psychological associate, nor did I like private practice. Although it was quite lucrative, I found it claustrophobic and solitary, and I missed nursing. I needed to get back to my roots.

I began to think about what I could do with my degrees, and in the mid-1980s, a private psychiatric hospital opened in town. I was hired to be the nurse-executive in charge of adolescent and child psychiatry in a 70-bed psychiatric hospital held by an investor-owned health care corporation. What joy it was to get back to nursing. What a joy to be surrounded by adolescents! Almost immediately into my tenure, I began to feel uneasy with certain aspects of the institution. The problems that I encountered included the following:

Clients and family members were not made aware of their rights under the mental health code when they were admitted or while they were hospitalized. Client and family rights were systematically ignored or violated. This took the form of withholding telephone or mail privileges, denying family or attorney visitation, using physical restraint when less restrictive interventions could have been used, failing to inform clients and families of potentially adverse side effects to neuroleptic medications, and refusing to allow clients to leave the hospital by request even though they were voluntary admissions and posed no threat to themselves or others.

The administrator and comptroller requested that we falsify documentation in charts to maximize or justify continued admission of clients. There were orders to falsify charts and records to reflect certain staffing patterns or treatments and therapies that never took place to comply with Medicare and JCAHO standards.

I saw adolescent clients placed on the same unit with adult clients with no regard to their special treatment needs to minimize the number of staffing requirements.

Other negative practices included coercive threats against clients and families, fraud in the form of admitting one person under the name and policy of another person, the use of unqualified individuals to screen and admit clients, and treatment that was structured around the dollar amount of the clients' insurance policy coverage.

I couldn't believe it! This was not the health care that I remembered. When I refused to participate in unethical practices and tried to improve conditions for the staff and clients, I was vilified by my colleagues in administration and labeled a "troublemaker," not a team player. After a particularly dangerous incident involving a loaded pistol, I resigned. After my foray into the world of big business, I worked for several years in a number of roles that included staff nursing and nurse-educator—all of them in the field of psychiatric-mental health nursing. I found that my medical-surgical and psychology background formed the basis of a comprehensive approach to clients that I thought was lacking in fields such as psychology and psychiatric nursing as it was being practiced.

I decided to invest the remainder of my career in nursing because I missed it and because it fits with my personality. Nurses are client advocates; they naturally side with the underdog. What better way for me to make a contribution than to devote myself to the most vulnerable, stigmatized underdog population—the mentally ill. I was hooked on research and writing, and I enjoyed adolescent populations. I thought the natural thing to do was to get my doctorate in nursing, continue to practice part time, and teach undergraduate students. I received my BSN and was admitted to the doctoral program at the University of Texas at Austin. When it came time to decide on a dissertation topic, the for-profit psychiatric hospital scandal had become front page news. I thought it was a natural topic for my dissertation. I had to overcome some obstacles: I had to convince people that this was a nursing issue, but I was very fortunate to have some visionaries on my side.

It was my great fortune to have my present mentor and chairman, Ann W. Burgess, take an interest in what I was doing and recruit me to the University of Pennsylvania. It was like a dream come true for me. I was hired to be the course director of psychiatric-mental health nursing for undergraduates. This gives me a great deal of time with young people, which I enjoy immensely. Also, I am continuing my research into the effects of unwarranted psychiatric hospitalization of children and adolescents and a number of other topics in child-adolescent mental health issues. I work closely with the National Alliance for the Mentally Ill to educate professionals about the experiences of people who are mentally ill and their families, a role that fulfills my basic need to advocate for the underdog. I have found that my experiences with the for-profit health system, although initially traumatic to me, have since become the basis for my interest in the topic of the commercialization of health care. They have also become the basis for my research career and present and future studies on the effects of commercialization on professionalism, client outcomes, and policy formation.

I have a number of personal reflections about my experiences in this matter and how they relate to where I am and what I do now. As I approached the writing of this section, I experienced a great deal of resistance that I had to force myself to overcome. The resistance is grounded in my profound suspicion for what I see as our faith in what I call "the cult of the expert." I am an expert in a very narrow area, and that does not necessarily give me a metacultural role to provide anyone with advice. Perhaps having said this, I should simply share with future nurses my own guidelines that have worked for me. Advising that you as future professionals should do this or that in your careers may be totally irrelevant tomorrow and may change across time and space, but principles are enduring.

◆ Mohr's Ten Commandments

- *Always* question and look at things from a variety of perspectives and argue from a devil's advocate position. This "oppositional imagination approach" invites creative thinking and keeps you from getting stale. At the same time, accept that you will not always be popular for going against conventional wisdom and ritual behaviors.
- *Never* take yourself too seriously. No one likes pomposity and narcissism.
- *Never* stop learning. Not only is it fun, but those who are always on new learning curves will never be left behind in a world that changes by the nanosecond.
- *Listen* to the clients. They are the experts. Not the doctors and not the nurses.
- *Always* remember that no matter how important you may think you and your accomplishments are, you will be remembered most fondly for how you treated the clients, the typist, and all those at the grass roots—not for how many papers you wrote.
- Life is *not* fair. Too bad. Get on with it.
- It truly *is* better to give than to receive.
- Empathy is a *practiced* life skill. Its capacity multiplies when you exercise it.
- Pick your battles carefully, but do the right thing. Life is not a popularity contest.
- Go with your intuition. It is your best friend.

Finally, I always like to point out to young nurses that none of us can go it alone in our careers, whether those careers are as staff nurses or as academicians. The future of nursing is poised as never before on the brink of challenge that will test us all. We cannot go it alone, and we cannot look only at our own narrow self-interests. The combined efforts of many working toward unselfish goals is where I see the future of nursing in all of its specialities. It must be that way. If we do not eschew the narrow self-interest that has characterized much of the "me generation," we are doomed as people and professionals. I often reflect on the vast number of people who have helped me to be a better nurse, teacher, and person. They include some of the nursing greats: Beverly A. Hall RN, PhD, FAAN; Ann W. Burgess RN, DNSc, FAAN; Jacqueline Fawcett RN, PhD, FAAN to name a few. They also include family members, staff nurses, and members of other professions without whom my own success would not have been possible. They were capable of going beyond themselves, and to all of them, I will always be profoundly grateful.

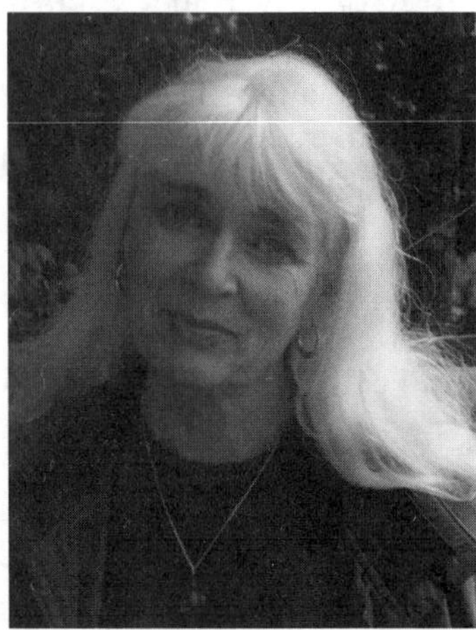

Nan Rich, RN, CS, PMHNP, PhD(c)
Clinical Specialist and Psychiatric Mental Health Nurse Practitioner, Bay Area Hospital, Coos Bay, Oregon

Analogous to the profession of psychiatric nursing, I am in a time of transition. I have recently left a position as a supervisor-nurse in a "secure residential treatment facility" with a population of 15 chronically mentally ill residents from the Oregon State Hospital. This facility was created to enable a small staff to focus intensely on rehabilitation in a relatively isolated rural setting. Although there are many similarities to a locked psychiatric unit, every effort is being made to change old patterns in staff and residents to establish a partnership that will be reciprocally empowering.

This is a pilot project in which psychiatric nurses may work as medication specialists, educators, and milieu managers. In the future, these small facilities may provide venues for psychiatric nurse-practitioners to manage medications and treatment planning. I have many mixed emotions about leaving, knowing I will miss the staff and residents there; we were a family.

I shall continue to work part time as a clinical supervisor for psychiatric-nurse practitioner students from an Oregon Health Sciences University outreach program in Southern Oregon. This relatively new and innovative role of psychiatric-mental health nurse practitioner is not recognized in all states. It requires graduate level education and imparts potential for fully independent practice, including diagnosis and prescriptive privilege.

I work with nine students residing in the crescent between Klamath Falls, Ashland, and Roseburg. They view their classes on an ednet system and are placed in clinical placements with psychiatrists and nurse-practitioners in their respective areas. I communicate with them by phone and e-mail, and I conduct clinical seminars at two different sites.

In my spare time, I am working on my doctoral dissertation at University of California, San Francisco. My dissertation work is on evaluating the ability of psychiatric nurses to gauge the emotional state of their clients using nonverbal clues in facial affect.

I am beginning to expand my own role as a psychiatric clinical specialist-nurse practitioner by moving to a hospital on the Oregon coast. I plan to use my training to assess the unit as a whole, to work with staff and clients, and to educate them about various aspects of mental illness and medication requirements. The hospital in my future endorses the concept of a facility "without walls," indicating the importance of integrating into the community. This is an idea particularly close to my core values of integrating systems of health care and through outreach, "normalizing" the functioning of the mentally ill in and out of acute settings.

I feel that I was chosen by the profession rather than choosing it. As a new graduate registered nurse, I relocated to the Bay Area and interviewed with a marvelous and dynamic head nurse at the Menlo Park Veteran's Administration. She became a role model for me in my subsequent years as a staff nurse, and I will never forget the blend of compassion, pragmatism, and humor that she displayed with the clients. I continue to evolve in the directions she initiated. I consciously use humor with clients and use their response as a guide for diagnosis and subsequent interaction. I remain in the field because I feel a sense of purpose with people who have diagnoses of mental illness. Their openness and trust in me require a challenging balance between personal intimacy and circumspect professionalism.

The most interesting part of working with the chronically mentally ill population is experimenting with novel ways of achieving familiarity with my clients, sorting out their multiple complaints, and avoiding falling back on old methods of coercion and control. I feel continually challenged in every setting to "do it differently," resolving to collaborate with my clients. It is crucial for enduring rehabilitation that clients have a trusting, collaborative relationship with the nurse.

My role as clinical supervisor for graduate students has challenged me to refine my vision of what is significant to psychiatric nursing in advanced practice. I have been considering the question of what differentiates the psychiatric-mental health nurse from that of the staff nurse on the psychiatric unit. I see the major division in degree of responsibility. The mental health nurse in the hospital or community setting can make recommendations, but the nurse in advanced practice writes orders, thereby assuming responsibility for their clients' future activities and mental health status. They are not only care providers, but also care directors.

In all of my work settings, the deepest rewards are from the personal relationships I have had with students and clients. I experience a profound sense of satisfaction when I connect with others on more than a superficial level. I feel joyful when my students are reflective about their practice and question me about my philosophy of psychiatric-nurse practitioner care. I feel a similar sense of joy when a client trusts me enough to share deeper feelings and insights. I enjoy interaction that helps me clarify my own core values.

It is essential to be firmly grounded in the physiology of the body before dealing with mental problems. Many people in crisis present with psychotic or delusional behavior. Differentiating among symptoms that are the result of an imbalance in the body, such as thyroid conditions; imbalance in brain chemistry, like bipolar disorder; or the side effects of a medication, such as restless behavior, requires substantial knowledge of body systems and medications. To understand the actions of the medications, one must be aware of which systems are impacted by the chemical activities in the body. It is impossible for a client to be focused and function well when his or her body is demanding attention secondary to physical discomfort or medication side effects and mental illness itself.

This flexibility is crucial in these times of rapid changes when psychiatric nurses may be required to float hospitalwide and to delegate some bedside care to unlicensed personnel. Astute choices must be made about the competency of the unlicensed staff and the requirements of the client. It is often a difficult judgment call and one on which continuing licensure balances.

Inpatient psychiatric nursing is becoming extremely limited in scope as insurance companies become more stringent about the number of days they will finance for mental health problems and hospitals respond by using unlicensed personnel to administer direct client care. The county hospitals continue to be transitional sites for the chronic mentally ill who are too sick to be in the community but have exhausted their resources; even their stay in the acute setting will be circumscribed by available money.

Emergent and crisis situations will always require knowledgeable staff people to provide assessments and interventions in the emergency room. There also is a great need for trained psychiatric nurses in forensic settings and certainly in community outreach situations as case managers or therapists. The need in these specialized situations mandates an increased professionalism among psychiatric nurses, for whom baccalaureate preparation may be seen as a prerequisite and master's degrees for independent practitioner status. In such settings, they may also be required to supervise or delegate care to aides after performing an initial assessment. Education of supportive personnel must be thorough and circumscribed.

It is urgent that psychiatric nurses give more than lip service to what are now being called alternative or supplementary therapies, such as massage and exercise. Advanced practice nurses can prescribe these type of therapies, but also psychiatric nurses in inpatient settings or the community can recommend them. Such stress-reduction techniques as yoga, meditation, and exercise have value supplementing the traditional cognitive therapies. Nurses are also role models, practicing these principles of vital living, so as a group, we must integrate these valuable routines and suggest them to others.

Living in accord with my personal beliefs, having thoughtfully and clearly articulated my core values, is possibly the most important component of my professional life. Not only does such a lifestyle help to avoid discomfort from cognitive dissonance, it gives me insight into problems others might encounter in changing their own patterns. It enables me to offer supportive suggestions from initial contact throughout the therapeutic process. I feel constantly challenged by the varieties of experience in mental health settings to affirm my core values of ethical and moral behavior.

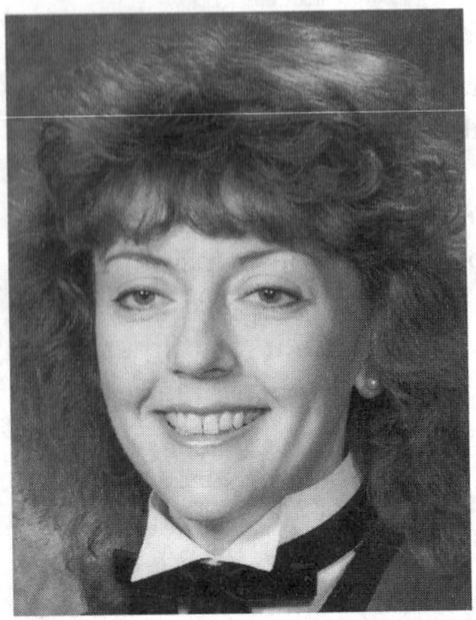

Cindy Lee Sherban, RPN, RN, BScN, CRPS
Coordinator, Substance Abuse Programs
Regional Co-trainer, OSAPP
Correctional Service of Canada
Regional Psychiatric Centre (Prairies)
Saskatoon, Canada

I chose the field of psychiatric-mental health nursing because I had a strong desire to help and to listen to people tell about their lives, their trials and triumphs, and their challenges, successes, and disappointments. Moreover, I am fascinated with the human mind, how it works, and why it works so differently for some.

In western Canada, there was a 2-year basic program in psychiatric nursing that led to a diploma; you were then eligible to write Registration Exams to be licensed. I knew general duty nursing was not for me because I was not interested in working with the physically ill. At the time, Bachelor of Arts degrees with a major in psychology were "a dime a dozen." Realistically, you needed at least a Master's degree to do any counseling. Added to this, there was still the lure of psychiatric illness. Schizophrenia, depression, and bipolar disorder all seemed to need more than simple counseling. So I began as a Registered Psychiatric Nurse.

As it turns out, I later obtained my diploma in general nursing and then completed a postdiploma Bachelor of Science (nursing) and a Business Administration certificate. This educational background has given me the opportunity to fill different roles and positions to gain a different perspective on the field.

I have never regretted my decision to work in this field. Because psychiatry is still a relatively new discipline, there is ongoing research and hence new implications for treatment. Improved technology that allows us to understand brain function has led us to new understandings and insights. Still, we can not forget the soft side—the caring, compassion, and empathy that are hard to teach, learn, or measure. This is one vital difference that technology cannot replace: the human factor. So for me, there is an interplay of the opportunity and challenge of ongoing learning and the necessity to focus on the human and humane aspect of our work.

I remain in the field because it is interesting, challenging, stimulating, and rewarding. It is a good fit with my needs and wants.

Within my role as a psychiatric-mental health nurse, there are many aspects and functions. I have usually functioned as part of a multidisciplinary team. However, I have a great deal of autonomy and independence despite being interdependent with others. I am a resource to the client, the team, the Correctional Service of Canada, and the community. We are not givers of direction (GODs). We guide, facilitate, and advocate to name a few. We act as liaison and referral agent. One of my favorite roles is that of teacher. In the field of mental health, there are so many skills we can teach to promote wellness and alleviate illness.

I have also worked in a management position. I was in charge of running the institution in the absence of the executive director. In this capacity, there was an overall coordinating function: All the information regarding the institution was filtered through me. I had to deal with situations as they arose and be prepared to manage a crisis situation until the crisis management team arrived. I learned a lot during that year about my organization, institution, and most of all, about me. While I handled the job well, I found that I did not derive the personal satisfaction from the job that I do when I have direct client contact. It is an important lesson to learn because I find I am being pulled and pushed and coaxed into administrative and managerial positions. With this in mind, I will make a different decision when the time comes.

Currently, I hold two positions. Within my institution, I am the Coordinator of Substance Abuse Programs. This entails assessing the severity of the substance abuse and matching the client to the appropriate level of program. I then deliver the programs, evaluate and report the outcome, and make recommendations for further programming. In addition, I act as liaison for the community volunteers who come into the institution to participate in the Narcotics Anonymous and Alcoholics Anonymous programs. I also take student placements from nursing, psychiatric nursing, correctional officer, and substance abuse worker programs. I do individual counseling, including relapse prevention. I am certified by the CENAPS Corporation in this function.

New to me is the role of Co-trainer in the Prairie region for the Offender Substance Abuse Prerelease Program. I now have responsibility for training staff to deliver this research-based program to offenders. I plan, coordinate, and deliver this training and then monitor functions, including viewing the videotapes of trainers delivering this program, to determine whether they will become a certified trainer. I also provide ongoing support and advice to this staff across the region. As a Regional Co-trainer, I also have some national responsibilities to fulfill.

Some of the things that keep my position interesting are the ongoing research, whether it be in the area of mental illness, sex offenders, violent offenders, new medications and treatment approaches, or new methods of doing things. The unique factors that led to our offenders' present situations are just that—unique. Sometimes their reality is so foreign to ours, it is hard to believe we grew up in the same city and time and perhaps even went to school together. For example, one man told me that when he was just 3 years old, his father and grandpa would put him through an open kitchen window. He would then open the door from the inside so that his father and grandpa could rob the house. Suspending our frame of reference and being nonjudgmental are necessary and at times, challenging.

I find it rewarding to teach people how to challenge irrational beliefs or to change the way they view a situation, including their past, and to have had a hand in facilitating new and effective behavior changes. Meeting a client who is now functioning at a more effective level and is able to live a more satisfying or less painful life is a joy. Watching them use new skills or behaviors gives me a sense of fulfillment. One of the painful things to see is the criminalization of the mentally ill. I wonder how things could be different so that these clients find their way into the health system rather than the legal system.

To those thinking of entering the profession, I would first say, "know yourself." Why do you want to work in this field; what is it you want to accomplish or achieve? I believe you must be strong and well balanced in your life and your approach to it. The work can be very demanding of you, mentally, emotionally, physically, and spiritually. Despite the rewards, there are countless heart- and soul-wrenching stories and situations. There are ethical and moral dilemmas, differences in approaches to treatment among staff, and differences in treatment outcome goals between you and the client. You must believe in yourself and know that you can and do make a difference.

You must be able to see achievement in small increments. Most of our clientele, especially in my area of corrections, are not good at or able to express gratitude or appreciation. At times there will be no obvious sign of improvement, and at times there really will be no change. A kind word, gentle smile, or simply acknowledging them as a fellow human with inherent worth and dignity may bring them joy and hope to continue to choose life. Such seemingly small gestures can have a tremendous effect.

I also caution you to know your limitations and to set limits. We cannot be all things to all people. We cannot be available to everyone all the time. You must have balance in your life so that you are fit and able to help others. Your effectiveness is in doubt if your own life is hanging in shreds or so tumultuous that there is nothing left for you to give or get out of your work. Do not open yourself to burnout. It saps all the joy out of work and the rest of your life. Additionally, you are in danger of venting your problems or negative attitudes on the client and reversing the roles of counselor and client. This is a terrible abuse of your position and wholly avoidable. Lastly, being a lifelong learner keeps the job changing and new. While some look at change as threatening, it is inevitable. If you can keep abreast of trends, you can anticipate and facilitate change. You can find new challenges and rewards to keep your life invigorating.

In the future, I see psychiatric-mental health nursing gaining more recognition and respect as a specialty within nursing. When you've chosen this field, you will hear a lot of, "How can you stand to do that? Isn't it depressing?" You will also hear, "I wouldn't do that in a million years." Once in a while, you will get a "Wow, you must be very special to work in that field." I think it takes a special person to work in any field. We each have unique characteristics and interests that make us better suited to one thing than another. If we find we do not fit our choice of career, then we can change it. We can damage ourselves and our clients by staying with a career poorly matched to our needs and wants. I believe new technology and developments will further enhance our knowledge and treatment of psychiatric-mental health clients. I also believe that no matter what technology does for us, we will still need the human face and touch that we bring to the practice of psychiatric-mental health nursing.

The world continues to change at a rapid pace. Jobs are being cut, and opportunities to work and achieve a decent livelihood are decreasing. Many of the factors currently in play lead to an increasing number of mental health problems. I foresee a greater need for promotion of mental health and prevention of mental illness. People need to learn effective coping strategies and skills. They need problem-solving skills to manage the demands of daily living problems. I believe we can serve a pivotal role. People need support, information, and education. These are but a few of the things we do so well. I believe there will be a continued demand for our profession for many years to come. I believe that our future will continue to be rewarding and challenging. As change continues or even increases, we will have to accompany people through the stresses. Thus, we as professionals must heed our own advice: Practice health promotion and live a balanced life.

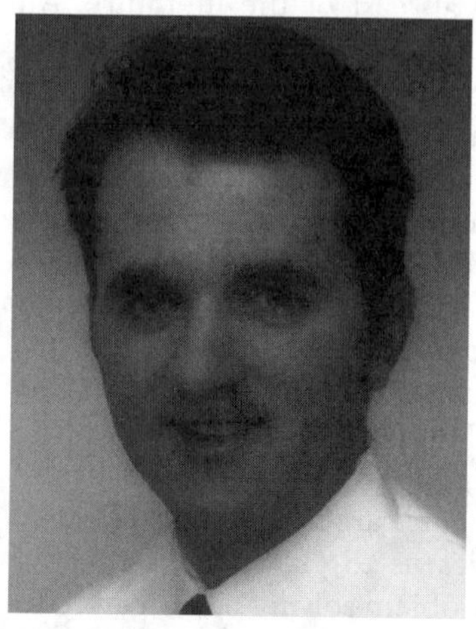

George Byron Smith, RN, C, MSN, CCM, CNAA
Director of Adult Psychiatric-Mental Health Services
Tampa General Healthcare-University Psychiatry Center
Courtesy Faculty College of Nursing
University of South Florida
Tampa, Florida

The current psychiatric-mental health care environment is experiencing "interesting times." There are new, changing, and innovative delivery systems, roles, and treatments. In the last 2 years, I have been the director of four inpatient adult psychiatric units. In this role, I provide leadership and administrative and clinical support. I work earnestly to develop staff as interdisciplinary teams and encourage them to work together in problem solving and managing change. It has been important in my role as leader to support and encourage staff. I've encouraged staff to retool for the future by developing new skills and expanding their knowledge base.

Psychiatric-mental health care, like other specialties, is moving from an acute care focus to community-care focus. Nurses will have to provide care and services to clients in the community, which will require us to think and practice differently. I believe the most successful nurses will be those who attempt to experience each level of the continuum of care from acute care to home care to community care. My next role will be providing or managing the home care of clients requiring psychiatric-mental health care in the community. To survive in these chaotic times, we all must be willing to change and grow into the future of health care.

In addition to psychiatric-mental health care nursing, I have been extensively involved in case management and critical pathway development. Prior to the position of director for adult psychiatric-mental health services, I was director of case management and special projects for a 174-bed acute care hospital in Tampa. There I developed the case management program. Within the case management program, I developed the role of nurse case manager-educator and coordinated the development of critical pathways. After developing and implementing the program, I had the opportunity to develop a niche in case management and critical pathways for psychiatry. At the time, very few critical pathways were being developed in psychiatry. I came to Tampa General Healthcare to manage the adult units and assist in developing the case management program and coordinating critical pathway implementation for clients with psychiatric illnesses. With this niche in case management and critical pathways for psychiatric-mental health care, I have written several continuing education courses, provided education to students and organizations, consulted with psychiatric-mental health care organizations, and provided workshops on how to develop, implement, and evaluate case management and critical pathways for psychiatric client populations.

At Tampa General Healthcare-University Psychiatry Center, we have downsized (or right-sized) the organizational structure and the number of client care units several times in the past few years. Within the last 2 years, I have experienced two layoffs, an organizational buy-out, and the turbulent times of psychiatry. Sometimes I wonder why I chose psychiatric-mental health care and why I choose to remain in the field. However, only psychiatric-mental health nursing can provide the prodigious opportunities and challenges of a changing health care system.

The decade of the brain has challenged us to rethink treatments and the quality of life of our clients. New treatments and medications have allowed us to move away from acute care models and into the living environments of those we serve. Changes in the delivery of mental health services have provided nurses with more opportunities to increase knowledge and skills.

With this increase in the different levels of care, psychiatric-mental health nurses have more opportunities than ever before to work in ambulatory care, home care, or community care.

Psychiatric-mental health nurses can use their knowledge and skills to lead the way in managing cost of care and quality outcomes. This is one area in which psychiatric-mental health nurses are not involved enough. We must do more to develop, evaluate, and research outcomes of clients across the continuum. Psychiatric-mental health nurses must be at the table to provide our perspectives and our experiences in managing mental illness. There is a dearth of research on how nurses and nursing practice impact the outcomes of the clients we serve. More research is need to validate nursing contribution to psychiatric-mental health care outcomes.

My advice to a novice nurse thinking of entering psychiatric-mental health nursing is fourfold. First, *know yourself.* Identify your strengths and weaknesses. In every interaction we have with clients and their families, we must be able to model healthy and adaptive behaviors. Our clients look to us for direction and guidance. The old adage, "walk your talk" is extremely important in psychiatric-mental health nursing. I believe we must use many of the tools we encourage our clients to use. My most successful moments in psychiatric-mental health nursing have been when I have shared my experience, strength, and hope with clients by demonstrating how techniques, strategies, or ideas work in real world terms.

Second, in addition to knowing effective communications and counseling skills, know the biological and neurological components of care and treatment of mental illness. Psychiatric-mental health care is evolving into a more holistic and complete specialty that requires our diligence to the complete person.

Third, read and stay abreast of the literature. An admired colleague once told me that to remain in the top 10% of any profession, one must read an article a day. I average about four to five articles a week. To remain a viable professional, you have to stay up on the latest developments, treatments, and techniques.

Finally, have fun. Life (and nursing) are meant to be fun. Enjoy what you are doing. If you don't enjoy working in psychiatric-mental health nursing (or any other specialty for that matter), get out. Nursing has so many different choices. However, I believe every nurse could benefit from working in psychiatric-mental health nursing at least once in their career. Psychiatric-mental health nursing challenges us to grow, learn effective communications and problem-solving skills, and develop a sense of humor about life and about the human race. Psychiatric-mental health nursing allows us to use all the nursing knowledge and skills we learned in nursing school and in our experiences to work with and improve the health and mental health of the clients and families we serve.

Psychiatric-mental health care is experiencing "interesting times." According to a Chinese proverb, interesting times are dangerous times. Psychiatric-mental health nursing is in dangerous times. We must assess the lay of the land, develop a plan of action, and forge ahead into the future of health care. One thing we all learn while working with our clients is that there are things we can control and things we cannot control. Let us all work together to take control of our future and continue to develop psychiatric-mental health nursing as a proud and valuable specialty in the future health care system.

DSM-IV Classification:
Axes I and II Categories and Codes

DISORDERS USUALLY FIRST DIAGNOSED IN INFANCY, CHILDHOOD, OR ADOLESCENCE

Mental Retardation

Note: These are coded on Axis II.

317 Mild Mental Retardation
318.0 Moderate Mental Retardation
318.1 Severe Mental Retardation
318.2 Profound Mental Retardation
319 Mental Retardation, Severity Unspecified

Learning Disorders

315.00 Reading Disorders
315.1 Mathematics Disorders
315.2 Disorder of Written Expression
315.9 Learning Disorder NOS

Motor Skills Disorder

315.4 Developmental Coordination Disorder

Communication Disorders

315.31 Expressive Language Disorder
315.31 Mixed Receptive-Expressive Language Disorder
315.39 Phonological Disorder
307.0 Stuttering
307.9 Communication Disorder NOS

Pervasive Developmental Disorders

299.00 Autistic Disorder
299.80 Rett's Disorder
299.10 Childhood Disintegrative Disorder
299.80 Asperger's Disorder
299.80 Pervasive Developmental Disorder NOS

Attention-Deficit and Disruptive Behavior Disorders

314.xx Attention-Deficit/Hyperactivity Disorder
.01 Combined Type
.00 Predominantly Inattentive Type
.01 Predominantly Hyperactive-Impulsive Type
314.9 Attention-Deficit/Hyperactivity Disorder NOS
312.8 Conduct Disorder
Specify type: Childhood-Onset/Adolescent-Onset
313.81 Oppositional Defiant Disorder
312.9 Disruptive Behavior Disorder NOS

Feeding and Eating Disorders of Infancy or Early Childhood

307.52 Pica
307.53 Rumination Disorder
307.59 Feeding Disorder of Infancy or Early Childhood

Tic Disorders

307.23 Tourette's Disorder
307.22 Chronic Motor or vocal Tic Disorder
307.21 Transient Tic Disorder
Specify if: Single Episode/Recurrent
307.20 Tic Disorder NOS

Elimination Disorders

—.- Encopresis
787.6 With Constipation and Overflow Incontinence
307.7 Without Constipation and Overflow Incontinence
307.6 Enuresis (Not Due to a General Medical Condition)
Specify type: Nocturnal Only/Diurnal Only/Nocturnal and Diurnal

Other Disorders of Infancy, Childhood, or Adolescence

309.21 Separation and Anxiety Disorder
Specify if: Early Onset
313.23 Selective Mutism
313.89 Reactive Attachment Disorder of Infancy or Early Childhood
Specify type: Inhibited/Disinhibited
307.3 Stereotypic Movement Disorder
Specify if: With Self-Injurious Behavior
313.9 Disorder of Infancy, Childhood, or Adolescence NOS

DELIRIUM, DEMENTIA, AND AMNESTIC AND OTHER COGNITIVE DISORDERS

Delirium

293.0 Delirium Due to . . .*
—.- Substance Intoxication Delirium**
—.- Substance Withdrawal Delirium**
—.- Delirium Due to Multiple Etiologies (code each of the specific etiologies)
780.09 Delirium NOS

Dementia

290.xx Dementia of the Alzheimer's Type, With Early Onset
.10 Uncomplicated
.11 With Delirium

NOS = Not Otherwise Specified

An *x* appearing in a diagnostic code indicates that a specific code number is required.

An **ellipsis** (. . .) is used in the names of certain disorders to indicate that the name of a specific mental disorder or general medical condition should be inserted when recording the name (e.g., 293 Delirium Due to Hypothyroidism).

* Indicate the General Medical Condition

** Refer to Substance-Related Disorders for substance-specific codes

*** Indicate the Axis I or Axis II Disorder

.12 With Delusions
.13 With Depressed Mood
Specify if: With Behavioral Disturbance
290.xx Vascular Dementia
.40 Uncomplicated
.41 With Delirium
.42 With Dulusions
.43 With Depressed Mood
Specify if: With Behavioral Disturbance
294.9 Dementia Due to HIV Disease
294.1 Dementia Due to Head Trauma
294.1 Dementia Due to Parkinson's Disease
294.1 Dementia Due to Huntington's Disease
294.10 Dementia Due to Pick's Disease
290.10 Dementia Due to Creutzfeldt-Jakob Disease
294.1 Dementia Due to . . . [Indicate the General Medical Condition not listed above]
—.- Substance-Induced Persisting Dementia**
—.- Dementia Due to Multiple Etiologies (code each of the specific etiologies
294.8 Dementia NOS

Amnestic Disorders

294.0 Amnestic Disorder Due to . . .*
Specify if: Transient/Chronic
—.- Substance-Induced Persisting Amnestic Disorder**
294.8 Amnestic Disorder NOS

Other Cognitive Disorders

294.9 Cognitive Disorder NOS

MENTAL DISORDERS DUE TO A GENERAL MEDICAL CONDITION NOT ELSEWHERE CLASSIFIED

293.89 Catatonic Disorder Due to . . .*
310.1 Personality Change Due to . . .*
Specify type: Labile/Disinhibited/Aggressive/Apathetic/Paranoid/Other/Combined/Unspecified
293.9 Mental Disorder NOS Due to . . .*

SUBSTANCE-RELATED DISORDERS

The following specifiers may be applied to Substance Dependence:

With Physiological Dependence/Without Physiological Dependence
Early Fully Remission/Early Partial Remission
Sustained Full Remission/Sustained Partial Remission
On Agonist Therapy/In a Controlled Environment

The following specifiers apply to Substance-Induced Disorders as noted:

[I]with Onset During Intoxication/[W]With Onset During Withdrawal

Alcohol-Related Disorders

Alcohol Use Disorders
303.90 Alcohol Dependence
305.00 Alcohol Abuse

Alcohol-Induced Disorders
303.00 Alcohol Intoxications
291.8 Alcohol Withdrawal
Specify if: With Perceptual Disturbances
291.0 Alcohol Intoxication Delirium
291.0 Alcohol Withdrawal Delirium
291.2 Alcohol-Induced Persisting Dementia
291.1 Alcohol-Induced Persisting Amnestic Disorder
291.x Alcohol-Induced Psychotic Disorder
.5- With Delusions[I,W]
.3 With Hallucinations[I,W]
291.8 Alcohol-Induced Mood Disorder[I,W]
291.8 Alcohol-Induced Anxiety Disorder[I,W]
291.8 Alcohol-Induced Sexual Dysfunction[I]
291. Alcohol-Induced Sleep Disorder[I,W]
291.9 Alcohol-Related Disorder NOS

Amphetamine (or Amphetamine-Like)-Related Disorders

Amphetamine Use Disorders
304.40 Amphetamine Dependence*
305.70 Amphetamine Abuse

Amphetamine-Induced Disorders
292.89 Amphetamine Intoxication
Specify if: With Perceptual Disturbances
292.0 Amphetamine Withdrawal
292.81 Amphetamine Intoxication Delirium
292.xx Amphetamine-Induced Psychotic Disorder
.11 With Delusions[I]
.12 With Hallucinations[I]
292.84 Amphetamine-Induced Mood Disorder[I,W]
292.89 Amphetamine-Induced Anxiety Disorder[I]
292.89 Amphetamine-Induced Sexual Dysfunction[I]
292.89 Amphetamine-Induced Sleep Disorder[I,W]
292.9 Amphetamine-Related Disorder NOS

Caffeine-Related Disorders

Caffeine-Induced Disorders
305.90 Caffeine Intoxication
292.89 Caffeine-Induced Anxiety Disorder[I]
292.89 Caffeine-Induced Sleep Disorder[I]
292.9 Caffeine-Related Disorder NOS

Cannabis-Related Disorders

Cannabis Use Disorders
304.30 Cannabis Dependence*
305.20 Cannabis Abuse

Cannabis-Induced Disorders
292.89 Cannabis Intoxication
Specify if: With Perceptual Disturbances
292.81 Cannabis Intoxication Delirium
292.xx Cannabis-Induced Psychotic Disorder
.11 With Delusions[I]
.12 With Hallucinations[I]
292.89 Cannabis-Induced Anxiety Disorder[I]
292.9 Cannabis-Related Disorder NOS

Cocaine-Related Disorders

Cocaine Use Disorders
304.20 Cocaine Dependence*
305.60 Cocaine Abuse

Cocaine-Induced Disorders
292.89 Cocaine Intoxication
Specify if: With Perceptual Disturbances
292.0 Cocaine Withdrawal
292.81 Cocaine Intoxication Delirium
292.xx Cocaine-Induced Psychotic Disorder
.11 With Delusions[I]
.12 With Hallucinations[I]

292.84 Cocaine-Induced Mood Disorder[I,W]
292.89 Cocaine-Induced Anxiety Disorder[I,W]
292.89 Cocaine-Induced Sexual Dysfunction[I]
292.89 Cocaine-Induced Sleep Disorder[I,W]
292.9 Cocaine-Related Disorder NOS

Hallucinogen-Related Disorders

Hallucinogen-Use Disorders
304.50 Hallucinogen Dependence*
305.30 Hallucinogen Abuse

Hallucinogen-Induced Disorders
292.89 Hallucinogen Intoxication
292.89 Hallucinogen Presisting Perception Disorder (Flashbacks)
292.81 Hallucinogen Intoxication Delirium
292.xx Hallucinogen-Induced Psychotic Disorder
.11 With Delusions[I]
.12 With Hallucinations[I]
292.84 Hallucinogen-Induced Mood Disorder[I]
292.89 Hallucinogen-Induced Anxiety Disorder[I]
292.9 Hallucinogen-Related Disorder NOS

Inhalant-Related Disorders

Inhalant Use Disorders
304.60 Inhalant Dependence*
305.90 Inhalant Abuse

Inhalant-Induced Disorders
292.89 Inhalant Intoxication
292.81 Inhalant Intoxication Delirium
292.82 Inhalant-Induced Persisting Dementia
292.xx Inhalant-Induced Psychotic Disorder
.11 With Delusions[I]
.12 With Hallucinations[I]
292.84 Inhalant-Induced Mood Disorder[I]
292.89 Inhalant-Induced Anxiety Disorder[I]
292.9 Inhalant-Related Disorder NOS

Nicotine-Related Disorders

Nicotine Use Disorder
305.10 Nicotine Dependence*

Nicotine-Induced Disorder
292.0 Nicotine Withdrawal
292.9 Nicotine-Related Disorder NOS

Opioid-Related Disorders

Opioid Use Disorders
304.00 Opioid Dependence*
305.50 Opioid Abuse

Opioid-Induced Disorders
292.89 Opioid Intoxication
Specify if: With Perceptual Disturbances
292.0 Opioid Withdrawal
292.81 Opioid Intoxication Delirium
292.xx Opioid-Induced Psychotic Disorders
.11 With Delusions[I]
.12 With Hallucinations[I]
292.84 Opioid-Induced Mood Disorder[I]
292.89 Opioid-Induced Sexual Dysfunction[I]
292.89 Opioid-Induced Sleep Disorder[I,W]
292.9 Opioid-Related Disorder NOS

Phencyclidine (or Phencyclidine-Like)-Related Disorders

Phencyclidine Use Disorders
304.90 Phencyclidine Dependence*
305.90 Phencyclidine Abuse

Phencyclidine-Induced Disorders
292.89 Phencyclidine Intoxication
Specify if: With Perceptual Disturbances
292.81 Phencyclidine Intoxication Delirium
292.xx Phencyclidine-Induced Psychotic Disorders
.11 With Delusions[I]
.12 With Hallucinations[I]
292.84 Phencyclidine-Induced Mood Disorder[I]
292.89 Phencyclidine-Induced Anxiety Disorder[I]
292.9 Phencyclidine-Related Disorder NOS

Sedative-Hypnotic-or Anxiolytic Related Disorders

Sedative-Hypnotic- or Anxiolytic Use Disorders
304.10 Sedative, Hypnotic, or Anxiolytic Dependence*
305.40 Sedative, Hypnotic, or Anxiolytic Abuse

Sedative, Hypnotic, or Anxiolytic-Induced Disorders
292.89 Sedative, Hypnotic, or Anxiolytic Intoxication
292.0 Sedative, Hypnotic, or Anxiolytic Withdrawal
Specify if: With Perceptual Disturbances
292.81 Sedative, Hypnotic, or Anxiolytic Intoxication Delirium
292.81 Sedative, Hypnotic, or Anxiolytic Withdrawal Delirium
292.82 Sedative-, Hypnotic-, or Anxiolytic-Induced Persisting Delirium
292.83 Sedative-, Hypnotic-, or Anxiolytic-Induced Persisting Amnestic Disorder
292.xx Sedative-, Hypnotic-, or Anxiolytic-Induced Psychotic Disorder
.11 With Delusions[I,W]
.12 With Hallucinations[I,W]
292.84 Sedative-, Hypnotic-, or Anxiolytic-Induced Mood Disorder[I,W]
292.89 Sedative-, Hypnotic-, or Anxiolytic-Induced Anxiety Disorder[W]
292.89 Sedative-, Hypnotic-, or Anxiolytic-Induced Sexual Dysfunction[I]
292.89 Sedative-, Hypnotic-, or Anxiolytic-Induced Sleep Disorder[I,W]
292.9 Sedative-, Hypnotic-, or Anxiolytic-Induced Disorder NOS

Polysubstance-Related Disorder

304.80 Polysubstance Dependence*

Other (or Unknown) Substance-Related Disorders

Other (or Unknown) Substance Use Disorders
304.90 Other (or Unknown) Substance Dependence*
305.90 Other (or Unknown) Substance Abuse

Other (or Unknown) Substance-Induced Disorders
292.89 Other (or Unknown) Substance Intoxication
Specify if: With Perceptual Disturbances
292.0 Other (or Unknown) Substance Withdrawal
Specify if: With Perceptual Disturbances
292.81 Other (or Unknown) Substance-Induced Delirium
292.82 Other (or Unknown) Substance-Induced Persisting Dementia
292.83 Other (or Unknown) Substance-Induced Persisting Amnestic Disorder
292.xx Other (or Unknown) Substance-Induced Psychotic Disorder
.11 With Delusions[I,W]
.12 With Hallucinations[I,W]
292.84 Other (or Unknown) Substance-Induced Mood Disorder[I,W]
292.89 Other (or Unknown) Substance-Induced Anxiety Disorder[I,W]
292.89 Other (or Unknown) Substance-Induced Sexual Dysfunction[I]
292.89 Other (or Unknown) Substance-Induced Sleep Disorder[I,W]
292.9 Other (or Unknown) Substance-Induced Disorder NOS

SCHIZOPHRENIA AND OTHER PSYCHOTIC DISORDERS

295.xx Schizophrenia

The following Classification of Longitudinal Course applies to all subtypes of Schizophrenia:

Episodic With Interepisode Residual Symptoms
(*Specify if:* With Prominent Negative Symptoms)/Episodic With No Interepisode Residual Symptoms/Continuous
(*Specify if:* With Prominent Negative Symptoms)
Single Episode in Partial Remission (*Specify if:* With Prominent Negative Symptoms/Single Episode in Full Remission
Other or Unspecified Pattern

.30 Paranoid Type
.10 Disorganized Type
.20 Catatonic Type
.90 Undifferentiated Type
.60 Residual Type

295.40 Schizophreniform Disorder
Specify if: Without Good Prognostic Features/With Good Prognostic Features
295.70 Schizoaffective Disorder
Specify type: Bipolar/Depressive
297.1 Delusional Disorder
Specify type: Erotomanic/Grandiose/Jealous/Persecutory Somatic/Mixed/Unspecified
298.8 Brief Psychotic Disorder
Specify if: With Marked Stressor(s)
Without Marked Stressor(s) With Postpartum Onset
297.3 Shared Psychotic Disorder
293.xx Psychotic Disorder Due to . . .*
.81 With Delusions
.82 With Hallucinations
—.- Substance-Induced Psychotic Disorder (refer to Substance-Related Disorders for substance-specific codes)
Specify if: With Onset During Intoxication/With Onset During withdrawal
298.9 Psychotic Disorder NOS

MOOD DISORDERS

Code current state of Major Depressive Disorder or Bipolar I Disorder in fifth digit

1 = Mild
2 = Moderate
3 = Severe Without Psychotic Features
4 = Severe With Psychotic Features
Specify: Mood-Congruent Psychotic Features/Mood-Incongruent Psychotic Features
5 = In Partial Remission
6 = In Full Remission
0 = Unspecified

The following specifiers apply (for current or most recent episode) to Mood Disorders as noted:

[a]Severity/Psychotic/Remission Specifiers/[b]Chronic/[c]With Catatonic Features/[d]With Melancholic Features/[e]With Atypical Features/[f]With Postpartum Onset

The following specifiers apply to Mood Disorders as noted:

[g]With or Without Full Interepisode Recovery/With Seasonal Pattern/[i]With Rapid Cycling

Depressive Disorders

296.xx Major Depressive Disorder,
.2x Single Episode[a,b,c,d,e,f]
.3x Recurrent[a,b,c,d,e,f,g,h]
300.4 Dysthymic Disorder
Specify if: Early Onset/Late Onset
Specify: With Atypical Features
311 Depressive Disorder NOS

Bipolar Disorders

295.xx Bipolar I Disorder,
.0x Single Manic Episode[a,c,f]
Specify if: Mixed
.40 Most Recent Episode Hypomanic[a,h,i]
.4x Most Recent Episode Manic[a,c,f,g,h,i]
.6x Most Recent Episode Mixed[a,c,f,g,h,i]
.5x Most Recent Episode Depressed[a,b,c,d,e,f,g,h,i]
.7 Most Recent Episode Unspecified[g,h,i]
296.89 Bipolar II Disorder[a,b,c,d,e,f,g,h,i]
Specify(current or most recent episode): Hypomanic/Depressed
301.13 Cyclothymic Disorder
296.80 Bipolar Disorder NOS
293.83 Mood Disorder Due to . . .*
Specify type: With Depressive Features/With Major Depressive-Like Episode/With Manic Features/With Mixed Features
—.- Substance-Induced Mood Disorder**
Specify type: With Depressive Features/With Manic Features/With Mixed Features
Specify if: With Onset During Intoxication/With Onset During Withdrawal
296.90 Mood Disorder NOS

ANXIETY DISORDERS

300.01 Panic Disorder Without Agoraphobia
300.21 Panic Disorder With Agoraphobia
300.22 Agoraphobia Without History of Panic Disorder
300.29 Specific Phobia
Specify type: Animal Type/Natural Environment Type/Blood-Injection-Injury Type/Situational Type/Other Type
300.23 Social Phobia
Specify if: Generalized
300.3 Obsessive-Compulsive Disorder
Specify if: With Poor Insight
309.81 Posttraumatic Stress Disorder
Specify if: Acute/Chronic
Specify if: With Delayed Onset
308.3 Acute Stress Disorder
300.02 Generalized Anxiety Disorder
293.89 Anxiety Disorder Due to . . .*
Specify if: With Generalized Anxiety/With Panic/Attacks/With Obsessive Compulsive Symptoms . . .*
—.- Substance-Induced Anxiety Disorder
Specify if: With Generalized Anxiety/With Panic Attacks/With Obsessive-Compulsive Symptoms/With Phobic Symptoms
Specify if: With Onset During Intoxication/With Onset During Withdrawal
300.00 Anxiety Disorder NOS

SOMATOFORM DISORDERS

300.81 Somatization Disorder
300.81 Undifferentiated Somatoform Disorder

300.11 Conversion Disorder *Specify type:* With Motor Symptom or Deficit/With Sensory Symptom or Deficit/With Seizures or Convulsions/With Mixed Presentation
307.xx Pain Disorder
.80 Associated With Psychological Factors
.89 Associated with Both Psychological Factors and a General Medical Condition
Specify if: Acute/Chronic
300.7 Hypochondriasis
Specify if: With Poor Insight
300.7 Body Dysmorphic Disorder
300.81 Somatoform Disorder NOS

FACTITIOUS DISORDERS

300.xx Factitious Disorder
.16 With Predominantly Psychological Signs and Symptoms
.19 With Predominantly Physical Signs and Symptoms
.19 With Combined Psychological and Physical Signs and Symptoms
300.19 Factitious Disorder NOS

DISSOCIATIVE DISORDERS

300.12 Dissociative Amnesia
300.13 Dissociative Fugue
300.14 Dissociative Identity Disorder
300.6 Depersonalized Disorder
300.15 Dissociative Disorder NOS

SEXUAL AND GENDER IDENTITY DISORDERS

Sexual Dysfunctions

The following specifiers apply to all primary Sexual Dysfunctions:

Lifelong Type/Acquired
Type Generalized Type/Situational Type
Due to Psychological Factors. Due to Combined Factors

Sexual Desire Disorders
302.71 Hypoactive Sexual Desire Disorder
302.79 Sexual Aversion Disorder

Sexual Arousal Disorders
302.72 Female Sexual Arousal Disorder
302.72 Male Erectile Disorder

Orgasmic Disorders
302.73 Female Orgasmic Disorder
302.74 Male Orgasmic Disorder
302.75 Premature Ejaculation

Sexual Pain Disorders
302.76 Dyspareunia (Not Due to General Medical Condition)
306.51 Vaginismus (Not Due to a General Medical Condition)

Sexual Dysfunction Due to a General Medical Condition
625.8 Female Hypoactive Sexual Desire Disorder Due to . . .*
608.89 Male Hypoactive Sexual Desire Disorder Due to . . .*
607.84 Male Erectile Disorder Due to . . .*
625.0 Female Dyspareunia Due to . . .*
608.89 Male Dyspareunia Due to . . .*
625.8 Other Female Sexual Dysfunction Due to . . .*
608.89 Other Male Sexual Dysfunction Due to . . .*

—.- Substance-Induced Sexual Dysfunction**
Specify if: With Impaired Desire/With Impaired Arousal/With Impaired Orgasm/With Sexual Pain
Specify if: With Onset During Intoxication
302.70 Sexual Dysfunction NOS

Paraphilias

302.4 Exhibitionism
302.81 Fetishism
302.89 Frotteurism
302.2 Pedophilia
Specify if: Sexually Attracted to Males/Sexually Attracted to Females/Sexually Attracted to Both
Specify if: Limited to Incest
Specify type: Exclusive Type/Nonexclusive Type
302.83 Sexual Masochism
302.84 Sexual Sadism
302.3 Transvestic Fetishism
Specify if: With Gender Dysphoria
302.82 Voyeurism
302.9 Paraphilia NOS

Gender Identity Disorders

302.xx Gender Identity Disorder
.6 in Children
.85 in Adolescents or Adults
Specify if: Sexually Attracted to Males/Sexually Attracted to Females/Sexually Attracted to Both/Sexually Attracted to Neither
302.6 Gender Identity Disorder NOS
302.9 Sexual Disorder NOS

EATING DISORDERS

307.1 Anorexia Nervosa
Specify type: Restricting, Binge-Eating/Purging
307.51 Bulimia Nervosa
Specify type: Purging/Nonpurging
307.50 Eating Disorder NOS

SLEEP DISORDERS

Primary Sleep Disorders

Dyssomnias
307.42 Primary Insomnia
307.44 Primary Hypersomnia
Specify if: Recurrent
347 Narcolepsy
380.59 Breathing-Related Sleep Disorder
307.45 Circadian Rhythm Sleep Disorder
Specify type: Delayed Sleep Phase/Jet Lag/Shift Work/Unspecified
307.47 Dyssomnia NOS

Parasomnias
307.47 Nightmare Disorder
307.46 Sleep Terror Disorder
307.46 Sleepwalking Disorder
307.47 Parasomnia NOS

Sleep Disorders Related to Another Mental Disorder

307.42 Insomnia Related to . . .***
307.44 Hypersomnia Related to . . .***

Other Sleep Disorders

780.xx Sleep Disorder Due to . . .*
.52 Insomnia Type
.54 Hypsomnia Type
.59 Parasomnia Type
.59 Mixed Type
— .- Substance-Induced Sleep Disorder (refer to Substance-Related Disorders for substance-specific codes
Specify type: Insomnia/Hypersomnia/Parasomnia/Mixed
Specify if: With Onset During Intoxication/With Onset During Withdrawal

IMPULSE-CONTROL DISORDERS NOT ELSEWHERE CLASSIFIED

312.34 Intermittent Explosive Disorder
312.32 Kleptomania
312.33 Pyromania
312.31 Pathological Gambling
312.39 Trichotillomania
312.30 Impulse-Control Disorder NOS

ADJUSTMENT DISORDERS

309.xx Adjustment Disorder
.0 With Depressed Mood
.24 With Anxiety
.28 With Mixed Anxiety and Depressed Mood
.3 With Disturbance of Conduct
.4 With Mixed Disturbance of Emotions and Conduct
.9 Unspecified
Specify if: Acute/Chronic

PERSONALITY DISORDERS

Note: These are coded on Axis II

301.0 Paranoid Personality Disorder
301.20 Schizoid Personality Disorder
301.22 Schizotypal Personality Disorder
301.7 Antisocial Personality Disorder
301.83 Borderline Personality Disorder
301.50 Histrionic Personality Disorder
301.81 Narcissistic Personality Disorder
301.82 Avoidant Personality Disorder
301.6 Dependent Personality Disorder
301.4 Obsessive-Compulsive Personality Disorder
301.9 Personality Disorder NOS

OTHER CONDITIONS THAT MAY BE A FOCUS OF CLINICAL ATTENTION

Psychological Factors Affecting Medical Condition

316 . . . [Specified Psychological Factor] Affecting . . .*

Choose name based on nature of factors:
Mental Disorder Affecting Medical Condition
Psychological Symptoms Affecting Medical Condition
Personality Traits or Coping Style Affecting Medical Condition
Maladaptive Health Behaviors Affecting Medical Condition
Stress-Related Physiological Response Affecting Medical Condition

Other or Unspecified Psychological Factors Affecting Medical Condition

Medication-Induced Movement Disorders

332.1 Neuroleptic-Induced Parkinsonism
333.92 Neuroleptic Malignant Syndrome
333.7 Neuroleptic-Induced Acute Dystonia
333.99 Neuroleptic-Induced Acute Akathisia
333.82 Neuroleptic-Induced Tardive Dyskinesia
333.1 Medication-Induced Postural Tumor
333.90 Medication-Induced Movement Disorder NOS

Other Medical-Induced Disorder

995.2 Adverse Effects of Medication NOS

Relational Problems

V61.9 Relational Problem Related to a Mental Disorder or General Medical Condition
V61.1 Partner Relational Problem
V61.20 Parent-Child Relational Problem
V61.8 Sibling Relational Problem
V62.81 Relational Problem NOS

Problems Related to Abuse or Neglect

(code 995.5 if focus of attention is on victim)

V61.21 Physical Abuse of Child
V61.21 Sexual Abuse of Child
V61.21 Neglect of Child
V61.1 Physical Abuse of Adult
V61.1 Sexual Abuse of Adult

Additional Conditions That May be Focus of Clinical Attention

V15.81 Noncompliance With Treatment
V65.2 Malingering
V71.01 Adult Antisocial Behavior
V71.02 Child or Adolescent Antisocial Behavior
V62.89 Borderline Intellectual Functioning
Note: This is coded on Axis II.
780.9 Age-Related Cognitive Decline
V62.82 Bereavement
V62.3 Academic Problem
V62.2 Occupational Problem
313.82 Identify Problem
V62.89 Religious or Spiritual Problem
V62.4 Acculturation Problem
V62.89 Phase of Life Problem

Additional Codes

300.9 Unspecified Mental Disorder (nonpsychotic)
V71.09 No Diagnosis or Condition on Axis I
799.9 Diagnosis or Condition Deferred on Axis I
V71.09 No Diagnosis on Axis II
799.9 Diagnosis Deferred on Axis II

Multiaxial System

Axis I Clinical Disorders
Other Conditions That May Be a Focus of Clinical Attention

Axis II Personality Disorders
Mental Retardation

Axis III General Medical Conditions

Axis IV Psychosocial and Environmental Problem

Axis V Global Assessment of Functioning

Answer Key

CHAPTER 1
Introduction to Psychiatric-Mental Health Nursing

1. Answer can include; self-governance/autonomy, orientation towards growth/self-realization, tolerance of uncertainty, self-esteem, mastery of the environment, reality orientation, stress management
2. Current trends include; care that is community based; brief therapies to effect crisis stabilization and return to optimal functioning. Care is based on integration of neurobiological theories and related treatments, particularly psychopharmacologic agents. Psychiatric-mental health nurses are engaging in health promotion/illness prevention activities, including working with high risk groups. Client and family education aims to provide information and foster understanding about mental illnesses, symptoms, and management & importance of various treatments, esp. adherence to medication regimes.
3. C
4. B
5. B
6. C
7. A

CHAPTER 2
Mental Health Promotion

1. C
2. B
3. A
4. D
5. C
6. B
7. A

CHAPTER 3
Conceptual Frameworks for Care

1. A
2. D
3. A

CHAPTER 4
Nursing Theory

1. D
2. B
3. B

CHAPTER 5
The Therapeutic Relationship

1. It is goal-directed, with the client's coping skills and growth as the goals; the nurse's supportive behavior and consistency provides the client with a basis for trust and a model of a positive relationship; the nurse unconditionally accepts the client as a person and reinforces their worth and dignity.
2. Allows client to identify their personal strengths and resources to improve coping skills and begin growth and change.
3. Increase client's awareness and perceptions of personal experiences
   Develop realistic self-concept and promote self-confidence
   Recognize areas of discomfort and verbalize feelings
   Make comparisons of ineffective behavior both within and without relationships
   Develop, implement, and evaluate a plan of action
   Assess readiness and provide opportunities for independent functioning
4. Termination is established in the initial phase of a therapeutic relationship; it may be necessary due to time restrictions or duration of contact with client.
5. Nurse can be consistent to provide role-modeling and a secure environment, can encourage clients to try new adaptive behaviors while giving emotional support, and can create a relationship in which clients share and have validated decision making.

CHAPTER 6
Communication

1. C
2. B
3. D

CHAPTER 7
Biological Bases for Care

7. C
2. A
3. D
4. C
5. B
6. A
7. D
8. B
9. B
10. D
11. C
12. A

CHAPTER 8
Assessment and Nursing Diagnosis

1. D
2. A
3. B
4. C
5. A
6. Use of an interpreter; knowledge of client's culture and individualism; using cultural considerations in review of body language, grooming.
7. Nursing diagnosis is a statement of the client's response pattern to a health disruption. It is obtained through accurate and holistic assessment of the client, family, and community, using as much data as possible. Causative factors are an essential part of a nursing diagnosis. A social worker's records about a client can contain valuable information towards creating nursing diagnoses, interventions, and goals for the client.
8. Risk for injury; Risk for violence; directed at self or others
9. Through nursing diagnoses, changes in behavior become the mechanism for evaluation. Goals, predicted and hoped-for changes in behavior, serve as the outcome criteria for this evaluation.
10. For the elderly client, briefer assessment tools are used, with emphasis on client observation rather than interview. For the child, assessment involves added attention to observing interaction, communication, and play.

CHAPTER 9
Planning, Intervention, and Evaluation

1. A
2. C
3. C
4. D

CHAPTER 10
Sociocultural Aspects of Care

1. A culture is a way of being, taught and learned from generation to generation, that represents a systemic blend of the real and the ideal norms or patterns of behavior.
2. Racial prejudice and cultural stereotypes influence psychiatric nursing practice and policy in several ways. European-American culture, with middle-class values, provides the basis for education, funding, and practice of nursing in the U.S., especially outside of urban areas. Frequent misdiagnosis of minorities' mental illnesses is reflected in the literature, which consistently reports diagnoses with a high frequency of psychosis and a low frequency of depression in ethnic minorities. In addition, stresses related to being a minority or of a different culture in this society may lead a need for mental health services. For example, African Americans experienced 1.8 times as many admissions to all types of mental health facilities as Caucasians.
3. Psychiatric nurses of color have contributed significant theoretical and research advances to psychiatric nursing. In addition, their own valuable diversity serves as a bridge to expand the cultural sensitivity of psychiatric nursing practice.
4. Issues regarding communication (spoken and body language), adapting both Western medicine and cultural healing into a care plan, differences in diet, avoidance of stereotypes, and need for sensitivity and openness to belief and practice orientations different from those of the nurse.
5. Care that accounts for cultural differences fosters the therapeutic relationship, provides respect for the client's culture and history, prevents misdiagnosis, and allows for development of a client care plan working with the client and family.
6. Curanderismo is a practice of folk healing that continues today in the Mexican-American community. In this system, healers, curanderas and curanderos, believe they are endowed with healing powers from God. Diseases are thought to be due to the will of God or to witchcraft.
7. Healers can serve as keepers of cultural information, providers of health care services, and providers of spiritual care and knowledge.

8. Take into full consideration the client's own perspective on his or her illness or need for care, family history, and beliefs, concerns, and fears about the illness. Collaborate with informal caregivers and other members of the client's culture to gain understanding of the individual's views on communication, space, time, and social organization.
9. In a cross-cultural nursing situation, family may serve as interpreters or communicators on the client's behalf, may have authority over the client's decisions within the family structure, may bring food or folk medicines from home, may provide contact with the rituals and healing practices of their culture, and may provide criticism or support for the Western medical system.

CHAPTER 11
Spiritual Aspects of Care

1. Individual essay.
2. C
3. A holistic approach views the client as a total being with physical, sociocultural, and emotional aspects. The spiritual aspect integrates these factors and is the core of the person, as well as impetus for a philosophical and emotional life. A non-holistic approach might not accomodate including spirituality in nursing practice.
4. B and D
5. C
6. Group and community spiritual care provides effective spiritual care through support and nurturing, socializing, and creating a space for spirituality with music, rituals, listening, or talking about personal concerns. These fulfil client needs for community and emotional support, as well as providing opportunities for growth.
7. C
8. Nurses' understanding of their own spirituality, in a holistic context, helps them to aid clients by respecting their religious pluralism, raising their awareness of the meaning of a spiritual quest, and giving them some personal background to deal with spiritual challenges, such as the difference between spirituality and religious concepts.

CHAPTER 12
Sexuality and Sexual Concerns

1. D
2. B
3. C
4. B
5. A comprehensive sexual assessment of a client includes a review of client records; a sex history (how client learned about sex, early sex experiences, etc.); means of showing affection in family of origin; client's feelings and attitudes about sex; information about present and past sexual relationships; sexual problem areas; influence of current health problem on sexual attitudes or behavior; self-image, body image and sexual image; current sexual habits and functioning; history of sexual abuse, harrassment, rape or sexual assault; and cultural influences on client perceptions of sexuality.
6. Medications may be used to treat sexual dysfunction; antianxiety medications for those whose anxiety interferes with their ability to engage in sexual activities; Prozac, tricyclic antidepressants, Haldol, Mellaril, Ativan and the MAOIs can prolong sexual activity in men with premature ejaculation; those with paraphilic disorders can be treated with medications to reduce sexual desire including Androcur and Provera.
7. Basic principles of sex therapy include careful assessment of the couple's sexual difficulties, clarification of each member's perceptions of the other and sexual activities, facilitation of communication between the partners, and acceptance of each other's feelings and attitudes.

CHAPTER 13
Grief and Loss

1. Grief: universal response to loss (process)
   Mourning: process of detachment (grief work)
   Bereavement; state of feelings, thoughts, responses which occur following a loss
2. Palliative care would focus on comfort and quality of life rather than treatment modalities for cure.
3. A
4. A
5. Denial, anger, bargaining, depression, acceptance
6. D
7. Contemporary research does not focus on time limitations of grief resolution as do the classic theories.
8. Create a memory packet (bracelet, pictures, footprints, lock of hair); provide appropriate grief literature and information on support groups; encourage family to see, hold, touch infant; encourage verbalization of feelings; discuss funeral arrangements; contact other members of health team (chaplain, social worker, visiting nurse)

CHAPTER 14
Milieu Therapy

1. B
2. C
3. C

CHAPTER 15
Individual Psychotherapy

1. C
2. D
3. B
4. D
5. A
6. B

CHAPTER 16
Groups and Group Therapy

1. D
2. D
3. B
4. B
5. A
6. A
7. A
8. D

CHAPTER 17
Families and Family Therapy

1. Two or more individuals who have commited to work together toward common goals.
2. Developmental stages of the family; family structure and function; family communications theory; family systems theory
3. Historical; lifestyle changes, changes in role and family structure, societal changes
   Developmental: birth of first child, adolescence, midlife crisis, older adulthood
   Role development and change; single parent families, blended families, teenaged parents
   Environmental: poverty, media, changing values, family violence, illness and disabilities
4. Optimal families; adequate families; midrange families; troubled families
5. Answer may include: Family coping; potential for growth, Ineffective family coping; compromised, Ineffective family coping; disabling.
6. Answer may include; family support, maintenance of family process, promotion of family integrity, family involvement, family mobilization, caregiver support, sibling support, and parent education.

CHAPTER 18
Behavioral Approaches

1. C
2. B
3. A
4. C
5. B
6. A
7. D

CHAPTER 19
Alternative Therapies

1. C
2. E
3. C
4. B
5. D

CHAPTER 20
Psychopharmacology

1. B
2. D
3. B
4. B
5. C

CHAPTER 21
Development of the Person

1. D
2. C
3. B
4. D
5. A
6. C
7. E

CHAPTER 22
Children

1. B
2. D
3. A
4. D
5. Areas include; functioning of family, communication patterns in family, family relationships, identification of problem including child's perceptions, sociocultural influences, child and family history, physical health, mental status, suicidal intent
6. B
7. Self-talk; to treat children with phobias or depression; Time out; to remove child with disruptive behavior from environmental reinforcement; Token economies; to reinforce positive behavior; Differential reinforcement; to teach language to children with autistic disorder; Parent training; to manage child's behavior.
8. D

CHAPTER 23
Adolescents

1. Primary changes of normal adolescence include biological/pubertal changes, psychological/cognitive changes, and social redefinition. Primary changes are universal across culture, occur prior to secondary changes, and have an impact on secondary changes via the contexts in which adolescents develop; family, peer, school, and work settings. The onset of pubertal changes among individuals and within the individual varies. Secondary changes include identity, achievement, sexuality, intimacy, autonomy, and attachment. Major psychological tasks of adolescence are the development of identity, decision-making about academic and occupational achievement, development of intimate friendships and mature sexuality, and establishment of emotional and behavioral autonomy without sacrificing attachment with primary caregivers. An example of the social consequences of early physical maturity is that a 14-year-old boy who is ahead of his peers in physical development may be preferred for involvement in athletic and social activities.
2. Piaget; Adolescence is the period of formal operational thinking where adult-level reasoning takes place. Adolescents who achieve such thinking abilities are able to think more abstractly and complexly, and are able to think realistically about the future. These cognitive changes influence parent-adolescent relationships, as adolescents discuss and argue about issues with their parents, see the flaws in their parents' arguments, imagine what different parents would be like, and think about their parents' marital relationship. Sullivan: Provides a stage theory for the development of peer relationships. He stresses the importance of interpersonal relationships and the differences between child-child and parent-child relationships. Sullivan describes the notion of "chumship" in adolescence and maintains that this same-sex frienship is a critical developmental accomplishment. This friendship is the basis for later close relationships.
3. The actual percentage is between 10% and 20%. Overdiagnosis and underdiagnosis can result from a lack of or erroneous knowledge of developmental norms. Those who believe that "storm and stress" are normal to adolescence tend to underdiagnose.
4. A. In adjustment disorder, multiple stressors, such as a move to a new city or a divorce, may overwhelm ability to cope and impair academic/social functioning. B. A child who has a difficult temperament and experiences parental rejection/neglect is at risk for conduct disorder. C. Parents who fail to acknowledge or confirm the developmental progress of their daughter and perceive her growth and development as her accomplishment, not theirs, increase the risk of their daughter developing an eating disorder.
5. All choices are risk factors for adolescent substance abuse.
6. Diagnosis is most likely ADHD. Assessment tools include Connors and Child Behavior checklist, clinical history and observational data from parents and teachers. Interventions for clients include; stimulant medications, client and parent education about the disorder, family therapy, behavior and cognitive therapy, and social skills training.
7. To develop self-awareness; A. Examine memories of own adolescence; B; evaluate to what extent you accomplished each of the adolescent growth tasks C; be honest with yourself and your client; D: be aware of potential reactions to adolescent behaviors.
8. The nurse may inadvertently encourage the adolescent to act out.

CHAPTER 24
Mental Health of the Aging

1. C
2. B
3. D
4. B
5. A

CHAPTER 25
Anxiety Disorders

1. D
2. A
3. C

CHAPTER 26
Somatoform Disorders

1. Somatization disorder is characterized by a history of many physical complaints over a period of several years and generally involves various bodily systems. Conversion disorder usually involves a disruption in one dimension of voluntary or motor function and is preceded by recent events that trigger conflict or stress. There generally is less long-term disability with conversion disorder than with somatization disorder. Body dysmorphic disorder features a specific preoccupation with an imagined deficit in appearance. Somatization conversion and body dysmorphic disorder have no biologic basis but serve to express psychological distress.
2. Responses to a client in this state include, "Tell me how that response makes you feel," "Talk

some about what you think about such remarks," and "I hear you talk of your suffering and I see you crying right now."

3. Be aware of your emotional response; respond supportively to client's fear and anger. Communicate empathy and dependability while giving feedback and setting limits. Share experience with other health team members.
4. With this answer, be sure and include awareness that the person's communication of physical symptoms must be unintentional and have no organic basis.
5. The person with hypochondriasis may be the "symptom bearer" of dysfunction within the family system. Possible stress and conflict within the family needs to be explored.

CHAPTER 27
Cognitive Disorders

1. A disruption of, or deficit in, cognitive functioning, which can include thinking, perception, and/or memory capabilities.
2. Growing geriatric population, in which most dementias are found; Increasing medical capabilities to increase the survivorship of clients with chronic diseases in which cognitive disorders occur; Increasing survivorship of clients entering acute care facilities.
3. A primary disease of the brain. 2. Systemic disease that secondarily influences brain functioning. 3. Reaction of brain tissue to introduction of an exogenous substance/pharmaceutical. 4. Reaction of brain tissue to withdrawal of an exogenous substance/pharmaceutical.
4. D

CHAPTER 28
Personality Disorders

1. B
2. B
3. B

CHAPTER 29
Depressive and Bipolar Disorders

1. C
2. B
3. C
4. C
5. A
6. B
7. A

CHAPTER 30
Schizophrenic Disorders

1. C
2. A
3. C
4. B
5. C
6. A

CHAPTER 31
Aggressive and Violent Behavior

1. B
2. C
3. D
4. A
5. B
6. D
7. C
8. B
9. C
10. A

CHAPTER 32
Dissociative Disorders

1. C
2. A
3. D
4. Absence from conscious awareness of some ordinarily familiar information, emotion, or mental function
5. C
6. A
7. Eating disorders/substance abuse
8. D
9. B

CHAPTER 33
Substance Abuse and Dependency

1. C
2. D
3. A
4. C
5. C
6. D
7. C
8. C
9. C
10. C

CHAPTER 34
Eating Disorders

1. D
2. D
3. A
4. A
5. A
6. D

CHAPTER 35
Codependency

1. C
2. A
3. D
4. D
5. A
6. C
7. B
8. A
9. B

CHAPTER 36
The Homeless Mentally Ill

1. Studies vary widely. Some study only shelter populations and miss those in domestic violence shelters, in abandoned buildings, in homeless "camps", and living as runaways. Even shelter studies have data influenced by noise level, conditions, and hesitancy to answer personal questions.
2. Homeless population is now younger, with more women, families, veterans, mentally ill persons and over-representation of African-Americans and Hispanics.
3. Personal hygiene, medication management, how to cope with side effects & symptoms, HIV and STD protection, measures to promote safety, protection from exposure, accessing social services, risks for chronic diseases, housing, substance abuse rehab and support, and measures to negotiate the mental health system.
4. The nurse should designate individualized, reasonable, attainable outcomes, taking into account local resources, acuity of symptoms, and client's perception of desired outcomes.
5. Sedation effects (impaired safety and lack of places to sleep), safety measures (storage of medicines and personal security), fluid intake needs (esp. with lithium), sun protection (lack of shelter, increased sun sensitivity due to phenothiazines) are all specific issues of medication management for the homeless.
6. Criteria for clinic eligibility can exclude homeless mentally ill persons by the following requirements; having an address, strict compliance with appointments, excluding clients who do not stay clean from drugs or alcohol.
7. A

CHAPTER 37
Mental Retardation

1. B
2. A
3. C
4. D
5. A

CHAPTER 38
Forensic Psychiatric Nursing

1. C
2. B
3. D
4. D
5. A

CHAPTER 39
Crisis Theory and Intervention

1. A
2. C
3. B
4. A, C, & D
5. B
6. C
7. C
8. A
9. A & B
10. All
11. All
12. A & B

CHAPTER 40
Rape and Sexual Assault

1. B
2. C
3. D
4. B

CHAPTER 41
Violence Within the Family

1. D
2. E
3. E

4. D
5. C

CHAPTER 42
Suicide

1. D
2. A
3. B
4. D

CHAPTER 43
Community Mental Health

1. F
2. D
3. A
4. G

CHAPTER 44
Psychosocial Home Care

1. C
2. B
3. D

CHAPTER 45
Community-Based Care and Rehabilitation

1. E
2. E
3. F
4. D

CHAPTER 46
Psychosocial Impact of Acute Illness

1. To deal with the stressful situation (problem-focused); to deal with emotional response to the situation (emotion-focused).
2. Material support; informational support; emotional support; comparison support.
3. Each illness situation carries its own unique combination of stressors, and each individual has his/her own coping skills and resources. No generalizations an be made as to which situation is more problematic; the nurse must assess the individual and plan interventions accordingly.
4. Control, which motivates individuals to seek information about their illness and to be involved in treatment decisions; Commitment, which motivates individuals to take an active role in treatment of their illness and recovery; and Challenge, since individuals who see stressors as a challenge and opportuhity for growth are able to mobilize coping resources.
5. A
6. C
7. C

CHAPTER 47
The Child at Risk: Illness, Disability, and Hospitalization

1. B
2. D
3. A
4. C
5. C

CHAPTER 48
The Client on the Human Immunodeficiency Virus Spectrum

1. The HIV invades the cells of the immune system which are responsible for defending against primitive invaders like fungi, yeasts, and other viruses. They usurp cellular function and instruct the cells to stop doing what they are supposed to, and to instead just produce the HIV. Then, the HIV teaches the cell how to wrap the new HIV in a lipoprotein coat which will help the new HIV find other cells to invade. The cell eventually dies after producing HIV; eventually, enough of these cells are destroyed that immune protection is weakened.
2. First, there is often a long latency period in which HIV positive patients feel and appear well. Since they don't feel ill, they might not seek contact with a reporting agency. Secondly, in most areas only a diagnosis of AIDS is reportable. Thus, the numbers of individuals who are HIV+ are underreported.
3. After exposure the the HIV, most individuals experience severe flu-like symptoms during which time their bodies are making antigens to defend against the HIV. The presence of these antibodies is proof that the individual has been exposed to the HIV.
4. Individuals who are in the early stages often use denial as a primary coping mechanism. In the middle stages, mechanisms include denial, and attempingt to control other elements of their lives—and their health. In the late stages, clients often reach realistic acceptance regarding their health and the uncertainty of the future.
5. When a patient believes that his or her condition is brought on as punishment for bad behavior, he or she may experience shame and diminished self esteem. When the nurse believes that a person with AIDS is getting what he or she deserves the countertransference prevents the nurse from providing the unconditional positive regard needed in each interaction.

6. The nurse's open and non-judgemental attitude, as well as the presence of relevant posters or literature will convey a willingness to discuss the client's fears about HIV.
7. The client's understanding of the meaning of the HIV test result, the client's coping mechanisms, and the suicide risk.
8. Anxiety is intensified by the uncertainty of the client's health status and fears associated with dying. Decreased self-esteem rooted in the client's inability to complete developmental tasks, and in shame associated with the stigmatization of being on the HIV spectrum.
9. As the client begins to experience a decline in health, coping mechanisms are tested more severely. The nurse is called upon to intervent with difficult psychosocial problems during the middle phase, and must also come to the realization that this relationship with the client will ultimately end in the client's death.
10. Direct Infection by HIV, Opportunistic Infections, Lymphomas, Toxic Effects of Treatments
11. The three main areas are intellectual function, sensorimotor function, and personality disturbances. The nurse must make individualized plans and adjust the way the care is provided, the nature of the interactions with the client, the expectations the nurse has of the client, and the environment in which the client operates.
12. The nurse must cull, through a mass of assessment data, those dysfunctional behaviors that were part of the client's baseline evaluation from those that result from inadequate coping in times of stress.

CHAPTER 49
Legal Implications of Psychiatric-Mental Health Nursing

1. A. Nurse has a duty to use due care toward plaintiff; B. Nurse's professional performance falls below the standard of care and is a breach of that duty; C. As a result, plaintiff is injured due to nurse's action which is the proximate cause of the injury; D. Act in which nurse engaged could forseeably have caused injury; 5; Plaintiff must show actual damages.
2. Reasonable Person test determines if the action is what the prudent nurse would have done under similar circumstances if that nurse came from the same or a similiar community.
3. Informed consent is not required if an emergency situation exists in which the patient poses a danger to self or others.
4. As a result of the Tarasoff Decision, therapists may have a duty to protect a erson who is threatened by the therapist's client.
5. Forensic psychiatry a specialty that provides mental health services to clients who are charged with criminal acts or who have been found not guilty by reason of insanity.
6. As a result of the Parham Decision, the Supreme Court held that juveniles can be authorized for psychiatric in-patient admission by their parents, but that accompanying the admission, some neutral fact finder should determine whether statutory requirements for admission are required.
7. ANA Standards focus nursing practice on the client's attainment and restoration of physical and mental health.

CHAPTER 50
Research in Psychiatric-Mental Health Nursing

1. C
2. A
3. D
4. B

Glossary

Acrophobia fear of heights

Acting in a kind of resistance that circumvents therapy through blocking, forgetting, changing the subject; trying to elicit the therapist's approval or disapproval while trying to recall or express feelings

Acting out the client substitutes some kind of action for feeling or thinking; common forms of acting out include running away, use of alcohol or drugs, sexual promiscuity, and aggressive behavior

ADC-AIDS dementia complex an array of problems related to central nervous system involvement

Addiction physical dependence, that is, a state manifested by withdrawal when the drug is removed

Adolescence the stage of development during which the physiologic changes of puberty, the emergence of the self-concept, and the integration of the biopsychosocial aspects of the individual occur

Affect mood or feeling tone

Affective instability shifts from normal mood to anger or depression with the return to normal mood in a short period of time

Aggression any behavior that expresses anger or its related emotions

Ageism a social stereotype that prevents the elderly from achieving fullness of living

Agoraphobia a marked fear of being alone or in a public place from which escape would be difficult or in which help would be unavailable in the event of suddenly becoming disabled

AIDS acquired immunodeficiency syndrome

Akathisia a syndrome characterized by motor restlessness

Ambiguity the experience of uncertainty

Ambivalence the experience of two strong, opposing feelings or wishes toward the same object or person resulting in conflict

Anal period late infancy or toddlerhood, the period from ages 2 to 3 or 4 years, during which the child is involved in the development of social, emotional and physiologic control

Anger a physical and emotional state in which a person experiences a sense of power to compensate for an underlying feeling of anxiety

Anorexia nervosa self-imposed starvation, a psychiatric disorder characterized by a voluntary refusal to eat

Antianxiety agents psychotropic drugs used in the treatment of overt anxiety

Anticipatory grief the progression through the phases of grief prior to the death of a loved one

Antidepressant agents psychotropic drugs used in the treatment of depression

Antipsychotic (or neuroleptic) agents psychotropic medication used primarily to treat psychoses, that is, severe emotional disorders

Anxiety the initial response to psychic threat, evidenced as feelings of discomfort, uncertainty, apprehension, dread, and restlessness

Anxiety disorder a psychiatric condition characterized by the emotion of intense terror

Assertiveness the employment of expressive, goal-directed, spontaneous, and self-enhancing behavior

Assessment the gathering, classifying, and categorizing of client information that forms the basis of nursing planning

Autocratic leadership the exercise of significant authority and control over group members, including the lack or rare use of input from the group and minimal group interaction and participation

Avoidance the management of anxiety-laden experiences through evasive behaviors

Battery the touching of another person without permission

Behavior a wide range of overt and covert responses that include emotions and verbalizations

Behavioral contract an agreement between client and psychiatric-mental health caregiver for a specific behavior

Behavioral rehearsal role playing, that is, the client rehearses new responses to problem situations after learning new adaptive responses portrayed through modeling

Behavioral therapy a form of treatment that deals with changing the individual's maladaptive behavior by a planned, objective approach, such as respondent conditioning

Bereavement the feelings, thoughts, and responses that occur following a loss

Bisexuality equal, or almost equal, preference for either sex as a sexual partner

Blackout resulting from persistent heavy drinking, a person appears to function normally while drinking, but later is unable to remember what happened

Blocking the client suddenly "blanks out" and is unable to finish a thought or an idea, that is, he represses painful knowledge and feeling

Body image a mental picture of one's body

Bulimia episodic, uncontrolled, rapid ingestion of large quantities of food over a short period of time, or binge eating, often accompanied by self-induced vomiting, obsessive exercise, or use of laxatives and diuretics

Catharsis the emotional re-experiencing of painful, frightening, or angry feelings that are associated with the client's symptom or behavior

Claustrophobia fear of closed spaces

Codependency a disorder involving loss of self; an aspect of the addictive process in which living is masked and the person's identity is not developed or is unknown to him

Coitus sexual intercourse, or penetration of the vagina by the penis

Collaboration working with others, as an equal, toward a common goal

Communication a personal, interactive system; a series of ever-changing, ongoing transactions in the environment

Community support system a systems model for the delivery of community-based mental health care, which includes rehabilitation, housing, physical and mental health services, educational and employment opportunities, and social networks

Compliance adherence to prescribed treatment regimens

Compulsions ritualistic behaviors that the individual feels compelled to perform either in accord with a specific set of rules or in a routinized manner and which are designed to prevent or reduce anxiety

Consciousness the perceptions, thoughts, and feelings existing in a person's immediate awareness

Coping mechanisms (also called ego defense mechanisms, mental mechanisms, and defense mechanisms) mechanisms that usually operate on an unconscious level to protect the ego from overwhelming anxiety

Countertransference an experience in which the therapist transfers his feelings for significant others onto the client

Crisis a turning point, a state of disequilibrium usually lasting 4 to 6 weeks

Crisis intervention a thinking, direct, problem-solving form of therapy that focuses only on the client's immediate problems

Cross-tolerance following tolerance to a drug, tolerance to other drugs in the same or related classes develops

Cryptic language abbreviated language, such as speaking aloud only every fifth or tenth word of one's thoughts

Cunnilingus oral-genital stimulation performed on a woman

Deinstitutionalization the discharge of large numbers of psychiatric clients from inpatient treatment centers to the community

Delusion a fixed, false belief that cannot be corrected by reasoning

Dementia clinical behavior manifested in the insidious development of memory and intellectual deficits, disorientation, and decreased cognitive functioning

Democratic leadership the encouragement of group interaction and participation in group problem solving and decision making; the group is marked by common goals, solicitation of opinions, ideas, and input and provision of feedback

Denial an unconscious coping mechanism wherein a person denies the existence of some external reality

Depression pathologically intense unhappiness

Development the orderly evolution of events moving from simple to more complex

Differentiation a tendency of living, open systems to increase in complexity over time

Discrimination a specific response occurring in a given situation

Disengagement a theory that proposes that the elderly or dying person acts voluntarily in giving up his roles in life, slowly loses interest in the active world, and withdraws from significant others

Displacement an unconscious coping mechanism through which a person transfers an emotion from its original object to a substitute object

Disqualifying an individual fails to attend to another's message by silence, ignoring it, or changing the subject

Dissociation the absence from conscious awareness of some ordinarily familiar information, emotion, or mental function

Distress damaging or unpleasant stress

Double-bind communication the sending of an incongruent message that includes a directive to do something and a nonverbal message to do the opposite, while the receiver of the message is not permitted to comment on it

DSM-III-R the American Psychiatric Association's *Diagnostic and Statistical Manual, Third Edition, Revised*

Dual diagnosis comorbidity, or coexistence of psychoactive substance dependence and major psychiatric disorder

Dyspareunia pain with sexual intercourse

Dystonia involuntary, jerking, uncoordinated body movements

Early latency the ages from 6 to 9 years, or early school-age years, during which the child focuses on learning, the acquisition of knowledge, the development of the social role outside the protection of home and family

ECT electroconvulsive therapy, a form of treatment for depression

Ego the structure of the human personality that has the greatest contact with reality

Ego-dystonic that which is unacceptable to the self

Ego-syntonic that which is acceptable to the self

Enculturation the process by which an individual learns the expected behavior of the culture

Enmeshment lack of clear boundaries between the parent and child subsystems and between individual family members

Entropy the tendency of a system to be closed to the environment

Erectile dysfunction (also called impotence) the inability to achieve or maintain erection sufficiently to perform coitus

Erogenous zones the areas of the body that are particularly sensitive to erotic stimulation, such as the neck, breasts, inner thighs, and genital areas

Ethnic group a group of people with a common origin

and holding basically similar values, beliefs, and means of communication

Evaluation the process of determining the value of something in the attainment of preset goals

Exhibitionism an erotic desire to expose one's genital or erogenous areas to others

Existential crisis a crisis in which the individual is faced with life in the form of aloneness, the absurdity of existence, and the responsibilities inherent in his attained freedom, and is confronted with a reorganization of the meaning of life

Extinction the withholding of reinforcers, thus reducing the probability of the occurrence of the response

Fading gradual reduction of the process of facilitation or accentuating the reinforcer

Family a primary group whose members are related by blood, marriage, adoption, or mutual consent, who interact through certain familial roles, and create and maintain a common subculture

Family structure the organization of the family

Family therapy a form of treatment based on the premise that the member of the family with the presenting symptoms signals the presence of pain in the whole family

Fantasy a coping mechanism through which a person engages in nonrational mental activity and thus escapes daily pressures and responsibilities

Fellatio oral-genital stimulation performed on a man

Female orgasmic dysfunction an inability to achieve or difficulty achieving orgasm

Fetishism a condition of recurrent sexual urges and sexually arousing fantasies by means of the use of nonliving objects alone or with a sexual partner

Flight of ideas a stream of thought characterized by a rapid association of ideas and play upon words

Folie à deux a delusional system shared by two persons, most commonly sisters

Forensic psychiatric nursing provision of psychiatric-mental health nursing care to mentally disordered offenders

Foreplay the petting and fondling activities engaged in during the excitement phase of the sexual response cycle

Formal group a group with structure, authority, and limited interaction, such as a business meeting

Free association a primary method of treatment in psychoanalysis, the free expression of thoughts and feelings as they come to mind

Frotteurism a disorder of recurrent, intense sexual urges and sexually arousing fantasies regarding rubbing against or touching a nonconsenting person; the touch, not the coercion, is the sexually exciting focus

Generalized anxiety disorder a disorder characterized by chronic anxiety that is uncomfortable to the point that it interferes with the individual's daily living

Gender identity how one chooses to view oneself as a male or female in interaction with others

Gender role how a person's gender identity is expressed socially, in behavior with others of the same and opposite sex

General Adaptation Syndrome (GAS) the body's manifestations of stress that evolve in three stages: alarm reaction, stage of resistance, and stage of exhaustion

Generalization the phenomenon by which adaptive behavior specific to one situation may occur in similar situations

Geropsychiatry the care of the aging psychiatric client

Grief a universal response to a loss

Grief work steps taken toward grief resolution

Group three or more persons with related goals

Group norm the development, over time, of a pattern of interaction within a group to which certain behavioral expectations are attached

Group therapy a form of treatment in which individuals explore their problems and styles of communication in a safe, confidential atmosphere where they can receive feedback from other groups members and undergo change

Habituation severe craving or compulsion to take a drug to feel good

Hallucination a false sensor perception, that is, without external stimuli, or a sensory perception that does not exist in reality, such as seeing "visions" or hearing "voices"

HIV human immunodeficiency virus

Homosexuality a male's preference for a male sexual partner, or a female's preference for a female sexual partner

Hostility a feeling of antagonism accompanied by a wish to hurt or humiliate others

Hypochondriasis unwarranted fear or belief of having a serious disease in the absence of significant pathology

Id the most primitive structure of the human personality; the site of the instincts

Identification a coping mechanism through which a person unconsciously adopts the personality characteristics, attitudes, values, and behavior of another person

Illusion a misinterpretation of a real sensory experience

Imagery a therapeutic approach in which the client pictures significant memories and present events that, combined with relaxation and role playing, increase awareness of events and behavior

Imitation the conscious process of identifying with another person

Informal group a group of members who are not dependent on each other, such as a hobby group

Informed consent the knowing consent given in a interaction or series of interactions between the treating physician and the client that allows the client to consider fully information about the treatment that is being proposed

Insight conscious awareness of the painful, angry, or socially unacceptable thoughts of feelings that the client repressed

Intellectualization an unconscious coping mechanism

through which a person uses his intellectual abilities such as thinking, reasoning, and analyzing to blunt or avoid emotional issues

Interpretation a person's insight or understanding of his feelings and behavior

Interview a purposeful, goal-directed interaction between two people

Laissez-faire leadership a style of leadership in which group members are free to operate as they choose

Latency the ages from 9 to 12 years, or late school-age years, during which the harmonization of various aspects of the self-concept, especially through clubs, sport teams, and scouts occurs

Latent content that content which is not discussed, which occurs on a feeling level, and which is seldom verbalized

Lesbianism a female's preference for a female as a sexual partner

Libido an energy source associated with the physiologic or instinctual drives such as hunger, thirst, and sex

Life review looking back over one's life and making peace with it

Listening focusing on all of the behaviors expressed by a client

Lithium carbonate a psychotropic drug used in the treatment of bipolar disorder (formerly termed manic-depressive illness)

Malingering conscious deception and communication of false symptoms

Malpractice a tort action brought by a consumer plaintiff against a defendant professional from whom the consumer plaintiff feels that he has received injury during the course of the professional-consumer relationship

Mania a mood disturbance characterized by elation, hyperactivity, agitation, and accelerated thinking and speaking

Manifest content the spoken words during an interaction

Masochism a paraphilia in which the person's preferred sexual object is the experience of pain

Masturbation self-stimulation of erogenous areas to the point of orgasm

Maturational (or developmental) crisis a crisis precipitated by the normal stress or development, such as pregnancy, birth, or adolescence

Melancholia depression, at one time thought to result from an excess of "black bile" in the body

Mental health a state of emotional well-being in which a person functions adaptively and comfortably within his society and is satisfied with himself and his achievements

Mental health team the groups of mental health caregivers, including nurses, occupational and recreational therapists, social workers, psychiatric nurse clinical specialists, dance and art therapists, psychologists, psychiatrists, pastoral counselors, and paraprofessionals, who work together to design and implement a therapeutic milieu for clients

Mental retardation a significantly subaverage general intellectual functioning existing concurrently with deficits in adaptive behavior and manifesting itself during the developmental period

Milieu environment or setting; in psychiatric-mental health nursing, the therapeutic milieu includes the people and all other social and physical factors in the 24-hour environment with which the client interacts

Milieu therapy a group therapy approach that uses the total living experience of a client to accomplish therapeutic objectives

Modeling imitation as a method of behavior change

Mourning the process of detachment from the loss

Negative reinforcer a harmful reinforcer that the client evades or avoids, thus strengthening or facilitating adaptive behavior

Negentropy a tendency toward openness to the environment, both inside and outside the family

Neologism new, private word with idiosyncratic meaning

Noncompliance the failure of the client and his family to adhere to prescribed treatment regimens, such as the failure to take prescribed psychotropic medication after discharge from the treatment facility

Nursing diagnosis a statement of a client's response pattern to a health disruption

Obsessions recurrent, persistent thoughts, ideas, images, or impulses

Obsessive-compulsive disorder a psychiatric condition in which the individual experiences recurrent obsessions or compulsions

Object constancy experience of security or stability; also known as object permanence

Objective data data or information that can be measured, observed, or validated

Oedipal period the preschool years, from age 3 or 4 to 6 years, during which stage the child's developmental needs include dealing with sexual and aggressive impulses and coming to terms with parental and societal demands

Oral period the first 2 years of life, or infancy, during which the personality structure of the individual is centered around the issue of impulsivity

Panic disorder an anxiety disorder characterized by recurrent, unpredictable anxiety attacks of panic proportions

Paraphilia the investment of an adult's sexual interest in objects, events, or particular types of people

Pedophilia recurrent and intense sexual urges and fantasies of sexual activity with prepubescent children

Perinatal loss the loss of a baby by miscarriage or stillbirth, or in the neonatal period

Personality an individual's consistent and stable pattern of behavior

Personality disorder a maladaptive personality style

Phobia a persistent, irrational fear attached to an object or situation that objectively does not pose a significant danger

Physical dependence (addiction) a state manifested by withdrawal symptoms after a drug is removed

Planning the structure of needs and problems in an orderly manner to achieve an end or goal

Pleasure principle the employment of pleasure-seeking behaviors that reduce tension when the physiologic or instinctual drives are released

Positive reinforcer a reward; that which strengthens a behavior

Post-traumatic stress disorder the development of characteristic symptoms after exposure to a traumatic life experience capable of psychologically harming most people

Preconscious that material which is not immediately accessible to a person's awareness

Primary gain an individual's symptom or behavior is defense against or reduction of the emotional pain associated with anxiety

Primary group a group of members with face-to-face contact and boundaries, norms, and explicit and implicit interdependent roles, such as a family

Primary prevention therapeutic approaches such as infant stimulation and parenting education programs that aim to prevent mental illness or disorder before it occurs

Primary process though processes deriving from the id and characterized by an illogical, confused form and preverbal, or preoperational, content

Problem solving using anxiety in the service of learning adaptive behavior

Projection an unconscious coping mechanism through which a person displaces his feelings, usually feelings perceived as negative, onto another person

Prompting the creation of a condition that facilitates or accentuates the reinforcer

Psychiatric nurse liaison mental health nursing, consultation, and education in a nonpsychiatric environment

Psychoanalysis a form of long-term therapy that uses strategies such as dream interpretation, hypnosis, and free association

Psychodrama a form of group therapy in which clients explore problems through dramatic methods

Psychoeducation a form of intervention aimed at the family members of individuals with psychiatric disorders that explores the families' reactions to mental illness of a member and provides families with information about, and ways to help the member with, an emotional disorder

Psychogeriatrics the special psychiatric care for clients in the over-65 age group

Psychological dependence (habituation) the expression of a severe craving or compulsion to take a drug in order to feel good

Psychopathology the difference or gap between the existing emotional developmental level of an individual and the expected emotional development level that corresponds to his chronological age

Psychopharmacology the use of psychotropic, or psychoactive, drugs to treat various emotional disorders

Psychosis an extreme response to stress that may be characterized by impaired reality testing, delusions, hallucinations, and affective, psychomotor, and physical disturbances

Psychosomatization the visceral or physiologic expression of anxiety

Psychotherapy the use of a group of techniques to modify feelings, attitudes, and behavior in people by means of understanding self and being understood by another, to achieve relatedness, and to relieve emotional pain

Punishment that which suppresses the maladaptive pattern of behavior

Rape a crime in which forcible penile-vaginal penetration of a female occurs without her consent and against her will

Rape trauma syndrome the process of adaptation in which the rape victim frees herself of overwhelming fear, redefines her feelings of vulnerability and helplessness, and regains control and equilibrium

Rationalization an unconscious coping mechanism through which a person substitutes socially acceptable reasons for the real or actual reasons motivating his behavior

Reaction formation an unconscious coping mechanism through which a person acts in a way opposite of how he feels

Reality principle the ability to delay pleasure in favor of more socially acceptable behavior

Reality testing the ability to perceive reality accurately

Reconstructive therapy deep psychotherapy or psychoanalysis that delves into all aspects of the client's life and may take 2 to 5 years or longer

Re-educative therapy psychotherapy that involves new ways of perceiving and behaving and exploring alternatives in a planned, systemic way, often requiring more than short-term therapy

Reframing putting information or beliefs into a different perspective

Regression an unconscious coping mechanism through which a person avoids anxiety by returning to an earlier, more satisfying or comfortable time in life

Reinforcer anything that increases the probability of a response

Relationship a state of being related; an affinity between two individuals

Repression a coping mechanism through which a person forces certain feelings or thoughts into his unconscious

Resilience ability of the personality to recover readily from or adjust to difficult situations and events and to mobilize coping resources

Resistance the client resists recalling information or recalling feelings

Ritual abuse a severe form of abuse in which a child is repeatedly physically and sexually abused in ceremonies by an organized group of perpetrators

Sadism a paraphilia in which the person's preferred sexual object is the act of inflicting pain on someone else

Safer sex general term for sexual practices which avoid contact with blood, feces, vaginal secretions, or semen and thus reduce the risk of contracting sexually transmitted diseases; includes limiting the number of sexual partners, using condoms, avoiding oral sex or French kissing with an unscreened partner, or using a glove or a finger cot when exploring anal or vaginal areas and touching the penis

Scapegoating the process in which a family tends to view one of its members as different and the cause of its trouble

Schizophrenia a severe disturbance of thought or association, characterized by impaired reality testing, hallucinations, delusions, and limited socialization

Secondary gain an individual's behavior or symptom relieves him of responsibility and provides extra attention or monetary rewards

Secondary group a group of members who do not have relationship bonds or emotional ties; an impersonal group such as a political party

Secondary prevention therapeutic approaches such as crisis intervention, counseling, and inpatient hospitalization that reduce prevalence of emotional disorders through early case finding and prompt intervention

Self-concept a composite of a person's beliefs and feelings about himself at a given time

Sex roles culturally determined patterns associated with male and female social behavior

Sexual identity the basic recognition of one's sex

Sexuality the expression and experience of the self as a sexual being

Shaping a behavioral reinforcement technique used to condition close approximations of some desired adaptive behavior

Simple phobia a persistent, irrational fear of, and compelling desire to avoid, exposure to a circumstance or class of thing other than those specific to agoraphobia or social phobia; common examples of simple phobias include claustrophobia and acrophobia

Situational crisis a crisis precipitated by a sudden traumatic event, such as divorce, job loss, or birth of a child with a congenital defect

Social phobia a persistent, irrational fear of, and compelling desire to avoid, situations in which exposure to the scrutiny of others may occur

Splitting the tendency to pigeonhole individuals into "all good" or "all bad" categories

Stress the nonspecific response of the body to any demand made on it, according to Hans Selye

Stressors stress-producing factors, including physiologic stressors such as failure, success, and loss

Subculture a group of people who may be distinguishable by ethnic background, religion, social status, or other similar characteristics, and simultaneously share certain features with larger segments of society

Subjective data data that reflects the client's feelings, perceptions, and "self talk" about his problems

Superego the structure of the human personality that contains the values, legal and moral regulations, and social expectations that thwart the free expression of pleasure-seeking behaviors

Supportive therapy psychotherapy that allows the client to express feelings, explore alternatives, and make decisions in a safe, caring relationship

Suppression a coping mechanism through which a person consciously excludes certain thoughts or feelings from this mind

Suspiciousness hypersensitivity, alertness, and hypervigilance

Tardive dyskinesia a late symptom associated with the long-term use of high-dose phenothiazine drugs; symptoms include buccolingual movements such as "fly catcher" movements, pursing of lips, jaw movements, and involvement of limbs and trunk

Termination the dissolution of a relationship

Tertiary prevention therapeutic approaches such as halfway houses and residential placements that aim to reduce long-term disability from emotional disorder through a program of rehabilitation, aftercare, and resocialization

Theory a conceptual system consisting of interrelated propositions that describe, explain, and predict selected phenomena

Therapeutic relationship a relationship in which the nurse and client participate with the goal of assisting the client to meet his needs and facilitate his growth

Time out a period of time during which the client is removed from any form of reinforcement

Token reinforcement a therapeutic approach that delays the use of direct reinforcers through the administration of tokens, which can then be redeemed for actual reinforcers

Tolerance a state in which an increased amount of a drug is necessary to obtain the desired effect or in which there is a decrease in the desired effect with regular use of the same amount of a drug

Transcendental self a self that exists beyond one's individual self-image, or a self in relation to the larger universe

Transference a tool or technique of psychotherapy whereby the client transfers feelings and attitudes held toward significant others onto the therapist

Transsexuality the belief that one is psychologically of the sex opposite his or her anatomical gender

Transvestitism a sexual desire to dress in the clothing, or adopt the mannerisms, of the opposite sex

Treatment alliance the ability to work together and to be invested emotionally in the task of therapy

Triangle a form of cross-generational clinging, such as a coalition formed by a mother and son against the father

Unconditioned response the response elicited by an unconditioned stimulus, for example, salivation is an unconditioned response in a hungry dog elicited by an unconditioned stimulus, food

Unconditioned stimulus that which elicits an unconditioned response, for example, food is an unconditioned stimulus that elicits an unconditioned response, salivation, in a hungry dog

Unconscious that material which is inaccessible to a person's awareness

Unresolved sexual trauma a state in which a person experiencing a sexual assault does not deal with the feelings or reactions to the experience

Vaginismus a spastic contract or tightening of the vagina before or during penetration for coitus

Voyeurism a desire to watch others in sexually vulnerable or erotic positions

Withdrawal the behavioral or psychological retreat from anxiety-provoking experiences

Working through a part of the final phase of therapy in which the client's insights are discussed and reworked over time

Index

Note: Page numbers in italics *indicate illustrations; those followed by b indicate boxed material; those followed by t indicate tables.*

◆ Lippincott's Quick-Access Psychopharmacology Disk

This software program has been designed to be used with an IBM or IBM-compatible computer and Microsoft Windows. This program enables you to access information on more than 75 psychopharmacologic drugs using either a generic or trade name. Once you have selected a drug, you can view the complete drug monograph, print the drug monograph, make an ASCII file, make your own drug cards, or create patient teaching printouts. If you choose to make an ASCII file, you will then be able to edit the drug information, using your own word processing program; change the information in any way that suits your needs; and print out edited information.

You Can Choose Either Print Option to Create Your Own Drug Cards!!!!

To start the program:

- insert the diskette into the floppy drive
- choose the Run command from the Windows Program Manager
- type A:QUIKDRUG and click OK. (or B:QUIKDRUG if your diskette drive is :>B:)
- view the Disk Title/Copyright Screen introducing *Lippincotts's Quick-Access Psychopharmacology Disk* and the drug disclaimer
- proceed by clicking OK

The generic drug name list will apear on your computer screen. You will now have seven (7) options:

- scroll through the list of drug names, using the mouse or UP and DOWN arrow keys
- view a monograph for a highlighted drug name
- switch from the generic drug name list to the trade drug name list
- search for a specific drug name
- print a drug monograph
- create an ASCII file
- exit the program

If you have selected to view a drug monograph, the monograph will appear on your computer screen. You now have four (4) options:

- scroll forward or backward through the monograph listing, using the mouse or the UP and DOWN arrow keys
- print the monograph
- create an ASCII file
- close the monograph and return to the drug name list

If you have selected to create an ASCII file:

- select and type in the drug file name using up to eight (8) characters
- click OK
- exit this program to use the file in your word-processing program

To exit the program:

- click Exit

(Sample Patient Teaching Printout)

Patient's Name: ______________________________

You should know the following information about the drug that has been prescribed for you:

Drug Name: lithium

How to Pronounce: ***lith' ee um***

Other names that this drug is known by: Carbolith (CAN), Duralith (CAN), Eskalith, Lithane, Lithizine (CAN), Lithonate, Lithotabs, lithium citrate

Instructions to follow for your safety:

** Take this drug exactly as prescribed, after meals or with food or milk.

** Eat a normal diet with normal salt intake; maintain adequate fluid intake (at least $2^1/_2$ quarts/d).

** Arrange for frequent checkups, including blood tests. Keep all appointments for checkups to receive maximum benefits and minimum risks of toxicity.

** The following side effects may occur: drowsiness, dizziness (avoid driving or performing tasks that require alertness); GI upset (frequent small meals may help); mild thirst, greater than usual urine volume, fine hand tremor (may persist throughout therapy; notify health care provider if severe).

** Use contraception to avoid pregnancy. If you wish to become pregnant or believe that you have become pregnant, consult your care provider.

** Discontinue drug, and notify care provider if toxicity occurs: diarrhea, vomiting, ataxia, tremor, drowsiness, lack of coordination or muscular weakness.

** Report diarrhea or fever.